Perspectives for Occupation-Based Practice

Perspectives for Occupation-Based Practice

Foundation and Future of Occupational Therapy

Edited by
Rita P. Fleming Cottrell, MA, OT/L, FAOTA

2ND EDITION

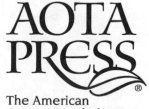

The American
Occupational Therapy
Association, Inc.

Vision Statement

AOTA advances occupational therapy as the pre-eminent profession in promoting the health, productivity, and quality of life of individuals and society through the therapeutic application of occupation.

Mission Statement

The American Occupational Therapy Association advances the quality, availability, use, and support of occupational therapy through standard-setting, advocacy, education, and research on behalf of its members and the public.

AOTA Staff

Frederick P. Somers, Executive Director
Christopher M. Bluhm, Chief Operating Officer
Audrey Rothstein, Group Leader, Communications

Chris Davis, Managing Editor, AOTA Press
Barbara Dickson, Production Editor

Robert A. Sacheli, Manager, Creative Services
Sarah E. Ely, Book Production Coordinator

Marge Wasson, Marketing Manager
Elizabeth Sarcia, Marketing Specialist

The American Occupational Therapy Association, Inc.
4720 Montgomery Lane
Bethesda, MD 20814
Phone: 301-652-AOTA (2682)
TDD: 800-377-8555
Fax: 301-652-7711
www.aota.org\

To order: 1-877-404-AOTA (2682)

Disclaimers

This publication is designed to provide accurate and authoritative information in regard to the subject matter covered. It is sold or distributed with the understanding that the publisher is not engaged in rendering legal, accounting, or other professional service. If legal advice or other expert assistance is required, the services of a competent professional person should be sought.

—*From the Declaration of Principles jointly adopted by the American Bar Association and a Committee of Publishers and Associations*

It is the objective of the American Occupational Therapy Association to be a forum for free expression and interchange of ideas. The opinions expressed by the contributors to this work are their own and not necessarily those of either the editor or the American Occupational Therapy Association.

ISBN: 1-56900-199-5

Library of Congress Control Number: 2004117604

Design by Sarah E. Ely
Composition by Laura J. Hurst, Grammarians, Inc.
Printed by Victor Graphics, Inc., Baltimore, MD

*To all past, current, and future occupational therapy
students, educators, practitioners, and scholars
who dare to withstand the pressure
to treat just a part of the person.*

*To all who respectfully consider all aspects of the
individual—physically, psychologically, socially,
culturally, spiritually, and politically—using
meaningful occupation to enable people with
disabilities to fully participate in life.*

To Christopher, the light of my life.

Contents

Part I: Occupational Therapy's Heritage: Historical and Philosophical Foundations for Best Practice

Part II: Theoretical Frameworks to Guide the Occupational Therapy Process

Part III: Contextual Considerations for Engagement in Occupation and Participation

Part IV: The Therapeutic Relationship: Joining With the Person

Part V: Guidelines for Best Practice Throughout the Occupational Therapy Process

Part VI: Current Realities and Future Directions for Best Practice in Occupational Therapy

Appendices

Preface

As some readers may know from my previous texts (Cottrell, 1993, 1996), my entry into the occupational therapy profession was deeply rooted in my personal life experiences. My life was forever changed and greatly enriched by my brother Kevin and his lifelong struggle with a degenerative neuromuscular disorder. Therefore, I begin this text by sharing our personal experience with the profession of occupational therapy, for it clearly highlights the meaningfulness of occupation and is a major precipitant for all of my publications and life work as an occupational therapist.

When I was a young child, my older brother Kevin was diagnosed with Friedreich's ataxia, a progressive neuromuscular disorder. Because we were only two years apart in age, his lifelong journey through the disease process became my journey also. Initially, my childhood naiveté prompted me to decide to become a physician who would cure my brother and all others with devastating illnesses. However, with age comes realism, and as I grew older I began to recognize that cures were infrequent, especially for such rare diseases as my brother's. While I realized that extensive research might one day find a cure (or at least an effective treatment), my brother needed something done during his lifetime to help him manage his progressive illness. Therefore, as an adolescent I began to explore the profession of physical therapy. Throughout high school I formalized my decision to become a physical therapist and subsequently entered New York University (NYU) as a "pre-PT" student. At this point, Kevin's disease had progressed significantly, and he could not participate in many activities of daily living. He was an avid reader and a music aficionado, but still many hours were filled with boredom and depression.

In my search to find ways to improve the quality of Kevin's life, I discovered the field of occupational therapy. It was a perfect match. Occupational therapy's holistic approach, which maximized abilities, minimized disabilities, and provided adaptive strategies and compensation methods to enable the individual to live a productive, satisfying life, was just what Kevin and I had been searching for.[1] I quickly changed my major to occupational therapy and became a "sponge" to absorb all of the information and skills we had been seeking for so many years (without even knowing what we had been looking for). With the field of occupational therapy finally discovered, I promptly had Kevin's physician refer him to an internationally known hospital for rehabilitation. The initial care he received seemed highly competent. He was given a customized wheelchair and scads of adaptive equipment. As an occupational therapy student, I was impressed with these obviously skilled practitioners and their thoughtful interventions. It quickly became evident, however, that Kevin's greatest needs were not being addressed by the rehabilitation team. Most striking was the total lack of interest in who Kevin was or what he wanted to achieve. As a 22-year-old living at home with no job or social network, Kevin clearly needed a complete occupational therapy evaluation. Unfortunately, his entire evaluation and treatment focused on his motor functioning, wheelchair mobility, and the self-care task of dressing. Increasing his strength and coordination were generally helpful to Kevin, but wheelchair mobility and dressing were difficult and extremely exhausting for him. Also, due to the nature of his illness, it was likely that these difficulties would increase as his disease progressed. Dressing in the morning took a frustrating 2 hours to complete and left him so fatigued that he could not even hold a book to read or put a record on his turntable. This was devastating to Kevin, because he was extremely intelligent and craved the fine literature and music that still filled his life with meaningful activity. To be so weary that one cannot enjoy life's pleasures is sad; to have this fatigue brought on by an ill-conceived treatment plan is tragic.

My brother's assertive nature fortunately remedied this unproductive situation. He quickly (and loudly!) refused to independently dress himself and threw out all of the adaptive equipment. This act of self-preservation was viewed by his occupational therapist and rehabilitation team as a clear indication that he was a "difficult, unmotivated" client, and he was promptly discharged from the occupational therapy program! (He was "allowed" to continue in the wheelchair clinic, "as needed.") Not once during the time he was involved with this treatment program did anyone fully assess his values, interests, or goals; they assessed only his muscle strength, range of motion, coordination, and sensory awareness.

Fortunately, I was continuing in my occupational therapy studies and developing a strong appreciation for the holistic and therapeutic use of occupation. After consulting with Kevin (and using him as a guinea pig for several of my school assignments), we decided that he would become a student at NYU during my senior year so that I would be available to assist him with his transition to independent living. His choice of a political science major, as he stated, was one of "pure selfish interest." It would have questionable use after graduation, but Kevin did not care, because the progressive nature of his

---

[1] Kevin had the unfortunate "luck" to be born before the development of childhood intervention programs and the expansion of occupational therapy into community, home care, and school settings; therefore, his childhood contact with therapists was nonexistent. It is hoped that, in this day and age, it would not take a lifetime for a family to obtain proper interventions for themselves and their loved ones.

illness precluded employment at the time (this was pre–Americans With Disabilities Act [ADA]). Kevin's primary goals for attending college were to be intellectually stimulated, to develop a social network, and to live independently. He accomplished all of these goals, with me serving as a novice occupational therapist and adapting his dorm and activities to meet his needs.

Kevin's success was truly a testament to his character, but I often found myself wondering what would have happened to him and his ability to attain his goals if his sister had not been an occupational therapist? Why was it so difficult for the occupational therapists working with him to see him as a whole person with interests, hopes, and dreams, not just a set of weak, uncoordinated muscles? Years went by, and Kevin pursued a successful academic career, typing his papers from memory with one finger while maintaining a B average! He obtained his bachelor's and master's degrees within 5 years, developed friendships, attended concerts, dined in restaurants, and traveled to England and a multitude of American states. A definite quality of life had replaced the boredom and depression of our "pre-OT" years.

Yet, the question about the lack of holism and the absence of occupation in actual occupational therapy clinical practice came back to haunt us many times. To preserve our sibling relationship, I tried not to act as Kevin's therapist, and periodically we obtained physician's referrals for occupational therapy to meet his needs as his disease progressed. During these forays into the rehabilitation world, I was always available as the family representative when a new therapist began working with Kevin. I never initially mentioned that I was an occupational therapist, for I was serving as a family member and not as a professional colleague. Invariably, each occupational therapist would competently assess Kevin's physical status, prescribe built-up handled utensils, and begin a morning dressing program. Only one occupational therapist ever asked Kevin what he did for leisure, work, or meaningful occupation. This same occupational therapist was the only one to question if there were any psychosocial needs that were not being met for Kevin and our family. Unfortunately, this gifted therapist did not stay in her position for long due to a lack of administrative support for her holistic approaches.

Kevin responded to all of these reductionistic occupational therapists by discontinuing treatment after only a few sessions because, as Kevin said, "it's pointless." This served to perpetuate his reputation as a difficult, unmotivated client. Invariably, I resumed my dual role of "sister–OT," adapting activities and modifying Kevin's environment according to his interests and needs. Again, we asked ourselves in frustration, "What if I weren't an occupational therapist?" "How could our family help Kevin manage a devastating progressive illness and maintain quality of life?" My occupational therapy professional literature was replete with holistic views about the therapeutic use of occupation and client-centered practices, but "Why did we see it in so few of my brother's occupational therapy interventions?"

Kevin passed away in 1989, but the lessons he taught me about life and the questions he raised about my profession continue to influence me and my teaching. In many respects, I cannot separate my personal self from my professional self because they were intertwined for so long. Therefore, I often use my brother and our life experiences as examples to underscore fundamental occupational therapy principles to my students. Thankfully, these examples are generally well-received, for I do not think I could teach occupational therapy any other way.

Kevin's life journey also taught me the critical need to be astute about the social, economic, and political issues that influence the reality of living with a disability in the United States. Therefore, the role of the occupational therapy practitioner as an advocate also is central to my teachings. Our parents' struggle to obtain basic medical care for Kevin because of our family's low socioeconomic status provided me with many early childhood memories that reflect societal inequities. My brother's battle to acquire an education that was equal to the education of students without disabilities enabled me, as a teenager, to appreciate the monumental significance of the Rehabilitation Act of 1973. In 1975, my brother and I celebrated the enactment of the Education for All Handicapped Children Act, which finally mandated free and appropriate education for all children, regardless of ability or disability. This act's passage was of special significance to our family because, as Staten Island residents, my parents were told that my brother should be institutionalized at the infamous Willowbrook State School (Riveria, 1972). Fortunately, my parents resisted the status quo, and as previously noted, my brother successfully attained a graduate degree from NYU. However, this path was fraught with obstacles, so we carefully followed all subsequent legislation related to disability rights.

Regrettably, my brother passed away before he could witness the passage of the ADA, but in 1990, I toasted this milestone in his honor. While this law is significant, the reality that it would not immediately alter the social, economic, and political barriers to full community participation had to be acknowledged. This realization has proven sadly true, as 15 years post-ADA, millions of Americans with disabilities remain institutionalized and segregated from society (Cottrell, 2003).

Recently, the American Occupational Therapy Association (AOTA) reaffirmed our profession's commitment to the promotion of full community participation for people with disabilities with the adoption of the *Occupational Therapy Practice Framework* (AOTA, 2002) and a revised definition of occupational therapy practice (Wilmarth, 2004; see Appendices A and C in this book). As an advocate, I was heartened to read that the *Framework* included political, economic, and institutional contexts that can support or hinder participation. The role of the occupational therapy practitioner in enabling individuals with disabilities to fully participate in their "desired roles, contexts, and life situations (AOTA, 2002, p. 2) in "home, school, workplace, community, and other settings" (Wilmarth, 2004, p. 7) is also strongly emphasized in these documents. It is my hope that the integration of the *Framework* and this definition, along with the seminal works in this text, will contribute to the personal and professional development of a new generation of occupational therapy practitioners who are committed to the use of occupation to attain and maintain quality of life for people with disabilities and their families. Based on my life experiences, this is the true purpose of authentic occupational therapy and the gift that my brother and I embraced many years ago. It is a legacy worth perpetuating.

References

American Occupational Therapy Association. (2002). Occupational therapy practice framework: Domain and process. *American Journal of Occupational Therapy, 56,* 609–639.

Cottrell, R. (1993). *Psychosocial occupational therapy: Proactive approaches.* Bethesda, MD: American Occupational Therapy Association.

Cottrell, R. (1996). *Perspectives on purposeful activities: Foundation and future of occupational therapy.* Bethesda, MD: American Occupational Therapy Association.

Cottrell, R. (2003, March 10). The Olmstead decision: Fulfilling the promise of the ADA: Implications for occupational therapists. *OT Practice,* pp. 17–21.

Riveria, G. (1972). *Willowbrook: A report on how it is and why it doesn't have to be that way.* New York: Random House.

Wilmarth, C. (2004, July 26). RA approves revised definition of OT practice. *OT Practice,* p. 7.

Note to Readers

This text is a second edition of the 1996 publication entitled *Perspectives on Purposeful Activity: Foundation and Future of Occupational Therapy,* published by the American Occupational Therapy Association (AOTA). The slight change in this new edition's title is to reflect the changes that have occurred in our profession's language in the ensuing years. As with the first edition, this text attempts to provide a philosophical yet practical link between occupational therapy's heritage, current practice realities, and future practice opportunities. To complete this publication, I have conducted an extensive literature review to gather the "best of the best" in the occupational therapy professional literature. Original occupational therapy literary classics along with thought-provoking recent works were selected to provide readers with a solid theoretical and philosophical foundation as well as realistic and relevant guidelines for best practice throughout the occupational therapy process. This resulting anthology can be considered an "at-your-fingertips" library and can save occupational therapy educators and students the time and effort needed to compile and access course packets and reserve readings.

Chapters are organized into topical parts with thought-provoking introductions that challenge readers to analyze their perceptions about person-directed, occupation-based practice. These reflective analyses can help readers integrate personal issues with their current knowledge and developing practice skills. While the chapters were judiciously selected to accurately reflect the philosophical foundations, contextual influences, and practical applications of occupation-based practice, there are realistic parameters to the text. Extensive reviews of occupational therapy frames of reference, models of practice, and evaluation methods are not provided, as there are several publications already available that provide in-depth information on these critical professional topics. Readers are urged to use the reference lists at the end of each chapter to study these topics and other relevant issues further. Readers also are encouraged to use these references and resources on an ongoing basis throughout their professional careers.

Readers should note that, because all the chapters in this text are reprinted from other sources, they vary in style. Due to the need to comply with copyright laws, all of the chapters in this text were reprinted as originally published. While editorial efforts were made to ensure grammatical accuracy and gender-neutral language, readers will note some inconsistencies in several chapters. These chapters contain relevant content, but their formats do not always adhere to the AOTA's publication guidelines. Areas of concern include various styles of referencing and usage, non-gender-neutral language, and potentially dated (or nonexistent) author credentials. In addition, because these writings have been culled from more than 80 years of occupational therapy professional literature, some concepts and terms will be understandably dated (e.g., "suffering" "schizophrenic patient"). These historical pieces were included because they were significant works during their respective time, and they remain a vital part of our profession's literary history and ongoing development.

While some individuals may maintain negative perspectives on occupational therapy practice in today's challenging health care system, this text will foster an increased awareness and appreciation of the relevance, variety, and richness of skilled, dynamic occupation-based practice. Using the philosophies and practices described in this text will enable readers to meet professional challenges positively and to develop a rich occupational therapy career, regardless of specialty choice.

Acknowledgments

I thank Christopher Gnad, Mary Ann Muraca, and Meghan Wolfe for their production assistance and the entire AOTA Press team, especially Barbara Dickson, Carrie Mercadante, and Chris Davis, for their assistance in bringing this project to fruition.

List of Figures, Tables, and Appendices

Appendix A

Appendix B

Occupational Therapy's Heritage: Historical and Philosophical Foundations for Best Practice

Introduction

Occupational therapy became a singular profession because its founders believed in the inherent healing power of occupation (Law, 2002; Quiroga, 1995). They emphasized the therapeutic value of occupation throughout their writings and in their work, providing us with a rich heritage and a strong foundation for occupation based practice. Over the years, this commitment to occupation has been challenged and weakened by reductionistic practices (Shannon, 1977; Whiteford, Townsend, & Hocking, 2000). Fortunately, many of our profession's leaders and best practitioners recognized the invaluable contribution occupational therapy can make to health and wellness, *if* it retained its unique legacy of occupation. Most recently, this commitment to occupation was re-affirmed when the American Occupational Therapy Association (AOTA; 2002; Appendix A in this volume) adopted the *Occupational Therapy Practice Framework: Domain and Process*. This *Framework* asserted that occupational therapy focuses on occupation and daily life activities and applies "an intervention process that facilitates engagement in occupation to support participation in life" (p. 608). This affirmation of the link between occupation and life participation holds the promise of assuring that current and future occupational therapy practice will reflect the core tenets and values of our profession as first put forth in the early 1900s.

An exploration of these founding principles and core beliefs is provided in this part's first five chapters. These chapters explore occupational therapy's philosophical base by presenting scholarly writings that examine the lives, times, values, and philosophies that influenced the development of our profession. Subsequent chapters by esteemed scholars build on this historical base to examine the danger of adopting conflicting ideologies and reductionistic approaches while supporting solid philosophical and practical arguments that support the therapeutic use of occupation. Many of these chapters are considered classics in the field, and it is an honor to include them in this text. It is hoped that thoughtful exploration of the richness of occupational therapy's heritage and a critical review of the missteps made during our profession's reductionistic periods will foster an appreciation for these timeless principles and develop an allegiance to the use of occupation in current and evolving practice (Law, 2002; Whiteford et al., 2000).

In Chapter 1, Peloquin begins this historical review by analyzing the writings of the founders of the National Society for the Promotion of Occupational Therapy. Her comprehensive literature review provides readers with an insightful inquiry into the contemporary historical events and the shared beliefs that influenced the founders of occupational therapy and resulted in the development of our multifaceted profession. She discusses the founders' understanding of service with respect to three primary agents: the person, the therapist, and the occupation. The interrelationships among these agents are emphasized throughout the chapter. The personal narratives, life stories, and unique perspectives of the founders are explored and supported by numerous quotes from their original writings, enabling readers to share their vision for a profession rooted in care and function.

This personalization of the early years of occupational therapy is continued in Chapter 2, which presents Adolph Meyer's landmark speech to the attendees of the Fifth Annual Meeting of the National Society for the Promotion of Occupational Therapy, in 1921. Although the profession was very young at that time and many years have since passed, readers will be struck by the timelessness of Meyer's "Philosophy of Occupation Therapy." His call for the individuation of activity based on the personal interests and the natural capacities of the person and the provision of opportunities for meaningful occupation, rather than the use of predetermined treatment prescriptions, has remained relevant despite the passage of many decades. Meyer's presentation traces the development of the therapeutic use of occupation from the 1890s to his time, and it looks toward a future in which all individuals will be able to engage in gratifying activity to productively use their time.

The next three chapters expand on this historical review by exploring two movements that began in the 18th century and greatly influenced the founders of occupational therapy in the early 19th century. The arts-and-crafts movement provided early occupational therapy practitioners with a theoretical base for the use of arts and crafts as treatment activities. In Chapter 3, Schemm explores the similarities and differences in the ideas and beliefs of the proponents of the arts-and-crafts movement and the founders of occupational therapy. She describes the historical, philosophical, political, and socioeconomic issues that lead to ideological conflicts within the field, underscoring the overwhelming influence the environment has on the development of a profession.

Peloquin further analyzes the tremendous impact that historical contexts and societal trends have on a profession's development in Chapter 4. Her presentation describes the moral treatment movement, its characteristics, and the course of its practice, detailing the successful therapeutic use of occupation within the asylums. The societal changes, ideological conflicts, and lack of leadership, which ultimately led to the demise of this movement, are clearly traced. The resulting inequity in treatment, the decrease in quality of care, and the often total lack of care are carefully considered, leading Peloquin to call for occupational therapy practitioners to reaffirm a humanistic view of practice that is committed to the effective use of occupation.

The influence of moral treatment on the development of the profession of occupational therapy is further explored by Bing in Chapter 5. In his 1981 Eleanor Clarke Slagle Lecture, Bing postulates that occupational therapy is a retitled form of moral treatment. He supports this viewpoint with a comprehensive analysis of the beginnings of moral treatment in Europe, its expansion in the United States, its disappearance in the last quarter of the 19th century, and its re-emergence in the early 20th century as occupational therapy. The occupation-based princi-

ples and definitions of occupational therapy identified by the founders of the profession are reviewed. This holistic occupation heritage is elaborated on in Bing's presentation of the second generation of occupational therapy practitioners, as exemplified in the life and work of Beatrice Wade. This chapter is replete with personal vignettes and quotes from the founders of occupational therapy and Wade, offering a unique perspective on the rich history of occupational therapy. Bing ends his historical analysis with a thoughtful summation of his views on the lessons current occupational therapy practitioners can learn from the first and second generation of our profession's leaders.

Bing's call to carefully consider our profession's "old values" when "charting new directions" and to learn from our history is taken up in Chapter 6 by Hooper and Wood. These authors provide a thought-provoking analysis of the influence that pragmatism and structuralism had on the development of occupational therapy as a profession. They present a clear historical and conceptual overview of these two discordant philosophies, highlighting their implications for occupational therapy practice. Readings in occupational therapy that reflect pragmatist and structuralist discourse are also reviewed. Hooper and Wood examine the pragmatist and structuralist assumptions about humanity and knowledge, which resulted in divergent and conflicting views about the purpose and focus, tools and methods, and goals and outcomes of occupational therapy intervention. They propose that following these two disparate discourses has contributed to an ongoing professional identity struggle for occupational therapy. Most importantly, they place this pragmatism–structuralism discourse into the broader contexts of society and culture. They conclude that practitioners must develop literacy to critically examine our assumptions about

knowledge and a consciousness about how what we know influences our practice. In addition, Hooper and Wood advocate for the development of cultural literacy to ensure that occupational therapy joins with an ethos that is congruent with our profession's varied practices, multiple theories, and numerous viewpoints so that occupational therapy practitioners' contribution to society is unequivocal and rich.

The negative impact of adopting a philosophy that is fundamentally incompatible with our profession's core values and founding beliefs is further explored by Friedland in Chapter 7. The incongruence between physical rehabilitation's stance that the disability itself is the defining problem that must be addressed, and occupational therapy's philosophy that the real problem is the person's difficulties with occupational performance is evident to those committed to occupation-based practice. However, this clarity of purpose was not always part of our profession's history, and as Friedland argues, the legacy of this inherent conflict is still evident in our profession's identity problems and reductionistic practices. She supports her position by providing a brief review of early philosophical influences on occupational therapy and reflecting on our emerging profession's commitment to occupation and activity. Friedland's discussion about the origins and history of our profession and the development of physical medicine underscores the inevitability of the conflict in values that resulted between occupational therapy and rehabilitation. Our profession's assumption, after World War II, of the physical rehabilitation model led to an erosion of our core values as evident in the abandonment of the use of occupation to achieve health and well-being. Friedland realistically discusses the contextual influences that contributed to the demise of occupation-based practices. She honestly discusses the complete lack of fit between authentic occupational therapy and the medical model and questions why we strive to fit into an environment that is intrinsically counter to our very being. She challenges practitioners to cease this abdication to the medical model and align ourselves with newer models of rehabilitation that emphasize social integration. Most significantly, Friedland concludes that our profession must reconnect to occupation-based practice if we are to uniquely contribute to health and well-being. I think if Friedland revisited her treatise today, the *Practice Framework* and its emphasis on occupation to achieve wellness and social participation would hearten her.

One of our profession's greatest leaders and scholars, Mary Reilly, would also likely feel a sense of renewal and relief in our profession's recommitment to our founding beliefs. Chapter 8 contains Mary Reilly's 1962 Eleanor Clarke Slagle Lecture in which she critically assessed the impact that practice specialization and the rehabilitation movement had on our profession's growth and development. She asks if occupational therapy has responded adequately and correctly to these changes and poses the question "Is occupational therapy a vital and unique service for medicine to support and for society to reward?" Her discourse in answer of this question is widely recognized in the field as a literary classic and contains perhaps the most widely quoted passage in our profession's literature. Reilly answers her query with a resounding "yes" in the form of her hypothesis "That man, through the use of his hands as they are energized by mind and will, can influence the state of his own health." Although over 40 years have passed since Reilly presented this lecture, her views on occupational therapy's unique body of knowledge and her concerns for future directions in the field remain relevant to this day.

Another classic in occupational therapy literature is presented in Chapter 9 by Fidler and Fidler, whose unique perspectives on occupational therapy remain pertinent today. Their exploration of sociological and psychological theoretical constructs provides a basis for a definition of "doing" and a foundation for the use of "doing" in occupational therapy. They define "doing" as purposeful action that enables one to become humanized. Prescribing interventions based on doing to develop performance skills, maintain health, and prevent pathology is strongly advocated by Fidler and Fidler. Their discussion provides readers with an understanding of the humanness of purposeful activity and its vital role in the development of adaptation.

The inherent value of doing and the impact of purposeful activity on adaptation are explored further in this section's last chapter by King, who proposes adaptation as a unifying concept for occupational therapy. In this seminal 1978 Eleanor Clarke Slagle Lecture, King recognizes the diverse areas of occupational therapy practice and the growth of specialization within the field. However, she also expresses concern that the lack of a shared theoretical framework for all occupational therapy practice will result in the increased fragmentation of our profession. In light of the subsequent reductionistic phase that our profession underwent, King's words are particularly relevant. To counter this trend, she offers adaptation as the foundation for a common theoretical structure for occupational therapy. She examines the characteristics of adaptation and analyzes developmental learning as an adaptive process. The maladaptive effects of sensory deprivation; the use of activity as an adaptive response to stress; and the role of occupational therapy in health maintenance, disease prevention, and health restoration are also explored. Her emphasis on these nonmedical model foci and her call on

readers to consider alternative models or to contribute to the construction of a science of adaptation remain pertinent almost 30 years later.

The intrinsic worth of occupation for adaptation, health, and wellness is emphasized by all of the authors in this section, from our profession's founders to our leading scholars. The historical writings, philosophical tenets, and theoretical frameworks presented here provide a wealth of thought-provoking writings on the foundations of occupation in our profession. It is hoped that critical reflection on this professional literature will facilitate readers' ability to develop a personal commitment to occupation that is congruent with the unique heritage of occupational therapy, cognizant of the missteps that our profession took when we forgot these core values and founding principles, and consistent with the *Practice Framework*'s support of society's need for full participation by all.

Questions to Consider

1. What were the historical trends, sociocultural issues, and sociopolitical forces influencing the development of the profession of occupational therapy? How did ideological conflicts influence this development? How do these trends, issues, forces, and conflicts continue to influence current occupational therapy practice?
2. What were the beliefs, values, and philosophies of the founders of occupational therapy? What are common views about the use of occupation and purposeful activity in occupational therapy practice that have stood the "test of time"?
3. How did the profession's adoption of structuralistic views and alignment with physical medicine and rehabilitation affect occupational therapy's development and identity? How could concepts put forth in the *Practice Framework* be used in reductionistic environments to

sustain the profession's core values and facilitate its unique contribution to society?

4. How would you define *occupation*? How would you explain the therapeutic value of occupation to consumers, families, health care professionals, reimbursers, and policymakers?

References

American Occupational Therapy Association. (2002). Occupational therapy practice framework: Domain and process. *American Journal of Occupational Therapy, 56,* 609–639. (Reprinted as Appendix A).

Law, M. (2002). Distinguished Scholar Lecture: Participation in the occupation of everyday life. *American Journal of Occupational Therapy, 56,* 640–649.

Quiroga, V. A. (1995). *Occupational therapy: The first 30 years—1900 to 1930.* Bethesda, MD: American Occupational Therapy Association.

Shannon, P. (1977). The derailment of occupational therapy. *American Journal of Occupational Therapy, 31,* 229–234.

Whiteford, G., Townsend, E., & Hocking, C. (2000). Reflections on a renaissance of occupation. *Canadian Journal of Occupational Therapy, 67,* 61–70.

Occupational Therapy Service: Individual and Collective Understandings of the Founders

CHAPTER 1

SUZANNE M. PELOQUIN, PHD, OTR

Florence Stattel (1977) pleaded for a comprehensive history of occupational therapy, because such a history would provide perspective for contemporary understanding and future growth. Her rationale was also that occupational therapists might, in formulating a history, seize the awareness that occupational therapy has "extended an idea" in the universe (p. 649). The present paper is an attempt to explore those beliefs held by occupational therapists in the earliest years of our history and to examine the personal understandings of service found in the occupational therapy literature between 1917 and 1930. This seems an apt place to start. Any idea, including the idea of service, rarely exists in the abstract, but emerges instead from the larger context of the understandings and experiences of the person who holds it.

Sutton wrote in 1925 that "service is, or should be, one of the stellar ideals of occupational therapy" (p. 54). In 1972, a special task force of the American Occupational Therapy Association (AOTA) issued a comprehensive definition of occupational therapy that included the statement, "occupational therapy provides service" (AOTA, 1972, p. 204). An early characterization of the occupational therapist was that "she must have a deep desire to serve" (Northrup, 1928, p. 267). Because service is an idea articulated by most professions, some unique character of service must account for occupational therapy's emergence as a profession distinct from others. The ideas held individually and collectively by our founders reflect contemporary values and norms, forces that shaped their understanding of how they might serve others in a unique manner.

An Idea Extended

The service particular to occupational therapy involves three primary agents: patient, therapist, and occupation. These agents interrelate; forces across time shape both their nature and their relationships. The character and quality of service provided to any person thus exist within a particular context shaped by contemporary trends. Our current understanding of practice acknowledges distinct patient-therapist-occupation interrelationships as well as the trends that shape them. If, for example, one considers a hand therapist in private practice, the image of service in this context differs from that of a therapist treating patients in an acute psychiatric setting, even though both situations include the patient, the occupational therapist, and some form of occupation. The characteristics of a therapist that shape the type of service provided include his or her personal traits, education and experiences, frame of reference regarding occupation and patient rapport, understanding of professional roles, position and authority held within the treatment environment, and degree of commitment to standards within the particular agency. Similarly, the particular patient and his or her occupational performance strengths and problems, expectations for service, goals for treatment, attitude toward therapy, and environmental circumstances shape the service received. The particular occupations selected from self-care, work, or play-related arenas, whether targeting functional increases in cognitive, psychological, neuromuscular, sensory integrative, or social interactional performances, also characterize the service provided. There can be many pictures of occupational therapy practice. Although no single picture of service exists, invariant features enable us to identify a practice as occupational therapy. The existence today of many forms of occupational service reflects the multifaceted yet singular understanding of our founders in 1917.

Historical inquiry discloses the invariant features of a service that may persist while also assuming different forms across time. A seminal idea can be extended while also being shaped in time. My particular inquiry aims to identify the founders' characterizations of the relationships among patient, therapist, and occupation, in order to better grasp their understanding of service in the earliest decades of occupational therapy practice. My search has constituted an attempt to "search out those unusual roots carefully planted and nurtured by our forebears" (Bing, 1983, p. 800). These roots intertwine with major forces that shaped early service: hospital treatment, industry, and war. Additional societal trends toward science, education, sex stereotyping, and professionalization nourished the subsoil that shaped our growth.

I hope that this inquiry will help therapists to estimate the value of our current reflections about caring. Yerxa (1980), for example, said that "caring means being true to our humanistic and functional heritage with its concern for the quality of daily living of our patients" (p. 534). She appealed for our allegiance to that heritage. Johnson (1981) (see Chapter 52) later cautioned against current forces that shape occupational therapy service into a form that might embarrass our forebears: "Part of the price we now pay is that our directions frequently seem to be predicated not upon the observations and concepts of our founders but upon external sources and influences" (p. 593). Many of us seem in this decade to regret the passing of a time in which we believe that it was somehow easier to care, to be humane, and to resist the forces that shape practice and service. The present inquiry aims to retrieve that time and to explore its influence in shaping the particular brand of caring that constituted occupational therapy.

Because the emphasis of this search is on the personal understandings that our founders had of the best way to serve in their time, a significant portion of the literature reviewed considers persons, personal stories, and personal philosophies. It seems apt to explore such narratives when researching a profession whose early aim was "not in the making of a product, but in the making of a MAN, of a man stronger physically, mentally, and spiritually than he was before" (Barton, 1920, p. 308). 1 also think it essential to consider, at least in broad strokes, what kind of world could want, shape, and nurture a service designed to reconstruct persons.

Crafting a New Service: Founders and Near Founders

In 1917, six persons gathered to found the National Society for the Promotion of Occupational Therapy: those attending the meeting at George Edward Barton and Dr. William Rush Dunton, Jr.'s, invitation were Thomas B. Kidner, Isabel G. Newton, Susan C. Johnson, and Eleanor Clarke Slagle.

Because Susan Elizabeth Tracy was teaching a new course in occupation and could not attend, she was listed as an incorporator instead of a founder. Because Barton did not accept Dunton's nomination of Dr. Herbert Hall, Hall was not included as a member of the founding group, but became an early member and later president of the Society. Tracy and Hall might thus be called *near founders*. Johnson (1981) (see Chapter 52) described the group:

> Our founders were physicians, architects, social workers, secretaries, teachers of arts and crafts, nurses.... Each brought a different perspective and came from a unique background and orientation, yet each observed the effects of occupation in their individual environments and believed in its curative powers. (p. 592)

Johnson (1981) (see Chapter 52) characterized the group as a gathering of specialists who supported the wide use of occupation as a curative service. Each founder shared life in the world of 1917, a world quite different from that which we experience today. Dr. Sidney Licht (1967) permitted a colorful glimpse of contemporary self-care, work, and play in that era when writing about the founding of occupational therapy. In 1917 there was neither television nor radio. For the first time that year, color movies ran in commercial theaters in New York. Admission to local movie houses was a dime for an adult and a nickel for a child. Children were not admitted unless accompanied by an adult. A loaf of bread cost a nickel; the annual cost of living for a family of four was $1,843. Dollar bills were longer and wider and obviously stretched farther. Homogenized milk had not been invented, but milk was delivered to homes 7 days a week by horse-drawn wagons. Neither electric refrigeration nor supermarkets existed. Oranges were prized Christmas stocking fillers, rare treats in winter. It cost a penny to send a postcard, a penny more to mail a letter. Most people who had telephones had party lines. There were no commercial flights. Ford's touring car sold for $360. There were no traffic lights and no parking meters; 729 people were killed in automobile accidents during that year. Street lamps were turned on each night by persons called *lamplighters*. In that year, Binet developed the IQ test; Dewey endorsed new educational techniques that proposed learning by doing. Sanitation was not particularly good. Most cities had a hospital for contagious diseases, and because antibiotics were nonexistent, a large part of medical practice was concerned with infection. A man with a bilateral inguinal herniorrhaphy was immobilized for 20 days. Houses were heated with wood or coal. The United States would enter its first world war, known then as the Great War. Though perhaps simpler because of fewer inventions and options, occupational tasks in 1917 were not easy by today's standards.

Beyond these daily exigencies, other societal concerns and trends greatly influenced the ideas of the founders of the National Society for the Promotion of Occupational Therapy. The major forces that shaped their perceptions of the need for occupational therapy emerge from their respective narratives; these forces include industry, war, educational reforms, and the nature of hospital care. A brief overview may prove helpful.

A recently industrialized society was increasingly aware of the adverse psychological and physical effects of mechanization. Arts-and-crafts societies emerged in a number of cities to restore pride in individual and quality workmanship against the increasing monotony and vanishing autonomy of factory work. Powerful machines maimed bodies at an alarming rate. Social workers such as Jane Addams of Chicago's Hull House recognized the negative effects of both industrialization and city living among poor persons and offered educational, recreational, and community-enhancing activities in neighborhood settlement houses. Advocates for reform in education, industry, and treatment of the ill used settlement houses as centers for generating changes in living and working conditions. Efficiency engineers such as Frank and Lillian Gilbreth promoted techniques to make persons and machines more effective on the job and at home. The crippling effects of war on neighboring countries and the ways in which their governments reconstructed their war heroes prompted a readiness in the United States to do the same. Hospital care was scrutinized. Inhumane conditions in state hospitals for "the insane" received public exposure, and the National Committee for Mental Hygiene sought to promote better treatment for institutionalized patients. Doctors, nurses, and patients increasingly criticized the failure of general hospitals to prepare patients for a society that valued effectiveness and productivity. Nurses and social workers strove for professional respect and credibility, often using contemporary pleas for reform as catalysts for changes in their practices. Each of our founder's conclusions about the kind of service that would be most helpful connects back to personal experiences with and personal understanding of these broader issues.

Changes occurring within medical settings during these early years seem particularly important, because much of the expressed need for occupation as therapy came from hospital workers:

> This was a time of significant medical advance. Medicine moved from a discipline concerned solely with treatment to one involved with preventing the occurrence and the recurrence of disease. However, as such infectious and epidemic illnesses as typhoid and small pox were being eliminated, new medical problems, which were to result in an increased number of chronic patients, became apparent. These included heart disease, arteriosclerosis, and diabetes. The number of the institutionalized mentally ill increased five times.... As more people were able to survive illness and accident due to rapid medical advances, more were left with lasting impairments. The war, a severe polio epidemic in 1916, industrial accidents, and the widening use of the automobile all contributed to the need for new methods of treating residual disabilities. (Woodside, 1971, p. 226)

Each founder of the Society drew a common understanding from this larger context of 1917: the right occupation might in some way help. Exploration of each founder's unique view of patients, therapists, and occupations clarifies the manner in which occupational therapy became multifaceted yet rooted in one basic idea.

George Edward Barton

George Edward Barton was a successful architect who originated the idea of founding a society to promote occupation as therapy. Because his background included a year's work in nursing and some studies in medicine, he had a working knowledge of medical matters (Staff, 1923). He was also knowledgeable of the patient's point of view. He spent a year in a sanitarium for treatment of tuberculosis and had recurrent attacks of the disease. Two of his toes, which had frozen and become gangrenous, were amputated after a trip during which he was investigating famine among farmers for the governor of Colorado. After his surgery he developed a hysterical paralysis on the left side of his body. He was sent to Clifton Springs Sanitarium in New York, where he counseled with the Reverend Dr. Elwood Worcester and developed an interest in occupation as therapy. Aware that he could not return to architecture, he was determined to spend the rest of his life "devoted to the subject of reclamation of the sick and crippled" (Barton, 1968, p. 340). He bought a small old house and barn and named them Consolation House, where in 1914 he opened a school, a workshop, and a vocational bureau for convalescents (Barton, 1914; Licht, 1967). Barton hired a secretary, Isabel G. Newton, who helped him in his work and whom he later married. She described his early efforts: "Paralyzed in his left side, he could scarcely do more than stand. With no motion possible in his left hand and arm, he used his own body as a clinic to work out the problem of rehabilitation himself" (Barton, 1968, p. 342). She remembered that his medical friends, appreciating his results, sent patients to him for help. These referrals launched his "first experimental practice of occupational therapy" (p. 342). In 1917, Barton invited Newton to become one of the founders of the Society. She agreed and became its first secretary. She worked alongside her husband, teaching occupation to convalescents until his death in 1923.

Barton's early views on the subject of occupational therapy are of considerable interest. In his earliest writings he called the therapy "occupational nursing" (Barton, 1915a, p. 335). He regretted that the work was "unfortunately called Occupational Therapy ... because the subject has so very many different sides that most people ... have such difficulty in making out what it is all about anyhow" (Barton, 1920, p. 304). He viewed occupational therapy's goal as the making of a person, that is, a productive individual. He was critical of the hospital's restricted role in treatment:

> To get the patient well has been the aim and the end of it all.... But if the hospital world expands, as the public is

demanding that it shall expand, so that to merely get the patient well is not the whole thing, but to get him well for something. (Barton, 1920, p. 305)

Barton (1920) argued that a man "is not a normal man just because his temperature is 98.6. A man is not a *normal* man until he is able to provide for himself" (p. 306). He believed that the hospital had lost a vital opportunity by becoming focused on the X ray and laboratory, thereby turning out "paupers instead of producers" (Barton, 1920, p. 307). He maintained that a patient fared better during the convalescent period with something to do (Barton, 1920). Occupying his or her mind with something worthwhile enabled that patient to sleep and heal at night. Barton thought that worthwhile activity meant activity with earning power. He reminded his audiences that concern over the inability to earn often impelled a patient to seize a nurse and say, "In God's Name, tell me what I'm going to do!" (Barton, 1915a, p. 335).

Barton (1920) believed that a "proper occupation" promoted physical improvement, "clarified and strengthened the mind," and could become "the basis or the corollary of a new life upon recovery" (p. 307). He believed that a person's spirit could resurrect in "greater strength and purity" to triumph over disability and despair (Barton, 1920, p. 308). He therefore chose a phoenix rising from the flames as the emblem for Consolation House. Barton recommended an extensive occupational diagnosis to include consideration of the patient's education and inclinations; present status, habits, and ambitions; and expectations. The diagnosis would suggest the prescription: the proper occupation in the proportion necessary to produce the desired physical, mental, and spiritual results. Barton believed that any prescription from *materia medica* (as cited by Barton, 1915b) could be translated into occupational terms. He explained that if medicine prescribed benzol to a patient as a leukotoxin for leukemia, occupational therapy would put the same patient to work in a canning factory where the fumes of hot benzine would "keep her in good health" while she supported herself (Barton, 1915b, p. 139). Each human activity could be associated with a physical effect. Barton's unique belief that every occupation had an effect analogous to that of a drug distanced some physicians and resulted in his being considered an extremist (Licht, 1948).

Barton thought that the teacher of the occupation must monitor its therapeutic effects. He called for scientific reeducation with an argument from Frank Gilbreth: "The teaching element is more important in this new phase of adequate placement than it has ever been before, because in every case a new or changed worker must be made useful, self-supporting, and interested" (as cited by Barton, 1920, p. 306). Gilbreth was himself elected to honorary membership in the Society at its founding meeting (Dunton, 1967).

Barton believed strongly that the teacher of occupation should be a nurse. He saw occupational work as an opportunity for the nursing profession to develop, expand, and become more important and useful (Barton, 1920). He exhorted nurses not to sit idly by while others took up this new line of work, leaving them to handle the "crescent basin" (Barton, 1915a, p. 338). Barton's commitment to occupational therapy's alliance with medicine is clear. He suggested that when Adam was cast from the Garden of Eden he was given a divine prescription to earn his bread by the sweat of his brow (Barton, 1915b). Barton used numerous medical analogies. One finds a now humorous medical reference in the paper entitled "Preparation of Patients for Inoculation [sic] of 'Bacillus of Work'" (as cited by Dunton, 1967, p. 287), which Barton read at the Society's founding meeting.

Barton was also the first secretary of the Boston Society of Arts and Crafts, a group allied with the arts-and-crafts movement against industrialization. He supported quality work crafted by conscientious persons. He was particularly fond of our Society's, if not our therapy's, name, including in his rationale a trait of the nonindustrialized worker:

> I am strongly in favor of the National Society for the Promotion of Occupational Therapy as a title. I know that it is long but it does tell the story and the S.P.O.T. suggests the ever alert "Johnnie." (as cited by Licht, 1967, p. 272)

Barton's understanding of occupational therapy was that the person providing occupation would be an advanced nurse who would be teaching scientifically from a medical and occupational knowledge base. This nurse-therapist would ensure harmony between occupational and medical treatments and use a frame of reference for treatment broader but parallel to that of medicine. The therapist would regard the patient as a mental, physical, and spiritual being and consider the patient's individual strengths, goals, and ambitions in these three realms when planning treatment. The addition of occupational therapy to hospital treatment would enable staff to remake a whole person who could lead a useful life.

Susan Elizabeth Tracy

Because Barton encouraged nurses to engage in occupational therapy, it seems fitting to next consider the legacy of one nurse who did: Susan Elizabeth Tracy. I refer to Tracy as a *near founder* because although not one of the founders, she was invited to the Society's founding session. Licht (1967) believed that "no one did more in this country to resurrect and establish occupational therapy than did Miss Tracy" (p. 275). Moodie (1919), herself a nurse, argued that "Occupational Therapy, in other words, the application of various forms of handicraft to meet the individual limitations of invalids and the physically handicapped was first brought into being by Miss Susan E. Tracy" (p. 313). During her training, Tracy had noticed that those patients on surgical wards who kept occupied seemed happier than those who remained idle (Licht, 1967). After completing her course work she became director of the nurses' training school at the Adams Nervine Asylum, Boston, where she initiated a program of manual arts. Her program was the first course in the United States designed to prepare instructors for patients' activities (Licht, 1948). Tracy also taught nurses in practice in the Boston area, including those at the city's Massachusetts General Hospital. One indication of her positive relationships with others and her ability to share her convictions is that an early surgical patient published her *Studies in Invalid Occupations* (Licht, 1967).

Tracy's (1913) book communicates her values and her ideas about service. She valued the support of physicians. In the chapter that introduces Tracy's ideas, Dr. Daniel H. Fuller of the Adams Nervine Asylum noted that "suitable occupation is a valuable agent in the treatment of the sick ... as an important adjunct to other forms of treatment, and sometimes it is quite all the treatment necessary" (Tracy, 1913, p. 1). Tracy no doubt perceived it important to include a physician's endorsement. She must have thought it also meritorious to include Fuller's characterizations of the quality of personal care required:

> Nurses are constantly being impressed with the fact that the technical and mechanical part of their work is but one aspect of their professional duty, that a broader conception must be attained—a sense of obligation to minister to the individual as well as to the disease. The value of wise human sympathy, of cheerfulness in work and mien, of tactful dealing with unreasonableness and irritability, of skillful diversion of thought from pessimistic channels ... are essential parts of the trained nurse's equipment to do her work. (Tracy, 1913, pp. 9–10)

Although Fuller saw occupation as helpful in meeting a physician's goals, he did not believe that a nurse had to be the provider. He believed instead in possession of the proper character:

> Without the constant cooperation of the teacher or nurse, without the daily expression of interest and the stimulus of example, the work is either never begun, or if begun, is thrown aside. The personality of the teacher and nurse therefore becomes an important factor. Her real enthusiasm and love for the work react most powerfully on the patient. (Tracy, 1913, p. 3)

In subtitling her book *A Manual for Nurses and Attendants,* Tracy also extended the role of providing occupation to those competent persons who had not been trained to nurse.

Tracy (1913) believed that a physician could prescribe work for the patient "whose physical, nervous, mental and moral characteristics he had made the object of keen observation and study" (p. 5). The result of such broad prescription was "cure in the broadest sense, in that the mental attitude toward life has been changed" (Tracy, 1913, p. 3).

Tracy (1913) used Dewey's definition of occupation as it related to education: "A mode of activity on the part of the child which runs parallel to some form of work carried on in the social life" (p. 13). She felt challenged to identify parallel occupations for hospitalized patients:

> The real problem of the nurse is to find means whereby she may initiate and actually lead and cooperate in forms of occupation suited to every invalid condition and any natural temperament. (Tracy, 1913, p. 18)

Tracy (1913) pleaded for a certain dignity and quality to the work, for employment of time on worthy materials and purposeful productions. She believed that although a handicraft teacher was perhaps suited to the hospital shop or workroom, sicker patients required special care: "When the shop is a sickroom, and the bed the bench, it is almost a necessity that the nurse be the teacher" (Tracy, 1913, p. 10). Whatever their background or training, Tracy (1913) believed that teachers of occupation in hospitals must have similar traits:

> They must possess resourcefulness, unfailing patience, quick perception of capacities and limitations, an enthusiasm which can anticipate for the patient the attractiveness of the finished product and the insight which substitutes a new piece of work or a new phase of the old before the patient is conscious of weariness or distaste.... The first requirement then in a teacher for this work is that she be able to understand abnormal conditions. (p. 18)

Tracy (1913) then proceeded to a chapter-by-chapter consideration of methods for the teaching of occupations to children and to patients in restricted positions, in quarantine, able to use only one hand, possessed of waning powers, without sight, and with clouded minds. Regardless of the patient's condition, Tracy believed that the teacher must be "thoughtful of the deeper needs of her patient" (Tracy, 1913, p. 10). She supported empathy because "in a large majority of the cases the trouble is local and the patient is like an animal caught in a trap" (as cited by Licht, 1948). Consideration of deeper needs would benefit patient and nurse alike:

> If a nurse can prove to the patient who chafes against his limitations that there is really a broad highway of usefulness opening before him of which he knew not, the mental friction is diminished and satisfaction steals in, while the whole physical organism prepares to respond by improved conditions. In this connection the effect upon the nurse herself must not be overlooked. She too will forget the tiresome routine. (Tracy, 1913, p. 171)

Almost a decade later, Tracy (1921) was calling occupational therapy a "healing force which should be used whenever possible" (p. 399). She personified occupational therapy:

> Suppose the door (to the hospital) is suddenly opened and Occupational Therapy is permitted to walk swiftly down the corridors to the wards. What is she looking for? If she is wise she is endeavoring to discover the human impulse for activity. It is certainly there. Here is a crowd of loafing, foot-swathed men on the veranda; no impulse to work visible. If work is proposed it may be, and often is, scouted. This is no signal for discouragement.

Of what is this crowd composed? A young house-painter who has fallen hurt from a staging and is pretty badly hurt.... Next a psychopathic patient in bed held in a restraining jacket.... Third a man who repairs furniture. Only one of his hands are [sic] available at present.... Then, a three-year-old baby with a new arm in place of the one crushed by an automobile.... Occupational Therapy sets down her basket.—There is always something interesting for each person. (Tracy, 1921, p. 398)

Tracy served as a nurse under the supervision of doctors and psychiatrists in hospital environments, and she was an instructor of other nurses. She had been exposed to multiple disabilities, she used occupation as a service provider rather than as a patient, and her training in occupations had been in the manual arts. These circumstances no doubt shaped her distinct perspective. She supported the use of occupation on wards with the more acutely ill and bedridden patients as a treatment well suited to a medical setting even in the earliest stages. She saw occupational treatment as a continuum along which the patient might move from bed to shop. She supported the physician's claim to authority in matters of the prescription for occupation, perhaps because the subordinate role in prescription writing was familiar or because the patients whom she wanted to treat were acutely ill. She must have recognized the slim chance of success for a hospital treatment that was not medically prescribed. Possibly, she also believed that her acknowledgment of their authority over occupation would enable physicians to admit, as did Fuller, that it was sometimes the only treatment required.

Tracy supported the employment of crafts teachers and attendants in hospital workshops. She valued occupation for the happiness and changed attitude that it produced and for that attitude's curative effect on disabilities. To Tracy, the *worthwhileness* of handicrafts referred to the quality and purposefulness of the end product, not to its earning power. She saw occupation as a means for the nursing profession to help and care for the whole patient. She emphasized interpersonal traits without which a nurse-teacher could not engage the patient successfully.

Barton and Tracy differed slightly in their understanding of how to provide occupations to patients; the differences relate largely to their respective life experiences. The narratives of other founders and near founders explain the additional facets of our heritage as reflections of their personal perspectives about how occupation might help.

William Rush Dunton, Jr.

Also concerned with the care of hospitalized patients, particularly with patients with mental illness, was William Rush Dunton, Jr., a psychiatrist whose contributions to the early Society can scarcely be enumerated. Dunton responded readily to Barton's suggestion that a national society be established. He was an organizer by nature, having himself founded both the Maryland Psychiatric Society and the Baltimore Physicians Or-

chestra (Licht, 1967). He was convinced of the merit of occupation in the treatment of persons with mental illness. Early in his 30-year career at Sheppard and Enoch Pratt Hospital, Towson, Maryland, he had discussed the value of occupation with its director, Dr. Edward Brush. In 1912, Brush appointed Dunton in charge of occupation; by 1915 Dunton had published a book on the subject.

Dunton described his early encounter with patients and occupation while he was an assistant physician. At that time, he organized dramatic performances for the patients, thus earning the "sobriquet of Charles Frohman Dunton" (Dunton, 1943, p. 245). He remembered an interaction with one patient:

At this period we had a scene painter as a patient and I was able by much bossing to make him paint some attractive sets. Each morning he would say: "Won't you let me off today?" And I would harden my heart and refuse.... It is probable that in later years I would not have been so brutal in my treatment of my scene-painter patient and I would have drawn him back to his vocation by easy stages, but experientia docet and I wanted new scenery. (Dunton, 1943, p. 245)

Dunton described his concurrent activities: "In order to interest patients I sought various craftsmen, such as bookbinders, leather toolers, and others who were kind enough to show me the rudiments of their craft so that I could by a little practice start a patient on a craft which attracted his interest and helped him on the way to recovery" (Dunton, 1943, p. 246). Dunton's personal experience with occupation deepened his commitment to moral treatment, a treatment practice used by psychiatrists many years before.

Of all the founders, Dunton articulated more than most the belief that his use of occupation constituted an earlier form of treatment that he was simply extending into a new period of history. His practice in a psychiatric hospital enabled his ready access to articles in the *American Journal of Insanity* about moral treatment in the 19th century. As a psychiatrist, he was perhaps eager to claim occupational therapy's roots among his forebears. Much of Dunton's (1919) writing included references to moral treatment. He regretted the passing of moral treatment toward the end of the 19th century:

It is a strange thing that the physician is so often willing, even anxious, to discard remedies which have proved efficacious in his practice and in that of others, for something new to him and perhaps hitherto untried, so that we have fashions in therapeutics, some of which seem quite as bizarre to us in after years as do those of costume. (p. 17)

Although Dunton accurately identified one factor that contributed to its discontinuance, there were multiple societal, professional, and institutional circumstances that contributed to the demise of moral treatment (Peloquin, 1989) (see Chapter 4). Because moral treatment's particular form is not so much at issue here as is the core of its service, my discussion will be broad and brief.

Dunton (1919) cited Sir James Connolly, who in 1813 caught the essence of moral treatment when speaking of the York Retreat in Pennsylvania:

> The substitution of sympathy for gross unkindness, severity, and stripes; the diversion of the mind from its excitements and griefs by various occupations, and a wise confidence in the patients when they promised to control themselves led to the prevalence of order and neatness, and nearly banished furious mania from this wisely devised place of recovery. (p. 21)

Stories of interactions among therapist, patient, and occupation contribute to an understanding of moral treatment. Leuret (1948) shared one:

> I had one patient, an old fiddler, whom I had not been able to draw out. He believed that he was being trailed by the police and consequently did not dare or care to budge. In order to make him rise, walk, or feed himself, entreaty and even compulsion were necessary. I was unable to make further progress with him until I thought of the violin. I led the patient into the bathing-room, turned on the shower, and at the same time gave him a violin. He had to choose between them. I greatly feared that he would choose the shower. He hesitated for quite some time but finally the memory of his calling returned; he took the violin and played a tune of his choice.... Two months after resuming his instrument he was discharged cured, to continue the practice of his calling and for his entire treatment I had used only music. (p. 30)

A more contemporary description of moral treatment is that it was "a grand scheme for activities of daily living, which placed the patient in a total program with the goal of arranging healthy living" (Kielhofner & Burke, 1977, p. 678). Bockoven (1971) indicated that the significant attitudinal features of moral treatment were "respect for human individuality and the rights of individuals... and respect for the need of every individual to be engaged in creative and recreational activity with his fellow citizens" (p. 223). Most recently, King (1980) argued that in moral treatment "caring for and caring about the patient was as implicit as occupation" (p. 523).

One must not unduly romanticize the practice of moral treatment. Asylum reports did verify that patients benefitted from individual attention, engagement in a wide variety of occupations, small patient–staff ratios, a family atmosphere, and a system that classified and treated patients according to severity of illness. But the patients' benefit was not the exclusive motivation for the practice. Moral treatment brought prestige to asylums and physicians alike. Systems for the classification of patients and for the involvement of patients in occupations reflected a class and sex bias: wealthy patients had carriage rides while poorer patients labored in the fields.

Conceptualizations of the good life were those held by upper-middle-class physicians who managed the asylums. Patient occupation was also a form of patient labor that helped to maintain the asylum. The particular form that moral treatment took lent itself to some distortions and to its eventual demise (Peloquin, 1989 [see Chapter 4]). Licht (1948) believed that "the disturbing element of this diminution is that it was world-wide, which points to a basic error in its conduct during that period" (p. 455).

Dunton warned always against repeating late-19th-century distortions of the use of occupation and in an issue of the *American Journal of Occupational Therapy* cited a cautionary segment written in 1892 by his former supervisor, Dr. Brush:

> Occupation is undoubtedly of very great importance in the treatment of the insane, but the idea of occupation which is satisfied by putting a row of twenty dements to picking hair or making fiber matts is as far short of the true aim of occupation as is the attempt to get labor out of cases of acute mania or melancholia already subject to exhaustive changes and waste ... a misconception of its true value. (as cited by Dunton, 1955, p. 17)

The ideal of moral treatment was that occupations of all kinds be used for the benefit of persons with mental illness. Shaw (1929) reflected early-20th-century thinking about this ideal: "By a new name, an old idea has had rebirth, and is called occupational therapy" (p. 199). The structural invariants of patient, therapist, and occupation mutually acting to improve the patient's condition constitute those strands of the 19th-century idea that Dunton believed the Society had extended into the 20th century.

The extension was timely. Clifford Beers, himself a patient in three mental institutions in Connecticut between 1900 and 1905, had framed a plea for the reform of contemporary abuses. Inhumane conditions after the demise of moral treatment had led Beers to organize the National Committee for Mental Hygiene. Through this organization, Beers (1917) advocated numerous hospital reforms, including individualized care of patients, occupations, recreation, and a more homelike atmosphere.

In the personal chronicle of his experiences, Beers maintained that he had contributed to his own cure through his initiative in engaging himself in reading, writing, and drawing. He often struggled against the system to procure materials with which to occupy himself. When reflecting about the origins of the use of occupation in treatment, Dunton (1921) admitted that "possibly the credit belongs to a number of patients, each one of whom found a tranquilizing influence in work casually undertaken and so continued it in the form originally begun, or in other ways" (p. 11). Dunton thus credited persons such as Beers with having influenced the development of occupational therapy.

The appendix to the 1917 edition of Beers's book details his organizational efforts for institutional reform. He included a letter from Julia Lathrop of Hull House, who had agreed to become an honorary trustee. Lathrop wrote that she had "felt for some time that a national society for the study of insanity and its treatment, from the social as well as the merely medical standpoint, should be formed" (Beers, 1917, p. 326). Lathrop's name is significant in the history of occupational therapy also because of her association with another founder, Eleanor Clarke Slagle. Another letter supporting Beers came from Dr. Adolph Meyer, Director of the Phipps Clinic at Johns Hopkins Hospital in Baltimore. Beers (1917) thanked Meyer, "who, because of his profound knowledge of the scientific, medical and social problems involved, helped more than anyone else" (p. 322). Meyer also worked to support the growth of occupational therapy in substantial ways. He presented a paper entitled "The Philosophy of Occupational Therapy" at the Fifth Annual Meeting of the Society, in which he said:

> A pleasure in achievement, a real pleasure in the use and activity of one's hands and muscles, and a happy appreciation of time began to be used as incentives in the management of our patients, instead of abstract exhortations to cheer up and to behave according to rules. The main advance of the new scheme was the blending of work and pleasure. (Meyer, 1922, pp. 2–3) (See Chapter 2.)

One passage from Beers's (1917) book resembles other passages in which he decried the lack of activity, even in the better institutions:

> For one year no further was paid to me than to see that I had three meals a day, the requisite number of baths, and a sufficient amount of exercise.... As I shall have many hard things to say about attendants in general, I take pleasure in testifying that, so long as I remained in a passive condition, those at this institution were kind, and at times even thoughtful. (p. 68)

When Dunton read his paper at the founding meeting of the Society for the Promotion of Occupational Therapy, it consisted of a history filled with references to the use of occupation in antiquity and to the practice of moral treatment. He encouraged the use of work, recreation, and exercise among persons with mental illness by invoking the success of an earlier time (Licht, 1967). Dunton thus responded to the need and push for hospital reform from persons such as Beers by proposing occupational therapy as a viable solution.

The Shaping Force of World War I

William Rush Dunton, Jr., became president at the Second Annual Meeting of the Society in 1918. At that meeting, he outlined the effectiveness of occupational therapy in treating shell shock, and he addressed the need for occupational workers in the war effort. He thought it important to articulate fundamental therapeutic principles, because many persons entering military service erroneously equated skill in handicrafts with occupational therapy (Dunton, 1919). Dunton's contemporaries were divided on the type of training required to teach occupations. Some considered craftsmen suited for the job; others believed that some form of medical training was necessary and that those most qualified were nurses (Licht, 1948). Dunton expressed his personal preference by establishing the first occupational training course for nurses.

Before discussing principles, Dunton (1919) classified occupational work into three types: invalid occupation, occupational therapy, and vocational training. *Invalid occupation,* primarily diversional, was the simplest form of occupational work. It helped recovery by promoting cheerfulness, rest, and freedom from worry. *Occupational therapy* described occupation whose primary object was to restore the patient's mental or physical function. *Vocational training,* although not occupational therapy per se, became so when used to restore function to persons with disabilities (Dunton, 1919). In all cases, Dunton argued that "the primary purpose of occupational therapy [is] cure" (p. 317). He enumerated nine curative principles that he believed essential to each type of occupational work:

1. The work should be carried on with cure as the main object.
2. The work must be interesting.
3. The patient should be carefully studied.
4. One form of occupation should not be carried to the point of fatigue.
5. It should have some useful end.
6. It preferably should lead to an increase in the patient's knowledge.
7. It should be carried on with others.
8. All possible encouragement should be given the worker.
9. Work resulting in a poor or useless product is better than idleness. (p. 320)

Dunton continued to propose that there were different types of occupational work, saying "there are many facets to the gem of occupational therapy and one of them has been humorously expressed" (Dunton, 1930, p. 349). He then recited a poem titled "Decorative Therapeutics," which linked medicine with occupation while also identifying occupational work as a primary therapeutic agent:

> Do you wish to lead a healthy, happy life?
> Be particular what furnishings you choose.
> For there isn't any question
> That these things affect digestion
> And have much to do with biliousness and blues.
>
> Old candlesticks are excellent for colds,
> And pewter is a panacea for pain;
> While a pretty taste in china
> Has been known to undermine a
> Settled tendency to water on the brain.

A highboy is invaluable for hives,
Or a lowboy if you're feeling rather low.
Colonial reproductions
Will allay internal ructions
And are splendid for a case of vertigo.

Old Chippendale is warranted for coughs.
And Heppelwhite is very good for nerves.
If your stomach is unstable
There is nothing like a table,
If it have the proper therapeutic curves.

Decorative therapeutics are the thing
If you happen to be feeling out of whack
We are happy to assure you
That these things are bound to cure you,
For there's virtue in the smallest bric-a-brac.
(Dunton, 1930, p. 350)

Dunton communicated his belief in the power of occupation with a creed that introduced his book on wartime reconstruction therapy:

That occupation is as necessary to life as food and drink. That every human being should have both physical and mental occupation. That all should have occupations which they enjoy. These are more necessary when the vocation is dull or distasteful. Every individual should have at least two hobbies, one outdoor and one indoor. A greater number will create wider interests, a broader intelligence. That sick minds, sick bodies, sick souls, may be healed through occupation. (Dunton, 1919, p. 17)

The philosophical grounding of this creed supports the use of occupation with persons who are well. The concept of health maintenance through occupation constitutes yet another facet of the early legacy.

Dunton (1921a) identified war as a catalyst for clarifying the principles of occupational therapy. Within months of the Society's founding, the United States entered World War 1. This event was important in that (a) the wartime need for occupational workers prompted the founders to more clearly articulate the service that they were promoting, (b) the war actively engaged three of the founders (Dunton, Slagle, and Kidner), and (c) the war validated the successes of occupational therapy. Dunton described the effect: "I can well remember the thrill experienced at the second annual meeting of the National Society for the Promotion of Occupational Therapy, in September, 1918, when it was announced that General Pershing had cabled to send over two thousand more aides as soon as possible" (p. 17).

The war also influenced an early understanding of what type of person was best suited to provide occupation. The first few wartime aides to go overseas had achieved much success. The circumstances of their recruitment and early engagement are fascinating. Dr. Frankwood Williams, then Associate Director of the National Committee for Mental Hygiene, want-

ed to include occupational workers on his staff for Base Hospital 117. He had gathered a group of women who were ready to serve, but he could not get Washington officials to appoint them. He then noticed openings for civilian aides—scrubwomen with no official connection to the army. He proposed that he get the recruits overseas by identifying them as scrubwomen, and they agreed (Myers, 1948). One of the original aides wrote the following:

The Aides were small in number, but large in optimistic plans for the work ahead—of which we knew practically nothing. Our unit did attend two or three lectures at the Academy of Medicine.... There were only four of us to teach handicrafts. (Myers, 1948, p. 209)

Myers (1948) also confirmed the aides' scrubbing tasks on Ellis Island. The nature of the task is important in light of the aides' backgrounds. Cordelia Myers had graduated from Columbia University in New York and was working in the occupational therapy department at Bloomingdale Hospital. Her "scrubwoman" companions were Eleanor Johnson, a psychologist; Amy Drevenstedt, a history teacher at Hunter College; Corrine Dezeller, a Columbia graduate; and Laura LaForce, a graduate nurse (Myers, 1948). Spackman (1968) described these women as skilled teachers of crafts or commercial subjects with no medical background. The aides who followed these pioneers were required to obtain a general education from a secondary school; normal school and college graduates were preferred. The age preference was between 25 and 40 years. Personal qualifications sought were those held by good teachers: knowledge and skill in the particular occupation; attractive, forceful personalities; sympathy; tact; judgment; and industry (Spackman, 1968).

Many schools opened to meet the war emergency and gave basic medical instruction. A sample course of studies lasted 4 months and included lectures on psychology, blindness, hearing problems, orthopedics, subnormal mental conditions, disorders of the central nervous system, and hospital etiquette (Spackman, 1968). Hospital practice was required for half a day per week. Spackman (1968) observed that "the occupational therapists so trained were equipped as teachers of arts and crafts, and not as therapists" (p. 68). Although she did not elaborate, she seemed to regret, as did Dunton, the aides' lack of understanding of curative principles and the superficiality of their medical training. Some courses were more accelerated than the one that Spackman criticized. The Chicago chapter of the Red Cross, for example, gave a 6-week course directed by Eleanor Clarke Slagle at the Henry B. Favill School of Occupations, Illinois Society for Mental Hygiene, Chicago. Twenty young women, most with training in social services or special work in sociology, attended (Dunton, 1919).

A comment from Dunton (1921a), made 3 years after his cautionary note about wartime training, clarified his initial concern:

There not being enough cafeterias to accommodate all the silly society girls who wanted to do war work, and there being a call for occupational therapists, a number of them took emergency training courses and proved their earnestness by sticking through and getting certificates. Those of us concerned with the training of this group found that as a rule they were not silly society girls at all, but were fine, earnest women despite their veneering of silly society girlism. (p. 18)

This comment identifies another force that shaped the determination of who should be occupational therapists at the time: The feeling that occupational therapy was women's work. Aides recruited for the war effort were women. Dunton (1921a) attributed a measure of their success in the war to their sex: "It had been found that the presence of energetic women who went through the wards of hospitals stimulating the patients to occupy themselves making things had had a wonderful effect in keeping up the morale of the patients" (p. 17).

Dunton was not alone in this belief. A writer for *Carry On,* a war journal reporting reconstruction efforts, argued that women alone could have a powerful effect on the recovery of injured soldiers:

> To prevent his losing hope, to keep his sense of responsibility is in the power of his womankind.... In every step the help of women is essential; not only in cheering him during the first stages, but in encouraging him to follow patiently and exactly the detail of his training....The recovery of our disabled soldiers—their return to a useful life— is in the control of the women of this country. (Miller, 1918, pp. 17–18)

The rationale for this endorsement of women was the belief that a man's state of mind reflected that of his wife or his mother. The writer was a woman expressing a common view that women created a moral refuge for their men, sustaining their spirits so that they could return refreshed to the world of men. These female reconstruction aides returned to the United States to join the ranks of other occupational therapists.

Few studies in the literature that I reviewed for this inquiry suggested that nurses complained that this advanced form of nursing had been snatched from them. Reverby (1987) noted that the scarcity of nurses during the war "brought nursing more damnation than blessings" (p. 163). Her reference, however, was not to a loss of the use of occupation, but to the war's having contributed to an increase in the number of country girls training as "subnurses" (p. 163).

The wartime shift away from a conviction that nurses made the best occupational workers may well have strengthened the belief that a physician should prescribe occupation; someone had to know medical conditions in depth. Dunton (1919) offered another reason for medical supervision:

> If the [occupation] director has not had medical training it has been found that there will be a lack of sympathy

between the medical staff and the occupational department so that this valuable therapeutic agent is not used so well as it should be.... For this reason alone, if for no other, it is believed that the director should be one of the senior physicians, who should at rounds, conferences, and elsewhere, instruct the juniors as to the value of occupation. (p. 55)

Dunton's argument for a physician's use and support of occupation reflected his role as the president of a society founded to promote occupation. His argument that the physician-director should train the staff and the teachers, arrange for the purchase of supplies, and supervise the shops seems consistent with a desire to replicate the managerial control held by physicians in the Moral Treatment era.

Dunton's (1919) estimation of the personal qualities required of the occupational director included tact, the "precious gift of inspiring others," knowledge of the psychology of everyday life, interest in occupation as therapy, "fertility of invention," and an artistic sense of form (pp. 43–45). These traits paralleled those thought necessary for occupational nurses and craft teachers. Physician-directors would provide a service centered on occupation and similar to that provided by nonphysicians.

The war also nurtured an idea of the kind of patient-therapist relationship that worked in occupational therapy. A soldier revealed the quality of the service that he as a patient experienced:

> I got a new vision of life.... I saw that men made unfit for the work of the past must be equipped for work in the future ... saw the dignity of labor made new and interesting, and even more powerful because of the handicap. (Cooper, 1918, p. 24)

The biography of Ora Ruggles, a reconstruction aide, chronicled this kind of service. Ruggles, a school teacher who had graduated from San Diego Normal School and had taken additional courses in the manual arts, responded to the war call for crafts experts. She quickly integrated the importance of engaging the interest and the heart of each patient. Physicians and administrators acknowledged her accomplishments. Ruggles's competence, warmth, and concern inspired awe, loyalty, and gratitude in her patients. She creatively adapted activities that allowed even patients with the most severe disabilities to succeed. Without having been trained to apply them, she understood many of the principles of occupational therapy:

> By now, Ora and the other reconstruction aides were keenly attuned to the word useful. It was a vital key to what they were trying to do. Whenever possible, they thought up projects that the patients could see had tangible use, particularly for the outside world, the world of the well. In this way they could literally work themselves to the level of the normal world. (Carlova & Ruggles, 1946, p. 81)

Ruggles summed up the essence of her view of service: "It is not enough to give a patient something to do with his hands. You must reach for the heart as well as the hands. It's the heart that really does the healing" (Carlova & Ruggles, 1946, pp. 249–250).

If the war shaped conceptualizations of the patient–therapist relationship, it acted similarly on the meaning of occupation. The founders' idea of prewar services was that occupation could be an effective treatment that would enable occupation after recovery. Occupation could serve both as the means and the goal of treatment. The wartime experience of occupational work affirmed this assumption while also emphasizing "the physical side of occupational therapy" (Dunton, 1919, p. 56). Wartime occupational therapy, often called *curative work*, was prescribed to "restore usefulness, overcome deformities or teach to the remaining portion of a limb or another member new functions" (Mock, 1919, p. 12). War injuries focused attention on the use of occupation to restore the patient to a functional condition.

During the war years, Frank Gilbreth had operationalized the efficiency principle of "fitting the machine to the man"; he designed numerous work adaptations that occupational therapists readily implemented as part of the goal of returning the patient to useful occupation (Dunton, 1919, p. 107). Dunton's (1919) book entitled *Reconstruction Therapy* contained several of Gilbreth's photographs of men wearing prostheses (e.g., the Amar claw, the Carnes artificial arm, and the Hanger leg). The book also included photographs of men using self-help devices for dressing, doing farm work, and driving a car. If the disabled person could be equipped with some adaptive device that would facilitate accomplishing the task, the occupational therapist would modify the instructions accordingly. The idea seemed a logical extension of the founders' views. If the prosthetic device were considered part of the person, and occupational therapy taught the whole person, then teaching its use became part of teaching the person. Conversely, if the device were considered a tool required to get the job done, then teaching its use would be inherent in teaching the occupation. One is struck by photographs of men wearing hooks and gadgets, crude by today's standards. The devices permitted a restorative role for the machine that otherwise excelled at maiming, wounding, or dehumanizing. The machine advanced into treatment to touch the patient.

The language of science peppered the occupational therapy literature during the war years. It had been there before, both in the group's plea that occupations be taught with the best scientific methods and in the scientific aims articulated by the original Society. The war experience operationalized this philosophy with methods that appeared to be scientific. Dunton (1919) mused about the many terms describing occupational therapy at the time and thought the term *ergotherapy* the best and the most scientific. He thought it "a very simple matter to trace the development of occupational therapy from simple tasks and amusements to the more scientific occupational

therapy or re-education applied to all forms of mental and physical disability" (p. 29). Dunton believed that a scientific evolution was evident in the growing number of studies on occupation, such as the one conducted by Kent at the Government Hospital in Washington, DC. Kent's study suggested that "definite practice effects can be obtained, by means of a short series of tests, from advanced cases of dementia praecox" among female patients (pp. 30–32).

The belief that occupational therapy's problems needed to be framed in a scientific manner appeared early in the literature. Dunton (1919) argued that much remained to be done before occupational therapy could be considered an exact science. He hoped that the task would attract the attention of the research worker:

> There are many difficulties to be encountered, chiefly centered about the emotional reaction of the patient. Why does one form of work, say carpentry, appeal to one man and not to another, when they are apparently of similar mental caliber and from the same social level?... In all probability the answer lies somewhere in the associative activities, but how can we most quickly stimulate the association which will give us the best co-operation of the patient? (pp. 30–31)

Occupational therapists were interested in answers to questions about how people learned; they were teachers of occupations. They were also concerned with human motivation because so much of their service consisted of interesting the patient in occupation (Mock, 1919, p. 13). Not surprisingly, much of the early literature about occupational therapy included discussions of recent developments in education and psychology. The war experience directed the application of occupations within the context of the growing body of knowledge in arenas related to teaching occupations and in the increasing use of technology designed to enhance individual functioning. The war challenged the founders to examine their service within this context in terms of both immediate applications and unanswered questions.

Eleanor Clarke Slagle

Eleanor Clarke Slagle completed a course given by Julia Lathrop at the Chicago School of Civics and Philanthropy. Lathrop had pursued Beers's (1917) cause for reform in treating persons with mental illness by designing a course in curative occupations and recreations for attendants and nurses in institutions and by resigning from the State Board of Control in Illinois in 1908 to protest poor conditions in that state. Most patients in Illinois state hospitals at that time sat idly through each day, with an able few engaging in hospital industries that consisted of monotonous work designed to help the hospital (American Occupational Therapy Association, 1940). After completing Lathrop's course in 1911, Slagle taught a similar course in Michigan. She then went to the Phipps Psychiatric Clinic of the Johns Hopkins Hospital, Baltimore, to direct the occupational therapy department under the supervision of Dr. Adolph Meyer.

Meyer had experienced occupational conditions similar to those seen by Slagle and had also supported Beers in his reform efforts. He described "industrial shops and work in the laundry and kitchen and on the wards…very largely planned to relieve the employees" (Meyer, 1922, p. 2 [see Chapter 2]). At the Phipps Clinic, he "secured the services of Mrs. Slagle," whose efforts he acknowledged as having positively contributed "to the level [then] represented at the Phipps Clinic" (Meyer, 1922, p. 4). While at the Phipps Clinic, Slagle gave 3-week courses on occupation to groups of nurses in training at the Johns Hopkins Hospital. The instructions included both occupations and the principles underlying their use (Dunton, 1921b). She discussed with Dunton her ideas about their new form of therapy (Licht, 1967).

Slagle returned to Chicago in 1915 to establish the Henry B. Favill School of Occupations and directed the school from 1918 to 1922. She had taken courses in social work and had worked with Meyer, who advocated "the creation of an orderly rhythm in the atmosphere" of the hospital (Meyer, 1922, p. 6 [see Chapter 2]). These influences shaped Slagle's perspective: She taught habit training through occupation. She selected severely regressed and chronically ill patients for her training program. It is not surprising that she started habit training with this group, because Meyer had characterized the patient with dementia praecox as "suffering from disorganized habits" (Wilson, 1929, p. 189). An original principle of occupational therapy permeates the concept of habit training: Occupations could be useful and curative by fostering their habitual use among patients with mental illness.

In habit training, small groups of patients were given close supervision throughout the day. They followed a carefully designed schedule that included self-care and personal hygiene, occupational class, walks, meals in small groups, recreational activities, and physical exercise. Each patient was encouraged to get into a routine and then to assume responsibility for that routine. Excerpts from one care report on a patient convey a sense of the personal service that Slagle initiated:

May 3, 1926—Admitted to habit training. Will not dress or undress self. Clothing untidy and unbuttoned. Mute. Will not wash self. Wets and soils the bed. Eats excessively. Masturbation frequent.

June to June 30, 1926—Washes and dresses self. Wets and soils less frequently. Polishes floor when continuously supervised. Does low-grade occupation.

July 10 to September 22, 1926—Speaks occasionally. Told superintendent that he was "slightly improved." Works on braid-weave rug. Helps attendant with cleaning and clears dishes from table at meals. Appetite more normal. (Wilson, 1929, pp. 196–197).

Physicians like Charles Vaux (1929) believed that habit training caused a "turning point that started [patients] on the road to recovery" (p. 329). He regretted that other physicians found it difficult to accept this "new viewpoint" and "work of reclamation" (p. 328). Slagle's reclamation work with occupation extended to those patients considered beyond the reach of contemporary treatments.

Slagle did not believe that the director of occupation had to be a physician, having herself assumed that role. She indicated that the "capability of such a person involved not only arts and crafts training, but, and most chiefly, personality and character" (Slagle, 1927, p. 126). Although she insisted on solid knowledge of materials and processes, she emphasized the personal element:

For, if lacking in this—in understanding, in give and take, in spiritual vision of the "end problem" of all too many of the cases, the craftsman may make some initial showing, but the work will eventually flag and be largely a failure. (Slagle, 1927, p. 126)

Given her early training in social work, Slagle's belief in the therapist's personal influence made sense. An early conceptualization in social work held that the social worker's (or friendly visitor's) character and his or her relationship with the patient together constituted the agent of change.

Although she did not believe that the director of occupations should be a physician, Slagle sought medical authority in occupational prescriptions. She believed that the physician should prescribe at least the kind of occupation needed, "such as stimulating, sedative, mechanical, intellectual, academic or varied" (Slagle, 1927, p. 128). She argued that all therapeutic measures were the responsibility of the physician in charge. Her definition of occupational therapy included a medical metaphor: "It is directed activity and differs from all other forms of treatment in that it is given in increasing doses as the patient's condition improves" (Slagle as cited by Hull, 1931, p. 219).

Slagle regarded her 3-week training courses as an orientation to nurses about the merits of occupation rather than training in what they might themselves do. She believed that although some nurses completed a period of service in an occupational therapy department, "this did not mean that the nurse would become a specialist…but that she would become acquainted with the nature and possibilities" of the therapy (Slagle, 1927, p. 129). Slagle included attendants in habit training, much as Tracy (1913) had endorsed their direct involvement in invalid occupation with medically stable patients.

Slagle was a leader. She was described as "a woman whose presence was felt by all who were in her company. She was regally tall and there were those who found that some of her pronouncements were in keeping with her appearance and bearing" (Licht, 1967, p. 271). Ruggles remembered Slagle's inspiring words during a personally difficult time. Slagle had told Ruggles that the occupational therapy movement needed her to "get behind it and push!" (Carlova & Ruggles, 1946, p. 113). This urging prompted Ruggles to return to service. Elected vice-president at the first Society meeting, Slagle eventually held every office in the Association and did so for a longer period than anyone else (Licht, 1967). She also agreed to direct occupational therapy for the Illinois Department of Mental Hygiene (Smith, 1929).

Slagle's leadership was exceptional. Men held the highest positions of authority in those early years. In treatment, occupational therapists deferred to physicians, who were predominantly men; in promotional and organizational efforts, men were most often elected to the highest position. The view that women were most effective with patients shaped a leadership pattern that placed men in administrative and supervisory roles and made Slagle's leadership remarkable. (Editor's note: See Appendix D for Adolf Myers' address in honor of Eleanor Clark Slagle.)

Herbert J. Hall

Licht (1967) reported that although Dunton had nominated Dr. Herbert J. Hall for inclusion at the founding meeting, Barton rejected his nomination. Because Hall was nearly selected, because his involvement with occupation was widely cited by the other founders, and because he assumed leadership roles early in the Society's history, Hall's views can be considered, like Tracy's, to be those of a near founder.

As early as 1904, Hall was prescribing occupation as a means of regulating his patients' lives (Hopkins, 1978). In 1906, Harvard University awarded him a grant to study the use of occupation in the treatment of neurasthenia. As a part of this grant project, Hall established an experimental workshop in Marblehead, Massachusetts. In a presidential address to the Society in 1921, he characterized the workshop as an experimental laboratory that addressed the technical problems of occupational therapy. The Society officially accepted his project as the Medical Workshop.

Hall's vision of service provided yet another understanding of the helping potential of occupation:

The writer of these chapters undertook ten years ago to meet in a small way the needs of a class of people who were not in actual want but who from illness or the overstrain of modern life had been obliged to give up their usual occupations. (Hall & Buck, 1915)

Hall reached out to single young people, "nervous invalids" who had "gone to pieces" from a lack of "depth and substance in their lives" (p. 57). Hall believed that these persons learned something of the dignity and satisfaction of "work with the hands" when engaged in occupation (Hall & Buck, 1915, p. 58). His goal was to simplify life through occupations that could rest the mind. One recognizes Hall's concurrence with contemporary criticisms of the "strain of modern life" (Upham, 1917, p. 409). One can also recognize Hall's support of a popular view of "women's work." He believed that the absence of home-like occupations and nurturing functions caused problems among single women; these could be remedied with occupations that substituted one means of creative satisfaction for another.

Another of Hall's unique views was that industries should be established specifically for persons with disabilities. Although he urged the development of workshops within hospitals, he believed that a further step was necessary. Because "the regular industries could not change their rules and systems for the sake of giving him employment ... the way out seems to lie in the establishing of special industries where the handicapped may be favored" (Hall & Buck, 1915, pp. xiii, xiv). Hall predicted a time when hospitals and sanatoriums would recognize the value of remunerative occupation for their patients and would conduct industries as adjunctive treatments (Hall & Buck, 1915). Hospital workshops and industries would help the patient take a first step toward later employment in special industries for disabled persons; there would be a continuum of restorative occupation. He described with deep feeling the patient who would otherwise face a life of idleness and dependence: "Put yourself in that man's place—imagine the despair and the final degeneration that must sap at last all that is brave and good in life" (Hall & Buck, 1915, p. viii).

Barton (1914) thought well of Hall's views because he thought that they represented a nonmedical orientation. Hall argued, however, for medical involvement in the use of occupations. He recommended the use of a prescription for occupation, providing illustrative models:

May 1, 1914
Occupation Work
Mrs. X—Room 50
Light occupation in bed
Basketry or knitting
Not more than 1 hour daily
[Physician's name], MD (Hall & Buck, 1915, p. 76)

Hall (1921) called occupational therapy the "science of prescribed work" (p. 245). He believed that there had previously been a "fatal gap" in medicine that had released the patient cured but "totally unfit because of weakness or discouragement, to take his place immediately among competitive labor" (p. 245). He believed that nurses and social workers needed training in the use of work as treatment and in 1908 provided such training at the Devereaux Mansion, Marblehead, Massachusetts (Hopkins, 1978).

Hall differed from other founders in his belief that the medical diagnosis and the patient's problems should remain unknown to the teacher of occupations. He argued that "work was one of the few normal habits left to the patient, and the nearer he could approach to health in his relations with the teacher the better" (Hall & Buck, 1915, p. 77). Only an unbiased teacher could relate normally with the patient. He further believed that medical information might be easily misunderstood and misapplied by nonmedical personnel. He argued that the ideal teacher would be a nurse serving under a craftsman, because the doctor could then share information necessary for dealing with the "whole problem" (Hall & Buck, 1915, p. 55).

Hall sought teachers with traits that enabled a low-conflict interpersonal approach. He thought that individualized teaching was important (Hall & Buck, 1915). He reasoned that "praise for effort should be given ungrudgingly; but praise of results should not be too lavish" (Hall & Buck, 1915, p. 87). He thought it wise to allow the patient a "liberty of choice" (Hall & Buck, 1915, p. 88). He believed that special effort was the hallmark of caring. As an example, he discussed the case of a choreic boy, aged 11 years, who had at first been dull and discouraged in occupation. The boy had eventually recovered the use of his hands. Hall associated his recovery with the fact that "the teacher took pains to show him exactly how to use his hands, and he gradually became quite expert in fretsawing and other crafts" (Hall & Buck, 1915, pp. 138–139). Special, individualized effort had made the difference. If a teacher had to address a patient's symptoms directly, as in the case of a neurasthenic patient, Hall (Hall & Buck, 1915) hoped that she would "use tact as well as skill" (pp. 138–139). She should also be flexible, using "common sense in the application of all rules" (Hall & Buck, 1915, pp. 168–169). Hall (1921) believed that this profile created a new field for women:

> We are at the beginning of a new profession for educated women. The actual work must be done for the most part by women. Feminine tact and perseverance alone can be depended upon to break down the barriers of prejudice, and to secure the cooperation of difficult patients. (p. 246)

Hall (1921) elaborated on his meaning, while also qualifying the nature of the prejudice he described:

> The theory is so divertingly simple that we may fall easily into error, and fail to realize that we are concerned with the very sources of human power.... Occupational therapy is a means to an end. Some of its proceedings may seem trivial, but they gain in importance through the opportuneness of their application. Practice in this field is not so simple as it looks. All the ingenuity in the world may not be sufficient to overcome the shiftlessness, the hopelessness, the lack of ambition, the evasion, the prejudice which stands in the way. (p. 245)

Hall joined the other founders in recognizing occupation as one of the sources of human power.

Susan Cox Johnson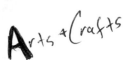

Susan Cox Johnson studied and taught high school arts and crafts in Berkeley, California. In 1912, she travelled in the Orient, eventually residing in the Philippines to teach crafts for 2 years. On her return, she accepted a position in the Hospital of New York City on Blackwell's Island and also agreed to direct the occupations committee for the Department of Public Charities of New York State. In this capacity, she aimed to prove that occupations could improve the mental and physical condition of patients and inmates in public hospitals and almshouses, that these persons could contribute to their self-support, and that occupation could be morally uplifting (Licht, 1967, p. 276). Her aim embodied her belief in the curative and restorative potential of occupation, a belief that was invariant among all the founders.

Johnson's work impressed Barton, who believed that she had "by all odds the most important job in the world, together with a very level head, a keen insight, good experience and a tremendous interest in the therapeutic side" (Reed & Sanderson, 1983, p. 196). Dunton had submitted Johnson's name for inclusion in the Society after Barton's rejection of Hall; Barton had readily agreed to her inclusion (Licht, 1967, p. 271). Shortly after the establishment of the Society and the United State's entrance into war, Columbia University in New York invited Johnson to teach occupational therapy in their nursing department. She accepted the position and soon directed the course (Licht, 1967). She simultaneously organized and directed an occupational therapy department at Montefiore Home and Hospitals, New York.

Five of Johnson's articles published in *Modern Hospital* addressed the training of personnel and the function of occupational therapy in the hospital (Reed & Sanderson, 1983). Her continued emphasis on the reeducational aspect of work and on the educational requirements for practitioners reflected her teaching background. Johnson shared the concerns of her cofounders about educational prerequisites. She regretted a "difference of opinion among those who are working with the same end in view" (Johnson, 1919, p. 221). She wrote:

> What seems to be a difference ... is often not a real difference at all, but is a misunderstanding due to our failure to keep always before us the several natural divisions of our work and the different purposes of each, as well as the fact that each must overlap and merge one into the other instead of being separate and aloof. No standards for training teachers can be set without the recognition of these different elements. (Johnson, 1919, p. 221)

Johnson (1919) believed that teaching occupations to invalids differed from other teaching; there was need to "plan with much greater consideration for the individual than is done in any system of instruction under normal conditions" (p. 221) . She outlined various training programs suitable for working with specific populations. She reasoned that persons teaching invalid occupations in a hospital needed more understanding and training in handling sick people, whereas those teaching in curative workshops or outpatient shops needed more educational courses, because their teaching would "fall into more nearly normal lines" (p. 222).

Johnson's arguments resembled Tracy's. She believed strongly that the educational curriculum mattered; the "great field of occupation would never bear full fruit until the dignity and importance of the position of the teacher in this field is recognized" (Johnson, 1919, p. 223). She thought it "dangerous" that the pendulum might swing toward "losing sight of the nursing aspect of the work of the teacher" (Johnson, 1919, p. 223). She predicted that there would "always be a problem keeping a definite middle path between the nursing and teaching aspects of this work" (Johnson, 1919, p. 223).

Johnson (1919) recognized that the debate over suitable therapists' qualifications had escalated during the war:

> The idea that it was desirable to have teachers specially trained for this work and that they could well be nonmedical people was just coming to be accepted when the avalanche of war necessity descended upon us. The great demand for nurses and the need for numbers of teachers in this field swept occupations out of the hands of the nurse without further discussion and made necessary either the absorption of a foreign group into the hospital regime or the discard of the whole idea of using occupation for a therapeutic purpose. (p. 221)

Johnson (1919) urged occupational workers to resolve the conundrum of suitable training, and in so doing to balance the need for specialized skills against the need for skills required across all settings. She believed that all teachers of occupation needed "an understanding of the psychology of both normal and abnormal minds" and a grounding "in the principles and methods of teaching the sick," regardless of their practice settings (p. 222).

Johnson argued that the product of the patient's work should be of high quality. Her emphasis on "maintaining high standards in the products of occupation" seems reasonable after so many years teaching and learning crafts (Johnson, 1919, p. 223). Recognizing that the field was in a "formative period," she cautioned against any hasty standardization, but encouraged the Society to instead provide "practical aid to the teacher in maintaining the best standards in products" (Johnson, 1919, p. 223). She perhaps supported the Society's establishment in 1920 of an occupational therapy bureau in Boston to investigate the market and the wholesale purchase of staples to sell at a low price to occupational therapy departments everywhere (Hall, 1921).

Johnson's background distinguished her from many other founders. Her views and questions, born of her personal competencies, pushed for a balanced view of occupational therapy as a part-medical, part-teaching function.

Thomas Bessell Kidner

Barton invited Thomas Bessell Kidner to the founding meeting because Kidner resided in Canada and thus would give the Society an international flavor (Reed & Sanderson, 1983). Kidner's foreign status was not the exclusive criterion for his selection, however. In 1915, he had been appointed Vocational Secretary to the Canadian Military Hospitals to develop a vocational rehabilitation system. Before that, Kidner had established a number of technical educational programs in various Canadian provinces. Dunton described Kidner's chief aims in life as being "to prevent the convalescent soldier from falling into habits of idleness and self-indulgence, to educate the crippled soldier in some vocation by which he can support himself " (Dunton, 1967, p. 288).

Like Barton, Kidner had been trained as an architect. He included several architectural drawings in his journal articles that detailed the planning of occupational therapy departments. Kidner served as president of the Society for six terms (Licht, 1967). Barton (1968) described Kidner as "outgoing in expressing his enthusiasm about the use of occupation, a fascinating personality, so very British, even the tailoring of his morning coat, striped trousers, winged collar and tie" (p. 345). During Kidner's presidency in 1923, the American Occupational Therapy Association (formerly known as the Society for the Promotion of Occupational Therapy) adopted an official insignia, which included a caduceus, and made this insignia ? available for use by Association members (Kidner, 1923; "Occupational Therapists Meet Again With A.H.A.," 1923). The pin symbolically fixed the affiliation of this new service to that of medicine.

Kidner (1923) spoke often about the progress of occupational therapy and the growing valuation of "curative work in practically every kind of disability" (p. 55). He reminded therapists that the Industrial Rehabilitation Act of 1920 had extended the use of occupation to many hospitals:

> Indeed, I think it is fair to say that many hospitals have had their attention drawn to the value of occupational therapy by the federal and state industrial rehabilitation authorities who are doing their best to place persons disabled by accident or disease in industry. (p. 500)

Kidner also credited the Act with introducing curative work into many new non-hospital-based service arenas. One new arena was the world of homebound persons, whom Kidner (1924) described as "the product of industrial accidents" (p. 500). Kidner (1923) estimated that the number of persons disabled by industrial and other accidents annually equaled the number of those who might be disabled in an army of 1.5 million men active in the field. He believed that the great number of disabled persons and the consequent "growth and development of occupational therapy naturally led to the evolution of standards" (Kidner, 1929b, p. 243).

In 1923, the year in which the standards were developed, the officers of the Association were mostly men; one of the three was a physician. Slagle was the only woman, reelected secretary–treasurer. Of the eight persons elected to the Board of Managers of the Association, five were physicians ("Occupational Therapists Meet Again With A.H.A.," 1923). In response to a growing interest in securing occupational therapists, "several doctors called the attention of the American Occupational Therapy Association" to the hurried wartime educational programs that gave "practically nothing more than instruction in simple manual arts" (Kidner, 1929b, p. 244). A committee that included physicians studied the problem of occupational therapy education; the membership then adopted a statement of minimum standards at their annual meeting (Kidner, 1930). These first educational standards for training in occupational therapy further shaped the early characterization of the occupational therapist.

The standards outlined prerequisites for candidates and curriculum content. Admission to a training course required at least a high school education or its equivalent. A year's special training in some related field such as applied art, crafts, social service, or advanced academic work was desirable. Successful employment or experience could replace time spent in training school or some other educational institution (Kidner, 1924). The training course had to last a minimum of 12 months, with no less than 6 hours of work and lectures daily. The year's course had to include no less than 8 months of theoretical and practical work and no less than 3 months of hospital practice training and supervision. The official statement required that adequate instruction be given in (a) psychology, normal and abnormal; (b) anatomy, kinesiology, and orthopedics; (c) mental diseases; (d) tuberculosis; and (e) general medical cases, including cardiac diseases. At least 1,080 hours were required in practical handiwork such as "woodworking, weaving, basketry, metal work and jewelry, drawing and applied design" (Kidner, 1924, p. 55). The standards also required lectures on work in several types of hospitals, the principles of hospital management, hospital ethics, the history and development of curative occupations, arts and crafts in relation to the development of civilization, modern industry and the factory system, and the relation of occupational therapy to vocational rehabilitation (Kidner, 1929b).

Course titles and recommended lectures did not specifically include the principles for use of occupation that had been endorsed by Dunton, then serving on the Board of Managers. Neither did the listing include occupations such as habit training or recreational activities. These omissions are of interest because Kidner (1923) mentioned that "the original group of incorporators of the association [except Barton, who was deceased] continued active in its affairs" ("Occupational Therapists Meet Again With A.H.A.," 1923, p. 500). Among those persons with the greatest investment in the inclusion of their own perspectives, none disputed the minimum

standards. Kidner (1924) did mention the existence of various views (p. 55) and suggested that the standards would warrant upcoming revisions, probably to increase their rigor. His summative statement that the standards "provided a fair and workable basis for the training of occupational therapists, and... represented the consensus of opinion on the subject of the great majority of those interested" (p. 55) suggests comfort with the standards. Kidner (1924) explained that "the board of managers endeavored to avoid the Scylla of placing the requirements so high that too few students would undertake the training, and, on the other hand, the Charybdis of lowering the standards of the work" (p. 55). Comprehensive requirements, although ideal, might stymie the development of a new group of therapists.

Whatever the rationale for the minimal curriculum, the standards purported to train the early therapist as both a medical worker and a crafts instructor, thereby resolving the question of which function, that of nurse or teacher, was more important. The occupational therapist had to be a bit of both. The therapist would understand the hospital world and the authority that the physician held in that world, and he or she would perform his or her service within that context. The therapist would be an instructor in crafts whose real end product would be a restored person.

Kidner (1924) detailed the end product of occupational therapy. He cautioned against misconstruing the value of occupation as the "making of a more or less useful and attractive object" for sale (p. 57). He reminded the membership that the "real value of curative work lay in the result obtained in the patient" (p. 57). He believed that to construe the "incidental products of occupational therapy to be the end and aim of treatment" was to not appreciate "the real meaning and significance of work" (Kidner, 1929b, p. 243). Although not acknowledged as such in the literature, Kidner's reminder might have constituted a redirection of members, trained primarily in handiwork, toward a valuation of the work process.

Kidner (1929a) spoke often of rehabilitation. When addressing graduating students, he shared his conception of the quality of service that they ought to provide:

> In your chosen field, a part of the noblest work of man— the care and relief of weak and suffering humanity—may you realize in increasing measure the value of certain spiritual things which are the real making of life, but which we call by many common names. Kindness, humanity, decency, honor, good faith—to give these up under any circumstances whatever would be a loss greater than any defeat, or even death itself. (p. 385)

Concern for the patient and for the quality of his or her personal relationship with the therapist wove through Kidner's statements on standards, medical affiliation, and the curative goal of occupation. Kidner contributed much to legacy. In a memorial tribute, Dunton (1932) characterized

Standards of OT

Kidner's connection with occupational therapy as a "bond of interest in advancing a body of knowledge of occupational therapy" that "grew into a firm friendship which death has ended" (p. 195).

National Society for the Promotion of Occupational Therapy

Each of the founders contributed a unique perspective to the multifaceted service that constituted occupational therapy. The founders also shaped the early service when acting collectively as the Society. Early signs of this collective shaping appeared at the first meeting. The certificate of incorporation of the National Society for the Promotion of Occupational Therapy identified its objectives for "the advancement of occupation as a therapeutic measure; for the study of the effect of occupation upon the human being; and for the scientific dispensation of this knowledge" (Reed & Sanderson, 1983, p. 272). Concerns for science, for humanity, and for the advancement of this new therapy were clear. To operationalize their objectives and to recruit additional members to the Society, the founders appointed each other to chair six district committees: Barton, the Committee on Research and Efficiency; Slagle, the Committee on Installations and Advice; Dunton, the Committee on Finance, Publicity, and Publication; Johnson, the Committee on Admissions and Positions; Tracy, the Committee on Teaching Methods; and Kidner, the International Committee (Dunton, 1967). Barton outlined the plan:

> Let each member, that is, each chairman of a standing committee select from his own acquaintances four others who will become members of the committee and of the society at the next meeting.... Then for the next step—let special subjects be assigned to each member of the society, or rather to the 20 new members, according to the strength, interest, and ability of the individual member. Then let each of these members secure from his personal friends four others to be members of his subcommittee.... Thus the work will "pyramid." (Barton as cited by Licht, 1967, p. 272)

The plan virtually assured the perpetuation of the varied perspectives of the founders as well as the common objectives of the Society. It enabled the growth of special interest groups with a central interest in promoting occupation as therapy.

In 1921, Hall, then president, had suggested that the name of the Society be replaced by the "crisper and more descriptive" American Occupational Therapy Association (Reed & Sanderson, 1983, p. 182). Simultaneously, the larger membership generated by the pyramid plan adopted a new constitution that established two governing bodies—a Board of Managers and a House of Delegates. The House of Delegates voted in 1922 to hold the meetings of the American Occupational Therapy Association in conjunction with those of the American Hospital Association so that hospital executives might better understand occupational

therapy (Reed & Sanderson, 1983). These joint meetings promoted occupational therapy while also sealing its affiliation with physicians and its practice in hospitals. The lectures on hospital management and ethics required by the 1923 standards affirmed this liaison.

In 1922, Hall articulated the goals of the Association and the service that it promoted:

> The association is a responsible, incorporated body with officers of large experience, and active committees encouraging research, collecting data and recommending standards. It seems reasonable to assert that here is a work of national importance, a human reclamation service touching vitally on matters of vast social and economic consequence. Mere encouragement, even placement in industry cannot restore men and women who have not learned through careful bedside training how to use their disabled bodies. The association is literally helping the helpless to help themselves. (pp. 164–165)

Much of the spirit and vitality of the individual founders permeates the statement.

When the official insignia was accepted in 1923, the House of Delegates also voted to establish a national registry, a measure that Kidner had promoted during his presidency. Numerous physicians had sought to secure the registration of occupational workers before 1921. The opinion of Dr. Salmon, a psychiatrist, is representative:

> We badly need a list of qualified workers in this field to which a hospital superintendent could refer with as much assurance in finding correct information with regard to an applicant for a position in an occupational therapy department as he could refer to the directory of the American Medical Association for the information regarding a doctor. (Salmon as cited by Kidner, 1929b, p. 245)

The Society's cooperation with physicians parallels that found in personal narratives of the founders. The early Association strived to cooperate with a number of groups. It endorsed a service that extended not only to the disabled patient and his or her family, but also to physicians, hospital managers, employers, and members of the scientific community. This accountability to many persons structured the Pledge and Creed for Occupational Therapists submitted by the Boston School and adopted by the Association in 1926:

> Reverently and earnestly do I pledge my wholehearted service in aiding those crippled in mind and body.
> To this end that my work for the sick may be successful, I will strive for greater knowledge, skill and understanding in the discharge of my duties in whatsoever position I may find myself.
> I solemnly declare that I will hold and keep whatever I may learn of the lives of the sick.
> I acknowledge the dignity of the cure of disease and the

safeguarding of health in which no act is menial or inglorious.

I will walk in upright faithfulness and obedience to those under whose guidance I am to work, and I pray for patience, kindliness and strength in the holy ministry to broken minds and bodies. (as cited by Welles, 1976, p. 45)

After an exploration of their personal understandings and stories, we can almost hear the voices of Barton, Tracy, Dunton, Slagle, Hall, Johnson, and Kidner reciting this creed.

Other than the writings of Barton, who was himself disabled, there was little written by patients about the early years of occupational therapy service. One article, "A Patient Looks at Occupational Therapy," written anonymously in 1930, is noteworthy. It coincides with what I consider the end of the early years. The patient wrote:

It is hard when the rudiments of many crafts must be mastered ... to keep the fuller vision of all that occupational therapy does and must mean if we are to be really helpful to those who need us.... The broader and more inclusive our outlook as to the wholesome interest in real things the more helpful and effective our work. (p. 277)

Conclusion

This inquiry has supported a broad view of the nature of occupational therapy's early service: that the right occupation could resolve many problems, and that the patient, therapist, and occupation could interrelate therapeutically. These understandings of the founders reflect their sensitivity to the problems and issues of their times, that is, hospital care, industrialization, and war. Also reflected are the founders' responses to contemporary trends toward science, education, sexual stereotyping, and professionalization. Both individual narratives and the collective activities of the Society support Yerxa's (1980) claim that the heritage of occupational therapy includes a focus on care and function. To use occupation as a way of helping persons live their lives in a way that is meaningful to them is to care about persons and about function.

The heritage of occupational therapy was shaped by numerous societal forces and historical events that enabled each founder to visualize occupation as helpful. Events in the early years affirmed the merits of the vision. Had there not been a need created by war; discomfort with the depersonalization and machine-maiming of industry; a push for hospital and other societal reforms; growing knowledge about teaching, psychology, and efficiency; and advances in medicine sufficient to permit a focus on chronic illness, one wonders whether the outcome might have been the same.

To regret the passing of the early 20th century as a time during which the founders resisted forces that threatened to undermine their essential idea constitutes a misreading of the time and a romanticizing of the founders. The founders, visionary and caring people with varied backgrounds and life experiences, shaped the unique, multifaceted character of occupational therapy. Although the idea of the use of occupation was not new, having been used before by psychiatrists, attendants, nurses, and social workers, the founding of a Society to name and promote occupational therapy extended that idea in time and into many places. The multifaceted character of occupational therapy practice today, when centered on occupation and relationships, rooted in a concern for care and function, and sensitive to broader societal issues and problems, extends the legacy into the 21st century.

References

American Occupational Therapy Association. (1940). History. *Occupational Therapy and Rehabilitation, 19*, 30.

American Occupational Therapy Association. (1972). Occupational therapy: Its definition and functions. *American Journal of Occupational Therapy, 26*, 204–205.

Barton, G. E. (1914). A view of invalid occupation. *Trained Nurse and Hospital Review, 52*, 327–330.

Barton, G. E. (1915a). Occupational nursing. *Trained Nurse and Hospital Review, 54*, 335–338.

Barton, G. E. (1915b). Occupational therapy. *Trained Nurse and Hospital Review, 54*, 138–140.

Barton, G, E. (1920). What occupational therapy may mean to nursing. *Trained Nurse and Hospital Review, 64*, 304–310.

Barton, I. G. (1968). Consolation house, fifty years ago. *American Journal of Occupational Therapy, 22*, 340–345.

Beers, C. W. (1917). A mind that found itself. New York: Longmans, Green.

Bing, R.K. (1983). Nationally Speaking—The industry, the art, and the philosophy of history. *American Journal of Occupational Therapy, 37*, 800–801.

Bockoven, J. S. (1971). Occupational therapy—A historical perspective: Legacy of moral treatment—1800s to 1910. *American Journal of Occupational Therapy, 25*, 223–225.

Carlova, J., & Ruggles, O. (1946). *The healing heart*. New York: Julian Messner.

Cooper, G. (1918). Re-weaving the web: A soldier tells what it means to begin all over again. *Carry On, 1*(4), 23–26.

Dunton, W. R. (1919). *Reconstruction therapy*. Philadelphia: Saunders.

Dunton, W. R. (1921a). The development of reconstruction therapy. *Trained Nurse and Hospital Review, 67*, 16–21.

Dunton, W. R. (1921b). *Occupational therapy: A manual for nurses*. Philadelphia: Saunders.

Dunton, W. R. (1930). Occupational therapy. *Occupational Therapy and Rehabilitation, 9*, 343–350.

Dunton, W. R. (1932). Thomas Bessell Kidner. *American Journal of Psychiatry, 89*, 194–196.

Dunton, W. R. (1943). How I got that way. *Occupational Therapy and Rehabilitation, 22*, 244–246.

Dunton, W. R. Jr. (1955). Today's principles reflected in early literature. *American Journal of Occupational Therapy, 9*, 17–18.

Dunton, W. R. Jr. (1967). Occupations and amusements: Organization of the National Society for Promotion of Occupational Therapy. *American Journal of Occupational Therapy, 21*, 287–289.

Hall, H. J. (1921). Forward steps in occupational therapy during 1920. *Modern Hospital, 16*, 245–247.

Hall, H. J. (1922). Editorial—American Occupational Therapy Association. *Archives of Occupational Therapy, 1*, 163–165.

Hall, H. J., & Buck, M. M. (1915). *The work of our hands*. New York: Moffat, Yard.

Hopkins, H. L. (1978). A historical perspective on occupational therapy. In H. L. Hopkins & H. D. Smith (Eds.), *Willard and Spackman's occupational therapy* (5th ed., pp. 3–23.) Philadelphia: Lippincott.

Hull, H. H. (1931). A survey of occupational therapy. *Occupational Therapy and Rehabilitation, 10,* 217–234.

Johnson, J. (1981). Old values—New directions: Competence, adaptation, integration. *American Journal of Occupational Therapy, 35,* 589–598. Reprinted as Chapter 52.

Johnson, S. C. (1919). Occupational therapy, vocational re-education, and industrial rehabilitation. *Modern Hospital, 12,* 221–223.

Kidner, T. B. (1923). Planning for occupational therapy. *Modern Hospital, 21,* 414–428.

Kidner, T. B. (1924). Occupational therapy in 1923. *Modern Hospital, 22,* 55–57.

Kidner, T. B. (1929a). Address to graduates. *Occupational Therapy and Rehabilitation, 8,* 379–385.

Kidner, T. B. (1929b). Standards of occupational therapy. *Occupational Therapy and Rehabilitation, 8,* 243–247.

Kidner, T. B. (1930). The progress of occupational therapy. *Occupational Therapy and Rehabilitation, 9,* 221–223.

Kielhofner, G., & Burke, J. P. (1977). Occupational therapy after 60 years: An account of changing identity and knowledge. *American Journal of Occupational Therapy, 31,* 675–689.

King, L. J. (1980). Creative caring. *American Journal of Occupational Therapy, 34,* 522–528.

Leuret, J. (1948). On the moral treatment of insanity. *Occupational Therapy and Rehabilitation, 27,* 27–33.

Licht, S. (1967). The founding and founders of the American Occupational Therapy Association. *American Journal of Occupational Therapy, 21,* 269–277.

Licht, S. L. (Ed.). (1948). *Occupational therapy source-book.* Baltimore: Williams & Wilkins.

Meyer, A. (1922). The philosophy of occupational therapy. *Archives of Occupational Therapy, 1,* 2–3. Reprinted as Chapter 2.

Miller, A. D. (1918). How can a woman best help? *Carry On, 1,* 17–18.

Mock, H. E. (1919). Curative work. *Carry On, 1*(9), 12–17.

Moodie, C. S. (1919). The value of occupational therapy to the nursing profession. *Hospital Social Service Quarterly, 1,* 313–315.

Myers, C. M. (1948). Pioneer occupational therapists in World War I. *American Journal of Occupational Therapy, 2,* 208–215.

Northrup, F. M. (1928). Work on wards: Methods, crafts and equipment. *Occupational Therapy and Rehabilitation, 7,* 267.

Occupational therapists meet again with A.H.A. (1923). *Modern Hospital, 21,* 499–502.

A patient looks at occupational therapy. (1930). *Occupational Therapy and Rehabilitation, 9,* 277–280.

Peloquin, S. M. (1989). Looking Back—Moral treatment: Contexts considered. *American Journal of Occupational Therapy, 43,* 537–544. Reprinted as Chapter 4.

Reed, K. L., & Sanderson, S. R. (1983). *Concepts of occupational therapy* (2nd ed.). Baltimore: Williams & Wilkins.

Reverby, S. M. (1987). *Ordered to care: The dilemma of American nursing, 1850–1945.* Cambridge, England; Cambridge University Press.

Shaw, C. N. (1929). Occupation as an aid to recovery. *Occupational Therapy and Rehabilitation, 8,* 199–206.

Slagle, E. C. (1927). To organize an "O.T." department. *Occupational Therapy and Rehabilitation, 6,* 125–130.

Smith, P. (1929). The value of occupational therapy from a medical inspector's standpoint. *Occupational Therapy and Rehabilitation, 8,* 331–334.

Spackman, C. S. (1968). A history of the practice of occupational therapy for restoration of physical function: 1917–1967. *American Journal of Occupational Therapy, 22,* 67–71.

Staff. (1923). Nurse's appreciation of George Edward Barton. *Modern Hospital, 21,* 658.

Stattel, F. M. (1977). Occupational therapy: Sense of the past— Focus on the present. *American Journal of Occupational Therapy, 31,* 649–650.

Sutton, B. (1925). Enthusiasm in occupational therapy. *Modern Hospital, 24,* 54.

Tracy, S. E. (1913). *Studies in invalid occupation: A manual for nurses and attendants.* Boston: Whitcomb & Barrows.

Tracy, S. E. (1921). Getting started in occupational therapy. *Trained Nurse and Hospital Review, 67,* 397–399.

Upham, E. G. (1917). Some principles of occupational therapy. *Modern Hospital, 8,* 409–413.

Vaux, C. L. (1929). Habit training. *Occupational Therapy and Rehabilitation, 8,* 327–329.

Welles, C. (1976). Ethics in conflict: Yesterday's standards—Outdated guide for tomorrow? *American Journal of Occupational Therapy, 30,* 44–47.

Wilson, S. C. (1929). Habit training for mental cases. *Occupational Therapy and Rehabilitation, 8,* 189–197.

Woodside, H. H. (1971). Occupational therapy—A historical perspective: The development of occupational therapy—1910–1929. *American Journal of Occupational Therapy. 25,* 226–230.

Yerxa, E.J. (1980). Occupational therapy's role in creating a future climate of caring. *American Journal of Occupational Therapy, 34,* 529–534.

Related Readings

Aims of the American Occupational Therapy Association. (1922). *Modern Hospital, 18,* 54.

Billings, F. (1919). Leaving too soon: The disabled soldier should remain in the hospital for full restoration, physical and mental. *Carry On, 1,* 8–10.

Boltz, O. H. (1927). The rationale of occupational therapy from the psychological standpoint. *Occupational Therapy and Rehabilitation, 6,* 277–282.

Bonner, C. A. (1929). Occupational therapy: Its contribution to the modern mental institution. *Occupational Therapy and Rehabilitation, 8,* 387–391.

Bowman, E. (1922). Psychology of occupational therapy. *Archives of Occupational Therapy, 1,* 171–178.

Brannan, J. W. (1922). Occupational therapy. *American Journal of Public Health, 12,* 367–376.

Carroll, R. S. (1910). The therapy of work. *Journal of the American Medical Association, 54,* 2032–2035.

Crane, B. T. (1919). Occupational therapy. *Boston Medical and Surgical Journal, 181,* 63–65.

Cromwell, F. S. (1977). Eleanor Clarke Slagle, the leader, the woman. *American Journal of Occupational Therapy, 31,* 645–648.

Cullimore, A. R. (1921). Objectives and motivation in occupational therapy. *Modern Hospital, 17,* 537–538.

Dunton, W. R. (1944). Some older occupational therapy literature. *Occupational Therapy and Rehabilitation, 23,* 138–141.

Dunton, W. R. Jr. (1913). Occupation as a therapeutic measure. *Medical Record, 83,* 388–389.

Durgin, D. D. (1923). The value of occupational therapy. *State Hospital Quarterly, 8,* 382.

Elton, F. G. (1924). Relationship of occupational therapy to rehabilitation. *Archives of Occupational Therapy, 3,* 101–108.

Gilfoyle, E. M. (1980). Caring: A philosophy of practice. *American Journal of Occupational Therapy, 34,* 517–521.

Gilligan, M. B. K. (1976). Developmental stages of occupational therapy and the feminist movement. *American Journal of Occupational Therapy, 30,* 560–567.

Grant, I. (1920). Practical side of occupational therapy. *Modern Hospital, 15,* 504–505.

Grant, I. (1928). Bedside, ward, porch, and shop methods. *Occupational Therapy and Rehabilitation, 7,* 95–98.

Gundersen, P. G. (1927). Dynamic occupational therapy. *Occupational Therapy and Rehabilitation, 6,* 131–135.

Haas, L. J. (1925). *Occupational therapy for the mentally and nervously ill.* Milwaukee: Bruce.

Hills, F. L. (1909). Work as an immediate and ultimate therapeutic factor. *Journal of the American Medical Association, 53,* 892.

Houston, I. B. (1928). Occupational therapy submerged. *Occupational Therapy and Rehabilitation, 7,* 413–415.

Kahmann, W. C. (1967). Fifty years in occupational therapy. *American Journal of Occupational Therapy, 21,* 281–283.

Kenna, W. M. (1927). Occupational therapy and hospital industries. *Occupational Therapy and Rehabilitation, 6,* 453–461.

Kielhofner, G., & Burke, J. P. (1983). The evolution of knowledge and practice in occupational therapy: Past, present, and future. In G. Kielhofner (Ed.), *Health through occupation: Theory and practice in occupational therapy* (pp. 3–54). Philadelphia: F. A. Davis.

Livingston, W. H. (1923). Useful occupational therapy vs. useless occupational therapy. *Modern Hospital, 21,* 51–52.

Mabie, H. R. (1919). A plea for occupational therapy. *Woman Citizen, 4,* 344.

Matthews, W. H. (1923). Work—The cure. *American Journal of Nursing, 24,* 164–167.

McNew, B. B. (1923). "Useless" versus useful occupational therapy. *Modern Hospital, 21,* 62–64.

Occupational therapy, vocational re-education and, industrial rehabilitation. (1919). *Modern Hospital, 12,* 221–223.

Occupational therapy. (1921). *Hospital Progress, 2,* 265.

Patients make attractive toys. (1921). *Modern Hospital, 16,* 42.

Patients to be trained. (1920). *Modern Hospital, 15,* 465.

Pennington, L. E. (1925). O.T. known for nearly 2,000 years. *Hospital Management, 19,* 37–38.

Reilly, M. (1962). Eleanor Clarke Slagle Lecture—Occupational therapy can be one of the great ideas of 20th century medicine. *American Journal of Occupational Therapy, 16,* 1–9. Reprinted as Chapter 8.

Robinson, G. C. (1919). Occupational therapy in civilian hospitals. *Modern Medicine, 1,* 159–162.

Sands, I. F. (1928). When is occupation curative? *Occupational Therapy and Rehabilitation, 7,* 115–122.

Second annual meeting of the National Society for the Promotion of Occupational Therapy. (1918). *Modern Hospital, 11,* 298.

Six "musts" for occupational therapy. (1921). *Modern Hospital, 16,* 169.

Slagle, E. C. (1921). To organize an "O.T." department. *Hospital Management, 12,* 43–45.

Spear, M. R. (1927). The value and limitations of attendants in occupational therapy departments in mental hospitals. *Occupational Therapy and Rehabilitation, 6,* 225–227.

Thayer, A. S. (1908). Work cure. *Journal of the American Medical Association, 51,* 1485–1487.

True occupational therapy. (1924). *Modern Hospital, 22,* 66.

Value of occupational therapy. (1921). *Hospital Progress, 2,* 316.

War brought wider recognition to O.T. (1923). *Modern Hospital, 20*(1).

What is occupational therapy? (1921). *Modern Hospital, 17,* 234.

Zamir, L. J. (1966). Editorial—Whither occupational therapy. *American Journal of Occupational Therapy, 20,* 195.

The Philosophy of Occupation Therapy

CHAPTER 2

ADOLF MEYER

There was a time when physicians and the public thought the art of medicine consisted mainly in diagnosing more or less mysterious diseases and "prescribing" for them. Each disease was supposed to have its program of treatment, and to this day the patient and the family expect a set of medicines and a diet, and a change of climate if necessary, or at least a rest-cure so as to fight and conquer "the disease." No branch of medicine has learned as clearly as psychiatry that, after all, many of these formidable diseases are largely problems of adaptation and not some mysterious devil in disguise to be exorcised by asfetida and other usually bitter and, if possible, alcoholic stuffs; and psychiatry has been among the first to recognize the need of adaptation and the value of work as a sovereign help in the problems of adaptation.

It so happened that in the first medical paper I ever presented, about December, 1892, or January, 1893—curiously enough before the Chicago Pathological Society, where one would least expect discussions of occupation—I asked my new neighbors and colleagues for suggestions as to the tastes and best lines of occupation of American patients. The proper use of time in some helpful and gratifying activity appeared to me a fundamental issue in the treatment of any neuropsychiatric patient. Soon after that, May 1, 1893, I went to Kankakee and found in that institution some ward work and shop work, and later, under the inspiration of Isabel Davenport, some gardening for the women in her convalescent cottages. But I also found there a little of a feeling which pervaded quite conspicuously much of the contemporary attitude toward this question.

Among a most interesting collection of abstracts from the history of American institutions put at my disposal by Dr. Wm. R. Dunton, I find a report on the employment of the insane by a committee from the Michigan institutions, dated 1822 and signed by Dr. Henry M. Hurd. The committee had visited European institutions and had been especially impressed by the use of occupation as a substitute for restraint. But they have a fear that the presence of *private* patients would interfere with the introduction of occupation. The conclusions contain the following statements:

> Employment of some sort should be made obligatory for all able-bodied patients …. (But) it would be feared that such measures would meet with much opposition from all quarters …. It might, consequently, be best to arrange at first for the employment of state patients and to procure legislative sanction of the step. If this works advantageously it will be comparatively easy to extend the system to other patients.

This represents the attitude of many hospital men of the time. Industrial shops and work in laundry and kitchen and on the wards were the achievements of that problem—very largely planned to relieve the employees.

A new step was to arise from a freer conception of work, from a concept of free and pleasant and profitable *occupation— including recreation and any form of helpful enjoyment as the leading principle.*

When in 1895 I was transplanted to Worcester, Mass., there was little in the atmosphere to foster interest in occupation: ward work and a few shops managed merely from the point of view of utility. Only the McLean hospital had the beginnings

This chapter was previously published in the *Archives of Occupational Therapy, 1,* 1–10.

This paper was originally read at "Fifth Annual Meeting of the National Society for the Promotion of Occupational Therapy" (now the American Occupational Therapy Association), held in Baltimore, Md., October 20–22, 1921.

of some organized recreative occupations. From 1902 it was my good fortune to have to work on Ward's Island in a division which then was under the immediate direction of an unusually active and enterprising man, Dr. Emmett C. Dent, always eager for therapeutic results and untiring in his development of hospital principles in the face of very cramped opportunities. In this new atmosphere I was greatly assisted by the wholesome human understanding of my helpmate, Mrs. Meyer, who under these conditions may have been one of the first, if not the first, to introduce a new systematized type of activity into the wards of a state institution.

She had become a great help to my patients in visiting them in my ward and had started the visiting of the homes, as probably the first social worker with a systematic program of help to patient, family, and physician, just before Miss Louise Schuyler urged the introduction of a very eleemosynary type of aftercare in November 1906. When in 1907 a real social worker, Miss Horton, was appointed, Mrs. Meyer turned her attention to the occupation and organized recreations of the patients on the ward, not only in the shops and amusement hall, but in the employment of the available time on the ward.

Shortly after that, in 1909, Miss Lathrop and the Chicago School of Civics and Philanthropy undertook a course of training in play and occupation for nurses, and Miss Wright was chosen to attend it and she returned to organize the work throughout the institution—with a wise balance between organized shopwork and more individual work on the wards.

It had long been interesting to see how groups of a few excited patients can be seated in a corner in a small circle of two or three settees and kept wonderfully contented picking the hair off mattresses, or doing simple tasks not too readily arousing the desire for big movements and uncontrollable excitement and yet not too taxing to their patience. Groups of patients with raffia and basket work, or with various kinds of handwork and weaving and bookbinding and metal and leather work, took the place of the bored wall flowers and of mischief-makers. A pleasure in achievement, a real pleasure in the use and activity of one's hands and muscles and a happy *appreciation of time* began to be used as incentives in the management of our patients, instead of abstract exhortations to cheer up and to behave according to abstract or repressive rules. The main advance of the new scheme was the blending of work and pleasure—all made possible by a wise supplementing of centralization by individualization and a kind of redecentralization.

When the Phipps Clinic was opened, we were able to secure the services of Mrs. Slagle, who, with her successors—Mrs. Price and Miss DeHoff, and Mrs. Marion, Mr. Russell, and Mr. Cass—brought us to the level you find now represented at the Phipps Clinic.

This contact with the evolution of occupation therapy gave a good opportunity to see this movement grow to a position which we now want to consider more closely.

Somehow it represents to me a very important manifestation of a very general gain in human philosophy. There is in all this a development of the *valuation of time and work* which is not accidental. It is part of the great espousal of the *values of reality and actuality* rather than of mere thinking and reasoning and fancy as characteristic of the 19th century and the present day.

As I said in my brief abstract, we feel today that the culminating feature of evolution is man's capacity of imagination and *the use of time with foresight* based on a corresponding appreciation of the past and of the *present*. We know more definitely than ever that the 24 hours of the day are the problem of nursing and immediate therapy, and not the medicines taken *t. i. d.* Somehow something apparently *self-evident* has taken its *proper position* in our attention. Just as in the medical aspects we have come to value an appreciation of the exceedingly *simple* facts of basal metabolism (that is, the simple measure of the amount of CO_2 we produce), so the simple fact of employment of *time* has become an important measure and problem for physician and nurse. The most important factor in the progress lay *undoubtedly* in the newer conceptions of *mental problems* as *problems of living*, and not merely diseases of a structural and toxic nature on the one hand or of a final lasting constitutional disorder on the other. The formulation in terms of habit-deterioration of even those grave mental disorders presently the serious problem of *terminal dementia*, made *systematic engagement of interest, and concern about the actual use of TIME and work an obligation and necessity.*

It is very interesting that the progress of all the fundamental sciences has shown the same trend during the last 30 years. The 90s of the 19th and the first decade of the 20th century marked the rise of <u>energetics</u> (so effectively brought home to all scientists by Professor Ostwald in his lectures in this country some 15 years ago)—a determination to replace the interest in *inert matter* by a broad conception of the world of physics and chemistry in terms of *energies,* which means literally "applications of *work.*" Similarly, during this same period the study of human and of animal life gave birth to the concept of *behaviorism* with its emphasis on performance as the fundamental formulation of what had figured up to that time on the throne of an abstract timeless psychology, curiously enough, first invaded by science in the form of studies in reaction *time*. Direct *experience* and performance were everywhere acknowledged as the fullest type of life. Thought, reason, and fancy were more and more recognized as merely a *step* to *action,* and mental life in general as the integrator of *time,* giving us the fullest sense of past, present, and future, but after all the best type of reality and actuality only in real *performance*. We all know how fancy and abstract thought can go far afield—undisciplined and uncensored and uncorrected; while performance is its own judge and regulator and therefore the most dependable and influential part of life. Our body is not merely so many pounds of flesh and bone figuring as a machine, with an abstract mind or soul added to it. It is throughout a live organism pulsating with its rhythm of rest and activity, beating time (as we might say) in ever so many ways, most readily intelligible and in the full bloom of its nature when it feels itself as one of those great self-guiding *energy transformers* which constitute the real world of living beings. Our conception of man is that of an organism that maintains and balances itself in the world of reality and actuality by being in active life and active use, i.e., using and living and acting its *time* in harmony with its own nature and the nature about it. It is the use that we make of ourselves that gives the ultimate stamp to our every organ.

This growing conviction that personality is fundamentally determined by *performance* rather than by mere good-will and good intention rapidly became the backbone of our psychology and psychopathology. It became a fair task for our ingenuity to *obtain* performance wherever it had failed to come *spontaneously* and thereby to serve the organism in the task of keeping itself in good form.

This philosophy of reality, of work and time, seen in all the sciences appeals to me because it expresses, with respect for fact, the simple and yet most valuable experiences of real life.

The whole of human organization has its shape in a kind of rhythm. It is not enough that our hearts should beat in a useful rhythm, always kept up to a standard at which it can meet rest as well as wholesome *strain* without upset. There are many other rhythms which we must be attuned to: the *larger rhythms* of night and day, of sleep and waking hours, of hunger and its gratification, and finally the big four—work and play and rest and sleep, which our organism must be able to balance even under difficulty. The only way to attain balance in all this is *actual doing, actual practice,* a program of wholesome living as the *basis* of wholesome feeling and thinking and fancy and interests.

Thus, with our *patients,* we naturally begin with a simple regime of *pleasurable* ease, the creation of an orderly *rhythm* in the atmosphere (a wise rule of using all our natural rhythms), the sense of a day simply and naturally spent, perhaps with some music and restful dance and play, and with some glimpses of activities which any one can hope to achieve and derive satisfaction from.

In this frame of rhythm and order of time, we naturally heed also the other factors—the personal interests and personal fitness. A large proportion of our patients present inferiority feelings, often over a sense of awkwardness and inability to use the hands to produce things worthwhile, i.e., respected by themselves or others. To get the pleasure and pride of achievement and use of one's hands and muscles, the feeling of worthwhileness of a little effort and of a well fitted use of time, is the basic remedy for the blase tedium that characterizes the indifference or the hopeless depression (that stands in the way of rallying thwarted personalities). I am convinced that a premium should be put on the production of things that are finished in one or a few sittings and yet have an independent emotional value. They must give the satisfaction of completion and achievement, and that in the eye of the maker and of those for whom he has tried to work. Performance and completion form also the backbone and essence of what Pierre Janet has so well described as the "fonction du real"—the *realization* of reality, bringing the very soul of man out of dreams of eternity to the full sense and appreciation of actuality.

Our role consists in giving *opportunities* rather than prescriptions. There must be opportunities to work, opportunities to do and to plan and create, and to learn to use material. There are bound to be valuable opportunities for timely and actually deserved approval and encouragement. It is not a question of specific *prescriptions,* but of opportunities, except perhaps where suggestions can be derived from the history of the patient and a minute study of the trends of fancy and even delusions reveals the lines of predilections and native longings—yet even here the physician would only exert his ingenuity to adapt *opportunities.*

In a meeting like this, the personal contact of many practical inspirers brings out an interchange of experiences and resources from the side of the instructors and helpers.

It takes rare gifts and talents and rare personalities to be real pathfinders in this work. There are no royal roads; it is all a problem of being true to one's nature and opportunities and of teaching others to do the same with themselves. I went through the occupation departments of a large institution the other day and was profoundly impressed by the wide differences of the personnel and the manifold ways of approach leading to success with the work. It takes, above all, resourcefulness and ability to respect at the same time the native *capacities and interests* of the patient. Freedom from premature meddling, and tact in avoiding false comparisons or undue expectations fostering disappointment, orderliness without pedantry, cheer and praise without sloppiness and without surrender of standard—these may be the rewards of a good use of personal gifts and of good training.

Somehow I see in all this profound importance extending far beyond our special field. Our efforts seem to me destined to be the soil for helps of much wider applicability. Present day humanity seems to suffer from a deluded craze for finding substitutes for actual work. It seems more difficult than ever to guide with the traditional preachments.

Our industrialism has created the false, because onesided, idea of success in *production* to the point of overproduction, bringing with it a kind of nausea to the worker and a delirium of the trader living on advertisement and salesmanship, instead of sound economics of a fair and sane distribution of the goods of this world according to need, and an education of the public as to where and how to find the best and worthiest.

The man of today has lost the capacity and pride of workmanship and has substituted for it a measure in terms of money; and now his money proves to be of uncertain value. A great deal of activity, to be individually and socially acceptable and exciting enough and mentionable for social exhibition of one's worth, has to be of the nature of conspicuous waste, a class performance like athletics and golf and racing about the country, and a display of rapidly changing fashions. Work and play, ambition and satisfaction, are apt to lose their natural contact with the natural rhythms of appetite and gratification, vision and performance, and finishable cycles of completion— of work and play and rest and sleep.

Our special work, which tries to do justice to special human needs, I feel is destined to serve again as the center of a great gain for the normal as well. It will work like the Montessori system of education. Grown out of the needs of defective children, it has become the source of inspiration and methods for a freer education for *all* children.

What satisfactions you may develop in the guidance in difficult conditions may bring out the best principles and philosophy for the ordinary walks of life.

We are often told, and I suppose it is largely true, that the world cannot and will not move back. A new sense of *uses of time,* new satisfactions from that inexhaustible fountain, that one thing, time, that will come and come, and only waits to become an opportunity used—that seems to me the gospel and salvation of the day. Human ideals have unfortunately and usually been steeped in dreams of timeless *eternity,* and they have never included an equally religious valuation of *actual time* and its meaning in wholesome rhythms. The awakening to a full meaning of time as the biggest wonder and asset of our lives and the valuation of opportunity and performance as the greatest *measure* of time; those are the beacon lights of the philosophy of the occupation worker. I have often felt that Dr. Herbert James Hall represents the true *religion* of work, leading us to a new sense of the sacredness of the moment—when fitted rightly into the rhythms of individual and social and cosmic nature. Another apostle of the Gospel is announced by Prof. Cassimir J. Keyser in his Phi Beta Kappa address in Science (September 9, 1921)— Count Alfred Korzybski's "Manhood of Humanity,"—the science and art of human engineering.

We might well sum up our philosophy in this way:

In the great process of evolution there is a great law of unfolding which shows in every new and higher step what we call the *integration* of the simpler phases into new entities. Thus the inorganic world continues itself into the plant and animal world. The laws of physics and chemistry expand into laws of growth and laws of function, still physical and chemical, but physical and chemical in terms of plans and in terms of the active animal, and finally in terms of more or less highly gifted man, with all that capacity to enjoy and to suffer, to succeed and to fail, to fulfill the life-cycle of the human individual happily and effectively or more or less falteringly. The great feature of man is his new sense of time, with foresight built on a sound view of the past and present. Man learns to organize time and he does it in terms of *doing* things, and one of the many good things he does between eating, drinking and wholesome nutrition generally and the flights of fancy and aspiration, we call *work and occupation*—we might call it the ingestion and digestion and proper use, and we may say a religious *conscience,* of *time* with its successions of *opportunities.*

With this type of background, we may well be able to shape for ourselves and our patients an outlook of sound idealism, furnishing a setting in which many otherwise apparently insurmountable difficulties will be conquered— and in which our new generations will find a world full of ever new opportunity and achievement in healthy harmony with human nature.

CHAPTER 3

The Influence of the Arts-and-Crafts Movement on the Professional Status of Occupational Therapy

RUTH LEVINE SCHEMM,
EdD, OTR/L, FAOTA

The arts-and-crafts movement ultimately came to be regarded as an oddity; yet in its beginnings, it was widespread and deeply influential. Its origins can be traced to the work of John Ruskin, a mid-19th-century British university professor.

Ruskin (1884b) maintained that machines and factory work limited human happiness. He urged a return to simpler ways of life where experience was "more authentic" because it was less complicated by modern bureaucratic and industrial structures. Ruskin was a romantic, looking back to similar ages when humankind purportedly was healthier because it was more connected with its environment, its work, and its religious values.

He found the Middle Ages especially attractive and lectured on facets of medieval life. Architecture especially interested him, and he pointed to the construction of Gothic churches as an example of how values were incorporated into people's lives: Workmen completed uplifting projects which gave a central meaning to their lives (Ruskin, 1884a). He also maintained that humans, not machines, completed objects; therefore, work was not abstracted from life but had a place at its very core. The manufactured goods of his own time he found to be both aesthetically and morally unsatisfying because the worker was treated like an extension of the machine, completing only a part of the finished product.

Ruskin's ideas were further refined by William Morris who criticized machine "gimcrackery" as threatening the foundation of civilized life (Rodgers, 1974, p. 77). These ideas struck a responsive chord in the United States as well as in Britain. They were most warmly received by the socially advantaged—not because of any widespread disaffection with the capitalist economic system, but because of a discomfort in some circles with excessive materialism and the shoddiness of mass production.

By the turn of the 20th century, the arts-and-crafts movement's advocates formed a network which reached across America. Proponents were eager reformers celebrating nature, authentic experience, and honest design. Like their British contemporaries, they displayed a patrician contempt for the system of mass production, which was keyed to lower class tastes. They advocated the use of natural materials and processes and the purchase and use of handmade items that were straightforward and simple in design. Indeed, for some advocates, the arts-and-crafts movement meant quality of design as much as quality of life.

In the United States, 25 arts-and-crafts societies appeared from 1895 to 1907 (Rodgers, 1974, p. 78). These handicraft clubs where filled with middle- and upper-middle-class Americans striving for self-improvement as well as social stability (Lears, 1981). Reverence for authentic objects and

This chapter was previously published in the *American Journal of Occupational Therapy, 41,* 248–253, under the name of Ruth Ellen Levine. Copyright © 1987, American Occupational Therapy Association.

simple but substantial designs for homes and furnishings testified to the good taste of arts-and-crafts proponents while at the same time conveying a comforting and traditional set of moral values (Wright, 1980). This was helpful in a world where strong ambitions threatened permanence and rapid social change heightened the need for stability.

Wiebe (1967) described late 19th century America as a "society without a core" (p. 12). Rapid social, economic, technological, civic, and cultural changes had created a "distended" society; yet people were still trying to understand the expanding American society in terms of their familiar, small-town environment. This simplistic orientation created even more problems because a larger vision of the future was required to deal with destabilizing forces such as westward expansion; millions of Eastern European immigrants; rising impersonal, industrialized work; technological advances that linked the country together; declining birth and death rates; changing roles of women; and economic instability.

The smug security of small-town America was ending, and local community members felt as if they were losing control over their lives, although the "enemy" was not always clear. People yearned for a slower paced life, governed by the old and authentic values. Thus, the arts-and-crafts movement rose in popularity, offering the promise of a more meaningful life-style.

The Transformation of Medicine

Medicine was in part responsible for the initial direction taken by occupational therapy. By the turn of the 20th century, American physicians were shifting to a scientific foundation. Disease was understood in terms of physiological processes rather than in terms of suffering or personal disorientation; specialists concerned themselves with organs and tissues rather than the whole patient; hospitals removed the sick from their environments and treated them as abstractions; and vital signs collected through such new instruments as the X-ray machine and interpreted by the laboratory obviated the need for the physician to listen to patients' complaints or win the patient's active partnership in treatment planning.

Yet some physicians, often those connected with the most prestigious institutions, believed that science, by itself, did not offer a complete answer to illness. They argued that earlier notions of mind–body unity were being overlooked in the new high-technology medicine.

Dr. Herbert J. Hall was one such dissenter. He was interested in neurasthenia, a medical problem that did not reduce itself easily to the limitations of the new medicine. This disease was not obviously physiological, its symptoms were diverse and could be linked to the strain of American life. The malady was identified in middle- and upper-class persons who complained of "morbid anxiety, unaccountable fatigue, irrational fears, and compulsive or inadequate sexual behavior" (Beard, 1881, pp. 7–8; also Lears, 1981, p. 50).

Hall (1910) developed a work cure to take the place of the commonly prescribed bed rest. He based his therapeutics squarely on the philosophy espoused by the arts-and-crafts enthusiasts. After securing financial backing from the prestigious Proctor Fund, he developed a sanatorium in Marblehead, Massachusetts, and began to validate the success of his work cure. Hall joined a network of likeminded physicians.

Two other physician dissenters who also became interested in curative occupations were Adolf Meyer and William Rush Dunton. Both searched for ways to humanize the care of chronically ill patients. Meyer was impressed with the results he saw at Worcester Massachusetts State Hospital where his wife, Mary Potter Brooks Meyer, a social worker, developed an occupations program for ward patients. Adolf Meyer, as a researcher, was usually removed from direct patient care. Mrs. Meyer, therefore, operationalized his ideas on adaptation and the therapeutic prescription of activities (Hopkins, 1979).

In Chicago, the collaboration between Meyer, a medical leader, and Julia Lathrop, a social worker and civic activist, resulted in the application of arts-and-crafts ideology to chronically ill mental patients. Lathrop studied bookbinding at Kelmscott Press under Morris. She wanted to improve the lives of the less fortunate by applying the principles of the arts-and-crafts movement to patient programs. She fulfilled this goal by using her influence as a member of the Illinois State Board of Charities and Correction. She and another Board member, Rabbi Emil Hirsch, in 1906 organized one of the earliest occupations training courses (Addams, 1935).

Dunton, who also came to believe in the curative effect of goal-directed activity, applied the occupations cure to his patients at the Sheppard and Enoch Pratt Asylum in Towson, Maryland, as early as 1895. By 1908, his observations of patients' undirected efforts led him to search for an arts-and-crafts teacher. Using *Studies in Invalid Occupations: A Manual for Nurses and Attendants* by Susan E. Tracy (1912), a nurse, Dunton established his own training program.

In her book, Tracy described an occupations training course she designed in 1906 for nurses working at Adams Nervine Hospital in Boston. The text, which is basically a craft book, offered teaching strategies, supply lists, and treatment rationales for a variety of settings, including the homes of advantaged and disadvantaged patients. These progressive physicians, Meyer, Hall, and Dunton, worked with social caretakers Lathrop and Tracy to link the holistic treatment of the past with modern, scientific approaches (Burnham, 1972). Combining ideas that were once important in medical practice with ideas from the arts-and-crafts movement, these individuals founded a new profession, which was later named occupational therapy.

The Arts-and-Crafts Origins in Occupational Therapy

Early occupational therapy practice combined the therapeutic and medical with the diversional and recreational use of activities. One of the earliest sources of overlap between these applications was the sheltered workshop. Hall and other physicians championed the development of sheltered workshops where patients produced carefully designed, well-made objects such as hand towels, ceramic vases, and cement pots. The craft objects were sold in shops that had three purposes—to employ talented people who could earn a living by making authentic objects, to give spiritual support to craftspeople who pursued crafts as an avocation, and to help employ the mentally and physically handicapped ("Craftsmanship," 1906; Evans, 1974; Roorbach, 1913; Simkhovitch, 1906). These purposes frequently overlapped, and it soon became difficult to separate rehabilitation goals from the aesthetic ideology of the arts-and-crafts movement.

Following Hall's lead, George Barton, an architect familiar with Morris, joined the Boston Society of Arts and Crafts in 1901. Barton was not a healthy man, and after a long struggle with tuberculosis he decided to move to Denver where he lost his left foot to frostbite in 1912. Depressed and ill, he returned to the East and sought the advice and counsel of both a physician and a minister who urged him to direct his energies toward a productive mission. Barton decided to help others instead of focusing on his own health problems and opened Consolation House in Clifton Springs, New York, in 1914. He received referrals from physicians and applied the principles of therapeutic arts and crafts to disabled individuals such as himself (Reed & Sanderson, 1983).

Barton joined a group of workshop managers who had to balance conflicting personnel and production goals. Goods had to be appealing, well made, and relatively cheap. Thus, the arts-and-crafts workshop proved a difficult venture even for nondisabled craftsmen because of the competition from mass-produced goods (Boris, 1984). The successful therapeutic workshop also had to address the additional factor of varied and inconsistent client needs. Above all, the goal of the therapeutic workshop was to move successful performers back into the workforce.

Solvent workshop endeavors were rare even if workers were nondisabled, skilled, and efficient. Machine-made goods proved to be stiff competition in the marketplace, lowering prices on workshop-produced goods and squeezing profits (Boris, 1984). To survive, workshops shifted their focus from therapeutics to cost-conscious ventures that would reap profits. The individualistic thrust of early occupational therapy was lost in this shift to economic considerations.

The early occupational therapy link to the arts-and-crafts movement did not end with the demise of the therapeutic workshop. This influence was still evident in the 1930s and 1940s, long after the ideas and beliefs of the proponents of the arts-and-crafts movement disappeared from the American culture. Evidence is plentiful: Black (1935) discussed the employment of sheep herders in the Arts and Crafts League of New Hampshire, Ash (1940) presented the use of handicrafts with blind and retarded patients, annual conferences included craft instructions, and the 1932 Annual Institute of Chief Occupational Therapists devoted 25% of its conference to a folk dance, a lecture, and a demonstration (Annual Institute for Chief OT's, 1932).

Glaser (1930) noted that the eye, hand, mind, and creative imagination are stimulated by arts and crafts. In line with this thinking, occupational therapy schools offered courses in needlework, weaving, metalwork, bookbinding, and leatherwork. The missions and philosophies of occupational therapy and the arts-and-crafts movement were so intertwined that few therapists would have disagreed with Will Levington Comfort when he remarked that "there is something holy in the crafts and the arts" (as cited by Glaser, 1930, p. 131).

Healthy individuals were drawn to the arts-and-crafts movement because involvement with arts and crafts promised to settle nervous lives. The occupational therapy founders creatively applied these ideas to a neglected group of chronically disabled patients. These applications were varied and creative and included the management of pain during recuperation, the redirection of the wandering minds of elders, and the diversion of self-indulgent thoughts of depressives. Therapists were slow to depart from the prescriptions of the founders who had argued that the "scientific" prescription of arts and crafts could cure a variety of chronic problems generally considered outside of the domain of medicine (Tracy, 1912; Hall & Buck, 1916; Dunton, 1918).

Changes in Social Values Create Conflicting Philosophies

Only a thin line divided the arts-and-crafts philosophy from occupational therapy. Arts-and-crafts persons were diversionists using an activity to achieve a cure; yet to them the craft product was as valued as the process. Therapists differed slightly, they focused more on the concept of function and were less concerned with the product, but they still used crafts.

Trained in specific modalities, many diversionists neglected the patient's interest in the activity at hand. Consistent with their crafts training, they searched for information about specific crafts rather than exploring why the occupation cure succeeded. Diversionists fervently believed that craftwork alone was curative. This belief was based on the work ethic. The differences between therapists and diversionists grew more and more obvious in the 1930s and 1940s.

The overlap between personal interests and professional roles and responsibilities was also confusing. Even Dunton demonstrated a mixture of personal and professional interests, displaying his quilt collection at an occupational therapy meeting held at the Baltimore Handicraft Club ("OT Notes,"

1930). This mixture of values proved difficult for early therapists who were trained in fine arts and specific crafts. To abandon their commitment to craftsmanship, to embrace the process over the end product was a violation of their cherished belief in the arts-and-crafts movement. Diversionists were so tied to the arts-and-crafts ideology that they overlooked the process by which the therapist elicits the patient's goals, values, and interest in the activity process (Dunton, 1928).

Furthermore, the professional occupational therapist was under severe strains. Health care's focus on the individual further eroded as the status of physicians rose and medicine was transformed into a specialty practice based on scientific principles. In this milieu, the holistic philosophy of early occupational therapy practice was increasingly compromised as diversionists continued to focus on specific craft concerns (Hall, 1922).

The Depression contributed to the changes in health care delivery. In some states, over 40% of the population subsisted on relief. The national income plummeted to less than half of what it had been in 1929 (Stevens, 1971). The bleak industrial situation created shortages in health services and providers. Physicians' incomes fell, nurses were unemployed, and hospitals developed insurance to guarantee payment. For many Americans, medical care became a luxury (Starr, 1982).

Occupational therapy survived using strategies such as "classes" to provide treatment to large numbers of patients. At the same time, leaders pushed therapists away from the values of the arts-and-crafts mission and toward the medical model (Mock, 1930; Munger, 1935). Occupational therapy leaders embraced functional concerns; arts-and-crafts values were subordinated to the functional orientation. Occupational therapy, like medicine, assumed responsibility for making decisions for the patient's welfare. Unlike the developing science of medicine, however, therapists had no technology to measure the accuracy of their prescriptions.

Occupational therapy was caught in a web of conflicting ideas. The scientific goals of medicine pulled against the holistic goals of the arts-and-crafts movement. Change did not come smoothly. In 1930, Eleanor Clarke Slagle, a prominent occupational therapy leader, felt obligated to warn new graduates of Sheppard and Enoch Pratt Hospital that "handiwork alone was insufficient" (p. 271).

Joseph Doane (1931), a physician and president of the American Occupational Therapy Association, was equally emphatic when he differentiated between two groups of occupational therapists: "There are those who believe that the occupationalist who diverts and amuses and who as a by-product perhaps spiritually improves the sick, contributes the greatest good to the community" (p. 365). Doane maintained that the "occupationalist" is likely to possess less vision and training than the therapist who uses supplies as a means to the performance end. Doane rejected the arts-and-crafts movement and promoted the science of occupational therapy. He noted that "Occupational therapy is not a fad which like many

others seizes the imagination of a community or country and then suddenly relinquishes its hold" (p. 364).

Dr. Horatio M. Pollock (1934) traced occupational therapy back to Galen in the 2nd century but noted that occupational therapy "has not yet won a place in the consciousness of a large part of the medical profession" (p. 362), In the same vein, Oscar M. Sullivan (1935), also a physician, predicted the future thrust of occupational therapy when he explained that although "craftwork constitutes the bulk of what is known as occupational therapy," there was no reason that "another kind of practical work should not develop quite as much" (p. 107). It was merely a matter of opportunity and facilities.

Thus, the profession struggled during the 1930s and 1940s and ultimately lost the momentum enjoyed during the initial years of organizing. Pulled by internal tensions regarding the focus of the occupation process, therapists were also influenced by shrinking health resources, the rising status of physicians, the limited roles of professional women, and most distressing, the doubts raised by patients who questioned the merit of craft therapy. In short, few therapists, physicians, or patients remembered the lofty mission of the forgotten arts-and-crafts movement.

Dr. Harry Steckel (1934) noted "it is quite possible that patients do not fully realize or recognize the true value of occupational therapy, even if they are not particularly interested in the project worked on by them" (p. 494). Steckel believed that occupational therapy could be improved by using a variety of projects with "more opportunity for personal choice, with a closer check upon the reaction of the patient to the type of work offered" (p. 498).

Thus occupational therapy survived the 1930s but was moored to the values of a forgotten social movement. Meanwhile, the medical profession had shifted from a holistic to a reductionist focus. During World War II, the occupational therapy profession struggled with the same unresolved tension between craft proponents and therapists, but the context had changed. Younger physicians no longer understood or valued the arts-and-crafts philosophy. Because occupational therapy practice did not seem scientific or theory based, they tended not to take it seriously. The example of a specific hospital offered below demonstrates that therapists changed little in their philosophy, theory, and therapeutic modalities during the first 35 years of practice. Few acknowledged that the context for health services had changed.

The Example of Norristown State Hospital

In 1884, Norristown State Hospital used occupations to control patients or as a "conspicuous feature of the management" ("Official Report," 1884, p. 35). A physician reported that it was not necessary to restrain patients because "employment and varied diversions of the mind" (p. 60) were prescribed. Overcrowding compromised this idealistic beginning. Only such production-oriented activities as farming; sewing dresses, shirts, and sheets; and housekeeping chores survived.

Overcrowding continued, and only a few patients were given occupations ("Sixth Annual Report," 1885).

In response to the arts-and-crafts influence, a craftsperson, Nancy Cresson, was hired in 1904 to teach Indian basket making. The focus on occupations was minimal until 1920 when the department for men's occupational therapy was used as a supplement to medical treatment, a means to get the mentally afflicted back into the work force ("41st Annual Report," 1920). That year, 52 men were so engaged. Yet at the same time, a nursing staff shortage caused the closing of the women's arts-and-crafts workroom. Activities were moved to the wards.

The male occupational therapy department was formally organized in 1924. Four therapists were assigned to over 4,000 patients. The department's year-end report contained the following facts for 1925: Activities included basketry, art, weaving, and sewing. The patients completed 245 rugs, 257 reed baskets, 324 raffia baskets, 27 leather items, 74 wood items, 92 embroidered objects, 97 lace objects, and 20 fiber mats (Norristown State Hospital, 1925). The arts-and-crafts focus is clear.

The hospital plant was in disrepair by 1930, and a drought also affected the farm. Yet occupational therapy thrived with four therapists and a supply and material budget. Physician turnover was problematic, but occupational therapy was even mentioned in the hospital mission although the main emphasis was on returning patients to the community. This was a time of opportunity when occupational therapists could have chosen to increase their influence because of the shortage of physicians and the limited status of other professionals. Therapists, nevertheless, were not prepared to take advantage of this opportunity.

Instead, the occupational therapists treated 600 patients during the year, producing 1,662 arts-and-crafts products. The occupational therapy department was described thus:

> Among the diversional methods of treating the mentally sick and hastening recovery is Occupational Therapy—the scheme of scientifically arranged activities which tend to improve the mental and physical health of patients. ("Fifty-Second Annual Report," 1931, p. 27)

The department organized two pageants and other forms of hospital entertainment. By 1934, occupational therapists used small ward groups to "prevent further deterioration in patients" ("Fifty-Fifth Annual Report," 1934, p. 30). Music, movies, bridge, French classes, and dance activities were also part of the department's responsibilities. An elaborate May Day pageant involved over 100 patients. Photos depict patients proudly posing in elaborate costumes and staging—activities for patients functioning at a high level. Annual reports and occupational therapy department reports mention only craft and diversional activities.

In the 1937 annual report ("Fifty-Eighth Annual Report"), nursing and occupational therapy were combined. The occupational therapy chief worked with six aides (therapists), and together they offered classes on nine wards. An average of 438 patients participated in occupational therapy programs, and the products were sold for a total of $1,178.23. Program changes in the department were minimal through the 1930s; the occupational therapy department basically continued the same work it had done in the 1920s.

On the other hand, psychologists, nurses, and other health professionals were paralleling the specialization of medicine in their own fields (Burnham, 1974). Occupational therapy was ill prepared to explain the activity process except in the idealistic language of the art-and-crafts movement. The resulting criticism from physicians and other professionals indicates that occupational therapists failed to explain the value of the activity process except in terms of a long forgotten social movement.

The Unresolved Conflict of Values

As the profession matured, confusion regarding our therapeutic mission, goals, and treatment techniques still remained. The use of arts and crafts boosted professional visibility during the early years of development, but the profession paid a price for capitalizing on a therapeutic form that was part of a lay health movement. In fact, occupational therapy became locked into treatment modalities that reflected the social values of a forgotten era. Arts-and-crafts proponents and therapists did not always have similar goals. Surprising evidence of these differences can be found in a telling exchange that took place in 1935.

In a letter to William Rush Dunton, the editor of *Occupational Therapy and Rehabilitation*, Susan Colson Wilson suggested that occupational therapists needed a patron saint. She selected St. Birgetta for the role of patroness. This seemed to upset Dunton, an occupational therapy founder and leader. In a 1935 editorial, Dunton responded sarcastically that

> St. Birgetta might be an admirable patron for the Needlework Guild of America, but her selection as a patron of occupational therapy seems to unduly emphasize a particular craft rather than the special object to be gained by use of any occupation. (p. 223)

Wilson, the chief occupational therapist at Brooklyn State Hospital, was an experienced therapist and an active member of the association. Her suggestion and Dunton's subsequent reply symbolize the conflicting philosophies that continued to surface between the arts-and-crafts proponents and the medically oriented therapists.

Summary

This paper traced the effects of changing health care demands on occupational therapy founders and arts-and-crafts proponents. The Founders were responding to the emerging needs of patients, whereas the proponents of the arts-and-crafts movement continued to focus on their original ideas. A study of past events underscores the overwhelming influence of the environment on professional practice. This influence must be recognized so that newly emerging public needs can be addressed.

Acknowledgments

I thank Morris Vogel, PhD, Professor of History at Temple University, Philadelphia, for his helpful comments on an earlier draft of this article and Doris Kaplan, OTR/L, Director of Occupational Therapy, Norristown State Hospital, Norristown, Pennsylvania, for lending supporting documents and artifacts.

References

Addams, J. (1935) *My friend Julia Lathrop.* New York: MacMillan.

Annual institute for chief OTs. (1932). *The Psychiatric Quarterly, 6,* 384–387.

Ash, F. (1940). The value of handicraft for the retarded blind. *Occupational Therapy and Rehabilitation, 19,* 339–343.

Beard, G. M. (1972). *American nervousness, its causes and consequences* [Reprint of 1881 ed.]. New York: Arno Press.

Black, W. D. (1935). League of arts and crafts of New Hampshire. *Occupational Therapy and Rehabilitation, 14,* 29–37.

Boris, E. (1984). *Art and labor: John Ruskin, William Morris, and the craftsman ideal in America 1876–1915.* Philadelphia: Temple University Press.

Burnham, J. C. (1972). Medical specialists and movements toward social control in the progressive era: Three examples. In J. Israel (Ed.), *Building the organizational society* (pp. 19–30). New York: Free Press.

Burnham, J. C. (1974). The struggle between physicians and paramedical personnel in American psychiatry, 1917–41. *Journal of the History of Medicine and Allied Science, 29,* 93–106.

Craftsmanship for crippled children. (1906). *The Craftsman, 9,* 667–677.

Doane, J. C. (1931). Presidential address. *Occupational Therapy and Rehabilitation, 10,* 363–368.

Dunton, W. R. (1918). The principles of occupational therapy. *Public Health Nursing, 10,* 316–321.

Dunton, W. R. (1928). *Prescribing occupational therapy.* Springfield, IL: Charles C Thomas.

Dunton, W. R. (1935). Editorial. *Occupational Therapy and Rehabilitation, 14,* 223.

Evans, P. (1974). *Art pottery of the United States: An encyclopedia of producers and their marks.* New York: Charles Scribner's Sons.

Fifty-eighth annual report of the Norristown State Hospital at Norristown, Pa., S. E. District of Pennsylvania for year ending May 31, 1937. (1937). Norristown, PA: Hospital Printing Office and Bindery.

Fifty-fifth annual report of the Norristown State Hospital at Norristown, Pa., for the year ending May 31, 1934. (1934). Norristown, PA: Hospital Printing Office and Bindery.

Fifty-second annual report of the Norristown State Hospital at Norristown, Pa., for the year ending May 31, 1931. (1931) Norristown, PA: Hospital Printing Office and Bindery.

Forty-first annual report of the State Hospital for the Insane, S. E. District of Pennsylvania, Norristown, Pa., for the year ending May 31, 1920. (1920). Norristown, PA: Hospital Printing Office and Bindery.

Glaser, L. (1930). Some notes on a St. Louis weaving shop. *Occupational Therapy and Rehabilitation, 9,* 127–131.

Hall, H. J. (1910). Work-cure. *JAMA, 54,* 12–14.

Hall, H. J. (1922). President's address. *Archives of Occupational Therapy, 1,* 435–442.

Hall, H. J., & Buck, M. M. C. (1916). *Handicrafts for the handicapped.* New York: Moffat, Yard, and Co.

Hopkins, H. L. (1979). *The status of occupational therapy: Implications for program development.* Unpublished doctoral dissertation, Temple University, Philadelphia.

Lears, J. T. (1981). *No place of grace: Antimodernism and the transformation of American culture.* New York: Pantheon.

Mock, H.E. (1930). The rehabilitation of the disabled. *JAMA, 95,* 31–34.

Munger, C.W. (1935). Fitting OT into the institutional scheme. *Occupational Therapy and Rehabilitation, 14,* 111–119.

Norristown State Hospital. (1925). *Report of occupational therapy for year ending June 1, 1925.* Norristown, PA: Author.

Official report of the trustees and officers of the State Hospital for the Insane for the S.E. District of Pennsylvania at Norristown, Pa., for the Year ending September 30, 1884. (1884). Allentown, PA: Allen W. Haines.

OT Notes. (1930). *Occupational Therapy and Rehabilitation, 9,* 253–258.

Pollock, H.M. (1934). The relation of occupational therapy to medicine. *Occupational Therapy and Rehabilitation, 13,* 361–366.

Reed, K.L. & Sanderson, S.R. (1983). *Concepts in occupational therapy.* Baltimore: Williams & Wilkins.

Rogers, D.T. (1974). *The work ethic in industrial America, 1850–1920.* Chicago: University of Chicago Press.

Roorbach, E. (1913). *Making pottery in the California hills.* The Craftsman, 24, 342–346.

Ruskin, J. (1994a). *Lectures on architecture and painting delivered at Edinburgh in November 1853.* New York: John Wiley & Sons.

Ruskin, J. (1884b). *Pre-Raphaelitism.* New York: John Wiley & Sons.

Simkhovitch, M.K. (1906). Handicrafts in the city—What their commercial significance is under metropolitan conditions. *The Craftsman, 11,* 363–365.

Sixth annual report of the State Hospital for the Insane for the S.E. District of Pennsylvania at Norristown, Pa., for the year ending September 30, 1885. (1885). Norristown, PA: Hospital Printing Office.

Slagle, E.C. (1930). Address to graduates. *Occupational Therapy and Rehabilitation, 9,* 271–276.

Starr, P. (1982). *The transformation of American medicine.* New York: Basic Books.

Steckel, H. (1934). Retrospective evaluation of therapy. *Psychiatric Quarterly, 8,* 489–498.

Stevens, R. (1971). *American medicine and the public interest.* New Haven: Yale University Press.

Sullivan, O.M. (1935). Relation of occupational therapy to state and federal rehabilitation service. *Occupational Therapy and Rehabilitation, 14,* 105–110.

Tracy, S.E. (1912). *Studies in invalid occupations: A manual for nurses and attendants.* Boston: Whitcomb & Barrows.

Wiebe, R.H. (1967). *The search for order, 1877–1920.* New York: Hill & Wang.

Wright, G. (1980). *Moralism and the model home, domestic architecture and cultural conflict in Chicago. 1873–1913.* Chicago: University of Chicago Press.

Moral Treatment: Contexts Considered

CHAPTER 4

Suzanne M. Peloquin, PhD, OTR

Moral treatment is intriguing in its emergence, its essence, and its decline. The fascination with moral treatment deepens when one encounters the 20th-century term *occupational therapy* used in historical commentaries about the 19th-century practice. Digby (1985), in discussing moral treatment, noted that "occupational therapy took a variety of forms" (p. 63). Bell (1980) and Grob (1973) both identified occupational therapy as a component of moral treatment. Although this identification is incorrect in the strict historical sense, it is perhaps apt in other ways.

Three views provide different representations of the nature of the relationship between moral treatment and occupational therapy. Bing (1981) (see Chapter 5), an occupational therapist, described the relationship as evolutionary: "Occupational therapy's roots are in the subsoil of the moral treatment developed in Europe during the Age of Enlightenment .... Moral treatment came to the U.S. as part of the Quaker's religious and intellectual luggage .... During the last quarter of the 19th century moral treatment disappeared. It re-emerged in the early decades of the 20th century as Occupational Therapy" (p. 499). In contrast, Bockoven (1971), a psychiatrist, insisted that "the history of moral treatment in America is not only synonymous with, but *is* the history of occupational therapy before it acquired its 20th century name of 'occupational therapy'" (p. 225). Engelhardt (1977), a philosopher familiar with Bockoven's work, suggested a similarity between moral treatment and occupational therapy in the attempt to "effect more successful adaptation to society through organizing certain activities for patients in special environments" (p. 668). These divergent views suggest that a clearer understanding of the nature of moral treatment is relevant for occupational therapy professionals. Such an understanding seems particularly valuable in light of the continued desire within the profession to clarify its identity and its lineage.

A Definition of Moral Treatment

Dr. Thomas Kirkbride (1880/1973), a physician and the superintendent of the Pennsylvania Hospital for the Insane from 1841 to 1883, described moral treatment in terms of daily efforts to provide "system, active movements, and diversity of occupation" to the patients (referred to then as "inmates") (p. 275). Dr. Amariah Brigham (1847), a contemporary of Kirkbride, interpreted moral treatment as "the removal of the insane from home and former associations, with respect and kind treatment upon all circumstances, and in most cases manual labor, attendance on religious worship on Sunday, the establishment of regular habits of self control, [and] diversion of the mind from morbid trains of thought" (p. 1).

More than 150 years later, Dain and Carlson (1960) characterized the theory and practice of moral treatment as the psychological medicine that constituted milieu therapy in the 19th century. Tomes (1984) believed that moral treatment was based on the assumption that one could appeal to the patient's innate capacity to live an ordered and rational existence. To allay any concern that moral treatment meant the enforcement

This chapter was previously published in the *American Journal of Occupational Therapy, 43,* 537–544. Copyright © 1989, American Occupational Therapy Association.

of moral standards, Bockoven (1963) argued that early psychiatrists used the word *moral* to mean *psychological* or *emotional*. He viewed moral treatment as "the first practical effort made to provide systematic and responsible care for an appreciable number of the mentally ill" (p. 12).

Other interpretations articulate various goals and principles underlying moral treatment. Several of these suggest that moral standards were, in fact, guiding principles. Grob (1973) described the goal of moral treatment as the "inculcation, through habit and understanding, of desirable moral traits and values" (p. 12). Rothman (1971) viewed the process of moral treatment as the arrangement of a disciplined routine that provided stability for a person suffering from environmentally generated ills. Bell (1980) considered moral treatment to be a distinct method of therapy that enabled the patient to understand right from wrong within a total therapeutic community. Through moral treatment, the physician manipulated both the environment and the patient to help the patient overcome past associations and to create an atmosphere in which natural restorative elements could assert themselves (Grob, 1983). The image of moral treatment emerging from these interpretations is one of a treatment of the mentally ill that occurred in virtually all institutions; it included humane treatment, a routine of work and recreation, an appeal to reason, and the development of desirable moral traits.

Moral Treatment Within Its Various Contexts

An understanding of certain 19th-century conditions is crucial to an appreciation of the significance of moral treatment's emergence. Two environments—the medical community and 19th-century society as a whole—did much to influence the characteristics of moral treatment and its emergence in institutions.

The medical community's perception of insanity greatly influenced the development of moral treatment. A shift in 19th-century thinking revolutionized medical thought: persons with mental disorders, then labeled "the insane," were capable of reason. Before this awareness, insane persons had been considered subhuman because they were believed to be devoid of reason (Deutsch, 1949). Torturous methods were used to treat insane persons. These methods were used not to inflict pain, but to frighten the irrational beast. Methods congruent with contemporary theory included chaining the patients, placing them in cold showers, and lowering them into water-filled wells. The physician's goal was to dominate patients to cure them (Carlson & Dain, 1960). Only when it was acknowledged in the early 19th century that insane persons retained intellectual and rational capacities could treatment methodologies change.

The new philosophy of insanity generated the first humane systems for treatment in Europe. Philippe Pinel, a physician in France, and William Tuke, a Quaker in England, established the specific regimen of moral treatment. Pinel first used the term *moral treatment* (*traitement morale*) in 1801, but it was not until 1817 that a hospital was founded in the United States expressly for the purpose of providing moral treatment. This hospital, built by Pennsylvania Quakers for members of their Society and patterned after Tuke's York Retreat in England, was named the Friend's Asylum. Within 7 years, three more privately endorsed mental asylums (called *corporate asylums*) were built: McLean Hospital in Massachusetts, Bloomingdale Hospital in New York, and the Hartford Retreat in Connecticut. All of these corporate asylums practiced moral treatment (Bockoven, 1963).

This humane system of moral treatment became identified with institutional care. Its character was shaped by the medical men of these early institutions. Scull (1981) called the first four asylums the "earlier generation of asylums" (p. 151). Many developments among this earlier generation significantly influenced later institutions. The first influence related to lines of authority for providing treatment. The Bloomingdale Hospital and the Friend's Asylum, which were patterned after the York Retreat in England, were initially managed by lay superintendents, a custom prevalent in Europe. These superintendents oversaw the provision of moral treatment, and resident physicians provided mild medical treatments for physical conditions. At the Hartford Retreat, a physician named Eli Todd was superintendent. Todd endorsed and supervised traditional therapeutics as well as an increasing use of opium and morphine to complement moral treatment. He campaigned for medical treatment at the other three asylums. As a result of his efforts, medical treatment came to figure more prominently at all of these institutions. Over time, an uneasy relationship developed between the medical leadership and the moral leadership. In 1850, the tension culminated in a codification: An asylum superintendent would be a well-qualified physician. This new role that combined moral and medical functions became the leadership model adopted by the second generation of asylums (Scull, 1981).

A second early asylum influence was the adoption of public relations measures in the community. Superintendents realized that the negative image of European "madhouses" was powerful. They made a point of using annual reports to communicate the advantages of asylum treatment. The widespread communication of these messages was continued by later superintendents.

A final measure through which early superintendents ensured their influence on second-generation asylums was their personal involvement in the establishment of the first state asylums: Worcester State Hospital and Utica Asylum. These two facilities, though designed more for public than for private use, were patterned after the early asylums. These second-generation asylums, in turn, became models for later state facilities. The consolidated physician–superintendent role, the public relations efforts, and the tutelage of second-generation superintendents solidified the manner in which moral treatment would be practiced. The setting would continue to be institutional, the overseers would be physicians, and the public would remain convinced of the utmost practicality of this arrangement.

Changing social patterns during the 19th century helped to place the practice of moral treatment in institutions. America was industrializing, and many people moved from farms to urban centers. The urban family clustered into smaller units and became less able to deal effectively with its ill members. Not surprisingly, the new view of insanity was linked to these changing social patterns of industrialization and urbanization. Dr. Isaac Ray (1861), superintendent of the Butler Hospital, noted that many of his patients displayed deranged moral faculties of the will and of the emotions, although their intellectual faculties remained apparently intact. Deranged moral faculties could be attributed to societal tensions and chaos in the community, which social observances and institutions of the time were unable to handle. The result, for some, was moral insanity (Rothman, 1971).

Given the environmental causes of insanity and the family unit's growing inability to keep a family member with insanity at home, upper- and middle-class members of the community saw the asylum as a new, less chaotic, and more effective environment that could first halt and then reverse the process of insanity. The acceptance of institutions was not a desperate measure. With physician–superintendents and asylum supporters advertising their effectiveness in curing insanity, families admitted the insane with a sense of optimism (Rothman, 1971). The community supported physicians in this new movement toward institutionalization of a class of the population heretofore treated at home. Poor persons, commonly housed in local jails and poorhouses, were minimally affected during the early years of moral treatment (Dain, 1964; Deutsch, 1949; Galt, 1846/1973).

American superintendents shaped the practice of moral treatment. In Europe, the prevalent belief was that moral treatment alone cured insanity; in the United States, some form of medical treatment accompanied moral treatment (Scull, 1981). Tomes (1984) claimed that American superintendents reworked Pinel's original concept of moral treatment to justify treatment by medical doctors. This reworking is evident in Brigham's (1844) writings. He believed that deranged moral and intellectual faculties were generally the result of a diseased brain, although he thought that emotions and great trials of affection could derange brain function and cause insanity. Treatment of insanity stayed within the province of medical practice because physicians continued to link insanity to a disease process. Additionally, moral treatment in the United States was considered most appropriate for recent cases of insanity; more chronic cases (often the long-standing cases among the poor) were considered less likely to be reversed. The chronicity of disease among the poor made them less suitable candidates for moral treatment. For the most part, the asylum community consisted mainly of upper-middle-class doctors treating upper- and middle-class patients.

The Asylum: Structuring a New Environment

American physicians became involved in the design of the new therapeutic environments. As asylum superintendents, they were responsible for individual patient care, management of daily operations, and supervision of asylum personnel. Largely from the upper middle class, they were said to prefer treating patients from their own social stratum (Bell, 1980). They enforced the admission policies specific to their asylums, although they sometimes made concessions to local authorities and accepted a few poor people. Admission policies varied widely. Many corporate institutions totally excluded the poor; others, such as the Quaker asylums, admitted them more freely.

The standards set by the private asylums also set the example for state institutions eager to attract curable patients (Tomes, 1984). The Pennsylvania Hospital for the Insane, a public institution that began receiving patients in 1841, has been called by much of the literature one of the best American mental institutions of that era. Superintendents of corporate asylums welcomed public institutions as an alternative for poor inmates. The previous two-tier treatment system of the asylum versus the poorhouse or jail was evolving into one of the private versus the state institution.

Appropriate construction was a critical factor. Kirkbride thought "a properly constructed building . . . indispensable for such an effect [cure]" (Dain, 1964, p. 76). The building design was also important because it had to appeal to the public. The typical state hospital of the 19th century was constructed according to the Kirkbride Plan, which was officially endorsed by the Association of Medical Superintendents of American Institutions for the Insane. The Kirkbride Plan called for a large central administration building, from which extended several long, straight wings for housing patients. The design of the wings, with windows spaced evenly, embodied the belief that insanity could be cured by an ordered and rational environment (Rothman, 1971).

The internal structure of the asylum was considered as important to the ability to effect a cure as was the external structure. Classification of patients was an essential component of moral treatment and was incorporated into the building's internal structure. In the 19th century, physicians classified insane patients as manic, melancholic, or demented. These categories continued to form one basis for their classification in the asylum. Inmates were also separated according to sex, behaviors, and degree of illness (Tomes, 1984). At the private Friend's Asylum, for example, quiet convalescent inmates were separated from more acutely ill, violent, and noisy patients. Asylums that admitted more heterogeneous populations housed and grouped their inmates according to classes as well. Tomes described the rationale: "Since, in a non-institutional setting, patients would have expected to see class distinctions in housing and employment, the asylum replicated these features of everyday life" (p. 126).

Classification dictated various levels of care. Private asylums usually gave paying patients better treatment than they gave poor patients; this meant better accommodations and more attention. Moral treatment methods for individual patients, then, varied according to their socioeconomic status, sex, degree of illness, and ability to gain admission to an asylum.

Occupations Within the Asylum Context

Pinel (1806/1962) said that silence and tranquility prevailed in the Asylum de Bicetre when the Parisian tradesmen supplied the patients with employment that held their attention. He noted that even "the natural indolence and stupidity of *ideots* [sic] might in some degree be obviated, by engaging them in manual occupations, suitable to their respective capacities" (p. 203).

American superintendents made daily routine and occupation a central component of moral treatment. They claimed that the ultimate results of these two components outweighed the considerable initial cost of the arrangements necessary for their implementation. Labor, or occupation, judiciously used, contributed not only to patient comfort but also to health and recovery (Kirkbride, 1880/1973). Asylum staff went to exceptional lengths to engage patients in manual tasks. Kirkbride encouraged his patients to do any task; the critical thing was to keep busy. The therapeutic rationale was that occupation inculcated the regular habits necessary for recovery (Rothman, 1971). Throughout each carefully structured day, men engaged in agricultural pursuits, carpentry, painting, and general maintenance. Women performed domestic chores and manual crafts. The superintendents agreed that productive labor was the most important element in moral treatment (Grob, 1973). A precise schedule and regular work characterized the best private and public institutions.

The superintendents assigned occupations according to a patient's classification. Not all occupations were considered suitable at all stages of illness; superintendents were cautious about overtaxing patients or exposing them to potentially hazardous situations. Brigham felt that the members of the curable class benefitted most from the rational engagement of the mind through reading, writing, drawing, music, and various studies and recreational pursuits. Patients viewed as incurable benefitted more from manual labor to preserve whatever mind they still possessed (Brigham, 1847). In some cases, hardworking patients could reduce their board payments or earn placement on the free list (Tomes, 1984). Cooperative and industrious behaviors could also result in the acquisition of special privileges or "advancement to a better gallery" (Galt, 1846/1973, p. 497). In most asylums, occupation was supplemented by religious exercises, regular physical exercise, and group amusements organized by the staff. The use of occupations reflected an awareness of individual differences, of comfort level, and of degree of illness, but it also revealed a class and sex bias.

Dr. Lee, the superintendent at McLean Hospital, described the results of occupation: "Give a man constant employment, treat him with uniform kindness and respect, and, however insane he may be, very little may be feared from him, either of mischief or indolence" (Galt, 1846/1973, p. 50). He said that bodily labor proved immeasurably superior to all other aspects of treatment with a large class of male patients. The asylum staff encouraged patients to engage in energetic labor as a way to work off irritability. Perseverance and ceaseless efforts resulted in a patient's return to industrious habits, even with chronic cases. In these cases, attendants often helped patients initially with the motion required for a task until it was mastered. Asylum reports touted the successes at length and in great detail. Labor helped to inculcate moral habits in the patients; as a secondary benefit, labor often helped maintain the asylum.

Besides occupation, other treatment operatives were used in the early asylum. The superintendents in all institutions invoked the use of kindness. The patient population was kept low to facilitate individual care, and doctors met with individual patients daily. The Hartford Retreat, for example, housed only 40 patients (Deutsch, 1949). The staff used restraints minimally, appealing instead to patients' rationality. A system of rewards and privileges replaced a system of punishments. Cooperative patients could be promoted in classification, which encouraged self-control (Galt, 1846/1973). Radical medical treatments such as bleeding and the use of purgatives and emetics were replaced by the use of tonics and narcotics such as opium (Galt, 1846/1973). Family members were discouraged, but not forbidden, from visiting, because new associations were essential. The attendants became the patients' constant companions, and each attendant cared for one to six patients. The superintendents were diligent in obtaining attendants and nurses of the best character (Galt, 1846/1973). Families were encouraged to commit patients for a minimum of 3 to 6 months, time enough to demonstrate some progress. Confinement in a new environment and isolation from previous associations marked the beginning of a cure for environmentally caused insanity (Rothman, 1971).

Early Successes

In the small early asylum, success meant a cure. Statistics from the Worcester State Hospital between 1833 and 1842 show recoveries in 70% to 75% of the patients admitted, and improvements in 3% to 8% of the patients. Dr. Eli Todd of the Hartford Retreat reported recovery in 90% of the patients admitted with mental illness of less than 1 year's duration (Bockoven, 1963). Kirkbride (1880/1973) described his clinical observations of patients' behaviors both before and after the introduction of evening amusements. He said that a comparison of results "leaves no room to question the importance and great superiority of the last" (p. 273). Countless case histories validated moral treatment's success. Many of these case histories appeared in Galt's *The Treatment of Insanity* (1846/1973) and in the asylum's annual reports. One man, for example, reportedly suffered violent fits at least once a month. After he took up gardening and became involved, he was subsequently free of attacks (Rothman, 1971).

Grob (1973) thought that the success of the early asylum rested on a series of circumstances: (a) the small number and homogeneous nature of patients, (b) the internal therapeutic atmosphere arising from the enthusiasm of the superintendent's personality, and (c) close interpersonal relationships. All this success resulted in a wild optimism that Deutsch called "the cult of curability" (Dain, 1964, p. 78).

The Demise of Moral Treatment

Moral treatment can perhaps be called a system. The systematization of moral treatment contributed in part to its own demise. Certain aspects of the practice and principles characterizing moral treatment made its survival incompatible with later 19th-century conditions.

Changes that led to the demise of moral treatment occurred first in 19th century society, and second, in the medical community. While the providers of asylum care were touting its curative effects, a social reform movement was pushing to extend humane care to all insane persons. The push was successful; thousands of persons were crowded into existing asylums. A Civil War-taxed economy could not provide the rapid institutional growth that was needed to house this influx of patients. Asylum conditions deteriorated both from overcrowding and from a radical change in the types of patients treated. Because it was almost impossible to provide moral treatment, custodial care prevailed. Curative moral treatment was eliminated. Meanwhile, medicine was committing itself to more scientific inquiry and somatic treatments of all illnesses. A shift in thinking had occurred: insanity was caused by lesions in the brain. Therefore, consideration of environmental causes or treatments for what was essentially a physiological problem was unnecessary.

This course of events contributed to the demise of moral treatment partly because of certain characteristics inherent in the moral treatment system. For all its successes, moral treatment had its problems from the outset. One significant problem was the early superintendents' reluctance to deal with the poor, whether because of class bias or because of a genuine belief that the advanced condition of their disease precluded a cure. The early asylum experience tended to validate the assumption that poor persons presented hopeless cases. This validation occurred in the following manner. Superintendents sometimes labored under financial limitations. Public officials capable of providing funds were less concerned with effectiveness of treatment than with convenience of placement. These officials pressured superintendents to accept less curable cases to the asylum in greater

proportions than had been recommended (Rothman, 1971). Additionally, it had been assumed that a therapeutic asylum would have a transient population because of a constant turnover of cured patients. In practice, a percentage of more chronic cases stayed at the asylum. This situation created a different type of institution from that originally envisioned (Grob, 1973). The poor and the chronically ill, because they stayed, validated physicians' assumptions about their hopelessness. This would create a major obstacle when larger numbers of poor persons were later admitted.

Given their original expectations, physicians embraced middle-class behaviors and values as the norm; their emphasis was on the order, moderation, and self-control inherent in a middle-class life-style (Rothman, 1971). The initial theoretical and practical groundwork of moral treatment (that insanity was curable and that moral treatment was the cure) could have inspired a vigorous progressive movement across all classes. Instead, asylums were small-scale experiments that reached only a select group. Moral treatment was isolated amid a scene of widespread stagnation begging for reform (Rothman, 1971). At the time, public provision for poor persons consisted of sending the "dangerous and violent" to prison; the harmless and mild "paupers" went to auction or the almshouse (Deutsch, 1949, p. 115). The asylum superintendents showed little desire to treat the very patients who were to dominate asylum populations after the reform movement.

Michel Foucault (1965), a harsh critic of institutions in any form, for any reason, described moral treatment of mentally ill patients as a gigantic moral imprisonment: a "structure that formed a kind of microcosm in which were symbolized the massive structure of bourgeois society and its values ... centered on the theme of social and moral order" (p. 274). Digby (1985) countered that any experience of moral imprisonment in the subjective estimation of patients would "turn on the extent to which they shared the moral values of the establishment" (p. 54). Real treatment successes would come from inducing self-control in patients sharing the values, assumptions, and objectives of their therapists. Those not sharing institutional values would only conform superficially; problems would surface with discrepancies in values (Digby, 1985). In fact, as Bell (1980) wrote, "When poor people having different values formed the majority of the patient population, moral treatment ran into difficulties" (p. 14).

Another problem of the moral treatment system was its administration by physicians. The patients might have fared better had asylums been under the direction of lay superintendents (Bockoven, 1963). Physician-superintendents focused on the cure. When scientific theory was to later challenge moral treatment's curative potential, physicians rejected their recovery statistics and early successes. Eager to join the mainstream of scientific medicine, they increasingly distanced themselves from the moral care of the institutionalized mentally ill patients (Grob, 1983). Bockoven described the situation as one in which psychiatry did not have the courage to pursue its original course.

Moral Treatment in Crisis

Moral treatment in the asylum meant cure. Social reformers thought that all insane persons should have access to asylum cure. A widespread reform movement in the 1830s and 1840s worked to improve the lot of persons who were blind, deaf, slaves, alcoholics, convicts, or insane. Dorothea Dix, using superintendents' annual reports as testimony, led state after state to construct asylums. Her dream, however, soon turned into a nightmare (Bell, 1980). New state laws mandated that dangerously insane persons be sent to asylums. Those insane persons previously housed in jails and almshouses also went to asylums. This rapid admission of large numbers of patients taxed superintendents and facilities prepared for small homogeneous patient groups. Psychiatrist-superintendents were largely unsuccessful in their protest against the influx and their suggestion that violent or chronic patients be segregated (Bockoven, 1963).

Overcrowding restricted the practice of moral treatment. Rooms used for leisure activities and workshops became sleeping quarters. Individualized patient care was no longer possible in the congested asylum maze. Overcrowding stressed the sewage, ventilation, and water systems; the health of the patients was compromised. Epidemics struck at numerous institutions (Bell, 1980). The superintendents became increasingly concerned with order, regularity, and control among growing numbers of patients. They reinstituted the use of restraints among patients who were noisy or violent. The attendants assumed responsibility for larger groups of eight to 15 patients each. Inmates were often appointed as temporary nurses and attendants because of the staff shortage. The most critical personal quality sought in an attendant shifted from kindness to obedience (Grob, 1973). Overtaxed institutional facilities provided fewer patients with meaningful work; idleness further complicated behavioral problems. The superintendents recognized a growing gap between their original theory and their practices; their powers to close the gap were diminishing.

The wide range of persons admitted to the asylum jeopardized adequate care. Older patients with dementia accounted for 10% of the number of admissions from 1830 to 1875, thereby complicating hospital management considerably (Grob, 1973). Insane criminals often required maximum security. Alcoholic patients, mentally retarded patients, and patients suffering from general paresis (resulting from the advanced stage of a syphilitic infection) or other organic diseases often required individual care at a time when none was possible. Under these conditions, chronic patients failed to respond to treatment. They became troublesome, engaging in disruptive behaviors, escapes, and physical violence that perpetuated the need for restraint (Tomes, 1984).

Poverty-stricken immigrants joined this influx in the post-Civil War years. American physicians had difficulty empathizing with "foreign insane paupers" (Bockoven, 1963, p. 25). Admitted to already deteriorating institutions, foreign patients quickly became apathetic, leading physicians to believe them less capable, less motivated, and less curable. A vicious cycle developed, with predictable consequences. Because they were thought to be incurable, poor patients received less care. Without care, these patients showed little improvement—this confirmed their incurability.

New theories about mental illness dealt moral treatment yet another incapacitating blow. One school of thought linked mental illness with heredity; another linked mental illness with a somatic, mechanical defect. Both views led to a decline in optimism about a cure and to a total disillusionment about moral treatment in the 1850s. By the 1870s, pessimism was the trend; by 1900, moral treatment was reduced to a minor form of therapy even in the most affluent of corporate asylums (Dain, 1964).

Emphasis on hereditary predisposition began to fill the psychiatric literature. Heredity was thought to predispose the poor person to poverty and insanity (Bockoven, 1963). Inferior biological stock was thought to produce conditions leading to insanity. Some physicians debated the logic of heredity as an explanation for insanity; they argued against the heredity explanation in defense of a somatic view (Bell, 1980). Although earlier in the century it had been understood that a weakening of the body's vital forces could damage the brain, microscopic lesions now found in the central nervous system of mentally ill patients upset previous environmental theories and confirmed the somatic cause of insanity (Bockoven, 1963).

The early successes of moral treatment were challenged. In 1877, Dr. Pliny Earle published a critique of pre-Civil War curability statistics and accused early superintendents of having exaggerated their figures (Bockoven, 1963). Earle questioned the validity of the high cure rates cited because in the 1870s corporate asylums could no longer replicate these cure rates. Some physicians argued in response that insanity was becoming less curable because society was becoming more chaotic. Others claimed that insanity had become more complex in the late 19th century; it was less curable because the categories of insanity, such as general paralysis, senile dementia, and hereditary insanity, had multiplied. Many thought that the physiological causes of insanity were intensifying: Organic alterations in the nervous system were more involved in producing insanity than before (Bockoven, 1963).

Conversion toward a more somatic view seemed inevitable. From 1840 to 1860, three men had been responsible for most of the psychiatric research in the United States: Luther Bell, Amariah Brigham, and Isaac Ray. Their work had largely involved data gathering, certainly not serious research by 20th-century standards. Even the curability statistics gathered between 1833 and 1842 by superintendent Samuel Woodward at Worcester State Hospital had failed to delineate criteria used to determine the recovery or improvement of patients. Those succeeding the early superintendents were deeply discouraged by the apparent failure of moral treatment and by their inability to validate its effectiveness scientifically. Articles in the *American Journal of Insanity* supporting the mechanical defect theory exhorted a move toward somaticism. Scientific medicine was gaining respect and credibility; any psychological approach to the treatment of insanity seemed outdated, illogical, and irrelevant. In 1894, Dr. Weir Mitchell, a neurologist, castigated physicians for having ever believed in some mysterious therapeutic influence (Bockoven, 1963).

Therapeutic regimens differed among asylums, depending on the superintendent's viewpoint. Moral treatment suffered in this respect as well. Bockoven (1963) attributed the demise of moral treatment to the lack of inspired and committed leadership after the death of its innovators. Only four of the original 13 founders of moral treatment survived the 1870s, and two of these founders had returned to private practice. Leaders seemed to have lacked foresight. They had failed to train moral therapists who might have been able to articulate or redefine moral treatment's efficacy in the face of social changes and scientific inquiry. This seemed a major failure.

The asylum, diverted from its original mission of treatment, and pressured into merely containing insane persons, sank into a mire of apathy and indifference (Bell, 1980). Moral treatment, once considered vital to the cure of persons with mental disorders, disappeared from psychiatric practice.

Conclusion

The complexity of moral treatment precludes the opposing views that it was a short-lived triumph of humanitarian zeal or that it was a rationalization of middle-class morality (Tomes, 1984). Moral treatment was neither of these stereotypes. One thing is clear: Moral treatment cannot be understood outside of the framework within which it developed and disappeared.

One can hope that occupational therapy practice today is free of the limitations that precluded the survival of moral treatment. One would hope to find, in this century, a freedom from class and economic bias, a freedom from a push for professional credibility that is blind to patient need, and a leadership committed to defend those humane aspects of practice only empirically validated.

One can also hope that occupational therapy practitioners understand the powerful forces that often define the character of occupational therapy practice. During the 19th century, the medical community and the society as a whole shaped several guiding principles and treatment concepts into the practice of moral treatment. These two communities cannot be underestimated in the 20th century; their demands shape the duration, direction, location, and quality of occupational therapy.

Preventive care, accountability, and documentation of measurable progress are but a few of the trends grounded in challenges from these two sectors.

Moral treatment's decline relates closely to a lack of inspired and committed leadership willing to articulate and redefine the efficacy of occupation in the face of medical and societal challenges. The desire to embrace the most current trend of scientific thought led to the abandonment of moral treatment in spite of its established efficacy. The failure to identify and address the social and institutional changes that had gradually made the practice and success of moral treatment virtually impossible led to the erroneous conclusion that occupation was not an effective intervention. The responsivity to trends supplanted any reaffirmation of basic assumptions.

Occupational therapists need to recommit, in this century and in the next, to the assumptions about man and occupation that inform the practice of occupational therapy. In the face of changing trends, therapists must continually redefine and rearticulate the value of a humane practice that transcends scientific validation and bureaucratic understanding.

Acknowledgments

Special thanks to Ellen More, PhD, whose flexibility and encouragement enabled the integration of course material with occupational therapy issues. Thanks also to Lillian H. Parent, MA, OTR, FAOTA, for her supportive suggestions.

References

Bell, L. V. (1980). *Treating the mentally ill.* New York: Praeger.

Bing, R. K. (1981). Occupational therapy revisited: A paraphrastic journey. *American Journal of Occupational Therapy, 35,* 499–518. Reprinted as Chapter 5.

Bockoven, J. S. (1963). *Moral treatment in American psychiatry.* New York: Springs Publishing.

Bockoven, J. S. (1971). Legacy of moral treatment—1800s to 1910. *American Journal of Occupational Therapy, 25,* 223–225.

Brigham, A. (1844). Definition of insanity—Nature of the disease. *American Journal of Insanity, 1,* 107–108.

Brigham, A. (1847). The moral treatment of insanity. *American Journal of Insanity, 4,* 1.

Carlson, E. T., & Dain, N. (1960). The psychotherapy that was Moral Treatment. *American Journal of Psychiatry, 117,* 519–524.

Dain, N. (1964). *Concepts of insanity in the United States: 1789–1865.* New Brunswick, NJ: Rutgers University Press.

Dain, N., & Carlson, E. T. (1960). Milieu therapy in the 19th century: Patient care at the Friend's Asylum, Frankford, Pennsylvania, 1817–1861. *Journal of Nervous and Mental Disease, 131,* 277–290.

Deutsch, A. (1949). *The mentally ill in America: A history of their care and treatment from colonial times.* New York: Columbia University Press.

Digby, A. (1985). Moral treatment at the Retreat, 1796–1846. In W. F. Bynum, R. Porter, & M. Shepherd (Eds.), *The anatomy of madness. Essays in the history of psychiatry* (pp. 52–72). New York: Tavistock.

Engelhardt, H. T. Jr. (1977). Defining occupational therapy: The meaning of therapy and the virtues of occupation. *American Journal of Occupational Therapy, 31,* 666–672.

Foucault, M. (1965). *Madness and civilization: A history of insanity in the Age of Reason.* New York: Vintage Books.

Galt, J. M. (1973). *The treatment of insanity.* New York: Arno Press. Original work published 1846.

Grob, G. N. (1973). *Mental institutions in America: Social policy to 1875.* New York: Free Press.

Grob, G. N. (1983). *Mental illness and American society, 1875–1940.* Princeton, NJ: Princeton University Press.

Kirkbride, T. S. (1973). *On the construction, organization, and general arrangements of hospitals for the insane.* New York: Arno Press. Original work published 1880.

Pinel, P. H. (1962). *A treatise on insanity.* New York: Harper Publishing. Original work published 1806.

Ray, I. (1861). An examination of the objections to the doctrine of moral insanity. *American Journal of Insanity, 18,* 112–139.

Rothman, D. J. (1971). *The discovery of the asylum.* Boston: Little, Brown.

Scull, A. (Ed.). (1981). *Madhouses, mad-doctors, and madmen.* Philadelphia: University of Pennsylvania Press.

Tomes, N. (1984). *A generous confidence: Thomas Story Kirkbride and the art of asylum keeping.* New York: Cambridge University Press.

Related Readings

Beers, C. W. (1917). *A mind that found itself.* New York: Longmans, Green, & Co.

Occupational Therapy Revisited: A Paraphrastic Journey

CHAPTER 5

1981 ELEANOR CLARKE SLAGLE LECTURE

ROBERT K. BING, EdD, OTR, FAOTA

Try as one might, it is impossible to recount the evolution of occupational therapy so that it resembles the cliff-hanging biographies of Butch Cassidy and the Sundance Kid. Masters and Johnson, as well as Kinsey, who took years to amass their stories, had something going for them that does not exist for us. Somewhat puckishly I was tempted to entitle this paper *Everything You've Ever Wanted to Know About Occupational Therapy, But Were Afraid to Ask*. That would not have been altogether misleading. Because of my part-German heritage, and true to that cultural bias and tendency, I thought I should take us back to the Thirty Years' War and bring everyone up to date. After all, it is important territory occupational therapy has won and lost.

The title, *Occupational Therapy Revisited: A Paraphrastic Journey*, prevailed because this paper is a tour to what should be familiar historical landmarks and progenitors. For some of us, it will renew old friendships and acquaintances. For others, it will be a second-hand account of certain ancestors, not unlike those stories that emanate from grandmothers. For some, it will only be like an endurance of those pictures that inevitably get projected on the screen by vacationers returning home.

Because of the relative youthfulness of those of us in practice (most have entered within the past decade), now seems the time to critically examine our ancestral roots and subsequent grafts to determine the nature of the present and to offer some speculations about why we (and the profession) developed as we did through several generations. This is not *the* history of occupational therapy nor of the Association that supports our endeavors. Nor is it *a* history like someone else might well find it. It is *not* a detailed, definitive account of how we multiplied, divided, and invaded several areas of medicine and health care. It is *one person's* way of telling the story of who we are and citing some lessons to be learned. That is important! After several months of submergence just off the coast of Texas (as my colleagues in Galveston will attest), I have at long last come up for air and am ready to declare my findings.

This is a statement of how an idea, born in a philosophical movement, became activated through *the good works of men and women* who inalterably believed in the ideal that those who are sick and handicapped can regain, retain, and attain some semblance of function within the fundamental limitations of the human organism and the expectations of the society in which all must exist: that this may occur through the most obvious means of all—*one's reorganization through occupation, through activity, through leisure, and through rest.*

This journey about occupational therapy, its evolution and development, presents vexation: one must accept a fair number of ambiguities, something some today consider a fundamental problem in occupational therapy; a more than reasonable amount of astonishment; and a certain degree of messiness, closely akin to what is created by the beginner in fingerpainting. What can it all mean? What was taking place at the time? Will the patient recover? Most significantly, does it make any difference? To answer these and related questions I wanted to conduct some scholarly research that could be equally interesting, helpful, and valuable to students, occupational therapists, and others who are interested in our profession. This is how I interpret the intent of the originators of the Eleanor Clarke Slagle Lectureship.

Such an historical presentation should be long enough to say something, yet short enough to be tolerated.

To give you some idea of the continuing dilemma I encountered these past several months in preparing the lecture and in limiting its scope and length, I wrote:

> There once was an historian named Dan,
> Whose prose no one could scan,
> When, once asked about it,
> He said, "I don't doubt it,
> Because I try to cram as many facts and dates into each sentence as I possibly can."

Significant Landmarks

Let us start this paraphrastic journey and take note of some significant landmarks along the way—those recurring patterns and themes of the past 200 years that give us today's relevance:

1. There is an inextricable union of the mind and the body; the employment of activity or occupation must be based on this precept, which is unique to occupational therapy. *- Holistic*

2. Activity, inherently, contains modes the patient may employ to gain understanding of and ascendancy over one's feelings, actions, and thoughts: these modes include the habits of attention and interest; the perceived usefulness of occupation; creative expression; the processes of learning; the acquisition of skill; and evidence of accomplishment. *multidimensional*

3. Activity provides a balance between the practical and intellectual components of experience; therefore, a wide variety of activities must be accessible to meet human objectives for work, leisure, and rest.

4. One's approach to the patient is as significant to treatment and rehabilitation as is the selection and utilization of an activity. *Client-centered / therapeutic use of self*

5. Essential elements of occupational therapy practice are continuous observation, experimentation, empiricism, and analysis. *research*

6. An appreciation of the pain that accompanies any illness or disability; a strong desire to reduce or remove it; a gentle firmness; and a knowledge of the patient's needs are fundamental characteristics of the provider of therapeutic occupations. *empathy*

7. Therapeutic processes and modes of treatment are synonymous with the processes of learning and methods of education. *Learning by doing*

8. The patient is the product of his or her own efforts, not the article made nor the activity accomplished.

Activity as means, not as an end.

A Theory of Experience

We could go back to the Garden of Eden to begin this story, if time permitted, since occupational therapy could well have started in that idyllic spot. Dr. Dunton, one of the founders of the 20th century movement, insisted that those fig leaves had to have been crocheted by Eve, who was trying to get over her troubles. They had something to do with her being beholden to Adam and his rib. We will unfortunately pass over all that and begin the modern epoch with a brief description of what was taking place in Europe approximately 200 years ago. *Wow — He REALLY went there?!*

It was the *Age of Enlightenment,* or, as some prefer, the *Age of Reason.* The roots of 20th century occupational therapy are visible in the empiricism of John Locke, an English philosopher and physician, who fostered confidence in human reason and freedom; in Etienne de Condillac, a French philosopher, who advanced the dualism of body and mind; and Pierre Cabanis, a French physician and theorist, who offered an explanation of the importance of the moral and social sciences in perfecting the art of medicine. These three, together with others, popularized the new ideas. Indeed, it was the *best of times,* a clear demarcation in the emergence of the modern world.

If one were to combine the thoughts of these three, one would arrive at a *theory of experience.* John Locke, in his famous *Essay Concerning Human Understanding,* published in 1690,[1] examines the nature of the human mind and the processes by which it learns about and comes to know the world. When born, the human is a blank tablet (tabula rasa). Because of an innate ability to receive sensations from the outside world, the human can assimilate and organize impressions. As contact with the environment stimulates the senses and causes impressions, the mind receives and organizes these into ideas and concepts. Since the human mind does not already contain innate ideas, all must come from without.[2(p287)]

There is a second source for the accumulation of experience, according to Locke. It is the mind itself: "… the perception of the operations of our own mind … (such as) thinking, doubting, believing, reasoning, knowing … this source of ideas every man has wholly within himself."[3(p74)] Locke strongly held that the body and mind exist as real entities and they interact. He spent a great deal of time developing his perspective. He spoke of the aim of education as the process of knowing and learning through experience and in striving toward happiness. Ideally, he contended, one should work toward a sound mind in a healthy body. To achieve this ideal, Locke advocated physical exercise as a hardening process, and an exposure to a wide variety of sensations from the physical and social worlds.

Condillac was Locke's apologist. He tried to simplify Locke's fundamental theory by arguing that all conscious experiences are the result of passive sensations: these sensations are the raw materials from which one forms complex and interrelated ideas. Learning is the noting of incomplete ideas, considering each separately, combining them into relationships, and ordering them. This process results in retaining the strongest degrees of association. Condillac asserted: "Then we shall grasp (ideas) easily and clearly and shall understand their origins entirely."[3(p7)]

Elsewhere in his writings Condillac presented his thoughts on analysis. One cannot have the proper conception of a thing until one is in a position to analyze it. "To analyze," claimed Condillac, "is nothing more than to observe in successive order the qualities of an object … the simultaneous order in which they exist."[4(p17)]

The third philosopher, Pierre Cabanis, tended to apply medicine to philosophy and philosophy to medicine. Cabanis considered illness and its impact upon the formulation of values and ideas. Through the social sciences, which emerged in the *Age of Enlightenment,* he explained *moral* as a psychological phenomenon on a physiological base. He concluded that moral impressions can have both physiological and pathological results. At last, there was a rational explanation for the psychological production of disease in which the so-called moral (emotional) passions play a significant part.[5(p37–38)] Cabanis contributed a socially based theoretical explanation of human experience that became the cornerstone for the moral management of the insane.

Age of Enlightenment and Moral Treatment

Moral treatment of the insane was one result of the *Age of Enlightenment.* It sprang from the fundamental attitudes of the day: a set of principles that govern humanity and society; faith in the ability of the human to reason; and the supreme belief in the individual. The rapid changes caused by this new philosophy advanced the disappearance of the notion that the insane were possessed of the devil. Mental diseases became legitimate concerns of humanitarians and physicians. The discontinuance of the idea that crime, sin, and vice were at the core of insanity brought forth humane treatment. Up to this time the insane had been housed and handled no differently than were criminals or paupers—often in chains.

Two men of the 18th century working in different countries, and unknown to each other, initiated the moral treatment movement. "No two men could possibly have been chosen out of all Europe at that time of whom it could be said more truly that they were cradled, and nursed, and educated among widely differing social, political, religious influences …"[6(p24–25)] Philippe Pinel was a child of the French Revolution, a physician, a scholar, and a philosopher. He is described as "…far exceeding the bounds of pure humanitarianism … to encompass the goals of a naturalist, … a reformer, a clinician, … and, above all, a philosopher."[7(Intro)] William Tuke was a devout member of the Society of Friends (Quakers).

Philippe Pinel: Physician-Reformer

Whenever Philippe Pinel's name comes up in a conversation among health professionals, he is immediately mentioned as the striker of the chains at two French hospitals. His efforts and contributions go way beyond that reformational act. As a physician, he began his most serious work in 1792 as superintendent of Bicêtre, the asylum for incurable males in Paris.

As a natural scientist, Pinel achieved exceptional skill in the observation of human behavior and the bringing of "…some order into the chaos of … treatment methods by means of critical and objective investigations."[5(p42)] Pinel says this about himself: Desirous of better information, I resolved for myself the facts that were presented to my attention; and forgetting the empty honors of my titular distinction as a physician, I viewed the scene that was opened to me with the eye of common sense and unprejudiced observation.[8(p109)] From his own experience, he urged that observations "…be the basis upon which (one) should decide what opinions to believe."[9(p74–75)] Throughout his work, he held constantly before him his own motto of independent thought: "Chercher à èviter toute illusion, toute prèvention, toute opinion adoptèe sur parole" (to seek to avoid all illusion, all prejudice, all opinion taken on authority)[10(p8–9)]

Pinel's descriptions of the mentally deranged provide insight into his own compassionate nature. For him, the loss of reason was the most calamitous of human afflictions. The ability to reason principally separates the human from other living forms. Because of mental illness, the human's "…character is always perverted, sometimes annihilated. His thoughts and actions are diverted…. His personal liberty is at length taken from him…. To this melancholy train of symptoms, if not early and judiciously treated … a state of the most abject degradation sooner or later succeeds."[8(p xv–xvii)]

What Pinel entitled *revolution morale,* or moral revolution, is the ultimate insight of the insane into the delusional and absurd nature of their experiences.[7(p256)] This, to him, was the basis for treatment. Some historians believe that he was stating that moral treatment is synonymous with the humane approach. His own writings do not bear this out. Pinel believed that each patient must be critically observed and analyzed; then treatment should commence. "To apply the principles of moral treatment, with undiscriminating uniformity, would be … ridiculous and unadvisable."[8(p66)] The moral method is well reasoned and carefully planned for the individual patient.

According to Pinel, moral management is a maintained continuity of approach; a predictable routine, infused with vigor by personnel who inspire confidence. Moreover, moral treatment calls for a constant, observed study of patient behavior and performance. It included a gentle, but firm approach. Each patient is given as much liberty within the institution as he or she can tolerate. The approach is designed to give the patient a feeling of security as well as a respect for authority. Pinel asserted: "The atmosphere should be the same as in a family where the parents are quite strict. To establish this relationship, the doctor must convince the patient that he wishes to help him and that recovery is a real possibility."[9(p76)]

Occupations figured prominently in Pinel's conception of moral treatment. He used activities to take the patients' thoughts away from their emotional problems and to develop their abilities. He considered literature and music as effective in altering patients' emotions. Physical exercise and work should be part of every institution's fundamental program and be employed in accord with individual tastes. He concluded: "The (occupations) method is primarily designed and intended to reach man at his best which…means human understanding, intelligence, and insight."[3(p63–64)]

The concept of _moral treatment_ belongs solely to Philippe Pinel. His fundamental belief was that its purpose is to restore the patient to himself, "…to use the patient's own emotions to balance his emotional excesses."[9(p76)] Truly, Pinel and his efforts, rooted in the _Age of Enlightenment_, mark the beginning of the modern epoch in the care of the mentally ill.

William Tuke: Philanthropist-Humanitarian

Across the channel, in England, things were astir at the same time. King George III, who was giving the American colonies fits, was himself in similar trouble. In 1788 it became public knowledge that the King was seized with mania. Questions arose about his fitness to continue ruling. Nevertheless, public sentiment was on his side. For the first time, insanity and its treatment formed a topic of public discussion: "The subject had been brought out of concealment in a way which defeated the conspiracy of silence."[11(p42)] This being the _Age of Enlightenment_, the public openly sympathized with the sufferer; there was no condemnation. No one suggested that the King was being visited by the Devil, or that he was being punished for his sins.

The Society of Friends, derisively called _Quakers_, originated in 17th century England and became one of the most distinctive movements of Puritanism: "They arose out of the religious unrest of England … and stood for a radical kind of reform within Christendom which contrasted sharply with Protestant, Anglican and Roman patterns alike."[12(p118)] George Fox, founder of the Society, discovered "…the spirit of the living Christ and knew that it was an experience open to all men. 'This was the true light that lighteth every man that cometh into the world!'"[13(p1)]

William Tuke, a devout Quaker, wealthy merchant, and renowned philanthropist, was made aware of the deplorable conditions in the insane asylum in York, England. There were tales of extreme neglect and possible cruelty. He was an unusual man, not given to listening to sensational reports and acting rashly.[14(p12)] In true Quaker fashion Tuke presented a concern at a Friend's Quarterly Meeting in the spring of 1792—that an institution for the insane be established in York under the direction of the Society. At first, he was met with considerable resistance by those who believed that there were too few mentally ill Quakers, and that no one would want them concentrated in such a lovely, quiet locale.[15(p58)]

The York Retreat

Initially, Tuke was disheartened; yet, he pressed on, and within 6 months _The Retreat for Persons_ afflicted with _Disorders of the Mind,_ or simply, _The Retreat_ came into being. Up until then the term _Retreat_ had never been applied to an asylum. Tuke's daughter-in-law suggested the term to convey the Quaker belief that such an institution may be "…a place in which the unhappy might obtain refuge; a quiet haven in which (one) … might find a means of reparation or of safety."[16(p20)] The cornerstone simply stated the purpose of the institution: "The charity or love of friends executed this work in the cause of humanity."[15(p19)]

William Tuke became the superintendent. Thomas Fowler, an unusually open-minded man, was appointed visiting physician. After a trial-and-error period, they came to believe that moral treatment methods were preferable to those involving restraint and use of harsh drugs. The new approach was a product of Tuke's humanitarianism and Fowler's empiricism.

Several fundamental principles became evident within a short time. The approach was primarily one of kindness and consideration. The patients were not thought to be devoid of reason, feeling, and honor. The social environment was to be as nearly like that of a family as possible, with an atmosphere of religious sentiment and moral feeling.[16(p35)]

Tuke and Fowler strongly believed that most insane people retain a considerable amount of self-command. Upon admission, the patient was informed that treatment depended largely upon one's own conduct. Employment in various occupations was expected as a way for the patient to maintain control over his or her disorder. As Tuke reported: "…regular employment is perhaps the most efficacious; and those kinds of employment … to be preferred … are accompanied by considerable bodily action."[16(p156)] The staff endeavored to gain the patient's confidence and esteem, to arrest the attention and fix it upon objects opposite to any illusion the patient might have. The fundamental purpose of employment and recreation was to facilitate the regaining of the _habit of attention,_ as Tuke called it. Various learning exercises were used, such as mathematical problems, to help the patient gain ascendancy over faulty habits of attention.

Tuke and Fowler determined that "indolence has a natural tendency to weaken the mind, and to induce ennui and discontent…"[16(p180–181)] A wide range of occupations and amusements was available. Patients not engaged in useful occupations were allowed to read, draw, or play various games. Tea parties, walks, and visitations away from the institution were planned regularly in preparation for the patients' returning home. All activities were closely analyzed through observation in order to individualize patients' needs. _8in to activity) analysis_

The pioneer work of William Tuke and his son, Samuel, who wrote the definitive treatise on _The Retreat,_ opened a new chapter in the history of the care of the insane in England. Mild management methods, infused with kindness, and building self-esteem through the judicious use of occupations, resulted in the excitation and elicitation of superior, human motives. Patients recovered, left *The Retreat,* and rarely needed to return for further care. The entire regimen was carefully patterned "...to accord (patients) the dignity and status of sick human beings."[17(p687)]

Moral Treatment Expansion

As soon as Pinel's major work on moral treatment (1801) and Samuel Tuke's description of *The Retreat* were published (1813), there was a rush toward implementing many reforms in other hospitals, particularly in England and the United States. In both countries occupations were introduced as an integral part of moral treatment.[18(p83-84)] Some unusual experiments were undertaken by Sir William Charles Ellis, a physician, who became the superintendent of a pauper lunatic asylum. The mainstay of his asylum management was useful occupations. He moved well ahead of mere amusements and "introduced a gainful employment of patients on a large scale and even had them taught a trade."[19(p62)] Ellis and his wife undertook other reforms. She organized the women patients into groups under the supervision of a *workwoman* to make useful and fancy articles.

Another Ellis innovation was the development of what would eventually be called *halfway houses.* Keenly aware of environmental and social influences on insanity, Ellis suggested "...after-care houses and night hospitals as a stepping stone from the asylum to the world by which ... the length of patients' stay would be reduced and in many cases the cure completed..."[17(p871)] He insisted that convalescing patients should go out and mix with the world before discharge. His proposals were made in the 1830s!

In the United States, few public and private asylums existed in the post-Revolutionary era; however, institutional reforms were needed. Any recounting of this period must include two very important individuals and their work: Benjamin Rush and Dorothea Lynde Dix. Their efforts did not overlap; they did not know one another; nor was one influenced by the other. Just as in the cases of Pinel and Tuke, no two individuals this side of the Atlantic could have been more unlike one another in background, education, or experience. Nevertheless, each recognized the hapless plights of the institutionalized insane and set out to alleviate dire conditions and the inauguration of moral treatment, including occupations and exercise.

Benjamin Rush: Father of American Psychiatry

Benjamin Rush, often referred to as the *father of American psychiatry,* was a Philadelphia physician in the latter half of the 1700s. Through his training in Europe and several visits there, he adopted many of Pinel's practices; however, Rush did not adopt moral principles until later. As a member of the staff of Pennsylvania Hospital, he was placed in charge of a separate section set aside for the insane, the first hospital in America to reserve such a section. He was appalled by the conditions and he appealed to the staff and the public for change. Change did come and humane treatment was instituted. Rush saw to it that "certain employments be devised for such of the deranged people as are capable of working..."[20(p257)] This approach was based upon his philosophical stance that man, by his very nature, is meant to be active; "Even in paradise (Garden of Eden) he was employed in the health and pleasant exercises of cultivating a garden. Happiness, consisting in folded arms, and in pensive contemplation...by the side of brooks, never had any existence, except in the brains of mad poets, and love-sick girls and boys."[21(p115-116)]

In his major writing, *Medical Inquiries and Observations Upon the Diseases of the Mind,* Rush clearly differentiates between goal-directed activity and aimless exercise: "Labour has several advantages over exercise, in being not only more stimulating, but more endurable in its effects;...it is calculated to arrest wrong habits of action, and to restore such as regular and natural..."[21(p224-225)]

Dorothea Lynde Dix: Humanitarian-Reformer

Dorothea Lynde Dix, a reform-minded humanitarian during the middle 1800s, vehemently pressed for improved conditions of the insane who were incarcerated in jails and almshouses. She presented a number of *Memorials* to state legislatures, believing that the public had an obligation to care for such individuals. By 1848 numerous states had responded to her efforts, and she decided to tackle a more formidable object—the federal government. Dix envisioned the sale of public lands to finance the building of a federal system of hospitals for the indigent blind, deaf, and mute, as well as the insane. For 6 years she wheedled and cajoled members of Congress. Finally, in 1854, the bill was ready for President Franklin Pierce's signature. He was a close friend of Miss Dix and she felt highly confident of the outcome. The President vetoed the bill claiming unconstitutionality: "...every human weakness or sorrow would take advantage of this bill if it became law.... It endangers states' rights."[22(p20)] Through her contacts with physicians in several states, Miss Dix embraced moral treatment as the most humane method. She strongly advocated "...decent care, quiet, affection and normal activity (as) the only medicine for the insane."[22(p11)]

United States: Individual Treatment, Occupations, Education

The Quakers brought moral treatment to the United States as part of their intellectual and religious luggage. Through published accounts about *The Retreat* in York, some private asylums were established in which moral principles were practiced. A number of public institutions altered their programs to include individualized treatment, occupations, and education. Those patients who had remained for years unimproved and listless, even on the verge of apathy "…are seen in encouraging instances, when transferred to attendants who have more disposition to attend to them,…to waken (them) from their torpor, to become animated, active and even industrious…."[23(p487–488)]

Moral management also was taking on a new facet: the influence of a sane mind upon the insane mind. Those who daily attended the sick were to impress upon the insane the influences of their own character, designed to specifically improve the patients' behavior. Personnel must possess a number of traits: observational skills to see the "…actual condition of the patient's mind…and a faculty of clear insight…."[23(p489)] Other traits: "…seeing that which is passing in the minds of (patients)….Add to this a firm will, the faculty of self-control, a sympathizing distress at moral pain, a strong desire to remove it…."[23(p489)]

Arguments appeared in the literature relative to the moral use of firmness and gentleness. Strong cases were made for both extremes; however, it took two alienists (the precursor to psychiatrist), John Bucknill and D. Hack Tuke, grandson of Samuel Tuke, in 1858 to settle the dispute: "The truth, as usual, lies between; and the (individual) who aims at success in the moral treatment of the insane must be ready to be all things to all men, if by any means he might save some."[23(p500)] They elaborate on their thesis by stating: "With self-reliance … it requires widely different manifestations, to repress excitement, to stimulate inertia, to check the vicious, to comfort the depressed, to direct the erring, to support the weak, to supplant every variety of erroneous opinion, to resist every kind of perverted feeling, and to check every form of pernicious conduct."[23(p500)]

Bucknill and Tuke also wrote that moral treatment included the gaining of the patient's confidence, fixing his or her attention on interesting and wholesome objects of thought, diverting the mind from introspection, and loosening the hold on concentrated emotion. They explain: "For (these) purposes useful occupation is far superior to any form of amusement. The higher the purpose, and the more appellant the nature of the occupation … the more likely it is to draw him from the contemplation of self-wretchedness, and effect the triumph of moral influences."[23(p493)]

The next step in institutional occupations emphasized education. Those occupations that require a process of learning and thought were determined far preferable, from a curative point of view, than those that require none. "Moral treatment is as wide as that of education; … it is education applied to the field of mental phenomena…"[23(p501)] Therefore, it was not unusual to find specific mental activities included with occupations. The purpose was to educate the individual in order to provide him or her with "the power of controlling his feelings, and his thoughts, and his actions.[24(p166–167)]

With continued experience, a number of alienists decided that occupations and amusements also could serve as a prophylactic against insanity. One interesting prescription for the return and maintenance of sanity was: "…rest in bed, occupation, exercise and amusements."[25(p14)] D. Hack Tuke declared: "If idleness is a curse to the sane, it is the parent of mischief and ennui to the insane, especially to the pubescent and adolescent."[26(p1315)] He urges that the same approach be taken with the sane and the insane: "Employment, Nature's universal law of health, alike for body and mind, is specially beneficial, … seeing that it displaces ideas by new and healthy thoughts, revives familiar habits of daily activity, restores (and maintains) self-respect while it promotes the general bodily health."[26(p1315)]

Decline of Moral Treatment

Moral management and treatment by occupations reached its zenith in the United States just before the outbreak of the War Between the States (Civil War). Corporate, private asylums continued to expand their efforts. State- and public-supported institutions withdrew their programs, so that by the last quarter of the 19th century, virtually no moral treatment was taking place.

Several reasons for this decline and eventual disappearance can be identified, including a nation at war with itself. Bockhoven cites others: 1. the founders of the U.S. movement retired and died, leaving no disciples or successors; 2. the rapidly increasing influx of foreign-born and poor patients greatly overtaxed existing facilities and required more institutions to be built with diminished tax support; 3. racial and religious prejudices on the part of the alienists, beginning to be called psychiatrists, reduced interest in treatment and cure; and 4. state legislatures became increasingly more interested in less costly custodial care.[27(p20–25)]

Essentially, there was no place in the public institutions for moral treatment. "The inferior physical plants and facilities, poorly trained and insufficient staff, … and, worst of all, overcrowding, prohibited any attempts to practice moral management."[28(p128)] A belief emerged that many insane were incurable. One eminent psychiatrist stated: "I have come to the conclusion that when a man becomes insane, he is about used up for this world."[29(p155)] Such pessimism was predominant for a century in this country. Custodial care had come to stay for a very long time.

As we shall see next, moral principles and practices emerged in the early years of the 20th century through the efforts of individuals, then by a group who founded an organization dedicated to those principles. This group, in collaboration with others, established a definition and fundamental principles that have carried over through several generations of specifically educated practitioners of occupational therapy.

Once again, as with Pinel and Tuke, Rush and Dix, the individuals who founded and pioneered the 20th century occupational therapy movement could not have been more diverse in their backgrounds, experience, and education. They included a nurse, two architects, a physician, a social worker, and a teacher.

Susan Tracy: Occupational Nurse

Susan Tracy was this country's first proponent of occupations for invalids. A trained nurse, she initiated instruction in activities to student nurses as early as 1905 as part of their expanding responsibilities. She also developed the term *occupational nurses* to signify specialization.[30(p401)] By 1912 she decided to devote all her energies to patient activities and she distinguished herself by applying moral treatment principles to acute conditions. As Tracy stated, "The application of this most rational remedy to ordinary, everyday sick people, as found in the general hospital, is almost unknown."[31(p386)] She strongly claimed that remedial treatments "are classified according to their physiological effects as stimulants, sedatives, anesthetics …, etc. Certain occupations possess like properties."[31(p386)] The physician may select stimulating occupations, such as watercoloring and paper folding; or sedative occupations such as knitting, weaving, basketry.

Throughout Tracy's many years of work she employed experimentation and observation to enhance her practice. Her carefully worded writings provide ample evidence of her intense desire to bring scientific principles to the application of invalid occupations. In 1918 she published a remarkable research paper on 25 mental tests derived from occupations; for example, by instructing the patient in using a piece of leather and a pencil, "require him to make a line of dots at equal distances around the margin and at uniform distances from the edge. This constitutes a test of *Judgement* in estimating distances."[32(p15)] Continuing with the same piece of leather, the patient is instructed to punch a hole at each dot. "In order to do this he must consider the two sides of leather, the two parts of his tool and bring these together thus making a *Simple Coordination* test."[32(p16)] Other tests in the fabrication of the leather purse include *Aesthetic Coordination and Rhythm, Differentiation of Form and Size, Purposeful Relation.* In all 25 tests, she stressed a completed, useful and "not unbeautiful" object.

Tracy's other writings state the value and usefulness of discarded materials to successful ward work.[33(p62)] She also emphasized high quality workmanship: "It is now believed that what is worth doing at all is worth doing well, and that practical, well-made articles have a greater therapeutic value than a useless, poorly made article."[34(p198)] A premium is placed upon originality and the "… adoption of the occupation to the condition and natural tastes of the patient."[35(p63)] Further, she believes that "… the patient is the product, not the article that he makes."[33(p59)]

Tracy's major work, *Studies in Invalid Occupation,* published in 1918,[36] is a revealing compendium of her observations and experiences with different kinds of patients, for instance: "the child of poverty and the child of wealth, the impatient boy, grandmother, the business man."

By 1921, Susan Tracy had adopted the term *occupation therapy* originally coined by William Rush Dunton, Jr., and defined it and differentiated it from vocational training. She felt this was necessary because of the arising confusion between the two concepts following World War I. She wrote: "What is occupation? The treatment of disease by occupation…. The aim of occupation is to get the man well; that of vocational training is to provide him with a job. Any well man will look for a job, but the sick man is looking for health."[37(p120)]

Throughout all of her writings she stated that nothing is "…too small to be pressed into the service of resourceful mind and trained hands toward … the establishment of a healthy mind in a healthy body."[33(p57)]

George Barton: Re-education of Convalescents

George Edward Barton, by profession an architect, contracted tuberculosis in his adult life. This plagued him for the remainder of his years. His constant struggle led him into a life of service to the physically handicapped. Out of his own personal concerns came the establishment of Consolation House, an early prototype of a rehabilitation center. He was an effective speaker and writer, often given to hyperbole; he gained his point with the listening or reading public.

Barton's central themes were hospitals and their responsibility to the discharged patient; the conditions the discharged patient faces; the need to return to employment; occupations and re-education of convalescents. These were intense concerns to him because of his own health problems.

His first published article, derived from a speech given to a group of nurses, points out a weakness he perceived in hospitals: "We discharge from them not efficients, but inefficients. An individual leaves almost any of our institutions only to become a burden upon his family, his friends, the associated charities, or upon another institution."[38(p328)] In the same article, he warms to his subject: "I say to discharge a patient from the hospital, with his fracture healed, to be sure, but to a devastated home, to an empty desk and to no obvious sustaining employment, is to send him out to a world cold and bleak…."[38(p329)] His solution: "…occupation would shorten convalescence and improve the condition of many patients."[38(p329)] He ended his oration with a rallying cry: "…it is time for humanity to cease regarding the hospital as a door closing upon a life which is past and to regard it henceforth as a door opening upon a life which is to come."[38(p330)]

Barton established Consolation House in Clifton Springs, New York. Those referred to his institution underwent a thorough review, including a social and medical history, and a consideration of one's education, training, experience, successes, and failures. Barton believed that "By considering these in relation to the condition (the patient) must presumably or inevitably be in for the remainder of his life, we can find some form of occupation for which he will be fitted…."[39(p336)] He claimed that Consolation House was "getting down to our social difficulties."[39(p337)]

By 1915, Barton had adopted Dunton's term, *occupation therapy,* but preferred the adjectival form: occupational therapy. He declared: "If there is an occupational disease, why not an occupational therapy?"[40(p139)] He expansively stated: "The first thing to be done … is for occupational therapy to provide an occupation which will produce *a similar therapeutic effect to that of every drug in materia medica*. An exercise for each separate organ, joint, and muscle of the human body. An exercise? An occupation! An occupation? A useful occupation! Then (occupational therapy) can fill the doctor's prescriptions… written in the terms of materia medica."[40(p139)] He even advocated a laxative by *occupation*.

Re-education entered Barton's terminology with the aftermath of World War I. He viewed hospitals as taking on a mission different from that previously adopted. A hospital should become "…a re-educational institution through which to put the waste products of society *back and into the right place*."[40(p139)] Using alliteration, he declared: "…by a catalystic concatenation of contiguous circumstances we were forced to realize that when all is said and done, what the sick man really needed and wanted most was the restoration of his ability to work, to live independently and to make money."[41(p320)]

Barton's major contribution to the re-emergence of moral treatment was the awakening of physical re-construction and re-education through the employment of occupations. Convalescence, to him, was a critical time for the inclusion of something to do. Activity "…clarifies and strengthens the mind by increasing and maintaining interest in wholesome thought to the exclusion of morbid thought … and a proper occupation…during convalescence may be made the basis of the corollary of a new life upon recovery…. I mean *a job, a better job, or a job done better* than it was before."[42(p309)] With Susan Tracy, Barton held that the major consideration of occupations "…should be devoted to the therapeutic and education effects, not to the value of the possible product."[43(p36)]

William Rush Dunton, Jr.: Judicious Regimen of Activity

Of the founders of the 20th century movement, William Rush Dunton, Jr., was the most prolific writer and the most influential. He published in excess of 120 books and articles related to occupational therapy and rehabilitation; served as president of the National Society for the Promotion of Occupation Therapy; and, for 21 years, was editor of the official journal. As a physician, he spent his professional career treating psychiatric patients in an institutional setting. Key to his treatment methods is occupational therapy, a term he coined to differentiate aimless amusements from those occupations definitely prescribed for their therapeutic benefits. Before embarking on what he called *a judicious regimen of activity*, he read the works of Tuke and Pinel, as well as the efforts of significant alienists of the 19th century.

From his readings and from observations of patients in Sheppard Asylum, a Quaker institution in Towson, Maryland, Dunton concluded that the acutely ill are generally not amenable to occupations or recreation. The acutely ill exhibit a weakened power of attention. Occupations at this time would be fatiguing and harmful. The prevailing prescription is "…to let the patient alone, meanwhile improve (his) condition, restore and revivify exhausted mental and physical forces…."[44(p19)] Later, activities should be selected that use energies not needed for physical restoration. Stimulating attention and directing the thoughts of the patient in regular and healthful paths would ensure an early release from the hospital. Dunton developed a wide variety of activities from knitting and crocheting to printing and the repair of dynamos, in order to gain the attention and interest, as well as to meet the needs, of all patients.

Dunton's proclivities for history and research led him to extensive readings and experimentations—all related to the human, his need for work, leisure, rest, and sleep; the causal factors of mental aberrations; various cures of mental illness. Each excursion brought him back to *a judicious regimen of activity* as the treatment of choice, regardless of whether the patient was mentally or physically ill. He became more and more convinced that attention and interest in one's work and play are as efficacious, if not more so, than the many and varied other medications available. He stated it this way: "It has been found that a patient makes more rapid progress if his attention is concentrated upon what he is making and he derives stimulating pleasure in its performance."[45(p19)]

At the second annual meeting of the National Society for the Promotion of Occupational Therapy (AOTA) in 1918, Dunton unveiled his nine cardinal rules to guide the emerging practice of occupational therapy, and to ensure that the new discipline would gain acceptance as a medical entity: 1. Any activity in which the patient engages should have as its objective a cure. 2. It should be interesting; 3. have a useful purpose other than merely to gain the patient's attention and interest; and 4. preferably lead to an increase in knowledge on the patient's part. 5. Curative activity should preferably be carried on with others, such as in a group. 6. The occupational therapist should make a careful study of the patient in order to know his or her needs and attempt to meet as many as possible through activity. 7. The therapist should stop the patient in his or her work before reaching a point of fatigue; and 8. encouragement should be genuinely given whenever indicated. Finally, 9. work is much to be preferred over idleness, even when the end product of the patient's labor is of a poor quality or is useless.[46(p26–27)]

The major purposes of occupation in the case of the mentally ill were outlined in Dunton's first book.[47(p24–26)] The primary objective is to divert the attention either from unpleasant subjects, as is true with the depressed patient; or from daydreaming or mental ruminations, as in the case of the patient suffering from dementia praecox (schizophrenia)—that is, to divert the attention to one main subject.

Another purpose of occupation is to re-educate—to train the patient in developing mental processes through "…educating the hands, eyes, muscles, just as is done in the developing child."[47(p25)] Fostering an interest in hobbies is a third purpose. Hobbies serve as present, as well as future, safety valves and render a recurrence of mental illness less likely. A final purpose may be to instruct the patient in a craft until he or she has enough proficiency to take pride in his or her work. However, Dunton did note that "While this is proper, I fear … specialism is apt to cause a narrowing of one's mental outlook…. The individual with a knowledge of many things has more interest in the world in general."[47(p26)]

Dunton continued to write and publish his observations, each one elaborating on a previous one. His texts became required reading for students preparing for practice. Even in his 90s, well beyond retirement from practice, he maintained an interest in our profession and continued to offer counsel.

Eleanor Clarke Slagle: Founder-Pioneer

Eleanor Clark Slagle qualifies as both a founder and a pioneer. She was at the birth of the Association in 1917. Before that time she had received part of her education in social work and had completed one of the early Special Courses in Curative Occupations and Recreation at the Chicago School of Civics and Philanthropy. Following this, she taught in two courses for attendants of the insane; directed the occupations program at Henry Phipps Clinic, Johns Hopkins Hospital, Baltimore, under Dr. Adolf Meyer; returned to Chicago to become the Superintendent of Occupational Therapy at Hull House. Later, Mrs. Slagle moved to New York where she pioneered in developing occupational therapy in the State Department of Mental Hygiene. In addition, she served with high distinction in every elective office of the American Occupational Therapy Association, including President (1919–1920) and as a paid Executive Secretary for 14 years.[48(p122-125); 49(p473-474); 50(p18); 51]

She found occupational therapy to be "…an awkward term…" but felt "… it has been well defined as a form of remedial treatment consisting of various types of activities … which either contribute to or hasten recovery from disease or injury … carried on under medical supervision and that it be *consciously* motivated." Further, she emphasized that occupational therapy must be "a *consciously* planned progressive program of *rest, play, occupation and exercise*…."[52(p289)] In addition, she explained it is "…an effort toward normalizing the lives of countless thousands who are mentally ill, … the normal mechanism of a fairly well balanced day."[53(p14)] She enjoyed quoting C. Charles Burlingame, a prominent psychiatrist of her day: "'What is an occupational therapist? She is that newer medical specialist who takes the joy out of invalidism. She is the medical specialist who carries us over the dangerous period between acute illness and return to the world of men and women as a useful member of society.'"[52(p290-291)]

Slagle placed considerable emphasis upon the personality factor of the therapist: "…the proper balance of qualities, proper physical expression, a kindly voice, gentleness, patience, ability and seeming vision, adaptability … to meet the particular needs of the individual patient in all things…. Personality plus character also covers an ability to be honest and firm, with infinite kindness…."[54(p13)]

The issue would constantly arise about the use of handicrafts as a therapeutic measure in the machine age. Her response is a classic: "…handicrafts are so generally used, not only because they are so diverse, covering a field from the most elementary to the highest grade of ability; but also, and greatly to the point, because their development is based on primitive impulses. They offer the means of contact with the patient that no other medium does or can offer. Encouragement of creative impulses also may lead to the development of large interests outside oneself and certainly leads to social contact, an important consideration with any sick or convalescent patient."[52(p292-293)]

Habit training was first attempted at Rochester (New York) State Hospital in 1901. Slagle adopted the basic principles and developed a far greater perspective and use among mental patients who had been hospitalized from 5 to 20 years and who had steadily regressed. The fundamental plan was "…to arrange a twenty-four hour schedule … in which physicians, nurses, attendants, and occupational therapists play a part…."[54(p13)] It was a re-education program designed to overcome some disorganized habits, to modify others and construct new ones, with the goal that habit reaction will lead toward the restoration and maintenance of health. "In habit training, we show clearly an academic philosophy factor…that is, the necessity of requiring attention, of building on the habit of attention—attention thus becomes application, voluntary and, in time, agreeable."[54(p14)]

The purposes of habit training were two-fold: the reclamation and rehabilitation of the patient, with the eventual goal of discharge or parole; and, if this was not reasonable, to assist the patient in becoming less of an institutional problem, that is, less destructive and untidy.

A typical habit training schedule called for the patient to arise in the morning at 6:00, wash, toilet, brush teeth, and air beds; then breakfast; return to ward and make beds, sweep; then classwork for 2 hours, which consisted of a variety of simple crafts and marching exercises. After lunch, there was a rest period; continued classwork and outdoor exercises, folk dancing, and lawn games. Following supper, there was music and dancing on the ward, followed by toileting, washing, brushing the teeth, and preparing for bed.[55(p29)]

Once the patient had received maximum benefit from habit training, he or she was ready to progress through three phases of occupational therapy. The first was what Slagle called *the kindergarten group*. "We must show the ways and means of stimulating the special senses. The employment of color, music, simple exercises, games and storytelling along with occupations, the gentle ways and means … (used) in educating the child are equally important in re-educating the adult…."[54(p14)] Occupations were graded from the simple to the complex.

The next phase was *ward classes in occupational therapy.* "…graded to the limit of accomplishment of individual patients."[56(p100)] When able to tolerate it, the patient joined in group activities. The third and final phase was the *occupational center.* "This promotes opportunities for the more advanced projects … (a) complete change in environment; … comparative freedom; … actual responsibilities placed upon patients; the stimulation of seeing work produced; … all these carry forward the readjustment of patients."[56(p102)]

This founder, this pioneer, this distinguished member of our profession provided a summary of her own accomplishments and philosophy by stating: "Of the highest value to patients is the psychological fact that the patient is working for himself…. Occupational Therapy recognizes the significance of the mental attitude which the sick person takes toward his illness and attempts to make that attitude more wholesome by providing activities adapted to the capacity of the individual patient and calculated to divert his attention from his own problems."[54(p290)] Further, she declared: "It is directed activity, and differs from all other forms of treatment in that it is given in increasing doses as the patient improves."[57(p3)]

Adolf Meyer: Philosophy of Occupation Therapy

Dr. Adolf Meyer is cited in this account of the evolution of occupational therapy because of his outstanding support and because his approach to clinical psychiatry was entirely consistent with the emerging occupational therapy movement.

Adolf Meyer, a Swiss physician, immigrated to the United States in 1892 and accepted a position initially as pathologist at the Eastern Illinois Hospital for the Insane in Kankakee. Over the next 14 years he held various positions in the United States and became professor of psychiatry at Johns Hopkins University in 1910. Throughout this period he developed the fundamentals of what was to become the psychobiological approach to psychiatry, a term he coined to indicate that the human is an indivisible unit of study, rather than a composite of symptoms. "Psychobiology starts not from a mind and a body or from elements, but from the fact that we deal with biologically organized units and groups and their functioning … the 'he's' and 'she's' of our experience—the bodies we find in action…."[58(p263)] Meyer took strong issue with those in medicine: "…who wish to reduce everything to physics and chemistry, or to anatomy, or to physiology, and within that to neurology…."[58(p262)] His enlightened point of view is that one can only be studied as a total being in action and that this "…whole person represents an integrate of hierarchically arranged functions."[59(p1317)]

His common sense approach to the problems of psychiatry was his keynote: "The main thing is that your point of reference should always be life itself…. I put my emphasis upon specificity…. As long as there is life there are positive assets—action, choice, hope, not in the imagination but in a clear understanding of the situation, goals and possibilities…. To see life as it is, to tend toward objectivity is one of the fundamentals of my philosophy, my attitude, my preference. It is something that I would recommend if it can be kept free of making itself a pest to self and to others."[60(p vi–xi)]

From the very beginning of his work in Illinois, he was concerned with meaningful activity. In time, it became the fundamental issue in treatment. "I thought primarily of occupation therapy," he stated, "of getting the patient to do things and getting things going which did not work but which could work with proper straightening out."[60(p45)] In a report to the Governor of the State of Illinois in 1895, Meyer wrote: "Occupation is, with good right, the most essential side of hygienic treatment of most insane patients."[60(p 59)]

By 1921, Meyer had become Professor of Psychiatry at Johns Hopkins University in Baltimore, and had extensive experiences with others, such as William Rush Dunton, Jr., Eleanor Clarke Slagle, and Henrietta Price, leaders in the occupational therapy movement. At the Fifth Annual Meeting of the National Society for the Promotion of Occupational Therapy in Baltimore, October 1921, Meyer brought together his fundamental concepts of psychobiology to produce his paper, *The Philosophy of Occupation Therapy* (see Chapter 2). Through time, this has become a classic in the occupational therapy literature. It bears study by all of us.

Psychobiology is clearly visible in his statement that "…the newer conceptions of *mental problems* (are) *problems of living,* and not merely diseases of a structural and toxic nature…."[61(p4)] The indivisibility and integration of the human are cited in this manner: "Our conception of man is that of an organism that maintains and balances itself in the world of reality and actuality by being in active life and active use…."[61(p5)]

Because of the nature of his paper, *The Philosophy of Occupational Therapy,* Meyer emphasized occupation, time, and the productive use of energy. Interwoven are the elements of psychobiology. He stated: "The whole of human organization has its shape in a kind of rhythm…. There are many … rhythms which we must be attuned to: the larger rhythms of night and day, of sleep and waking hours…and finally the big four—work and play and rest and sleep, which our organism must be able to balance even under difficulty. The only way to attain balance in all this is actual doing, actual practice, a program of wholesome living is the basis of wholesome feeling and thinking and fancy and interests."[61(p6)]

According to Meyer, a fundamental issue in the treatment of the mentally ill is "…the proper use of time in some helpful and gratifying activity…."[61(p1)] He expands on this precept by stating: "There is in all this a development of the *valuation of time and work,* which is not accidental. It is part of the great espousal of the *values of reality and actuality* rather than of mere thinking and reasoning…."[61(p4)] The introduction of activity is "… in giving opportunities rather than prescriptions. There must be opportunities to work, opportunities to do and to plan and create, and to learn to use material.... It is not a question of specific prescriptions, but of opportunities ... to adapt opportunities."[61(p7)] He concluded his philosophic essay by returning once again to time and occupations: "The great feature of man is his new sense of time, with foresight built on a sound view of the past and present. Man learns to organize time and he does it in terms of doing things, and one of the many things he does between eating, drinking and ... the flights fancy and aspiration, we call work and occupation."[61(p9–10)]

Near the end of his working life, Meyer summed up his major efforts. He wrote of dealing with individuals and groups from the viewpoints of *good sense;* of *science,* "...with the smallest numbers of assumptions for search and research..."; of *philosophy;* and of *religion,* "... as a way of trust and dependabilities in life."[62(p100)]

Occupational Therapy Definitions and Principles

As the founders and pioneers were experimenting with and writing their concepts, a definition of occupational therapy was emerging. It is remarkable that so early in the formation of the 20th century movement, a definition could be developed and stand for several decades and several generations of occupational therapists. Many of us were required in school to immortalize it through needlepoint, embroidery, and even printing.

H.A. Pattison, M.D., medical officer of the National Tuberculous Association, advanced his view at the annual conference of the National Society for the Promotion of Occupational Therapy in Chicago, September 1919. It was also adopted by the Federal Board of Vocational Education: "Occupational Therapy may be defined as any activity, mental or physical, definitely prescribed and guided for the distinct purpose of contributing to and hastening recovery from disease or injury."[63(p21)] Twenty-one years later, in 1931, John S. Coulter, M.D., and Henrietta McNary, OTR, added one phrase: "...and assisting the social and institutional adjustment of individuals requiring long and indefinite periods of hospitalization."[64(p19)] This was inserted in order to recognize occupational therapy's involvement in chronicity.

By 1925, a committee, made up of four physicians including William Rush Dunton, compiled an outline for lectures to medical students and physicians.[65(p277–292)] Though their document never received the official imprimatur of the AOTA, it nevertheless served for several years as a guide for practice.[66(p347)] Fifteen principles were enunciated: "Occupational therapy is a method of training the sick or injured by means of instruction and employment in productive occupation; ... to arouse interest, courage, confidence; to exercise mind and body in...activity; to overcome disability; and to re-establish capacity for industrial and

social usefulness."[65(p280)] Application called for as much system and precision as other forms of treatment; activity was to be prescribed, administered, and supervised under constant medical advice. Individual patient needs were paramount.

The outline stressed that "employment in groups is ... advisable because it provides exercise in social adaptation and stimulating influence of example and comment...."[65(p280)] In selecting an activity, the patient's interests and capabilities were to be considered and as strength and capability increased, the occupation was to be altered, regulated, and graded accordingly because "The only reliable measure of the treatment is the effect on the patient."[65(p280)]

Inferior workmanship could be tolerated, depending upon the patient's condition, but there should be consideration of "...standards worthy of entirely normal persons ... for proper mental stimulation."[65(p281)] Articles made were to be useful and attractive, and meaningful tasks requiring healthful exercise of mind and body provided the greatest satisfaction. "Novelty, variety, individuality, and utility of the products enhance the value of an occupation as a treatment measure."[65(p281)] While quality, quantity, and the salability of articles made could be of benefit, these should not take precedence over the treatment objectives. As adjuncts to occupations, physical exercise, games, and music were considered beneficial and fell into two main categories: gymnastics and calisthenics, recreation and play.

One last principle spoke of the qualities of the occupational therapist: "...good craftsmanship, and ability to instruct are essential qualifications; ... understanding, sincere interest in the patient, and an optimistic, cheerful outlook and manner are equally essential."[65(p281)]

Occupational Therapy's Second Generation

The die was cast. Practice rapidly expanded in a phenomenal number of settings following the establishment of the founders' principles and definition. A *second generation* of therapists emerged during the late 1920s and the 1930s. They were the practitioners and educators who elaborated, codified, and applied the initial theory upon which present-day practice is based. A chronicle of their efforts would offer a highly valuable and valued study in itself. The names of Louis Haas, Mary Alice Coombs, Winifred Kahmann, Henrietta McNary, Harriet Robeson, Marjorie Taylor, and Helen Willard would figure prominently in such an account.

For the purpose of *this history,* a composite of these and others is drawn into one individual who exemplifies the spirit and deeds of the *second generation* of occupational therapists—those whose efforts are lasting and ensure our present and future education and practice.

Understandably, it would be a woman. She would devote her professional career to either teaching, practicing, or administering. Quite possibly she would combine two or more of these. She would acquire an expertise in one area of practice, such as the mentally ill.

Her belief in the treatment of the total patient would guide her thoughts and actions. Occupational therapy, she would declare, "since its founding has concerned itself with the basic tenet—the treatment of the total patient. This approach is unique to occupational therapy among the … health disciplines…. There has always existed a strong component concerned with the behavior of the physically ill or disabled, as well as the mentally sick; with the entirety of man and his functioning as a patient. This occupational therapy concept," she would continue, "prevented (as has occurred in medical practice) an undesired separation of the psychiatric therapist from those who develop knowledge and skills centered in the treatment of the physically disabled."[67(p1)] Stated another way, "The major emphasis in occupational therapy is not the body *as such* but the individual *as such*. The therapist's background is strongly weighted in an understanding of personality adjustment and reactions to social situations; … and in the patients' attitudes toward an adjustment to acute and chronic disabilities."[68(p9)]

At some point in her work, she would be asked to serve as a consultant to one or more medical facilities, possibly a state hospital system. In time, she would produce a report and restate her definition of occupational therapy. It might well go this way: "The goal of all treatment in a modern mental hospital is the physical, social and economic rehabilitation of the patient…. The accepted function (of occupational therapy) … is the scientific utilization of mental and physical activities for the purpose of raising the patient to the highest level of integration; to assist him in making his initial adjustment to the hospital; to sustain him while his body responds to physical treatment and his mind to psychotherapy; or to assist him in making a satisfactory adjustment to chronic illness."[69(p24)]

In the report she would also call for an atmosphere as normal as possible, where a patient could be encouraged to respond in as normal a manner as possible: a balanced program of work and play, with flexibility to meet individual needs: "There must be organized a succession of steps through which the patient will be gradually led to his highest level of integration…. At each level … the patient experiences a feeling of success and self-respect. One cannot overemphasize the importance of careful planning … in order that there be a systematic progression up this ladder of integration."[69(p24)]

In another context, supportive care, as a vital concern to the therapist, would also be described, particularly in the care of the physically disabled: "To name only a few of its treatment objectives, occupational therapy may function as a diagnostic evaluative instrument; as corrective treatment; … or a design for effecting prevocational evaluation. Incorporated in each … is a treatment phase referred to as supportive care. This is a most fundamental and yet less definitive and indeed the least spectacular element of the total rehabilatory program. In supportive care, the occupational therapist (is concerned) with the behavioural factors which have and will affect the patient's response to the rehabilitation program…." Convincingly, she would say: "…it can be said with conviction that successful rehabilitation can be effected only when the patient has attained a true state of rehabilitation 'readiness.'"[70]

Not just a woman of words, she would find one or more ways to activate her philosophy. She might well become active with a group of former patients and assist in organizing an association of and for individuals who have been hospitalized—for instance, the mentally ill. Such an endeavor would be the first of a kind. Through such an experience, she would conclude: "One difficulty which presented itself again and again was the need to instill in these (former) patients a philosophy toward their own rehabilitation: … an organized effort beyond the hospital which would offer special training, guidance and professional evaluation of their potentials."[71(p3)]

This would lead her to even greater endeavors on behalf of a whole category of patients. As an example, she would find that the 1920 Federal Vocational Rehabilitation Act excluded former psychiatric patients. In the manner of Dorothea Lynde Dix, whom she probably emulated, she would wage a relentless battle to right such a wrong. By enlisting the assistance of physicians' associations and veterans' groups she would see the legislation change. As part of her campaign she would write: "The former mental patient, in his struggle for economic rehabilitation, incurs the burden imposed on the physically handicapped 'plus' the stigmatization based on the popular misconception of mental disease. He must cast aside self-pity or the idea that the world owes him a living. The world does owe him understanding and guidance."[72(p114)] Finally, amendments to *Public Law 113* were passed and signed by President Franklin Roosevelt. Psychiatric patients could now qualify for the benefits of the vocational rehabilitation act.

With such efforts the therapist's personal beliefs about emotional illness become even more strongly felt: "The majority of mentally ill are (sick) through no fault of their own … any more than one who has contracted a physical illness. Persons suffering from mental disease are generally ill as a result of an accumulation of unsuccessful efforts…to adjust to his environment."[72(p83)]

Two continuing concerns of all occupational therapists would be commented upon: the qualifications of the therapist and the use of media. One is as significant as the other. "The personality of the therapist," she would say, "must command respect, admiration, hope and confidence, … for no therapy is better than the therapist who directs it."[72(p83)] Therapeutic media have a number of inherent qualities, such as providing a vehicle for objectively recording patient performance, and, for the patient, affording opportunities for "…creative expression and evidence of accomplishment. The therapist should have a wide variety of activities (available) in accordance with the interests, aptitudes, and mental state of the patient. A craft track mind had no place in preparing such a program," she would state.[72(p103)]

The accumulation of experiences as a clinician, and educator, or an administrator, or possibly a combination of these, would lead this *therapist of the second generation* to arrive at a new definition of occupational therapy. It would precede by several years an altered definition by the national organization. It would incorporate the social and behavioral sciences, with a diminished emphasis upon medicine. Human development would appear for the first time as a focus for the treatment of physical and psychosocial dysfunction. She would declare: "Occupational therapy's function is to provide skilled assistance in influencing human objectives; its approach is inextricably conjoined with the behavioral factors involved. It is interested in how the process of growth and development is modified by hospitalization, chronic illness or a permanent handicap."[73(p2)]

This re-focus was quite explainable and understandable to her since occupational therapy, and its ancestral emphasis, has always been the totality of the human organism. She would say, "It was inevitable, therefore, that there evolve an ever increasing emphasis in occupational therapy … a greater understanding of the part that the developmental process plays in the preventive and therapeutic factors of this form of treatment."[74(p3)]

The foregoing has been a descriptive composite of a whole generation of therapists and assistants. The composite is actually the story of one individual; her observations alone have been cited. That individual is *Miss Beatrice D. Wade, OTR, FAOTA.*

The story is far from finished. Without a doubt, someone sometime will chronicle the lives and works of those who are still making contributions from that era to the present generation. Among them are Marjorie Fish, Virginia Kilburn, Mary Reilly, Ruth Robinson, Clare Spackman, Ruth Brunyate Wiemer, Carlotta Welles, and Wilma West. Each one, together with many others, continues to serve us well as clarifiers and definers of reasonable and reasoned alternatives. As counselors, they confirm old values and clearly point out *new directions* as well as our faithfulness or infidelity to those timeless principles established by our professional ancestors.

Lessons From Our History

The history of occupational therapy is the most neglected aspect of our professional endeavors. Seemingly, *old values* are least considered when charting *new directions*. On occasion we have been accused of taking leave of our historical senses. More to the point is that we have no historical sense. The problem primarily lies in not taking the time to assiduously locate our profession's diggings, to excavate what is relevant, and, then, to learn from what has been unearthed.

Archival materials from the past 200 years have been abundantly used in the development of this paper. Location and excavation has been difficult at times; however, it is reassuring to note that records and accounts still exist that are extremely relevant to today's endeavors. Lessons can be learned and they must. May I encourage each of you to determine for yourself what you have learned from this paraphrastic journey to our profession's diggings. To assist in this endeavor, may I cite a few lessons I have gained.

Mind and Body Inextricably Conjoined

No less than our professional ancestors, we must refuse to accept any alternative to the belief in the wholeness of the human—that the mind and body are inextricably conjoined. Illness, treatment, and the return to a healthful state simultaneously affect the physiological and emotional processes. Indeed, should these processes ever become separated, then occupational therapy would be of no value. The patient has died!

The Natural Science of the Human

The inextricable union of the human leads to another lesson. The science fundamental to our practice is the natural science of the human. No amount of neurophysiology, psychology, sociology, or child development alone can determine the differential diagnosis, treatment, or prognosis of the patient undergoing occupational therapy. The current trend toward specialization, with its varying emphases upon one or another science, to the neglect of other human sciences, and indeed to the neglect of other nonscientific aspects of occupational therapy, borders on superstition and mythology. It is the continuous acquisition and scientific synthesis of the ingredients of the human organism and its surround that guarantees authentic occupational therapy.

The Human Organism's Involvement in Tasks

Occupational therapy is the only major health profession whose focus centers upon the *total* human organism's involvement in tasks—a making or doing. In spite of the many grafts we have effected, our roots remain in the subsoil of the *art,* the *craft*: a paradigm of the total activity of the human. Just as those who have come before us, we think of ourselves and others fundamentally as makers, as users, as doers, as tools. We look at: "…craft as a way in which man may create and cross a bridge within himself and center himself in his own essential unity."[75(p vii)] The procedures one goes through in rearranging and reassembling the basic elements in art or craft operate upon and within the doer: "… his material modifies him as he modifies it, in proportion to his openness, his awareness of the exchange that is taking place."[75(pvii)] The procedure one goes through in rearranging and reassembling the basic elements in art or craft operate upon and within the doer: "… his material modifies him as he modifies it, in proportion to his openess, his awareness of the exchange that is taking place."[75 (px)]

The Differentiation of Occupational Therapy

Any definition, any description, any differentiation between ourselves and other health providers must have as its major theme occupation and leisure. Without it, we become a blurred copy, a xerography of a host of others.

Without the dynamics of human motion inherent in purposeful activity, we become quasi-physical therapists. Without the interaction between human objects and the objects of work and leisure, we become quasi-social workers, psychologists, or nurses. Without the demonstrated and proven interrelationships between healthful, normal growth and development, activity, and the pathology of illness and disabling conditions, we become quasi-physicians and psychiatrists.

The more we intermingle our fundamental philosophy and our treatment techniques with others, the more likely we will become enfeebled, the more likely we will degenerate, the more likely we will eventually disappear.

A Refusal to Accept the Common Verdict

As Hugh Sidey has noted, "History is a marvelous collection of stories about men and women who refuse to accept the common verdict that certain achievements (are) impossible."[77(p18)] The history of occupational therapy is the story of the ideals, deeds, hopes, and works of *individuals.* Changes and advancements came from those who eliminated inhumaneness, which prevented or discouraged the sick and disabled from achieving their potential. These same individuals were willing to assume the care and responsibility for those *who were not highly valued by the society:* the mentally ill and retarded, the severely disabled—all those defined as "non-producing, … an economic burden."[65(p277)]

In numerous places and on countless occasions these same individuals were derided, hated, or, at best, ignored, because they pressed for change in the human condition. Yet, they persevered, knowing there was nothing innately unusual about themselves or what they wished to achieve. Few ever saw their names inscribed on monuments.

They were a *cast* quite diverse in character, and largely obscure because of the immensity of the saga being enacted. A few received *speaking parts,* primarily through reporting their own clinical findings. Only very few were singled out to be stars. None ever became members of the *audience,* passively observing events. All were *actors.*

The very same can be said of the present occupational therapy generation. We are actors, not observers. We continue to willingly strive on behalf of those who are not highly valued by the society. We refuse to see this as a burden. Rather, we perceive it as an obligation, as an opportunity, as a way of life.

Legacy of Experience

Too often we are disposed to think that those lessons another generation learned do not apply to the present generation. We should be mindful that there are two ways to learn: by our own experience and from those who have made discoveries, regardless of how long ago they were made. The experience of others is a magnificent heritage, and the more we learn from them, the less time we waste in the present, proving what already has been proved.

Those of us who are teachers and clinicians have a special obligation to pass on the legacy of experience, the knowledge of timeless principles and practices that do not change merely because times change.

Who They Were, What They Did

The legacy of experience suggests one more lesson. So often we are caught up in our daily activities we tend to forget what it is we owe those who came before us. All probably agree that each occupational therapy generation seemingly acquires a sense of self-sufficiency. It is true that we of the present occupy the positions that once were filled by others.

It is, however, of great import that we realize we are influenced by those who came before us more than we can truly know. Who they were and what they did has immeasurable bearing upon what we are and what we do. No generation is capable of isolating itself from its past. The past, plus what we are and what we do, greatly assists in fashioning our future.

The archives, the portraits and photographs, the published accounts, the personal memorabilia and scrapbooks are records of considerable moment. At the least, they are a profound reminder of the possibility that someday, someone may be looking back and may be wondering who we were and what we did.

Conclusion

It is altogether fitting and proper to conclude this lecture with the observations of two former Presidents of the Association, Mr. Thomas B. Kidner and Mrs. Eleanor Clarke Slagle. In 1930, Mr. Kidner offered a personal impression of the state of occupational therapy at the annual meeting of the Connecticut Occupational Therapy Society. In part, he said: "May we, therefore, look on occupational therapy—with the increased faith as the years go by—as a natural means of aiding in the restoration of the sick and disabled to health and working capacity (which means happiness) because it appeals to all our human attributes."[57(p11)]

Mrs. Slagle, a year after she retired in 1937, made this observation: "The story of the profession of occupational therapy will never be fully told, nor will that of the patients who have so abundantly appreciated the opportunities of the service. There has been no fanciful crusading 'for the cause'; it has meant that a few have perhaps borne many burdens, but in the slow process that make permanent things of great value, it can be said that there is a fine body of professional workers, experienced and well trained, coming forward and being welcomed to a really great human service, that of helping to show the way to the person with large disabilities to make the best of his incomplete self."[78(p382)] Finally, in an editorial "From the

Heart," she concluded: "The integrity of your profession is in your hands. I bid you all Godspeed in your work."[79(p345)]

Acknowledgments

A study of this nature and scope is not possible without the valuable and valued assistance of numerous individuals and sources. I wish to recognize the incomparable services provided by the staffs of the Moody Medical Library, The University of Texas Medical Branch at Galveston; the Quine Library, University of Illinois at the Medical Center, Chicago; the McGoogan Library of Medicine, University of Nebraska Medical Center, Omaha; and the Archives, Shapiro Developmental Center (Eastern Illinois State Hospital), Kankakee.

Finally, I wish to recognize Frances Sawyer, COTA, and the Board of Directors, The Texas Occupational Therapy Association, Inc., who placed my name in nomination for this exalted honor. My gratitude to them is immeasurable.

Dedication

I wish to dedicate the 1981 Eleanor Clarke Slagle Lectureship to my parents, who provided me with those cumulative experiences and values that inevitably led me to the decision to become an occupational therapist; to a very great woman, Beatrice D. Wade, OTR, FAOTA, who has been my valued teacher and beloved mentor for more than 30 years; to my cherished colleagues, Lillian Hoyle Parent and Jay Cantwell, both occupational therapists, who constantly stimulate me and insist on a high level of constructive activity; to Charles H. Christiansen, OTR, FAOTA, whose personal and professional qualities and insistence on excellence from himself and others assure me of the future of occupational therapy.

Without the examples, teachings, guidance, counseling, and friendship of these individuals, I could never have achieved this exalted opportunity.

References

1. Locke J: *An Essay Concerning Human Understanding* (Two Volumes). New York: Dover Press, 1894F

2. Frost SE: *Basic Teachings of the Great Philosophers*, New York: Barnes and Noble, Inc., 1942

3. Riese W: *The Legacy of Philippe Pinel: An Inquiry into Thought on Mental Alienation*, New York: Springer Publishing Co., 1969

4. Condillac EB de: *Oeuvres Philosophiques de Condillac*, Paris: Presse Universataires de France, 1947

5. Ackerknecht EH: *A Short History of Psychiatry*, New York: Hafner Publishing Co., 1968

6. Tuke DH: *A Dictionary of Psychological Medicine* (Vol One). Philadelphia: P Blakinston, Son & Co., 1892

7. Pinel P: *Traité Médico-Philosophique sur 'Alienation Mentale*, Paris: Richard, Caille & Rover, 1801

8. Pinel P: *A Treatise on Insanity In Which Are Contained the Principles of a New and More Practical Nosology of Maniacal Disorders*, Translated by DD Davis. London: Cadell & Davis, 1806 (Facsimile published by Hafner Publishing Co., New York, 1962)

9. Mackler B: *Philippe Pinel: Unchainer of the Insane*, New York: Franklin Watts, Inc., 1968

10. Folsome CF: *Diseases of the Mind: Notes on the Early Management, European and American Progress*, Boston: A. Williams & Co., Publishers, 1877

11. Jones K: *Lunacy, Law, and Conscience: 1744–1845: The Social History of Care of the Insane*, London: Routledge & Kegan Paul, Ltd., 1955

12. Dillenberger J, Welch D: *Protestant Christianity: Interpreted Through Its Development*, New York: Charles Scribner's Sons, 1954

13. Philadelphia Yearly Meeting of the Religious Society of Friends: *Faith and Practice*, Philadelphia: Philadelphia Yearly Meeting, 1972

14. Tuke DH: *Reform in the Treatment of the Insane. Early History of the Retreat, York; Its Objects and Influence*, London: J & A Churchill, 1872

15. Tuke DH: *Reform in the Treatment of the Insane: An Early History of the Retreat, York: Its Objects and Influence*, London: J & A Churchill, 1892

16. Tuke S: *Description of The Retreat, An Institution Near York for Insane Persons of the Society of Friends: Containing an Account of Its Origins and Progress, The Modes of Treatment, and a Statement of Cases*, York, England: Alexander, 1813

17. Hunter R, Macalpine I: *Three Hundred Years of Psychiatry, 1535–1860: A History Presented in Selected English Texts*, London: Oxford University Press, 1963

18. Connolly J: *The Treatment of the Insane Without Mechanical Restraints*, London: Smith, Elder & Co., 1856 (Facsimile copy published by Dawson's of Pall Mall, London, 1973, with introduction by R Hunter and I Macalpine)

19. Ellis WC: *A Treatise on the Nature, Symptoms, Causes, and Treatment of Insanity*, London: Holdsworth, 1838

20. Goodman N: *Benjamin Rush: Physician and Citizen, 1746-1813*, Philadelphia: University of Pennsylvania Press, 1934

21. Rush B: *Medical Inquiries and Observations Upon the Diseases of the Mind* (4th Edition). Philadelphia: J Grigg, 1830

22. Buckmaster H: *Women Who Shaped History*, New York: Macmillian Pub. C., 1966

23. Bucknill JC, Tuke, DH: *A Manual of Psychological Medicine*, New York: Hafner Pub. Co., 1968 (Facsimile of 1858 Edition)

24. Barlow J: *Man's Power Over Himself to Prevent or Control Insanity*, London: William Pickering, 1843

25. Skultans V: *Madness and Morals: Ideas on Insanity in the Nineteenth Century*, London: Routledge & Kegan Paul, 1975

26. Tuke DH: *A Dictionary of Psychological Medicine*: Volume Two, Philadelphia: P Blakiston, Son & Co., 1892

27. Bockhoven JS: *Moral Treatment in American Psychiatry*, New York: Springer Publishing Co., Inc. 1963

28. Dain N: *Concepts of Insanity in the United States, 1789–1865*, New Brunswick, NJ: Rutgers University Press, 1964

29. Deutsch A: *The Mentally Ill in America: A History of Their Care and Treatment from Colonial Times* (2nd Edition). New York: Columbia University Press, 1949

30. Tracy SE: The development of occupational therapy in the Grace Hospital, Detroit, Michigan. *Trained Nurse Hosp Rev* 66:5, May 1921

31. Tracy SE: The place of invalid occupations in the general hospital. *Modern Hosp* 2:5, June 1914

32. Tracy SE: Twenty-five suggested mental tests derived from invalid occupations. *Maryland Psychiatr Q 8:* 1918

33. Barrows M: Susan E. Tracy, RN. *Maryland Psychiatric 16:* 1916–1917

34. Tracy SE: Treatment of disease by employment at St. Elizabeths Hospital. *Modern Hosp* 20:2, February 1923

35. Parsons SE: Miss Tracy's work in general hospitals. *Maryland Psychiatr Q 6:* 1916–1917

36. Tracy SE: *Studies in Invalid Occupation*, Boston: Witcomb and Barrows, 1918

37. Tracy SE: Power versus money in occupation therapy. *Trained Nurse Hosp Rev* 66:2, February 1921

38. Barton GE: A view of invalid occupation. *Trained Nurse Hosp Rev* 52:6, June 1914

39. Barton GE: Occupational nursing. *Trained Nurse Hosp Rev* 54:6, June 1915

40. Barton GE: *Occupational therapy. Trained Nurse Hosp Rev* 54:3, March 1915

41. Barton GE: The existing hospital system and reconstruction. *Trained Nurse Hosp Rev* 69:4, October 1922

42. Barton GE: What occupational therapy may mean to nursing. *Trained Nurse Hosp Rev* 64:4, April 1920

43. Barton GE: *Re-education: An Analysis of the Institutional System of the United States.* Boston: Houghton Mifflin Co., 1917

44. Sheppard Asylum: *Third Annual Report of the Sheppard Asylum,* Towson, MD: 1895

45. Dunton WR: The relationship of occupational therapy and physical therapy. *Arch Phys Ther* 16: January 1935

46. Dunton WR: *The Principles of Occupational Therapy. Proceedings of the National Society for the Promotion of Occupational Therapy: Second Annual Meeting,* Catonsville, MD: Spring Grove State Hospital, 1918

47. Dunton WR: *Occupational Therapy: A Manual for Nurses,* Philadelphia: WB Saunders, 1915

48. Komora PO: *Eleanor Clarke Slagle. Ment Hyg* 27:1, January 1943

49. Pollock HM: In memoriam: Eleanor Clarke Slagle, 1876–1942. *Am J Psychiatr* 99:3, November 1942

50. American Occupational Therapy Association: *Then and Now, 1917–1967,* New York: American Occupational Therapy Association, 1967

51. Loomis B, Wade BD: *Chicago…Occupational Therapy Beginnings: Hull House, The Henry B. Favill School of Occupations and Eleanor Clarke Slagle.*

52. Slagle EC: Occupational therapy: Recent methods and advances in the United States. *Occup Ther Rehab* 13:5, October 1934

53. Slagle EC: History of the development of occupation for the insane. *Maryland Psychiatr Q 4:* May 1914

54. Slagle EC: Training aids for mental patients. *Arch Occup There 1:*1, February 1922

55. Slagle EC, Robeson HA: *Syllabus for Training of Nurses in Occupational Therapy,* Utica, NY: State Hospital Press, date unknown

56. Slagle EC: A year's development of occupational therapy in New York State Hospitals. *Modern Hosp* 22:1, January 1924

57. Kidner TB: Occupational therapy, its development, scope and possibilities. *Occup Ther Rehab* 10:1, February 1931

58. Meyer A: The psychological point of view. In *Classics in American Psychiatry,* JP Brady, Editor. St. Louis: Warren H Green, Inc., 1975 (Also, In *The Problems of Mental Health,* M Bentley, EV Cowdey, Editors. New York: McGraw-Hill, 1934)

59. Arieti S: *American Handbook of Psychiatry* (Vol Two), New York: Basic Books, Inc., Publishers, 1959

60. Lief A: *The Commonsense Psychiatry of Dr. Adolf Meyer: Fifty-two Selected Papers, Edited with Biographical Narrative.* New York: McGraw-Hill Book Co., 1948

61. Meyer A: The philosophy of occupation therapy. *Arch Occup Ther 1:*1, February 1922. Also in Am J Occup Ther 31(10): 639–642, 1977. Reprinted as Chapter 2.

62. Meyer A: The rise to the person and the concept of wholes or integrates. *Am J Psychiatr 100:* April 1944

63. Pattison HA: The trend of occupational therapy for the tuberculous. *Arch Occup Ther 1*(1): February 1922

64. Coulter JS, McNarry H: Necessity of medical supervision in occupational therapy. *Occup Ther Rehab* 10(1): February 1931

65. An outline of lectures on occupational therapy to medical students and physicians. *Occup Ther Rehab* 4(4): August 1925

66. Elwood, ES: The National Board of Medical Examiners and medical education, and the possible effect of the Board's program on the spread of occupational therapy. *Occup Ther Rehab* 6(5): October 1927

67. Wade BD: Occupational Therapy: A History of Its Practice in the Psychiatric Field. Unpublished paper presented at 51st Annual Conference, American Occupational Therapy Association, Boston, October 19, 1967

68. Advisory Committee in Occupational Therapy: The Basic Philosophy and Function of Occupational Therapy. *University of Illinois Faculty—Alumni Newsletter of the Chicago Professional Colleges.* 6:4, January 1951

69. Wade BD: A survey of occupational and industrial therapy in the Illinois state hospitals. *Illinois Psychiatr* 2(1): March 1942

70. Wade BD: Supportive care, *Bull Rehab Inst Chicago,* date unknown

71. Wade BD: Supportive care. Bull Rehab Rehabilitation of the Mentally Ill. Unpublished paper presented to the Department of Public Welfare, State of Minnesota, June 26, 1958

72. Willard HS, Spackman CS: *Principles of Occupational Therapy* (First Edition). Philadelphia: JB Lippincott Co., 1947

73. Wade BD: The Development of Clinically Oriented Education in Occupational Therapy: The Illinois Plan. Unpublished paper presented at 49th Annual Conference, American Occupational Therapy Association, Miami, November 2, 1965

74. Wade BD: Introduction. *The Preparation of Occupational Therapy Students for Functioning with Aging Persons and in Comprehensive Health Care Programs: A Manual for Educators,* Chicago: University of Illinois at the Medical Center, 1969

75. Dooling EM: *A Way of Working,* Garden City, NY: Anchor Press/Doubleday, 1979

76. Sidey H: The presidency. *Time 116*(22):December 1, 1980

77. Slagle EC: Occupational therapy. *Trained Nurse Hosp Rev* 100(4): April 1938

78. Slagle EC: Editorial: From the heart. *Occup Ther Rehab* 16(5): October 1937

Pragmatism and Structuralism in Occupational Therapy: The Long Conversation

BARB HOOPER, MS, OTR
WENDY WOOD, PHD, OTR/L, FAOTA

The history of occupational therapy may be understood as a continual transaction between two cultural discourses: pragmatism and structuralism. *Pragmatism* is a way of thinking that presupposes humans are agentic by nature and knowledge is tentative and created within particular contexts. *Structuralism* is a way of thinking that assumes humans are composites of recurring general frameworks and that knowledge is objective and can be generalized to multiple contexts. Early in the field's history, both pragmatist and structuralist assumptions about the human and knowledge produced different readings, or interpretations, of what constituted the appropriate tools, methods, and outcomes for occupational therapy. Consequently, occupational therapy adopted an interesting mix of pragmatist language regarding the human and structuralist approaches to knowledge, resulting in professional identity problems still experienced today. However, recent developments offer an opportunity for occupational therapists to correct old identity problems through critically evaluating incompatible assumptions and carefully reading the prevailing cultural ethos.

That occupational therapists have historically struggled with issues of professional identity is clear. Why occupational therapists have struggled and the consequences of that struggle for the profession's future viability are matters of much murkiness, complexity, and debate. This article enters into occupational therapy's long-standing foray into its identity by focusing on the role that discourse has played in the profession's evolution. A discourse is composed of a recurrent pattern of language that both shapes and reflects a profession's intellectual commitments by being the medium through which its practices are constituted (Tinning, 1991). In other words, how practitioners "read" the problems, tools, and desired outcomes of their services—and, consequently, the particular ways they eventually come to practice and the particular professional identity they eventually hone—are shaped partly by the discourses in which they participate. As Mattingly and Fleming (1994) observed in their landmark study of clinical reasoning, occupational therapy practitioners often work within "two different discourses" (p. 302): one that concentrates on restoring persons to satisfying lives and another that concentrates on fixing body parts. We propose herein that these discourses reflect those of pragmatism and structuralism, respectively; moreover, they have coexisted in various ways since occupational therapy's inception. Additional discourses, such as moral, humanist, feminist, and performance-dominated, have helped to pattern occupational therapy's practices and language and deserve historical analysis. However, we make a case that the profession's intellectual history may be conceived as one long conversation, at times conflictual, between the two divergent discourses of pragmatism and structuralism.

The basic purpose of this article is to analyze how pragmatist and structuralist discourses emerged and came to be expressed in occupational therapy. The larger purpose is to develop implications of this analysis for the profession's future. Our first consideration addresses the historical background of pragmatist and structuralist discourse and their guiding assumptions about the human and about knowledge. We targeted these assumptions because they represent the core intellectual commitments of a professional discourse (Kielhofner & Barrett, 1998; Tinning, 1991); consequently, they have been used in occupational therapy to show how pretheoretical assumptions influence clinical reasoning (Hooper, 1997), in occupational science to construct an occupational theory of health (Wilcock, 1998), and in philosophy as elements of theories of human nature (Stevenson & Haberman, 1998). Our second consideration pertains to how each discourse "reads" occupational therapy. As used here, reading refers to the interpretations or meanings that people attach to things. We propose that pragmatism engenders a particular reading of practice largely discordant with that of structuralism; that is, the two discourses highlight different phenomena as well as relegate different phenomena to the background of concern or edit them out altogether. Our analysis then proceeds to how these discourses have been negotiated and shaped, not as dichotomies, but as ratios and conjoined assumptions. Lastly, we pose ways in which this long conversation offers guidance to the future.

The method for this analysis included both historical and discourse analysis. Discourse analysis seeks to reveal the realities individuals or groups have forged, and continue to forge, through language and practice (Denzin & Lincoln, 2000). Accordingly, original historical texts of early and contemporary pragmatists were coded for theories of human nature (Stevenson & Haberman, 1998). After these theories were constructed, we used them as conceptual grids for analyzing language patterns in occupational therapy texts. Our emphasis throughout is on prominent works, as we presume that they have been especially influential in shaping the profession's discourses. Our analysis is also situated in the United States and, thus, although most likely germane to occupational therapy in other countries, is not intended as a broad generalization about the field's evolution on multinational levels.

Pragmatism: Historical and Conceptual Overview

In the late 19th century, America faced an intellectual crisis due to the impact of new scientific discoveries, Darwinism, new biblical criticism, and the emergence of the social sciences. Taken-for-granted religious explanations of knowledge, human nature, and reality were being vigorously debated, with pragmatism posed as one alternative to traditional religious views (Hodge, 1872/1997; Peirce, 1878/1995; Sumner, 1881/1997; Ward, 1884/1997). As a dominant intellectual discourse in the early 20th century, pragmatist tenets were adopted by many disciplines, such as law (Holmes, 1920/1997), anthropology (Mead, 1928/1997), sociology (Ward, 1884/1997), and business (Lippman, 1914). Core intellectual commitments of occupational therapy were likewise being constructed from a pragmatist perspective at that time (Breines, 1986; Serrett, 1985).

Pragmatist Views of the Human

The philosophy of pragmatism promoted particular assumptions about human beings that these disciplines embodied. Fundamentally, the pragmatist view of the human was holistic given its rejection of anything that sublimated people to anything less than their total experiences. Early pragmatists thus rejected dichotomies like mind–body, thought–action, rational–practical, and function–structure that presumed people could be divided into parts (Dewey, 1908/1995; Leys, 1990). Additionally, because people were seen as agentic and in possession of potentials to cultivate their environs (Emerson, 1883/1995), the individual occupied the foreground of pragmatic discourse. Thus did Dewey (1915/1944) write that children are endowed with "native tendencies to explore, to manipulate tools and materials, to construct, to give expression to joyous emotion" (p. 195). Also conveying pragmatism's celebration of human agency, James (1907/1995b) observed that because every department of life bears the stamp of human power and imagination, "the trail of the human serpent is thus over everything" (p. 60).

Early pragmatists also delimited human agency in three ways having to do with other qualities of being human. First, humans were seen as teleological, meaning that they envisioned desired futures and directed action toward realizing those futures (Leys, 1990). Hence, part of human nature is to apply tools, technology, art, and knowledge toward a telos or vision of "the good." Yet because human activity also could be confined by what was seen as desirable, one "telos" could occlude views of other equally desirable or beneficial futures. Second, inextricable ties with biology, the physical environment, and society were seen to delimit human agency (Dewey, 1930; James, 1892/1985, 1907/1995a). Humans were seen as so interwoven into the fabric of their social and physical environs that Dewey (1939/1973) described this connection as "intercourse with our surroundings" (p. 571). Biology, environment, and society thus worked in tandem to both direct and constrain human activity in particular ways. Third, human agency was delimited by the sensory-reliant nature of people. Human understandings of the world (i.e., opinions, ideas, conceptions of "fact") were seen as molded from direct sensory experiences that shaped particular habits of mind and, in turn, guided future perceptions and actions (James, 1892/1985). Experiences that were novel to established habits of mind were thus difficult to assimilate and often ignored, even when potentially positive.

Pragmatist Views of Knowledge

The pragmatist view of the human not only is congruent with, but also informs and is informed by its view of knowledge. Because pragmatists believed that experiences undertaken with forethought and intentionality were needed to reveal the fluid truths of phenomena, they were skeptical of discourses that presumed absolutes and certainty in knowledge. Pragmatists instead promoted a view of knowledge as flexible, fallible, and contingent (Cherryholmes, 1999). Knowledge was flexible because it was determined in the making and doing of direct experience and, therefore, could not be "found" or become fixed. Knowledge was fallible because it was always being overturned by better ways of explaining or understanding things. As Emerson (1883/1995) expressed, "There is not a piece of science but that its flank may be turned tomorrow" (p. 28). Knowledge was likewise contingent because it issued from an iterative process between action and particular contexts. As Dewey (1908/1995) noted, "All knowledge issues in some action which changes things to some extent" (p. 82). Given these suppositions, pragmatic method was experimental in nature on the basis of critical inquiry into practical consequences. Emerson (1883/1995) captured this spirit of inquiry by proclaiming, "No facts are to me sacred; none are profane; I simply experiment, an endless seeker" (p. 31). James (1907/1995b) later stipulated that the key to pragmatic inquiry was its dedication to ascertaining, "What difference would it practically make to anyone if this notion rather than that notion were true?" (p. 54).

The pragmatist view of knowledge has mistakenly been interpreted as doing what works. Yet pragmatism stresses active inquiry far beyond mere expediency. Such inquiry scrutinizes not only the practicality of an action and its main or intended consequence, but also all of its effects (Dewey, 1939/1964; Peirce, 1878/1995). Knowledge is seen as continually being made through habits of reflection and inquiry regarding the consequences of chosen actions in light of a coveted future. Thus, pragmatist discourse recently has been associated with a nonfoundational approach to knowledge, the aim of which is to "arrive temporarily at warranted assertions" via continual engagement in a rich critical inquiry (Cherryholmes, 1999, p. 34). Such inquiry presumes that because ideas and theories (and other human creations) are socially embedded in the present and products of past discourses, they cannot be held to be theoretically neutral, timeless, or independent of particular historical or political contexts.

Pragmatist Readings of Occupational Therapy

One of the primary routes by which occupational therapy inherited its pragmatist discourse was from John Dewey and William James via their friend and colleague Adolf Meyer (Serrett, 1985). James's and Dewey's pragmatism played a large role in shaping Meyer's practice of psychobiology. This practice highlighted pragmatist themes by stressing the indispensability of understanding people in context of their environs, life histories, and ways of acting in the world (Leys, 1990; Meyer, 1933/1948; Muncie, 1939/1985). Meyer (1922) relied heavily on his psychobiology in writing *The Philosophy of Occupation Therapy*, possibly the most cited work in occupational therapy literature ever (see Chapter 2). The following classic quote from this work reveals how Meyer's view of the human accentuated certain clinical problems as critical, certain therapeutic tools as most helpful, and certain outcomes as most desirable:

> Our body is not so many pounds of flesh and bone figuring as a machine with an abstract mind or soul added to it. It is throughout a living organism pulsating with its rhythm of rest and activity, beating time (as we might say) in ever so many ways, most readily intelligible and in the full bloom of its nature when it feels itself as one of those great

self-guiding energy-transformers which constitute the real world of living beings. Our conception of man is that of an organism that maintains and balances itself in the world of reality and actuality by being in active life and active use, i.e., using and living and acting its time in harmony with its own nature and the nature about it. (p. 5). (See Chapter 2.)

Meyer's (1922) reading of occupational therapy may be one of the field's cleanest examples of pragmatic discourse (see Chapter 2). His reading highlighted problems related to the suppression of natural experiences in total life contexts and to disturbances in self-efficacy and natural rhythms of time; it elaborated on tools of practice that dealt with the particularities of each case, such as providing opportunities to plan, do, and create according to patients' skills and interests; and it elaborated on outcomes that restored temporal rhythms and natural connections among work and play, ambition and satisfaction, and desires and performance. Conversely, Meyer's reading edited out clinical problems that were not problems of action, clinical tools that were generic or prescriptive, and clinical outcomes that did less than empower "the individual to face his or her own deficiencies and deploy his or her own resources" (Leys, 1990, p. 50). Also edited out were ideas that did not situate people in their environs or that divided them into physical–psychological or function–structure dichotomies.

Yerxa's 1966 Eleanor Clarke Slagle lecture, another frequently cited work, points out the agreement between occupational therapy and existential thinkers who see humans as agents involved in the process of becoming more authentically their true selves (Yerxa, 1967). Congruent with this view of the human, Yerxa (1967) used strong pragmatist themes to depict how occupational therapists help people become more authentic. That is, because occupational therapy clients needed to act in the world of reality as their own agents, her reading of practice highlighted problems of action, methods that supported patients' self-initiation, and outcomes pertaining to patients' self-actualization and realistic perceptions of themselves and their environs. This reading also highlighted knowledge as being constructed from within professional experience and supported by continuous inquiry. More recently, Clark's 1993 Slagle lecture promoted a pragmatist reading by emphasizing the individual case over general principles and the importance of nurturing "the human spirit to act" by empowering persons to define and solve their problems through a healing process of occupational storytelling and storymaking (Clark, 1993, p. 1076).

Pragmatic discourse regarding the human has more than endured in occupational therapy across the 20th century, but perhaps pragmatic discourse regarding knowledge has not—a situation that we traced to the field's earliest educational practices. Although herself educated in England, Wilcock (1998) characterized occupational therapy's educational practices in the late 1950s and early 1960s as "didactic and authoritarian" (p. 4). She further posed that such educational practices did not prepare practitioners to "defend the value of occupation to health when medicine adopted an increasingly reductionistic, scientific and technological stance from the late 1960s onward" (p. 4). Similarly, Reilly (1962) (see Chapter 8) and West (1992) vehemently argued, 30 years apart from one another, that occupational therapists needed to develop far greater comfort and capacity for critical analysis if the field was to evolve into legitimate professionalism. Ultimately, the degree to which pragmatist views both of the human and of knowledge were adopted may have been thwarted by the early challenge of structuralism (Serrett, 1985), another powerful discourse with views of the human and knowledge that are largely discordant to those of pragmatism.

Structuralism: Historical and Conceptual Overview

Like pragmatism, structuralism was an interdisciplinary movement that sought new ways to establish truth following the rise of science and the secularization of society. Structuralists shared pragmatists' concerns with meaningful connections and, thus, rejected the disconnected and atomistic ideas produced by radical empirical science (Merquior, 1986; Sturrock, 1986). But unlike pragmatism, structuralism rejected Enlightenment liberal–rational values that privileged nature, natural experiences, and the rational individual over society (Harland, 1987). Guided by linguistics, structuralism instead treated underlying structures as ultimate. Thus, the analogy of a kaleidoscope has been used to describe the structuralist perspective. Although a kaleidoscope seems to consist of many different forms, it is actually only "a matrix composed of just a few recurring elements" (Merquior, 1986, p. 191). Likewise, how the structure of a whole building can be explained by its parts was seen as analogous to the anatomical, psychological, and social structures of people (Dosse, 1997). Given its explanatory power, structuralism was adopted by most social sciences by the mid 20th century and went on to produce "a veritable revolution" held akin to a powerful "scientific baptism" (Dosse, 1997, p. xxii).

Structuralist Views of the Human

As suggested by the analogy of the kaleidoscope, a structuralist perspective was one in which humans were viewed as composites of recurring general frameworks, thus placing emphasis on static parts rather than on dynamically assembled action that is contextual, volitional, and self-transforming. Structuralism, consequently, was far less preoccupied with human agency than pragmatism (Sturrock, 1986). Rather, the quality of being human derived from general frameworks that precede experience and to which experience conformed (Andi, 1999; Harland, 1987). Structuralist discourse thus downplayed the agentic and holistic individual, stressing instead general systems in which people act, general structures common to all people, and general internal systems of all people.

Structuralist Views of Knowledge

As in pragmatism, the structuralist view of the human both informed and was informed by its view of knowledge. Hence, structuralist discourse minimized the relevance of context, subjectivity, or case-specific particulars to the development of knowledge. Instead, knowledge was seen as being composed of various timeless, universal, and objectively verifiable structures and mechanisms, be they biological, sociological, or anthropological (among other possibilities) in nature (Harland, 1987). Moreover, because such structures and mechanisms were divorced from experience, they could be applied to most episodes of human behavior; likewise, their deliberate manipulation or unmasking was precisely what generated new knowledge. This allure of scientificity attracted numerous social sciences to structuralism in the 20th century (Dosse, 1997). Accordingly, structuralist discourse has been viewed as being consistent with a foundational approach to knowledge. This foundational approach presumes that various phenomena possess independent essences that can be objectively secured (Cherryholmes, 1999). Assuming that knowledge is foundational, structuralist inquiry seeks to represent a phenomenon as it "truly" is according to its fixed essence. Deciphering whether something represents a particular phenomenon is then accomplished by referring to that phenomenon's "objectively" established structure.

Structuralist Readings of Occupational Therapy

Because structuralism conveys very different intellectual commitments about the human and knowledge than does pragmatism, its produces very different readings of practice. The following quote from Fiorentino's 1974 Slagle lecture reflects a rather pure structuralist reading of practice; significantly, it also manifests a developmental model that has dominated pediatric practice in occupational therapy for many years (Coster, 1998):

> In the areas of gross and fine motor development, we cannot accept, as a goal of treatment, functional use of the hands without first attaining stability of everything to which the hand is attached. Development is cephalo–caudal, proximal–distal, medial–lateral, gross to fine. This is how treatment should progress if we are to give children their maximal functional potential. Also, we should place our emphasis on normal developmental sequences of CNS [central nervous system] development: for example, learning on a subcortical basis, followed by cortical, voluntary learning, finally reaching the stage of spontaneous automatic movements. (Fiorentino, 1975, p. 20)

Fiorentino's (1975) reading of practice relegated to the background of clinical consideration concern with the historical particularities of each case as well as with persons' subjective experiences and whole performances of doing. Conversely, highlighted were clinical problems related to disturbances in structures underlying performance, clinical tools that sequentially applied universal procedures, and clinical outcomes that could verify that children with disabilities were developing "on time" with and in the same ways and sequences as their peers without disabilities. Fiorentino's view of the human focused on internal systems that were presumed to be universal; likewise, she understood knowledge to derive from general and timeless principles of human development.

Similar themes in other structuralist readings of practice include using decontextualized clinical techniques as prerequisites for doing things "naturally" in ordinary rhythms of time and applying general cases to individuals. For example, Reed traced in her 1986 Slagle lecture the evolution of crafts as clinical media in occupational therapy (see Chapter 46). Reed's (1986) research suggested that practitioners gradually shifted from seeing bilateral sanding blocks as woodworking tools to seeing them as tools for facilitating upper-extremity integration and strength. Once a "therapist-reader" brought the motion of sanding out in the foreground, the next step was easy to have patients sand "without sand paper on an incline plane made of Formica" (p. 602) as a prerequisite to complex occupational engagement. This clinical strategy is rooted in a historic reliance on a priori, fixed knowledge of human movement in an ideal general case. Licht (1957), a mid-century physician and influential writer in occupational therapy, detailed a kinesiologic approach to craft analysis that was predicated on how a skilled crafter would work, including exact types of muscle contraction, amounts of joint movement, and total energy used by each joint. Paisley (1929), an early occupational therapist, similarly executed very tight control over how children with cerebral palsy did craftwork, assuming that they ought to strive for "normal" movement as determined by the standard of children without disabilities.

Because a structuralist reading of practice views client problems as problems of underlying structures or mechanisms, such as muscle strength, muscle tone, or developmental age, it elaborates on clinical tools that address such structures and mechanisms as progressive resistive exercise, neurodevelopmental techniques, or linear sequences of developmental tasks. Although such a reading of practice can use activity as a therapeutic tool, it presumes that activity "works" by changing underlying structures and processes. Thus, a structuralist reading places into its background of concern persons' subjective experiences as they do things, their unique ways of doing things, and contextual influences on what they do and how.

Foundations of the Pragmatist–Structuralist Conversation

If both pragmatist and structuralist readings of practice have coexisted throughout occupational therapy's history, then on what bases have these discourses been negotiated and shaped? To answer this question, we examined the pragmatist–structuralist conversation in two ways that we believe shed some light on the field's persistent struggles over

professional identity: (a) parallels in the shifting discourses of occupational therapy and the culture at large and (b) an internal incongruence between a pragmatist view of the human and a structuralist view of knowledge.

The Larger Cultural Ethos

Whereas pragmatism was a widely recognized and valued discourse in American society in the early 20th century, structuralism asserted its dominance by mid-century. Today, however, scholars argue that a revival of pragmatism and a shift to a poststructural discourse has occurred in the culture at large (Merquior, 1986; Putnam, 1990/1995; Rorty, 1992/1995). Therefore, nonfoundational knowledge, a critical stance toward language and power, and inquiries into the efficacy of actions to produce desired futures are once again prevalent in contemporary society (Cherryholmes, 1999; Kloppenberg, 1996). These reciprocating shifts in the culture at large have their parallel shift within occupational therapy, not in discrete phases, but in alternating ratios. Configuring the discourses as a ratio suggests that both remain present but in alternating proportions of dominance and influence.

The Early-20th-Century Conversation

Attesting to the early influence of pragmatism on occupational therapy, Slagle and Robinson (1941) described the field as a service that sought to "arouse interest, courage, and confidence; to exercise body and mind in healthful activity; to overcome disability; and to re-establish capacity for industrial and social usefulness" (p. 5). Habit training, a specific practice endorsed by Slagle, was described in words borrowed directly from James's work on habits: "There is no *general* habit, no *general* memory, that is common to all mankind. It is *individual* habit and memory. Everyone builds his or her own" (p. 33). The use of such pragmatist discourse that highlighted, like Meyer (1922) (see Chapter 2), the human capacity to restore oneself to usefulness and health through occupation was pervasive in the field's literature from about 1900 to 1940 (Kielhofner & Burke, 1983). Yet, on closer inspection of how some early practitioners actually provided services, structuralist approaches to clinical problems and methods are evident. Indeed, Slagle's habit training program consisted of a highly prescriptive regime of daily activity that a group of patients, after having been assigned to the program by a physician, were meticulously made to follow from the time they rose until just before bedtime (Slagle & Robinson, 1941). Thus, though described in bold pragmatist terms and certainly built around a balance of activity and rest at its core, the program concurrently evidenced structuralist themes of generalized procedures, standardization, and uniformity. Although infrequent, these structuralist themes and the idea that therapy "worked" by changing presumably universal internal structures or processes are evident in how other early occupational therapists provided services to other clinical populations in the 1920s and 1930s (e.g., Hurt, 1934; McNary, 1934; Paisley, 1929).

The Mid-Century Conversation

By mid-century, this ratio of pragmatist-to-structuralist discourses in occupational therapy was well under way to reversing itself along with the larger cultural shift toward structuralism. Thus, by the 1960s and 1970s, practitioners had mostly come to represent their profession and to base their methods on a view of humans that highlighted the ultimate importance of internal neurologic, psychic, or kinesiologic workings (Kielhofner & Burke, 1983; see also Ayres, 1963; Huss, 1977; Moore, 1976). Nevertheless, some strong pragmatist readings of practice were evident, such as Yerxa's (1967) as already noted. Additionally, pragmatist themes kept repeatedly "popping up" in what were otherwise strong structuralist readings of practice. For example, Rood's 1958 Slagle lecture promoted the structuralist practice of applying a priori knowledge of presumably universal developmental patterns to all persons' "emotional, intellectual, and professional development as well as physical growth" (Rood, 1958, p. 328). Yet, by titling her lecture, "Every One Counts," and by stressing that people, whether patients or occupational therapists or their students, ought to be supported in setting their own goals, Rood (1958) simultaneously showed that she, like the pragmatists, valued human agency.

The Late-20th-Century Conversation

By century's end and, again, consistent with the general culture, the ratio of pragmatist-to-structuralist discourses in occupational therapy was reversing itself once again, and pragmatist readings of practice were ascending in dominance. Contemporary constructs of lifestyle redesign, conditional and narrative reasoning, and client-centered practice advanced a view of the human as agentic, teleological, and socially interdependent (Jackson, Carlson, Mandel, Zemke, & Clark, 1998; Law, 1998; Mattingly & Fleming, 1994). Likewise, new assessments urge continual evaluation of whether or how therapy helps persons do what they want and need to do given the particular circumstances of their lives, thus advancing a view of knowledge as flexible, fallible, and contingent (e.g., Coster, 1998; Law, 1998). Moreover, not only Clark's (1993), but also every other Eleanor Clarke Slagle lecture of the 1990s has placed pragmatist themes in the foreground: how resilience and a unique inner life can "transform...traumas into varying degrees of triumph" (Fine, 1991, p. 493); why "meaningfulness and purposefulness are key therapeutic qualities of occupation" (see Chapter 25) (Trombly, 1995, p. 960) (see Chapter 16) ; why "occupation...is so basic to human health yet so flexible" (Nelson, 1997, p. 11 [see Chapter 12]); how occupation enables "people to seize, take possession of, or occupy the spaces, time, and roles of their lives" (Fisher, 1998, p. 509 [see Chapter 14]); or how occupation is "the principal means through which people develop and express their personal identities" (Christiansen, 1999, p. 547 [see Chapter 42]). Perhaps Grady's 1994 Slagle lecture is the most telling of the field's shifting discourses given her correction of her own past practice theory for wrongly emphasizing "ways therapists

could influence the child's development rather than ways in which the environment could be prepared to accommodate the child's function" (Grady, 1995, p. 305 [see Chapter 30).

Even as pragmatist discourse is again being loudly spoken in occupational therapy, structuralist discourse is far from mute. At times, the conversation between the two has been loud and impassioned. For example, the American Occupational Therapy Association's (AOTA's) 1991 debate over practitioners' use of physical agent modalities manifested a heated clash between pragmatist and structuralist readings of practice, unfolding just as a renewed pragmatist discourse was ascending in the field and eclipsing some of the esteem once reflexively attributed to structuralist practices (e.g., Ahlschwede, 1992; West & Wiemer, 1991). At other times in the conversation, structuralism has remained the louder voice of the two, especially when practitioners work within a biomedical culture. It was within this culture that Mattingly and Fleming (1994) found that practitioners straddle two discourses: one that concentrated on restoring persons to satisfying lives and another that concentrated on fixing body parts. Of considerable significance, many practitioners in their study experienced "an unease at the heart of their practice" as related to the field's self-portrayal as a service that treats "the whole person" (p. 296). That is, pragmatist values about holism, action, and natural experiences in the everyday world went "underground" (p. 296), meaning that practitioners did not speak too loudly of these values, if at all, during formal professional communications. Rather, to gain credibility in a culture that saw patients, their problems, and treatments in biomedical terms, the chart-talk, body-as-biomechanical-machine language of medicine predominated.

A Pragmatist View of the Human but a Structuralist Approach to Knowledge

With the parallels between cultural and professional discourses duly noted, the pragmatist–structuralist conversation within occupational therapy did not, however, unfold in such equal exchanges. Indeed, a pragmatist view of the human was promoted early on in the field, but in tandem with a structuralist view of knowledge as objectively fixed, theoretically neutral, context free, universal, and derived from external authority. Hence, occupational therapy started cultivating at its inception a basic and problematic incompatibility between its oft-stated pragmatist view of the human and its structuralist approach toward knowledge.

The Evolution of Discordant Assumptions

We date these incompatible views of the human and knowledge at least to the start of World War I when early occupational therapists had a moral philosophy and a moral imperative to train more practitioners but no knowledge base of their own with which to educate them or much of any status or expertise with which to argue for particular educational practices. This vacuum was largely filled by deference to medical authorities. As Presseller (1984) noted in a historical study of the field's educational practices and policies, emergency war courses taught anatomy and kinesiology as core subjects to prepare reconstruction aides for their work with wounded soldiers. Also under the strong influence of physicians, basic medical sciences and applied medical lectures occupied more and more of the field's core curricula over ensuing decades. Of more significance than this core content per se (which is significant in and of itself), early pedagogical practices simulta-? neously embodied structuralist views of knowledge.

The Effects of Discordant Assumptions

Specifically, in approaching knowledge of the human body and disease as "core" professional knowledge received from medical authorities, occupational therapists were socialized early on into passively accepting knowledge as objectively "true" and inviolable. One cannot help but note the irony that as Meyer and Dewey were actively promoting richly experiential, self-exploratory, critically evaluative, and process-oriented pedagogic approaches for medical students and young children alike (Dewey, 1915; Muncie, 1939/1985), occupational therapy was being built on an educational foundation that all but forbade challenging medical authority and made virtually no room for critical inquiry (e.g., Quiroga, 1995; Serrett, 1985). This foundation presumed—contrary to the pragmatic method but in accord with the role of women at the time— that because male physicians would tightly control the work of female occupational therapists, the latter did not need to learn to evaluate and question received content for its coherence, implied actions, or the varying consequences of those actions across different life contexts. Hence, according to Presseller (1984), medical sciences, theory, and techniques were taught as subjects disconnected from one another and from their applications to practice in early educational programs. This lack of integration furthermore promulgated an immediate rupture between theory and clinical methods. Presseller blamed this rupture for many of the profession's identity issues and, therefore, for why practitioners could express "a commitment to activity" but could not connect theory to practice and would "use whatever technique was at hand" (p. iv). In our view, long-standing disconnections among basic academic content, theory, and techniques coupled with pedagogic methods that discouraged critical inquiry allowed a view of the human as a decontextualized biological system of presumably universal structures and functions to take root in occupational therapy and later thrive.

Beyond formal educational practices, structuralist approaches to knowledge are also evident in various clinical tools and ways of describing practice. In the 1930s and 1940s, occupational therapy faced increasing pressure to house its holistic conception of occupation in a container that could satisfy medicine's questions of efficacy and scientificity according to medical epistemology (Rogers, 1982). Licht's (1957) approach to activity analysis, a core clinical tool throughout the field's history, responded to and promoted this pressure by its kinesiologic formula of how movement ought ideally occur.

As noted previously, by the 1960s and 1970s, practitioners commonly appropriated the language of kinesiology, neurology, and psychoanalysis to describe their methods and outcomes. In all cases, the structuralist analogy of a kaleidoscope as a matrix of a few recurring parts was advanced; that is, occupational behavior, a seemingly complex phenomenon, consisted "truly" of relatively few parts and mechanisms that could be fully enumerated.

Structuralist assumptions about how complex behavior is conceptualized continue to be evident today. *Uniform Terminology*, an influential document in practice and education, dates to 1979 when the field made an effort to define its domain of concern, clinical methods, and outcomes in standardized and theoretically neutral terms that captured "typical" practices irrespective of context (AOTA, 1979). By emphasizing performance components, all editions of the document have analogized, however tacitly, occupational performance to the structuralist kaleidoscope (AOTA, 1979, 1989, 1994). Moreover, although theory and context are acknowledged in the most recent edition, practice and occupational performance are still depicted with relatively few uniformly defined constructs that are presumably theoretically "neutral." It is furthermore presumed that these concepts can be readily interrelated using a preestablished grid with little regard to how various contingencies might influence or possibly even contradict implied relationships.

The Conversation Continues: Guideposts for the Future

Viewed as a whole, the intellectual history of occupational therapy may, in some important respects, be understood as a long conversation between pragmatist and structuralist discourses: Pragmatist readings of practice were first privileged over but did not silence structuralist readings, then the ratio of that privileging reversed itself, then reversed itself again, all in accord with the most compelling cultural ethos at hand. Moreover, this conversation has been characterized by numerous tensions, many of which remain unreconciled partly because of dynamics that took root early on and remain viable today. Specifically, a pragmatist view of the human was being spoken and clinically applied even as a structuralist approach to knowledge was instantiated in the earliest educational programs to legitimize the fledgling field. This incompatibility laid the groundwork, albeit not alone, for structuralist readings of practice to rise into eventual dominance. Structuralist views of knowledge as foundational, universal, and objectively securable contributed to an unease over critical evaluation of discordant professional practices. These dynamics speak to the profession's identity conundrum that has persisted for almost 100 years. Although its practitioners have portrayed their work as dedicated to treating patients holistically in accord with their personal interests and goals, they have struggled greatly in how best to realize and to match their clinical approaches to that portrayal.

If our interpretation of the profession's evolution is reasonably sound, then guideposts for navigating onward are suggested. These guideposts resonate with the more recent shift toward pragmatism in the larger culture: a state of affairs that we think is conducive to occupational therapy's best interests and offers practitioners great opportunities to author the profession's future. To exploit these opportunities, we propose that two new forms of literacy be cultivated.

Reading and Speaking the Language of Assumptions

One form of literacy concerns occupational therapists' capacities to apprehend the assumptions about humans and knowledge embodied in their readings of practice and, hence, how they interpret clinical problems, select media and methods, and conceive outcomes. With direct implications for the profession's internal and public identity, this form of literacy would allow occupational therapists to examine how the view of humans embedded in our shared language—"treating the whole person," "functional," or "meaningful occupation"—aligns with the view of humans embedded in actual professional methods. In complementary fashion, the capacity to examine assumptions about knowledge would raise occupational therapists' consciousness about what knowledge claims and whose knowledge claims inhabit their practice and on what bases they habitually grant legitimacy to claims of what is "core" or "truth" or "fact" in their practice. This consciousness would stimulate occupational therapists to adopt an appropriate skepticism toward categorical assertions about media and methods until the multifold consequences of those media or methods on persons' lives were credibly traced.

In effect, we are arguing on behalf of occupational therapists developing disciplined habits of mind that will spur their own conversations with themselves, ones that recurrently ask such questions as: What assumptions about the human are embedded in my therapy? What assumptions about knowledge dominate the criteria I use to legitimate my practice? On what evidence, on whose evidence, do I decide that my therapy actually helps persons do what they want and need to do given the particular hopes and challenges of their lives? Finally, do my clinical actions consequentially carry my patients to results that support the viability of occupational therapy?

Reading, Entering, and Shaping the Cultural Discourse

The second form of literacy has to do with cultural literacy. We refer specifically to occupational therapists' abilities to read the cultural ethos in which their practices (clinical, educational, research) are situated with respect to what values and ways of doing things are most privileged therein. Such cultural literacy would allow occupational therapists to discern when a particular ethos is in accord with the profession's best interests (as

we believe is now the case with the pragmatist discourse) or significantly foil those interests (as we believe occurred during structuralism's dominance). Discernment of such matches and mismatches will be necessary to avoid passive absorption of cultural discourses and, instead, to decide proactively which forces to join, which to support or try to influence, and which to reject and resist outright.

These two forms of literacy would allow for the possibility of rich conversations not just within individual occupational therapists, but also among occupational therapists and the entire profession. Such literacy would help occupational therapists ensure that both disciplinary and interdisciplinary discourses are critically examined according to their capacity to deliver a particular coveted future: one that has transcended occupational therapy's identity confusions even as its eclectic array of media and methods have at times scattered in a helter-skelter of directions. We speak of the profession's dedication to helping people do what they want and need to do each day in ways that maximize their occupational capacities and health: key domains of the contemporary interdisciplinary construct of quality of life to which we believe occupational therapists can contribute enormously (Albert & Logsdon, 2000; Wilson & Cleary, 1995). In calling for these conversations, we stand in agreement with Kloppenberg (1996), a contemporary pragmatist, and Dewey who each regarded critical inquiry in social communication as the indispensable medium for clarifying and resolving disputes and instilling cooperation.

Were occupational therapists individually and collectively to resume a conversation started by Meyer and his pragmatist colleagues in which discordant views of humans and knowledge are understood to engender fundamentally different calls to action and ends, we believe that a number of desired outcomes would be facilitated. Consistent with the philosophy of pragmatism, a multiplicity of theories, viewpoints, and practices would be not only tolerated, but also generated by the communal process of anticipating how specific ideas and actions help usher in occupational therapy's particular coveted future: helping people do what they want and need to do each day in ways that maximize quality of life. Uncritical, unreflective, and uninformed practices would be explicitly eschewed because occupational therapists would skillfully draw crucial distinctions among divergent theories, assumptions, and practices with respect to whether and how well each serves this coveted future. Also with respect to this future, incompatibilities among a wide array of professional practices would be carefully scrutinized to ferret out those that were obstructive and to advance those that were progressive. Likewise, discussion and debate would be deliberately carried forward so that questions of great consequence to the profession's identity, and hence distinctive service to society, could be clarified and resolved. Three such questions in our view are these: What academic content and pedagogical practices best empower occupational therapists to ascertain discourses and their corresponding claims about human nature and knowledge that shape professional practices? How do educators avoid the historical reliance on foundational knowledge and instead design curricula consistent with nonfoundational approaches to knowledge? What research questions and methods are relevant and conducive to a future where occupational therapists expertly address the occupational capacities of people and societies? If occupational therapists were to engage passionately and astutely in critical inquiry of present professional practices, and if they were to develop the kinds of literacy needed to identify influential discourses, the profession may begin to resolve its identity issues internally and within the culture at large and thrive as an autonomous academic profession whose value to society is both clear and great.

Acknowledgments

We thank Charles Cooper, PhD, Professor of History, University of North Carolina at Chapel Hill, for his review of an earlier draft of this article.

This article grew from Barb Hooper's original research into the core assumptions of occupational therapy that she completed in partial fulfillment of requirements for a doctoral cognate in occupational science undertaken in the Division of Occupational Science, University of North Carolina at Chapel Hill. Because both authors contributed equally to the article, order of authorship was determined alphabetically.

References

Ahlschwede, K. (1992). The Issue Is—Views on physical agent modalities and specialization within occupational therapy: A rebuttal. *American Journal of Occupational Therapy, 46,* 650–652.

Albert, S., & Logsdon, R. (Eds.). (2000). *Assessing quality of life in Alzheimer's disease.* New York: Springer.

American Occupational Therapy Association. (1979). *Occupational therapy product output reporting system and uniform terminology for reporting occupational therapy services.* Rockville, MD: Author.

American Occupational Therapy Association. (1989). Uniform terminology for occupational therapy (2nd edition). *American Journal of Occupational Therapy, 43,* 808–815.

American Occupational Therapy Association. (1994). Uniform terminology for occupational therapy—Third edition. *American Journal of Occupational Therapy, 48,* 1047–1054.

Andi, R. (Ed.). (1999). *The Cambridge dictionary of philosophy* (2nd ed.). Cambridge, MA: Cambridge University Press.

Ayres, A. J. (1963). The development of perceptual-motor abilities: A theoretical basis for treatment of dysfunction, 1963 Eleanor Clarke Slagle lecture. *American Journal of Occupational Therapy, 17,* 221–225.

Breines, E. (1986). *Origins and adaptations: A philosophy of practice.* Lebanon, NJ: Geri-Rehab.

Cherryholmes, C. H. (1999). *Reading pragmatism* (Vol. 24). New York: Teachers College Press.

Christiansen, C. H. (1999). Defining lives: Occupation as identity: An essay on competence, coherence, and the creation of meaning, 1999 Eleanor Clarke Slagle lecture. *American Journal of Occupational Therapy, 53,* 547–558. Reprinted as Chapter 42.

Clark, F. (1993). Occupation embedded in a real life: Interweaving occupational science and occupational therapy, 1993 Eleanor Clarke Slagle lecture. *American Journal of Occupational Therapy, 47,* 1067–1078.

Coster, W. (1998). Occupation-centered assessment of children. *American Journal of Occupational Therapy, 52,* 337–344.

Denzin, N. K., & Lincoln, Y. S. (Eds.). (2000). *Handbook of qualitative research.* Thousand Oaks, CA: Sage.

Dewey, J. (1915). *Democracy and education: An introduction to the philosophy of education.* New York: Macmillan.

Dewey, J. (1930). *Human nature and conduct: An introduction to social thought.* New York: Modern Library.

Dewey, J. (1964). The continuum of ends–means. In R. D. Archambault (Ed.), *John Dewey on education: Selected writings* (pp. 97–107). Chicago: University of Chicago Press. Original work published 1939.

Dewey, J. (1973). Having an experience. In J. J. McDermott (Ed.), *The philosophy of John Dewey* (pp. 554–573). Chicago: University of Chicago Press. Original work published 1939.

Dewey, J. (1995). Does reality possess practical character? In R. B. Goodman (Ed.), *Pragmatism: A contemporary reader* (pp. 79–93). New York: Routledge. Original work published 1908.

Dosse, F. (1997). *History of structuralism* (D. Glassman, Trans.). Minneapolis, MN: University of Minnesota Press.

Emerson, R. W. (1995). Circles. In R. B. Goodman (Ed.), *Pragmatism: A contemporary reader* (pp. 22–34). New York: Routledge. Original work published 1883.

Fine, S. B. (1991). Resilience and human adaptability: Who rises above adversity? 1990 Eleanor Clarke Slagle lecture. *American Journal of Occupational Therapy, 45,* 493–503. Reprinted as Chapter 25.

Fiorentino, M. R. (1975). Occupational therapy: Realization to activation, 1974 Eleanor Clarke Slagle lecture. *American Journal of Occupational Therapy, 29,* 15–21.

Fisher, A. G. (1998). Uniting practice and theory in an occupational therapy framework, 1998 Eleanor Clarke Slagle lecture. *American Journal of Occupational Therapy, 52,* 509–521. Reprinted as Chapter 14.

Grady, A. P. (1995). Building inclusive community: A challenge for occupational therapy, 1994 Eleanor Clarke Slagle lecture. *American Journal of Occupational Therapy, 49,* 300–310. Reprinted as Chapter 3.

Harland, R. (1987). *Superstructuralism: The philosophy of structuralism and post-structuralism.* New York: Methuen.

Hodge, C. (1997). Selection from systematic theology. In D. Hollinger & C. Capper (Eds.), *The American intellectual tradition* (Vol. II, pp. 6–12). New York: Oxford University Press. Original work published 1872.

Holmes, O. W. (1997). Natural law. In D. Hollinger & C. Capper (Eds.), *The American intellectual tradition* (Vol. II, pp. 123–126). New York: Oxford University Press. Original work published 1920.

Hooper, B. (1997). The relationship between pretheoretical assumptions and clinical reasoning. *American Journal of Occupational Therapy, 51,* 328–338.

Hurt, S. (1934). Occupational therapy in traumatic conditions. *Archives of Physical Therapy, X-ray, and Radium, 15,* 673–675.

Huss, A. J. (1977). Touch with care or a caring touch? 1976 Eleanor Clarke Slagle lecture. *American Journal of Occupational Therapy, 31,* 11–18.

Jackson, J., Carlson, M., Mandel, D., Zemke, R., & Clark, F. (1998). Occupation in lifestyle redesign: The well elderly study occupational therapy program. *American Journal of Occupational Therapy, 52,* 326–336.

James, W. (1985). Habit. *Occupational Therapy in Mental Health, 5*(3), 55–67. Original work published 1892.

James, W. (1995a). Pragmatism and humanism. In R. B. Goodman (Ed.), *Pragmatism: A contemporary reader* (pp. 65–75). New York: Routledge. Original work published 1907.

James, W. (1995b). What pragmatism means. In R. B. Goodman (Ed.), *Pragmatism: A contemporary reader* (pp. 53–64). New York: Routledge. Original work published 1907.

Kielhofner, G., & Barrett, L. (1998). Meaning and misunderstanding in occupational forms: A study in therapeutic goal setting. *American Journal of Occupational Therapy, 52,* 345–353.

Kielhofner, G., & Burke, J. P. (1983). The evolution of knowledge and practice in occupational therapy: Past, present, and future. In G. Kielhofner (Ed.), *Health through occupation: Theory and practice in occupational therapy* (pp. 3–54). Philadelphia: F. A. Davis.

Kloppenberg, J. T. (1996). Pragmatism: An old name for some new ways of thinking? *Journal of American History, 83*(1), 100–138.

Law, M. (1998). Client centered occupational therapy. Thorofare, NJ: Slack.

Leys, R. (1990). Adolf Meyer: A biographical note. In R. Leys & R. B. Evans (Eds.), *The correspondence between Adolf Meyer and Edward Bradford Titchener* (pp. 39–57). Baltimore: Johns Hopkins University Press.

Licht, S. (1957). Kinetic occupational therapy. In W. R. Dunton & S. Licht (Eds.), *Occupational therapy: Principles and practice* (pp. 53–83). Springfield, IL: Charles C Thomas.

Lippman, W. (1914). *Drift and mastery: An attempt to diagnose the current unrest.* New York: M. Kennerly.

Mattingly, C., & Fleming, M. H. (1994). *Clinical reasoning: Forms of inquiry in a therapeutic practice.* Philadelphia: F. A. Davis.

McNary, H. (1934). Anatomical considerations and technique in using occupations as exercise for orthopedic disabilities: Part III—Wrist and fingers. *Occupational Therapy and Rehabilitation, 13*(4), 24–29.

Mead, M. (1997). Selection from coming of age in Samoa. In D. A. Hollinger & C. Capper (Eds.), *The American intellectual tradition* (Vol. II, pp. 197–204). New York: Oxford University Press. Original work published 1928.

Merquior, J. G. (1986). *From Prague to Paris.* London: Verso.

Meyer, A. (1922). The philosophy of occupation therapy. *Archives of Occupational Therapy, 1,* 1–10. Reprinted as Chapter 2.

Meyer, A. (1948). Spontaneity. In A. Lief (Ed.), *The commonsense psychiatry of Dr. Adolph Meyer: Fifty-two selected papers* (pp. 576–589). New York: McGraw-Hill. Original work published 1933.

Moore, J. C. (1976). Behavior, bias, and the limbic system, 1975 Eleanor Clarke Slagle lecture. *American Journal of Occupational Therapy, 30,* 11–19.

Muncie, W. (1985). Historical and philosophical bases of psychobiology. *Occupational Therapy in Mental Health, 5*(3), 77–100. Original work published 1939.

Nelson, D. L. (1997). Why the profession of occupational therapy will flourish in the 21st century, 1996 Eleanor Clarke Slagle lecture. *American Journal of Occupational Therapy, 51,* 11–24. Reprinted as Chapter 12.

Paisley, A. (1929). Occupational therapy treatment for a group of spastic cases: Children under twelve years of age. *Occupational Therapy and Rehabilitation, 8*(2), 83–94.

Peirce, C. S. (1995). How to make our ideas clear. In R. B. Goodman (Ed.), *Pragmatism: A contemporary reader* (pp. 34–49). New York: Routledge. Original work published 1878.

Presseller, S. R. (1984). Occupational therapy education: Yesterday, today, and tomorrow (Doctoral dissertation, Boston University, 1984). *Dissertation Abstracts International, 45*(12B), 3777.

Putnam, H. (1995). A reconsideration of Deweyian democracy. In R. B. Goodman (Ed.), *Pragmatism: A contemporary reader* (pp. 183–205). New York: Routledge. Original work published 1990.

Quiroga, V. A. M. (1995). *Occupational therapy: The first thirty years, 1900–1930.* Bethesda, MD: American Occupational Therapy Association.

Reed, K. (1986). Tools of practice: Heritage or baggage? 1986 Eleanor Clarke Slagle lecture. *American Journal of Occupational Therapy, 40,* 597–605. Reprinted as Chapter 46.

Reilly, M. (1962). Occupational therapy can be one of the great ideas of 20th century medicine, 1961 Eleanor Clarke Slagle lecture. *American Journal of Occupational Therapy, 16,* 1–9. Reprinted as Chapter 8.

Rogers, J. C. (1982). The spirit of independence: The evolution of philosophy. *American Journal of Occupational Therapy, 36,* 709–715.

Rood, M. S. (1958). Every one counts, 1958 Eleanor Clarke Slagle lecture. American Journal of Occupational Therapy, 12, 326–329.

Rorty, R. (1995). Feminism and pragmatism. In R. B. Goodman (Ed.), *Pragmatism: A contemporary reader* (pp. 125–149). New York: Routledge. Original work published 1992.

Serrett, K. D. (1985). Another look at occupational therapy's history: Paradigm or pair-of-hands? *Occupational Therapy in Mental Health, 5(3),* 1–31.

Slagle, E. C., & Robinson, H. A. (1941). *Syllabus for training of nurses in occupational therapy* (2nd ed.). Utica, NY: State Hospital Press.

Stevenson, L., & Haberman, D. L. (1998). *Ten theories of human nature.* New York: Oxford University Press.

Sturrock, J. (1986). *Structuralism.* London: Paladin.

Sumner, W. G. (1997). Sociology. In D. Hollinger & C. Capper (Eds.), *The American intellectual tradition* (Vol. II, pp. 29–38). New York: Oxford University Press. Original work published 1881.

Tinning, R. (1991). Teacher education and pedagogy: Dominant discourses and the process of problem setting. *Journal of Teaching in Physical Education, 11*(1), 1–20.

Trombly, C. A. (1995). Occupation: Purposefulness and meaningfulness as therapeutic mechanisms, 1995 Eleanor Clarke Slagle lecture. *American Journal of Occupational Therapy, 49,* 960–972. Reprinted as Chapter 16.

Ward, L. F. (1997). Mind as social factor. In D. Hollinger & C. Capper (Eds.), *The American intellectual tradition* (Vol. II, pp. 39–47). New York: Oxford University Press. Original work published 1884.

West, W. (1992). Ten milestone issues in AOTA history. American Journal of Occupational Therapy, 46, 1066–1074.

West, W. L., & Wiemer, R. B. (1991). The Issue Is—Should the Representative Assembly have voted as it did, when it did, on occupational therapists' use of physical agent modalities? *American Journal of Occupational Therapy, 45,* 1143–1147.

Wilcock, A. A. (1998). *An occupational perspective of health.* Thorofare, NJ: Slack.

Wilson, I. B., & Cleary, P. D. (1995). Linking clinical variables with health-related quality of life. *Journal of the American Medical Association, 273,* 59–65.

Yerxa, E. J. (1967). Authentic occupational therapy, 1966 Eleanor Clarke Slagle lecture. *American Journal of Occupational Therapy, 21,* 1–9.

Occupational Therapy and Rehabilitation: An Awkward Alliance

CHAPTER 7

JUDITH FRIEDLAND,
PHD, MA, DIP. P&OT

In the preface to his book *Rehabilitation Medicine: A Textbook on Physical Medicine and Rehabilitation*, Rusk (1958) noted the objectives of the newly founded field of rehabilitation medicine. The first was:

> to eliminate the physical disability if that is possible; the second, to reduce or alleviate the disability to the greatest extent possible; and the third, to retrain the person with a residual physical disability to live and work within the limits of the disability but to the hilt of his capabilities. (p. 7)

Rusk went on to say that, although effective rehabilitation depended on the skills and services of members of many professions, "the physician, however, *by the very nature of the problem* [italics added], must be the leader of the team" (p. 7).

This chapter was previously published in the *American Journal of Occupational Therapy, 52,* 373–380. Copyright © 1998, American Occupational Therapy Association.

The phrase "by the very nature of the problem" provides the clue to the difficulty for occupational therapists in rehabilitation as well as the theme for this article. If the very nature of the problem *is the disability itself* and efforts are directed at eliminating it, then occupational therapists are at a disadvantage, because for us, the very nature of the problem *is not the disability but the occupational performance of the person with the disability.* We must then consider the possibility that some of the difficulties we have with our roles and with the content of our curricula are a result of there being more in the paradigm of rehabilitation that *conflicts* with occupational therapy than complements it.

In this article, I argue that rehabilitation is only a part of occupational therapy; that it *is an aspect but not the essence of occupational therapy,* that embracing rehabilitation in the way that we have has contributed to our identity problems; and that, although occupational therapy has enhanced the field of rehabilitation, rehabilitation has not helped the profession of occupational therapy to the same extent. I briefly review early influences on occupational therapy and reflect on some philosophical ideas about activity and occupation. I examine the role of occupational therapy as treatment both in Canada and in the United States during the first part of this century and then trace the incorporation of occupational therapy into rehabilitation. Finally, I reflect on the influence that rehabilitation has had on our core values and note recent changes that hold some promise for our future directions.

Early Influences in Occupational Therapy

Articles that describe the use of occupation to promote or restore health (e.g., Bing, 1981 [see Chapter 5]; Engelhardt, 1977; Haas, 1944; Kielhofner & Burke, 1977; Peloquin, 1991a, 1991b [see Chapter 1]) often begin with ancient Egypt and work through biblical times to Greece and Rome, where the virtues of activities and pastimes (e.g., art, music, exercise, dance) were extolled. These chronicles tend to skip several centuries to reach the Moral Treatment Era of the early 1800s, where a caring environment and the notion of work were added to activities as a means of promoting health (Bockhoven, 1972). With World War I (WWI), the arts-and-crafts movement became well established (Levine, 1987), as did curative workshops (Robinson, 1981), and occupational therapy as we know it began to unfold. No longer do we see the profession as embedded in other movements; rather, it has become a separate entity (Peloquin, 1991a, 1991b [see Chapter 1]). In the late 1930s and early 1940s, the profession began to take a biomedical turn and pretty much stayed there for the next four decades, with periodic visits back to core concepts through contributions from, among others, Reilly (1962 [see Chapter 8]), Keilhofner and Burke (1977), Fidler and Fidler (1978 [see Chapter 9]), Gilfoyle (1984), and West (1984). It is as though the core concept of occupation as a means of promoting health and well-being was somehow elusive and, in not being well enough articulated, became dissipated.

Philosophical Ideas About Activity and Occupation[1]

For all the histories of the profession that have traced the idea of occupation, very few have grappled with what it is that is so therapeutic about occupation and why its value has persisted over the centuries. Philosophical ideas have contributed to the importance we attach to the concept of activity while also fostering its elusiveness. Plato came closest to noting what we consider the inherent need for activity when he suggested that "in every man and woman there is born the instinct to make and to do" (as cited in Bruce, 1933, p. 6).[2] The implication for occupational therapy is that although injured or ill in some way, people still need to make and to do. This idea is probably the closest we come in philosophical terms to the essence of occupational therapy.

Plato also spoke about *therapeutic arts,* which could be considered to include rehabilitation, and noted their different components:

> In the state of all [such] therapeutic arts, the corrective portion is more apparent but less important, while the regulative portion is largely hidden but far more essential. [Hence] there is grave danger lest "prevention" and "maintenance," the real work of the art, be overlooked, and attention exclusively be devoted to the correction of diseases already there, a mere by-product of the art. (Wild, 1946, p. 65)

Thus, in Plato's terms, because occupational therapy's role in rehabilitation does not cure disease or remove disability (i.e., the corrective portion of therapeutic arts) but, instead, works to develop or maintain occupational performance *despite* disease or disability (i.e., the regulative and essential portion of therapeutic arts), its importance is often overlooked.

Aristotle (trans. 1925) wrote about pursuing well-being. He saw well-being of the soul *(eudaimonia)* as the end result of desirable and satisfying activity or action *(praxis).* In *The Nicomachean Ethics,* he expounded on the notion that "of all things that come to us by nature, we first acquire the potentiality and later exhibit the activity." He said that "the things we have to learn before we can do them, we learn by doing them,"

and although his comment that "states of character arise out of like activities" (p. 28) refers to how man becomes virtuous, it also reflects the notion that only by doing can one become. Adler (1991) commented on Aristotle's view that both practical thinking and productive thinking are required to carry out purposeful activity and noted that Aristotle believed that "until making and doing actually begin, productive thinking and practical thinking bear no fruit" (p. 71).

In distinguishing between basic needs and wants, Aristotle noted that everyone has the same basic needs. These "needs" (for food, for shelter, for love, etc.) were called the "external goods," and like Maslow, Aristotle said that they must be met in order to approach the fulfillment of all our human capacities. The "wants" in life can also be met as long as they do not interfere with our abilities to satisfy our needs or fulfill our capacities. Occupational therapists facilitate their patients' abilities to meet their needs and wants and recognize the necessity of enacting thinking to achieve those ends.

Aristotle also examined the meaning of happiness and the ways in which it could be achieved. For him, happiness was in and of itself an activity; more specifically, happiness existed when one was engaged in "virtuous" activity. It was Aristotle, perhaps, who started the debate on the relationship between work and leisure when he stated that "happiness is thought to depend on leisure; for we are busy that we may have leisure." His ideas about reaching a sense of self through activity that develops our capacity and makes us happy and fulfilled in the process are certainly echoed within occupational therapy (e.g., Reilly, 1962 [see Chapter 8]; Yerxa, 1993) and psychology (Csikszentmihalyi, 1991; White, 1971).

Voltaire, whose works appeared in the middle and late 1700s, also thought about the meaning of occupation. For Voltaire, activity was a means of bringing relief to much of the unhappiness that life brought: "Man is born for action...not to be occupied and not to exist amount to the same thing" (as cited in Waterman, 1942, p. 40). Thus, at the very least, to support existence, one must be occupied so as to see evidence of existing. Occupational therapists who have worked with persons who are severely depressed know the glimmer of hope that comes to one who has been occupied and has seen that something qualitatively different can be experienced that is outside of despair. Indeed, labeling such engagement as positive is a cornerstone of cognitive therapy for depression (Beck, Rush, Shaw, & Emery, 1979).

John Stuart Mill (1859/1947) wrote in *On Liberty* about the importance of encouraging and celebrating individuality in the activities that people undertake. Provided no harm was done to others, individuality could bring human beings nearer to the best thing they could be and could have a cumulative effect on the whole human race. Mill said, "In proportion to

---

[1]Philosophical discussions refer primarily to activity but seem to use the term to mean what we would call occupations (e.g., "groups of activities and tasks of everyday life" [Townsend, 1997, p. 34]).

[2]A primary source for this quote by Bruce (1933) has not been found despite an extensive search; it may not have originated with Plato.

---

the development of his individuality each person becomes more valuable to himself, and is therefore capable of being more valuable to others" (p. 63). Therapists who assume a client-centered approach to enabling occupation help their clients to develop their individuality and increase their opportunities for self-fulfillment.

Philosophical ideas about occupation seem to have centered on, at the very least, making life bearable (Voltaire); maintaining health (Plato); being responsible for happiness (Aristotle); and at the highest level, being self-actualized (Mill, 1859/1947). These ideas can readily be seen in the roots of our profession (Friedland, 1988; Peloquin, 1991a, 1991b [see Chapter 1]) where it was believed that occupation could relieve despair (e.g., of persons who were mentally ill) and could contribute to overall well-being (e.g., of soldiers during WWI). It was also thought that lack of meaningful activity could make one more ill or dysfunctional (e.g., as with persons recovering from tuberculosis) and that the right type and level of activity could bring one to a state of mastery. Johnson (1996) noted the importance of these ideas remaining central to our profession: "The greater our understanding of occupations and how they maintain, enhance, and promote health and well-being, the greater will be our ability to link this knowledge with practice and education of future therapists" (p. 393).

Occupation as Treatment: The United States and Canada (1900–1940)

In the United States, an early rationale for occupation as treatment was simply that patients did better and were less restless if they were engaged in activity. Nurse Susan Tracy started using occupations as treatment in 1905 and is credited with providing the first course in occupations in 1906 (Reed & Sanderson, 1983). Other early courses in occupational therapy were prompted by similar reasoning; for example, the course at the Chicago School of Civics and Philanthropy in 1908 was instigated by two members of the State Board of Control in protest against the idleness they saw on the wards of the state hospitals (Dunton, 1918). Indeed the formation of the National Society for the Promotion of Occupational Therapy (NSPOT) was itself prompted by George Barton's experience of being ill with tuberculosis and finding that manual activities hastened his recovery. It is interesting to note the professions of the founders of NSPOT and to consider their perspectives on occupations. For psychiatrist William Rush Dunton, architects Thomas Kidner and George Barton, social worker Eleanor Clarke Slagle, teacher Susan Johnston, secretary Isabel Newton, and nurse Susan Tracy, the key idea was that the right occupation could help persons in need (Peloquin, 1991b [see Chapter 1]). Although they spoke of occupation as curative, it was not in relation to medical or psychiatric conditions but rather to the human condition, to harnessing occupation for what Hall called one of the "sources of human power" (as cited in Peloquin, 1991b, p. 739 [see

Chapter 1]). Schwartz (1992) emphasized the similarities between Dewey's ideas on the importance of occupations in education and occupational therapy's use of occupations to facilitate healthy development in patients. Similarly, Schemm (1994) noted that the arts-and-crafts movement, which greatly influenced early practice in occupational therapy, saw activity as a means of improving society; it was a way "to socialize less accepted members of society such as disabled, mentally ill, impoverished, and underachieving persons in insane asylums and manual training programs" (p. 1083).

Although Adolph Meyer was not considered an official founder of occupational therapy, his influence in psychiatric circles of the day meant that his ideas on the importance of occupation carried considerable weight. Meyer (1922/1977) (see Chapter 2) promoted the value of occupation, including work-like activities, and his words on the subject have become very familiar to occupational therapists: "The proper use of time in some helpful and gratifying activity appeared [to me] a fundamental issue in the treatment of any neuropsychiatric patient" (p. 639). Meyer stressed the need for "giving opportunities rather than prescriptions... opportunities to work, opportunities to do and to plan and create, and to learn to use material" (p. 641).

In Canada at the turn of the century, C. K. Clarke was prominent among those advocating occupation in the Ontario Hospitals for the Insane. Clarke, who was a noted psychiatrist, wrote of his experiences at the Rockwood Asylum in Kingston, Ontario, where he incorporated a wide range of activities (e.g., painting, carpentry, music, work, sports) into the daily regime. At that time, there was great concern over the need to restrain patients. Clarke noted that nonrestraint had become an established practice at Rockwood, and he (like Meyer) credited this fact to the use of occupation. Clarke (1922) stated:

> No one comforted himself with the belief that occupation was a panacea for all the ills that the mind is heir to, but we did realize that intelligently supervised occupation was a tremendous factor not only in aiding cure in recent cases, but in making happy and improving the most unfortunate class in our community. (p. 13)

In 1918, the University of Toronto offered the first course in occupations in Canada (Robinson, 1981). These short courses were established in the faculty of applied science at the request of Herbert Haultain, a professor of engineering, and Norman Burnette, the head of a workshop at a military hospital. Both men saw the need for occupations for soldiers who, on returning from WWI, were confined to bed. Professor C. H. C. Wright of the department of architecture was in charge, and Winifred Brainerd, an American occupational therapist, was brought from New York to teach. Kidner, the Canadian architect who had also been a founder of NSPOT, was then vocational secretary of the Canadian Military Hospitals Commission, and he helped to organize the venture. Within the year, some 350 women had graduated from one of these short courses, and most of them went on to work with soldiers returning from the war (Robinson, 1981).

C. B. Farrar (1940b), a noted psychiatrist who was later to become the first superintendent of the Toronto Psychiatric Hospital, wrote about occupation as treatment for war neuroses and psychoses during WWI. He stated that "congenital and systematic occupation should be given foremost place in any scheme of treatment. Idleness… should be reduced to the uttermost minimum" (p. 16). He elaborated on this idea, noting that:

> there is the benefit of occupation as such, common to practically all cases; and there is the possible benefit of an awakened and sustained interest in an employment which is new, and which affords a pleasing relief from a former distasteful or humdrum occupation. Here we have occupation-therapy passing over into vocational re-training, with the latter perhaps completing the cure begun by the former. (Farrar, 1940a, p. 23)

At Government House in Ottawa in 1925, Farrar was among those who spoke at an open meeting of the newly formed Ontario Society of Occupational Therapists. A prominent newspaper of the time reported his comments as follows:

> Next to proper housing and proper feeding, occupational therapy is the most important factor in the cure of nervous patients. The rest cure, so long ordered for these patients, has been supplanted by work, and occupational therapy provides this most necessary employment and effects the cure. ("Is Practical Christianity," 1925)

This link between occupations and work had been important since the Moral Treatment Era and has continued throughout our history.

In summary, the main focus of occupational therapy in the early part of the century, both in the United States and in Canada, was on the person and on the activity. The approach did not address pathology, which at the time was primarily mental illness; rather, it focused on interests and abilities and worked around the pathology to engage the person in occupations. It was engagement in occupation that could have an effect on the person and could, over time, be transformative. Engagement in occupation was made possible by the therapist's knowledge and understanding of the patient's condition and came from within the therapeutic relationship that had been established. As the profession continued to develop, occupational therapists began to work with persons with physical disabilities, for example, those who were injured in industrial accidents. The goal of therapy was to return them to productive lives, economic independence, and social usefulness (Ambrosi & Schwartz, 1995a). By the early 1920s, curative workshops were established in both the United States (Baldwin, 1919) and Canada (LeVesconte, 1935) where work-like activities were designed to prepare patients for employment.

The largest population of persons with physical injuries had been the soldiers returning from WWI, and, with them, began a gradual shift in occupational therapy toward a focus on medical outcomes and away from earlier humanitarian and social benefits (Ambrosi & Schwartz, 1995b). During this early period, different philosophies of occupational therapy for persons with physical disabilities began to be seen. In the United States, Wilson H. Henderson was one of the first physicians to apply occupational therapy to physical disabilities. He thought that occupational therapy for men with war-time injuries should require technical rather than physical strength, more mental than physical activity, and enough general exercise to stimulate recovery (Reed & Sanderson, 1983). Referring to Canadian war-time experience, Goldwin Howland (1944/1986), physician and first president of the Canadian Association of Occupational Therapists, delineated five forms of occupational therapy: diversional, physical, recreational, psychological, and preventive. All but the second of these (physical) were directed at maintaining interest and morale.

Graded activity, which had been widely used with patients with tuberculosis in both countries to improve overall physical endurance and maintain morale, soon became more focused and was directed to improving range of motion and strengthening muscle groups (Creigton, 1993). The psychologist Baldwin tried to use both a holistic approach and the scientific method in designing activities for WWI veterans attending his occupational therapy department at Walter Reed Hospital (Wish-Baratz, 1989). He stated that the purpose of occupational therapy was to "help each patient find himself and function again as a complete man, physically, socially, educationally and economically" (Baldwin, 1919, p. 447). However, the means of achieving that purpose was through remedial exercises that required "a series of specific voluntary movements involved in the ordinary trades or occupations, physical training, play, or the daily routine activities of life" (p. 448). By the 1940s, Sidney Licht, a physician and editor of the journal *Occupational Therapy and Rehabilitation* was promoting "kinetic" and "metric" occupational therapy (i.e., muscle strengthening, joint mobilization, coordination training) and increasing the amount of work completed in a unit of time or the number of times an activity was completed in a calendar unit (Reed & Sanderson, 1983).

Occupational Therapy and Rehabilitation

By 1937, occupational therapy practice patterns, as reported by the American Medical Association (AMA), which registered all American occupational therapists at that time, showed that 36 occupational therapists worked in orthopedics, 456 in general hospitals, and 1,809 in mental hospitals (Reed & Sanderson, 1983). These numbers reflect the state of health care at the time, that is, the high numbers of persons with mental illness who were institutionalized and the fact that people were not surviving the serious illnesses and injuries that were later to be seen with the development of modern medicine. However, the numbers also reflect the fact that the profession was still strongly focused in mental health.

It was not until after WWII that the shift in focus for occupational therapy from occupation as a means of developing or maintaining health to occupation as a means of enhancing medical outcomes became firmly established. The change came with the development of the new specialty of "physical therapy physicians" and the subsequent development of departments of physical medicine and rehabilitation. This medical specialty area, which had been developing since the turn of the century, had been based primarily on an interest in the use of "medical electricity," later called electrotherapy (Gritzer & Arluke, 1985).

Rusk, who was a major figure in the development of this new medical specialty, recalled that he had created programs in air force hospitals for making good use of convalescent time. He said that "gradually, the concept of rehabilitation came to me as I found out how much really could be done for these men" (as cited in Gritzer & Arluke, 1985, p. 91). After several years of battling with the AMA, orthopedic surgeons, the Department of Veterans Affairs, and the Office of Vocational Rehabilitation, physical therapy physicians were finally allowed to call themselves physiatrists and to call their field physical medicine and rehabilitation. One of their early acts was to bring physical therapy and occupational therapy training programs, such as those at Columbia University and the University of Illinois, under their authority (Gritzer & Arluke, 1985). At the University of Toronto, a department of physical medicine and rehabilitation was created in 1950 that actually combined the educational programs for physical therapists and occupational therapists into one and brought the new program, for "P&OTs," under the control of physiatry. During this same period, many hospitals in the United States and Canada developed departments of physical medicine and rehabilitation. As Brintnell, Cardwell, Robinson, and Madill (1986) pointed out, "The development of physical medicine was to influence the services provided by occupational therapy for years to come" (p. 27). (See also Colman [1992] for a description of occupational therapy's struggle to maintain its roots and autonomy as physical therapists and physiatrists came to dominate the field.)

In his chapter on the role of occupational therapy in rehabilitation, Rusk (1958) had delineated three areas of therapy: supportive (psychologic), prevocational (vocational), and functional (physical). Supportive therapy was intended to maintain morale by helping the patient to realize his or her abilities and was to be closely coordinated with the psychiatrist and psychologist. Prevocational therapy was designed to assess and train the patient in preparation for a return to work and was to be a joint effort with the vocational counselor. The functional component of occupational therapy was directed to exercise in which the patient used his or her disabled part in the course of some constructive procedure,

such as woodworking. Principles of therapeutic exercise were followed, starting with active-assistive exercises for those muscles that had a muscle-testing grade of poor plus or better and working toward active and active-resistive activities. For Rusk, the activity had become the means, and improving joint range, muscle strength, and motor skill the end. Brintnell et al. (1986) summed up the period during which these practices were followed in Canada, stating that "the fifties and sixties saw the emergence of the rehabilitation movement and with it, mixed blessings for occupational therapy. The physical aspects of treatment gained prominence over psychological concerns" (p. 33).

Gradually, the role of occupation as central to maintaining health and well-being began to erode. The pressure for occupational therapists to be a part of rehabilitation as it was conceived and practiced was too hard to resist. To modify the concept and practice of rehabilitation to better suit occupational therapy was too difficult, given the small size of the profession and its perceived lack of power and credibility (Froehlich, 1992). Equally important was the fact that *rehabilitation* was a glamorous term. The medical model, complete with its uniforms and jargon, gave occupational therapists what was considered a loftier status. Rehabilitation was more respected and better understood than occupational therapy, and it caught the public eye. Persons with physical disabilities had the public's sympathy (certainly more so than persons who were mentally ill), and if we were helping them in such obvious and concrete ways as getting stronger, moving faster, or gaining a fuller range of motion, well, then we must be good too.

Another pressure away from the meaning and value attributed to occupation came in work with children with cerebral palsy and persons with polio. During this period, occupational therapists became fixated on the value of independence (Froehlich, 1992) and worked with their patients to achieve it despite the time away from occupations that might have been more meaningful, such as being a student. The focus on dressing as an end in and of itself rather than as the means to an end continues to this day in many settings. Of course, there were exceptions, and many facilities still engaged their patients in occupations. One interesting example of where meaningful activity continued to be important was in the craft work that occupational therapists did with Native North American populations with tuberculosis (Staples & McConnell, 1993).

So for many years we have devoted a large part of our energies to fitting in with the medical model, where occupational therapists were never intended to be (West, 1984). As occupational therapists continued to compete in the reductionist environment of medicine, we found that our qualifications were generally not as good as others who could fix broken parts. And although *no one else* could do what we did, no one, including ourselves, seemed to value that. No one, including ourselves, seemed to notice that we had abdicated our role in developing and maintaining health and well-being through occupation in order to join the ranks of the reductionists. Meanwhile, physical therapists, who most of us would agree are the better "fixers," grew in number and stature so that, today, in North America, there are twice as many physical therapists as occupational therapists. Some would support Yerxa (1992) in saying that in our efforts to align ourselves more closely with medical values and medical thinking, we have become more like physical therapy in the role we play in rehabilitation. It is ironic that we should be competing with physical therapists when, on the basis of the backgrounds of those who created our profession, one would have predicted that we would be competing with nurses, engineers, architects, social workers, or teachers.

Newer Models of Rehabilitation

Over the years since Rusk's initial description of rehabilitation, the concept of rehabilitation has broadened, and its definition is now somewhat more in tune with the foundations of occupational therapy. Instead of focusing only on restoring function, the field now recognizes other important outcomes. For example, the World Health Organization's 1981 definition stated that:

> rehabilitation includes all measures aimed at reducing the impact of disabling and handicapping conditions, and at enabling the disabled and handicapped to achieve social integration. Rehabilitation aims not only at training disabled and handicapped persons to adapt to their environment, but also intervening in the immediate environment and society as a whole in order to facilitate their social integration. (p. 9)

Such a definition recognized the end result of social integration, a broad category that could be considered to subsume occupations. It sharpened the focus of rehabilitation on reducing the impact of disability and handicap, thus opening the door to interventions in the environment.

More recently, the *Research Plan for the National Center for Medical Rehabilitation Research* (U.S. Department of Health and Human Services, 1993) has suggested that "the successful process of rehabilitation restores the individual to maximal functioning *and provides a foundation for a fulfilling, productive life following rehabilitation* [italics added]" (p. 29). Note that the definition is still tied to function, and rehabilitation needs only to provide the foundation for a fulfilling, productive life. It is as though somehow after rehabilitation these attributes of life will magically occur. However, the document further stated:

> Activities which enhance productivity and give a sense of purpose and enjoyment to life must be possible; these may include employment, education, recreation, family, and community involvement. This participation should provide meaning and dignity to life so that people with disability have a reason to live, not merely to exist. (p. 29)

So perhaps at last, we are beginning to see some of our occupational therapy values coming to the forefront in rehabilitation and that the field is richer for the role that we can play. Moreover, in this role, we can use our understanding of medical thinking without adopting the medical paradigm (Yerxa, 1992). And from a pragmatic point of view, if "social integration and fulfillment" become outcome measures in rehabilitation—as indeed they should—then our special skills and core values could become very important in this era of evidence-based practice. But how do we go from the *ifs, shoulds,* and *coulds* to the (re)enactment of our core values?

Friedson (1994) suggested that:

> the competition between professions for jurisdiction over a particular area may be analyzed as conflicting definitions of the *nature of the problem or activity* [italics added] each is seeking to control, and claims about the way they can best be solved or carried out. (p. 70)

Rusk and the founders of rehabilitation thought that the very nature of the problem was the disability itself, and in practice, they focused their efforts on restoring function to the person with the disability where our role was helpful, though limited. The founders of occupational therapy incorporated philosophical views about the importance of activity and determined that the very nature of the problem was a person's intrinsic need for occupation that was thwarted by illness or disability. Social integration, productivity, meaning, and dignity in life are outcomes of rehabilitation that are consonant with the core values of occupational therapy. Knowing how to enable persons with disabilities to achieve these outcomes is the special knowledge and skill that, in sociological terms, make occupational therapy a profession (Friedson, 1994).

Future Directions

Our profession has its own view of what the issue in rehabilitation is and how it is solvable; that is, we have our own paradigm within which to operate. Both in the United States and in Canada, there appears to be a growing consensus in occupational therapy that a return to our core values is needed (e.g., Kielhofner & Burke, 1977; Polatajko, 1992; Townsend, 1997; West, 1984; Yerxa, 1992). As a profession, occupational therapy must now be prepared to champion that cause and to advance its aims.

However, there is a deep concern that as a profession we may not be up to the task. In 1966, Thelma Cardwell, the first occupational therapist to hold the position of president of the Canadian Association of Occupational Therapists (which since its inception in 1926 had a male physician as president) stated:

> We are too diffident a group, both individually and collectively. We are much too timid in bringing our work to the attention of others. In short, we are ineffective in selling our profession. It is time we learned to be vocal, to be enthusi-

astic, to be competent, in representing the professional point of view of our discipline and in interpreting our aims and functions. These, with an added degree of confidence, can do an immeasurable amount in establishing the personal and professional reputation and respect that our profession warrants. (Cardwell, 1966, p. 139)

Others have made this plea before (Reilly, 1962 [see Chapter 8]) and since (Johnson, 1996). We know what to do; the question is will we do it? Will we undertake the research needed to study occupation and expand our understanding of the concept? Will we develop a core body of knowledge regarding occupation? Will we redesign our curricula to reflect our focus on the centrality of occupation? Will we demand the liberal arts background for entry to our programs that this focus requires? Will we instill confidence in our students about the value of our focus, and can we establish the competence to underpin that confidence? Finally, can we move on from the education of our students to the reeducation of practicing therapists who for too long have supported narrow views of our role in rehabilitation? Only then will we have a strong enough voice to undertake the social and political activity that is required. For as Friedson (1994) noted:

> The maintenance and improvement of the profession's position in the market-place, and in the division of labour surrounding it, requires continuous political activity. The profession must become an interest group to at once advance its aims and to protect itself from those with competing aims. (p. 68)

Conclusion

We are the only health profession that can focus on occupation; others can focus on function but not on occupation. As philosophers noted centuries ago, activity is what defines the lives of human beings. With illness or disability, this route to meaning is often threatened. It is the mission of occupational therapists, alone among health professionals, to keep that route open. When we define ourselves exclusively as "rehab professionals"—even with the most modern of definitions— we limit our ability to make that unique contribution.

There is clearly a common denominator, a unifying theme, in all that we do, and as has been said in many different ways, occupation is it. Occupation is what explains the "jack of all trades" epithet that makes us so uncomfortable. It is why we can help persons with all kinds of disabilities and at all ages. In occupation, we have had, and do have, a unique and powerful tool not to cure, but to positively influence health and well-being. However, we must get on with it and not continue to be lured away. For to paraphrase that great contemporary philosopher Will Rogers, we may be on the right track, but if we just sit on it, we will be run over by the train.

Acknowledgments

This article was originally prepared for the 1995 spring institute at the Department of Occupational Therapy, Dalhousie University, Nova Scotia, Canada. I thank the faculty members for inviting me to speak and the participants for their stimulating discussion. I also thank two students: Joanne Brady, whose final year major paper in this area added further insight, and Mary Liang, who assisted in the preparation of the final manuscript.

References

Adler, M. (1991). *Aristotle for everybody.* New York: Collier.

Ambrosi, E., & Schwartz, K. B. (1995a). Looking Back—The profession's image, 1917–1925, part 1: Occupational therapy as represented in the media. *American Journal of Occupational Therapy, 49,* 715–719.

Ambrosi, E., & Schwartz, K. B. (1995b). Looking Back—The profession's image, 1917–1925, part 2: Occupational therapy as represented by the profession. *American Journal of Occupational Therapy, 49,* 828–832.

Aristotle. (trans. 1925). *The Nicomachean ethics.* Oxford, U.K.: Oxford University Press.

Baldwin, B. T. (1919). Occupational therapy. *American Journal of Care for Cripples, 8,* 447–451.

Beck, A. T., Rush, J., Shaw, B., & Emery, G. (1979). *Cognitive therapy of depression.* New York: Guilford.

Bing, R. K. (1981). Occupational therapy revisited: A paraphrastic journey, 1981 Eleanor Clarke Slagle lecture. American Journal of *Occupational Therapy, 35,* 499–518. Reprinted as Chapter 5

Bockhoven, J. S. (1972) *Moral treatment in community mental health.* New York: Springer.

Brintnell, S., Cardwell, T., Robinson, I., & Madill, H. (1986). The fifties and sixties: The rehabilitation era: Friend or foe. *Canadian Journal of Occupational Therapy, 53,* 27–33.

Bruce, H. (1933). An address. Third Annual Convention of the Canadian and Ontario Occupational Therapy Associations. *Canadian Journal of Occupational Therapy, 2,* 6–9.

Cardwell, T. (1966). President's address. *Canadian Journal of Occupational Therapy, 33,* 139–140.

Clarke, C. K. (1922). *Statement of Dr. C. K. Clarke re: occupational therapy in Ontario Hospitals for the Insane.* Unpublished manuscript.

Colman, W. (1992). Maintaining autonomy: The struggle between occupational therapy and physical medicine. *American Journal of Occupational Therapy, 46,* 63–70.

Creighton, C. (1993). Looking Back—Graded activity: Legacy of the sanatorium. *American Journal of Occupational Therapy, 47,* 745–748.

Csikszentmihalyi, M. (1991). *The psychology of optimal experience.* New York: Harper & Row.

Dunton, W. R. (1918). *Occupation therapy: A manual for nurses.* Philadelphia: Saunders.

Engelhardt, H. T., Jr. (1977). Defining occupational therapy: The meaning of therapy and the virtues of occupation. *American Journal of Occupational Therapy, 31,* 666–672.

Farrar, C. B. (1940a). Rehabilitation in nervous and mental cases among ex-soldiers. *Canadian Journal of Occupational Therapy, 7,* 17–25.

Farrar, C. B. (1940b). War neuroses and psychoses. *Canadian Journal of Occupational Therapy, 7,* 5–16.

Fidler, G. S., & Fidler, J. W. (1978). Doing and becoming: Purposeful action and self-actualization. *American Journal of Occupational Therapy, 32,* 305–310. Reprinted as Chapter 9.

Friedland, J. (1988). The Issue Is—Diversional activity: Does it deserve its bad name? *American Journal of Occupational Therapy, 42,* 603–608.

Friedson, E. (1994). Professions and the occupational principle. In E. Friedson (Ed.), *Professionalism reborn: Theory, prophecy, and policy* (pp. 61–74). Chicago: University of Chicago Press.

Froehlich, J. (1992). The Issue Is—Proud and visible as occupational therapists. *American Journal of Occupational Therapy, 46,* 1042–1044.

Gilfoyle, E. M. (1984). The transformation of a profession, 1984 Eleanor Clarke Slagle lecture. *American Journal of Occupational Therapy, 38,* 575–584.

Gritzer, G., & Arluke, A. (1985). *The making of rehabilitation: A political economy of medical specialization, 1890–1980.* Berkeley: University of California Press.

Haas, L. J. (1944). *Practical occupational therapy.* Milwaukee, WI: Bruce.

Howland, G. (1986). Occupational therapy across Canada. *Canadian Journal of Occupational Therapy, 53,* 18–26. Original work published 1944.

"Is Practical Christianity" Occupational Therapy Praised. (1925, May 1) *The Evening Telegram* (Toronto), p. 14.

Johnson, J. (1996). Occupational science and occupational therapy: An emphasis in meaning. In R. Zemke & F. Clark (Eds.), *Occupational science: The evolving discipline* (pp. 393–397). Philadelphia: F. A. Davis.

Kielhofner, G., & Burke, J. P. (1977). Occupational therapy after 60 years: An account of changing identity and knowledge. *American Journal of Occupational Therapy, 31,* 675–689.

LeVesconte, H. (1935). Expanding fields of occupational therapy. *Canadian Journal of Occupational Therapy, 3,* 4–12.

Levine, R. E. (1987). Looking Back—The influence of the arts-and-crafts movement on the professional status of occupational therapy. *American Journal of Occupational Therapy, 41,* 248–254. Reprinted as Chapter 3.

Meyer, A. (1977). The philosophy of occupation therapy. *American Journal of Occupational Therapy, 31,* 639–642. Original work published 1922. Reprinted as Chapter 2.

Mill, J S. (1947). *On liberty.* New York: Appleton-Century Crofts. Original work published 1859.

Peloquin, S. M. (1991a). Looking Back—Occupational therapy service: Individual and collective understandings of the founders, part 1. *American Journal of Occupational Therapy, 45,* 352–360. Reprinted as Chapter 1.

Peloquin, S. M. (1991b). Looking Back—Occupational therapy service: Individual and collective understandings of the founders, part 2. *American Journal of Occupational Therapy, 45,* 733–744. Reprinted as Chapter 1.

Polatajko, H. (1992). Naming and framing occupational therapy: A lecture dedicated to the life of Nancy B. *Canadian Journal of Occupational Therapy, 59,* 189–199.

Reed, K., & Sanderson, S. (1983). *Concepts of occupational therapy.* Baltimore: Williams & Wilkins.

Reilly, M. (1962). Occupational therapy can be one of the great ideas of 20th-century medicine, 1961 Eleanor Clarke Slagle lecture. *American Journal of Occupational Therapy, 16,* 1–9. Reprinted as Chapter 8.

Robinson, I. (1981). The mists of time, 1981 Muriel Driver memorial lecture. *Canadian Journal of Occupational Therapy, 48,* 145–152.

Rusk, H. (1958). *Rehabilitation medicine: A textbook on physical medicine and rehabilitation.* St. Louis, MO: Mosby.

Schemm, R. L. (1994). Bridging conflicting ideologies: The origins of American and British occupational therapy. *American Journal of Occupational Therapy, 48,* 1082–1088.

Schwartz, K. (1992). Looking Back—Occupational therapy and education: A shared vision. *American Journal of Occupational Therapy, 46,* 12–18.

Staples, A. R., & McConnell, R. L. (1993). *Soapstone and seed beads: Arts and crafts at the Charles Camswell Hospital, a tuberculosis sanatorium* (Special publications no. 7). Alberta: Provincial Museum of Alberta.

Townsend, E. (Ed.). (1997). *Enabling occupation: An occupational therapy perspective.* Ottawa, Ontario: CAOT Publications ACE.

U.S. Department of Health and Human Services. (1993). *Research plan for the National Center for Medical Rehabilitation Research* (NIH Publication No. 93-3509). Washington, DC: Author.

Waterman, M. (1942). *Voltaire, Pascal, and human destiny.* New York: King's Crown Press.

West, W. L. (1984). A reaffirmed philosophy and practice of occupational therapy for the 1980s. *American Journal of Occupational Therapy, 38,* 15–23.

White, R. W. (1971). The urge toward competence. *American Journal of Occupational Therapy, 25,* 271–274.

Wild, J. (1946). *Plato theory of man.* New York: Octagon.

Wish-Baratz, S. (1989). Looking Back—Bird T. Baldwin: A holistic scientist in occupational therapy's history. *American Journal of Occupational Therapy, 43,* 257–260.

World Health Organization. (1981). *Disability, prevention, and rehabilitation* (Technical report series 668). Geneva, Switzerland: Author.

Yerxa, E. J. (1992). Some implications of occupational therapy's history for its epistemology, values, and relation to medicine. *American Journal of Occupational Therapy, 46,* 79–83.

Yerxa, E. J. (1993). Occupational science: A new source of power for participants in occupational therapy. *Occupational Science, 1,* 3–10.

CHAPTER 8

Occupational Therapy Can Be One of the Great Ideas of 20th-Century Medicine

1962 Eleanor Clarke Slagle Lecture

MARY REILLY, EdD, OTR

Specifying the Theme

As an occupational therapist honored by her peers, I join my Eleanor Clarke Slagle predecessors in feeling the awesome responsibility of the award. The occasion, it seems to me, makes it obligatory for an awardee to objectify a lifetime experience and then speak of an issue of concern to all. With this in mind, I have elected to present an issue which impinges upon the very root meaning of our existence. In developing the idea, I have sought to reflect it against the changing background of the world in which we live. My hope is that its exploration will add to an understanding of the profession which we practice.

o Fundamentals of Neuro, etc. should be involved.

o Man, through the use of his hands as they R energized through mind + will, can influence the state of his own health.

o 2° principle – To grow + be productive. – what about alz. pts.? – TBI pts.?

o Active in environment.

The question I would like to speak to is one which each one of us has asked at some time or other in our professional lives. Some of us have asked it many times. It has been raised in different ways and expressed in different words, both within and outside our field. In all probability, it will continue to be asked by those who follow us. I am referring to an anxiety about our value as a service to sick people. This theme I have identified by the question, *Is occupational therapy a sufficiently vital and unique service for medicine to support and society to reward?*

The anxiety begins in a primitive form when we stand before our first patient and sense the enormous demands that a treatment problem makes upon the occupational therapy brush, hammer, or needle. The wide and gaping chasm which exists between the complexity of illness and the commonplaceness of our treatment tools is, and always will be, both the pride and the anguish of our profession. Anxiety accumulates as we become increasingly involved in treatment, teaching, and research, and even more sophisticated questions tend to arise from that same source to plague us.

The theme of today's presentation is focused, therefore, on the critical appraisal of the essential worth of occupational therapy. I say critical because the technique of criticism will be the method by which the issue will be explored. The subject was selected because I found from my experience that the value of occupational therapy exists in a controversial state. Among any group of my colleagues who have practiced long and well, I found that this question of value constituted a continuous and almost lifelong dialogue.

The Theme Converted to a Hypothesis Test

Where and how does one begin to make dependable and hence usable judgments about value? Taking full advantage of the freedom inherent in the Slagle lectureship, I reasoned that the idea most basic to our practice ought to be searched out and then converted into a kind of a question which might be answerable to some degree. This search, I further reasoned, should begin in the time of our earliest days. I began there and found that there was a single root idea embedded deep in our foundation and this deeply imbedded belief is what we call occupational therapy. In the stormy years between then and now, I found that there were few opportunities given to examine the roots of our foundation and to consider the growth which sprang from it.

My re-examination of our early history revealed that our profession emerged from a common belief held by a small

This chapter was previously published in the *American Journal of Occupational Therapy, 16,* 2–9.

group of people. This common belief is the hypothesis upon which our profession was founded. It was, and indeed still is, one of the truly great and even magnificent hypotheses of medicine today. I have dared to state this hypothesis as: *That man, through the use of his hands as they are energized by mind and will, can influence the state of his own health.* This is the inherited occupational therapy hypothesis passed on for proof by the early founders.

The splendor of its vision goes far beyond rating it as an idea conceived once in a lifetime or even once in a century. Rather, it falls in the class of one of those great beliefs which has advanced civilization. Its magnificence lies in the optimistic vote of confidence it gives to human nature. It implies that there is a reservoir of sensitivity and skill in the hands of man which can be tapped for his health. It implies the rich adaptability and durability of the central nervous system which can be influenced by experiences. And more than all this, it implies that man, through the use of his hands, can creatively deploy his thinking, feelings, and purposes to make himself at home in the world and to make the world his home.

For a profession organized around this hypothesis it sets few limits to its growth. It merely endows a group with the obligation to acquire reliable knowledge leading to a competency to serve the belief. Because this is a hypothesis about health, it requires that this knowledge be made available for the guidance of physicians and that it be made applicable to a wide range of medical problems.

The Role of Criticism

Before preparing a brief for its validation I would like to make a detour into a description of the method whereby the issue will be explored. The method is in harmony with my temperament because, by choice, I am neither a conservative nor am I a conformist. I am a devout and practicing, card-carrying critic. Because criticism as a technique of public discussion has yet to emerge in our association affairs, I feel a need to define and describe it. Its philosophy, techniques, and tactics will constitute the point of view from which I will speak.

The public use of criticism by a profession has been spelled out best by Merton[1] who sees it as a prevailing spirit within a group necessary to maintain a group's progress. Its greatest usefulness is that it acts to repudiate a smugness which assures that everything possible has already been attained. Its presence commits an association to keeping its members from resting easily on their oars when they are so inclined. In general, Merton finds that criticism stings a profession into a new and more demanding formulation of purpose and maintains a policy position of divine discontent with the state of affairs as they are.

A disciplined person in either the sciences or the professions uses critical thinking as a personal tool of reality testing and problem solving. When a professional organization as a whole accepts criticism as the dominating mode of thought,

then indeed, theorizing flourishes and the intellectual atmosphere of their gatherings is characterized by sweeping controversies. In this atmosphere of controversy, progress becomes somewhat assured.

But a card-carrying critic must do more than merely engage in critical thinking. Judgments made by a critic must emerge from a discreet use of techniques which are difficult to master and dangerous to apply. Basically, the skill is dependent upon an ability to analyze, interpret, and synthesize. A critic must have a sharply developed capacity to see deficiencies in data and fallacies in interpretation. The best stock in trade that any critic has is a discerning eye for trends and an ability to pattern and verbalize them. Whether a critic is worth listening to is usually decided by an ability to use language well, by a creativeness in synthesizing new relations, and by courage to propose provocative hypotheses. Ultimately, however, a good critic rests his case upon how well he has been able to restructure the issue so that the necessary powers for its resolution can be freed. These idealistic but difficult standards are the ones I hope to follow in restructuring the issue of how valuable is occupational therapy.

Design of the Presentation

Having discussed the point of view from which I will speak, it is now necessary to describe the plan of attack which will be made on this global theme. For the sake of this presentation let us suppose that the hypothesis I have proposed is the wellspring of our profession and that it is worth proving. It would not follow necessarily from this that it is provable. A large part of the power to act on the hypothesis, of course, resides with us, the members of the American Occupational Therapy Association. But the society in which our profession lives holds power too and can rule on its growth. Even before we begin the validation, we must look at the probability that this idea may not be capable of proof in this century. I plan to ask first whether the American culture can tolerate such a hypothesis. Next I shall question whether the 20th century is the right time for the test. The most crucial aspect of the presentation will be an attempt to identify the point at which the process of proof ought to begin. This will be followed by an attempt to identify the basic pattern of our service by which the hypothesis will be proven. Finally, I shall comment on some ongoing crises which the hypothesis is undergoing and then leave for history its continuing proof.

Is America the Place to Test the Hypothesis?

Let us first consider the tolerance in America for the occupational therapy idea. In his social history, Max Lerner[2] identified certain dynamic forces which impelled the greatness of this country. He cited in the American mind two crucial images present since the beginning. One was the self-reliant craftsman, whether pioneer, farmer, or mechanic. He was the man who could make something of the American resources, apply his strength and skill to nature's abundance, fashion new tools and machines, imagine and carry through new constructions. Without taking himself over-seriously, Max Lerner's American has generally regarded the great engineering, business, government, and medical tasks as jobs to be done. Progress in technology was seen simply as agenda for the craftsman.

The second image Lerner drew was from the American environment. It was that of a vast continent on earth, as in space, waiting to be discovered, explored, cleared, built-up, populated, and energized. Lerner contends that our culture is dominated by an American spirit which hates to be confined. A drive toward action, he postulated, is a part of the American character.

This drive toward action seems to me to make reasonable the American idea of a patient. Our cultural concept of the man of action suffers little change when an American moves into a hospital community. It has been supported by a series of principles which merged and fused into what we now call rehabilitation. Early in this century, there emerged the principle in medical management that patients were easier to handle when they were occupied with mild tasks. Later when it was found that an active patient tended to recover faster, early ambulation became an acceptable principle of physiology and blended well with the principal of patient occupation. Concern for the psychological nature of patients brought forth the widespread acceptance of craft, recreation, and work programs in hospitals. The need to train patients in self-care became almost a crusade to ensure the rights of patients to be independent. Within the community, laymen cooperated in ventures to assure the handicapped's right to return to work. Now we are implementing in full swing the socioeconomic principle that it is good business for society to support such programs with public monies.

There are some obvious things which can be concluded about America's tolerance for the occupational therapy hypothesis. It would seem almost axiomatic that the American society in general, and medicine in particular, has need of a profession which has as its unique concern the nurturing of the spirit in man for action. In every way it knows how, America has said that this spirit must be served and served in a special kind of way when it has been blocked by physical or emotional ills. That this need will be persistent in American culture seems fairly certain. That occupational therapy will persist is not quite so certain. It is true, however, that if we fail to serve society's need for action, we will most assuredly die out as a health profession. It is also most assuredly true that if we did dissolve from the scene, in a decade or so, another group similarly purposed and similarly organized and prepared would have to be invented. I believe, therefore, that the occupational therapy hypothesis is a natural one to be advanced in America.

Is the 20th Century the Time?

The timeliness of the hypothesis is the next question I should like to raise. Are we the people and these the times for the test? We are all deeply entangled in the forces and events of the century in which we live. But if this entanglement commits our energies to the endless treadmill of survival, then the hypothesis cannot get off the ground. The social scientists tell us that the world we live in is in a state of indigestion from too much change. We have yet to absorb the disorganizations brought on by a depression, two wars, and an ongoing massive technological revolution. This change is being reflected by society into all its component institutions. It follows naturally that we feel its reflection in our professional lives.

But our state of turmoil was not always so, because occupational therapy was born in the quieter times of this century. In the first several decades of our existence, medicine offered us a tranquil and supportive setting. Our literature reveals that physicians tended to nurture the development of our schools and clinics. In these earlier times we were helped to meet the challenges of contributing to the ongoing medical scene. The last several decades, however, have put excessive stress for expansion upon a profession whose role had been barely defined. We have seen our practice organized into specialty fields by the demands of World War II. Our clinicians have only recently been systematized into team behavior by the pressures of rehabilitation. Now in the 60s we are confessing to a mounting sense of confusion and voicing a need for direction. We are keenly aware of the conflicting demands being made upon our practice. The problems that our schools face in digesting the accumulating technical knowledge which practice demands is a matter of growing distress. Caught up in these forces, how free can we be to control our growth?

If we are anxious today, the social scientist offers the explanation that it is because we are now aware that the hopes we had cultivated in gentler times of the past are being threatened by the pace of the world around us. Historians, however, are quick to counter that when times of great change appear, they are forecasting a death to the old and a birth to a new way of life. It is inconceivable that we or any other group with organized intelligence would stand idly by and permit the random destruction of the old and encourage blind birth to the new. Fortunately, most institutions have centralized their action for controlling change through planning groups variously called the Task Force, Master Plan Committee, or the Role Definition Study. Our national association has not remained aloof from such efforts and is currently involved in three change-controlling studies. As many of us know well, the studies involve professional curriculum and clinical practice, the functions of the organization, and the future development of the profession.

We may conclude that we have shown by our action that we have felt the buffeting of great change and are attempting to control it. But how can we know whether the efforts we are making are sufficient and are of the right kind? This difficult question has some partial answers. One common sense answer is that we must recognize the fact that we have grown and have changed as we grew. In our 40 years of existence our sense of purpose, our anchorage points have shifted. It is only logical to reason that we will not rediscover a sense of purpose by merely reflecting within our professions the problems of the larger society in which we exist. Few rewards are granted to those who are content to reflect on problems. Society demands that its problems be answered. Therefore, to any group which aspires to be a profession, there is placed before it a clear-cut mandate. This mandate says that if we wish to exist as a profession we must identify the vital need of man which we serve and the manner in which we serve it.

I contend that this is the point at which the proof of the occupational therapy hypothesis begins. The reality of our profession depends upon an identification of the vital need of mankind that we serve. How free we are in these troubled times to reconstruct our thinking at this basic level I do not know. But I do know that the crucial nature of our service cannot be spelled out in the loosely constructed way that it is today. I personally have little trust that we can continue to exist as an arts-and-crafts group which serves muscle dysfunction or as an activity group which serves the emotionally disabled. Society requires of us a much sharper focus on its needs. As the next step in the development of the theme it becomes necessary to make a critical examination of what, if any, vital need we serve.

What Vital Need Is Served?

As the first order of the business at hand we ought to have it clearly in mind what constitutes a vital need. Of all the descriptions of the need states of man which I have heard I like Eric Fromm's[3] the best. He says that needs are an indispensable part of human nature and imperatively demand satisfaction. The need we serve must fall within this category. He says further that they are rooted in the physiological organization of man and consist of hunger, thirst, and sleep and that in general they all belong to self-preservation. He proposes a simple, forthright formula of self-preservation which is directly applicable to occupational therapy. According to Fromm, when man is born the stage is set for him. He has to eat, drink, sleep, and protect himself from his enemies. Therefore, for his self-preservation he must work and produce. Work, in the Eric Fromm sense, is a physiologically conditioned need and therefore a need to work is postulated as an imperative part of man's nature.

In our 40 years of practice we have accumulated some fascinating odds and ends of understanding about the need to work. For example, early in my training I was taught that work was good for people. All people needed to work and sick people even more so. This kind of justification of service reminds me of the old story about the man who died and woke up surrounded by all kinds of delights which were his for the mere bend of the finger. After he had satiated himself

well, he called for the headman, expressed his appreciation for the manner in which he was treated, and then said, "Now that I have pleasured myself well, it is my wish to do something. My good man, what is there for me to do in this paradise?" The answer given to him was, "You are doing it now." "But," replied our man, "I must do something or else my stay in heaven will be intolerable." "Who" replied the headman firmly, "said that you were in heaven?" In the past I have been guilty of believing and having my patients persuaded that work was good and heaven would prove me right. The rationale that man works because it is good for him, regardless of comfort to us, makes little contribution to our understanding of work as a basic need.

During the 30s, the economic depression gave us an unparalleled opportunity to learn that when able people could not find work, certain psychological disorganization occurred. These changes were deemed to be over and above the changes which could reasonably result from economic loss. We are able to generalize from the depression that human nature does not thrive in idleness. In the last several decades we have accumulated a few more broad generalizations. One is that the stress of work produces psychosomatic conditions in modern businessmen. Another generalization which is now being formulated is that when people retire from their work, they retire from life itself.

A vital need to be occupied however, is not to be inferred from such global generalizations. It is being left to the more rigorously controlled experimentations to do this. Now under laboratory conditions man's need-state for action is being rigorously investigated. In the United States and Canada basic research is going on in an area called sensory deprivation. The work began in reaction to the Russian brainwashing attempts. The research was designed on the principle of restricting man's interaction with the ongoing world of reality. Under controlled conditions of isolation man was found to suffer profound disturbances of his thought processes. In isolation men regressed to unrealistic and prelogical modes of behavior. The sensory deprivation findings suggest strongly that the concepts of man's response to his environment must be sharply revised. The behavioral aberrations which were observed in the idleness of depression and retirement, and the stress of overwork, appear to have been confirmed by the laboratory-induced sensory deprivations. The data were checked out by neurologists, psychiatrists, biochemists, pharmacologists, mathematicians, and engineers.

The final sensory-deprivation report sums up to a concept that the mind cannot continue to function efficiently without constant stimuli from the external world. The central nervous system is now seen as a complex guessing machine oriented outward for the testing of ideas. The experimenters postulate that each individual constructs a different development pattern with respect to strategies for dealing with reality. Jerome Brauner[4], as one of the researchers, concluded that early sensory deprivation prevents the formation of adequate models and strategies for dealing with the environment. Later sensory deprivation in normal adults, he suggests, disrupts the vital evaluation process by which one constantly monitors and corrects the strategies one has learned to employ in dealing with the environment.

To summarize at this point, it seems to me that the American drive toward action as identified by Max Lerner and the human drive toward work as identified by Fromm have been verified in the laboratories. I believe that we are on safe ground right now to say that man has a vital need for occupation and that his central nervous system demands the rich and varied stimuli that solving life problems provides him and that this is the basic need that occupational therapy ought to be serving.

What Is the Unique Service?

A profession, however, must do more than identify the need it serves. There is a twin obligation to spell out its unique pattern of service. The next gigantic task which this presentation faces and with some trepidation, because of the limitation of time, is an attempt to identify the basic pattern of our service by which the hypothesis may be proven. The charge is gigantic because it makes it obligatory to define the occupational therapy body of knowledge, its treatment process, and techniques.

A search for valid content, process, and methods has been my preoccupation in the past 10 years of reading, study, and practice. If I had the ability to do all this with any degree of clarity, I would not be here talking about it. I would be in a clinic doing it. However, I am now admitting to a rising sense of satisfaction in the project and a receding sense of frustration. At no time in technological history have the behavioral scientists been producing so much knowledge directly applicable to our field as they are now. The material is emerging from sources as divergent as neurological theory, animal psychology, developmental and personality theory, and from psychologists as diverse as Allport, Murphy, Harlow, Hebb, Goldstein, Piaget, and Schlachtel.

In order to plunge directly into this material I am going to have to make use of a device in logic known as a First Principle. For if we were to have a First Principle in occupational therapy it would provide us with a way to specify our knowledge. To those who may not be familiar with the meaning of First Principle, it is a device in reasoning to account for all that follows. For instance, the idea of God is a First Principle which accounts for the Universe. There has been a First Principle postulated to explain the nature of man. We are told that the first duty of an organism is to be alive. Medical science derives its premise from this first law of life. If it were not desirable to cure disease and prolong life, the rules of science and the skills and practice of medicine would be irrelevant. The second duty of an organism is to grow and be productive. Occupational therapy ought to derive its premise from the second law of life. If it were not desirable to be productive, the skills and practices of occupational therapy would be irrelevant.

These two laws merge into a concept of function which asserts that both the existence and the unfolding of the specific powers of an organism are one and the same thing. This concept of function is expressed as: the power to act creates a need to use the power, and the failure to use power results in dysfunction and unhappiness. The validity of the First Principle is easily recognizable in the physiological functions of man. Man has the power to talk and move, therefore, if he were prevented from using the power, severe physical discomfort would result. Freud utilized this First Principle to build a powerful theoretical position from which emotional illness was so successfully attacked. He accepted man's biological necessity to produce and generalized that when sexual energy was blocked, neurotic disturbances resulted. He endowed sexual satisfaction with all-encompassing significance. He developed his theory of sexual satisfaction into a profound symbolic expression of the fact that man's failure to use and spend what he has is the cause of sickness and unhappiness. The Freudian theory that human action is primarily sexually based has thrown a strong but restrictive shadow over other behavioral fields. It has been only lately that attention has been given to human productivity in non-sexual areas. Occupational therapy's focus, it is asserted here, lies in the non-sexual area of human productivity and creativity.

In Gardner Murphy's[5] brilliant defense of human productivity he makes us aware that there is a distinct path which leads to becoming human. This path is not seen as being sexually directed. The direction lies largely in the enrichment and elaboration of the sensory and motor experience and the life of symbolism which depends upon them. He maintains that the sheer fact that we have a nervous system, the sheer fact that we can learn, means that we can prolong and complicate sensory and motor satisfactions, can make them richer, can give them more connections, can avoid boredom, can recombine them, can feed upon them, can become immersed in them and make them a part of ourselves. In all these respects, Murphy says man is most completely human. His primary thesis is that man achieves satisfaction in using what he has, in using the equipment that makes him human; and this entails not only the sensory and motor equipment but that central nervous system upon which the learning and thinking processes depend.

Murphy's spirited description of the conditions necessary for being human can provide the basis for an occupational therapy First Principle. This logic constitutes our mandate to discover and organize our body of knowledge; to develop a treatment process; and to devise techniques for its application to the health of man. The logic of occupational therapy rests upon the principle that man has a need to master his environment, to alter and improve it. When this need is blocked by disease or injury, severe dysfunction and unhappiness results. Man must develop and exercise the powers of his central nervous system through open encounter with life around him. Failure to spend and to use what he has in the performance of the tasks that belong to his role in life makes him less human than he could be. With this principle in mind I would like to summarize my thoughts of the last several years of work on our body of knowledge, our treatment process, and techniques.

Regarding the Body of Knowledge

Because our profession is focused on influencing the health of people there will always be a need to include in our body of knowledge the fundamental material of anatomy, neurophysiology, personality theory, social processes, and the pathological states to which these functional areas are subject. However, I do not feel this is our unique content. We should have as a special contribution a profound understanding of the nature of work.

Knowledge of work capacity lies scattered over many behavioral fields. We do know, for instance, that man's ability to work has been developed in the long evolutionary process. It began when man hunted and fished for his food and continued as he grew his food and fabricated objects for his comfort. The lot of man was considerably improved when he freed himself from arduous labor through tools and machinery. His comfort was immeasurably assured by the social institutions he built and operated with increasing skill over the centuries. It is my contention that this evolutionary process, plus a bit more, is present, symbolically expressed in today's culture. The concept of work capacity as being an outgrowth of an evolutionary process I call the phylogenesis of work. I believe that cultural history of work ought to be deeply embedded in the occupational therapy body of knowledge and its phylogenetic nature considered particularly in program building.

We know that as a child grows, he recapitulates the history of his race in the stages through which he himself must pass enroute to maturity. The need to pass through phylogenetic experiences in work is necessary for mature work capacity to be developed. There is historical evidence that a child's ability to play, to explore his environment, to exercise his motor skills are the foundation for his later school experiences. The problem-solving processes and the creativity exercised in school work, craft, and hobby experiences are the necessary preparations for the later demands of the work world. Because we know that the random movements of the infant progress in developmental sequence toward the job competencies of the mature adult, I postulate an ontogenesis of work. I believe that the ontogenetic nature of work ought to be considered in the case-study approach to each treatment problem.

The occupational therapy body of knowledge should include therefore, an understanding of the developmental nature of the sensory-motor systems; the patterning of aptitudes, abilities, and interests; and the nature of the learning process involved in the acquisition of skills. It should include also an understanding of the developmental nature of the problem-solving process and process of creativity. My epistemological conclusion is that the biological, psychological, or social knowledge we select as part of our thinking content must be intermeshed deliberately with the knowledge of work–phylogenesis and work–ontogenesis.

Regarding the Treatment Process

The capacity to work develops in the long socialization process through which a child becomes an adult. It proceeds along the path of growth as man learns to intermesh his motor with his intellectual functions and adapt this integration to the tasks of his life which satisfy his need to control his environment. Work capacity, in this sense, can be said to develop out of the struggle with gravity for motor control, the struggle with learning for manual and mental skills, and the struggle with people and people purpose for economic and social control. When the struggle is great, the personal involvement is high; although conflict and frustration are high, so, too, is work satisfaction high. It follows, too, that when involvement is low, work satisfaction is low. The occupational therapy process becomes primarily concerned with that special aspect of the socialization process called work satisfaction. Its approach in treatment is biographical because work satisfaction is, by its nature, the result of past experiences expressed in the present ability to cope with the environment. Its focus is on the meaningful involvement in problem-solving tasks or creative performances. The parameters of its concern are the ability to experience pleasure in achievement, to tolerate the frustrations of struggle, to sustain the burden of routine tasks, and to maintain the level of aspiration within the reality level of work skills. The goal of the process is to encourage active, open encounter with the tasks which would reasonably belong to his role in life. The process is paced and guided by the supervision of the prescribing physician.

Regarding treatment techniques. Techniques which would emerge from the body of knowledge and the professional process as just described would be concerned with program and treatment execution. Methods would include all those administrative techniques of program building which would provide a laboratory setting for human productivity. The treatment technique would be all those procedures associated with modifying sensory-motor dysfunctions, perceptual difficulties, and the difficulties inherent in coping with the world of play, work, and school. It is suggested in terms of today's thesis that in the merging of our content, process, and methods, the unique pattern of our function will be spelled out. If this pattern is focused strongly on man's need to be occupied productively and creatively, the hypothesis will grow stronger.

Major Tests of the Hypothesis

Of all the ongoing tests of the occupational therapy hypotheses, I have selected a few major ones upon which to comment. The first and obvious one is whether a need to accumulate substantial knowledge about human productivity and creativity will be recognized and acted upon in our schools and clinics. The problem of balancing our knowledge has been with us for some time. Until now our attention has been preoccupied with the medical science which supports the application of our craft knowledge to medical conditions. But medical science knowledge is a means for the application of our service and not an end in itself. A profound knowledge of human dynamics of productivity and creativity is the end to which our knowledge ought to be designed. As far as our practice today is concerned, we have more medical science knowledge than we know how to apply and we are applying more knowledge about human productivity than we actually have on hand.

The second, and not so obvious test, is the delimiting effect that psychoanalytical practice has on the promotion of a non-sexual concept of human productivity. The fundamental doctrine of the Freudian pleasure principle is that the essential movement of a living organism is to return to a state of quiescence and that primary pleasure is sought in sensual gratification. A fundamental principal of work is that primary pleasure can be sought through efficient use of the central nervous system for the performance of those ego-integrating tasks which enables man to alter and control his environment. In this sense psychoanalytical theory is seen to focus on subjective reality while work theory becomes largely concerned with objective problem-solving reality. It is not that these points of view run counter to each other. They simply do not meet or interact except under very special conditions of intimate supervision by a psychoanalyst.

In 1943 Hendrick[6] raised this issue in the *Psychoanalytic Quarterly*. He argued that the psychosocial activities of the total organism are not adequately accounted for by the pleasure and reality principles when these are defined, in accordance with Freudian tradition, as immediate or delayed response, respectively, to the need for sensual gratification. He suggests that work is not primarily motivated by sexual need or associated aggressions, but by the need for efficient use of the muscular and intellectual tools, regardless of what secondary needs (self-preservation, aggressive, or sexual) a work performance may also satisfy. Hendrick postulated a need for a work principle which asserts that primary pleasure is sought by efficient use of the central nervous system for the performance of well-integrated ego functions which enable the individual to control or alter his environment.

In psychoanalytic practice today sexual satisfaction is seen as being influenced by ontogenetic, phylogenetic, and biographical considerations while no such considerations are seen needed for work satisfaction. Although many analysts have agreed that sexual capacity correlates highly with work capacity, the idea has not been developed much beyond the statement. Work is seen as a kind of experience a patient ought to have and whatever satisfaction he derives from it will be dependent upon his subjective state. As a result, extensive activity programs have grown up around psychiatric treatment which have been designed for participation, but not specifically for ego involvement. These programs are now being called activity programs and those implementing them are called activity therapists.

Such activity programs encourage the participation of large groups and usually appeal to the automatic, learned patterns of behavior. However, activity programs so designed, deny the dignity of a human being to struggle, to control his environment as witness the fact that they tend to make man quiescent within the hospital community. They tend to depersonalize, institutionalize, and, in general, debase human nature. The occupational therapy hypothesis makes the assumption that the mind and will of man are occupied through central nervous system action and that man can and should be involved consciously in problem solving and creative activity. It is believed that psychoanalytical theory and the occupational therapy hypothesis can profitably co-exist if a work principle is postulated and executed. This will be even more true if occupational therapy deepens its understanding of the phylogenetic and ontogenetic nature of work and makes a case-study approach to ego involvement of patients. It is not so possible, however, that activity therapy and occupational therapy can co-exist. It is believed that the major crisis in the proof of our hypothesis will not be how to co-exist with psychoanalytical theory but to know the difference between activity and occupation and to act on the knowledge of this difference.

The last major test which I will discuss has to do with the physical disability field. In this specialty we have been placing heavy emphasis upon muscle efficiency and enabling devices. There is a long, perilous, and complex ladder to be scaled between neuro-muscular efficiency and work satisfaction. The ontogenetic reconstitution of motor behavior is a tedious process and must be done step by step. It begins at the reflex muscle action stage and proceeds to the development of complex patterns of motor skills which are utilized in a rich variety of work skills. These, in turn, must be disciplined to a sustaining level of tolerance for routine labors. It is upon this broad pattern that human tolerance for working with people in people affairs is built. If any of these steps are missing, they must be refashioned and the whole pattern reshaped accordingly. The proof of the occupational therapy hypothesis in the physical disability field will depend upon how much we know about the process of restoring work capacity. It cannot be done from prescriptions based upon a narrow understanding of human productivity. It cannot be done in cramped clinics dependent upon scrap material. Nor can it be done from our present ignorance of the world of industry for which we believe we are preparing patients. The challenge to the hypothesis in this area is severe, yet provocative. The technical literature of our profession is indicating that this challenge is not being ignored.

Summary and Conclusion

In summarizing the many ideas I have touched or expanded upon in this thesis, I once again return to my original question: *Is occupational therapy a service vital and unique enough for medicine to support and society to reward?* In answering it, I have said that we have had a magnificent hypothesis to prove, and if it could be proven, even to some degree, the answer would be that we are valuable to medicine and to society. The hypothesis that I presented for evidence of proof was that *man, through the use of his hands, as they are energized by mind and will, can influence the state of his own health.* I asked if this were a kind of idea that America could subscribe to and to that I replied with a resounding yes. I wondered about the stress that the terrible 20th century was putting on this idea and worried some about the energy left to us to advance it. I suggested the hypothesis would begin its proof when we identified the drive in man for occupation and would continue as we shaped our services to fill that need. I speculated on some of the crises the hypothesis was now undergoing and left the decision not in the lap of the gods but in our own laps for us to think and act upon in our daily practice.

I have said that our profession has a magnificent medical purpose. Whether we shall fulfill it or whether it shall ever be fulfilled I have not said because I do not know. But this I can say from personal experience, that we belong to a profession that requires the mind to look at the history of man's achievements throughout civilization. It requires the spirit to respond to the wonders of what man has accomplished with his hands. It gives us a mandate to apply this knowledge and more to help man influence the state of his own health.

Bibliography

1. Merton, Robert K. "The Search for Professional Status." *American Journal of Nursing*, March, 1959.
2. Lerner, Max. *America as a Civilization*. New York: Simon and Schuster, 1957.
3. Fromm, Eric. *The Fear of Freedom*. London, England: Routledge and Kegan Paul Ltd., 1960.
4. Solomon, Philip, & etc. *Sensory Deprivation*. Cambridge, Massachusetts: Harvard University Press, 1961.
5. Murphy, Gardner. *Human Potentialities*. New York: Basic Books, 1958.
6. Hendrick, Ives. "Work and the Pleasure Principle." *Psychoanalytic Quarterly*, Vol. VII, No. 3, 1943.

Bibliographical Notes

Work has been studied from the viewpoint of economics, philosophy, sociology, and psychology, and although the literature is considerable, and is being added to constantly it is a comparatively recent focus for scholars. So far no general study of work has been written, but to some extent a student in this field need not be left entirely without guidance. He needs to remember, however, that the literature is too extensive for one individual to investigate thoroughly. This bibliography noting is designed to serve as an introductory guide. Many of the recommended writings also include full bibliographies of the topic with which they are concerned.

Anyone who seeks to be a student of human occupation should attempt first to build a historical perspective of the field. A History of Technology, edited by Charles Singer, E. J. Holmyard and A. R. Hall, is a massive five-volume series published by Clarendon Press in Oxford from 1954 to 1958 and provides a general historical background as far as science, economics, and technology is concerned. An account of the effect of labor and technology on the culture of the west is set forth at another series titled The History of Civilization, edited by C. K. Ogden and published in New York by Alfred A. Knopf, 1926 to 1929.

The sociological nature of work may be approached through a study of the socialization process and the field of industrial social psychology. This aspect of study is excellently covered in The Handbook of Social Psychology, edited by Gardner Murphy and published in two volumes by Addison-Wesley Company in 1952. A recent perceptive and illuminating view of the social and economic nature of work and the worker is presented by Theories of Society Vol. I and II, edited by Parsons, Stills, Naegele, and Pitts published by the Free Press of Glencoe, Inc., in 1961.

The specific classics regarding human occupations are exemplified by: Theodore Caplow's The Sociology of Work, (Minneapolis: The University of Minnesota Press, 1954); Eli Ginzberg's Occupational Choice: An Approach to a General Theory (New York: Columbia University Press, 1951); Anne Roe's The Psychology of Occupations (New York: John Wiley and Sons, 1956); Donald Super's The Psychology of Careers: An Introduction to Vocational Development (New York: Harper and Brothers, 1957); and John Darley and Theda Hagenah's Vocational Interest and Measurement: Theory and Practice (Minneapolis: The University of Minnesota Press, 1955).

The classics concerned with human creativity are: Vikor Lowenfeld's Creative and Mental Growth, revised edition (New York: The Macmillan Company, 1952); Edwin Ziegfeld's Education and Art: A Symposium (Paris: 19 Avenue Kleber, United Nation's Educational, Scientific, and Cultural Organization, 1953), and Harold Anderson's Creativity and its Cultivation (New York: Harper and Brothers, 1958).

The author further recommends: Robert Gagne and Edwin Fleishman's Psychology and Human Performance (New York: Henry Holt and Company, 1959); Ernest Schachtel's Metamorphosis (New York: Basic Books, 1959); Gordon Allport's Personality and Social Encounter (Boston: Beacon Press 1960); Hannah Arendt's The Human Condition (New York: Doubleday Anchor Books, 1959); Erich Fromm's Man for Himself; (New York: Rinehart and Company, 1945); Gerald Gurin, Joseph Veroff, and Sheila Feld's Americans View Their Mental Health: Number Four (New York: Basic Books, 1960); and Frederick Herzberg, Bernard Mausner, and Barbara Snyderman's The Motivation to Work (New York: John Wiley and Sons, 1959).

Doing and Becoming: Purposeful Action and Self-Actualization

CHAPTER 9

GAIL S. FIDLER, OTR, FAOTA

JAY W. FIDLER, MD

A ristotle made the following observations: "Now we realize our being in action (for we exist by living and acting) and the man who has made something may be said to exist in a manner through his activity. So he loves his handiwork because he loves existence. It is part of the nature of things. What is potential becomes actual in the work which gives it expression."

- Humans R dependant upon social + cultural environments.

- Sense of accomplishment

- Innate human drive to explore + muster environ.

- 1's sense of competence is verified + given value by others
*   - efficacy + value as a human is confirmed*

- Sensorially impoverished environment loses control of his mental functions.

- By doing we are "reality testing" - feedback.

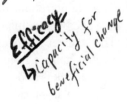

Efficacy, biapacity for beneficial change

During the intervening centuries the behavioral sciences have contributed little to the elaboration of the relationship between handiwork and individual development. Belief in the value of activity for the mentally ill has nevertheless been sustained for many years and is reflected in the universal use of activity programs in community mental health and psychiatric hospital services. However, despite the historical use of activity experiences for patients, understanding it has remained limited. Human action and doing continue to be viewed as peripheral components of intervention. Motivation for such programming seems to be to avoid immobility, rather than for providing positive help. When aftercare programs emphasize medication, psychotherapy, and social service as having priority over the development and improvement of those functional skills that make it possible to achieve a sense of mastery of self and the environment, services remain tangential to mental health or human needs. Also, when services consist of activity programs characterized by single techniques such as art, dance, music, or poetry, a comprehensive perspective on human productivity is sacrificed.

If health professionals are to assume a major responsibility for designing environments and experiences for the prevention of illness, for the maintenance and restoration of health, they need to achieve a more sophisticated understanding of doing. The word doing is selected to convey the sense of performing, producing, or causing. It is purposeful action in contrast to random activity in that the action is directed toward the intrapersonal (testing a skill), the interpersonal (clarifying a relationship), or the nonhuman (creating an end product). Doing is viewed as enabling the development and integration of the sensory, motor, cognitive, and psychological systems; serving as a socializing agent, and verifying one's efficacy as a competent, contributing member of one's society.

All organisms are born to act. Although lower forms of animals come equipped with behavioral patterns enabling them to cope with the external world, humans are dependent upon their social and cultural environments for learning and developing the action patterns necessary for both survival and satisfaction. That action is essential to human existence has been known and pursued by philosophers for many years, although the fields of medicine and psychiatry, with few exceptions, have viewed action (in the sense of doing) as peripheral to the human condition. Today, developments in social psychiatry, ethology, brain research, and developmental psychology reflect a growing sophistication in understanding the relationship of mental activity to motor behavior. There is an accumulation of significant data to support the thesis that the drive to action, transformed into the ability to "do," is fundamental to ego development and adaptation.

Becoming—"I"

The ability to adapt, to cope with the problems of everyday living, and to fulfill age-specific life roles requires a rich reservoir of experiences gathered from direct engagement with both human and nonhuman objects in one's environment. Doing is a process of investigating, trying out, and gaining evidence of one's capacities for experiencing, responding, managing, creating, and controlling. It is through such action with feedback from both nonhuman and human objects that an individual comes to know the potential and limitations of self and the environment and achieves a sense of competence and intrinsic worth.

The play of childhood is a striking manifestation of the natural drive to action in the service of learning—of exploration and discovery about the body, the self, and the external world. Bruner's studies of perception and learning emphasize the need for ongoing engagement with the world of reality as the means by which behavioral patterns and strategies for dealing with the environment are learned. His recent explorations into the meaning and uses of play (1) provide impressive evidence of the critical value of all aspects of play in individual development and evolution. Piaget's (2) observations about play and other exploratory behaviors led him to define these as the processes by which the child assimilates experiences while accommodating to the world. His remarkable studies continue to expand the body of knowledge regarding adaptive human action in a world of objects. Reilly (3) views play as a "connectivity" phenomenon leading to competence and adult "workmanship." She makes some valuable observations about the development of adaptive function and productivity. Erickson continues to emphasize the value of doing in achieving a sense of mastery, personal integrity, and in successfully participating in one's external world. His psychoanalytic background and ego psychology orientation are reflected in his focus on the expressive aspects of play (4) and on doing in the process of self-actualization and acculturation. (5)

In his study of the nonhuman environment, Searles (6) convincingly argues that relatedness to nonhuman objects is a significant force in the development of the sense of self as human, as differentiated from the nonhuman. He describes how involvement with one's nonhuman environment is a means for learning about self and others, and for both symbolically and realistically dealing with one's affective states, needs, and ideations.

In another work, the authors (7) hypothesize that when an activity relates both realistically and symbolically to an individual's needs and personal characteristics, it is an agent for learning and growth. Doing within this context is seen as a means for communicating feelings and ideas, expressing and clarifying individuality, and achieving gratification. The authors and Edelson (8) emphasize that doing in this sense can mediate between one's inner and outer world, nurture the capacity to invest, teach realistic responses to success and failure, provide concrete evidence of one's capacities and limitations, test the reality base of fantasy and perceptions, and validate the ability to achieve and influence one's environment.

The writings of John Dewey articulate the criticality of doing for developing a sense of "I" and in accumulating a store of action experiences essential for human functioning. Becker (9) explores how the sense of self is developed by and sustained in action. He adds dimension to Dewey's earlier hypothesis, emphasizing the significance of the inherent feedback loop process in doing. He views such action as essential for coming to know the realities of self and the world and for testing out the truth of one's perceptions and mental images. Becker's thesis considers schizophrenia and other psychiatric disorders as occurring when internal and external factors limit or preclude an individual's acting on— trying out—an idea or thought.

In defining "objective orientation," Black (10) states that the process of acting enables knowing or "taking account of" the presence of independent, material objects, and emphasizes that it is such action processes that make possible the distinction between reality and illusion.

Neurophysiologic theory seems to be converging on a similar description of behavior. In Karl Pribram's (11) intriguing use of the holographic paradigm, an organism perceives a reality, conceives an intended reality or goal, and learns what motor activity is needed to achieve the goal through a constant series of "tests" to define each increment of change in perceived reality.

A counterpoint to doing as the means for defining reality is made by Don Juan as he explains not-doing to Castaneda. The sorcerer discovers a separate or nonordinary reality by freeing himself from consensual reality. Don Juan explains, "that a rock is a rock because of all the things you know how to do to it—I call that 'doing.'—A man of knowledge— knows the rock is a rock only because of 'doing,' so if he doesn't want the rock to be a rock, all he has to do is—not-doing." (12, p. 227)

In another context, each individual has personal evidence of the sense of well-being, the excitement of challenge, the satisfaction of achievement that comes, for example, from a particular job success: mastering the calculator, planting the garden, repairing the carburetor, "teeing off" in form, or painting a landscape. Whatever limitations there may be in the "artistry" of the end product from the viewpoint of the "expert," there is a keen satisfaction and sense of competence in having accomplished it from one's own resources. Such gratification, the joy of being a cause, can be understood within the context of the human being's innate drive to master the environment.

Robert W. White (13) for a number of years has articulated the thesis that there is an innate human drive to explore and master the environment and that this drive can best be understood as motivation toward competence. White views a sense of competence and efficacy as emerging from direct encounters with and mastery of the environment. He further suggests that gratification from such mastery is intrinsic "in the sense that strictly speaking it requires no social reward or ratification from others. The child acts on the intention, for instance, to climb a stone wall; the outcome of the ensuing struggle between his muscles, hard surfaces, and the law of gravity is brilliantly clear to him even if no one is around to pronounce upon it." (14, p. 273)

White urges that the "helping" professionals become more knowledgeable about the phenomenon of competence and more alert to the patient's sense of competence. He suggests that to become "as sensitive to the client's feeling of competence as we are to anxiety, defensiveness, love and hate, would open a wide additional channel to being of help." (14, p. 274)

When one's accomplishments, one's sense of competence is verified and given value by others, one's efficacy and value as a human being is confirmed. If, for example, climbing the stone wall has no relevance to the child's social group, the intrinsic gratification may be short lived, or limited as an exploratory learning experience. The meaning and worth of one's doing or mastery is appreciably determined by the views and values of significant others. Humans are inextricably dependent upon others for learning and thus for the feedback that verifies that something has been learned and that the new function has value to others. Self-esteem can therefore be understood as evolving from the intrinsic gratification of accomplishment and the feedback from others regarding the achievement.

The significance of doing and feedback from others in developing a realistic sense of competence and efficacy was illustrated in one of the author's experience with a patient group. The group was composed of patients who persistently refused any aspect of occupational therapy programming. With few exceptions, they acted out provocatively in the community and in the hospital. Their actions were random. A decision was made to see them in a talking group and to move cautiously toward action with a purpose. It became evident that action planned toward productivity and achievement generated tremendous anxiety. Their nonverbal behavior in this setting and the groups' reflections on the experiences strongly suggested that "to do" was to risk verification of their incompetence, lack of control over self and the environment, inability to master the environment, and of their "nonhumanness." Subsequently, several members of the group were able to describe that. Their expectations were that what they produced, the "fruits" of their actions, would replicate what they

were. Their appallingly limited "action-learning" experiences and the negative or nonexistent feedback from the environment had left them with few action alternatives.

Action leading to achievement is in contrast to random activity. Action is both the product of a mental image that sets the objective and the creator of a mental image. The mental image that is created includes the refinement of strategies for achieving the objective and an affective evaluation of the achievement. The actor builds a self-image as a competent actor, confronts the realities of the results of the action, finds the boundaries for reasonable objectives, and learns the social relevance of competent actions. When the motivation or ability to act on mental images or ideation is blocked or inhibited by forces in the environment or by sensorimotor deficits, coping behaviors and adaptive skills are not learned.

Becoming—"A Social Being"

Humanization, becoming part of human society, may be defined as the process whereby the individual, beginning life as a biologic organism, becomes a person whose primitive actions are gradually transformed into behavior that concomitantly satisfies individual needs as well as contributes to societal development. In this sense humanization can be viewed as the process of learning about self and one's world, of developing those perspectives and related performance skills essential to a functional society and a functional individual with satisfaction to both.

Mead (15) suggests that social roles are learned through the activity of play and games. Game playing teaches a perspective about the significant other and begins the process of internalization of social roles and values. Let us return again to White's child and the stone wall. As the child struggles to master the hard surface, the pull of gravity, the child is exploring, testing, and developing age-appropriate motor planning, physical skills, and agility. If peers share in the climbing experience, there is additional exploration and learning about "the significant other." If the activity becomes a game, it is reasonable to assume that the rules for playing the game will be defined according to the cognitive, psychologic, and social learning needs appropriate to the developmental level of those participating and congruent with their culture. If significant adults applaud the achievement, then the efficacy of the action is reinforced and verified as socially significant.

The task-oriented groups described by one of the authors (16) are based on such hypotheses regarding doing, with the group providing consensual validation of the efficacy of action and interpreting social/cultural norms: the choices of tasks and the action process per se both reflect and meet the individual's developmental and learning needs.

Moore and Anderson (17) hypothesize that all societies have created "folk models" for dealing with the most critical features of their relationship with the environment. These models can be understood as games, the rules of which teach the necessary perspectives and skills. The authors identify first the nonrandom aspects of nature; second, the random or chance elements: third, interactional relations with others; and fourth, the normative aspects of group living. These are correlated with four types of games: puzzles, which teach a sense of agency, the joy of being a cause; games of chance, which teach a relationship to events over which one has no control; games of strategy, which teach the individual to attend to the behavior and motivation of significant others; and aesthetic entities, or art forms, which teach people to make normative judgments and evaluations of their experiences. Learning experiences planned from this folk model are thus structured to include activities that incorporate varying aspects and characteristics of these models, and are matched with the developmental level and personal characteristics of the learner.

As reviewed here, such perspectives about doing bring into focus two critical dimensions for determining the value of any activity for a given individual. First, the activity or doing must match the individual's sensory, motor, cognitive, psychologic, and social maturation, as well as their developmental needs and skill readiness. Second, it must be recognized by the social, cultural group as relevant to their values and needs.

The information that is available from the various social sciences for research is impressive. However, what is not known about doing and human productivity and what is not being investigated is even more impressive.

Constraints on Doing

Middle class values place great significance on verbal skills. Professionals frequently reinforce the priority of this value in both their educational and treatment orientations and practices regardless of what they know about learning and human functioning.

In mental health practice, there is the familiar problem posed by those patients who, with impressive verbal skill, can describe the psychodynamics of their difficulties and articulate the psychotherapeutic process, but are much less able to act on such cognitive awareness. These are most frequently the clients who disdain activity programs and view action and doing as irrelevant to their needs, problems, or life style. As community mental health programs have broadened the base of psychiatric services, practice has come to include those persons whose culture and learning experiences place a priority on action. These persons most frequently view talking as oblique to their needs, problems, and life style.

There is a need to pursue investigation into the neurological, perceptual, and social components of action in relation to mental health. Simultaneously, conscious efforts need to be made toward breaking down the stereotypes regarding priorities on introspection and talking in isolation of doing. Both the quality and variety of doing is critical for ego development and adaptation.

Social change and technological development have altered the interaction of the person and the world. Direct life-supporting and life-threatening contacts with flora and fauna are almost eliminated. Communication and information are dramatically extended. People hear of events immediately but do not interact with them. The accuracy of reality testing is always dependent upon one's neurological idiosyncrasies, perceptual distortions, the results of prior actions, and social responses. Contemporary psychopathology is fashioned by the current demands on all neurologic functions, on perceptual accuracy, on reduced opportunity for learning through action, and by the enlarged input of information and language.

One can, for instance, easily visualize the different possibilities in the world of John who lives on a farm near a wooded hillside with his parents, grandparents, three siblings, and an uncle. He is expected to be responsible for a number of chores to maintain the household. He is free to endlessly explore nature with all manner of physical skills. He gets direct and consistent response from several generations while also observing them in their work roles. He receives indirect response from family members reacting with value judgments to each other. Finally, he has the direct and indirect responses available to all children at school.

Compare John to Peter who lives in an apartment in a city with two working parents, a cat, and a neighborhood that holds personal threat during much of the 24 hours. He may have some chores but they may not be viewed as critical to the maintenance of family life. He is given very limited freedom to explore. He receives some direct response from two people whose work he does not observe except in the housework about which they complain. He gets vestigial, indirect response from his parents and many hours of passively received indirect response from television or radio. Finally, he has the direct and indirect responses available to all children at school. Once Peter has learned to manipulate his predictable toys he is limited to exploring the behavior of his cat, which is limited in its own behavioral possibilities. A sense of mastery, especially for the new and unexpected, is difficult to achieve. A sense of value and social role identity is even more difficult. Feelings, actions, and meanings do not become integrated.

It can be hypothesized that the prevalence of senseless, purposeless violence by children and adolescents who show no remorse can be generated by hours of viewing television violence that has no relation to their behavior and that is not accompanied by action on their own part. When action does not follow thought, perception is distorted and the critical learning that comes from confronting the consequences of an act is precluded. This dissociation of thought, affect, and action so characteristic of schizophrenia can follow this process of "learning without action." Schizophrenic dissociation can occur when neurologic and perceptual deficits preclude action and when the nature of one's environment inhibits doing or does not support doing in a variety of contexts. The limited learning of functional, adaptive skills that occur when there is a paucity of opportunity for doing is emphasized by Winn (18). She discusses the faulty reality testing, loose distinction between illusion and reality, and the passivity of response evident in children whose daily hours are filled with TV viewing as opposed to psychomotor activity.

There is increasing evidence that limited action experiences are no less significant for the adult. Speaking to the role of activity in maintaining normal human functioning and the consequences of sensory deprivation, Bruner points out that "an immobilized human being in a sensorially impoverished environment soon loses control of his mental functions." (19, p. 7) Greenberg quotes Stainbrook commenting on thrill seeking as reflecting a search for individual mastery, "So much of our life has become sedentary, inhibitive action. There has been an over-emphasis on cerebration—thrill seeking behavior is expressing an almost desperate need for active, assertive mastery at something. We are programmed for action,—but where there is so much less adaptive behavior which requires physical action, there is an insidious anxiety about the concept of mastery. We need to restore a sense of physical mastery and assertion; a sense of control, of self doing rather than merely thinking." (20, p. 21)

Prescribing Intervention

The complexities of a rapidly expanding, industrialized society make it imperative for the health professions to attend to those factors that preclude or inhibit doing. A reduction in doing generates pathology. When pathology is identified, doing must be used in the service of personality integration. If treatment is heavily biased toward verbal communication, and if treatment responds to symptoms rather than to performance skill development and reinforcement, then it will have a limited effect. Likewise, when activity programs fail to relate to the specific development of performance skills, their impact is more like random activity and much of their potential benefit is lost. The extent of carry over of learning and changes from the treatment setting to the home environment is frequently determined by the degree to which treatment modalities are relevant to the adaptive and performance skill demands and expectations of the home setting.

Programming for the prevention of ill health or for the remedy of dysfunction must reflect an appreciation for and understanding of the internal relationship between internal and external systems in the generation and shaping of human behavior. Selective attention to one system, one skill area or component of coping, fragments the totality of the human being.

The question then is how to elaborate concepts about doing to create plans or prescriptions to enhance critical human functions? Different periods in the life cycle demand different configurations of skills, both those relating to the internal realities and those relating to the external realities. Performance can be understood as the ability, throughout the life cycle, to care for and maintain the self in a more independent manner, satisfy one's personal needs for intrinsic gratification, and contribute to the needs and welfare of others. The balance among these performance skill clusters, that is, the proportion of time, attention, and energy allocated to each, is critical in achieving and maintaining a way of life that is satisfying to self and others and is health sustaining.

The level and kind of skills and the balance among them at any one point are determined by age, developmental level, unique biology, and culture. For example, what is an adequate level of independent self care and what are appropriate self-care activities will vary in accordance with age as well as with cultural norms. Likewise, what is considered a healthy balance among caring for self, pursuing personal need gratification, and caring for others, changes with the different stages of life and varies according to one's culture.

Planning for intervention requires an initial assessment of the nature and level of the individual's intact skills, skill limitations, and balance among performance skill clusters. Once such assessments have been made, it is necessary to identify those components or subsystems of performance that inhibit or prevent skill development. This description includes evaluations of the sensory, motor, psychologic, and social deficits as well as identification and assessment of those human and nonhuman factors in the environment that impact on being able to do.

Concepts regarding the components of doing make it possible to analyze activities or doing experiences in relation to skill acquisition. Planning therefore requires that activities be understood and analyzed in terms of the level and kind of motor skill requirements, sensory integrative components, psychologic meaning, cognitive requisites, interpersonal and social elements, and cultural relevance and significance. Such knowledge then makes it possible to match activity experiences to the individual's deficits, learning readiness, intact functions, and values. On the basis of such data and planning, doing can be designed to provide the action-learning experiences necessary for the development of the critical components of performance and for skill acquisition.

Each human action calls on some neurologic function. It is done within some social context and has various potential values and meaning. Understanding the nature and relevance of doing to human adaptation should make it possible to plan intervention programs to facilitate learning and change, increase the chances of helping others maintain a state of health, contribute to a better understanding of the basis of pathology or dysfunction and, thus, hopefully develop more effective prevention strategies.

Acknowledgment

This article is adapted from a paper presented to the Sixth International Congress of Social Psychiatry, Opatjia, Yugoslavia, October 1976.

References

1. Bruner JS, Jolly A, Sylva K (Editors): *Play, Its role in Development and Evolution,* New York: Basic Books, 1976.
2. Piaget J: *Play, Dreams, and Imitation in Childhood,* New York: W.W. Norton, 1962.
3. Reilly M (Editor): *Play as Exploratory Learning,* Beverly Hills, CA: Sage Publications, 1974.
4. Erickson EH: Play and actuality. In *Play, Its Role in Development and Evolution,* JS Bruner, A Jolly, K Sylva, Editors. New York: Basic Books, 1976.
5. Erickson EH: *Childhood and Society,* New York: W.W. Norton, 1963.
6. Searles HF: *The Nonhuman Environment,* New York: International University Press, 1960.
7. Fidler GS, Fidler JW: *Occupational Therapy: Communication Process in Psychiatry,* New York: MacMillan, 1964.
8. Edelson M: *Ego Psychology, Group Dynamics, and the Therapeutic Community,* New York: Grune and Stratton, 1964.
9. Becker E: *The Revolution in Psychiatry,* New York: The Free Press, 1964.
10. Black M. The objectivity of science. *Bull Atomic Scientist 33:* 55–60,1977.
11. Pribam KH: *Languages of the Brain,* Englewood Cliffs, NJ: Prentice Hall, 1971.
12. Castaneda C: *Journey to IXTLAN,* New York: Simon and Schuster, 1972.
13. White RW: Motivation reconsidered: the concept of competence. *Psychol Rev 66:*297–333,1959.
14. White RW: The urge toward competence. *Am J Occup Ther 25:* 271–274, 1971.
15. Mead GH: *Mind, Self, and Society,* Chicago: University of Chicago Press, 1934.
16. Fidler GS: The task-oriented group as a context for treatment. *Am J Occup Ther 23:* 43–48, 1969.
17. Moore OK, Anderson AR: Some principles for the design of clarifying educational environments. In *Handbook of Socialization Theory and Research,* D Goslin, Editor. Chicago: Rand McNally, 1968.
18. Winn M: *The Plug-in Drug,* New York: Viking Press, 1977.
19. Bruner JS: *On Knowing—Essays for the Left Hand,* Cambridge, MA: The Belknap Press of Harvard University Press, 1962.
20. Greenberg PF: The thrill seekers. *Human Behav 6:*17–21, 1977.

CHAPTER 10

Toward a Science of Adaptive Responses

1978 ELEANOR CLARKE SLAGLE LECTURE

LORNA JEAN KING, OTR/L, FAOTA

An "asset almost peculiar to occupational therapists is their high tolerance for puzzlement, confusion and frustration." (1) Ten years ago this was the opinion of Dr. J. S. Bockoven, one of our profession's most vocal admirers. Today one might argue about the tolerance, but who could dispute the puzzlement, confusion, and frustration as we look back on a good many years of effort to define practice, to structure theory, and to build philosophies of occupational therapy.

[Handwritten margin notes:]
- *Adaptation – unifying principle of OT*
- *Utilize real life environ.*
- *4 characteristics of Adaptive Response*
  1. *Demands a positive role*
  2. *It's called forth by the environ.*
  3. *most efficiently organized subcortically*
  4. *It's self-reinforcing*

Need for a Comprehensive Theory

And, as we look toward an era of increasing specialization, we are soberly aware that, without a unifying theory to ensure cohesiveness, specialization could easily become fragmentation. In fact, back at the time when the profession's definition began "Occupational therapy is any activity, mental or physical, ... ," (2) recreation, art, music, and dance all fell under the rubric of occupational therapy. The responsibility for the fact that these modality-based specialties have become separate professions can be assigned in large measure to the lack of unifying theory.

It seems readily apparent that splintering into small professions results in watering-down of job development effectiveness, the scattering of progressively scarcer financial resources for education, and the loss of political "clout." The economics of the health care delivery system will not indefinitely support professional proliferation and duplication of effort. To allow future specialization to result in further fragmentation might well be suicidal. Therefore, we need a framework that will give specialists the bond of a common structure.

We must also cope with the fact that today's consumers, far more sophisticated than in the past, expect to understand what they are paying for. They will no longer accept "on faith" what they are told. This underscores the need for a coherent theoretical model understandable, not just to the professional initiate, but also to the consumer. We may develop complex theories, but, to be really useful, they will need to be based on a straightforward structure that can be widely understood, and is clearly related to the client's life functions.

Difficulties in Constructing a Science of Occupation

As a prelude to an attempt to identify a usable theoretical framework, let us look at the roots of some of our difficulties in achieving a science of occupation. One of the difficulties is related to the fact that occupational therapy was born of common sense; and common sense is, by definition, "what everyone knows." Everyone knows that it is a good thing to keep busy. There is the old proverb, "The devil finds mischief for idle hands." Carlyle said it with great feeling, "An endless significance lies in work; in idleness alone is there perpetual despair." (3) One must reach far down on the evolutionary ladder to find organisms that are not active, that simply exist. Occupation, or employment, or activity, is quite literally bred in our bones. Occupational therapy, then, deals with purposeful behavior—with people *doing*. But isn't this what people are engaged in during most of their waking hours? It is hard to see what is significant about such a commonplace fact of life, and that is precisely the problem, or one of them—something so ever present is hard to grasp conceptually. Whitehead is credited with saying that the more familiar something is to us, the more difficult it is to subject it to scientific inquiry (4). As a commonplace example, consider how many eons must have gone by before Man even thought to wonder about the nothingness that surrounded him. A great many more eons probably passed before Man realized that it was *not* nothingness, and named it atmosphere. I am suggesting, then, that the very universality of the filling or occupying of time with purposeful behavior has made it difficult to form concepts that would help us to construct a theory or science of occupation.

Who has not had the experience of trying to explain occupational therapy to someone, only to realize that people think they know all about it because, of course, they have *experienced* occupation and activity. They are thinking about it in everyday terms, and the therapist is, hopefully, thinking about it scientifically and analytically. So, although words are exchanged, frequently no communication takes place.

Another problem in constructing models is the difficulty that therapists sometimes have in communicating with each other because of the many levels on which purposeful behavior can be organized. One can talk about the effects of activity on the biochemistry of cells, or about its place as an essential component of neurodevelopment. Purposeful behavior is also basic to cognitive processes; and on the still broader scale of cultural anthropology, an individual's role in the cultural milieu can be thought of as determining purposeful behavior. Conversely, behavior may determine cultural roles. So, whether one looks at biochemical Man; psychological Man; social, economic, or ecological Man, purposeful behavior is inextricably woven into the total fabric of human function. However, if one therapist looks at occupation solely in terms of its psychological implications, while another looks only at the cognitive issues, and a third describes chiefly the neurophysiological consequences, a situation results much like that of the blind men examining the elephant. One described the leg, another the ear, and another the trunk. Finally, they were convinced that they could not possibly be talking about the same creature. Certainly an outsider would be hard-pressed to find a principle unifying work simplification, sensory integration, hand splints, and acceptable outlets for aggression, to name just a few of the topics with which therapists may be concerned.

Naturally, attempts have been made to deal with this disparity of viewpoints. Development frameworks are appropriate for many clients, but are not particularly helpful with the normally developed adult who is suddenly faced with trauma or disabling disease. Other models deal with occupation in terms of chronic conditions or the sequelae of disease—a rehabilitative context. These are not readily applicable to developmental problems or acute, as contrasted with chronic, conditions. Few models that I am aware of have spelled out what it is that is peculiar to occupational therapy as contrasted with physical therapy or vocational counseling, for example. What *is* that factor which makes occupational therapy so uniquely valuable that, as Dr. Reilly says, if the profession were to disappear tomorrow, it would have to be quickly reinvented? (5)

General systems theory teaches that systems share common features, that large inclusive systems tend to recapitulate the features found in more specific units. As Laszlo says, "A system in one perspective is a subsystem in another." (6) It seems, then, that our task in finding a theoretical frame for occupational therapy is to identify a level of system that is not so specific as to shut out some of our areas of specialization, nor yet so general as to include a great many more areas than are applicable.

In short, to satisfy the profession's current needs, a theory or science of occupational therapy should provide:

1. A unifying concept that will apply to all areas of specialization;
2. A framework that will clearly distinguish occupational therapy theory and techniques from those of other disciplines;
3. A model that is readily explainable to other professionals and to consumers; and
4. A theory that is adequate for scientific elaboration and refinement.

Adaptation as a Unifying Concept

While mulling over some of these considerations, I read Konrad Lorenz's recent book, *Behind the Mirror, A Search for a Natural History of Human Knowledge* (7). Lorenz deals essentially with the evolutionary and individual processes of adaptation that are involved in Man's active acquisition of knowledge and techniques. I was struck with the implications of his work for occupational therapy. Then Kielhofner and Burke's recent review of the ideological history of occupational therapy (8) drew my attention to Dr. Ayres' phrase, "eliciting an adaptive response," (9) which seemed a succinct and accurate description of what an occupational therapist does. I was at this time going over the occupational therapy literature, and suddenly the words *adaptation* and *adaptive* seemed to leap out from almost every page. In fact, few of our professional articles fail to mention adaptation, regardless of the author's specialty or point of view. I was struck, like Cortez, with "a wild surmise" (10); could the *adaptive process* be an adequate synthesizing principle for our profession? Is it too nebulous a concept to be useful? Surely it is too simple an idea—or is it? Has its very familiarity, like that of the word *occupation* blinded us to its true significance?

Certainly the words *adaptation* and *adaptive* are well known to us. We advertise on bumper stickers that occupational therapists are adaptive; we have large investments in adaptive equipment; and assumptions about adaptation are implicit in our literature. Adolph Meyer began his treatise on "The Philosophy of Occupation Therapy," in 1922, by defining disease and health in terms of adaptation (11) (see Chapter 2). But I have not found evidence that we have rigorously analyzed the concept or used it consciously to explain our functions in any broad sense. Perhaps it is time that some of our implicit assumptions about adaptation be made explicit. Only when these assumptions are articulated can their validity be examined through research.

At the outset we must distinguish between adaptation as an evolutionary concept and the process of individual adaptation. Evolutionary adaptation refers to changes in the structure or function of an organism or any of its parts that result from the process of natural selection (12). Natural selection, in turn, is the process by which a differential survival advantage is transmitted to successive generations. The process of evolutionary adaptation is very slow, requiring at the minimum hundreds of thousands of years for significant changes in form or function to occur.

Individual adaptation refers to adjustments made by the individual that primarily enhance personal rather than species survival, and secondarily contribute to actualization of personal potential. Tinbergen says, "Adaptedness is a certain relationship between the environment and what the organism must do to meet it." (13)

The idea of using adaptation as a model in a health-related profession is reinforced by Dr. Rene Dubos in his book, *Man Adapting* (14). He says "states of health or disease are the expressions of the success or failure experienced by the organism in its efforts to respond adaptively to environmental challenges."

Rappaport, the general systems theorist, says "Science is clearly a systematized search for simplicity." He adds, "Seek simplicity, and distrust it." (15) I would invite you, then, to keep a healthy skepticism as we explore the concept, a relatively simple one, that the adaptive process constitutes the core of occupational therapy theory, and that specific attributes of adaptation are also the significant and characteristic attributes of occupational therapy. This will make explicit and specific and testable some of our heretofore unexamined assumptions.

Characteristics of the Adaptive Process

Initially, let us discuss four specific features of individual, as opposed to evolutionary, adaptation. The first characteristic of adaptation is that it demands of the individual a positive role. The adapting person is defined as "adjusting himself to different conditions or environments." (12) In doing this he is acting, not being acted upon. An adaptive response cannot be im-

posed, it must be actively created. To quote Nobel prize-winning ethologist Tinbergen again, "Living things do not move passively through the physical processes of the environment; they do something against it." (13) Active participation of the client in the treatment process has long been recognized as characteristic of occupational therapy.

Alexei Leontiev, Chairman of the Psychology Faculty of the University of Moscow, reminds us that "Even seemingly simple human functions develop as an interaction between sensory stimulation from the environment and the *person's own activity*." (16) (Italics by this author [King])

Even unprofitable or maladaptive adjustments to change are actively entered into. Withdrawal, for example, which is often considered a negative condition, is actually an active response, sometimes appropriate, sometimes maladaptive.

Secondly, adaptation is called forth by the demands of the environment. The challenge of something the individual needs or wants to do—obstructed by change or deficit in the self or the environment—calls forth a specific adaptive response. We could say that occupational therapy consists of structuring the surroundings, materials, and especially the demands, of the environment in such a way as to call forth a specific adaptive response. Another way of saying this is that occupational therapy uses the demands of tasks or other goal-oriented activities in a specially structured environment to trigger the unfolding of a needed adaptation.

Among the healing sciences, occupational therapy is unique in its utilization of the demands of the real-life environment. An adaptive response cannot truly be said to have occurred until the individual consistently carries it out in the course of ordinary activities. Thus an amputee may practice opening the hook of the prosthesis over and over, but has not truly adapted to it until the prosthesis is used habitually in a daily routine. The occupational therapist uses this knowledge by providing the amputee with many real-life activities in which to use the prosthesis. The therapist knows that pure exercise, no matter how repetitive, often does not generalize into daily activities, and therefore fails to be adaptive.

This brings us to the third characteristic of the adaptive response, namely that it is usually most efficiently organized subcortically, and, in fact, often can *only* be organized below the conscious level. Conscious attention to a task or an object permits the subconscious centers to integrate and organize a response. Dr. Yerxa, in her 1966 Slagle Lecture (17), gave an example that can hardly be improved upon. She said, "A year ago I helped evaluate a brain damaged client's function. She was asked to open her hand. No response occurred, except that she was obviously trying. Next she was moved passively into finger extension while the therapist demonstrated the desired movement. This time the client responded with increased finger flexion. In frustration she cried, 'I know, I know.' Finally she was offered a cup of water. As the cup was perceived, her fingers opened almost miraculously to grasp it."

It would be hard to overemphasize the importance of the therapist's using his or her cognitive powers to structure situations that will elicit a subcortical adaptive response from the client. We tend to rely too much on the client's cognitive processes.

Another example of the importance of subcortical adaptive learning is less familiar to the therapist, but popular with the sports enthusiast. It is to be found in such concepts as "inner tennis." Gallweg, author of *The Inner Game of Tennis* (18), says, "There is a far more natural and effective process for learning and doing almost anything than most of us realize. It is similar to the process we all used but soon forgot as we learned to walk and talk. It uses the so-called unconscious mind more than the deliberate 'self-conscious' mind, the spinal and mid-brain areas of the nervous system more than the cerebral cortex. This process doesn't have to be learned, we already know it. All that is needed is to unlearn those habits which interfere with it, and then to just let it happen." This approach recognizes the frequently *disorganizing* effects of analyzing consciously what should be automatic sequences of movement.

I stress this point because it is another essential reason why occupational therapists use purposeful activity instead of exercise: namely, that tasks, including crafts, or other goal-directed activities, such as play (where the goal is fun), focus attention on the object or outcome, and leave the organizing of the sensory input and motor output to the subcortical centers where it is handled most efficiently and adaptively. I am suggesting, then, that the distinguishing characteristic of occupational therapy, derived from a similar truth about adaptation, is that *there is always a double motivation:* first, the motivation of the activity itself—catching the ball, creating the vase, making the bed; and the second motivation, recovering from illness, maintaining health, preventing disability—in short, adapting. Now no *animal* recognizes the need to "adapt." It sets out to do something specific—escape a pursuer, or find food. The immediate objective provides the motivation. Adaptation is a secondary and unrecognized goal. But in dealing with humans we need to recognize that the double motivation of therapeutic activity may or may not need to be brought to the client's awareness, depending on age, cognitive function, and so forth. The therapist should see to it, however, that other professionals and the client's family are made aware of *both* motivations, and of how the direct motivation of the activity subserves the indirect, but *primary* motive of therapy.

The implications of the foregoing definitions of the nature of occupational therapy practice are important in light of certain current problems. As mentioned earlier, the profession has been concerned with role definition—how to delimit the boundaries that separate our practice from that of physical therapy or other professions. In a recent report of an American Occupational Therapy Foundation board meeting, to which Washington area therapists were invited, concern was expressed about occupational therapists "infringing on" exercise, the territory of physical therapy (19). And well may we

be concerned, for it is *our* professional identity that will be diluted by this infringement, not theirs. Obviously all disciplines that are working with a client should work together cooperatively, but it seems equally obvious that it is uneconomic if there is duplication of function. Exercise has its important place, so also does purposeful activity as a producer of adaptive responses, and this latter is the realm of the occupational therapist. We need to be able to explain in terms of the principles outlined above why purposeful behavior can elicit adaptive responses that exercise alone cannot. Defining our role in this way will be much more satisfactory than the old way of dividing the patient in the middle and giving the top half to the occupational therapist and the bottom half to the physical therapist.

The *fourth* characteristic of the adaptive response is that it is self-reinforcing. In animal behavior the reward for successful mastery of environmental demand is survival, and the penalty for failure is death. In humans the results are seldom so immediate and stark. Nevertheless, mastery of environmental demand is a powerful reinforcer and Maslow lists the drive to master the surroundings as one of Man's innate needs (20). Mastery of one demand is rewarding and serves as a stimulus for attention to the next necessary response at a higher level of challenge. This is the genius of occupational therapy—that, as the old adage has it, "nothing succeeds like success." As the occupational therapist plans and structures successful efforts, each success serves as a spur to a greater effort. Exercise, psychotherapy, behavior modification are all means to an end. But with purposeful activity, the activity itself is an end, as well as being a means to a larger end, therapy or adaptation, hence the double motivation mentioned before.

To summarize the thesis thus far, I am implying that the essential purpose of occupational therapy is to stimulate and guide the adaptive processes through which an individual may best survive and develop. I have suggested that the basic characteristics of occupational therapy derive from the corresponding elements of adaptation; *first,* that it is an active response; *second,* that it is evoked by the specific environmental demands of needs, tasks, and goals; *third,* that it is most efficiently organized below the level of consciousness, with conscious attention being directed to objects or tasks; and *fourth,* that it is self-reinforcing, with each successful adaptation serving as a stimulus for tackling the next more complex environmental challenge.

Having tried to identify the basic characteristics of the adaptive process from which the significant features of occupational therapy derive, let us look at some familiar aspects or categories of practice in the light of adaptation, and also at the adaptive process as an organizing principle in two newer or less familiar areas of practice.

In broad general terms we can divide individual adaptation, on the one hand, into the phase that is synonymous with developmental learning, and, on the other hand, the process of adjusting to change or stress.

Developmental Learning as an Adaptive Process

The organizing of sensory input into information, and the subsequent integration of an appropriate motor response, is a continuous adaptive process. As mentioned earlier, Leontiev suggests that human functions consist of the interaction of sensory input and individual activity. For example, we learn to see by seeing. The visual figure-ground skills of a child raised in the green leafy lights and shadows of the jungle will be different from those of the child raised in the clear light and great vistas of the Navajo reservation. Each child begins with similar, basic visual equipment, but the process of learning to see in each environment is a process of adaptation in which available stimuli, combined with active sorting and filing, produce patterned vision.

There are a number of theoretical frames for considering the adaptive processes of early childhood, and the occupational therapy profession can be proud of the several outstanding developmental theorists among its ranks. It is not the intention here to recapitulate developmental theories, but to emphasize the fact that "eliciting an adaptive response," in Dr. Ayres' apt phrase, is, in essence, eliciting goal-directed or purposeful behavior. This may be as basic as enticing an infant to lift its head to look at a toy, or more complex, such as suggesting to a child that he shovel sand into a wheelbarrow to trundle across the playground to a sandbox. The child's goal is playing with the sand; the therapist's goal is stimulating co-contraction, heavy work patterns, and so forth, in the service of integrating and organizing sensory input and motor behavior.

The role of the occupational therapist in stimulating this sequence of integration and response appears deceptively simple to the consumer who cannot be expected to understand, without explanation, that it takes considerable knowledge and professional finesse to know which adaptive response is needed and to provide the proper setting and stimuli for a given action at the opportune moment when the individual's development makes it possible for him to make a successful response.

We have been considering the well-known field of developmental learning in children. However, it is not only in childhood that one must organize sensory data and respond appropriately. This process goes on throughout life. Afferent, or incoming impulses, particularly those characterized as proprioceptive feedback, play a crucial role in sensory integrative processes in adults as well as in children. The key concept is that sensory input is the raw material for adaptation at *any* age. If developmental adaptation does not take place normally in childhood, the adult will show various disabilities ranging, as an example, from mild motor planning problems to severe disabilities such as process schizophrenia. Recent studies, suggesting that the adult brain is relatively plastic, give some hope that even in adulthood developmental adaptations can be facilitated.

The role of sensory data in the adult has been strikingly illuminated in the last 25 years by a large number of sensory deprivation studies, which have, as a matter of fact, strengthened the theoretical base for sensory integration theory. However, the critical relationship between these studies and the health of the average citizen is just beginning to be appreciated. As an example, consider the scenario for an all too familiar tragedy that goes something like this. An elderly man, in somewhat precarious health, must undergo major surgery. As a precaution, he is kept somewhat longer than usual in the intensive care unit. When he is moved to a room, he is kept very quiet, sedated, curtains drawn, and visitors restricted. Somewhere between the third and fifth day, post-surgery, the nurse's notes show that the patient appears to be confused and disoriented. The following day he is hallucinating and has to be restrained because he is trying to get out of bed. There are no family members who are willing to care for him in his apparently deranged state, so he is transferred to a nursing home where he continues in a state of relative sensory deprivation, and his mental and physical condition deteriorates rapidly.

The tragedy is that this kind of occurrence is often preventable. And in the instances where confusion or disorientation occur in spite of precautions, it is important to note that it is often reversible if suitable sensory input is provided. Lipowski, whose studies (21) suggest the reversibility of deprivation-caused psychiatric symptoms, also warns that around age 55 vulnerability to the effects of sensory deprivation increases quite sharply. Thus it is apparent that it is not just the very old who are at risk.

It is also important to note that the effects of deprivation are cumulative, and that the more sensory modes that are understimulated, the faster confusion and disorientation result. One of Lipowski's most significant findings appears to be that immobilization is the most disabling form of deprivation, and that, if added to other sensory losses, is very likely to produce psychiatric symptoms in the vulnerable.

In terms of the emphasis of this discussion on adaptation, we may think of confusion and disorientation as *dis*-adaptation—failure of organization and response. Hallucinatory and delusional phenomena, on the other hand, represent *mal*-adaptation; the sensory data is organized, but incorrectly, and therefore, of course, the response seems inappropriate. So-called unpatterned stimuli are as bad or worse than complete absence of stimuli. "White noise," such as the constant hum of a motor, is an auditory example, while the test pattern on a television set is an instance from the visual domain. Kornfeld, Zimberg, and Malm, in a paper on psychiatric complications of open heart surgery (22), report that "The patient might first experience an illusion involving, for example, sounds arising from the air conditioning vent or the reflection of light from the plastic oxygen tent. Many experience a rocking or floating sensation. These phenomena were often not reported to the staff and could then develop into hallucinatory phenomena and associated paranoid ideation." Kornfeld and his group confirm the harmful effects of immobilization, noting that many patients interviewed after recovery remembered as one of their chief discomforts not being able to move. Let us emphasize again that *sensory input is the raw material for adaptation*. Without adequate sensory data, the individual's adaptive capacity is greatly curtailed.

Motivational loss is another aspect of hospital-induced sensory deprivation that is of critical importance in rehabilitation or therapy. Zubek, in a report on electroencephalographic correlates of sensory deprivation (23), reports that not only were alpha frequencies progressively decreased during 14-day deprivation experiments, but this was also accompanied by severe motivational losses. The abnormal encephalograms persisted for a week after the subjects returned to normal living conditions, *but the motivational losses lasted even longer.* These findings have profound implications for all medical personnel who are trying to motivate patients toward independence. Perhaps the cart has been ahead of the horse! Perhaps the first thing to do is to provide sensory stimulation, particularly of the proprioceptors, through whatever degree of mobility is possible. Then motivation for independent behavior might follow more quickly and spontaneously.

I am indebted to Lillian Hoyle Parent for discussing with me some of the material on sensory deprivation, and, as she points out in her recent helpful summary of the deprivation studies (24), occupational therapists are better prepared than any other health care professionals to make use of this information. A dozen exciting research projects come readily to mind in reference to hospital-induced deprivation. For example, a control group receiving the usual post-operative care could be compared with an experimental group receiving systematic meaningful sensory stimulation under an occupational therapist's supervision. Comparisons could be made of number of hospital days post-surgery, incidence of complications, and amounts of pain and sleep medications.

We have suggested that sensory input and motor output are the essentials of individual adaptation as seen in the familiar field of developmental learning, and we have looked at the less familiar concept of sensory deprivation as a prime factor in *dis*-adaptation or *mal*-adaptation.

Therapeutic Adaptation to Change or Stress

The *second* general category of adaptive response is adaptation to change or stress. One aspect of response to change is represented by a very active current field of specialization in occupational therapy, namely the field of physical disabilities. This field concerns itself with the individual's adaptation to physical change.

Changes within the person can be of many kinds; what they have in common is the demand that the individual alter habitual responses. Arthritis, heart disease, amputations, spinal cord injuries, stroke, and blindness are a few examples. The use of adaptive equipment, work simplification, splinting,

development of strength, and skill in residual body segments are among the adaptive considerations in this area of practice. Sometimes the acquiring of appropriate adaptive responses may actually be a matter of survival, as with the cardiac client. More often adaptation means the possibility of actualizing potential that would otherwise be wasted.

While the concepts of adapting to physical change are very familiar to us as therapists, we have had less direct experience with the relatively new field of adaptation as it relates to stress medicine. The role of activity in adapting to or coping with stress is an old idea whose scientific time has come. Dr. Hans Selye, who is considered the "father" of stress medicine, comments, "The existence of physical and mental strain, the manifold interactions between somatic and psychic reactions, as well as the importance of defensive-adaptive responses, had all been more or less clearly recognized since time immemorial. But stress did not become meaningful to me until I found that it could be dissected by modern research methods and that individual tangible components of the stress response could be identified in chemical and physical terms." (25) Dr. Selye called this stress response the "general adaptation syndrome." Today few literate people are unaware of the fact he demonstrated: that any stimulus which appears to pose a threat to survival elicits a response that includes the secretion of the cortico-steroids which prepare the body for a fight or flight reaction. The heightened blood pressure, pulse, and respiration that follow a danger signal had a distinct survival value when the appropriate reaction was running, or climbing, or hand-to-hand combat. In our present cultures, running, climbing, or fighting are seldom considered appropriate responses, and threats are often perceived as long continued, like the danger of losing one's job, or the daily stress of driving through rush-hour traffic. There are well-known stress diseases such as ulcers, high blood pressure, and heart disease, to mention the most common, that follow chronic stimulation of cortico-steroid secretion. The current vogue for jogging, marathon running, and other strenuous sports owes part of its very real usefulness as a health maintenance measure to the fact that exercise metabolizes and renders harmless the stress hormones that otherwise might accumulate and cause permanent damage to the body.

What is not so often considered is the effect of either subtle or overt stress on an already over-taxed system. A person who is already feeling ill is told he must enter the hospital. Whether it is for surgery or for tests, or for nursing care, everything about the experience spells danger: the strangeness, the uncertainty, the painful or uncomfortable procedures, but most of all the feeling of helplessness. Stress hormones are poured into a system that not only is already reacting to the stress of illness, but also has few opportunities for activity that might help to metabolize and dissipate the cortico-steroids. Stress hormones can make the sick person sicker and can retard recovery.

It is often assumed that *rest* is what is needed in the hospital, but, as Dr. Selye points out, unless the organism is completely exhausted, activity of some sort is much more appropriate to stress dissipation than too much rest. Many years ago an occupational therapist frequently stepped into a hospital room and made available purposeful, goal-directed activities that allowed the patient an adaptive response to stress. If we had known then what we know now, we might have called it *stress management* or *stress reduction therapy.* Instead, someone used the word *diversional,* with the result that the whole area of human needs has been virtually abandoned, and the word diversional has become the equivalent of profanity. In fairness we must point out that few third-party reimbursement agents are willing to pay for something labeled *diversional.*

To turn to another aspect of this subject, before the stress hormones and their physiological effects had been identified by Dr. Selye, we often spoke of *tension,* and in the mental health field were able to recognize the usefulness of activity, even though the reasons were vague. Dr. Roy Grinker writes of the treatment of *battle fatigue* or *war neuroses* (26) and says, "In their free time physical activities are encouraged in order to dissipate accumulated tensions. Enforced idleness and rest are bad therapy for these states." Later he comments, "The patients are busy the whole day with physical and mental activities and various aspects of occupational therapy."

The high hopes held for the usefulness of the psychotropic drugs led to the serious curtailment of other forms of treatment such as those described by Grinker. Now that there is widespread disillusionment with the major tranquilizers, which seem to cause almost as many problems as they solve, perhaps the efficacy of what might be called *adaptational therapy* will be rediscovered.

The psychiatric disorders provide excellent examples of the interrelatedness of the various aspects of the adaptive process. In some instances, as in autism or in process schizophrenia, we are probably dealing with inadequate developmental adaptive learning and the attendant severe problems in perception and communication. These problems inevitably produce stress and the concomitant physical changes produced by the stress hormones. These, in turn, probably further derange the sensory-integrative processes. Many of the symptoms seen in the psychoses represent either disadaptations or maladaptive behavior. As the therapist is able to facilitate adaptive development, that is, sensory integration, coping behaviors improve. Activity also helps to metabolize stress hormones and thus increases the client's feeling of well-being. Though basic biochemical causes may ultimately be found for some of the major psychoses, there will probably always be a need for facilitating adaptive or coping skills in a society that seems increasingly stressful.

Psychologists Gal and Lazarus, it seems to me, have made the strongest case for activity as an adaptive response to stress. Their article, "The Role of Activity in Anticipating and Confronting Stressful Situations," (27) spells out the physio-logical correlation of activity with the reduction, or metabolism, of the stress hormones. They point out that while activity which is related to the cause of the stress is best, activity of any kind is better than none. Their useful analysis of the literature concludes with these words: "Regardless of the interpretation, it seems quite evident that activity during stressful periods plays a significant role in regulating emotional states. We are inclined to interpret activity as being a principal factor in coping with stress. As has been repeatedly argued by Lazarus a person may alter his/her psychological and physiological stress reactions in a given situation simply by taking action. In turn this will affect, his/her appraisal of the situation, thereby ultimately altering the stress reaction."

To summarize, we may divide adaptation in response to change or stress into three major components of concern to the occupational therapist:

1. Adaptation to physical change (which includes a component of adaptation to stress because the physical changes are in themselves stressors);
2. Adaptation to the stress of hospitalization or acute illness;
3. Adaptation to reduce stress reactions in psychiatric conditions.

We have engaged in a lengthy exploration of stress and adaptation because it seems that in the foreseeable future coping with or adapting to stress is going to be one of the major health challenges facing humanity. Toffler, in his book *Future Shock,* (28) makes a good case for the thesis that the extremely rapid rate of change in almost all of our cultural institutions is a significant cause of stress for large segments of humanity, certainly including our own. Ethologist Tinbergen warns, "The amounts of strain now imposed on the individual may well overstretch man's capabilities to adjust." (13) If it is true that stress is a major health problem for modern man, and if, as Gal and Lazarus propose, activity is of major importance in stress adaptation, then occupational therapy has a major role to play in health maintenance and disease prevention as well as in health restoration.

One of my colleagues (Roene Shortsleeve) once drew a cartoon that expressed this rather well. She drew a bearded figure in the white robes of a prophet. In his hand was a placard which read, "The world is NOT coming to an end; therefore, you had better come to occupational therapy and learn to cope."

Conclusion

I have attempted to demonstrate in this paper that the adaptive process can provide a theoretical framework for occupational therapy that meets the criteria suggested at the outset: that it can be applied to all the specialty areas as a unifying concept; that it will differentiate occupational therapy from other professions; that it is readily explainable to other professionals and to consumers; and that it is adequate in depth to allow for scientific elaboration and refinement.

The adaptive process is probably not the only tenable model for occupational therapy. If this paper spurs others to articulate a more suitable theory, it will have served its purpose.

Toffler, in concluding *Future Shock*, comments that, as yet, there is no science of adaptation. Is it too ambitious to suggest that occupational therapists are uniquely prepared to begin constructing *a science of adaptive responses?* It is a challenge worthy of our best.

References

1. Bockoven JS: Challenge of the new clinical approaches. *Am J Occup Ther 22:*24, 1968.
2. Dunton WR: *Prescribing Occupational Therapy,* Springfield, IL: Charles C Thomas, 1947.
3. Carlyle T: *Past and Present,* Boston: Houghton Mifflin, 1965, p 196.
4. Thayer L: Communications systems. In *The Relevance of General Systems Theory,* E Laszlo, Editor. New York: Braziller, 1972, p 96.
5. Reilly M: The educational process. *Am J Occup Ther 23:*300, 1969.
6. Laszlo E: *The Systems View of the World,* New York: Braziller, 1972, p 14.
7. Lorenz K: *Behind the Mirror: A Search for a Natural History of Human Knowledge,* New York: Harcourt Brace Jovanovich, 1977.
8. Kielhofner G, Burke JP: Occupational therapy after 60 years; An account of changing Identity and knowledge. *Am J Occup Ther 31:*657–689, 1977.
9. Ayres AJ: *Southern California Sensory Integration Tests Manual,* Los Angeles: Western Psychological Services, 1972.
10. Keats J: On first looking Into Chapman's Homer. In *Century Readings in English Literature,* JW Cunliffe, Editor. New York: The Century Company, 1920, p 639.
11. Meyer A: The philosophy of occupation therapy. *Arch Occup Ther 1:*1–10, 1922. Reprinted as Chapter 2.
12. Stein J (Editor): *Random House Dictionary of the English Language,* Unabridged. New York: Random House, 1966.
13. Tinbergen N, Hall E: A conversation with Nobel prize winner Niko Tinbergen. *Psychol Today,* March 1974, pp 66, 74.
14. Dubos R: *Man Adapting,* New Haven: Yale University Press, 1965, p xvii.
15. Rappaport A: The search for simplicity. In *The Relevance of General Systems Theory,* E Laszlo, Editor. New York: Braziller, 1972, pp 18, 30.
16. Leontiev AN, cited by Cole M, Cole S: Three giants of Soviet psychology, conversations and sketches. *Psychol Today 10:*94, 1971.
17. Yerxa E: Authentic occupational therapy. *Am J Occup Ther 21:*2, 1967.
18. Gallweg WT: *The inner Game of Tennis,* New York: Random House, 1974, p 13.
19. The Foundation. *Am J Occup Ther 31:*114, 1978.
20. Maslow AH, Murphy G (Editors): *Maturation and Personality,* New York: Harpers, 1954.
21. Lipowski ZJ: Delirium, clouding of consciousness, and confusion. *J Nerv Ment Dis 145:*227–255, 1967.
22. Kornfeld DS, Zimberg S, Malm JR: Psychiatric complications of open-heart surgery. *New Engl J Med 273:*287–292,1965.
23. Zubek JP: Electroencephalographic changes during and after 14 days of perceptual deprivation. *Science 139:*490–492,1963.
24. Parent LH: Effects of a low-stimulus environment on behavior. *Am J Occup Ther 32:*19–25,1978.
25. Selye H: *The Stress of Life,* New York: McGraw-Hill, 1956, p 263.
26. Grinker R: Men *Under Stress,* 2nd edition. New York: McGraw-Hill. 1962, pp 30, 218.
27. Gal R, Lazarus RS: The role of activity in anticipating and confronting stressful situations. *J Human Stress 4:*4–20, 1975.
28. Toffler A: *Future Shock,* New York Random House, 1970.

PART II

Theoretical Frameworks to Guide the Occupational Therapy Process

Introduction

Lorna Jean King concluded the first part of this text with a call for a unifying theory to ensure cohesiveness within our profession. Her appeal was based on her valid concern that increased specialization within occupational therapy would lead to fragmentation and a lack of consumer understanding about the value of occupation. King acknowledged that her adaptive process theoretical framework was not the only tenable model to address these concerns. She expressed hope that her presentation spurred others to explore occupational therapy's philosophical foundations and professional practices to develop additional coherent models of practice. In the 30 years since King put forth this challenge, many of our profession's best scholars have responded. Several seminal works have been published (Bruce & Borg, 1993; Kielhofner, 2004) that meet King's criteria for theory that is "based on a straightforward structure that can be widely understood and is clearly related to the client's life functioning."

This section provides readers with several leading theoretical frameworks put forth by prominent occupational therapy scholars to clarify the link between theory and practice. Although these models differ in content, structure, and format, all emphasize the use of occupation and a person-centered approach throughout the occupational therapy process. It is important to note that a complete presentation of practice models and frames of reference is beyond the scope of this text. However, a thoughtful review of selected practice

models that reflect our profession's core commitment to occupation can help readers develop a theoretical mindset for person-centered, occupation-based practice. These frameworks can be particularly helpful in the assessment of a person's occupational profile, the analysis of his or her occupational performance, and the design of an intervention plan based on the concepts and principles identified in the *Occupational Therapy Practice Framework* (American Occupational Therapy Association, 2002). The use of a clear, well-developed practice model can ensure that our philosophical foundations and core values are actualized in practice and that occupational therapy intervention facilitates the person's engagement in occupation to support life participation in context.

Schkade and Schultz begin this section by echoing King's concern about the impact increased specialization has had on our ability to provide occupation-based intervention. They propose that their Occupation Adaptation frame of reference will facilitate an integrative approach to clinical reasoning that will decrease the fragmentation of occupational therapy because it is reflective of the core values of our profession. They review underlying assumptions and key concepts of this model, emphasizing that Occupation Adaptation provides a holistic framework that considers the person, his or her occupational environment, and the interaction between the person and the environment as equally important. They explore the model's three main components (e.g., the person, environment, and interaction) in depth. The

person is viewed as a configuration of sensorimotor, cognitive, and psychosocial systems that desires occupational mastery. The environment is comprised of physical, social, and cultural subsystems that place demands for mastery on the person. While the interaction between the person and the environment results in a press for mastery that creates an occupational challenge and corresponding occupational role expectations, the person's perception of this challenge generates an adaptive response that can be classified as existing, modified, or new. Occupation Adaptation is therefore viewed as a normal developmental process that leads to competence in occupational functioning. A schematic of the Occupation Adaptation process is presented and thoroughly explained, with practice examples provided to assist readers in the clinical application of this model.

Chapter 12 by Nelson further explores key concepts related to occupation and its therapeutic application. In this 1996 Eleanor Clarke Slagle Lecture, Nelson reviews his lifework of seeking to adequately define occupation, which has culminated in the development of the Conceptual Framework for Therapeutic Occupation (CFTO). In this framework, Nelson defines occupation as a relationship between occupational form and occupational performance. The multidimensional nature of occupational form and its relationship with occupational performance is presented. The meaningfulness and purposefulness of occupation to the individual is examined. Nelson explores the dynamics of occupation and the impact of occupational performance on the environment, the individual, and his or her occupational adaptation. He proposes that the occupational therapy practitioner who understands the possibilities of different occupational forms and who collaborates with the person to design therapeutic intervention that uses personally purposeful and meaningful forms will elicit the power of therapeutic occupation. Nelson emphasizes that this occupational therapy specialty in occupation synthesis is the reason occupational therapy will thrive in the 21st century.

The significance of the use of occupation synthesis to elicit meaningful and purposeful occupational performance is supported by Nelson's analysis of past, current, and potential future models of practice. As he notes, these models all have differing viewpoints, but they all share an emphasis on essential occupation-based principles, validating the importance of occupation synthesis to society. Key principles of the CFTO are presented, and several examples are provided throughout Nelson's treatise to illustrate the practical application of these concepts and support our profession's unique contribution to human health. Nelson concludes with a call for research to examine the power of therapeutic occupation. He advocates that all occupational therapy practitioners embrace and use the term *occupation* in our literature and interactions with the public to ensure that society recognizes our professional ownership of the use of occupation as therapy.

A model that supports Nelson's stance that occupational synthesis is occupational therapy's unique professional domain is discussed in Chapter 13 by Fidler, who presents her Lifestyle Performance Model. In this practice model, Fidler provides an organized, holistic framework for knowing and understanding a person's lifestyle and activity repertoire within the context of his or her human and nonhuman environment. The functions, underlying principles, and major hypotheses of

this model are reviewed, providing a basis for conceptualizing the interrelatedness of person, environment activity profile, and quality of life. Fidler emphasizes that the assessment of an individual's interests, capacities, patterns of daily living, and the analysis of potential activities and environmental contexts is essential before defining and prioritizing intervention. This assessment ensures that the plan of occupational therapy treatment is motivating to the individual and pertinent to his or her lifestyle. Fidler poses five fundamental questions that are highly congruent with the *Practice Framework*. The answers to these questions can be used to develop an occupational profile and plan and implement occupational therapy intervention. Four primary interrelated domains of performance that are relevant throughout the life span are also described. According to Fidler, the use of personally, socially, and culturally relevant activities that are designed to create and enhance the facilitative elements of the environment provides congruence among the person, activity, and environment, thereby increasing treatment efficacy and enhancing quality of life.

The need for practice models that consider the whole person is further explored in Chapter 14, which presents the 1998 Eleanor Clarke Slagle Lecture. Fisher begins her presentation by contrasting reductionistic, therapist-directed practice to occupation-based, person-driven practice and reflecting on her personal development as a practitioner and scholar with a strong belief in the value of occupation as a therapeutic agent. Fisher defines occupation as a noun of action, for it conveys the powerful essence of our profession and enables people to seize; take possession of; or occupy the space, time, and roles of their lives. She reflects that our profession's uniqueness lies in our use of occupation as a therapeutic agent. However, this unique focus on occupation is not always evident in practice. In response

to this gap, Fisher developed her Occupational Therapy Intervention Process Model to guide clinical reasoning so that occupational therapy intervention is based on a client-centered performance context. She presents four continua—ecological relevance, source of purpose, source of meaning, and focus of intervention—which can be used to evaluate the characteristics of activities used in occupational therapy intervention. Based on an analysis of occupational therapy practice according to these continua, she identifies four main activities (e.g., exercise, contrived occupation, therapeutic occupation, and adaptive occupation) that are typically used in intervention. Of these, Fisher argues that therapeutic occupation and adaptive occupation are the legitimate activities of occupational therapy. She describes the interrelated dimensions of context and provides clear guidelines for using a top-down approach to evaluation and for implementing intervention for the purposes of compensation or remediation. A case example supports the clinical application of each step in this model.

Fisher's emphasis on a top-down approach to the occupational therapy process that focuses on occupation and collaboration is upheld in Chapter 15 by Gray, who begins by exploring the disconnect that can occur when holistic practice models are not used to plan intervention. She openly discusses the difficulty many occupational therapy practitioners experience when they emphasize client factors and performance skills rather than occupation as the core of their therapeutic intervention. Gray reflects that this reductionism results from and contributes to our profession's identity crisis. She proposes that embracing the concepts of occupation as ends and occupation as means provides a guide to intervention planning. Each concept is defined and analyzed for its historical significance and its applicability to current therapeutic problems. Useful guidelines to assist occupational therapy practitioners in their clinical decision-making and to facilitate their understanding and expression of our profession's unique occupational expertise are provided. A case example that includes realistic complexities faced by individuals that receive occupational therapy services is presented to support the application of occupation as ends and occupation as means in evaluation and intervention.

Gray's discussion provides a clear overview of Trombly's 1995 Eleanor Clarke Slagle Lecture. Chapter 16 presents this seminal lecture in its entirety. In this influential presentation, Trombly puts forth her Model of Occupational Functioning, which conceptualized occupational performance as a descending hierarchy of roles, tasks, activities, abilities, and capacities. Each component of her model is clearly defined and supported by pertinent examples and relevant research. Trombly distinguishes occupation as a treatment end-goal from occupation as a means to remedial impairment, but she emphasizes that both are therapeutic *if* purposeful and meaningful. She hypothesizes that purposefulness organizes behavior, and meaningfulness motivates behavior; she then analyzes their relationships to both forms of therapeutic occupation. She recognizes that these aspects of occupation require exploration, clarification, and interpretation through research and proposes several highly relevant research questions. A comprehensive literature review of research related to the use of occupation in the motor domain is presented; however, it is apparent that more definitive research is needed. Trombly expresses her hope that her model will spark an explosion of research to further clarify and strengthen the link between occupation and therapeutic outcomes.

Questions to Consider

1. Explain the relevance of theory to occupational therapy practice. How do frames of reference and practice models help link theory to practice? What key theoretical principles guide the use of purposeful activity in occupational therapy evaluation and intervention?
2. Consider an area of practice that most interests you. Which model is most congruent with this practice area? How could this model be used to guide program development and the occupational therapy process?
3. What are the commonalities in language between the *Practice Framework* and the different theoretical models put forth in this section? What models seem most congruent with the domain and process of occupational therapy as defined and described in the *Practice Framework*?
4. How can each model be used to develop a person's occupational profile as described in the *Practice Framework*? Are there gaps in these models that would require the use of another theoretical framework to adequately complete an occupational profile?
5. How can each model be used to design an intervention plan that is person-centered and occupation-based in accordance with the *Practice Framework*?

References

American Occupational Therapy Association. (2002). Occupational therapy practice framework: Domain and process. *American Journal of Occupational Therapy, 56,* 609–639.

Bruce, M. A., & Borg, B. (1993). *Psychosocial occupational therapy: Frames of reference for intervention* (2nd ed.). Thorofare, NJ: Slack.

Kielhofner, G. (2004). *Conceptual foundations of occupational therapy* (3rd ed.). Baltimore: Williams & Wilkins.

Occupational Adaptation: Toward a Holistic Approach for Contemporary Practice, Part 1

CHAPTER 11

JANETTE K. SCHKADE, PHD, OTR
SALLY SCHULTZ, PHD, OTR

A theoretical perspective designed for clinical application and based on fundamental occupational therapy principles is offered. This perspective, the occupational adaptation frame of reference, is presented as an articulation of (a) a normal developmental process leading to competence in occupational functioning; (b) the process through which the benefits of occupational therapy occur; and (c) a perspective that promotes holistic practice. The person is viewed as operating occupationally through an idiosyncratic configuration or sensorimotor, cognitive, and psychosocial systems, all of which are inevitably involved in each occupational response. This occupational functioning is described as occurring through interaction of the person with a work, play and leisure, or self-care context that has distinctive physical, social, and cultural properties (i.e., the occupational environment). Occupational adaptation is a perspective that can influence practice, education, and research.

Occupational therapy is a profession in which practitioners view themselves as treating the whole person. However, the current trend toward increased specialization in health care has led to narrowing of this view and consequently to a more limited scope of intervention. As occupational therapists, we frequently tend to represent ourselves as psychosocial therapists, physical disabilities therapists, hand therapists, or sensory integration therapists. Although this array of designations reflects the diverse areas in which occupational therapists practice, such labels suggest a departure from, rather than adherence to, our holistic perspective (Heater, 1992). The purpose of this paper is to describe the conceptualization of a process that we believe to be fundamental to both human experience and the philosophical underpinnings of the profession. This process is referred to as *occupational adaptation*. We believe that the clinical application of the principles presented in this paper can foster an integrative way of thinking that will reduce fragmentation of not only our professional identity but also our approach to those persons we treat. The concepts and assumptions proposed are intended to complement, not supplant, the work of others who are engaged in the process of enhancing our understanding of occupation and its power in the lives of human beings (e.g., Clark et al., 1991; Kielhofner, 1985; Nelson, 1988). Yerxa (1992) stated, "Occupational therapy needs to develop fresh models and frames of reference for practice that create intelligibility and that are generative rather than positivistic" (p. 81). It is in this spirit that the occupational adaptation framework presented here is offered.

The doctoral planning committee at Texas Woman's University, Denton, Texas, through its deliberations in the planning process, selected the concept of occupational adaptation as the focus for basic and applied research (Texas Woman's University, School of Occupational Therapy, 1989). It was determined by the committee that this research focus should reflect the core concepts of occupational therapy in its unique explanation of therapeutic intervention. One of the most important features of the occupational adaptation perspective is integration of the constructs of occupation and adaptation into a single interactive construct.

Assumption: Occupation provides the means by which human beings adapt to changing needs and conditions, and the desire to participate in occupation is the intrinsic motivational force leading to adaptation. Occupational adaptation reflects the interdependence of these two constructs for occupational therapists. This framework is intended to be readily applicable to a normative process of adaptation as well as to situations in which that normative process has been disrupted through illness or trauma.

Assumption: Occupational adaptation is a normative process that is most pronounced in periods of transition, both large and small. The greater the adaptive transitional needs, the greater the importance of the occupation adaptation process, and the greater the likelihood that the process will be disrupted. The construct of occupational adaptation and its therapeutic implications will be introduced in two parts. In this paper, Part 1, the basic framework explaining the occupational adaptation process is described. In a subsequent paper, Part 2, treatment implications will be addressed.

Theoretical Background

Both occupation and adaptation have been accepted as critical concepts within the discipline of occupational therapy since its origin (American Occupational Therapy Association, 1979; Kielhofner & Burke, 1985; Meyer, 1922 [see Chapter 2]). Both constructs have been the subject of several Eleanor Clarke Slagle lectures (e.g., Bing, 1981 [see Chapter 5]; Fine, 1991 [see Chapter 25]; Gilfoyle, 1984; Johnson, 1973; King, 1978 [see Chapter 10]; Llorens, 1970; Reilly, 1962 [see Chapter 8]). The relationship between the two constructs in the provision of occupational therapy has been explored by many others (e.g., Breines, 1986; Clark, 1979; Fidler, 1981; Fidler & Fidler, 1978 [see Chapter 9]; Kleinman & Bulkley, 1982; Lindquist, Mack, & Parham, 1982; Llorens, 1984, 1990; Mosey, 1968; Nelson, 1988; Reilly, 1962 [see Chapter 8], 1969; Yerxa, 1967, 1989) and by several occupational therapy theorists as an essential component of their theories. Four theories that have similarity with the proposed construct of occupational adaptation are the theory of spatiotemporal adaptation (Gilfoyle, Grady, Moore, 1981, 1990); a model of adaptation through occupation (Reed, 1984); the model of human occupation (Kielhofner, 1985); and the model of occupation (Nelson, 1988).

In the theory of spatiotemporal adaptation, as proposed by Gilfoyle et al. (1981, 1990), adaptation is presented as the process that human beings experience in developing the skills necessary for performing within the context of their environment. The environment is conceptualized as a primary stimulus for development. Spatiotemporal adaptation focuses on the sensorimotor adaptations essential to functional skills. Adaptation is represented schematically as a spiral-like developmental phenomenon progressing from primitive to mature neurological responses.

In Reed's (1984) model, adaptation through occupation, occupation is conceptualized as the means by which adaptation may occur both internally and externally. She described occupation as being adaptive, maladaptive, or nonadaptive. Reed also chose to conceptualize her proposed model as a developmental spiral. She emphasized the importance of the external environment, which she described as the social setting for work and play, as either a facilitator or a hindrance to occupational adaptation. Reed stated that "occupational adaptation and adjustment" are the outcomes of the adaptation through occupation process (p. 498).

Kielhofner and Burke (1985) proposed a hierarchical relationship between occupation and adaptation. In the Model of Human Occupation, they espoused that human adaptation is the more global construct under which occupational function and dysfunction is a subcategory. They concluded that the unique concern for occupational therapy is the adaptation of the person specific to his or her level of occupational functioning. Adaptation is conceptualized in the model as an outcome dependent upon both personal satisfaction and satisfaction of the environmental demands. Barris, Kielhofner, Levine, and Neville (1985) described the environment as consisting of four hierarchical layers: (a) objects, (b) tasks (work, play, and self-care activities), (c) social groups and organizations, and (d) culture. The model of human occupation emphasizes that occupational performance is the outcome of the interactions between persons and their unique environment.

Nelson's (1988) model of occupation presents adaptation as a change that occurs within the person's developmental structure as the result of occupation. Such adaptation occurs not only as a result of the environment's demand for performance, but also because of the effect the person has on those demands. Nelson asserted that occupational performance is a result of both the person's unique developmental capacities and perceived meaning attached to the external expectation. Nelson conceptualized the dynamics of occupation as a continuous interactive loop made up of external demands, performance, and the resultant effect (adaptation).

Each of these four theories provides an explanation of the relationship between occupation and adaptation, and their conceptualizations have both similarity and divergence. The occupational adaptation framework also has similarities with these theoretical perspectives; however, we believe that the conceptual model and treatment approach in this perspective represent a different emphasis. First, occupation and adaptation are conceptualized as more than interrelated concepts. The term *occupational adaptation* refers specifically to how occupation and adaptation become integrated into a single internal phenomenon within the patient. Occupational adaptation is a process-based, nonhierarchical, and non-stage-specific explanation of this phenomenon. Second, this framework emphasizes the patient's experience of self in relevant occupational contexts. This holistic approach gives equal importance to the occupational adaptation experience, and that will promote the ability to perform occupations with greater efficiency, effectiveness, and satisfaction. Third, the occupational adaptation frame of reference focuses treatment on the patient's internal adaptation process and the use of meaningful occupations to affect that phenomenon as opposed to outward measures of performance (Schultz & Schkade, [Chapter 48]). Fourth, the assumptions that serve to ground this perspective are clearly stated, and the essential constructs are operationally defined to facilitate both practice and research. Although the construct of occupational adaptation has been previously addressed in the occupational therapy literature (Llorens, 1990; Reed, 1984; "Research Priorities," 1984), we propose in this paper a unique explanation of their construct that is not only congruent with the evolution of occupational therapy theory, but also can add a new dimension to current practice.

Occupational Adaptation: The Basic Framework

The three basic elements of the occupational adaptation process are seen as the *person*, the *occupational environment*, and the *interaction* of the two as they come together in occupation. The hypothesized occupational adaptation process is represented schematically in Figure 11.1. This representation follows the general systems depiction of an open loop where the feedback following an event influences the subsequent input of that system into future events. Most persons cycle through this process continually. Many of these cycles proceed rapidly; others are more protracted. In addition, multiple cycles can be operating simultaneously. The isolation of the process components in the figure is artificial but necessary for an understanding of these components.

The Occupational Adaptation Constants

Each of the three occupational adaptation elements (person, occupational environment, and interaction) is believed to be consistently influenced by a respective constant (see Figure 11.1). The constant for the person element is viewed as a desire for mastery in occupational situations. This results in an occupational challenge. The constant in the occupational environment element is the demand for mastery from the person in these occupational situations. These two constants interact and result in a press for mastery, which is the constant in the interaction element. The notion of a press for mastery is pervasive in the developmental literature, particularly the writings of Piaget (Flavell, 1963; Piaget & Inhelder, 1969). Before proceeding with a discussion of the occupational adaptation process flow, we must present four essential definitions: occupations, adaptation, and occupational adaptation as both a state and a process of occupational functioning.

Occupations are activities characterized by three properties—active participation, meaning to the person, and a product that is the output of process. The product may be tangible or intangible. *Adaptation* is a change in functional state of the person as a result of the movement toward relative mastery over occupational challenges. *Occupational adaptation (the state)* is a state of competency in occupational functioning toward which human beings aspire. The existence and strength of this state in a person is a function of the extent to which occupational responses have been effective in producing relative mastery over occupational challenges and the extent to which they have successfully generalized in a variety of occupational challenges. *Occupational adaptation (the process)* is the process through which the person and the occupational environment interact when the person is faced with an occupational challenge calling for an occupational response reflecting an experience of relative mastery.

We must also further describe the conceptualization of the person and the occupational environment elements from an occupational adaptation perspective. These conceptualizations are based on the traditional domains in which occupational therapists have operated. This is not to suggest that other ways of viewing persons and environments do not exist. These conceptualizations evolved through an effort to develop a framework that is consistent with occupational adaptation concept as described.

The *person* is viewed as being made up of three systems: sensorimotor, cognitive, and psychosocial.

Assumption: All three systems are present and active in every occupational response. Each of the systems is active to varying degrees, depending on the particular occupational challenge and response. The person systems are uniquely configured for each person as the result of genetic, environmental, and experiential and phenomenological subsystems that contribute to the makeup of each person system.

The *occupational environment* (as distinguished from other environments) is one that calls for an occupational response. Occupational environments are contexts in which occupations occur. These contexts are work, play and leisure, and self-maintenance. Just as the person systems are uniquely configured by subsystems that contribute to their makeup, so are occupational environments. The subsystems that contribute to the nature of a particular occupational environment are physical, social, and cultural. These subsystem designations are based on the work of Spencer (1987). The physical subsystem is made up of nonhuman factors. The social subsystem is made up of the nonhuman factors. The social subsystem consists of the persons who are present and influencing a particular occupational environment through their social predispositions, attitudes, and actions. Both formal and informal social networks are part of this subsystem. The cultural subsystem reflects the ways that the physical and social subsystems come together in serving the mission or purpose of the occupational environment. The cultural subsystem is made up of the procedures, methods, rituals, values, and constraints of the work, play and leisure, or self-maintenance context.

The Process Flow

The following discussion of the occupational adaptation process is intended to reflect the process in a single cycle. As stated earlier, this isolated account is presented for the purpose of clarification and analysis only. It does not represent the complexity of simultaneously occurring events that take place in day-to-day functioning.

The flow of the occupational adaptation process begins with the occupational challenge and proceeds to a perception

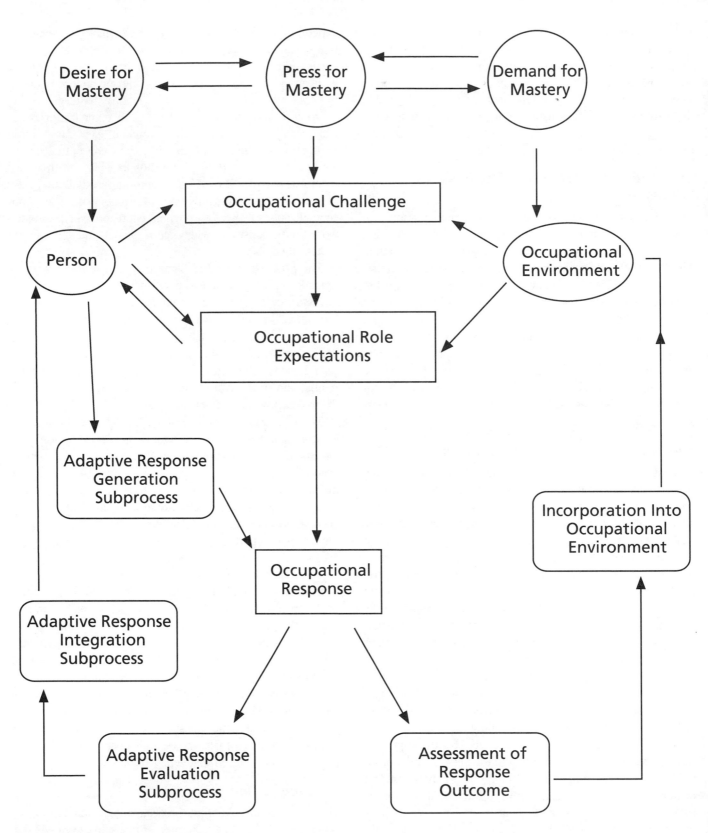

Figure 11.1. Schematic of the occupational adaptation process.

of the internal and external expectations for occupational performance. On the basis of these perceptions, the person generates an occupational response, evaluates the outcome, and integrates feedback from the response for subsequent use. At the same time, evaluation and feedback integration functions are taking place in the occupational environment element. The process is repeated as another occupational challenge emerges.

As shown in Figure 11.1, both the person and the occupational environment contribute to the nature of a particular occupational challenge. Some challenges are the result primarily of personal selection, whereas others are primarily chosen by the occupational environment. Still other reflect mutual selection:

A toddler wants a cookie but sees the cookie jar out of reach on top of a kitchen cabinet. In this self-maintenance occupational environment, the physical subsystem contributes to the challenge through the height of the cabinet and the presence of a chair nearby. A parent in an adjoining room is busy attending to another child (the social subsystem). The cultural subsystem (parental rules) are that cookies are given out of parental discretion.

Each occupational challenge carries with it certain expectations for the person. Occupational challenges occur within roles played by the person. Thus the expectations of a particular challenge will vary as a function not only of the specific environment, but also of a particular role. With the existence of an occupational challenge, expectations for the person's performance also exist. These expectations are an interaction of the person's contribution and that of the occupational environment:

A kindergartner is in her first day of the student role. Her personal history of success experiences (relative mastery) in responding to occupational challenges typical of early childhood development has led her to view herself as a capable person, and her expectation is that she will succeed in school. As she is oriented to the classroom, she perceives that the hanger for her coat is of a height that requires her to stand on tiptoe and that the floor and chairs on which she sits are different from those at home. She further notes that there are some children with whom she has already made friendships; others she already does not like. She finds that she is expected to take care of her materials, to listen to and follow the teacher's directions, and to take turns being leader. Thus the student as well as the physical, social, and cultural subsystems in her occupational environment contribute to expectations of how she will carry out her occupational role of student as she responds to the various occupational challenges with which she will be presented.

Thus far we have described situations in which the person is confronted with an occupational challenge and has perceived a set of occupational role expectations.

Subprocesses of the Occupational Adaptation Framework

Assumption: Because of the desire for mastery, the person intends to produce a response to the occupational challenge that will be adaptive and therefore will lead to mastery. Three subprocesses are available to the person for use: the adaptive response generation subprocess, the adaptive response evaluation subprocess, and the adaptive response integration subprocess. The output of these subprocesses will subsequently affect the state of occupational functioning.

Adaptive Response Generation Subprocess

With the occupational challenge and the role expectations perceived, the person generates the response. This feed-forward portion of the occupational adaptation process is represented by the *adaptive response generation subprocess.* The subprocess is characterized by two components—an adaptive response mechanism that functions to select energy levels, methods (modes of patterns), and behaviors and an adaptation gestalt that configures the output of the adaptive response mechanism into a plan for the sensorimotor, cognitive, and psychosocial involvement. The gestalt becomes manifested as an occupational response. The two components of selection mechanism and gestalt, acting in concert, constitute the adaptive response generation subprocess.

The *adaptive response mechanism* determines the type of adaptation energy to be used and selects from a repertoire of adaptive response modes or patterns and adaptive response behaviors. The occupational adaptation conceptualization of *adaptation energy* was influenced by the work of Selye (1956) as presented in the research on the effects of stress. Selye concluded that unremitting stress led to excessively high usage of the adaptive capacity (adaptation energy) of endocrinological systems in laboratory animals and to premature death. He posited a general adaptation syndrome that described this process in humans. If Selye's conclusions have validity, there is a compelling rationale to assert that one's supply of adaptation energy is limited and that careful management of that supply will enhance occupational functioning.

Assumption: Adaptation energy is a finite although adequate supply of energy present at birth, the bounds of which are idiosyncratic to each person. This assumption implies a need to manage energy wisely and to promote efficient use of what is believed to be a limited resource. The assumption of a bounded energy supply should not be construed to a mean *small.* Instead, it should be interpreted as a supply adequate for a lifetime of adaptation needs if it is not depleted prematurely or injudiciously. Consistent with this assumption, occupational adaptation posits an approach to making better use of this energy that is consonant with fundamental occupational therapy notions regarding the influence of a balanced lifestyle on health and well-being.

Assumption: Adaptation energy operates at two levels of awareness. The primary level is a focused, higher awareness level. Excessive use of primary-level adaptation energy depletes the supply more quickly than use of the secondary level energy. Although this lower awareness level is more sophisticated and creative, it requires less of the energy supply to operate and therefore depletes energy reserve more slowly. The information processing notion of *simultaneous* or *parallel processing* (Posner, 1973) was a major influence on this assumption. A second influence was the literature regarding creative problem solving (Whetton & Cameron, 1984). Creative problem solving involves methods for seeking alternatives to existing approaches ("breaking set") when those approaches fail to produce solutions. Implications for adaptive problem solving are that a person who becomes stuck after working at a primary level may shunt the task to the secondary level for more efficient and effective processing. When returning to the problem at a primary level, the person will be farther along toward a solution with less energy expenditure. The person may, in fact, have identified a solution when the problem-solving task was processed at the secondary level:

A 6th-grade boy must develop a science project from a set of materials that do not seem to have any relationship. He has been thinking about the project without success for several days. Feeling discouraged, he goes to the skating rink and spends a Saturday afternoon playing hockey with his friends. He comes home, looks at the science project materials, and has an idea for his project.

The repertoire of *adaptive response modes* or adaptive patterns (Spencer & Davidson, 1992; Spencer et al., 1992) has developed over the person's experience with occupational challenges. These modes can be classified as existing, modified, and new. This conceptualization is influence by Gilfoyle et al. (1981, 1990).

Assumption: It is common for persons to respond to occupational challenges with existing modes whether or not they are appropriate to the task. Only as these modes fail to produce relative mastery outcomes do modified or new modes develop. Adaptive response behaviors can be characterized by hyperstability (primitive), hypermobility (transitional), and blended mobility and stability (mature). The three classes of behaviors can be identified for all three person systems—sensorimotor, cognitive, and psychosocial. Hyperstabilized or primitive behaviors in the sensorimotor system are seen in frozen postures and nonfluid movement. They are manifested cognitively by rigidity of thinking or in less advanced forms of reasoning such as transductive reasoning. They are seen in the psychosocial system with primitive defense mechanisms that interfere with psychosocial movement. Regardless of the particular person system, hyperstabilized behaviors interfere with adaptive movement.

Assumption: When confronted with an occupational challenge that is beyond the person's current capabilities, engagement in primitive behavior is normative when used as a temporary balance-restoring strategy.

As in the case of hyperstabilized behaviors, hypermobile or transitional behaviors can be seen in all three person systems. Hypermobile behaviors are characterized as unmodulated, unsystematic, frequently random, and uncoordinated. For example, hypermobile sensorimotor behaviors might include high levels of activity without focus or clear goal direction. Hypermobile cognitive behaviors could include high levels of activity without focus or clear goal direction. Hypermobile cognitive behaviors could include faulty attention, that is, attention to irrelevant cues and lack of attention to relevant cues. Problem-solving efforts are active but disorganized. Psychosocial hypermobility can be seen in interpersonally intrusive or presumptive behavior. It can also be seen in psychosocial activity where there is a lack of appreciation for consequences. In general, hypermobility behaviors are action for the sake of action rather than adaptive movement.

Assumption: Hypermobile behaviors offer more promise than hyperstable behaviors because they provide variability. This variability may ultimately produce a response that results in a successful outcome. Behaviors that demonstrate blended mobility and stability (mature behaviors) are most likely to produce occupational response that will promote relative mastery. Such behaviors represent an exploratory strategy that is systematic and solution-oriented while being grounded in realistic perception of the task. Sensorimotor behaviors are reasonably coordinated with a magnitude and direction likely to achieve relative mastery. Cognitive behaviors show attention to relevant cues and more systematic consideration of options. Psychosocial behaviors are neither bound by primitive defenses nor the result of ill-considered impulsivity.

Assumption: Expression of mature behaviors in response to one occupational challenge does not guarantee mature behaviors in subsequent situations. Human beings use all three classes of behaviors as a function of the nature of the challenge, the person's experience with similar challenges, and the difficulty of the challenge as perceived by the person. The adaptive response mechanism offers a structural explanation of the way persons begin to produce a response that is intended to meet an occupational challenge with relative mastery:

A 15-year old girl is learning with her mother's help to make her own clothes. This is the only way she can afford the clothes she would like. She has thus far used fabrics that have no wrong side. After saving her money, she has purchased fabric for a much-desired velveteen jacket. She has been cautioned to wait for assistance before cutting the fabric. She has never cut fabric, without her mother's assistance (existing mode), is afraid to begin, and is angry with her mother because she is not at home (hyperstabilized behavior). She is using a high level of primary energy. Her desire to begin overcomes her reluctance, and she decides to try (new mode). Aware that she must cut the fabric differently but not knowing how, she places the pattern pieces randomly and incorrectly (hypermobile behavior). She continues to use high levels of primary energy. She concludes that the fabric is too expensive to risk. She can achieve part of her desire to begin by studying the pattern instructions, laying the pieces in place, and waiting for her mother to assess her work (modified mode, blended mobility, and stability behavior). She decides to shampoo and roll her hair while she thinks about it some more (secondary energy).

The *adaptation gestalt* reflects the organizational balance of the person systems as it programs the person systems into a plan for carrying out the adaptive response. In a holistic plan, all person systems are present and participating to some degree. Ideally, the plan is appropriately balanced for the occupational challenge; for example, tasks that are primarily cognitive will require more from the cognitive system and less vigorous sensorimotor participation than tasks emphasizing sensorimotor activity. The psychosocial involvement is also involved in cognitive activity and must be incorporated into the gestalt at a level that facilitates cognitive processing rather than interfering with it. Each task associated with responding to an occupational challenge requires a different person systems gestalt:

> A 19-year-old high school graduate is enrolled in a trade school to learn the repair of electronic equipment. He is reasonably well coordinated but experiences difficulty in fine motor tasks when he demonstrates the repair of a unit. His anxiety level is very high (high psychosocial involvement), he is reading the specifications incorrectly (low cognitive involvement), and his hands are shaking significantly (low sensorimotor involvement). Thus, the effect of the excessive psychosocial programming in this instance reflects an imbalance in his adaptation gestalt. The adaptation gestalt is not appropriately balanced to meet this particular occupational challenge.

When the adaptation response generation subprocess has resulted in an occupational response, an evaluation of the effect of that response takes place. Evaluation occurs in both the person and the occupational environment in question.

Adaptive Response Evaluation Subprocess

This subprocess is offered as an explanation of the evaluation phenomenon. It is activated by the person through comparison of the adaptation gestalt to the effect of the occupational response. It is in the evaluation subprocess that the person assesses the experience of relative mastery.

Assumption: Relative mastery is the extent to which the person experiences the occupational response as efficient (use of time and energy), effective (production of the desired result), and satisfying to self and society; that is, it is pleasing not only to the self but also to relevant others as agents of the occupational environment:

> A 32-year-old professional woman is juggling a career and a family composed of a husband and two children (a preschooler and a second grader). The cultural subsystem in this family is that the wife has most of the child-care responsibilities and the husband bears most of the physical maintenance responsibilities. The woman often brings work home to avoid spending long hours at her office that interfere with family time. The present occupational challenge is to prepare a program proposal that she must present to her board of directors the next day. She has previously gathered necessary background information and materials and has thought about her presentation approach. She lacks the final preparation, which she is doing at home. Her evening consists of integrating her parental responsibilities with her professional responsibilities. She alternates among working, mediating sibling disputes, assisting the second grader with homework, reading to the preschooler, doing laundry, making carpool arrangements, and other tasks. After the children are in bed, she concentrates on finalizing her presentation. She discovers in short order that (a) part of her material was left at the office; (b) she needs one more overhead transparency to make her presentation really effective; and (c) her husband forgot to retrieve her favorite presentation attire from the cleaners. She makes as much progress as she can, plans to arrive at the office 2 hours early to complete her presentation, and changes her plan for clothing to a backup choice, which requires that she wash and iron necessary blouse. She does not feel well prepared for her presentation but manages to be persuasive enough to have the proposal approved. She reflects on the outcome of this presentation and concludes that it was inefficient, basically effective, but not satisfying to her in the worker role or to her work environment because her performance was below internal and eternal expectations. It was satisfying to her and others in her self-care environment because her parental role and expectations had been addressed.

Assumption: With evaluation, the occupational event is placed at some point on a continuum from occupational dysadaptation to occupational adaptation with homeostasis as a midpoint. The woman described in the example above might place this event on the occupational adaptation side of the continuum but not far beyond homeostasis. She did manage to have her proposal approved but realized that the overall picture was not consistent with her view of herself as personally and professionally competent.

An occupational environment evaluates an occupational event according to its own performance expectations. These expectations are based on the physical, social, and cultural subsystems and their performance implications. The occupational environment, when integrating the outcome of its evaluation, may be influenced to modify the expectations through relaxation of the expectations or through intensification of them. The expectations may also remain essentially the same.

Adaptive Response Integration Subprocess

At this point in the occupational adaptation process flow, the person has generated the adaptive response, executed it in the occupational response, and evaluated the occupational event in terms of relative mastery and placement on the occupational adaptation continuum. The final subprocess, the adaptive response integration subprocess, now comes into play. Here the learning that has taken place becomes integrated into the person's systems and modifies those systems accordingly.

Assumption: The person's state of occupational functioning is changed as a result of an occupational event. One of the three states of occupational functioning is reinforced as a result: occupational adaptation, homeostasis, or occupational dysadaptation.

> A 40-year-old man has sustained a minor eye injury while engaged in his favorite woodworking hobby because he failed to wear protective glasses. He did not experience relative mastery with occupational event and placed it well on the occupationally dysadaptive side of the continuum. However, learning has resulted in his purchase of good-quality eyewear, which he now wears whenever he engages in woodworking. As a result, the state of occupational functioning that has been reinforced is that of occupational adaptation, although the event itself was assessed as occupationally dysadaptive.

Those persons whose adaptive response evaluation and adaptive response integration subprocess are functioning marginally will experience the greatest difficulty in times of major adaptive transition needs. In contrast, those persons with well-functioning subprocesses with have more efficient, effective, and satisfying responses to major adaptive transition needs.

The adaptive response integration subprocess represents the final step in the occupational adaptation process flow. The cycle begins again with the next occupational challenge. One should remember that the process flow represented in this paper represents a type of freeze-frame approach. In real time, occupational adaptation process will often proceed rapidly and with multiple occupational challenges confronted and addressed simultaneously.

Summary

Occupational adaptation has been presented as a normative process, internal to the person, by which competence in occupational functioning develops. Occupation is seen as an interaction of the person and the occupational environment. Fundamental are the assumptions that (a) the person with sensorimotor, cognitive, and psychosocial systems desires to behave adaptively and masterfully, and (b) the work, play and leisure, or self-care occupational environment (with physical, social, and cultural subsystems) demands and expects adaptation and mastery. Occupational adaptation is further presented as a holistic perspective that requires that all three person

systems are involved in every occupational response. The person uses three subprocesses to generate, evaluate, and integrate the responses to occupational challenges. The person's state of occupational functioning is the cumulative effect of that person's occupational adaptation process activity.

Occupational adaptation, like any concept with therapeutic implications, must be subjected to research. Both basic and applied research are necessary to validate or disconfirm essential ideas. Basic research on the concept of occupational adaptation is proceeding with both qualitative and quantitative methods. One major line of research has been initiated to study the fundamental nature of adaptive transition and what role it plays in community reintegration after cardiovascular accident (Spencer & Davidson, 1992; Spencer et al., 1992). Other research is focused on a longitudinal study of adaptive transition patterns after spinal cord injury (Spencer & Davidson, 1992). The adaptive transitional patterns of well elderly persons are also being investigated. An important aspect of this work is the investigation of cultural and ethnic influences (V. White, personal communication, January 31, 1992). Each of these studies should enhance the understanding of adaptive patterns (modes) used by persons in various circumstances and how such modes are important in the overall occupational adaptation process. The adaptation gestalt construct is the focus of another research effort. This research will attempt to identify patterns of person system involvement in the adaptation gestalt as a function of the occupational role expectations (Burros, 1991).

Applied research studies have also been initiated. Specific practice models have been developed for a variety of therapeutic settings, including acute care, hand rehabilitation, gerontic rehabilitation, and mental health. Outcome studies will be designed to assess the ability and use of occupational adaptation as a model for therapeutic intervention.

Acknowledgments

We acknowledge the impetus, support, and challenging critical comments provided by the doctoral planning committee at Texas Women's University: Grace Gilkeson, EdD, OTR, FAOTA; Adelaide Flower, MA, OTR; Carol Freeman, MA, OTR; Harriet Davidson, MA, OTR; Nancy Griffin, EdD, OTR; Nancy Nashiro, PhD, OTR; Jean Spencer, PhD, OTR (Chair); and Virginia White, PhD, OTR. We also appreciate the input from Lela Llorens, PhD, OTR, FAOTA; Anne Henderson, Phd, OTR, FAOTA; and Kathlyn Reed, PhD, OTR, FAOTA, who critiqued earlier versions of this paper.

References

American Occupational Therapy Association. (1979). The philosophical base of occupational therapy. *American Journal of Occupational Therapy, 33,* 785.

Barris, R., Kielhofner, G., Levine, R., & Neville, A. (1985). Occupation as interaction with the environment. In G. Kielhofner (Ed.), *A model of human occupation: theory and application* (pp. 42–62). Baltimore: Williams & Wilkins.

Bing, R. K. (1981). Eleanor Clarke Slagle Lectureship—1981—Occupational therapy revisited: A paraphrastic journey. *American Journal of Occupational Therapy, 35,* 499–518. Reprinted as Chapter 5.

Breines, E. (1986). *Origins and adaptations: A philosophy of practice.* Lebanon, NJ: Geri-Rehab.

Burros, I. (1991). *Research method proposal for the adaptation gestalt construct of the occupational adaptation frame of reference.* Unpublished professional paper, Texas Woman's University, Denton.

Clark, F. A., Parham, D., Carlson, M. E., Frank, G., Jackson, J., Pierce, D., Wolfe, R. J., & Zemke, R. (1991). Occupational science: Academic innovation in the service of occupational therapy's future. *American Journal of Occupational Therapy, 45,* 300–310.

Clark, P. N. (1979). Human development through occupation: A philosophy and conceptual model for practice, Part 2. *American Journal of Occupational Therapy, 33,* 577–585.

Fidler, G. S. (1981). From crafts to competence. *American Journal of Occupational Therapy, 35,* 567–573.

Fidler, G. S., & Fidler, J. W. (1978). Doing and becoming: Purposeful action and self-actualization. *American Journal of Occupational Therapy, 32,* 305–310. (Reprinted as Chapter 9).

Fine, S. (1991). Resilience and human adaptability: Who rises above adversity? 1990 Eleanor Clarke Slagle Lecture. *American Journal of Occupational Therapy, 45,* 493–503. Reprinted as Chapter 25.

Flavell, J. (1963). *The developmental psychology of Jean Piaget.* Princeton, NJ: Van Nostrand.

Gilfoyle, E. (1984). Eleanor Clarke Slagle Lectureship, 1984: Transformation of a profession. *American Journal of Occupational Therapy, 38,* 575–584.

Gilfoyle, E., Grady, A., & Moore, J. (1981). *Children adapt.* Thorofare, NJ: Slack.

Gilfoyle, E., Grady, A., & Moore, J. (1990). *Children adapt* (2nd ed.). Thorofare, NJ: Slack.

Heater, S. L. (1992). The Issue Is—Specialization or uniformity within the profession? *American Journal of Occupational Therapy, 46,* 172–173.

Johnson, J. A. (1973). The Eleanor Clarke Slagle Lecture—1972—Occupational therapy: A model for the future. *American Journal of Occupational Therapy, 27,* 1–7.

Kielhofner, G. (Ed.). (1985). *A model of human occupation: theory and application.* Baltimore: Williams & Wilkins.

Kielhofner, G., & Burke, J. P. (1985). Components and determinants of human occupation. In G. Kielhofner (Ed.), *A model of human occupation: theory and application* (pp. 12–36). Baltimore: Williams & Wilkins.

King, L. J. (1978). Toward a science of adaptive responses—1978 Eleanor Clarke Slagle Lecture. *American Journal of Occupational Therapy, 32,* 429–437. Reprinted as Chapter 10.

Kleinman, B. L., & Bulkley, B. L. (1982). Sonic implications of a science of adaptive responses. *American Journal of Occupational Therapy, 36,* 15–19.

Lindquist, J. E., Mack, W., & Parham, L. D. (1952). A synthesis of occupational behavior and sensory integration concepts in theory and practice, Part I, theoretical foundations. *American Journal of Occupational Therapy, 36,* 365–374.

Llorens, L. A. (1970). Facilitating growth and development: The promise of occupational therapy, 1969 Eleanor Clarke Slagle Lecture. *American Journal of Occupational Therapy, 24,* 93–101.

Llorens, L. A. (1984). Theoretical conceptualizations of occupational therapy: 1960–1982. *Occupational Therapy in Mental Health, 4*(2), 1–14.

Llorens, L. A. (1990). Foreword. In E. Gilfoyle, A. Grady, & J. Moore (Eds.), *Children adapt* (2nd ed., pp. xi–xii). Thorofare, NJ: Slack.

Meyer, A. (1922). The philosophy of occupational therapy. *Archives of Occupational Therapy, 1,* 1–10. Reprinted as Chapter 2.

Mosey, A. (1968). Recapitulation of ontogenesis: A theory for practice of occupational therapy. *American Journal of Occupational Therapy, 22,* 426–432.

Nelson, D. (1988). Occupation: Form and performance. *American Journal of Occupational Therapy, 42,* 633–641.

Piaget, J., & Inhelder, B. (1969). *The psychology of the child.* New York: Basic.

Posner, M. I. (1973). *Cognition: An introduction.* Glenview, IL: Scott, Foresman.

Reed, K. (1984). *Models of practice in occupational therapy.* Baltimore: Williams & Wilkins.

Reilly, M. (1962). Occupational therapy can be one of great ideas of 20th-century medicine. *American Occupational Therapy, 16,* 1–9. Reprinted as Chapter 8.

Reilly, M. (1969). The educational process. *American Journal of Occupational Therapy, 23,* 299–307.

Research priorities for the 1990s. (1984, November 1). *Occupational Therapy News.* p. 12.

Schultz, S., & Schkade, J. K. (in press). Occupational adaptation: Toward a holistic approach for contemporary practice, Part 2. *American Journal of Occupational Therapy.* Reprinted as Chapter 48.

Selye, H. (1956). *The stress of life.* New York: McGraw-Hill.

Spencer, J. (1987). Environmental assessment strategies. *Topics in Geriatric Rehabilitation, 3,* 35–41.

Spencer, J., & Davidson, H. (1992). A program of research based on the concept of occupational adaptation. In the American Occupational Therapy Foundation's *Proceedings of the Second Annual Research Colloquium on the Concept of Occupation.* Rockville, MD: Author. (Available from the American Occupational Therapy Foundation, 1383 Piccard Drive, PO Box 1725, Rockville, MD 20849-1725.)

Spencer, J., Davidson, H., Cameron, S., Crow, M., Stokes, D., & Giles, J. (1992). *Development and initial evaluation of the Community Adaptive Patterns Assessment.* Submitted for publication.

Texas Woman's University, School of Occupational Therapy. (1989). *Proposal to establish a doctoral program.* Denton, TX: Author.

Whetton, D. A., & Cameron, K. S. (1984). *Developing management skills.* Glenview, IL: Scott, Foresman.

Yerxa, E. (1967). Authentic occupational therapy, 1966 Eleanor Clarke Slagle Lecture. *American Journal of Occupational Therapy, 21,* 1–9.

Yerxa, E. (1989, October 30). What is this thing called occupation? *Advance for Occupational Therapists,* p. 5.

Yerxa, E. (1992). Some implications of occupational therapy's history for its epistemology, values, and relation to medicine. *American Journal of Occupational Therapy, 46,* 79–83.

CHAPTER 12

Why the Profession of Occupational Therapy Will Flourish in the 21st Century

1996 ELEANOR CLARKE SLAGLE LECTURE

DAVID L. NELSON,
PhD, OTR, FAOTA

Welcome to this celebration of our profession! Eighty-eight years ago, a young woman named Eleanor Clarke Slagle attended a course that explored the potentials of occupation as a therapeutic medium (Quiroga, 1995). Convinced of the power of occupation to enhance human life, Slagle went on to help found our profession. In her name, I am honored to present the 35th Eleanor Clarke Slagle Lecture.

Occupational therapy as a profession will flourish over the next century for the same reason that it has flourished over the past century. Real human beings needed therapeutic occupation in the days of Eleanor Clarke Slagle; they need therapeutic occupation in our times; and they will continue to need it beyond our days. Our service of occupational therapy is so sound because the idea of therapeutic occupation is so basic: The human being can attain enhanced health and quality of life by actively doing things that are personally meaningful and purposeful; in other words, through occupation. We are the profession uniquely devoted to helping persons help themselves through their own active efforts.

This chapter was previously published in the *American Journal of Occupational Therapy, 51,* 11–24. Copyright © 1997, American Occupational Therapy Association.

The Need for a Historical Perspective

To appreciate the core of occupational therapy and its importance for human health and quality of life over the next century, we need a macroscopic point of view. I am not referring to the immediate time frame of next year's health legislation in Congress, the year 2000, or even the year 2050. My time frame is approximately the year 2096, a good time for someone, certainly not me, to be summing up the second century of organized occupational therapy just as we are now in a position to sum up its first century.

What the 20th century teaches us is that apparently reliable trends on which people make predictions break down categorically in totally unforeseeable ways. Who in the progressive early 1900s could have predicted the horrors of World War I, the beginning of which was marked by soldiers on horseback and the end of which marked by mechanized trench warfare where combatants were at risk for instant death from distant unseen forces? Who could have predicted the Russian revolution; the worldwide economic depression; or the rise of Fascism, genocide, and World War II with its unprecedented millions of dead, including civilians? Who could have predicted the nuclear terror of my generation or the rise of Pax Americana amidst the sudden, implosive collapse of the Soviet empire?

It will be at least as hard for us to predict the 21st century as it was for the first occupational therapists to predict the 20th century. We can do our best to extrapolate current trends into the future, but the trends that are visible now will break down categorically just as the optimistically progressive trends of 1900 broke down over the past century. We will be surprised. Our descendants will be surprised. I put it this way because this is the larger context from which we should view the profession. Only those things will endure that are both fundamental to human nature and adaptable to a changing world. I believe that one of those things is occupational therapy.

The profession of occupational therapy was founded for one reason: To use occupation as a therapeutic method. The original articles of incorporation of the National Society for the Promotion of Occupational Therapy (1917) clearly stated the purposes of this new organization: "the advancement of occupation as a therapeutic measure," "the study of the effect of occupation on the human being," and "the scientific dispensation of this knowledge" (p. 1). It is important to note that the founders thought of occupation as a method, not just a goal. They believed that occupation could have therapeutic effects on the human being, and they wanted to document these effects through scientific research.

Mores have changed dramatically since the founding of our profession, and they will change in the future in ways that are unimaginable to us now. When we look at photographs of early occupational therapy (e.g., Howe & Schwartzberg, 1986), we see starched uniforms, serious and even stern facial expressions, military-like decorum, and highly structured crafts that required many sessions to complete. Those early photographs reflect a different era of America and of occupational therapy. It was a different culture, and the therapeutic occupations of those times reflected that culture. In like manner, occupational therapists 100 years from now will look back at the archives documenting today's occupational therapy and see quaintness in our dress, our mannerisms, and our speech. Yet, they will recognize their essential connectedness to us. Therapeutic occupations change with the times and with the culture, but the underlying idea of occupation as therapy remains constant.

Defining Occupation

Given our title as *occupational* therapists and given our reason for being, it is ironic that we have not spent much effort in defining occupation. This curious omission has been pointed out by advocates of occupation as therapy (e.g., Christiansen, 1990; Gilfoyle, 1984). Much of my work has focused on the definition of the term *occupation* (Nelson, 1988, 1994, 1996). Occupation is defined as the relationship between an *occupational form* and an *occupational performance* (see Figure 12.1). Occupational performance means the doing. Occupational form means the thing, or the format, that is done. For example, consider the occupation of a boy making potato pancakes (latkes) in December during the Jewish holiday of Hanukkah. His occupational form has physical features, such as the way those potatoes soak up oil and fry crispy on the outside, yet a little soggy on the inside. His occupational form also has sociocultural features, including its connection to his religious heritage and that the chef's hat he wears once belonged to his grandfather. The handle of the frying pan (part of the occupational form) elicits the occupational performance of grasping. Other aspects of his occupational performance include his speech, gaze, smile, and posture.

OCCUPATION

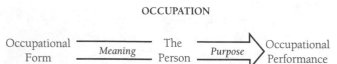

Figure 12.1. Occupation as the meaningful, purposeful occupational performance of a person in the context of an occupational form.

Occupational form and performance are objectively observable; we can see and analyze the boy's environment and movement patterns. But occupation also has subjective, experiential elements that are not directly observable. These subjective aspects of occupation are *meaning* and *purpose*. Meaning is the person's active interpretation of the occupational form. Meaning has to do with making sense of things perceptually; for example, the boy has a basic awareness that he is not too close to the fire. Meaning also has to do with interpreting the symbols in his occupational form, for example, the words of others and the idea of Hanukkah as a playful holiday. Meaning is also affective: The boy is having fun.

After meaning is present (i.e., the person makes sense of the occupational form), then purpose is possible. Purpose is the person's goal orientation; it is what the person wants or intends. For example, what does the boy making latkes want? Does he want to make his sister laugh? Does he want to make tasty latkes that he can douse with applesauce and eat or share with his family? Does he want to participate in a family tradition? At any given moment, a human being typically has multiple purposes—some immediate, such as wanting to hold onto the spatula, and some long term, such as wanting to belong within a family. It is characteristic of an occupational approach to consider both the immediate and the ultimate purposes of the person engaged in occupation.

Occupation influences the world around the person (see Figure 12.2). This influence is called *impact*. The human being is not just a passive respondent who is always under environmental control. The person can affect his or her own future occupational forms. The boy in the example actively changes his occupational form: The latkes are cooked and the kitchen is somewhat of a mess. The cooking occupation sets up the next occupation—eating.

Another dynamic of occupation is that a person can literally change his or her own nature by engaging in occupation. This is called occupational *adaptation*. Active doing, or occupation, can lead to changes in sensorimotor abilities, cognitive abilities, and psychosocial abilities. As we do, so we become. For example, consider the occupation of a healthy 8-month-old boy playing peek-a-boo with his mother. The boy's occupational form includes a piece of cloth first placed over his face and later over his mother's face. By putting the cloth over her own face, the mother gives the boy an opportunity to have an impact through active occupational performance. He is rewarded by her smiling face and her animated talk when the cloth is removed. There is an established game that is present in the occupational form: Our culture makes available to us the game of peek-a-boo. The boy's occupational performance involves complex patterns of reaching, grasping, trunk rotation, posture, laughing, facial expression, and prespeech sounds. This occupational form is meaningful to the boy perceptually, symbolically, and affectively. He is full of purpose as he tries to reestablish eye contact with his mother by attempting to remove the cloth from her face. We can infer multiple sensorimotor adaptations, such as posture, reach, and grasp, but perhaps more importantly, there are cognitive and psychosocial adaptations. For example, the boy is learning the rules of reciprocal play. Additionally, object permanence is being established, and the boy is learning that important things, like mother, do not go away just because they cannot be seen temporarily.

Brief occupations such as these are the dynamics that while interacting with physiological maturation power human development. These brief occupations are nested within higher-level occupations. Indeed, large roles in life are occupations that consist of thousands of brief occupations. For example, consider the reciprocal occupations of a father and daughter on a roller coaster at an amusement park. The man is smiling, however terrified. The girl raises her hands in adolescent bravado. For the girl, the roller-coaster ride is nested within a series of amusement park occupations over many years from the merry-go-round of her toddlerhood to the ultimate goal of going to the amusement park with friends, including boys (no parents needed, thank you). The ride on the roller coaster is also nested within all the summer and family vacations of the girl's life. Given past adaptations, she is ready to go on to new occupations and adventures. From the father's point of view, his daughter is an immediate part of his occupational form, but he would not be there on that screaming roller coaster with his 48-year-old vestibular system if it were not because this occupation is integrally connected to all the occupations of fatherhood. The artful interlocking of successive levels of a person's occupations, bound together by corresponding levels of purpose, connects the present moment to the life span. It would be just as reductionistic to ignore brief moments of occupation as it would be to ignore occupational roles that span decades. We cannot really understand the long-term occupations without understanding the short-term occupations that make them up and vice versa.

Occupational adaptation marks every age of the developing person. Consider the occupations of happy elderly newlyweds singing at a microphone. Their occupational form is the small town wedding celebration. In the basement hall of the American Legion with Old Glory in the background and long wooden tables decorated with balloons and banners, the newlyweds take their turn at the microphone. More than 200 people are present, including new in-laws getting to know each other, townspeople discussing their views on local events, young children racing through the aisles, and teenagers trying to sneak off to the parking lot. The occupational form of marriage means something profound to each marriage partner. Their purposes are both to sing a pretty good tune (pertaining to the immediate occupation) and to start a life together (pertaining to their long-term occupations). Growing beyond their recent roles as

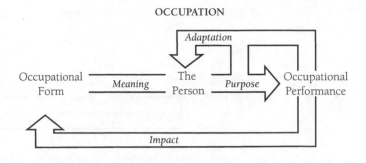

Figure 12.2. Occupation depicted with the occupational dynamics of impact and adaptation.

widow and widower, they adapt to new occupational roles. Occupational forms, the gifts of nature and of culture, not only sustain us, but also challenge us to engage in the continuous adaptations that constitute life.

A Conceptual Framework for Therapeutic Occupation

Given the power of occupation in healthy human development, it makes great sense to have founded a profession on the idea of occupation as therapy. We as a profession believe that a person can affect the quality of his or her life through occupation. We also believe that the person can be helped through this process by another person—an occupational therapist.

At the Medical College of Ohio, we advocate a Conceptual Framework for Therapeutic Occupation (CFTO; see Figure 12.3). The occupational therapist understands the potentials of various occupational forms and is willing to collaborate in synthesizing occupational forms that are meaningful and purposeful to the person. The occupational therapist hopes and predicts that the occupational form will be perceptually, symbolically, and emotionally meaningful to the person; that the occupational form and the meanings the person actively assigns to it will result in a multidimensional set of purposes (when therapy is best, the person is full of purpose); and that the person will engage in a voluntary occupational performance.

Consider the occupation of an older man who has had a stroke on the right side of his brain that led to left hemiparesis, perceptual problems, and left neglect. In the rehabilitation hospital, he was continuously told to do things with his left hand. "Use your left hand." "Look at your left hand." "Watch out for your left hand." But he did not understand why until he hurt it in the spokes of his wheelchair. The man's therapeutic occupational adaptation occurs in the occupational therapy bathroom where he is given a comb in front of a mirror. Here the occupational form is full of salient cues for what is expected. Though there are many cues, the situation as a whole suggests a unified response: It is time to comb hair. The occupational form is immediately meaningful to him, words are really not necessary He knows that the water should be

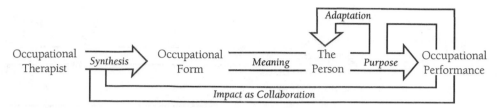

Figure 12.3. A Conceptual Framework for Therapeutic Occupation (for therapeutic adaptation). The occupational therapist collectively synthesizes an occupational form and makes a prediction concerning the person's meaning, purpose, occupational performance, and adaptation.

turned on, so he independently does so. He combs his hair in his accustomed way; that is, his left arm rises in synchrony and coordination with his right hand as he straightens his hair. Embedded in this occupation are left shoulder flexion and external rotation accompanied by elbow flexion with wrist, hand, and finger control. This coordinated pattern of movement takes place outside his visual range, hence guided by proprioceptive input. This occupation is an excellent intervention for his motor control, left neglect, and problems of body scheme. Of course, a single occupation does not result in dramatic gains, yet dramatic gains are impossible without a series of therapeutic occupations like this one.

Sometimes the person's problem is resistant to occupational adaptation. Hence, compensatory occupation is the goal (see Figure 12.4). In compensation, the therapist collaborates with the person in synthesizing an atypical or alternative occupational form. As always, the therapist hopes and predicts that the occupational form will be meaningful and purposeful. However, in compensation, the goal is to have a successful impact as a result of a substitute occupational performance or as a way around the problem.

Consider an older man who is holding his cafeteria tray with a myoelectric prosthesis. The prosthesis is an atypical part of an otherwise typical occupational form. However, the prosthesis has meaning to the man (he knows how to operate it), and it has purpose to him (he wants to operate it). The substitute occupational performance is that he contracts or relaxes the remaining segments of his upper arm muscles to control the device. The comparable impact is that the tray is held while he uses his dominant right hand to scoop the food. This is successful occupational compensation. Frequently, compensation depends on prior adaptations or learning how to use the compensatory device. In this example, the role of the occupational therapist was to help the man learn how to manipulate the prosthetic elbow and wrist joints and how to match his muscle contractions to the electronics of the prosthesis so that objects could be picked up without dropping or crushing them. Hence, adaptations led to successful compensations.

Occupational adaptation and adaptational compensation are different but dynamically interacting processes. Both depend on *occupational synthesis,* or design, of forms that are meaningful and purposeful to the person. Occupational synthesis is what we occupational therapists do for a living. Our specialty is to know about occupational forms in all their variety and to perceive the special capabilities of persons so that a therapeutic match can be made. Sometimes this involves highly naturalistic, everyday forms. But often, there is an element of simulation involved. Consider a boy with cerebral palsy whose occupational form involves virtual reality equipment and a new power wheelchair with an unfamiliar joystick. The meaningfulness and purposefulness of the occupational form to him can be inferred from his occupational performance: He manipulates the joystick in a sustained way and his gaze is set on the feedback device. His occupational adaptation is his learning how to operate the joystick that will control his wheelchair. This will provide him with compensatory mobility in the future.

The virtual reality in this example is "high tech," but we occupational therapists have always used virtual reality, or simulation, whether high tech or low. For example, the occupational therapy kitchen is a treatment area that simulates the homes of many patients while providing the possibility of special safety features and assistive devices. In some cases, the occupational therapy kitchen provides the ideal location; in others, a home visit would be more therapeutic. Much of occupational therapy clinical reasoning and program development depend on judgments about the suitability or unsuitability of simulated versus naturalistic occupational forms. Simulation can involve great creativity and technology, as with virtual reality or electronic work simulators. But the naturalistic occupational forms provided by our culture are the starting points for our ingenuity.

The Flexibility of Therapeutic Occupation: Diverse Models of Practice

Therapeutic occupation, the common core of occupational therapy, is a robust construct capable of accommodating many different approaches to intervention. Mosey (1970) introduced the term *theoretical frame of reference* to describe systematic guidelines for occupational therapy practice that are grounded in theoretical statements about the nature of the

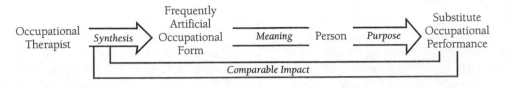

Figure 12.4. A Conceptual Framework for Therapeutic Occupation (for therapeutic compensation). The occupational therapist collaboratively synthesizes an occupational form (often somewhat atypical socioculturally). The resulting occupational performance substitutes for the typical way of doing things but leads to a comparable impact.

person and his or her relations to the world. Others, including Kielhofner (1992), have used the term *conceptual model of practice* to denote the diversity of theory-based approaches to occupational therapy.

My idea of model of practice has two main parts: (a) a theoretical base describing healthy and unhealthy occupation and (b) principles and techniques for occupational syntheses. The theoretical base draws from one or more disciplines. It is a coherent description of the potentials and pitfalls of human occupation, including the nature of the person, the role of occupational forms, the types of meanings and purposes experienced by the person, and the dynamics of successful and unsuccessful occupational performances. Basic research is cited as available. The second part of a model of practice provides principled yet practical guidelines for occupational syntheses that are consistent with the theoretical base. How does the therapist conduct occupational syntheses in the evaluation process? How does the therapist use occupational analysis in the goal-setting process? How does the therapist collaborate with the person in synthesizing occupational forms for adaptation or compensation? Applied research is cited as available.

There currently are many models of practice in occupational therapy. Some are more carefully worked out than others; all are works in progress. Consideration of selected occupational therapy models of practice from the past can enhance appreciation of today's diverse models of practice. In discussing these models, I will apply the same occupational terminology introduced earlier in this article (e.g., *occupational form, occupational performance*) to the diverse ideas expressed by various authors. I believe that this terminology provides a systematic way to compare and contrast occupational therapy models of practice.

Slagle's Habit Training Model of Practice

Slagle (1922) was a proponent of one of the first models of practice in occupational therapy. She drew from many different theoretical sources, including John Dewey's Chicago-school philosophy of pragmatism; William James's psychology of attention; Ruskin's arts-and-crafts movement; the Society of Friends's moral treatment; and Adolph Meyer's ideas about holism, mental hygiene, and use of time. Slagle theorized that

habit reactions largely constitute the lives of most people. The healthy person engages each day in a rich succession of habit occupations—a balance of productive work, self-reliance, rest, and activation of what Slagle called the "play spirit" (p. 16). Underlying all habits is the necessity for attention; indeed attention itself is a habit that can be built.

Unlike the well-organized habits of healthy persons, the habits of persons with mental disorders are deteriorated and disorganized. Attention drifts restlessly and irrelevantly. Neither the joy of productivity nor the joy of play is experienced. Grandiosity on the one hand and passivity on the other are poor substitutes for actual occupation. Given this theoretical base of healthy and unhealthy occupation, what kinds of occupational syntheses are called for in the Slagle model of practice? The main occupational form that Slagle described was a 24-hour-per-day schedule that provided a balance of self-care, physical exercises, work, and play (Kidner, 1930). Specifically noted were instructional periods for self-care (e.g., shoe lacing, teeth cleaning, toileting). Work occupations were to be individually graded from simple to complex. Stimulating music with clearly evident rhythm was recommended to accompany the physical exercises. Moving pictures, folk dancing, storytelling, and simple competitive games rounded out the day. After the basic habit occupations were attained, the patient could progress to the *occupational center,* also called the *curative workshop.* Here patients engaged daily in major crafts or preindustrial groups that required sustained attention over many sessions. The developmental structure of the discharged patient was enhanced by adaptations in the attentional mechanisms and habit reactions.

Baldwin's Model of Practice for the Restoration of Movement

Another early model of practice focused on different aspects of the developmental structure from those focused on by Slagle. Baldwin's (1919) model of practice was designed to restore movement abilities in young soldiers wounded in World War I and drew into occupational therapy concepts from kinesiology, biomechanics, and psychology. He detailed the relationships among various occupational forms and joint range of motion, strength, and endurance. He saw coordination as a high-level skill involving complex series of movements across several joints, and he believed that this high-level skill is inextricably linked to everyday occupations. Movement skill was viewed not just in terms of immediate learning but also in terms of what can be "transferred to another occasion or to other types of movements" (p. 7). Although he focused on the patient's motor abilities, Baldwin also cited "interest, "attention," "initiative," "inspiration," "optimism," and "cheerfulness" (pp. 6-9) as factors that affect the overall quality of the patient's occupations. Baldwin specifically identified social factors that typically inhibited the development of self-responsibility among disabled veterans, including the military's discouragement of the initiative typical of civilian life and the public's misdirected sympathy. Baldwin also considered the patient's intelligence and vocational aptitude when synthesizing therapeutic occupational forms.

Given this view of the person's developmental structure, the main guideline for occupational synthesis was to provide occupational forms that naturalistically challenge the identified problems of range, strength, endurance, and coordination. In Baldwin's (1919) own terms:

> Occupational therapy is based on the principle that the best type of remedial exercise is that which requires a series of specific voluntary movements involved in the ordinary trades and occupations, physical training, play, and the daily routine activities of life. (p. 5)

Occupational forms were analyzed in terms of their typical challenges for the purposes of grading from easy to hard and providing options to different patients, depending on their interests. The end-products, or the impacts, of the work were thought to enhance meaning and purpose; impact also provided direct feedback about the patient's progress. Baldwin favored the use of everyday occupational forms, including, but not restricted to, crafts. The advantages of naturalistic occupational forms were (a) the allowance for personal initiative, (b) the incentives provided for sustained effort, (c) the development of coordination, (d) the transfer of skills, and (e) the opportunity for membership in a social group of fellows working on parallel projects. Baldwin was a strong proponent of research that documented the effects of everyday occupational forms on motor abilities. Much of my research today (e.g., Nelson et al., 1996) investigates principles identified in Baldwin's model of practice that was described more than 75 years ago.

Other Early Models of Practice

It is important to realize that those who helped found the profession espoused different approaches to the use of therapeutic occupation. Each model of practice had its own conceptualization of healthy and unhealthy occupation, and each had its guidelines for synthesizing occupational forms. For example, Tracy (1910) presented a model for bedside occupations for hospitalized patients. The focus was on preventing the negative psychosocial consequences of bedrest so that the patient could be a full partner in his or her medical treatment. Synthesized occupational forms varied depending on the age of the patient, the nature of the disability, and interest. It is interesting to note that all three of the authors cited so far included calisthenics as a potentially valuable type of therapeutic occupation.

A fourth example of an early model of practice in occupational therapy is Hall's work cure for persons with what was then called neurasthenia. In a letter from Hall (1917) to William Rush Dunton, Hall expressed expertise in only one area of what he called therapeutic occupations. Is this not an early expression of specialization by model of practice while remaining cognizant of one's integral link to other models through the organizing framework of therapeutic occupations? Another early letter, however, makes clear that proponents of different models did not always accept or appreciate each other's differences. In a letter to Dunton, Barton (1916), the first president of the National Society for the Promotion of Occupational Therapy and an opponent of Hall's model of practice, expressed the hope that Hall "not put cyanide in our tea" (p. 2) to avenge his exclusion from the deliberations of the charter officers of the society. This facetious remark reflects an ongoing struggle among adherents of different approaches to the use of therapeutic occupation.

The Psychodynamic Model of Practice

How flexible is the concept of therapeutic occupation? Let us consider the change that accompanied American psychology and psychiatry in the 1930s and 1940s when the Freudians advocated a new and controversial view of the person. At that time, Fidler (1948), who has become one of the most influential leaders in the history of the profession, proposed the adoption of a psychodynamic approach in occupational therapy. How do dynamic theorists view the person and occupation, and given this viewpoint, what kinds of occupational forms are synthesized for therapy? In this model of practice, the most important meanings and purposes underlying occupation are unconscious reflections of biological drives. These powerful libidinal and aggressive impulses are theorized to be the products of psychosexual development in early childhood. With maturation, the ego defends itself against anxiety via a variety of unconscious mechanisms, some of which are relatively adaptive and some maladaptive.

Given this view of the occupational structure of the person, the early stages of occupational therapy involved a close, nonthreatening match between carefully selected occupational forms and individual personality. For example, the patient who is unconsciously aggressive is provided with clay to pound or with wood to cut, and the person who is compulsively neat is provided with an occupational form such as weaving, which requires much repetition and involves little waste. Over time, the therapist gradually introduces occupational forms that facilitate relatively mature defense mechanisms.

Humanistic Models of Practice

An illustration of how the profession can accommodate new models of practice can be seen in Fidler's ongoing developments. We can compare and contrast the Fidler and Fidler (1978) article, "Doing and Becoming: Purposeful Action and Self-Actualization," (see Chapter 9) with the Fidler (1948) psychodynamically inspired article we have just discussed. The title of Fidler and Fidler's article indicates the sweeping changes occurring in the 1970s in American psychology and psychiatry. Humanism and existentialism were discovered and adopted as philosophical positions. Instead of conceptualizing the person as conflict laden due to unconscious drives, as in Freudianism, the humanist views the person as a consciously choosing, self-determining being with created values and interests. The person is looked on optimistically in terms of his or her ability to change self or to adapt via occupational performance. Self-actualization is viewed as a person's highest achievement.

The ideas of humanism have strongly influenced many leaders within the profession, including Reilly (1962 [see Chapter 8]), Yerxa (1967), and Kielhofner (1995). Kielhofner's Model of Human Occupation conceptualizes the person's occupations in terms of personal causation, values, interests, internalized roles, and habit patterns in addition to many different skills. Recently influenced by dynamic systems theory, Kielhofner currently emphasizes the volitional processes of attending, experiencing, and choosing, as well as the processes underlying changes in roles and habits. The person is the creator of a life story, a narrative. Given this viewpoint of the person, Kielhofner's occupational forms emphasize naturalistic options and the opportunity for success. Naturalistic options in the occupational form make choices with high levels of symbolic meaning possible. Intrinsic purpose in occupation is most highly valued. The occupational therapist's verbal responsiveness is also a critical aspect of the occupational form because the client and therapist collaboratively synthesize occupational forms. This model of practice has an optimistic viewpoint of the person's ability to adapt and take control of his or her own life, regardless of residual impairments.

The Sensory Integrative Model of Practice

Humanism was not the only great idea influencing Western civilization in the 1960s and 1970s. Another set of ideas with a profound effect on the development of occupational therapy models of practice has come through the advent of neuroscience. Consider Ayres's (1972) sensory integrative model. As with all the other occupational therapy models of practice we have and will discuss, most of the foundational ideas for sensory integration were taken from sources outside occupational

therapy. Ayres conceptualized the person in neurological terms. The first words of her classic book were: "Learning is a function of the brain; learning disorders are assumed to reflect some deviation in neural function" (p. 1). In Ayres's original work, the brain is conceptualized phylogenetically and hierarchically, with higher level cognitive centers in the cerebrum that depend on lower level centers, especially those governing somatosensory input, including vestibular, tactile, and proprioceptive sensation. Ayres hypothesized that many children with learning disorders do not integrate somatosensory input with visual and auditory processing. She also hypothesized that children have an inner drive for mastery in occupation.

Given this conceptualization of the developmental structure, Ayres (1972) created some of the most fascinating occupational forms in the history of our profession: rolling and tumbling forms such as scooter boards and carpeted barrels that support or envelop the child while eliciting somatosensory meanings and bolsters, nets, and swings that hang from the ceiling and provide vestibular input in the occupational context of a game. These occupational forms that elicit whole-body occupational performances are prerequisites to the highly structured occupational forms of education, which assume adequate visual and auditory comprehension necessary for advanced cognition. Like humanistic models of practice, this neurologically based model of practice is optimistic about the person's ability to adapt via occupational performance.

Allen's Model of Cognitive Disabilities

A very different model of practice is also rooted in a neuroscientific conceptualization of the person. In Allen's (1985) model of cognitive disabilities, certain neurological disorders are considered intractable. Although the person's interests and sensorimotor abilities are considered, the focus of this model is on cognitive levels, which are viewed hierarchically from an unresponsive coma state to an advanced level of deductive reasoning. Given that progress from one cognitive level to the next cannot occur through occupation (but might occur in some disorders through the physiological healing of the brain), the emphasis in this model of practice is on evaluation and compensation. What kinds of occupational forms are used? The Allen Cognitive Levels test uses selected crafts (e.g., various forms of leather lacing) to challenge cognition. Crafts are readily recognizable in our society yet are not threatening in the way that many tests are. The materials provide definite structure across space and time, and the craft product (an impact) is an objective indicator of the quality of occupational performance. Hence, the occupational therapist can monitor changes along the cognitive dimension tested as the brain heals. In addition, the occupational therapist can synthesize compensatory occupational forms designed to match the patient's cognitive level. For example, the person who learns only by trial and error will need supervision for safety's sake in everyday occupational forms.

Toglia's Multicontext Approach to Perceptual Cognitive Impairments

An emerging model of practice that posits the adaptational capacity of persons with neurological impairment has been put forward by Toglia (1991). Drawing on knowledge from modern neuropsychology, Toglia hypothesized that metacognition and cognitive processing strategies can be enhanced through a variety of naturalistic occupational forms—a multicontext approach that uses everyday situations as the crux of therapy. Everyday situations from the supermarket to the bus line provide similar cognitive challenges yet provide sufficient variations for generalized learning to occur. Consistent with occupational therapy history, Toglia suggested that the everyday world of our communities can be the occupational therapist's clinic. As we encounter our everyday occupational forms, so we become.

Motor Control and Motor Learning Models of Practice

One of the fascinating events of the past 10 years has been the change in focus within the motor control models of practice. One way of describing this revolution is that theorists and therapists are focusing more on occupational synthesis. In the past, the emphasis was on the patient's physiology and movements (e.g., muscle tone, symmetry, isolation of movement patterns). While remaining sophisticated about the patient's physiology, therapists today are also becoming more sophisticated about the other half of the therapeutic equation: the occupational forms that the patient needs in order to engage in active occupational performance. Symbolic of this revolution is Trombly's (1995) Eleanor Clarke Slagle Lecture in which she cited research, theory, and practical experience in favor of occupational forms that are meaningful and purposeful to the person (see Chapter 16). Whether guided by the neurodevelopmental model of practice (Levit, 1995) or a contemporary approach drawing from dynamic systems theory (Mathiowetz & Haugen, 1995), therapists today are synthesizing naturalistic occupational forms of work, play, and self-care, with the active collaboration of the patient in the choice of those forms.

Selected Other Models of Practice

To suggest the tremendous range of potential applications of our core concept of therapeutic occupation, I will briefly mention a few of the many other occupational therapy models of practice. Occupational models of practice are being refined for persons with Alzheimer's disease and their caregivers (American Occupational Therapy Association [AOTA], 1994), and some models are being developed for the handwriting problems of schoolchildren (Amundson, 1992). Als's conceptualization of the premature infant is compatible with an occupational therapy model of practice geared toward both the emerging occupations of the infant and the occupations of parents (Vergara, 1993). A fourth area in which the special skills of occupational therapists are needed is hospice care (Pizzi, 1993), where meaningful and purposeful occupation is a reflection of the value placed on human life. Although these are but a few samples of the many areas in which therapeutic occupation is contributing to quality of life, my experience tells me that creative occupational therapy practitioners will continue to develop new models of practice that meet the real needs of real persons for therapeutic occupations—therapy by doing.

Beyond Direct Service Models

A commitment to the use of occupation as the method of occupational therapy does not commit us to direct service models as opposed to educational models or consultative models. The occupational therapist can play an essential and cost-effective role in the collaborative synthesis of occupational forms, even though the therapist will not be physically present when the person engages in the occupational form. Because the therapist has expertise in occupational forms—their physical and sociocultural complexity—he or she can advise the daughter of a woman with Alzheimer's disease about least restrictive environments (AOTA, 1994), a teacher or nurse about proper positioning (Dunn & Campbell, 1991), or the foreman of a workstation with a high rate of carpal tunnel syndrome about repetitive trauma disorders (AOTA, 1992). Such advice is a collaborative occupational synthesis. For the same reason, a truly occupational model of practice is used when the therapist advises patients with diseases of the hand about occupations in the home, at work, and at play (Kasch, 1990).

Occupational Therapy Models of Practice in the Future

What future roles will the occupational therapist play in the health-care system? Readers 100 years from now will no doubt be aware of occupational therapy practice that we cannot dream of today. And I am sure that there will be an occupational therapy reader 100 years from today because of the fundamental power of occupation and its adaptability to new circumstances.

Independent Living Movement

One current trend that may well grow in the future is the independent living movement in which persons with disabilities see themselves as consumers of health-care services. As consumers, they make decisions about their lives and rehabilitation with professional help but without the authoritarianism that sometimes accompanies the medical model. This approach is in tune with the principles of occupational therapy (AOTA, 1993; Yerxa, 1994). The problem is not to be thought of as lying in the consumers (their developmental structures), but in the everyday occupational forms they encounter, such as barriers to restaurants, workstations, and fields of play. Given this philosophy, the occupational therapist emphasizes collaborative occupational synthesis and compensatory strategies from ramps to robots and from social acceptance to political power. The consumer who takes control of his or her life within an insensitive society could not do better than to have an occupational therapist as an advocate.

Technology

The independent living movement dovetails nicely with another identifiable trend for the future: new technologies that promote successful and personally satisfying occupation. As Mann and Lane (1991) pointed out, the occupational therapist "can—and should—be the professional who takes responsibility for assembling the appropriate assistive technology team" (p. 26). The occupational therapist has the knowledge and experience to take a leadership role in working with the consumer in making the best possible match between the multiple factors in technologically oriented occupational forms and the multiple capacities of the consumer's developmental structure. We need to think of assistive devices as parts of the occupational forms that have meaning and purpose to the person, not as mechanical extensions of a mechanical person.

Wellness Models of Practice

Another trend is the move toward an increased emphasis on wellness, health promotion, and disease prevention. With the brave new world of capitation, managed care, primary care, efficacy, and efficiency, the health-care system may at last get serious about wellness. Wellness pays. Nothing could be more positive for the profession of occupational therapy. Theorists within the profession have been preparing us for the advent of a health-care system that emphasizes health as opposed to illness (Johnson, 1986; Rosenfeld, 1993). Occupational therapists working with persons who already have disabilities have long emphasized the importance of healthy occupational profiles and disease prevention to their patients, even though those efforts have not always been reimbursable. The wellness models of practice are in place and only await general funding.

Models for Public Health

Another role for the future of occupational therapy is in the solution of some of our society's chronic social and public health problems, such as drugs, violence, unprepared motherhood, unemployment, and homelessness. A problem of special interest for me is the development of an occupational therapy model of practice for the prevention of childhood obesity. Obesity has devastating lifelong consequences, with sensorimotor, cognitive, and psychosocial impairments and impoverished occupational patterns. A comprehensive model of therapeutic occupation needs to be tested for this major problem of public health. Occupational therapy leaders, such as Baum (1991), have found ways to fund occupational models of practice, even in a pessimistic sociopolitical environment where social programs are mistrusted. I call this America's 1990s

regression to the social Darwinism of the 1890s. But sooner or later, the profession of Eleanor Clarke Slagle will provide occupational models of practice for homeless people with schizophrenia and occupational models of practice for persons in so-called nursing homes. (Let us call them homes for therapeutic occupation!) The mark of a great civilization is not its store of consumer goods but the meaningfulness and purposefulness of the everyday occupations of all its citizens.

Hospital-Based Models

I believe that occupational therapy will continue to play an essential role in the acute-care hospital and in other medically related facilities from the rehabilitation hospital, to subacute sites, to extended-care facilities, to the facilities of the future. It is true that hospitals are downsizing, and patients are being discharged more and more quickly. It is also true that the ideal health-care system of the future will promote wellness as its highest goal. Nevertheless, people will continue to become ill; they will continue to go to the hospital, however downsized, for acute care. Many of these people will continue to need an occupational approach at one or more stages of their illness and recovery (Torrance, 1993). With increasing technology and quicker discharge, the need for therapeutic occupation increases, not decreases. Occupational therapists will be needed to work with patients in problem-solving self-care occupations amidst the constraints of the tubes, monitors, and fixators; to activate patients at risk because of the deleterious effects of bedrest; to help patients and caregivers plan realistically for what the patients will do and for how the patients will live and care for themselves after discharge but before healing; and to assess patients' quality of life before and after hospitalization.

For an example of the importance of therapeutic occupation in an acute-care setting, consider a 5-month-old girl born with a neuromuscular disease of unknown etiology. The disease is characterized by the total absence of many of the proximal muscles, including those responsible for respiration. Picture her with multiple intubations for respiration and nutrition and with life-support monitors. The occupational therapist carefully removes her from the crib and bounces her gently while talking to her in high-pitched, rhythmical tones. In response to this occupational form, the infant's adaptations are to learn to use the muscles controlling her vocal cords as she imitates the therapist; to learn to use the remaining muscles in her left arm as she grabs the therapist's keys; and most of all, to begin to learn that she too has a legitimate place in the human family. The therapist next places a piece of cloth playfully over the child's face, as in our prior example of the importance of peek-a-boo in healthy development. Like the healthy infant, this baby also removes the cloth and laughs. Despite the high-technology setting, this baby also needs to encounter the occupational form of peek-a-boo in order to develop a sense of self and a sense of other. I believe that occupational models of practice will be needed for the acute-care hospital for patients at all points on the life span as much as they are needed for community-based care.

Models of Practice and the Great Ideas of the 20th Century

Therapeutic occupation is a remarkably powerful yet flexible idea. Consider all the different philosophies and branches of science that have washed across the 20th century and that have become the theoretical bases of occupational therapy models of practice: the moral treatment initiated by members of the Society of Friends; the arts-and-crafts movement initiated by the British socialist Ruskin as an antidote to the negative effects of industrialism; the philosophy of pragmatism; the holistic medicine of Meyer; James's psychology of attention; principles of kinesiology and biomechanics; the dynamic theories of the Freudians, neo-Freudians, and ego psychologists; behaviorism and learning theory; developmental theory; humanism and existentialism; neuroscience and neuropsychology and their many schools; efficacy and competency theory; systems theory and dynamic systems theory; the social psychology of groups; ecological psychology; motor learning and motor control theories; cultural anthropology and ethnography; and narrative analysis. (For discussion of these topics and their influences on occupational therapy models of practice, see Breines, 1995; Christiansen & Baum, 1991; Kielhofner, 1992.) These schools of thought reflect many of the majestic ideas in the intellectual history of the 20th century. Even though every one of them originated from outside the occupational therapy profession, each has contributed essential theory to our models of practice. Across every model of practice, the core of therapeutic occupational synthesis can be identified: form, meaning, purpose, performance, evaluation, adaptation, and compensation. This robust flexibility at the core of our profession is the basis for my saying that therapeutic occupation will flourish in the 21st century.

Two Recommendations

Research

My first recommendation is research—research for occupational therapists conducted by occupational therapists and those who understand occupation as therapy. Our primary focus should be to examine the power of occupation as therapy. My vision for the 21st century is that occupational therapy will take its rightful place among the major professions in our society. The powers and complexities of occupation justify the sanctioning of a major profession. This will be especially true if the society of our descendants devotes increased attention to the actual occupations of daily life, to the meanings of life, and to the qualities of existence. Should there not be a Nobel prize for occupational therapy?

But to be a major force in research, we must examine our basic principles in highly systematic ways—ways that are accepted by the larger research community. If we do not

examine the great ideas of occupational therapy, some other group will. For decades, occupational therapists have used common, everyday occupational forms and hands-on doing to enhance what Dunton (1945) called the "mental processes of reasoning or judgment or remembering" (p. 11). Recently cognitive researchers, mainly psychologists, have developed a body of knowledge about the effects of subject-performed tasks (SPTs) on human cognition (e.g., Backman, 1985). The basic idea of SPTs is that hands-on doing, with its added sensory input and opportunity for feedback, is a greater cognitive stimulant than demonstration or other teaching techniques that do not involve hands-on experience. The problem is that the cognitive psychologists pursuing this line of research have not cited occupational therapy authors, who have advocated this principle since the beginning of the profession. Our problem here is that we have not done the research necessary to establish our special expertise in the area of hands-on doing, or occupation.

In like manner, we are only beginning to do the research that establishes our expertise in the area of occupationally embedded movement. Carr and Shepherd (1987) have written eloquently and at length about how everyday situations, such as a glass of water, can elicit therapeutic patterns of movement, such as a good hand path, in patients with neuromuscular disorders. However, these authors, neither of whom are occupational therapists, do not once cite occupational therapy or its history of using everyday occupational forms to promote therapeutic patterns of movement.

My point is that persons from other professions are coming late to the table and claiming credit for some of the great ideas of occupational therapy These ideas deserve the most careful philosophical and scientific scrutiny As occupational therapists, we need to own these ideas while enlightening other disciplines as to their usefulness.

Equally needed are basic research examining the nature of occupation and applied research examining models of practice. Academically respected quantitative and qualitative research methodologies should be used. One approach to research in occupational therapy is what I have called the experimental analysis of therapeutic occupation (Nelson, 1993). Here, occupational forms are contrasted to each other in terms of participants' occupational performances, impacts, adaptations, or reported meanings and purposes. A different approach, termed *occupational science,* has been proposed by Clark et al. (1991). These authors have recommended qualitative methods for studying the multiple dimensions of naturally occurring occupations. It is critical that the profession encourage different types of inquiry at least until there is a broad consensus that a single type of inquiry satisfactorily deals with all the research problems of the profession. I predict that no such consensus will ever develop.

To support the research enterprise, funding will be essential. A specific goal of the AOTA should be the establishment of study sections specifically devoted to occupational therapy research in federal grants management agencies, as is the case with nursing. Only those with considerable knowledge of the profession of occupational therapy can appreciate and nurture the full potential of occupational therapy knowledge. In the interim, the AOTA and the American Occupational Therapy Foundation, which is to say all of us, should make special efforts to support research that is specifically occupational. A priority is the further development of doctoral programs devoted to the development of occupational therapy knowledge. More than anything else, a sound doctoral program is a socialization experience toward a new identity as a scholar in a particular field. Although scholars of diverse backgrounds have made great contributions to knowledge in occupational therapy, a true profession requires the intense engagement at its core, which is expected in doctoral programs devoted to the development of occupational therapy knowledge.

Occupation, Not the A Word

My second recommendation is for all of us to embrace and own the idea of occupation as therapy. Wilma West (1984) not only urged us to use the term *occupation* with pride, but also wrote that the term *occupation* "is infinitely more expressive and encompassing than 'purposeful activity'" (p. 22). Nothing is more important to this profession. We are called *occupational* therapists, and the essence of our profession is the use of occupation as a therapeutic method. In contrast, the term *activity* lacks the connotation of intentionality. The term *activity* denotes motion, for example, *volcanic activity, molecular activity,* and *gastric activity,* not occupation that is replete with meaning and purpose.

Another major problem with the use of the word *activity* is that we confuse the public. Slagle (1922) wrote about her "system of occupational analysis" (p. 16). Neither she nor we need to say activity analysis. If the essence of our profession is activity, then why are we not called activity therapists (Darnell & Heater, 1994)? We need to be able to explain occupation and things occupational to many different audiences from fellow professionals to payers, from persons with immaturities to persons with various disabilities, from journalists to the arts media, and from our students to ourselves. If we explain clearly that occupational therapy involves the active doing of things (occupations) for the sake of enhanced health, our public relations problem and our so-called identity problem will disappear immediately. We have the power to influence standard usage. There are more than 50,000 of us in this country and tens of thousands more in other English-speaking countries. If we are clear and forthright about the essential nature of our service—the use of occupation as method—then society will accommodate us. New words and new professions come into the language system all the time. This problem is entirely within our control.

Over time—keep in mind that we are talking about the next century—society and fellow health care professionals will adopt new terms that are related to what we call occupation. For example, since the founding of occupational therapy the terms *rehabilitation, allied health, deinstitutionalization, function, functional outcomes,* and *inclusion* have come into favor for very good reasons. As occupational therapists, we need to promote the good that is represented in these terms. Yet, we need to resist the temptation to redefine ourselves with every new trend in health care. We are not rehabilitation professionals—we are occupational therapists whose mission is much more basic and enduring than even the rehabilitation movement. Nor are we functional therapists or functional outcomes therapists. The term *function* is reflective of the mechanistic, business-oriented climate of these times. Automobiles function, toasters function, and livers function. Human occupation is far richer than the term *function* can possibly connote. In our era, every health professional from the surgeon to the dietitian must document so-called functional outcomes if they are going to be paid. What makes us unique is not that we document functional outcomes but that we use occupation as the method to achieve positive outcomes.

We are occupational therapists, and we are aptly named. Indeed we are named more aptly than many of the professions with which we work. We need to explain this clearly and assertively to the world, but a good starting point will be to explain this clearly and assertively to each other. Occupation as therapy is inclusive enough for all the occupational therapy models of practice. There is no reason to be afraid of cyanide in the tea.

Conclusion

To summarize, occupation is a powerful force in the development of the human being. The essence of our profession is the use of occupation as therapy whose core flexibly accommodates various past, present, and future models of practice drawn from historically important theories that originated outside the profession. I proposed a CFTO, including definitions of occupational form, occupational performance, developmental structure, meaning, purpose, impact, adaptation, compensation, and occupational synthesis. The CFTO highlights the core of therapeutic occupation across diverse models of practice and provides an analytical method for comparing and contrasting different models of practice.

Basic and applied research that investigate principles of occupation are necessary not only for the standing of the profession among other disciplines, but also for the sake of our own integrity. The ultimate statement of pride and confidence in the profession will be the full adoption of the term *occupation* in the language of the profession, with each occupational therapist taking personal responsibility for explaining to the world why we are called occupational therapists.

Acknowledgments

I thank all the colleagues, students, and loved ones who have contributed so much to the content and spirit of this lecture. My children, my sisters, and my mother say that they enjoyed being with us at the lecture.

This lecture included audiovisual themes that cannot be reproduced in article format; therefore, this article makes use of examples and explanations suited for the printed page as opposed to the lecture stage.

References

Allen, C. K. (1985). *Occupational therapy for psychiatric diseases: Measurement and management of cognitive disabilities.* Boston: Little, Brown.

American Occupational Therapy Association. (1992). Statement: occupational therapy services in work practice. *American Journal of Occupational Therapy, 46,* 1086–1088.

American Occupational Therapy Association. (1993). Statement: The role of occupational therapy in the independent living movement. *American Journal of Occupational Therapy, 47,* 1079–1080.

American Occupational Therapy Association. (1994). Statement: Occupational therapy services for persons with Alzheimer's disease and other dementias. *American Journal of Occupational Therapy, 48,* 1029–1031.

Amundson, S. J. C. (1992). Handwriting: Evaluation and intervention in school settings. In J. Case-Smith & C. Pehoski (Eds.), *Development of hand skills in the child* (pp. 63–78). Rockville, MD: American Occupational Therapy Association.

Ayres, A. J. (1972). *Sensory integration and learning disorders.* Los Angeles: Western Psychological Services.

Backman, L. (1985). Further evidence for the lack of adult age differences on free recall of subject-performed tasks: The importance of motor action. *Human Learning, 3(1),* 53–69.

Baldwin, B. T. (1919). *Occupational therapy applied to restoration of movement.* Washington, DC: Commanding Officer and Surgeon General of the Army, Walter Reed General Hospital.

Barton, G. E. (1916, December 20). *Letter to W. R. Dunton, Jr.* (Available from the American Occupational Therapy Archives, Box 1, File 12, Wilma L. West Library, 4720 Montgomery Lane, PO Box 31220, Bethesda, MD 20824-1220)

Baum, C. (1991). Professional issues in a changing environment. In C. Christiansen & C. Baum (Eds.), *Occupational therapy: Overcoming human performance deficits* (pp. 804–817). Thorofare, NJ: Slack

Breines, E. B. (1995). Understanding 'occupation' as the founders did. *British Journal of Occupational Therapy, 58,* 458–460.

Carr, J. H., & Shepherd, R. B. (1987). A motor learning model for rehabilitation. In J. H. Carr & R. B. Shepherd (Eds.), *Movement science: Foundations for physical therapy in rehabilitation.* Rockville, MD: Aspen.

Christiansen, C. (1990). The perils of plurality. *Occupational Therapy Journal of Research, 10,* 259–265.

Christiansen, C., & Baum, C. (Eds.). (1991). *Occupational therapy: Overcoming human performance deficits.* Thorofare, NJ: Slack

Clark, F. A., Parham, D., Carlson, M. E., Frank, G., Jackson, J., Pierce, D., Wolfe, R. J., & Zemke, R. (1991). Occupational science: Academic innovation in the service of occupational therapy's future. *American Journal of Occupational Therapy, 45,* 300–310.

Darnell, J. L., & Heater, S. L. (1994). The Issue Is—Occupational therapist or activity therapist—Which do you choose to be? *American Journal of Occupational Therapy, 48,* 467–468.

Dunn, W., & Campbell, P. H. (1991). Designing pediatric service provision. In W. Dunn (Ed.), *Pediatric occupational therapy* (pp. 139–159). Thorofare, NJ: Slack.

Dunton, W. R., Jr. (1945). *Prescribing occupational therapy* (2nd ed). Springfield, IL: Charles C Thomas.

Fidler, G. S. (1948). Psychological evaluation of occupational therapy activities. *American Journal of Occupational Therapy, 2,* 284–287.

Fidler, G. S., & Fidler, J. W. (1978). Doing and becoming: Purposeful action and self-actualization. *American Journal of Occupational Therapy, 32,* 305–310. Reprinted as Chapter 9.

Gilfoyle, E. M. (1984). Eleanor Clarke Slagle Lectureship, 1984: Transformation of a profession. *American Journal of Occupational Therapy, 38,* 575–584.

Hall, H. J. (1917, February 23). *Letter to W. R. Dunton, Jr.* (Available from the American Occupational Therapy Archives, Box 2, File 15, Wilma L. West Library, 4720 Montgomery Lane, PO Box 31220, Bethesda, MD 20824-1220)

Howe, M. C., & Schwartzberg, S. L. (1986). *A functional approach to group work in occupational therapy.* Philadelphia: Lippincott.

Johnson, J. A. (1986). *Wellness: A context for living.* Thorofare, NJ: Slack.

Kasch, M. (1990). Acute hand injuries. In L. W. Pedretti & B. Zoltan (Eds.), *Occupational therapy practice skills for physical dysfunction* (pp. 477–506). St. Louis, MO: Mosby.

Kidner, T. B. (1930). *Occupational therapy: The science of prescribed work for invalids.* Stuttgart, Germany: Kohlhammer.

Kielhofner, G. (1992). *Conceptual foundations of occupational therapy.* Philadelphia: F. A. Davis.

Kielhofner, G. (1995). *A model of human occupation: Theory and application* (2nd ed.). Baltimore: Williams & Wilkins.

Levit, K. (1995). Neurodevelopmental (Bobath) treatment. In C. A. Trombly (Ed.), *Occupational therapy for physical dysfunction* (4th ed., pp. 446–462). Baltimore: Williams & Wilkins.

Mann, W. C., & Lane, J. P. (1991). *Assistive technology for persons with disabilities: The role of occupational therapy.* Rockville, MD: American Occupational Therapy Association.

Mathiowetz, V., & Haugen, J. B. (1995). Evaluation of motor behavior: Traditional and contemporary views. In C. A. Trombly (Ed.), *Occupational therapy for physical dysfunction* (4th ed., pp. 157–185). Baltimore: Williams & Wilkins.

Mosey, A. C. (1970). *Three frames of reference for mental health.* Thorofare, NJ: Slack.

National Society for the Promotion of Occupational Therapy. (1917, March 15). *Certificate of Incorporation of the National Society for the Promotion of Occupational Therapy.* (Incorporated in the District of Columbia and notarized by James A. Rolfe in Clifton Springs, New York)

Nelson, D. L. (1988). Occupation: Form and performance. *American Journal of Occupational Therapy, 42,* 633–641.

Nelson, D. L. (1993, June). The experimental analysis of therapeutic occupation. *Developmental Disabilities Special Interest Section Newsletter, 16(2),* 7–8.

Nelson, D. L. (1994). Occupational form, occupational performance, and therapeutic occupation. In C. B. Royeen (Ed.), *AOTA self-study series: The practice of the future: Putting occupation back into therapy, lesson 2* (pp. 9–48). Rockville, MD: American Occupational Therapy Association.

Nelson, D. L. (1996). Therapeutic occupation: A definition. *American Journal of Occupational Therapy, 50,* 775–782.

Nelson, D. L., Konosky, K., Fleharty, K., Webb, R., Newer, K., Hazboun, V. P., Fontane, C., & Licht, B. (1996). The effects of an occupationally embedded exercise on bilaterally assisted supination in persons with hemiplegia. *American Journal of Occupational Therapy, 50,* 639–646.

Pizzi, M. (1993). Environments of care: Hospice. In H. L. Hopkins & H. D. Smith (Eds.), *Willard and Spackman's occupational therapy* (8th ed., pp. 853–864). Philadelphia: Lippincott.

Quiroga, V. A. M. (1995). *Occupational therapy: The first 30 years, 1900–1930.* Bethesda, MD: American Occupational Therapy Association.

Reilly, M. (1962). Occupational therapy can be one of the great ideas of 20th-century medicine, Eleanor Clarke Slagle Lecture. *American Journal of Occupational Therapy, 16,* 1–9. Reprinted as Chapter 8.

Rosenfeld, M. S. (1993). *Wellness and lifestyle renewal.* Rockville, MD: American Occupational Therapy Association.

Slagle, E. C. (1922). Training aides for mental patients. *Archives of Occupational Therapy, 1,* 11–17.

Toglia, J. P. (1991). Generalization of treatment: A multicontext approach to cognitive perceptual impairment in adults with brain injury. *American Journal of Occupational Therapy, 45,* 505–516.

Torrance, M. (1993). Acute care occupational therapy. In H. L. Hopkins & H. D. Smith (Eds.), *Willard and Spackman's occupational therapy* (8th ed., pp. 771–783). Philadelphia: Lippincott.

Tracy, S. E. (1910). *Studies in invalid occupation: A manual for nurses and attendants.* Boston: Whitcomb & Barrows.

Trombly, C. A. (1995). Occupation: Purposefulness and meaningfulness as therapeutic mechanisms. 1995 Eleanor Clarke Slagle Lecture. *American Journal of Occupational Therapy, 49,* 960–972. Reprinted as Chapter 16.

Vergara, E. (1993). *Foundations for practice in the neonatal intensive care unit and early intervention: A self-guided practice manual.* Rockville, MD: American Occupational Therapy Association.

West, W. L. (1984). A reaffirmed philosophy and practice of occupational therapy for the 1980s. *American Journal of Occupational Therapy, 38,* 15–23.

Yerxa, E. J. (1967). Authentic occupational therapy, 1966 Eleanor Clark Slagle Lecture. *American Journal of Occupational Therapy, 21,* 1–9.

Yerxa, E. J. (1994). Dreams, dilemmas, and decisions for occupational therapy practice in a new millennium: An American perspective. *American Journal of Occupational Therapy, 48,* 586–589.

CHAPTER 13

Lifestyle Performance:
From Profile to Conceptual Model

GAIL S. FIDLER, OTR, FAOTA

The Life Style Performance Model evolved from the Life Style Performance Profile originally conceptualized in the mid-1970s (Fidler, 1982, 1988b). The purpose of the profile was to identify and then relate the activity-focused aspects of daily living to the fundamental biopsychosocial needs of the human being. The profile represented an effort to discern the personal and interpersonal dimensions of daily living activities, articulate more clearly the relevance of such activities to each person's quality of living and, thus, avoid the ambiguities and stereotypes inherent in the generalized terms of work, play, leisure, and self-care.

The profile proposed that a lifestyle that sustains health and enables life satisfaction includes a culturally relevant, age-specific harmony among four activity domains. These domains were identified as those occupations or activities concerned with self-care and self-maintenance and personally referenced pleasure and intrinsic gratification, societal contribution, and interpersonal engagement. The term *daily living activities*, within the context of the profile, refers to all of the activities that compose a person's daily life, not simply self-care. The Life Style Performance Profile provided the format for obtaining and organizing information that reflected a patient's personal and socially determined interests, skills, and limitations in each domain (see Appendix G for the profile). The profile was expected to provide both the patient and therapist with a view of the patient's characteristic activity patterns of daily living and the harmony–disharmony or balance among them and then serve as a guide in defining occupational therapy interventions (Fidler, 1982, 1988b).

Exploration of the viability of these tenets, first in mental health practice and then in geriatrics and physical disabilities, led to the development of the model presented in this chapter. The questions that guided this development included

- Can activity patterns of daily living be explained in more personally meaningful terms than is possible in the traditional general categories of self-care, leisure, play, and work?
- Is it possible to explicitly describe and evaluate the relationship between a person's patterns of daily living and his or her quality of living?
- Can a format be designed that would facilitate arriving at more personally relevant treatment goals or interventions?
- What are the environmental elements that notably affect patterns of activity?
- Are such themes applicable to occupational therapy practice?

During maturation and socialization, each person develops a configuration of activity patterns that can be characterized as a life-style. These patterns of doing—these ways of engaging and being engaged in doing—emerge through the interplay of the person's intrinsic needs, desires, capacities, and unique expectations of the environmental context of living (Fidler & Fidler, 1978 [see Chapter 9], 1983). An overall sense of satisfaction and well-being depends on the sum of positive benefits derived from such interplay. A resulting sense of harmony, or life-style balance, then emerges from the congregate experiences of active engagement, gratifying emotional expression, evidence of personal achievement, societal contribution, positive response from significant others, and membership in a chosen group or groups. Development and maintenance of a repertoire of activity patterns that enable and support such experiences are essential to the quality of a person's life.

The existing strengths and limitations of a person's sensory processing, motor patterns, cognition, psychologic structure, and interpersonal perceptions are important variables in the development of activity patterns. Any impediment to these systems causes a temporary or long-lasting disruption of a person's physical integrity, psychologic structure, or interpersonal orientation. Likewise, achievement of a state of harmony or a sense of well-being is frequently disrupted or made unlikely when the external world presents barriers or limitations on either the development or the maintenance of positive activity configurations.

Occupational therapy practitioners are called upon to intervene when one or more domains of a person's life-style performance are deemed to be deficient to a degree that produces distress in that person or in those who are part of that person's social matrix. Thus, in addition to addressing a specific disability or dysfunction, establishing outcome objectives for occupational therapy requires working with a person to develop, or redevelop, a life-style pattern of activities that will enhance the quality of his or her way of living. In some instances, this process means establishing a more satisfactory life-style. In others, it is restoring a previously achieved life-style.

Function of the Model

Thus, building on the descriptive outline of the Life Style Performance Profile (see Appendix G), a practice model has evolved that offers a framework for defining individually relevant, wellness-generating, as well as remedial goals of occupational therapy interventions. The Life Style Performance Model provides a way of describing and examining the interacting, multiple dimensions of doing and living from an organized, holistic framework applicable to all ages, cultures, and persons. The configuration of the model makes it possible to identify the relationship of activity patterns to the pursuit of a person's unique needs to achieve a personal identity, to know self as a contributing member of society, and, thus, to confirm self as acceptably human. It provides a focus for study and practice of occupational therapy as a many faceted process of enabling a way of living that is intrinsically gratifying as well as socially contributory. The model extends the parameters of occupational therapy beyond reducing disability, shifts the focus of practice beyond the realm of our traditional daily living activities, and establishes as a top priority the development of an individualized life-style profile as both a first step in defining intervention goals and an outcome focus of practice.

A fundamental concept on which the model is based is that dysfunction and remedial interventions are definable only from the perspective of what constitutes a given person's state of health and well-being. The model therefore stresses an initial focus on individual interests, capacities, and customary patterns of daily living as the basis for defining and prioritizing any intervention. An inherent belief underlying the model is that quality of life is the single most important theme in human performance. Wellness and a sense of well-being are understood as a state of being that is optimally satisfying to self and to significant others. It is hypothesized that such satisfaction is gleaned from personally and socially relevant activities that focus on and maximize individual strengths, capacities, and interests. Most important is the concept that intrinsic motivation is elicited and sustained when there is congruence between the characteristics of an activity and the biopsychosocial characteristics of the person. An important function of the model is to facilitate such a match.

Although themes related to the holistic perspective of occupational therapy have repeatedly appeared in the literature, they are frequently an elusive goal for practice. There is a marked gap in efforts to specifically connect intervention activities with the quality of a person's way of living and, thus, with what holds personal meaning and is intrinsically gratifying for that person. Current practice environments, issues of reimbursement, and reduced lengths of stay all exert pressures that most often result in reductionistic practices. The need for a model or format that encourages and readily fosters a broader, more holistic perspective for our study and practice is evident.

Christiansen (1993) cautioned that we need to understand and consider the meaning of disability and the intervention process from the patient's point of view. Addressing the focus of assessments, he called for approaches that "better [reflect] the context (including the environment) of the patient's everyday life" (p. 258). "Without this context," Christiansen asserted, "interpretations of the meaning of assessment data will have limited validity and may lead to irrelevant goals for intervention" (p. 258).

Likewise, Trombly (1993) suggested that an initial "inquiry into role competency and meaningfulness would clarify the purpose of occupational therapy" (p. 253). She advised that "those roles that are important to the person, especially those that he or she engaged in prior to illness or trauma, become the focus of inquiry" (p. 253). Trombly conjectured that if a discrepancy among the past, present, and future role performance becomes evident, it serves to clarify the purpose and relevance of an occupational therapy intervention. More recently, Trombly (1995) (see Chapter 16) has expressed the need to find more personally relevant terms to describe what we have traditionally generalized as work, play, and leisure occupations. She has cited studies that ranked the importance given to daily living activities by patients and therapists. Such studies, she reported, indicated that occupational therapists were not always good judges of what is important to the patient.

Although the importance of the environment has become an increasing focus in occupational therapy literature, there are marked lags in the application of such perspectives to practice. Addressing issues of person–environment interactions, Kielhofner (1993) cautioned that the evaluation criteria we traditionally have used may "unwittingly rob individuals of both voice and power to determine the direction of their own lives" (p. 249). He stated that too frequently we assume that the problem resides in the person, and, thus, "issues [such as] environment or workplace conditions and incentives are largely ignored" (p. 249). In a similar context, Law (1993) emphasized the critical importance of understanding and relating a person to the environmental context. She stated that most occupational therapy assessments, for example, do not consider the patient's culture and roles or the environment in which he or she lives. Furthermore, she contended that occupational therapists "do not routinely consider balance in occupational performance over a day or across a person's life-style" (p. 235).

Underlying Principles of the Model

The Life Style Performance Model facilitates the practitioner's address of these concerns, bridging the gaps among current practice, our philosophic constructs of holism, personal relevance, and quality of life. Traditionally, the goal of occupational therapy is to improve function and enhance the ability of a person to perform. The question now is: To what end? The Life Style Performance Model proposes that the outcome of occupational therapy intervention is to enable a way of living that allows persons to develop and bring into harmony a configuration of daily living activities that have personal, social, and cultural relevance for them and their significant others.

The frames of reference underlying the Life Style Performance Model incorporate the basic principles and philosophic constructs of the occupational therapy profession. The relationship of a sense of well-being, self-fulfillment, and adaptation to active participation in one's world is one principle that has been explored throughout the history of occupational therapy as well as within other disciplines. The innate drive to explore and cope with one's environment is viewed as essential to human existence and adaptation not only as a means of survival, but most importantly as enabling personal and social development (Erickson, 1950; Fidler & Fidler, 1978 [see Chapter 9], 1983; White, 1971).

In occupational therapy, this perspective has led to the construct that the drive toward action, when channeled into personally and socially relevant occupational behavior, is fundamental to the development of a positive self-regard, coping, adaptation, and health (Fidler & Fidler, 1978 [see Chapter 9], 1983; White, 1971). Additionally, the profession has embraced the concept that the sense of competence and self-agency gained through occupational performance carried out in relation to others encompasses social role learning and societal contribution (Fidler, 1988a; Fidler & Fidler [see Chapter 9], 1978, 1983; Kielhofner, 1985; Reilly, 1971). From these perspectives, purposeful activity, as used in the Life Style Performance Model, means a personally referenced action that is concerned with testing a skill, ability, or level of competence or an activity that is focused on clarifying a relationship and discerning the nature of one's relatedness to another person (or persons) or to one's nonhuman world (Fidler & Fidler [see Chapter 9], 1978). In a related sense, an *activity* is understood to reference any act or series of interconnected acts requiring the active engagement of a person's mind and body in the pursuit of a discernible outcome. In the current construction of this model, *purposeful activity* and *occupation* are viewed as interchangeable terms.

I have offered several hypotheses regarding the motivational, developmental, sociocultural, and restorative potential of occupations and activities (Fidler, 1981). I suggested that

- Mastery and competence in those activities that are valued and given priority in one's society or social group have greater meaning in defining one's social efficacy than competence in activities that carry less social significance
- A total activity and each of its elements have symbolic as well as reality-based meanings that notably affect individual experience and motivation
- Mastery and competence are more readily achieved and the sense of personal pleasure and intrinsic gratification is more intense in those activities that are most closely matched to one's neurobiologic and psychologic structure
- Competence and achievement are most readily seen and verified in the end-product or outcome of an activity, thus, the ability to do, to overcome, and to achieve becomes obvious to self and others.

These factors all play a major role in eliciting motivation and engagement and in defining personal meaning to the person.

Becoming part of human society has been described as the process that transforms primitive actions into behaviors that both satisfy personal needs and contribute to the development of society (Fidler & Fidler, 1978 [see Chapter 9], 1983; Moore & Anderson, 1968). The importance of doing—of occupational performance—in this transformation and in the consequent configuration of an individual pattern of daily living activities is a fundamental focus of occupational therapy and of the Life Style Performance Model. Understanding the relevance of occupational performance—of purposeful activity—to human development, health restoration, and the quality of life involves complex mixes of anthropologic, historic, physical, psychologic, sociocultural, political, and economic variables. It is from these multidimensional dynamics that the scientific base of occupational therapy must seek to explain how doing or being occupied relates to the dimensions of physical integrity, psychologic structure, and social relatedness. The scientific base, furthermore, must seek to explain how such relationships then generate a person's ability to fulfill personally relevant activities and roles of everyday living in ways that are mutually satisfying to self and significant others. The Life Style Performance Model offers a framework for the study, practice, and testing of such undertakings.

Because the model is concerned with identifying and describing a contextual configuration of daily living activities that optimize individual wellness and quality of life, and from which idiosyncratic dysfunction can be defined, two major components are addressed. First, the model seeks to identify and describe the nature and critical doing elements of an environment that supports and fosters achievement of a satisfying, productive life-style. Second, it proposes a way of looking at and categorizing those activity clusters, their contextual dynamics, and interrelationships that compose the critical activities of everyday living.

The Environmental Context of the Model

The importance of the interaction between persons and environment has been studied in many professions. Literature in the fields of anthropology, psychology, sociology, psychiatry, and, more recently, occupational therapy provide a rich resource for conceptualizing the impact of both the human and nonhuman environment on human behavior. The era of Moral Treatment, for example, demonstrated the importance of the environment in shaping the behavior of persons with mental illness (e.g., Stanton & Schwartz, 1934). During the period of renewed interest in this philosophy, numerous studies were undertaken to define and create a treatment environment that would maximize the therapeutic potential of the mental hospital (Greenblatt, York, & Brown, 1955; Jones, 1953; Stanton & Schwartz, 1934). Moos's (1974) evaluation of treatment environments further influenced the design of institutions; Goffman's (1963) work contributed considerably to understanding the influence of institutions on behavior; Searles' (1960) offered impressive evidence of the role of the nonhuman environment both in health and in mental illness; and Wolfensberger's (1972) initiatives in describing the normalizing aspects of an environment transformed institutions and homes for persons with developmental disabilities. Anthropologic studies added dimension to the growing awareness of the dynamics of an environmental context in shaping patterns of behavior and, in turn, communicating values, customs, and beliefs (Benedict, 1934; Geertz, 1973; Langor, 1942; Mead, 1964; Schwedor & LeVine, 1986).

Environmental psychology has complemented the people focus of studies through research on the impact of the physical environment on behavior (Holohan, 1986; Prohansky, Ittleson, & Rivlin, 1970). Building on the seminal work of Dewey (1916), numerous studies evaluated the impact of the environmental context on learning (Bruner, 1962, 1989; Jarvis, 1992; Moos, 1979). Moore and Anderson (1968) identified environmental elements that they considered essential for maximizing individual potential for social role learning and personal development. More recently, Fidler and Bristow

(1992) described the structure and process of creating a total institutional environment that maximized the competence of both staff members and patients. Similarly, in the field of management, there is a plethora of studies attesting to the influence of environmental factors on workers' performance and productivity (Bennis, 1989; Bolman & Deal, 1984; Hersey & Blanchard, 1982; Kantor, 1983; Senge, 1990).

Looking at the phenomenon of environmental congruence, Murray (1938) explored the relationship between persons and environment, coining the phrase *environmental press*. Kahana (1975) offered an intriguing perspective in her study of the necessary fit between environmental settings and individual preferences of older persons. Yarrow, Rubinstein, and Pederson (1975) explored the congruence of environment and infant cognitive and motivational development. Fidler and Bristow's (1992) Community-Family-Individual Resource Format addressed the issue of synergy between persons and environment by looking at a number of factors and characteristics of the family or family surrogate, the community, and the person. In this context, the relationship between a person's skills, limitations, and expectations and the characteristics, values, and expectations of the family and community is seen as defining the dimensions of congruence between the person and the environment.

The influence of the environment on performance has been a consideration in occupational therapy for some time (Barris, 1982; Dunning, 1972; Kiernet, 1990; Law, 1991; Llorenz, 1984; Parent, 1978). Further evidence of the extent to which the profession considers the environment to be a critical dynamic can be found in Christiansen and Baum (1991). In this publication, several authors explore the influence of public policy and the social, cultural, and physical environments on performance. Most recently, the challenging work of Dunn, Brown, and McGuigan (1994) (see Chapter 17) offered a framework for investigating the relationship between environment and performance. These authors considered such study essential to the development of a broadened perspective and studied approach to occupational therapy intervention.

Relationship of Self, Doing, and the Environment

The Life Style Performance Model presents a view of a person's environment as comprising the interactive dimensions of interpersonal, societal, cultural, physical, and temporal elements in which that person lives and acts. It contends that an environment can maximize individual performance to the extent that it includes, emphasizes, and ensures, by the nature of its structure, its operations and interpersonal practices, those doing experiences that optimize the following:

*   *Autonomy*—to be self-determining, gain a sense of being in control of one's life, and be as self-dependent as personal needs and capacities define
*   *Individuality*—to be self-differentiating, see and know one's uniqueness, verify the existence and identity of

oneself, distinguish self from others, and confirm the entitlement of one's interests, skills, and differences
- *Affiliation*—to have evidence of belonging; be part of a dyad, group, or cluster; have associations with others; and know interdependence
- *Volition*—to have alternatives, access to sufficient information, and latitude to make and act on one's choice
- *Consensual validation*—to have feedback from one's activity and from other persons that verify one's perceptions and reality and to be part of reciprocal exchanges that clarify and acknowledge one's contributions and actions
- *Predictability*—to discern and evaluate cause and effect, be able to predict, limit ambiguity and chanciness, give order to one's world, and experience the comfort of predictables
- *Self-efficacy*—to have evidence of one's competence, of being able to cope and manage one's everyday life, of being a cause, and of making things happen
- *Adventure*—to seek and try out the new, the unknown; to explore; to look beyond the here and now; and to discover, experiment, and dare to risk
- *Accommodation*—to be free from physical and mental harm and to function in an environment that is responsive to individual capabilities while compensating for individual limitations
- *Reflection*—to have respite from activity, ponder on the meaning of things, and review and contemplate recent and past events.

These elements have relevance to hospitals, institutions, and residential settings as well as to living arrangements within the home and community. They provide a base from which guidelines can be developed for evaluating, creating, adapting, or managing a living or treatment environment. For example, although the positive impact of a hospital or nursing home environment on recovery is theoretically acknowledged, many institutional environments fail in this regard. Too frequently, the occupational therapist's singular focus on the patient's functional deficit precludes attention to the context in which services are being provided. The efficacy of intervention strategies is maximized when the occupational therapy process includes activity designed to create and enhance the elements of the environment as described in the previous paragraph. The life-style of any one person is a multidimensional, dynamic phenomenon created by the inner self shaping and being shaped by the unique characteristics and dynamics of that person's human and nonhuman external world.

Structure of the Model: Four Domains

As stated earlier, achievement of social efficacy, personal satisfaction, and a way of living that is more satisfying than not to self and significant others relates directly to achieving and maintaining an age-specific, culturally relevant synergy among four primary domains of performance:

- Taking care of one's self and maintaining one's self in as self-dependent a manner as personal needs and capacities determine
- Pursuing personally referenced pleasure, enjoyment, and intrinsic gratification
- Contributing to the need fulfillment and welfare of others
- Developing and sustaining reciprocal interpersonal relationships.

These domains form the structure of a Life Style Performance Profile (Fidler, 1982) (see Appendix G) and are seen as composing an occupational or activity repertoire that encompasses the patterns of daily living activity.

Because these domains represent the principal focus of daily living activities, they are viewed as relevant throughout the life span. What may be described for any one person, at any point in time, as an adequate, relevant, and balanced lifestyle depends on the age, cultural orientation, and neurobiologic endowment of that person as well as the values and resources of that person's social matrix. Performance skills and life-style expectations change with different stages of life and vary in accordance with cultural and social norms.

Although each of the activity domains is characterized as having a distinct purpose, the domains are not independent entities. Rather, they are interrelated parts of a life-style, a way of living that has meaning in defining and expressing a personal and social identity and a self-regard.

The Domain of Self-Care and Self-Maintenance

Self-care is both an expression of self and a self–other link. Our commercial world and its advertising offer ample testimony to the importance of dressing, grooming, and related activities as both social and personal statements. The unique dress codes that regularly emerge among each new generation of adolescents, ethnic dress and grooming styles, the arrangement and decoration of living spaces, food choices, and cooking methods are only a few examples of how such activities are part of one's theme of personal identity as well as a link with others. Christiansen (1994) stated that self-care activity has importance as a "foundation for enabling a shared existence with others and as part of the continuing search to understand who we are and to make meaning of our existence" (p. i).

The care and maintenance of self in as self-reliant a manner as possible also addresses the universal human need to achieve and sustain a sense of autonomy. For example, the child's need to experience self as increasingly independent frequently is first manifested in dressing and other personal care activities. The need to express one's uniqueness, one's differentiation from others, is a strong force that is expressed during these early years in many self-care and self-maintenance activities. Only later is there a beginning discovery that the autonomously unique self is not lost in affiliation, but rather strengthened by it. Thus, one's ways and manner of caring for and maintaining the self play out the paradox of the need for individuality and affiliation with others. "Self care is part of an intimate, ego invested portrait, a powerful narrative of one's self and one's relationship with others" (Fidler, 1994, p. v).

The Domain of Intrinsic Gratification

Engagement in an activity for the sheer joy of the experience is an essential part of defining self and one's personal worth. Developing an activity repertoire with no strings attached except for the fun and enjoyment in the doing is one important dimension of getting to know self; developing an awareness of one's skills, capacities, ability to commit; caring about self; and discerning one's capacity for joy and pleasure. Csikszentmihalyi (1990) observed that "when we act for the sake of action rather than for ulterior motives, we learn to become more than what we are" (p. 42). Fidler and Fidler (1978 [see Chapter 9], 1983) called attention to the importance of the sense of pleasure, the joy of doing, and being a cause. To acknowledge and legitimize one's uniquely personal interests and needs is an important theme in shaping the quality of one's way of living. Only as we know the dimensions of self can we come to know another; only as we are able to freely care about and treasure self can we care for and value another. We are reminded by Devereaux (1984) that "the ability to develop caring relationships with others is in direct proportion to the ability to care for self" (p. 795). Searles (1960) pointed out that it is "through engagement with one's non-human world that we become more deeply human, more committed to our status as a human being" (p. 89). This domain is therefore concerned with exploring patterns of activity related to the pursuit of one's personal interests, pleasure, and joy.

The Domain of Social Contribution

Contributing to the need fulfillment and welfare of others is another critical dimension in the evolution of a mutually satisfying way of living. The identity of self as a productive member of society is molded through social and economic contributions to one's society. Engagement in those activities that are necessary for the survival and well-being of a group in society enables a sense of self as essential and verifies such contribution. The child's delight in helping with household tasks and assisting with adult chores and the stature of volunteerism or community service in American society are testimony to the importance of activities that embody social contributions and adult responsibility (Fidler & Fidler, 1978 [see Chapter 9]; Kelly & Godbey, 1992; Mosey, 1986). The dimensions of a person's social roles, such as wage earner, homemaker, student, family member, and volunteer, are themes to be explored within this domain.

The Domain of Interpersonal Relatedness

Perhaps one of the most simple and fundamental constructs about human behavior is that one becomes human through association with humans. A sense of personal acceptability, of human and interpersonal worthiness, emerges through encounters and relationships with other human beings. The importance of mutually satisfying interpersonal relationships in all aspects of living has been studied and verified well beyond question. It is axiomatic to acknowledge that a repertoire of activity patterns focused on development and maintenance of reciprocal human relationships is essential to achieving a life-style that is mutually satisfying to self and to those with whom one shares living. Verifying one's humanness and connectedness with others is a critical theme of daily living, and engagement in reciprocal human relationships is a principal dynamic in that process. Jarvis (1992) stated that "only in reciprocal relationships can being and becoming be maximized" (p. 112). The description of the nature and extent of a person's activity repertoire that enables and sustains reciprocal patterns of relating, enabling friendships, intimacy, family relationships, and peer and group affiliations are all important components of the focus of this domain.

Application of the Model

A first priority in application is coming to know and understand what is or has been a person's characteristic way of living and how that way reflects or does not reflect personal and social needs and expectations. It must again be emphasized that any deficit or dysfunction can be defined, understood, and allocated meaning only within the context of a person's life-style needs and expectations. An occupational therapy plan for either prevention or remediation therefore includes

- The development of a Life Style Performance Profile that reflects what is and has been the person's typical life-style activity pattern
- A description of current performance skill strengths and limitations relative to each of the four activity domains
- The performance expectations and preferences in each of these domains in relation to self-interest and the needs of significant others
- The balance or imbalance of harmony among the domains within the context of age and social and cultural norms and interests
- The dimensions of the family and community's social and cultural values, performance expectations, interests, economic resources and limitations, and environmental resources and constraints
- Evaluation of those components of performance that notably affect performance
- Individual characteristics, interests, values, and attitudes that shape performance
- The design of a recommended Life Style Performance Profile that reflects current capacities, interests, and needs relative to each activity domain.

An occupational therapy intervention plan for either prevention or remediation is designed in response to five fundamental questions. First, what does the person need to be able to do—that is, what performance skills are essential and at what level? Second, what is the person able to do—that is, what are the strengths, capacities, and interests of the person and of the external environment that can be used to enable successful intervention? Third, what is the person unable to do—which internal and external factors interfere, and how should these be addressed? Fourth, what interventions must be undertaken and in what order of priority so that the person will be able to move toward fulfilling relevant life-style performance needs and expectations? Finally, what are the characteristics and patterns of activity and the environment that will enhance the quality of this person's living?

Summary

The use of personally relevant activity, of occupation, in the development and restoration of performance skills has been the hallmark of occupational therapy since its inception. It is this focus that distinguishes the profession from other disciplines in the health or behavioral sciences. Questions surrounding the relationship of occupation to performance in daily living, coping and adaptation and the meaning and quality of life have consistently been a principal concern of practice and inquiry in occupational therapy. More recently, society's interest in wellness and in defining health as more than the absence of disease has far-reaching importance for occupational therapy. Thus, the questions for occupational therapy have broadened and become more complex. Further exploration and critique of the Life Style Performance Model should lead to our ability to raise increasingly sophisticated questions and pursue such inquiry.

Acknowledgment

This article was developed during the author's tenure as Scholar-in-Residence, Occupational Therapy Program, College Misericordia, Dallas, Pennsylvania.

References

Barris, R. (1982). Environmental interactions: An extension of the model of occupation. *American Journal of Occupational Therapy, 36,* 637–644.

Benedict, R. (1934). *Patterns of culture.* Boston: Houghton Mifflin.

Bennis, W. (1989). *Why leaders can't lead.* San Francisco: Jossey-Bass.

Bolman, L. G., & Deal, T. E. (1984). *Modern approaches to understanding and managing organizations.* San Francisco: Jossey-Bass.

Bruner, J. S. (1962). *On knowing: Essays for the left hand.* Cambridge, MA: Harvard University Press.

Bruner, J. S. (1989). *Acts of meaning.* Cambridge, MA: Harvard University Press.

Christiansen, C. (1993). The Issue Is—Continuing challenges of functional assessment in rehabilitation: Recommended changes. *American Journal of Occupational Therapy, 47,* 258–259.

Christiansen, C. (Ed.). (1994). *Ways of living: Self care strategies for special needs.* Rockville, MD: American Occupational Therapy Association.

Christiansen, C., & Baum, C. (Eds.). (1991). *Occupational therapy: Overcoming human performance deficits.* Thorofare, NJ: Slack.

Csikszentmihalyi, M. (1990). *Flow: The psychology of optimal experience.* New York: Harper & Row.

Devereaux, E. B. (1984). Occupational therapy's challenge: The caring relationship. *American Journal of Occupational Therapy, 38,* 791–798.

Dewey, J. (1916). *Democracy and education.* New York: Free Press of Glencoe.

Dunn, W., Brown, C., & McGuigan, A. (1994). The ecology of human performance: A framework for considering the effect of context. *American Journal of Occupational Therapy, 48,* 595–607. Reprinted as Chapter 17.

Dunning, H. (1972). Environmental occupational therapy. *American Journal of Occupational Therapy, 26,* 292–298.

Erickson, E. (1950). *Childhood and society.* New York: Norton.

Fidler, G. S. (1981). From crafts to competence. *American Journal of Occupational Therapy, 35,* 567–573.

Fidler, G. S. (1982). The life style performance profile: An organizing frame. In B. Hemphill (Ed.), *The evaluation process in occupational therapy.* Thorofare, NJ: Slack.

Fidler, G. S. (1988a). *Examining the knowledge base of occupational therapy.* Unpublished manuscript, American Occupational Therapy Foundation.

Fidler, G. S. (1988b). *The life style performance profile. In focus: Skills of assessment and treatment.* Rockville, MD: American Occupational Therapy Association.

Fidler, G. S. (1994). Foreword. In C. Christiansen (Ed.), *Ways of living: Self-care strategies for special needs* (pp. v–vi). Bethesda, MD: American Occupational Therapy Association.

Fidler, G. S., & Bristow, B. (1992). *Recapturing competence: A systems change for geropsychiatric care.* New York: Springer.

Fidler, G. S., & Fidler, J. W. (1978). Doing and becoming: Purposeful action and self-actualization. *American Journal of Occupational Therapy, 32,* 305–310. Reprinted as Chapter 9.

Fidler, G. S., & Fidler, J. W. (1983). Doing and becoming: The occupational experience. In G. Kielhofner (Ed.), *Health through occupation: Theory and practice in occupational therapy.* Philadelphia: F. A. Davis.

Geertz, C. (1973). *Interpretation of culture.* New York: Basic.

Goffman, E. (1963). *Asylums.* New York: Doubleday.

Greenblatt, H. M., York, R. H., & Brown, E. I. (1955). *From custodial to therapeutic care in mental hospitals.* New York: Russell Sage Foundation.

Hersey, P., & Blanchard, K. (1982). *Management of organizational behavior.* Englewood Cliffs, NJ: Prentice Hall.

Holohan, C. J. (1986). Environmental psychology. *Annual Review of Psychology, 37,* 381–407.

Jarvis, P. (1992). *Paradoxes of learning.* San Francisco: Jossey-Bass.

Jones, M. (1953). *The therapeutic community.* New York: Basic.

Kahana, E. (1975). Matching environment to the needs of the aged—A conceptual schema. In J. F. Gubrium (Ed.), *Communities and environmental policy.* Springfield, IL: Charles C Thomas.

Kantor, R. (1983). *The change masters.* New York: Simon & Schuster.

Kelly, J. K., & Godbey, G. (1992). *Sociology of leisure.* State College, PA: Venture.

Kielhofner, G. (1985). *A model of human occupation: Theory and application.* Baltimore: Williams & Wilkins.

Kielhofner, G. (1993). The Issue Is—Functional assessment: Toward a dialectical view of person–environment relations. *American Journal of Occupational Therapy, 47,* 248–251.

Kiernet, J. M. (1990). Considering the environment. In C. B. Royeen (Ed.), *AOTA Self Study Series: Assessing Function* (Lesson 6). Rockville, MD: American Occupational Therapy Association.

Langor, S. (1942). *Philosophy in a new key.* Cambridge, MA: Harvard University Press.

Law, M. (1991). The Muriel Driver Lecture: The environment: A focus for occupational therapy. *Canadian Journal of Occupational Therapy, 58,* 171–180.

Law, M. (1993). Evaluating activities of daily living: Directions for the future. *American Journal of Occupational Therapy, 47*, 233–237.

Llorenz, L. A. (1984). Changing balance: environment and individual. *American Journal of Occupational Therapy, 38*, 29–34.

Mead, M. (1964). *Continuities in cultural evolution.* New Haven, CT: Yale University Press.

Moore, O. K., & Anderson, A. R. (1968). *Some principles for the design of clarifying educational environments.* Pittsburgh: University of Pittsburgh, Research and Development Center.

Moos, R. H. (1974). *Evaluating treatment environments: A social ecological approach.* New York: Wiley.

Moos, R. H. (1979). *Evaluating educational environments: Procedures, methods, findings and policy implications.* San Francisco: Jossey-Bass.

Mosey, A. (1986). *Psychosocial components of occupational therapy.* New York: Raven.

Murray, H. R. (1938). *Explorations in personality.* New York: Oxford University Press.

Parent, L. H. (1978). Effects of a low-stimulus environment on behavior. *American Journal of Occupational Therapy, 32*, 19–25.

Prohansky, H. M., Ittleson, W. H., & Rivlin, L. G. (Eds.). (1970). *Man and his physical settings.* New York: Holt, Rinehart & Winston.

Reilly, M. (1971). The modernization of occupational therapy. *American Journal of Occupational Therapy, 25*, 243–246.

Searles, H. (1960). *The non-human environment.* New York: International Universities Press.

Senge, P. (1990). *The fifth discipline.* New York: Doubleday.

Schwedor, R. A., & LeVine, R. A. (Eds.). (1986). *Culture theory and essays on mind, self and emotion.* New York: Cambridge University Press.

Stanton, A. H., & Schwartz, M. S. (1934). *The mental hospital.* New York: Basic.

Trombly, C. (1993). The Issue Is—Anticipating the future: Assessment of occupational function. *American Journal of Occupational Therapy, 47*, 253–257.

Trombly, C. (1995). Occupation: Purposefulness and meaningfulness as therapeutic mechanisms—1995 Eleanor Clarke Slagle Lecture. *American Journal of Occupational Therapy, 49*, 960–972. Reprinted as Chapter 16.

White, R. W. (1971). The urge towards competence. *American Journal of Occupational Therapy, 25*, 271–274.

Wolfensberger, W. (1972). *The principles of normalization in human services.* Toronto: National Institute of Mental Retardation.

Yarrow, L. G., Rubinstein, J. L., & Pedersen, F. A. (1975). *Infant environment: Early cognitive and motivational development.* New York: Wiley.

CHAPTER 14

Uniting Practice and Theory in an Occupational Framework

1998 ELEANOR CLARKE SLAGLE LECTURE

ANNE G. FISHER, ScD, OTR

The roots of this lecture began years ago in the late 1960s, when I was an occupational therapy student. Occupational therapy was in the midst of what Kielhofner (1997) has termed the *mechanistic paradigm.* My physical dysfunction theory courses had a heavy focus on exercise and the neurophysiologic approaches of the Bobaths (Semans, 1967), Brunnstrom (1970), and especially Margaret Rood (as interpreted by Stockmeyer, 1967). While on my affiliations, I was guided by some of my supervisors to use weight lifting to strengthen the wrist extensors of clients with spinal cord injury. During my psychiatric affiliation, I was encouraged to give clients with unconscious hostility opportunities to act out their emotions through metal hammering. All of these clients did these activities whether they wanted to or not.

But there was another side to my early experiences. I remember vividly working with a young man who had quadriplegia as a result of a spinal cord injury. He was fascinated with electronics, and he wanted to explore the possibilities of being able to build electronic devices. I went to the local electronics store and bought a do-it-yourself radio kit filled with resistors, capacitors, circuit boards, and tiny nuts and bolts. I also bought solder and a soldering iron. Together, we worked on developing strategies he could use to manage the tools and materials. He had no active movement in his fingers, but because he wore wrist-driven flexor hinge splints, he was able to hold on to many of the objects. When he had difficulty, we worked together to create alternative strategies.

He built the radio, not I. And in the end, he had a radio he could listen to; he had the satisfaction that comes from accomplishment; and he had learned that he could develop for himself compensatory strategies when confronted with challenging circumstances. But that is not all he gained. As an indirect consequence of his participation in meaningful and purposeful activity, the muscles in his upper limbs became stronger, and his fine motor coordination improved. Although I regret that I do not remember this young man's name, I am grateful that he was included among the clients I worked with who have taught me the value of occupation as a therapeutic agent.

A few years later, I began working on a project with Lyla Spelbring. I remember Spelbring telling me about her philosophy of when occupational therapy practitioners should be involved with clients during the continuum of care that begins in the acute-care phase and extends through discharge and into the community. Spelbring proposed that occupational therapy practitioners have an initial role in the early part of the acute-care phase, addressing issues of self-care and the provision of assistive devices. Then, she said, we should let physical therapy take over to develop the clients' physical capacity. Only when the clients are strong enough to engage in occupation should we re-enter and work with them during the latter part of their rehabilitation stays and as they transition back into the community.

Spelbring seemed to be saying that, throughout our involvement, our focus should be on enhancing occupational performance and not the remediation of underlying impairments. Her ideas felt radical, and with my own interest in neurophysiological techniques designed to remediate neuromotor impairments, I was not at all ready to hear the intent of her

Occupation

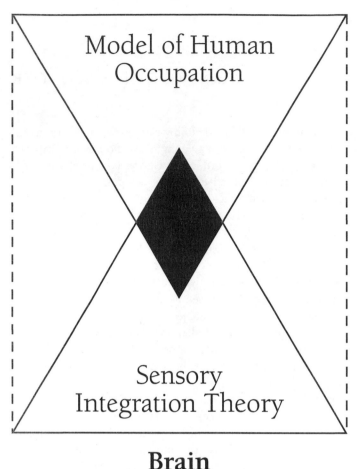

Model of Human Occupation

Sensory Integration Theory

Brain

Figure 14.1. Schematic relationship between the Model of Human Occupation and sensory integration theory.

message. But still, I remember it, and now I realize she may have been right.

Soon thereafter, I went to graduate school. My master's thesis had to do with the effects of the inverted head position on alpha and gamma motor neuron activity in the upper extremity. Obviously, the mechanistic paradigm remained alive and well.

Catherine Trombly was my major advisor. Under her mentorship, I learned about, and came to value, the need for research that supports (and fails to support) the theories and intervention methods we use in occupational therapy. I also observed in her someone who has always valued the use of purposeful activity as a therapeutic mechanism.

Still later, after completing my doctorate, I began teaching with Gary Kielhofner. We worked together on a number of projects. With some resistance, I learned about, and ultimately became immersed in, the Model of Human Occupation. At the time, I was editing a textbook on senso-

ry integration (Fisher, Murray, & Bundy, 1991). Kielhofner drew a figure of how he visualized the interrelationship between sensory integration and the Model of Human Occupation (see Figure 14.1). The figure was like an hourglass constructed of two overlapping triangles. The top triangle was inverted to show that the Model of Human Occupation stressed occupation and barely acknowledged the role of the brain in occupational behavior (Kielhofner, 1985). The lower triangle was upright to show that sensory integration theory stressed brain functioning, with minimal discussion of the occupational nature of humans (Ayres, 1972). About this figure, Kielhofner said that if we can bridge the gap and fill in the void so as to construct a rectangle, we will have a richer view of occupational therapy.

I believed strongly in the value of occupation as a therapeutic agent. I had not forgotten the man with the spinal cord injury who wanted to build a radio. And I had not forgotten Spelbring's view that we should return physical restoration to the physical therapists. No doubt, she would also have us return remediation of psychiatric impairments to the psychiatrists, the psychologists, and the social workers. Trombly helped me to recognize the importance of implementing research to validate occupational therapy theory and practice. But, even with all that, I still lacked a vocabulary to explain to others what I did, how what I did was unique, and how my role could be clearly differentiated from that of the physical therapist, the nurse, the social worker, and so on. My work with Kielhofner on the Model of Human Occupation paved the way for me to finally conceptualize the unique contribution of occupational therapy within the health-care arena and to articulate the important role of occupation as a therapeutic agent (Fisher, 1994, 1995, 1997d).

Occupation: A Noun of Action

I came to realize the incredible power of the term *occupation*. The term occupation is a noun of action. Occupation is defined as *the* action of seizing, taking possession of, or occupying space or time. It is also defined as *the* holding of an office or position, such as one's role. Finally, in the sense of action, occupation refers to *the* being engaged in something (*The Oxford English Dictionary*, 1989).

As I have argued elsewhere, occupational therapy practitioners enable their clients to seize, take possession of, or occupy the spaces, time, and roles of their lives (Fisher, 1994). When we speak of the action of seizing, taking possession of, or occupying space, we can think of the actions our clients must perform to occupy their homes, their schools, their workplaces, and the places where they engage in recreation or leisure. Similarly, when we speak of the action of seizing, taking possession of, or occupying time—and being engaged in something—we can think that as our clients engage in task performances, they engage in a course of action that unfolds over time. We can also think about our client's need to occupy time, not just in the sense of "being busy" but also in a sense that connotes the action of doing a mental, physical, or social task that is meaningful to the person. Lastly, when we speak of the action of seizing, taking possession of, or occupying roles, we can think about the performances our clients must enact in order to assume their life roles.

Occupation is a wonderful word. Think of it—a noun of action—it is about "doing!" It conveys the powerful essence of our profession—enabling people to perform the actions they need and want to perform so that they can engage in and "do" the familiar, ordinary, goal-directed activities of every day in a manner that brings meaning and personal satisfaction (American Occupational Therapy Association [AOTA], 1993, 1995; Clark et al., 1991; Evans, 1987; Kielhofner, 1997; Rudman, Cook, & Polatajko, 1997)

Occupation: Purposeful and Meaningful Activity

I believe that we must view occupation as not just any activity, not even just any purposeful activity but as activity that is both meaningful and purposeful to the person engaged in it. As I use the term here, *meaning* pertains to the personal significance of the activity to the client (see Figure 14.2). Meaningfulness is important as it provides a source of motivation for performance (Trombly, 1995a [see Chapter 16]). As I use the term *purpose*, it pertains to the client's personal aim, reason for doing, or intended goal. Purposefulness is important as it helps organize the client's performance (Trombly, 1995a).

I believe that purpose can be derived from the meaning one makes of a situation (Nelson, 1988), but I also believe that meaning can be derived from one's purpose for engaging in the activity (Fisher, 1994). Meaning and purpose, when considered in relation to occupation, are inextricably interrelated.

Consider the following example. Ken is a minister. Each Sunday, he puts on slacks and dress shoes instead of his usual jeans and tennis shoes. Over that he dons his vestments and a cross. He does this for "appearance"—to be socially appropriate and to wear the "correct" attire. But he also wears them to make a statement about who he is and what he believes. For Ken, they are tied to tradition, and they are symbolic of his Christian faith. Ken's purpose and Ken's meanings are virtually inseparable.

But why does Ken wear the particular cross he does? Ken wears the cross he does because of the symbolism embedded within its design. The design is that of a desert rose. Imagine a rose blooming in the desert—a rose growing out of nothing. For Ken, this is a symbol of the Resurrection—in the darkest part of our lives we can bloom; we can heal and grow. This is a belief tied to his Christian faith, but the significance of Ken's wearing of this cross is also very personal.

Ken was very ill. He had to give up his position as senior pastor and discontinue all physical activity. He went on

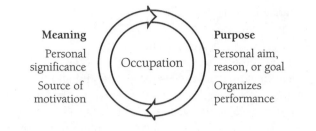

Figure 14.2. Interrelationship between meaning and purpose when applied to occupation.

Note: Copyright © 1998 by Anne G. Fisher. Reprinted with permission.

disability. He had excruciating pain and was heavily medicated. He says, "I was like a zombie." He could not talk, and he could only eat through a straw. He became even more ill and had to be hospitalized. There was concern that Ken might not live. But then he was given a new medication. He went into remission. With guidance from others, he developed strategies to deal with his residual disability. Six months ago, Ken resumed his ministry. Last week he went skiing. He has plans to begin rollerblading once again this spring.

Ken wears the cross he does as a symbol of his own life transition:

> I went from being a responsible professional, working 70 hours a week, to basically nothing. I went from 7 days a week being busy to having no purpose or meaning in life. I went from that to getting it all back.

The point is: Purposefulness is important, but it is not enough. Occupation is both purposeful and meaningful. If we can identify activities that have potential to be meaningful to the person, we can use them to increase motivation and a sense of purpose. In this process, we cannot confuse our purposes or meanings with those of our clients.

Defining Occupation Within a Practice Context

As I have traveled internationally, I have continued to be confronted with an apparent paradox—occupational therapy practitioners who know, implicitly, that they possess unique and important expertise but who have difficulty, just as I have had, articulating their uniqueness. Moreover, they often use evaluation and intervention methods that are so similar to those of their colleagues in physical therapy, neuropsychology, social work, and nursing that any distinctions between occupational therapy and these professions become blurred and even abolished.

Since the beginning of our profession, occupation has been viewed as both a means and an end (Clark, 1917; Dunton, 1928; Gritzer & Arluke, 1985; "Occupational Therapy in the General Hospital," 1917; Quiroga, 1995; Upham, 1917). Our uniqueness has been in the use of occupation as a curative or restorative force as well as in the view that enhanced occupational performance is the desired goal of therapy. These beliefs continue to be reflected in current official statements from within our profession. According to the AOTA (1997), occupational therapy practitioners use purposeful and meaningful activities in two ways: to restore underlying capacities and to develop meaningful occupations.

As I have talked with occupational therapy practitioners both here in North America and abroad, I have found that we indeed share an understanding of occupation, but that understanding often seems to be detached from what I observe in their daily practice. Our unique focus on occupation is not always obvious in practice.

Common Intervention Methods

To clarify what I mean, I will describe the intervention methods occupational therapy practitioners currently use in their everyday practice. The focal point here will be the characteristics of the activities in which clients are engaged. As I introduce the general activity types, the astute reader will no doubt think of activities that do not fall neatly within one of these groups. It may help, therefore, to begin by thinking of four continua (see Figure 14.3).

The first continuum indicates that an activity may be more contrived or offered as exercise, or the activity may be more naturalistic and offered as occupation. The second and third continua indicate that the purpose and the meaning of the activity, respectively, may be generated more by the practitioner or generated more from within the client. Finally, the focus of the intervention may be more on remediation of impairments or more on enhanced occupational performance. These four continua can be used to evaluate the characteristics of any activity we might use as intervention. As I proceed to describe each of the major activity groups, certain key characteristics of the activities will move from left to right along one or more of the continua.

The first group of activities I have termed *exercise*. The most salient feature of this type of activity is that the client is engaged in rote exercise or practice. The activity may have a purpose or goal, but more often than not, the purpose originated with the practitioner and not the client. In all probability, therefore, the exercise has little or no meaning to the client. Finally, the focus of the exercise is on the remediation of impairments. Examples of exercise include having the client draw a series of straight vertical lines on lined paper to develop eye-hand coordination, stretch Thera-Band®[1] or lift weights to develop strength, or stack cones to develop reach.

The second group of activities I have termed *contrived occupation*. Contrived occupation includes exercise with "added purpose" and occupation with a "contrived" component. Again, there may be a purpose or a goal, but if there is, the purpose most likely originated with the practitioner and not

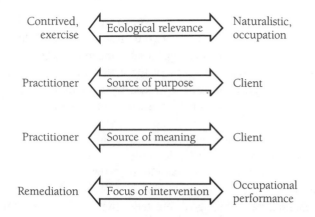

Figure 14.3. Four continua that can be used to evaluate the characteristics of any activity used as occupational therapy intervention.

Note: Copyright © 1998 by Anne G. Fisher. Reprinted with permission.

the client. Because the purpose originates with the practitioner, the meaningfulness of the activity to the client remains minimal. Finally, as with exercise, the focus is on the remediation of impairments.

Exercise with added purpose is exercise embedded in an activity in which both task objects and any potential meanings or purposes are contrived. One example would be to have a woman practice picking up golf balls from the floor with a reacher and placing them in a nearby bucket. Another example would be to have a man place cones on a shelf, telling him that he should pretend that they are glasses and that he is putting the dishes away. The key element is that golf balls and cones have little relevance to the actual tasks that are being simulated.

In *occupation with a contrived component,* the objects are real and not simulated. Having a boy pound nails into a board, encouraging him to pretend that he is going to build a birdhouse, is one example. The objects are real and relevant to the *practitioner-specified* purpose, but there is to be no real birdhouse. Asking a girl to throw bean bags at a target without her engagement in a game is another example. In both of these examples, the purpose and the meaning have been contrived; they are more those of the practitioner than they are those of the children.

The third group of activities I have termed *therapeutic occupation.* A critical characteristic of therapeutic occupation is that the client actively participates in occupation. They are activities the client identifies as purposeful and meaningful. And, to the greatest extent possible, the occupational performance is naturalistic and contextual. The client performs the activities using real objects in natural environments. The focus of therapeutic occupation remains on the remediation of impairments.

---

[1]Thera-Band Products, The Hygenic Corporation, 1245 Home Avenue, Akron, OH 44310.

An example of therapeutic occupation would be to use *graded occupation* to treat impairments of balance or reach. For example, Lillian loves to read. She has expressed concern that she is experiencing difficulty maintaining her balance while reaching for objects, including books, from shelves. Together, we decide to go to her library and work on her problem areas. By progressively grading the task in terms of the challenges to her balance or the extent of reach required, engagement in an activity that has purpose and meaning to the client can be used to remediate her underlying impairments that are limiting her occupational performance. As her underlying abilities improve, she can begin to retrieve from or return to higher shelves books that are heavier.

Another example of therapeutic occupation involves *direct intervention* of impairments in the context of occupation. Here, the occupational therapy practitioner might work on social abilities while a group of adolescents makes a cake for one of their mothers. Or the practitioner might attempt to remediate attentional deficits as the person engages in a favored card game.

The final group of activities I have termed *adaptive or compensatory occupation*. As with therapeutic occupation, a critical characteristic is the client's active participation in occupations that are chosen by the client. Again, the activities are purposeful and meaningful to the client, and the occupational performance is naturalistic and contextual. In fact, the major distinction between adaptive occupation and therapeutic occupation is that adaptive occupation is focused on improved occupational performance and not on the remediation of impairments. When we use adaptive occupation, we provide assistive devices, teach alternative or compensatory strategies, or modify physical or social environments. No attempt is made to remediate the underlying impairments.

An example of adaptive occupation might involve engaging Roy, who has lung cancer and resultant low endurance, in a desired grocery shopping task. While he is shopping for his needed groceries, the occupational therapy practitioner would use education to teach him alternative ways to manage his shopping. One strategy might be to teach him to put only a limited number of items into a bag. Another might be to teach him to use a cart to transport his groceries. The key characteristic of adaptive occupation is the use of adaptation to alter or change the activity so that the client can perform it successfully (Mosey, 1986). The goal is not to improve Roy's endurance.

Legitimate Activities for Occupational Therapy

What then are the legitimate activities for occupational therapy? Kielhofner (1997) has argued that the emerging paradigm of occupational therapy requires that we recognize occupation as the level of intervention. I believe that this should be true whether the intervention involves engaging the person in therapeutic occupation for purposes of remediation or engaging the person in adaptive occupation to directly enhance occupational performance. Certainly, if we tie current practice to our philosophical base, then the clear *emphasis* must be therapeutic occupation and adaptive occupation. At the same time, we must heed Spelbring's advice and return exercise and most of our use of contrived occupation to their legitimate "owners."[2]

We do not like to think that what we are doing is not legitimate occupational therapy. But, whether we want to admit it to ourselves or not, there are still many occupational therapy practitioners here in the United States and internationally who continue to *emphasize* the use of exercise or contrived occupation to remediate impairments, justifying their programs to themselves and others by stating that their *ultimate* goal is improved occupational performance. We are challenged to ask ourselves, how are these programs any different from those of physical therapy, neuropsychology, and others?

Conceptualizing an Occupational Therapy Intervention Process Model

How can we make the philosophical foundations of our profession a reality of everyday practice? I believe that we do that by uniting practice and theory in an occupational framework. That is, we must conceptualize and implement practice in a manner that explicitly ties what we do to our unique focus on occupation as a therapeutic tool. If we are to remain a viable profession and avoid the risk of being viewed as redundant, we must continue the move away from the mechanistic paradigm and reconnect to our philosophical foundations.

In the remainder of this lecture, I will propose the Occupational Therapy Intervention Process Model as a structure for realizing this objective (see Figure 14.4). This model stresses the use of a top-down approach to evaluation. It also provides a framework to guide professional reasoning that leads to implementation of adaptive occupation for purposes of compensation as well as therapeutic occupation for purposes of remediation.

---

[2] I believe that there is some justification for the *occasional* use of contrived occupation, especially with clients who lack motivation or who are too fearful to engage in activities that we might believe are more relevant to their daily life needs. In this case, group, craft, or play and leisure activities may be used early in the intervention in an attempt to facilitate the client's active participation and to increase motivation. The client may initially "go through the motions" of implementing the task performance, but his or her sense of purpose and meaning in relation to the activity likely is minimal. The hope is that purpose and meaning will emerge. If, however, the use of such activities has no apparent therapeutic benefit, and the client remains unwilling to engage in occupation, then perhaps we should turn the intervention over to other professionals whose methods and focus may be more appropriate.

Establish the Client-Centered Performance Context

The first step of the Occupational Therapy Intervention Process Model is to establish the client-centered performance context. The client-centered performance context provides the framework for understanding, evaluating, and interpreting the person's occupational performance. Occupational performance unfolds as a transaction between the person and the environment as he or she enacts a task (see Figure 14.5). Therefore, the person's motivational characteristics, roles, and capacities are just as critical as the task and the features of the environment for providing the framework that is needed to understand why, and how, a person performs the tasks he or she does and why certain aspects of the task performance may result in the person experiencing difficulty or dissatisfaction. This view is in contrast to

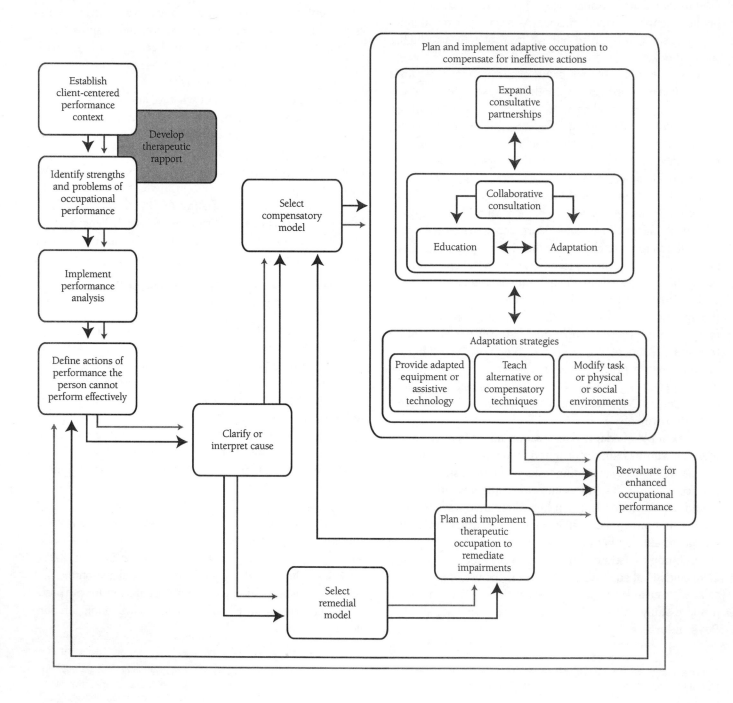

Figure 14.4. Schematic representation of the Occupational Therapy Intervention Process Model.
Note: Copyright © 1998 by Anne G. Fisher. Reprinted with permission.

the view that defines the context as being limited to the environment or all that is external to the person (Christiansen & Baum, 1997; Dunn, Brown, & McGuigan, 1994 [see Chapter 17]; Haugen & Mathiowetz, 1995).

The following interrelated dimensions define the client-centered performance context:[3]

1. The *temporal dimension* places the client's occupational performance within context of his or her past; present; and possibilities, priorities, and hopes for the future.

2. The *environmental dimension* includes the persons who are present, the objects that are present, and the physical spaces where the task performances occur.

3. The *cultural dimension* pertains to the shared beliefs, values, and customs of one's cultural group that influence where one performs tasks, what tasks one performs, how one performs them, and what tools and materials are used.

4. The *societal (institutional) dimension* includes one's available community resources, relevant economic factors, and implicit or explicit rules and regulations, including medical precautions.

5. The *social dimension* includes one's connections and relationships with others as well as the extent of collaboration that occurs between the client and others during occupational performance.

6. The *role dimension* pertains to the relationship between one's roles and the related collection of task performances that must unfold in a logical, timely, and socially appropriate manner. We must understand the person's perceived roles and any incongruities between his or her role behavior and the role behavior that is expected by society or desired by the person.

7. The *motivational dimension* pertains to one's values, interests, and goals that give meaning to activity and provide a source of motivation.

8. The *capacity dimension* pertains to the clients' diagnosed condition and the broad clinical picture of his or her neurologic, musculoskeletal, cognitive, and psychosocial capacities and impairments we gain through our initial observations and interview with the client. These are the *initial* impressions we have of a client that *begin* to inform us about the client's potentials for change, delimiters to progress, and precautions we might need to consider during intervention.

9. The *task dimension* includes both the task to be performed and the constraints that define that task. The

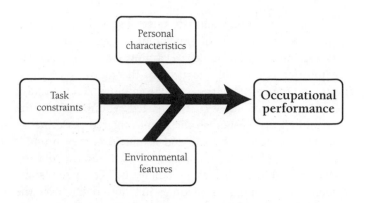

Figure 14.5. Schematic representation of occupational performance unfolding as a transaction between the person and the environment as he or she enacts a task. *Note:* Copyright © 1998 by Anne G. Fisher. Reprinted with permission.

task constraints are a set of culturally defined task characteristics that result in shared recognition that "this" person is performing "this" task (Fisher, 1997c). These culturally defined task characteristics specify the appropriate context, the tools and materials to be used, the norms or rules for the performance, and the necessary temporal order of the task actions. They are a component of what Nelson (1988) has called *occupational form*. When a person does not enact the specified occupational form, we recognize such deviations as errors. Such errors may reflect inefficiencies in organizing time or space, inappropriate or unsafe object use, inappropriate actions that are irrelevant to the specified form, unsafe actions that place the person at risk, and so on. The important point here is that within the context of occupational therapy, we recognize "problems of performance" through the recognition that some aspect of what we observe the client doing is "out of form."

Establishing the context begins with an initial referral and perhaps a chart review. Then we meet the client. Through interview, observation, and the use of life stories (Clark, 1993; Kielhofner, 1995; Spencer, Davidson, & White, 1996), we begin to construct the client-centered performance context. The use of structured interviews, such as the Occupational Performance History Interview (Kielhofner & Henry, 1988) or the Canadian Occupational Performance Measure (Law et al., 1994), provides a structure to gathering information and identifying the client's goals.

---

[3]The dimensions included within the client-centered performance context may be likened to what Christiansen and Baum (1997) termed *performance enablers*. In fact, their term, *performance enablers,* is preferred to the term *performance components* (AOTA, 1994b). The use of the term *performance components* tends to imply small (component) units of the enactment of a task performance rather than the intended underlying supporting framework. The small, goal-directed units of a task performance are *actions,* not the person's underlying capacities. For that reason, I have deliberately avoided referring to performance components during this lecture, substituting instead terms such as *capacities, abilities, limitations,* and *impairments.*

The meaningfulness and relevance of specific task performances to the client are of critical importance in the evaluation and intervention process. Learning about the tasks that are most important to the person, the meaning of those tasks, and the nature of the contexts within which those task performances are likely to be enacted requires taking the time and effort to establish the client-centered performance context. This step is critical, and it must occur, even under the pressures of cost containment, reduced duration of care, staff cuts, and increased accountability. In fact, there is some evidence that taking more time, initially, to establish the client-centered performance context will result in overall outcomes being enhanced and overall costs reduced (Bowen, 1996; Neistadt, 1995).

Consistent with a top-down approach, it is important to point out that we do not begin to formally assess the person's underlying capacities and abilities until later (Fisher & Short-DeGraff, 1993; Trombly, 1993). Rather, at this stage in the evaluation process, we consider only the person's diagnosed condition and what we learn through informal observation and interview.

For example, before I actually met Jim, I was aware that he had sustained a brain injury several years ago and that he was experiencing difficulty finding satisfying employment. This information led me to suspect that he might have either physical or cognitive limitations, but if he did, they were unlikely to change. My first contact with him was by telephone. During our conversation, I became aware that he has expressive aphasia but that he is able to communicate most of his ideas in a manner that I could understand.

Later, when I met Jim, I noticed that he does not use his right arm. He allows it to hang at this side. As Jim and I began to talk, I quickly learned that he is bilingual—he knows both American Sign Language and English. Jim cues himself visually, using sign language, when he has difficulty verbalizing what he wants to say. During our conversation, I sensed that Jim has good comprehension and no major memory deficits. He is outgoing and appears to have good social skills. Things he said also led me to infer that he likely has good self-awareness and problem-solving abilities. But a critical feature here is that I did not formally test any of Jim's capacities. I did not ask him to move his right arm. I did not ask him to tell me the meaning of a saying like "a rolling stone gathers no moss." I did not ask him to remember and repeat number sequences or count backward from 100 by 7s.

Instead, I learned about his history, his interests, his values, and his goals. Jim is 28 years old. He sustained a brain injury in an automobile accident 12 years ago as he was driving to diving practice. He had been a champion diver in state competition. He has had occupational therapy and speech therapy. He learned how to use a variety of assistive devices. He loves music and has taught himself to play both acoustic and electric guitar one-handed. When I asked him how he did it, he said, "Practice, practice, practice." He writes music, paints, and composes poetry. He is currently working on an album where his poetry will be set against his music. He speaks poignantly through his poetry:

> I am angry...
>> Where is the blame.
> I am alive...
>> If I find the treasure of life.
> I am alone...
>> Communications breakdown. (Cacciatore, 1994)

Jim is highly motivated to work and earn an income so that he can live on his own, but all of his past jobs have been low paying. He has worked as a companion for another young man with a brain injury. He tried working as a cashier, but found the work too stressful. He currently has a job gathering carts from the parking lot of a large warehouse department store. He has good work skills; he is friendly, on time, and able to carry out routine sequences. He has a small T-shirt company. He uses a computer to design the graphics and adds his own words. Jim wants to be a graphic designer, but he lacks the needed skills. He went to a local community college to study graphic design but did not complete the final course in English as it was too difficult. He did not earn the degree.

He says about himself, "I've adapted—I take a 'don't worry, be happy' attitude." He has maintained hope, but still he is concerned about work and wants very much to move out of his parents' home and live independently in his own apartment.

Develop Therapeutic Rapport

As I talk with Jim, I not only establish the client-centered performance context, but also begin the critical step of developing therapeutic rapport (Tickle-Degnen, 1995). "Rapport is the process of establishing and maintaining a comfortable, unconstrained relationship of mutual confidence and respect between a practitioner and client" (Mosey, 1981, p. 96). This is the beginning of a collaborative (consultative) partnership between Jim and myself that will continue to develop throughout the time we work together (depicted by the lighter gray line in Figure 14.4). Collaboration with the client *throughout the intervention process* is required by the AOTA's (1994a) *Code of Ethics*. Effective goal setting and treatment planning demands the development of a collaborative partnership between the practitioner and the client. The practitioner brings to this partnership expertise related to available intervention strategies and knowledge related to potential outcomes. The client brings his or her values, interests, goals, and priorities. If the collaborative partnership is to be effective, there must be open sharing of each other's motivations and rationales (Bowen, 1996).

Identify Strengths and Problems of Occupational Performance

As I progress downward and narrow the focus of the evaluation, I identify tasks that are currently supporting or hindering Jim's role behavior. Task performances that support Jim's role behavior are Jim's strengths. Those that he experiences as problematic or that hinder his role behavior are his problems of occupational performance. In the process of narrowing the focus of the evaluation, I remain alert to potential discrepancies between my estimation of Jim's potential problem areas and those actually identified by him. I will include those tasks among those I will observe Jim performing. For example, Jim indicated that playing guitar is a strength; I wanted to verify his ability. I suspected that preparing meals that are not ready made may pose a problem, even though Jim did not identify cooking as a problem area. I also wanted to know more about his computer and graphic design skills.

Develop a Performance Analysis

As I proceed downward to the next step of the evaluation process, I implement a performance analysis (Fisher, 1997a, 1997d). Performance analysis is defined as the observational evaluation of a person's task performance to identify discrepancies between the demands of a task and of the person. The person's problems and strengths are described in terms of the quality of the goal-directed actions that comprise the occupational performance, not the client's underlying capacities and impairments. Perforce analyses should not be confused with task or activity analyses, which are intended for purposes of identifying the underlying impairments that limit occupational performance or the inherent therapeutic value of a task for remediating those impairments (AOTA, 1993; Hagedorn, 1995, 1997; Llorens, 1993; Trombly, 1995b; Watson, 1997).

Implementing a performance analysis requires that we observe the quality of the transaction between the client and the environment as the client performs a task that is similar, meaningful, purposeful, and relevant. The Assessment of Motor and Process Skills (AMPS) (Fisher, 1997b) is a standardized performance analysis. The performance analysis also can be accomplished through informal observation of a person's occupational performance.

Because I used the AMPS to evaluate Jim, I will describe a few of its key features. The AMPS skill actions are small units of the enactment of a daily life task. An important feature of the skill actions is that they are goal directed. Most frequently, the goal of the AMPS skill action pertains to an action or step embedded within the overall task performance—*reaching* for and *lifting* the jar from the shelf or *gathering* the lettuce to the table. For other AMPS skill actions, the goal pertains more to the overall task performance—*heeding* the client-specified goal (i.e., the client's doing what the client said he or she would do) or *sequencing* the steps of the task in a logical manner such that the person-environment transaction unfolds as a coherent and recognizable routine.

An important feature of scoring an AMPS observation is that no judgment is made regarding the person's underlying capacities. That is, a person may be assigned a low score on the AMPS skill action *Sequences* for reasons other than decreased sequencing capacity. Similarly, a high score on the AMPS skill action *Lifts* would not necessarily mean that the person has good lifting capacity. Because the AMPS is a test of the quality and effectiveness of a person's occupational performance (and not underlying capacities), the person is scored on the basis of what was observed—the transaction of the person with the environment as he or she performs a familiar and chosen task. More specifically, the quality of the performance is what is graded, not the "quality" of the person's underlying capacities nor the "quality" of the environment or task objects with which the person interacts. Those judgments are deferred to the interpretation stage (i.e., Clarify or Interpret Cause), where the practitioner uses professional reasoning and perhaps further assessment to determine person, environmental, task, or sociocultural factors that may be limiting performance.

Define Actions of Performance That the Person Cannot Perform Effectively

Having observed Jim perform tasks, I proceed to define the actions that he can and cannot perform effectively. When I implemented an informal performance analysis and observed Jim set up and play his guitars, I learned that he is able to do so and, indeed, he is able to play very well using a hammer and "draw" method. When I used the AMPS and observed him prepare toast and coffee, I learned that he is able to lift, transport, and grip task objects effectively. He chose and used appropriate tools and materials, and he heeded the goal of the client-specified task. He had moderate difficulty, however, with effectively stabilizing the toast while buttering it, organizing his workspace, and adapting to problems he encountered during his task performance. Plans are under way to evaluate Jim's computer and graphic skills.

Clarify or Interpret Cause

Having identified the actions that Jim cannot perform effectively, I proceed to clarify or interpret the underlying cause of his ineffective performance. In Jim's case, the underlying cause was obvious. He has hemiplegia, and, during his task performance, he did not use any of the many assistive devices he had received earlier in his rehabilitation. Part of clarifying the cause of Jim's ineffective performance, however, will be to inquire as to why he did not use any assistive devices.

In other cases, as we seek to understand the underlying cause of a person's ineffective occupational performance, we can think in terms of impairments (e.g., John cannot put his arm into the sleeve of his shirt because of limitations in range of motion at the shoulder). We can think in terms of physical environments (e.g., Mary cannot reach the glasses from the cupboard shelf because they are too high). We can think in terms of social environments (e.g., Steven does not finish his school work tasks because the classroom environment is noisy and chaotic). We can consider societal constraints (e.g., Lillian must not bend her hip beyond 90 degrees and reach to put on her shoes because of total hip precautions). And finally, we can consider societal expectations (e.g., Bill's work performance is not acceptable because his low productivity affects company profits).

When the underlying cause is not clear, the occupational therapy practitioner may choose to implement further assessment. Selected practice models, such as the Model of Human Occupation (Kielhofner, 1995) or the Ecology of Human Performance framework (Dunn et al., 1994), provide conceptual structures for assessing characteristics of the person or the environment that limit and support occupational performance. Occupational therapy practitioners are never at a loss for tests of the person's underlying neurologic, musculoskeletal, cognitive, or psychosocial capacities. Finally, a wide range of environmental assessments also are available (Letts et al., 1994).

Select Compensatory Model

Now that I have clarified Jim's problems and the reasons for his limitations, I am ready to select one or more intervention models. I select the remedial model when I believe that restoration of underlying capacities will result in improved occupational performance. I select the compensatory model when I believe that remediation is unlikely to affect occupational performance significantly; when remediation will be "too costly in terms of time, energy or money" (Trombly, 1993, p. 255); or when I am directed by legislation to focus on occupational performance and role behavior. I also can implement both model types simultaneously. Because I suspect that remediation will not benefit Jim, I select the compensatory model.

Plan and Implement Adaptive Occupation to Compensate for Ineffective Actions

Once the compensatory model is chosen, the next step is to plan and implement adaptive occupation. The desired outcome is the design of adaptive occupation to compensate for the client's ineffective actions. Specific details have been published elsewhere (Duran & Fisher, in press; Fisher, 1997a; Trombly, 1995c), but I will present an overview here so as to demonstrate the process of implementing the compensatory model.[4]

Consultative partnerships. When we first meet a client and begin to develop therapeutic rapport, we develop a collaborative (consultative) partnership with the client. Once we know that we will be implementing adaptive occupation, we also must enter into shared *consultative partnerships* with those persons who have access to needed information or who will be affected by the proposed changes. For example, members of the client's family who are living with him or her, or persons who will be providing the client with assistance, are important members of the consultative partnership.

Collaborative consultation, education, and adaptation. Once the members of the consultative partnership are identified, the practitioner implements methods of collaborative consultation (Fisher, 1997a), education (teaching-learning) (Mosey, 1986; Trombly, 1995c), and adaptation (Fisher, 1997a; Trombly 1995c). Through collaboration with the client and his or her family, client-centered goals are established. Then, building on the development of collaborative relationships, the members of the consultative partnership work together to propose and develop strategies for intervention that are based on the principles of adaptation. Finally, the members of the consultative partnership responsible for implementing the interventions are trained in how to do so on the basis of the principles of education. These persons may include the client, caregiver, service extender, or another professional.

Adaptation strategies. As I noted earlier, adaptation includes providing adapted equipment or assistive technology, teaching the client alternative strategies or compensatory techniques, and modifying the task or the physical or social environment. Maria uses a special keyboard and mouse to lessen the effects of repetitive motion. Jim has learned to tie his shoes one-handed. He has also taught himself how to play his guitar, using a one-handed hammer and "draw" method. Ken was taught to use lists to remember which of his many medications to take when. He use a stool to sit and preach because one of his medications has caused peripheral neuropathy in his feet. Because of continued safety risk, Lillian requires standby assistance when standing and transferring to and from her wheelchair: For occupational therapists, who are experts in adaptation, the list of possibilities is endless.

Re-evaluate for Enhanced Occupational Performance

Once the adaptations have been implemented, the client's occupational performance is re-evaluated. We again use performance analyses to verify whether the client has met his or her goals. Finally, documentation of the effectiveness of our occupational therapy interventions is a critical step toward

---

[4]The compensatory model has been called the *rehabilitation* (compensatory) model by Trombly (1995c) and the *expanded rehabilitation* model by Fisher (1997a). In this lecture, I have chosen to call it the compensatory model as the term *rehabilitation* implies physical restoration and remediation of impairments. When the compensatory model is used in isolation of the Occupational Therapy Intervention Process Model, it includes all steps included in Figure 14.4, except Select Remedial Model and Plan and Implement Therapeutic Occupation to Remediate Impairments (Duran & Fisher, in press; Fisher, 1997a).

communicating the unique role of occupational therapy as well as justifying payment of occupational therapy services by health-care payers.

Redefine Actions of Performance That the Person Cannot Perform Effectively

If the performance analysis implemented during the re-evaluation results in the identification of additional problems, the actions the person cannot perform effectively must be redefined, and the cycle of clarifying the cause, selecting a model, and so on, is repeated.

Select Remedial Model—Plan and Implement Therapeutic Occupation to Remediate Impairments

In the event that the occupational therapy practitioner judges the client to be a good candidate for remediation, the practitioner can select one of many remedial models (e.g., biomechanical, sensory integration). Activity analysis and synthesis (Mosey, 1986) are then used to design therapeutic occupations to remediate the person's impairments that are limiting occupational performance. Ideally, the practitioner re-evaluates for enhanced occupational performance, documents changes in performance, and re-enters the cycle if further intervention is indicated. If the remediation not effective, or if recovery plateaus, the practitioner can abandon the use of therapeutic occupation and select the compensatory model.

Conclusions

I realize that we all face the ongoing challenges of changing health care. Many of you, especially those of you affected by managed care and prospective payment, will view what I say as idealistic. I disagree. I believe that my view is the more realistic one. As Karen Selley DeLorenzo (personal communication, March 15, 1998) has so clearly articulated, there will be reduced monies available for rehabilitation services. We will no longer have the luxury of providing intervention for as long as functional gains can be documented. Therefore, we must make every effort to enable our clients to achieve maximum gains within the limited time available. The only way to do this is to introduce adaptive occupation and consultation from day one. Remediation is time consuming, and there is growing evidence that remediation may have limited effects on functional outcomes.[5]

These challenges also provide us with opportunities. In an environment where we are expected to provide quality service in less time, we face a critical need to communicate who we are, why we are important, and that what we do is unique. Case managers and teachers should be the primary targets of these educational efforts. We need to make a philosophical shift. We may need to let go of the type of thinking that is *driven* by a focus on remediation of impairments. Instead, we need to focus on what the person wants and needs to do and work with the person to enable him or her to perform tasks that are meaningful to the person and in a manner that brings satisfaction. This means that we need to rethink what is really important from the perspective of the person—occupational performance or his or her impairments. We need to rethink the evaluation process, using a top-down approach that focuses on occupation. We need to revise our intervention strategies and focus more on adaptation, education, and collaborative consultation and less on remediation. Focusing on occupational performance instead of remediation does not mean that remediation will not occur. The man who built the radio developed better strength and coordination even though that was neither his goal nor mine. Restoration of self-esteem, interests, and values also can, and should, occur through participation in adaptive occupation. When we do focus on remediation, we need to tie our interventions to our philosophical base through the application of therapeutic occupation. And, although I have said little about it during this lecture, I will add that we need to recognize the need to set goals and document efficacy in terms of occupational performance and not impairments or performance components.

Are you prepared to heed Jim's final words?

I will accept and go on.
It is my problem, not you.
What are you going to do about it? (Cacciatore, 1994)

Acknowledgments

I thank my many colleagues and students, here and abroad, who have contributed so much to the development of this lecture through their support and assistance. Many of them have also provided constructive feedback either in the context of the classroom or through ongoing dialogues that, in some

[5]I base this assertion on research that has not demonstrated a strong enough relationship between underlying impairments and occupational performance to support the basic assumption that if the underlying cause (i.e., neuromuscular, biomechanical, cognitive, or psychosocial impairments) of limitations in occupational performance can be identified and treated, then the effects will generalize to improved occupational performance (Bernspång, Asplund, Eriksson, & Fugl-Meyer, 1987; Jongbloed, Brighton, & Stacey, 1988; Lichtenberg & Nanna, 1994; Pincus et al., 1989; Reed, Jagust, & Scab, 1989; Skurla, Rogers, & Sunderland, 1988; Teri, Borson, Kiyak, & Yamagishi, 1989). I also make this assertion despite the fact that some researchers (Judge, Schechtman, Cress, & the FICSIT Group, 1996) continue to claim strong relationships between discrete physical performance measures and instrumental activities of daily living performance even though 75 percent of their observed relationships were $r < .50$ (< 25 percent explained variance) and 100 percent of their observed relationships were $r < .60$ (< 36 percent explained variance). Additional evidence to support my assertion lies in studies that indicate that the effectiveness of remedial approaches may be limited (Benedict et al., 1994; Fetters & Kluzik, 1996; Hutzler, Chacham, Bergman, & Szeinberg, 1998; Kaplan, Polatajko, Wilson, & Faris, 1993; Law et al., 1997; Nakayama, Jørgensen, Raaschou, & Olsen, 1994; Neistadt, 1992).

cases, have gone on for years. This feedback has played a critical role in the evolution of my thinking about occupation and occupational therapy. I also thank Carol Wassell, Coordinator, Instructional Services, Colorado State University, for her preparation of the figures included in this lecture.

References

American Occupational Therapy Association. (1993). Position paper: Purposeful activity. *American Journal of Occupational Therapy, 47,* 1081–1082.

American Occupational Therapy Association. (1994a). Occupational therapy code of ethics. *American Journal of Occupational Therapy, 48,* 1037–1038.

American Occupational Therapy Association. (1994b). Uniform terminology for occupational therapy—Third edition. *American Journal of Occupational Therapy, 48,* 1047–1054.

American Occupational Therapy Association. (1995). Position paper: Occupation. *American Journal of Occupational Therapy, 49,* 1015–1018.

American Occupational Therapy Association. (1997). Statement— Fundamental concepts of occupational therapy: Occupation, purposeful activity, and function. *American Journal of Occupational Therapy, 51,* 864–866.

Ayres, A. J. (1972). *Sensosy integration and learning disorders.* Los Angeles: Western Psychological Services.

Benedict, R. H. B., Harris, A. E., Markow, T., McCormick, J. A., Nuechterlein, K. H., & Asarnow, R. F. (1994). Effects of attention training on information processing in schizophrenia. *Schizophrenia Bulletin, 20,* 537–546.

Bernspång, B., Asplund, K., Eriksson, S., & Fugl-Meyer, A. R. (1987). Motor and perceptual impairments in acute stroke patients: Effects on self-care ability. *Stroke, 18,* 1081–1087.

Bowen, R. E. (1996). The Issue Is—Should occupational therapy adopt a consumer-based model of service delivery? *American Journal of Occupational Therapy, 50,* 899–902.

Brunnstrom, S. (1970). *Movement therapy in hemiplegia: A neurophysiological approach.* New York: Harper & Row.

Cacciatore, J. (1994). *Head injury aggression.* Unpublished poem.

Christiansen, C., & Baum, C. (1997). Person-environment occupational performance: A conceptual model for practice. In C. H. Christiansen & C. M. Baum (Eds.), *Occupational therapy: Enabling function and well-being* (2nd ed., pp. 47–70). Thorofare, NJ: Slack.

Clark, F. (1993). Occupation embedded in a real life: Interweaving occupational science and occupational therapy, 1993 Eleanor Clarke Slagle Lecture. *American Journal of Occupational Therapy, 47,* 1067–1078.

Clark, F. A., Parham, D., Carlson, M. E., Frank, G., Jackson, J., Pierce, D., Wolfe, R. J., & Zemke, R. (1991). Occupational science: Academic innovation in the service of occupational therapy's future. *American Journal of Occupational Therapy 45,* 300–310.

Clark, F. P. (1917). The beneficial effects of work therapy for the insane. *Modern Hospital, 8,* 392–393.

Dunn, W., Brown, C., & McGuigan, A. (1994). The ecology of human performance: A framework for considering the effect of context. *American Journal of Occupational Therapy 48,* 595–607. Reprinted as Chapter 17.

Dunton, W. R. (1928). *Prescribing occupational therapy* Springfield, IL: Charles C Thomas.

Duran, L., & Fisher, A. G. (in press). Occupational therapy assessment and treatment of a client with disorder of executive abilities. In C. Unsworth (Ed.), *Cognitive and perceptual dysfunction: A clinical reasoning approach to assessment and treatment.* Philadelphia: F A. Davis.

Evans, K. A. (1987). Nationally Speaking—Definition of occupation as the core concept of occupational therapy. *American Journal of Occupational Therapy, 41,* 627–628.

Fetters, L., & Kiuzik, J. (1996). The effects of neurodevelopmental treatment versus practice on the reaching of children with spastic cerebral palsy. *Physical Therapy, 76,* 346–358.

Fisher, A. G. (1994). Functional assessment and occupation: Critical issues for occupational therapy. *New Zealand Journal of Occupational Therapy 45(2),* 13–19.

Fisher, A. G. (1995). *Assessment of Motor and Process Skills.* Fort Collins, CO: Three Star Press.

Fisher, A. G. (1997a). An expanded rehabilitative model of practice. In A. G. Fisher, *Assessment of Motor and Process Skills* (2nd ed., pp. 73–86). Fort Collins, CO: Three Star Press.

Fisher, A. G. (1997b). *Assessment of Motor and Process Skills* (2nd ed). Fort Collins, CO: Three Star Press.

Fisher, A. G. (1997c). Background information. In A. G. Fisher, *Assessment of Motor and Process Skills* (2nd ed., pp. 11–34). Fort Collins, CO: Three Star Press.

Fisher, A. G. (1997d). Introduction. In A. G. Fisher, *Assessment of Motor and Process Skills* (2nd ed., pp. 1–9). Fort Collins, CO: Three Star Press.

Fisher, A. G., Murray, E. A., & Bundy, A. C. (1991). *Sensory integration: Theory and practice.* Philadelphia: F. A. Davis.

Fisher, A. G., & Short-DeGraff, M. (1993). Nationally Speaking—Improving functional assessment in occupational therapy: Recommendations and philosophy for change. *American Journal of Occupational Therapy, 47,* 199–202.

Gritzer, G., & Arluke, A. (1985). *The making of rehabilitation.* Berkeley, CA: University of California Press.

Hagedorn, R. (1995). *Occupational therapy: Perspectives and processes.* Edinburgh, Scotland: Churchill Livingstone.

Hagedorn, R. (1997). *Foundations for practice in occupational therapy* (2nd ed.). New York: Churchill Livingstone.

Haugen, J. B., & Mathiowetz, V. (1995). Contemporary task-oriented approach. In C. A. Trombly (Ed.), *Occupational therapy for physical dysfunction* (4th ed., pp. 510–527). Baltimore: Williams & Wilkins.

Hutzler, Y., Chacham, A., Bergman, U., & Szeinberg, A. (1998 Effects of a movement and swimming program on vital capacity and water orientation skills of children with cerebral palsy. *Developmental Medicine and Child Neurology, 40,* 176–181.

Jongbloed, L., Brighton, C., & Stacey, S. (1988). Factors associated with independent meal preparation, self-care and mobility in CVA clients. *Canadian Journal of Occupational Therapy, 55,* 259–263.

Judge, J. O., Schechtman, K., Cress, E., & the FICSIT Group (1996). The relationship between physical performance measures and independence in instrumental activities of daily living. *Journal of the American Geriatrics Society, 44,* 1332–1341.

Kaplan, B. J., Polatajko, H. J., Wilson, B. N., & Faris, P. D. (1993). Re-examination of sensory integration treatment: A combination of two efficacy studies. *Journal of Learning Disabilities, 26,* 342–347.

Kielhofner, G. (1985). *A model of human occupation: Theory and application.* Baltimore: Williams & Wilkins.

Kielhofner, G. (1995). *A model of human occupation: Theory and application* (2nd ed.). Baltimore: Williams & Wilkins.

Kielhofner, G. (1997). *Conceptual foundations of occupational therapy* (2nd ed.). Philadelphia: F. A. Davis.

Kielhofner, G., & Henry, A. D. (1988). Development and investigation of the Occupational Performance History Interview. *American Journal of Occupational Therapy, 42,* 489–498.

Law, M., Baptiste, S., Carswell, A., McColl, M. A., Polatajko, H., & Pollock, N. (1994). *Canadian Occupational Performance Measure* (2nd ed). Toronto, Ontario: CAOT Publications.

Law, M., Russell, D., Pollock, N., Rosenbaum, P., Walter, S., & King, G. (1997). A comparison of intensive neurodevelopmental therapy plus casting and a regular occupational therapy program for children with cerebral palsy. *Developmental Medicine and Child Neurology 39*, 664–670.

Letts, S., Law, M., Rigby, P., Cooper, B., Stewart, S., & Strong S. (1994). Person-environment assessments in occupational therapy. *American Journal of Occupational Therapy, 48*, 608–618.

Lichtenberg, P. A., & Nanna, M. (1994). The role of cognition in predicting activities of daily living and ambulation functioning in the oldest-old rehabilitation patients. *Rehabilitation Psychology, 39*, 251–262

Llorens, L. A. (1993). Activity analysis: Agreement between participants and observers on perceived factors in occupation components. *Occupational Therapy Journal of Research, 13*, 198–211.

Mosey, A. C. (1981). *Occupational therapy: Configuration of a profession.* New York: Raven.

Mosey, A. C. (1986). *Psychosocial components of occupational therapy.* New York: Raven.

Nakayama, H., Jorgensen, H. S, Raaschou, H. O., & Olsen, T. S. (1994). Compensation in recovery of upper extremity function after stroke: The Copenhagen Stroke Study. *Archives of Physical Medicine and Rehabilitation, 75*, 852–857.

Neistadt, M. E. (1992). Occupational therapy treatments for constructional deficits. *American Journal of Occupational Therapy, 46*, 141–148.

Neistadt, M. E. (1995). Methods of assessing clients' priorities: A survey of adult physical dysfunction settings. *American Journal of Occupational Therapy, 49*, 428–436.

Nelson, D. L. (1988). Occupation: Form and performance *American Journal of Occupational Therapy 42*, 633–641.

Occupational therapy in the general hospital. (1917). *Modern Hospital, 8*, 425–427.

Pincus, T., Callahan, L. F., Brooks, R. H., Fuchs, H. A., Olsen, N. J., & Kaye, J. J. (1989). Self-report questionnaire scores in rheumatoid arthritis compared with traditional physical, radiographic, and laboratory measures. *Annals of Internal Medicine, 110*, 259–266.

Quiroga, V. A. M. (1995). *Occupational therapy: The first1, years, 1900 to 1930.* Bethesda, MD: American Occupational Therapy Association.

Reed, B. R., Jagust, W. J., & Seab, J. P. (1989). Mental status as a predictor of daily function in progressive dementia. *Gerontologist, 29*, 804–807.

Rudman, D. L., Cook, J. V., & Polatajko, H. (1997). Understanding the potential of occupation: A qualitative exploration of seniors' perspectives on activity. *American Journal of Occupational Therapy, 51*, 640–650.

Semans, S. (1967). The Bobath concept in treatment of neurological disorders. *American Journal of Physical Medicine, 46*, 732–785.

Skurla, E., Rogers, J. C., & Sunderland, T. (1988). Direct assessment of activities of daily living in Alzheimer's disease: A controlled study. *Journal of the American Geriatrics Society, 36*, 97–103.

Spencer, J. C., Davidson, H. A., & White, V. K. (1996). Continuity and change: Past experiences as adaptive repertoire in occupational adaptation. *American Journal of Occupational Therapy, 50*, 526–534.

Stockmeyer, S. A. (1967). An interpretation of the approach of Rood to the treatment of neuromuscular dysfunction. *American Journal of Physical Medicine, 46*, 900–956.

Teri, L., Borson, S., Kiyak, H. A., & Yamagishi, M. (1989). Behavioral disturbance, cognitive dysfunction, and functional skill: Prevalence and relationship in Alzheimer's disease. *Journal of the American Geriatrics Society, 37*, 109–116.

The Oxford English dictionary (2nd ed.). (1989). Oxford, UK: Clarendon.

Tickle-Degnen, L. (1995). Therapeutic rapport. In C. A. Trombly (Ed.), *Occupational therapy for physical dysfunction* (4th ed., pp. 277–285). Baltimore: Williams & Wilkins.

Trombly, C. (1993). The Issue Is—Anticipating the future: Assessment of occupational function. *American Journal of Occupational Therapy, 47*, 253–257.

Trombly, C. A. (1995a). Occupation: Purposefulness and meaningfulness as therapeutic mechanisms, 1995. Eleanor Clarke Slagle Lecture. *American Journal of Occupational Therapy; 49*, 960–972. Reprinted as Chapter 16.

Trombly, C. A. (1995b). Purposeful activity. In C. A. Trombly (Ed.), *Occupational therapy for physical dysfunction* (4th ed., pp. 237–253). Baltimore: Williams & Wilkins.

Trombly, C. A. (1995c). Retraining basic and instrumental activities of daily living. In C. A. Trombly (Ed.), *Occupational therapy for physical dysfunction* (4th ed., pp. 289–318). Baltimore: Williams & Wilkins.

Upham, E. G. (1917). Some principles of occupational therapy. *Modern Hospital, 8*, 409–413.

Watson, D. E. (1997). *Task analysis: An occupational performance approach.* Bethesda, MD: American Occupational Therapy Association.

Putting Occupation Into Practice: Occupation as Ends, Occupation as Means

CHAPTER 15

JULIE MCLAUGHLIN GRAY, MA, OTR

A recent conversation with a client yielded the following description of his past experiences with occupational therapy: "Pick that up there and put it over here." It was clear from the client's description that he was referring to some type of upper-extremity retraining. I found this conversation disheartening—this description of occupational therapy—yet very poignant. It struck me as a powerful example of how sometimes occupational therapy so heavily emphasizes performance components that it ceases to be occupational in terms of the client's perceptions and the overall emphasis of treatment planning. By *occupational* I mean interventions that have the following characteristics to varying degrees: purposefulness, or goal-directedness; meaningfulness to the individual; wholeness or finiteness, an inherent beginning, middle, and end; and the multidimensionality possessed by an activity in context, the human and his or her multiple systems—emotional, cognitive, perceptual, physical—interacting with the environment.

The client's portrait of occupational therapy seems a sad but honest reflection of the struggle faced by many occupational therapists and the profession as a whole—the struggle to provide occupation-centered treatment. I have prescribed similar activities with the intent of improving upper-extremity function. These activities provided structured, repetitive practice but seemed void of characteristics I had been taught to associate with occupational therapy, such as purposefulness, meaning, and holism. At times, I left these sessions questioning my unique role in the client's recovery, as well as whether or not I was meeting his or her occupational needs.

Despite a professional commitment to occupation-centered treatment, I have not found it an easy task either in the experiences described by my colleagues and students, nor in my own practice. Recent discussions with students returning from Level I fieldwork revealed observations by several that "no one is doing occupation out there." Worse, some received feedback from clinical preceptors that they were "trying to be too creative." One student was discouraged from participating in an outdoor gardening activity with a client who was very interested in "getting out" and gardening, because of role delineations at the facility. I have also observed interns and new therapists who leave the classroom with wonderful ideas of how to organize treatment around occupation, but limit themselves to the use of self-care, pure exercise, or purposeful activities that have no relevance to the client's interests or developmental level.

My own career path has involved a great deal of time and energy pondering the uniqueness of occupational therapy as well as how to incorporate occupation into treatment with adults with neurological disorders. I am a practicing clinician of 13 years, and I continue to work with clients, therapists, and interns in a hospital-based rehabilitation setting. My strong sense of dedication to our profession has been coupled with a strong sense of frustration about inadequate professional identity and recognition. In addition to clinical work, I have spent the last several years studying two areas in depth: neurodevelopmental treatment (NDT) and occupational science. Despite my concurrent interest in both of these areas and a sense of needing more information in both to work effectively with clients, I have often felt internal pressure to limit my focus to one or the other and have been unclear about how to integrate the two approaches effectively. Nevertheless, my solution has been to spend many hours reflecting on how they might best fit together in practice and how we as occupational therapy practitioners might best communicate to our clients and other health-care professionals the purpose of our services. Making the leap from classroom learning to working with adults with physical disabilities, from exercise and remedial training to the use of occupation as the therapeutic medium, is difficult for many therapists in many settings.

In this article, based upon my struggle, readings, observations, and conversations with colleagues, I will propose and analyze some problems that occupational therapists experience in upholding occupation-centered approaches to treatment, describe a possible solution to these difficulties by expanding upon the concepts of occupation as ends and occupation as means presented by Trombly (1995a) in her Slagle lecture, and apply that solution to an authentic case. In doing so, I hope to provide a framework that encourages and assists occupational therapists to become more occupational in our respective approaches. (See Chapter 16.)

The Nature of the Problem

The history of occupational therapy has been discussed by several scholars and is a helpful adjunct to an analysis of current difficulties in keeping occupation at the center of practice. In Kielhofner and Burke's (1983) overview of paradigms and paradigm shifts within occupational therapy, they described the early paradigm of occupational therapy as one that strongly emphasized occupation as central to practice. Beginning circa the late 1930s, however, occupational therapists were influenced by the medical model to shift away from this paradigm to an emphasis on "inner mechanisms" (p. 30), manifested in several approaches, such as the neurologic, kinesiologic, and psychodynamic approaches, that addressed the dysfunction treatment of components underlying occupation. This emphasis on inner mechanisms offered the benefit of an intensified scientific foundation for practice in occupational therapy, but brought the simultaneous detriment of a shift away from occupation as the central, unifying focus within theory and treatment (Kielhofner & Burke, 1983).

Component-Driven Practice

This shift away from occupation persists today (Wood, 1998). The client's comment quoted above represents the most common deterrent to occupation-centered treatment with physically disabled adults: the reduction of treatment goals to components. That is, clients' underlying problems are identified and therapists select exercises and purposeful or nonpurposeful activities specifically geared toward improving strength, range of motion, coordination, visual perception, problem solving, balance, attention, and so forth. Often the "activities" are chosen on the basis of what is typically available in the occupational therapy clinic or within the facility. Materials (e.g., pegs, cones, parquetry boards) are chosen for their potential to provide repetitive, structured practice of a specific component. Although therapists may improve underlying

performance components, a number of problems may nevertheless persist.

One problem is that component-driven approaches bear the assumption that changing underlying components will automatically create changes in occupational performance. This is especially problematic when these approaches are imported without correlation to a larger, occupational framework. The goal of treatment becomes improvement of the underlying neurologic, kinesiologic, or psychodynamic components without analysis of their relationships to the client's occupational health and recovery. This approach has facilitated a "bottom-up" approach to treatment, described by Trombly (1995b) as "treatment to enable the person to accomplish the tasks of his life... preceded by treatment to increase strength and other capacities and abilities that contribute" (pp. 15-16). It is established knowledge that improvement of underlying performance components may not lead to desired changes in engagement in occupation (Trombly, 1995b). The client may leave occupational therapy with unaddressed occupational problems. To assume that changing performance components will automatically yield occupational outcomes represents adherence to a hierarchical view of order, disorder, and change. According to dynamic systems theory, change in complex organisms interacting with the environment is non-hierarchical in nature (Prigogine & Stengers, 1984). Occupation can be viewed as the output of a complex system interacting with the environment in which change cannot always be predicted by a hierarchical arrangement of multiple variables. Approaches based on remediation of component deficits have limited value in achieving occupational outcomes (Gray, Kennedy, & Zemke, 1996; Trombly, 1995b).

A second problem is that the client may be learning decontextualized skills that do not easily or readily transfer to his or her daily activities. This type of learning emphasizes the distinction between remediative and adaptive approaches that warrants scrutiny. The influence of the rehabilitation movement, in combination with the emphasis on inner mechanisms, has led to the categorization of treatment as either remediative, that is, geared toward improving components of performance, or adaptive, focused on changing the task or the environment to enable performance of occupations within current limitations. Quintana (1995a, 1995b) discussed remediation and adaptation in terms of cognitive and perceptual treatment and outlined some of the problems associated with the approaches, particularly remediative, that must be addressed in today's treatment strategies. Parallels can be drawn between her analyses and the remediation of neurologic, kinesiologic, and psychodynamic mechanisms interfering with occupation.

A recognized problem with the traditional remediative approaches is lack of generalizability (Quintana, 1995a, 1995b). Although clients may demonstrate progress in the performance of a given subskill, there is no substantial research that shows these skills are transferred to their daily occupations. Quintana summarized, "The results of much of the research presented seem to indicate that there is little generalization from one treatment task to another or from more remedial tasks to function" (p. 536). Motor learning research has revealed similar characteristics in the acquisition of motor skills (Mathiowetz & Haugen, 1995). Quintana (1995a, 1995b) and others (Toglia, 1991) recommended a different form of remediative approach, namely methods that help to bridge the gap between the skill being learned, whether cognitive, perceptual, or motor, and its incorporation into function. Occupation as a treatment modality, when given careful activity analysis and therapeutic structuring by an occupational therapist, can be the perfect venue for establishing more generalizable skills. More research is needed on the application of occupation as a treatment modality in this way (Trombly, 1995a). (See Chapter 16.)

Experience with persons with disabilities has also informed us that the choice between remediative and adaptive approaches is often much more ambiguous than it seems. People are not always ready to just "accept" that their physical bodies are not going to improve and therefore do not always readily accept or express interest in adaptive approaches, particularly early on in treatment. For many clients, adaptation seems to symbolize finality in terms of progress. People often want to be able to perform occupations in ways they previously performed them. The adaptation involved in occupational recovery takes time and is a process about which we, as occupational therapists, need more research. If occupational goals, developed in conjunction with the client, are at the center of treatment planning, decisions about how to integrate adaptation and remediation might become more clear.

A third problem with component-driven practice is that the client has been deprived of the other beneficial outcomes of an occupational treatment. Namely, occupation, when it is applied as activity with wholeness, purpose, and meaning to the person, can also affect him or her psychologically, emotionally, and socially in ways that purposeful activity unrelated to the person cannot. As Wood (1995) stated, "Engagement in meaningful occupations has a kind of multiplicative impact, not merely an additive one, upon a person's state of health" (p. 47). And finally, the client may still not have a clear understanding of the expertise of occupational therapy, which could lead to a lack of future inquiries or referrals should occupational problems ensue.

Narrowing of Occupation to Basic Activities of Daily Living (ADL)

In many rehabilitation facilities, occupational therapists are encouraged by team members and standardized outcome assessments to focus treatment planning on feeding, bathing, toileting, grooming, hygiene, and dressing. Although these self-care occupations are familiar and can be important to the client, they are often reflexively used without analysis of their therapeutic impact. Self-care occupations are therapeutically applied only when they have been identified as activities of importance and value to the client, are incorporated as personal rituals approximating the normalized context as much as possible, emphasize not only independence but also active engagement and possibilities for interdependence, and are structured to provide the "just-right challenge" in light of underlying physical and psychosocial impairments. Moreover, because self-care occupations can be uninteresting to many clients and overly threatening to others, they should not be the *only* occupations considered in occupational therapy at any time. Occupational therapists should feel free to use other occupations from the client's history, such as home and leisure occupations, to address the client's needs and should feel compelled to address all domains of the occupational person (Baum, 1997).

The above discussions of component-driven practice and the narrowing of occupation outline the primary difficulties occupational therapists have in maintaining an occupational perspective in treatment, particularly with adults with physical disabilities. Several treatment approaches exist, both remediative and adaptive, some conflicting, which therapists are compelled to apply in rehabilitation facilities without an overarching theoretical perspective that relates those approaches to occupation. As one solution, therapists may choose one treatment approach and apply it solely, focusing exclusively on components or basic ADL. In the meantime, research is exposing the limitations of these traditional hierarchical approaches. The climate is ripe for new perspectives; however, integrating occupation with the traditional approaches is not easy! Guidance on how to place occupation at the center of treatment may be needed.

The Solution: Occupation as Ends, Occupation as Means

In her Eleanor Clarke Slagle lecture, Trombly (1995a) (see Chapter 16) discussed *occupation as ends* and *occupation as means* as two ways we "consider" occupation or two "uses" of occupation. Her descriptions parallel the adaptive and remediative approaches. Trombly's discussion has value for occupational therapy. In extending her discussion, I offer below a slightly different analysis of the two concepts, using the work of several theorists within occupational therapy and occupational science. I believe that occupation as ends and occupation as means are not only ways in which occupational therapists use occupation in treatment, but also represent the unique realm of occupational therapy's expertise.

Occupation as Ends

Trombly (1995a) described *occupation as ends* as situations in which "occupation (is) the goal to be learned" (p. 963) (see Chapter 16). She linked *occupation as ends* with the performance of activities, tasks, and roles toward a functional goal within the individual's capacities and abilities and likened it to the adaptive or rehabilitative approach. It is similar to *performing functional daily tasks* in the bottom-up treatment approach (Trombly, 1995b). According to Trombly, *occupation as ends* does *not* involve the use of occupation or purposeful and meaningful activity to improve performance components.

I believe occupation as ends need not be limited to the goal or desired outcome of an occupation-centered treatment, but rather can be the over-arching goal of all occupational therapy interventions. In the current health-care arena, it is difficult at times to establish any one rehabilitation professional as the expert in functional outcomes. Insurance companies are requesting results in the form of functional gains, and all disciplines must be concerned with the effect of their interventions on a client's ability to function. Nevertheless, I believe that occupational therapists have the strongest backgrounds of all rehabilitation specialists for analyzing, from a multidimensional perspective, an individual's ability to perform functional activities in context. Relative to occupation as ends, in other words, occupational therapists are experts in analyzing a person's ability to function in his or her environment, and thus to participate in personally satisfying, organized daily routines of culturally and developmentally relevant activities: occupation. Maintaining a focus on occupation as ends directs our concern toward a client's occupational health and requires that our assessments and treatment modalities reflect that overarching purpose.

What can occupational therapists draw upon to assert and reinforce our expertise in the area of occupation as ends? The literature within the profession, and specifically within occupational science (Zemke & Clark, 1996), provides a knowledge base for occupational therapy's concern with occupation as ends. A helpful conceptual resource is Rogers' (1982) analysis of the differences between medicine's and occupational therapy's determination of a state of order or disorder in an individual. Rogers contended that occupational therapists must recognize that the phenomena they analyze and treat are different from the phenomena addressed by many other health-care professionals. She proposed the "occupational therapy diagnosis" (p. 33), which reflects the occupational therapist's perspective on states of order and disorder in the human, and how to bring about change from disorder to order. She described the state of order, or "ends," toward which occupational therapy is directed as occupational performance or engagement. Occupational performance includes competence in self-care, work, and play "activities" (p. 30) and involves "integration of the biopsychosocial dimensions" (p. 30) of the human. Kielhofner and Burke (1983) also encompassed a reference to occupation as an intended outcome of treatment, in terms of occupational roles, in their discussion of the goals of early occupational therapy. They presented the first paradigm of occupational therapy as having a strong emphasis on occupation as ends and occupation as means without categorizing it as such. In applying this perspective to occupational therapy today, Burke (1983) described occupation as ends as follows:

The issues to be confronted in the occupational therapy clinic are no longer just those related to increasing functional abilities, but are more precisely defined according to the goals and objectives that will serve the client in reestablishing and selecting new methods for continuing their chosen occupational lives. (p. 126–127)

Under this analysis of occupation as ends, everything that is done in occupational therapy evaluation and treatment should be directed toward the ultimate outcome of restoring client's "occupational lives." Therapists are called upon to analyze not only a client's performance of given occupations, but also his or her overall use of time, daily habits and routines, activities in relation to the developmental continuum, and need as an occupational being for creativity, competence, and challenge. A complex arrangement of any number of variables, including the environment, may be reinforcing or interfering with that person's ability to engage. It is the occupational therapist's charge to analyze that complexity and determine which variables must be altered to effect a change in the entire system. Once those variables are identified, the occupational therapist structures intervention to achieve the goal of occupation as ends. Many times, ideally, an occupation or an aspect of an occupation is used as the means to that ends.

Occupation as Means

Occupation as means, according to Trombly's (1995a) analysis, "refers to occupation acting as the therapeutic change agent to remediate impaired abilities or capacities" (p. 964) (see Chapter 16). She described occupation as means as "limited to simple behaviors" (p. 963) and gave examples of purposeful, repetitive activity designed to enhance a particular motor component of performance, such as muscle imbalance or incoordination. The question arises: If the occupation as means is "limited to simple behaviors," is it still occupation; or might these simple behaviors be viewed instead as exercise or physical modalities to be used as adjuncts to occupation? I would suggest that often they are precursors to occupation, necessary for the enhancement of underlying components interfering with occupation, but are *not* occupation. Similar to physical agent modalities, these "simple behaviors" should not replace occupation, but should be used in preparation for and in conjunction with occupation (American Occupational Therapy Association, 1994).

I propose that *occupation as means* refers to the use of therapeutic occupation as the treatment modality to advance someone toward an occupational outcome. This may include the adaptation and practice of the intended occupation or the employment of thoughtfully structured occupation to alter relevant performance components. The critical difference between my analysis and Trombly's analysis concerns the definition of occupation and results in the observation that once you apply occupation as redefined, occupation as ends and occupation as means begin to merge together in the therapeutic context. Occupation as means, in my analysis, is not limited to simple behaviors, but rather refers to using activities that have the following criteria—perceived as "doing"; pertaining to the client's sense of self; goal-directed, personally meaningful; and culturally and developmentally relevant (Christiansen, 1994; Clark et al., 1991; Gray, 1997)—to "treat" physical, cognitive, and psychosocial components of performance. Occupation, in this sense, cannot be effectively used as treatment without completion of a thorough occupational history to determine what activities fit these criteria for a given individual, as well as to gain some perspective on the typical physical, temporal, and social context of the person's occupations.

As with occupation as ends, there are numerous accounts of the notion of occupation as means within occupational therapy literature, often with different terminology. Reilly (1958) described a curriculum for occupational therapy that would isolate and focus upon the unique contributions of the profession as "occupational therapy is treatment with activity" (p. 296). Trombly (1995a) (see Chapter 16) referred to the work of Cynkin and Robinson (1990) in her discussion of occupation as means. Cynkin (1979) discussed the emphasis within occupational therapy on activities as "occupational therapy undertakes remedy by means of activities" (p. 6), and she discussed the question of "what makes activities therapeutic" (p. 29). According to her analysis, the profession of occupational therapy began with the use of activities as a therapeutic tool, initially with arts and crafts and then, influenced by the rehabilitation movement, with ADL in the areas of self-care, work, and leisure.

Using occupation as the therapeutic modality to affect performance components interfering with engagement in occupation and to enhance a person's recovery from any type of disabling condition may steer us away from what I have described in this paper as component-driven practice. It is not that occupational therapists should ignore components. An important aspect of the occupational therapist's evaluation is careful examination of all of the elements that may be interfering with occupational performance to ensure outcomes that endure and relate to the individual's life. Occupational therapists also need, however, to reconsider the power of occupation to treat those components. Rather than completing an assessment and using problem areas (components) to decide which activities to use for treatment (e.g., macrame is great for coordination, parquetry puzzles are assumed to help visual perceptual deficits), the occupational therapist has the added challenge of looking into the client's occupational history and selecting activities related to the client's occupations and interests that can be modified and structured to improve coordination and visual perception. Perhaps that particular client enjoyed waxing the car, making fried chicken, or playing with his or her nieces. The occupational therapist could, with a little creativity and ingenuity, tailor those occupations to treat the very same coordination or visual perceptual deficits.

When occupation is used in this way, it has more relevance to the person's life, it more clearly emphasizes the expertise of occupational therapy to clients and health-care team members, and it has the benefit of overlapping cognitive, perceptual, kinetic, and psychosocial dimensions that a puzzle or purely motor task may not offer. Instead of being two distinct conditions as Trombly (1995a) described, occupation as ends and occupation as means exist simultaneously within the above treatment examples (see Chapter 15). Perspectives that separate "treating underlying components" and "performing functional daily tasks" as mutually exclusive categories seem to neglect this essential element of treatment and to suggest that occupation is incapable of affecting performance components; I propose a use of occupation as means that recognizes the powerful impact of therapeutic occupation on both component and occupational recovery.

Occupation, applied in this manner, is a unique contribution to a client's recovery. It is not, however, easy to do. Clients sometimes resist engaging in activities that may actually illuminate their weaknesses. Other health-care professionals often do not see the value of and scientific expertise behind the everyday tasks involved in therapeutic occupation. Clients and family members may subscribe to the widely held belief that if the body is healed, everything else will fall into place. Trombly (1995a) also identified the problem of the inconsistencies that arise among different therapists in analyzing the components of occupation for their therapeutic potential (see Chapter 15). All of these observations have some truth, but ignore the reality that occupation can be a valuable tool in a person's recovery that does not have to take the place of the healing of the body, but can actually supplement and enhance it, or even be the catalyst for healing. That using occupation in this way might present problems in terms of quantifying performance and progress should not be seen as a reason for not using occupation, but rather an area requiring more investigation by occupational therapists and occupational scientists. Using occupation to affect performance components is generally supported by current motor learning research, which suggests the need to practice skills with more variety in a more natural context (Mathiowetz & Haugen, 1995). The need for more research is clear. To apply occupation as means effectively, the occupational therapist must understand the complexity of action in the environment and the involvement of a number of systems in normal action.

Case Application: Alejandro
Top-Down Approach to Evaluation

As in all my cases, an initial outpatient occupational therapy evaluation was completed for the case of Alejandro to determine the occupational therapy diagnosis and to outline, in terms of long- and short-term goals, the desired occupational outcomes (occupation as ends). The occupational evaluation followed a top-down approach (Trombly, 1993), beginning with a thorough occupational history, followed by evaluation of occupational performance, then relevant performance components. The occupational history reflected the work of Mattingly and Fleming (1994) on the narrative nature of clinical reasoning in occupational therapy and Clark's (1993) occupational storytelling and story making and revealed Alejandro's occupations and interests before and since his injuries. The key areas of occupation addressed included self-care, home management, community activities and involvement, avocations and leisure, work, and daily routine and use of time. Alejandro's goals were discussed and incorporated into his treatment plan.

Occupational and Medical History

Alejandro is 50 years old and has been living with his parents in a house in South Central Los Angeles after rehabilitation from an assault in 1982. Before that assault, Alejandro was living alone. He is divorced. He was married for approximately 20 years and has four grown children. Before his injuries, Alejandro worked full-time for several years for a sign-making company as a factory mechanic. During his free time, often spent with his son, he played soccer and pool and enjoyed watching sports with his children.

Alejandro's initial injury occurred on his way home from work. He took the bus to and from work, and his usual shift ended in the middle of the night. Alejandro was waiting for the bus when he was mugged and attacked by a couple of men, who hit him over the head with a baseball bat. He was immediately hospitalized and underwent brain surgery, then subsequently transferred to another hospital for additional surgery and rehabilitation. He was discharged from inpatient rehabilitation to live with his parents and, in his words, it "works well for everyone" because they are older and benefit from having him around.

Alejandro indicated that he was in a wheelchair for a year after his injury and that his recovery had been taking a long time. He reported becoming very depressed at the reality of spending all that time in the wheelchair and not being able to do many things he did before the assault. It took Alejandro a long time to get to the point where he was able to leave the house to participate in activities with family members again. He still experienced a great deal of fear related to the incident. Family relations were strained at times, and he could not always rely on family members for transportation or other assistance.

In 1995, 13 years after his original accident, Alejandro was hit by a car as he was crossing the street. He suffered multiple injuries, including a possible closed-head injury, and was hospitalized again. His right upper and lower extremities were in casts, and his physical mobility was significantly limited. After hospitalization, Alejandro was again discharged to live at home with his parents, but described that everything was much more difficult than the first time. He was no longer able to get around, and he experienced significant pain and difficulty using his right side. He did not leave the house for

any activities and, in addition to the decline in his overall ability to move and to do things for himself, the anxiety and depression that he had been experiencing since his initial assault had become nearly overwhelming for him. Once he was able get around a little, he resumed appointments at a county medical clinic for psychiatric consults and medications for anxiety and depression. It was via these appointments that the rehabilitation medical director encountered Alejandro and noted that he had significant restrictions in terms of his mobility and had not overcome the decline in functional status resulting from the second accident. He admitted Alejandro for another course of inpatient rehabilitation from August 9 to September 6, 1996, which included occupational, physical, and speech therapies.

When Alejandro left the rehabilitation unit, he was able to walk with an assistive device and was able to do his personal care and some simple homemaking activities. He had made many friends on the inpatient unit and enjoyed spending time straightening the rehabilitation day room when he was not in therapy. He was discharged home with outpatient physical therapy. The physical therapist realized that Alejandro was experiencing difficulties in a number of areas and recommended outpatient speech therapy and occupational therapy as well.

During the occupational therapy evaluation, Alejandro expressed difficulty in various occupational areas. He was performing all self-care without problems. He sometimes participated in the home management, preparing meals or portions of meals, and especially liked to be involved in housecleaning. It was eventually disclosed that he did have some difficulties, however, in the kitchen, particularly with leaving a burner on and burning himself or food on occasion. He described consistent criticism that he received from his parents about his errors and his slowness at home. They did not seem to understand the nature of his mistakes and their relation to his brain injury. When questioned, Alejandro was certain that they would not be available for or interested in any type of family training or education.

In terms of community occupations, Alejandro's primary involvement was at a county hospital, where he attended numerous medical appointments, and at our facility, where he had become well-known during his inpatient stay and seemed to feel comfortable and attached. He did some errands on foot in his neighborhood but revealed that he would often make errors, such as buying two of one item at the market and none of something else that his mother had listed. He avoided all family gatherings. He did not drive or participate in any leisure or work activities. He was taking the bus to therapy, which took 2 hours each way, and reported incidents of extreme anxiety and fear about interactions with other passengers. At times, Alejandro would come to therapy and barely speak. When we attempted to discuss what was going on with him, he would describe a situation in which he had been scolded by his parents for making a mistake, had left a burner on, or had accidentally bumped someone on the bus with his cane and they had made a nasty remark to him. He seemed to live in almost constant, often disabling fear. When we discussed Alejandro's goals and the occupations he had enjoyed in the past, he would frequently comment on being extremely depressed.

Establishing Alejandro's Goals

Alejandro wanted to be able to "do everything" for himself, without problems, and was very interested in doing things for others. His ultimate goal was some sort of work, but initially he frequently discussed the idea of becoming a volunteer, preferably at the hospital, to "give back" what he had received. The "occupational end" toward which Alejandro's occupational therapy program was structured incorporated these long-term goals:

1. Independent and safe participation in home management tasks
2. Independent management of his daily schedule, incorporating use of a day planner and memory tool (in coordination with speech therapy)
3. Independent involvement in some type of support group addressing the psychosocial and emotional needs of individuals recovering from brain injury
4. Identification of leisure interests and beginning participation in one or two leisure activities as identified by the client
5. Exploration of and involvement in alternate transportation, preferably the county-provided transportation for people with disabilities
6. Involvement in a volunteer position, preferably closer to his home and community, providing some variation among his community outlets

I felt that all of these occupations, if engaged in on I regular basis with success, could have a positive impact on Alejandro's overall state of fearfulness and perception of himself.

Identifying Performance Assets and Impairments

Subsequent to the occupational history, performance components were evaluated to determine which variables were most *limiting* Alejandro's ability to participate in desired occupations and which variables were *contributing* in a positive way to his overall engagement. Physical, cognitive, and emotional components of performance were addressed.

Motor Control and Upper-Extremity Functional Use

Evaluations of range of motion and motor control were performed after observation of Alejandro's functional use of his upper extremities. He presented with limited shoulder range of motion, pain in his right upper extremity, and difficulty with rapid control. He was, however, able to use the right upper extremity functionally in any activity that did not require reaching overhead. He was receiving physical therapy and, after conference with occupational therapy, it was decided that physical therapy would address his right upper-extremity range and pain problems. This way, the occupational therapy time could be spent on issues more directly related to his occupations, because his upper-extremity status was not a major limiting variable. Alejandro's physical mobility was generally functional for his desired home, community, and work-related occupations, and was considered an asset.

Cognition and Visual Perception

Cognition and visual perception were evaluated during observation of functional performance. Alejandro presented with moderate difficulties in his new learning and short-term memory, including recall of daily events. He had a memory book that he was beginning to use in speech therapy, and he required maximum cuing to incorporate the information into his daily routine and activities. He demonstrated good selective attention to structured tasks but difficulty with alternating or divided attention (hence the frequent accidents while cooking). He also demonstrated the ability to learn new tasks, starting at two to three steps at a time, but required maximum assistance with organization, planning, and problem solving. Alejandro's ability to learn new tasks with repetition and to recall global daily events were assets; however, cognition overall, in terms of memory for specific details and higher-level attentional and organizational skills, was significantly limiting his ability to participate in desired occupations. Vision and visual processing were functional for reading and other daily activities.

Psychosocial and Emotional Factors

An absolutely essential discovery during Alejandro's evaluation was the realization that his anxiety, depression, and negative images of himself were playing a large part in his ability or inability to function on a daily basis. From Alejandro's accounts, these emotions were often debilitating. He would, in his words, "close down," unable to be around people or talk to anyone, if he had an awkward encounter with a stranger or became lost or confused in any way. Consequently he would miss appointments, remain lost, and so forth. He was seeing a psychiatrist monthly and receiving medications; however, he had no daily or weekly support for these issues.

On the positive side, when he was not emotionally distressed about something, Alejandro was and is an extremely well-liked, polite, and considerate person. He made several acquaintances on the rehabilitation unit, and everyone had nothing but positive comments to make about him. He was somewhat reserved, but he demonstrated a high level of concern for others. This led to the sense that most difficulties Alejandro might have in social situations might be due to his inner life rather than his interactions with other people.

Alejandro's Occupational Therapy Program

I have seen Alejandro two to three times weekly in outpatient occupational therapy for approximately 9 months. The team worked together to establish a comprehensive and consistent program for Alejandro. He has been seen for an extraordinary length of time, but it has been justified based upon continued progress and remaining functional goals. Treatment included occupations or related activities that were either part of Alejandro's life or his occupational goals. The occupations were structured to influence the above performance components. In other words, every occupation was graded to challenge Alejandro's memory, planning, and organizational skills, as well as to provide a successful outcome to promote feelings of competence, mastery, and self-esteem. The following examples of occupation used in treatment with Alejandro are organized around the above long-term goals as well as chronologically.

Home Management

Alejandro planned a cooking activity of preparing a Mexican soup, an occupation that related to his environment and interests, which led to the discovery of difficulties he was having with his memory book. He planned to bring items for the soup and left them twice, once by the door at home and once on the bus. When all items were available, Alejandro performed well with this cooking activity, and the level of challenge was increased.

Next, Alejandro planned to make taquitos and guacamole. This occupation took several sessions to complete and involved opportunities for problem solving, practicing organizational skills, and using the memory book. Alejandro wanted to bring the chicken and guacamole from home so that we would not have to make both items in our 1-hour session. Within treatment, he made a menu and grocery list then went to a nearby market. We incorporated compensatory strategies, and Alejandro successfully purchased all but one item on the list without assistance. In the following session we made taquitos, incorporating a timer as another memory tool. An important goal of this occupation as the means of intervention was to influence the emotional components of Alejandro's performance. Alejandro was teaching me during these sessions. I had never made taquitos before, and he was obviously an expert. We spent a few sessions practicing the same tasks until Alejandro needed only occasional cuing for safety or use of the timer. The taquitos and guacamole were a hit! Everyone wanted his recipe for the guacamole. He spent additional sessions writing down the recipe and demonstrating, for several clients and staff members, how to make the guacamole. Again, all of these tasks required Alejandro to plan and organize; thus the occupation was used as a treatment for cognitive and emotional components.

Daily Schedule and Memory Book

As we attempted to expand his occupational repertoire, Alejandro had difficulty keeping track of changes and new activities that required action away from the hospital. A system was developed by the speech therapist, Alejandro, and myself that simplified his memory book and added space for daily "to do" lists. It was incorporated in treatment each visit to assist Alejandro in planning ahead for activities that could not be accomplished in the same day, such as recalling items he needed to bring for therapy or phone calls he needed to make. Alejandro was also involved in the tasks of making the new book, many of which were similar to work-related occupations. He photocopied the pages to go in the book and dated the new pages, again addressing cognitive components.

Community Support Group

Alejandro agreed that a brain injury support group might be helpful in dealing with his emotional and interpersonal difficulties. We looked at the list of local groups, and Alejandro chose one close to his home. We planned to attend the group together. Alejandro made the telephone calls to inquire regarding details of the group and arranged his own transportation. I was unable to attend the first session, and Alejandro decided to go on his own, which was a big step. Alejandro came to his next therapy session raving about the group. He had spent a long time in front of the group telling his story and everyone had clapped at the end. It was a very positive experience for him, and he has continued to attend independently.

Leisure

Alejandro explored his leisure interests in occupational therapy through discussion and completion of the Interest Check List (Matsutsuyu, 1969). There may not be enough therapy time (in terms of reimbursement) to pursue this area further, but I speculate that if other occupational areas are intact and Alejandro has good community support and reliable transportation, he may eventually pursue this on his own.

Transportation

Alejandro was involved in all of the steps of applying for county-provided transportation for individuals with disabilities. He completed, addressed, and mailed the application, partly in therapy and partly on his own, and I added information on Alejandro's cognitive and emotional difficulties, with his approval. Alejandro then called for a personal interview, recording necessary information into his memory book. He attended the interview on his own and was granted services. We reviewed the criteria for use of the services, including how and when to call for a pickup. He initially used the service to attend the brain injury support group because he did not want to take the bus in the evening. He was dropped off at the group on time, but unfortunately waited a couple of hours after the group for his ride home, which instilled some fear about using the service. He has used it again, with hesitance, to attend the support group, but not to attend therapy due to fear he will be late.

Vocational or Volunteer Work

Occupations performed in the above areas addressed performance components necessary for success in a volunteer position, such as organizational skills and effective use of a memory tool in daily tasks. Alejandro was also given prevolunteer activities, specifically two-to-three-step repetitive tasks that involved new learning and could be completed within one session. He was encouraged to evaluate his own performance at the end of each session. The tasks were graded for more difficulty and either additional steps were added, unfamiliar tasks were used, or Alejandro was assigned responsibility for task set-up and organization as well as completion. Examples of tasks are assembly of soft charts for outpatient therapies, photocopying, collating, filing, and making deliveries.

Alejandro demonstrated the ability to learn new activities of up to three to four steps with a significant amount of repetition but consistently required a moderate amount of assistance to set up and organize those tasks He could not switch among different activities without assistance. He also had a difficult time evaluating his performance in a balanced way. If he made no errors, his performance was good; otherwise he focused on mistakes and could not evaluate in detail his problems and improvements. Toward the end of this process, Alejandro worked on these tasks with only distant supervision and was responsible for contacting the therapist when he became confused or had a problem or question about his work. He needed to become accustomed to gauging his own performance and working without constant monitoring by someone else.

Alejandro remained insistent upon volunteering at our facility. I contacted the director of volunteers and made an appointment for Alejandro and me to meet her during one of his sessions. We discussed the general requirements of volunteering as well as Alejandro's goals, abilities, and limitations. I proposed a transition to volunteering that would include the occupational therapist as a "job coach." We decided that Alejandro would begin at the front desk with the tasks of delivering mail, packages, and flowers. He was given instructions regarding the necessary steps of application, most of which he completed outside of therapy time. Alejandro began volunteering during his occupational therapy sessions, and continues his volunteering as this article is being written. At his suggestion, he is now doing 1 of 3 days without coaching and is progressing toward being discharged from occupational therapy.

The above outlines the primary occupations used in treatment with Alejandro. These included planning a snack, cooking Mexican soup and taquitos, grocery shopping, making a memory book, photocopying, making telephone calls, making deliveries within the hospital, attending a brain injury support group, and applying for public transportation. Of course, as sessions progressed, there were also opportunities for troubleshooting in relation to Alejandro's daily activities. He asked the therapist to make phone calls for him (e.g., to his dentist when his tooth was bothering him, the front desk regarding transportation) and he was required and assisted in therapy to make those arrangements himself. He had to make a decision about a shower chair because he had bought a used one that was unsafe. Modifications were made to his backpack strapping because it exacerbated his right shoulder pain. He worked with speech therapy on organizing and labeling his medications. The emphasis remained, in any activity, on Alejandro's ability to use memory tools, solve problems, and organize to ensure successful outcomes. and to promote feelings of competence and mastery. There were many times when all therapists working with Alejandro needed to discuss his psychosocial issues. I attempted to link those discussions to his performance in occupations and to the interpersonal and communication skills he would need for his goal of becoming a worker in the future.

Conclusion

The above discussion and case presentation are intended to provide occupational therapists with a practical solution to the difficulty many experience in keeping occupation at the center of treatment. I believe that recognizing and analyzing *occupation as ends* and *occupation as means* as the unique focus within occupational therapy can help guide treatment planning. The case of Alejandro provides an example. Alejandro's occupational goals—home management, community involvement, and work or volunteerism—guided treatment planning. We worked on the performance components that most strongly interfered with these goals, namely cognition and emotion, through the structuring and grading of several occupations, activities that were relevant to Alejandro's goals and interests. These sessions also provided opportunities for practice and adaptation toward Alejandro's occupational goals. When treatment is structured in this way, emphasizing the client's occupational goals and providing structured occupation to achieve those goals, remediation and adaptation, occupation as ends and occupation as means, begin to merge together in a single occupational therapy session. Treatment more closely relates to the client's life, providing greater opportunities for transference. The complexity of everyday occupation in context is recognized and addressed.

Such a grounding in occupation that is clearly manifested in treatment can, in turn, influence occupational therapy's reputation and collective spirit. The survival of the profession may seriously rest in each occupational therapist's ability to give coherent and attractive answers to the prevailing questions: "What is occupational therapy?" and "What do occupational therapists do that is different from other health care professionals?" Baum (1997) suggested that "the occupational therapy practitioner must see himself or herself as having expertise to address the self-care, productivity, and leisure needs of clients and their families" (p. 2). I would like to modify Baum's suggestion to include *the occupational therapy practitioner must see himself or herself as having expertise*. . . period. We know how to assess functional performance, how to communicate with clients to determine their interests and goals, and how to analyze activities and patterns of activity for problems and adaptive benefits. All these skills indicate occupational therapy's expertise in human engagement in purposeful and meaningful activity. Other health-care team members do not possess this occupational expertise.

Many people may not ascribe to the expanded definition of occupation that our profession uses but would rapidly begin to understand our focus if our treatment, documentation, and other reporting centered around the client as an occupational being and our concern for his or her ability to participate in meaningful, productive, and satisfying daily routines of self-care, work, rest, and play, at any stage of the developmental continuum. In this way, what we do and what we discuss with our clients would correspond to the name of our profession. Reilly's (1962) prediction (see Chapter 8) made over 35 years ago that "society will require that we occupational therapists grow up to our name" (p. 224) is most apt in the current health-care climate.

Acknowledgments

I thank Dr. Wendy Wood for her mentorship and support in the preparation of this article and Jaynee Taguchi for her encouragement and assistance via numerous conversations on the above ideas. The occupational science faculty at the University of Southern California have greatly influenced my ability to understand occupation and, therefore, my clinical practice, over the last several years. I also thank the individual, who shall remain anonymous, who willingly allowed me to share his story in order that others may benefit and learn.

References

American Occupational Therapy Association. (1994). *A guide for the preparation of occupational therapy practitioners for the use of physical agent modalities.* Rockville, MD: Author.

Baum, C. (1997). The managed-care system: The educator's opportunity. *Education Special Interest Section Quarterly, 7*(2), 1–3.

Burke, J. P. (1983). Defining occupation: Importing and organizing interdisciplinary knowledge. In G. Kielhofner (Ed.), *Health through occupation: Theory and practice in occupational therapy* (pp. 125–138). Philadelphia: F. A. Davis.

Christiansen, C. (1994). Classification and study in occupation: A review and discussion of taxonomies. *Journal of Occupational Science (Australia), 1*(3), 3–21.

Clark, F. (1993). Occupation embedded in real life: Interweaving occupational science and occupational therapy, 1993 Eleanor Clarke Slagle lecture. *American Journal of Occupational Therapy, 47,* 1067–1078.

Clark, F. A., Parham, D., Carlson, M. E., Frank, G., Jackson, J., Pierce, D., Wolfe, R. J., & Zemke, R (1991). Occupational science: Academic innovation in the service of occupational therapy's future. *American Journal of Occupational Therapy, 45,* 300–310.

Cynkin, S. (1979). *Occupational therapy: Toward health through activities.* Boston: Little, Brown.

Cynkin, S., & Robinson, J. M. (1990). *Occupational therapy and activities health: Toward health through activities.* Boston: Little, Brown.

Gray, J. M. (1997). Application of the phenomenological method to the concept of occupation. *Journal of Occupational Science (Australia), 4*(1), 5–17.

Gray, J. M., Kennedy, B. L., & Zemke, R. (1996). Application of dynamic systems theory to occupation. In R. Zemke & F. Clark (Eds.), *Occupational science: The evolving discipline* (pp. 309–324). Philadelphia: F. A. Davis.

Kielhofner, G., & Burke, J. P. (1983). The evolution of knowledge and practice in occupational therapy: Past, present, and future. In G. Kielhofner (Ed.), *Health through occupation: Theory and practice in occupational therapy* (pp. 3–54). Philadelphia: F. A. Davis.

Mathiowetz, V., & Haugen, J. B. (1995). Evaluation of motor behavior: Traditional and contemporary views. In C. A. Trombly (Ed.) *Occupational therapy for physical dysfunction* (4th ed., pp. 157–186). Baltimore: Williams & Wilkins.

Matsutsuyu, J. S. (1969). The Interest Check List. *American Journal of Occupational Therapy, 23,* 323–328.

Mattingly, C., & Fleming, M. H. (1994). *Clinical reasoning. Forms of inquiry in a therapeutic practice.* Philadelphia: F. A. Davis.

Prigogine, I., & Stengers, I. (1984). *Order out of chaos: Man's new dialogue with nature.* New York: Bantam Books.

Quintana, L. A. (1995a). Remediating cognitive impairments. In C. A. Trombly (Ed.), *Occupational therapy for physical dysfunction* (4th ed., pp. 539–548). Baltimore: Williams & Wilkins.

Quintana, L. A. (1995b). Remediating perceptual impairments. In C. A. Trombly (Ed.), *Occupational therapy for physical dysfunction* (4th ed., pp. 529–537). Baltimore: Williams & Wilkins.

Reilly, M. (1958). An occupational therapy curriculum for 1965. *American Journal of Occupational Therapy, 12,* 293–299.

Reilly, M. (1962). Occupational therapy can be one of the great ideas of 20th century medicine. *American Journal of Occupational Therapy, 16,* 1–9. Reprinted as Chapter 8.

Rogers, J. C. (1982). Order and disorder in medicine and occupational therapy. *American Journal of Occupational Therapy, 36,* 29–35.

Toglia, J. P. (1991). Generalization of treatment: A multicontext approach to cognitive perceptual impairment in adults with brain injury. *American Journal of Occupational Therapy, 45,* 505–516.

Trombly, C. A. (1993). The Issue Is—Anticipating the future: Assessment of occupational function. *American Journal of Occupational Therapy, 47,* 253–257.

Trombly, C. A. (1995a). Occupation: Purposefulness and meaningfulness as therapeutic mechanisms, 1995 Eleanor Clarke Slagle lecture. *American Journal of Occupational Therapy, 49,* 960–972. Reprinted as Chapter 16.

Trombly, C. A. (1995b). Theoretical foundations for practice. In C. A. Trombly (Ed.), *Occupational therapy for physical dysfunction* (4th ed.). Baltimore: Williams & Wilkins.

Wood, W. (1995). Weaving the warp and weft of occupational therapy: An art and science for all times. *American Journal of Occupational Therapy, 49,* 44–52.

Wood, W. (1998). Nationally Speaking—It is jump time for occupational therapy. *American Journal of Occupational Therapy.*

Zemke, R., & Clark, F. (Eds.). (1996). *Occupational science: The evolving discipline.* Philadelphia: F. A. Davis.

Occupation: Purposefulness and Meaningfulness as Therapeutic Mechanisms

1995 ELEANOR CLARKE SLAGLE LECTURE

CHAPTER 16

CATHERINE A. TROMBLY,
ScD, OTR/L, FAOTA

I chose the topic of therapeutic occupation because that was what attracted me to the profession, and it is the concept about which I have thought most. I became an occupational therapist because I liked arts and crafts and "medical things." When I was about 11 years old, my friend's sister came home with paintings and jewelry and other things she had made at college. She was enrolled in the occupational therapy program at the University of New Hampshire and told me she was preparing to work in a hospital using arts and crafts to help people get better. I decided then and there that that was the profession for me. So eventually I went to the university and enjoyed learning all those activities. Those were the days when a large proportion of the curriculum was devoted to developing knowledge and skill in crafts. We learned technique from artists and theory in our occupational therapy classes. We learned that activities were therapeutic because they were purposeful; that is, they demanded certain responses that might be deficient in people who had a disease or injury, and that by doing activities, people improved their skills and abilities. We learned how to adapt activities to change the demands as the person changed. We also learned that because the person got to choose from several activities that demanded similar responses, the chosen activity was meaningful and kept the person interested and working. These beliefs were based on anecdotal observations passed down from early occupational therapists.

This chapter was previously published in the *American Journal of Occupational Therapy, 49,* 960–972. Copyright © 1995, American Occupational Therapy Association.

These beliefs are still taught, but have hardly been researched. Current economic and scientific forces in our society require us to provide support for the hypothesis that engagement in purposeful and meaningful occupation improves impaired abilities or produces occupational functioning. It would be to our advantage also to discover *how* therapeutic occupation brings about those changes so that we can treat more effectively.

Because I have always felt the need to know more about what made occupation therapeutic, I took the opportunity of this lecture to attempt to sort out some concepts concerning therapeutic occupation for myself and to pull together evidence for whether and how occupation is therapeutic. My goal is to spark an explosion of research concerning therapeutic occupation.

If there is novelty in this lecture, to paraphrase White (1959), it lies in examining pieces that already lie before us, in seeing how to fit those pieces into a larger conceptual picture, and in determining what new pieces are needed to complete the picture.

Occupation

In the early days of occupational therapy, crafts were as diversions, as general methods of recovery from disease and injury (Llorens, 1993; Slagle, 1914), and for their utilitarian value because products were produced that could be sold (Haas, 1922). The purpose of the craft was to keep the patient occupied so that manic or depressive thoughts would be replaced (Dunton, 1914). Replacement happened because one cannot think about two things at once and occupation compelled attention. Believed prerequisite to the therapeutic value of the craft were the patient's feelings of interest and personal pride, which the instructor needed to instill if not evoked by the activity itself (Purdum, 1911). It was Susan Tracy who moved occupational therapy into the general hospital (Barrows, 1917; Editorial, 1929). She emphasized that the product was the patient, not the article he or she makes, and thereby changed the focus of occupation from a money-making enterprise to a specific therapeutic one (Barrows, 1917; Parsons, 1917). Occupation was primarily prescribed to remediate impairment (Barrows, 1917; Swaim, 1928), although there is a report that Tracy developed what we now call a *universal cuff* to enable persons to feed themselves (Cameron, 1917). By 1930, therapists were being invited to move beyond remediation to join the rehabilitation effort. The philosophy of

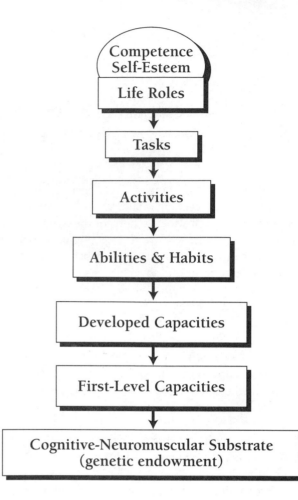

```
        ╭─────────────╮
        │ Competence  │
        │ Self-Esteem │
        ├─────────────┤
        │ Life Roles  │
        └─────────────┘
              │
              ▼
        ┌─────────────┐
        │    Tasks    │
        └─────────────┘
              │
              ▼
        ┌─────────────┐
        │ Activities  │
        └─────────────┘
              │
              ▼
        ┌──────────────────┐
        │ Abilities & Habits│
        └──────────────────┘
              │
              ▼
        ┌─────────────────────┐
        │ Developed Capacities│
        └─────────────────────┘
              │
              ▼
        ┌──────────────────────┐
        │ First-Level Capacities│
        └──────────────────────┘
              │
              ▼
 ┌───────────────────────────────────┐
 │ Cognitive-Neuromuscular Substrate │
 │      (genetic endowment)          │
 └───────────────────────────────────┘
```

Figure 16.1. Conceptualization of occupational performance.

rehabilitation is to focus not on what is lost, but on what capabilities remain, to prepare the person for return to the fullness of life's activities (Lowney, 1930). Occupation came to include activities of daily living (ADL) and prevocational training.

In the past several years papers have been written and several conferences held to discuss occupation, but consensus about what occupation is and is not continues to elude us. Nelson (1988) presented a detailed conceptualization of occupation in which he defined occupation as the relationship between occupational form and occupational performance. By *occupational form* he meant the task demands and environmental context. By *occupational performance* he meant the act of doing. According to his view, *therapeutic occupation* is the synthesis of an occupational form by the occupational therapist that either enables the patient to compensate to achieve a goal activity or produces an adaptive change in what Nelson called the person's developmental structure (1990). In this conceptualization, any voluntary activity a person does of *whatever complexity* is considered occupation as long as the occupational form of the activity has meaning from the person's point of view and the performance is based on a sense of purpose. According to this conceptualization,

reaching for something of interest and preparing one's lunch are both occupations.

Occupation is limited to complex activity sequences by others. Clark and her colleagues (1991) defined occupation as "chunks of culturally and personally meaningful activity in which humans engage that can be named in the lexicon of the culture" (p. 301). By that they meant such things as doing one's job, dressing, cooking, and gardening. Christiansen and Baum, as reported by Christiansen (1991), defined *occupation* as all goal-oriented behavior related to daily living, including spiritual and sexual activities. In their view, the basic unit of occupation is activity. They defined *activity* as specific goal-oriented behavior directed toward the performance of a task. Bathing is an example of a task; filling the bathtub and washing one's self are examples of activities. They acknowledged that abilities are required to engage in activities and tasks, but did not seem to include this level in their characterization of occupation. *Occupation,* as defined by Clark and her colleagues and by Christiansen and Baum, seems to assume ability to perform. For those who treat patients with physical impairments, occupation thus defined is problematic because most of our patients cannot perform.

A Model of Practice for Physical Dysfunction

I want to suggest a different way of considering therapeutic occupation, but first I need to tell you how I view the practice of occupational therapy for adults with physical dysfunction and define some terms. I am limiting my examples to physical dysfunction because that is what I know best, although the ideas apply to many areas of practice. The model I am presenting is not my original idea. I think it has been used since the inception of the application of occupational therapy to this population, but I have named it the model of occupational functioning (Trombly, 1993). This model of practice parallels a certain conceptualization of occupational performance. This conceptualization of occupational performance is a descending hierarchy of roles, tasks, activities, abilities, and capacities (see Figure 16.1).

In the model of occupational functioning, the goal of occupational therapy is to develop a sense of competency and self-esteem. A competent person has sufficient resources to interact effectively with the physical or social environments and to meet the demands of a situation (White, 1959). A sense of competency is highly associated with feelings of self-efficacy (Abler & Fretz, 1988; Bandura, 1977), a belief that one is capable of accomplishing a goal. To be competent means to be able to satisfactorily engage in one's life roles (or to voluntarily reassign a role to another). The American Occupational Therapy Association (AOTA) (1994) categorized roles into the three performance areas of work, play and leisure, and activities of daily living. However, I prefer to categorize roles from the point of view of the person (Trombly, 1993)—for example, roles that relate to self-achievement or productivity; roles that are essentially self-enhancing or that add pleasure or joy to one's life; and roles that maintain the self, which in my view includes family preservation and home maintenance.

Any categorization, however, is deceptive in that it implies that particular roles can be unequivocally classified into one category or another. They cannot. A particular person may categorize one role as an achievement-productivity role, whereas someone else may classify the same role as an enhancement-recreational role. The example that comes quickest to mind is the role of shopper. For some persons shopping is recreation and adds joy to their lives; for others, shopping is a chore done simply to acquire the raw materials needed for living. The category depends upon the meaning that the role has for the person. This fact becomes readily apparent when we note the results of a study by Yerxa and Locker (1990). They examined how 15 subjects with spinal cord injury categorized their daily activities. They found that the same activity was often placed into different categories. For example, eating was categorized by different subjects as self-maintenance, rest, play, and "other."

In order to engage satisfactorily in a life role, a person must be able to do the tasks and activities that make up that role within the natural context. Some tasks are essential to the role and must be mastered by whoever chooses the role. For example, the role of bus driver requires that the person be able to do the activity of steering the bus on a city street. Other roles are defined by the person so that the same role may be constituted in terms of different tasks by different persons. For example, one woman might consider the task of helping with homework an essential aspect of her mother role, whereas another, like the patient with chronic back pain interviewed by Nelson and Payton (1991), might consider roughhousing with her children as very important to that role. The patient, or a significant other, decides which roles the patient should work toward resuming. Furthermore, the person decides which tasks and activities constitute particular roles according to his or her values as well as sociocultural mores and expectations.

To go on with the description of the occupational functioning model, tasks are composed of *activities*, which are smaller units of behavior. For example, peeling a potato is an activity within the task of meal preparation. To continue further down the hierarchy, in order to be able to do a given activity, one has to have certain sensorimotor, cognitive, perceptual, emotional, and social abilities. *Abilities* are skills that one has developed through practice and that underlie many different activities—for example, eye–hand coordination. Abilities emanate from developed capacities that the person has gained through learning or maturation. *Developed capacities* are refinements, gained through maturation and learning, of biologically based capacities. Graded grasp to accommodate the size and shape of an object is an example of a developed capacity. Developed capacities depend upon first-level capacities. *First-level capacities* are reflex-based responses or subroutines that underlie voluntary movement and derive from a person's genetic endow-

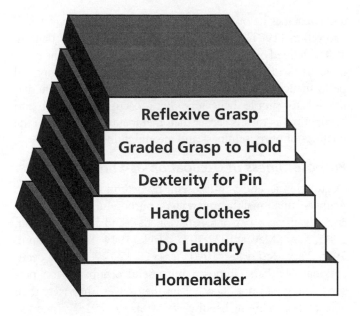

Figure 16.2. Nesting of levels of occupation.

ment or spared organic substrate. For example, reflexive grasp and reflexive release, which underlie the higher capacity of graded grasp, are first-level capacities.

In this conceptualization, complex occupations, such as maintenance of one's clothes, have progressively simpler occupations nested within them (see Figure 16.2) (e.g., doing the laundry, hanging clothes on a clothesline, fastening the clothespin, grasping the clothespin). This nesting contributes to our quandary in characterizing what is, and what is not, occupation and in building a theory of therapeutic occupation. A second dimension that makes occupation difficult to define is time: occupations comprise a range of time from brief moments to the entire lifespan (Nelson, 1988; Yerxa et al., 1990). So not only does occupation have a vertical dimension, complexity, as I have just described, but it also has a horizontal dimension, time.

Another Look at Occupation

For me, one way to begin the characterization of occupation was to notice, in the process of thinking about the occupational functioning model, that in some situations we consider occupation as the goal to be learned and in other situations we consider occupation as the change agent. I have termed these *occupation-as-end* and *occupation-as-means*. I suggest this distinction because I think the goals and therapeutic processes of these two forms of occupation are different. Furthermore, there is historical basis for this separation because these two uses of occupation came into occupational therapy practice at different times. I equate the idea of occupation-as-end to the levels of activities, tasks, and roles in the occupational functioning model. At each of these levels, the person has a functional goal and tries to accomplish it by using what abilities and capacities he or she has. I think this is close to how Clark and others (1991) and Christiansen and Baum (Christiansen, 1991) defined occupation. Occupation-as-means, on the other hand, is *the therapy* used to bring about changes in impaired performance components. Occupation at this level often is limited to simple behaviors. Both occupation-as-end and occupation-as-means garner their therapeutic impact from the qualities of purposefulness and meaningfulness.

Purposefulness in Occupation-as-End

Occupation-as-end is purposeful by definition. According to many occupational therapy writers, purposeful occupation-as-end organizes a person's behavior, day, and life (Kielhofner, 1985, 1992; Meyer, 1922/1977; Slagle, 1914; Yerxa & Baum, 1986; Yerxa & Locker, 1990; Yerxa et al., 1990). Early occupational "workers" imposed purposeful occupation on persons who could not choose it for themselves; they were then able to act in more healthy ways (Slagle, 1914). Time-use studies indicate that people who are mentally able to envision goals distribute their awake time among occupational tasks and activities. The studies also indicate that this distribution is affected by age (McKinnon, 1992) or disability (Yerxa & Baum, 1986; Yerxa & Locker, 1990). For example, Yerxa and Baum found that the number of hours that community-living subjects with spinal cord injury devoted to particular occupations differed significantly from the number of hours their friends without disabilities devoted to those occupations. The subjects with spinal cord injury worked fewer hours and devoted more hours to occupations categorized as "other," which for some subjects included shopping, going to church, eating, or watching television. The problem with this study, for our purposes, is that subject-designated categories were used as the data. Subjects categorized the same occupation (e.g., eating) differently. Further research is needed concerning purposefulness in occupation-as-end. Time-use studies inform us that persons fill their time with activities and tasks that they can name and categorize. However, I found no studies in our literature on how occupation-as-end organizes persons' lives. One paradigm that might be fruitful is to examine how persons without mental illness, who are recently retired, in extreme circumstances such as in prison or lost in the wilderness, or even on extended lazy vacations try to impose organization on their lives by planning and carrying out purposeful occupations of various complexities.

Meaningfulness in Occupation-as-End

Occupation-as-end is not only purposeful but also meaningful because it is the performance of activities or tasks that a person sees as important. Only meaningful occupation remains in a person's life repertoire. Meaningfulness as a therapeutic aspect of occupation derives from our belief in the mind-body connection. The actions of the body are guided by the meaning ascribed to them by the mind (Bruner, 1990). Meaningfulness of occupation-as-end is based on a person's values that derive from family and cultural experiences. Meaningfulness also derives from a person's sense of the importance of participating in certain occupations or performing in a particular manner; or from the person's estimate of reward in terms of success or pleasure; or perhaps from a threat of bad consequences if the occupation is not engaged in.

Meaning is individual (Bruner, 1990) and although the occupational therapist can guess what may be meaningful based on a person's life history, he or she must verify with each patient that the particular occupation is meaningful to that person *now* and verify that the person sees a value in relearning it. The therapist cannot substitute his or her own values in selecting appropriate occupational goals for the patient. Two studies concerning differences in valuing between therapist and patient come to mind. In 1974, Taylor reported that the values attached to goals by 19 occupational therapists differed significantly from those of 44 patients with spinal cord injuries. The patients valued development of work tolerance most, followed by bladder and bowel control. They did not value ADL skills highly. The therapists valued development of adapted devices and ADL skills most and bowel and bladder control least. Chiou and Burnett (1985) surveyed 26 patients living at home after stroke to determine the relative importance of 15 ADL tasks to each of them. Then the researchers paired each patient with one or more of 10 visiting occupational therapists and physical therapists who were treating these patients, to form 29 pairs. Patients and therapists, independently, ranked the 15 items from not at all important to very important for the particular patient. Scores for each patient and therapist pair were correlated. Only one of the 29 pairs yielded a significant correlation, and that was only of moderate strength [.57]. These results seem to indicate that therapists were not good judges of the value ascribed by patients to particular ADL tasks.

The meaningfulness of occupation-as-end is so profound that people at least partially define life satisfaction in terms of competent role performance. For example, in the study by Yerxa and Baum (1986) of 15 subjects with spinal cord injuries and their 12 friends without disabilities, a significant, moderate correlation of $r = .44$ was found between satisfaction with performance in home management and overall life satisfaction. A slightly higher correlation of $r = .62$ was found between satisfaction with performance of community skills and overall life satisfaction. Bränholm and Fugl-Meyer (1992) surveyed 201 randomly selected 25- to 55-year old northern Swedish persons without disabilities to determine what value they attached to certain roles in relation to their perceived level of life satisfaction. Roles associated with vocation, family life, leisure, and home maintenance correctly classified 62 percent to 78 percent of the subjects in terms of satisfaction with life. Smith, Kielhofner, and Watts (1986) studied 60 persons with a mean age of 78 years, half of whom were institutionalized, to determine the relationship between engagement in daily occupations and life satisfaction. They found that those subjects who were classified into the high-satisfaction category engaged in recreation and work significantly more and in ADL and rest significantly less than those classified in the low-satisfaction category.

Therapeutic Achievement of Occupation-as-End

I think that occupation-as-end is brought about by teaching the activity or task directly, using whatever abilities the patient has at his or her disposal or providing whatever adaptations are necessary. It is the Rehabilitative Approach (Trombly, 1995a) or skills training approach (Rogers, 1982). In this approach, occupations are analyzed to ensure that they are within the capabilities of the patient, but are not used to bring about change in those capabilities, per se. The patient learns, with the help of the therapist as teacher and as adaptor of the task demands and context. In the therapeutic encounter, the therapist organizes the subtasks to be learned so that the person will succeed, provides the feedback to ensure successful outcome, and structures the practice to promote improved performance and learning. The purpose of the activity or task is readily apparent to the patient and, if the therapist has allowed patient goals to guide treatment, it is meaningful. Therapeutic principles for this approach derive from cognitive information processing and learning theories.

Occupation-as-Means

Occupation-as-means refers to occupation acting as the therapeutic change agent to remediate impaired abilities or capacities. Various arts, crafts, games, sports, exercise routines, and daily activities that are systematically selected and tailored to each person (Cynkin & Robinson, 1990) are examples of occupations-as-means. Occupation in this sense is equivalent to what is called *purposeful activity* (AOTA, 1993). Purposeful activity demands particular, more circumscribed responses than occupation-as-end.

The therapist analyzes the occupation to determine that it demands particular responses from the person and that the responses demanded are slightly more challenging than what the person can currently easily produce. The therapist provides the opportunity to engage in the potentially therapeutic occupation (Meyer, 1922/1977), and as the person makes the effort and succeeds, the particular impairment that the occupation-as-means was chosen to remediate is reduced.

Although occupation is provided, therapy may be absent. What makes occupation-as-means therapeutic? First, the activity must have a purpose or goal that makes a challenging demand, yet has a prospect for success. Second, it must have meaning and relevance to the person who is to change so that it motivates the will to learn and improve (Cynkin & Robinson, 1990). The therapeutic aspects of occupation used

as a means to change impairments, then, are purposefulness and meaningfulness.

Purposefulness in Occupation-as-Means

Occupation-as-means is based on the assumption that the activity holds within itself a healing property that will change organic or behavioral impairments. We have further assumed that those inherent therapeutic aspects can be reliably identified through the activity analysis process (Llorens, 1986, 1993). However if that assumption were true, therapists should fairly unanimously identify the inherent characteristic components of particular activities. But Tsai (1994), who surveyed 120 therapists experienced in the treatment of stroke, found poor consensus on the sensorimotor, cognitive-perceptual, or psychosocial components demanded by five particular activities that are commonly used in the treatment of patients who have had a stroke, such as stacking cones, putting on a shirt, and making a sandwich. Neistadt, McAuley, Zecha, and Shannon (1993) also reported discrepancies among therapists in identifying components required to do common activities.

Research Related to Purposefulness of Occupation-as-Means in the Motor Domain

When analyzing activities to remediate motor impairments, we have assumed that there are inherent aspects of an activity that elicit particular muscular responses. However, this assumption is not supported by electromyographic evidence. If the therapeutic benefit were inherent in the activity, then whenever any person did that activity, the effects should be similar from trial to trial and similar from person to person, especially in those with normal biomechanical and neuromuscular systems. However, a colleague and I completed an electromyographical study some years ago that examined the responses of hand muscles of 15 persons without disabilities when they were doing 16 different occupational therapy hand activities (Trombly & Cole, 1979). I had assumed in designing this study that if the goal was the same (e.g., "open this lock with this key"), and placement of objects was the same from subject to subject, and if each subject was positioned the same in relation to the objects (i.e., if the task demands were the same), then the same muscles would be used at similar levels by the various subjects. However, the results indicated that each subject used his or her own muscle activation pattern and amount of muscle activity. This finding was contrary to my expectations, but fully in agreement with predictions of Bernstein (1967).

Bernstein theorized that neuromuscular variability between trials is due to the redundancies in the musculoskeletal systems. Such redundancies allow the same goal to be accomplished effectively by a wide variety of muscle combinations and movement patterns (Horak, 1991; Morasso & Zaccaria, 1986; Newell & Corcos, 1993). Bernstein's ideas,

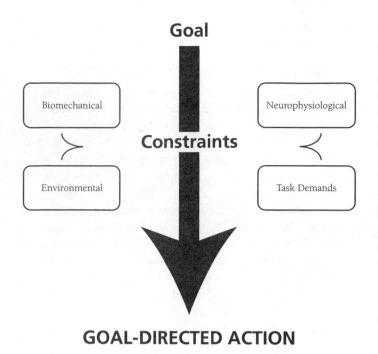

Goal

Biomechanical

Neurophysiological

Constraints

Environmental

Task Demands

GOAL-DIRECTED ACTION

Figure 16.3. Dynamical systems theory of motor control hypothesizes that goal-directed action emerges from a synthesis of goal or purpose and personal and contextual constraints.

and the evidence that supports them, contributed to the paradigm shift to the dynamical systems theory of motor control. The term *dynamical systems* refers to any area of concern in which order and pattern emerge from the interaction and cooperation of many systems (Hawking, 1988). Applied to motor behavior, dynamical systems refers to movement patterns that emerge from the interaction of multiple systems of the person and performance contexts to achieve a functional goal (see Figure 16.3) (Mathiowetz & Haugen, 1994, 1995; Haugen & Mathiowetz, 1995).

According to Bernstein's hypothesis, the central nervous system temporarily yokes muscles together to constrain the number of degrees of freedom to within its capability of control at the moment, given the current resources of the person and the particular demands of the context. This synergic coupling, or coordinative structure, forms as needed at the moment and then dissolves. The next time the person does the same thing, his or her muscles may be more warmed up, or there may be a slight difference in placement of task object in relation to the active limb, so a new coordinative structure evolves. That is, different muscles may be recruited, or the same muscles used before may be more or less active in order to accomplish the movement goal in the most efficient way. The motor goal is constant or invariant and requires a constant, invariant response, but this response can be fulfilled by a varying set of muscular contractions (Luria, 1973). The goal or purpose seems to

organize the most efficient movement, given the constraints of person and context (see Figure 16.3).

What evidence is there that purpose organizes behavior? Motor commands issued to moving segments are not accessible to an experimenter and must be inferred from study of the limb trajectories that they ultimately produce (Jeannerod, 1988). Limb trajectories are recorded with instruments designed to track the spatial-temporal aspects of movement. Different spatial-temporal patterns, which are indicative of differences in movement organization, emerge for particular goals (Jeannerod, 1988). Movement organization can be detected from the shape of the velocity profile (Georgopoulos, 1986; Kamm, Thelen, & Jensen, 1990) that changes depending on goal (Nelson, 1983). The goal of reaching to a large target that does not demand accuracy produces a unimodal and bell-shaped velocity profile. The goal of reaching precisely to a target, which requires accurate, guided movement, on the other hand, has a left-shifted velocity profile because more time is spent in deceleration than in acceleration.

In 1987, Marteniuk, MacKenzie, Jeannerod, Athenes, and Dugas demonstrated for the first time the impact of goal on the organization of movement. They found that five university student subjects used a different movement organization when they reached for the same object for two different purposes. One goal was to pick up a 4-centimeter disk and place it in a slot; the other goal was to pick up the same disk and throw it into a basket. The task demands and the context were exactly the same. Only intent after the reach was different. The different purposes produced two different velocity profiles (see Figure 16.4), indicating different movement organizations, for the reaches to the disk. Reaches before placing the disk into a slot produced a left shift of velocity profile in which a significantly greater percentage of total reach time was spent in the deceleration phase and the acceleration phase was significantly shortened as compared to reaches before the throwing condition.

Mathiowetz (1991) tested whether the same motor organization was elicited when 20 subjects with multiple sclerosis performed functional tasks in natural, impoverished, partial, and simulated conditions. In one of the experiments, the subjects actually ate applesauce with a spoon in the natural condition; pretended to eat applesauce, with no applesauce, spoon, or dish present in the impoverished condition; pretended to eat applesauce with a dish and spoon, but no applesauce present in the partial condition; or did, in the simulated condition, the feeding subtest of the Jebsen-Taylor Hand Function Test (Jebsen, Taylor, Trieschmann, Trotter, & Howard, 1969) that requires the subject to pick up kidney beans with a spoon and transfer them to a can placed in front of him or her. The outcomes of each trial were described qualitatively in phase plane diagrams in which velocity is graphed against displacement. These should be replicable from trial to

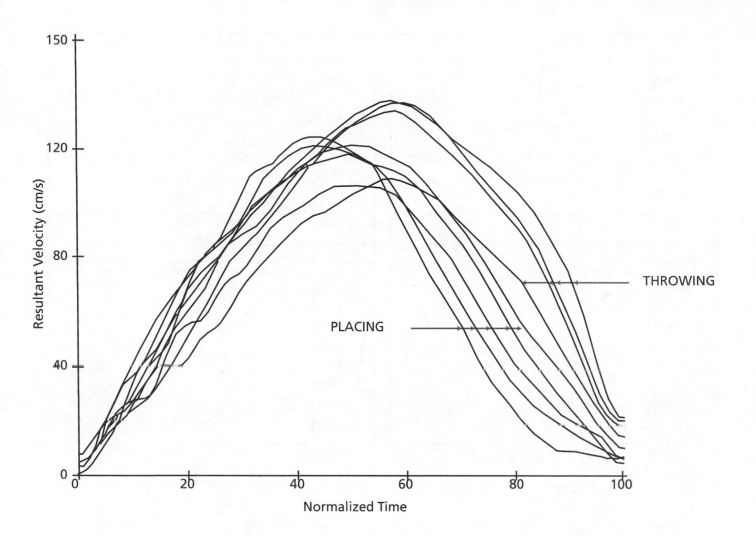

Figure 16.4. Velocity profiles for reaches to a 4-centimeter disk, after which the goal was to fit the disk into a slot or to throw it into a basket.

Note: From Marteniuk, R. G., MacKenzie, C. L., Jeannerod, M., Athenes, S., & Dugas, C. (1987). Constraints on human arm movement trajectories. *Canadian Journal of Psychology, 41*(3), 365–378. Used with permission.

trial if the subject is using the same movement organization. However, the phase planes were judged, by experienced judges, to be different among the four conditions. Figure 16.5 depicts two trials of two conditions, the natural and the simulated, by one subject. The repeated trials are similar, but the two conditions are different. Because subjects produced unique phase planes for each condition, Mathiowetz concluded that subjects perceived each condition as a unique activity, having a different goal.

In another test of differences in goal situation, Van der Weel, van der Meer, and Lee (1991) tested nine children of average intelligence, aged 3 to 7 years, who had right hemiparesis. They measured the children's range of supination and pronation movement when moving a drumstick back and forth in the frontal plane with the instruction "to move as far as you can" (the abstract condition). The children had previously experienced the full range of movement passively. Range

was also measured when the children were told to use the same drumstick to "bang the drums" which were placed to require full range of motion (the concrete condition). Movement range was significantly greater ($t_8 = 6.75$, $p < .0001$) for the concrete task of banging the drums than for the abstract task, which had a vague goal.

Wu (Wu, 1993; Wu, Trombly, & Lin, 1994) investigated whether actually reaching for a pencil to write one's name, reaching the same distance for an imagined pencil, or reaching forward in a biomechanically similar way would produce different outcomes in terms of the organization of movement. In the sample of 37 college-aged subjects without disabilities, the materials-based occupation of reaching for an actual pencil elicited significantly different and more efficient organization of movement than imagery-based occupation of reaching for a pretend pencil or exercise. The reach was faster

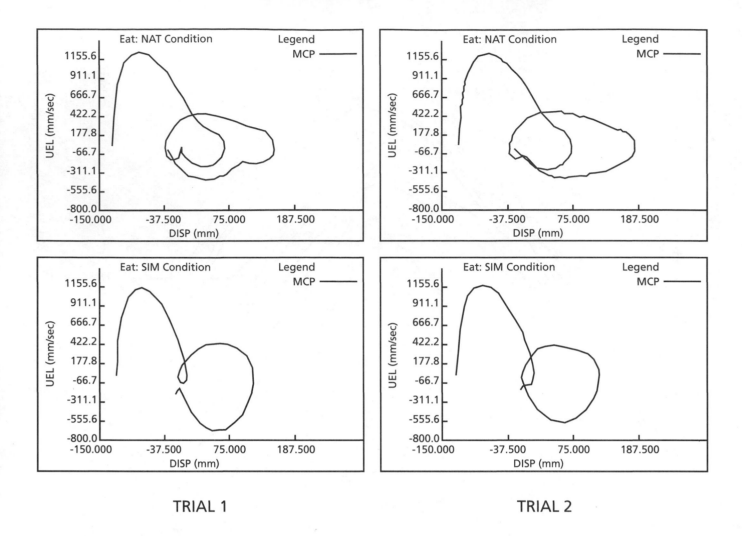

TRIAL 1   TRIAL 2

Figure 16.5. Phase planes (velocity x displacement) of two trials of two conditions (natural and simulated) by one normal subject.

Note: From Mathiowetz, V. G. (1991). *Informational support* and *functional motor performance.* Unpublished doctoral dissertation, University of Minnesota, Minneapolis. Used with permission.

($F_{2,62}$ = 20.44, $p < .001$) and straighter ($F_{2,62}$ = 23.25, $p < .001$), was more preplanned ($F_{2,62}$ = 22.13, $p < .001$), and used less force ($F_{1,62}$ = 6.13, $p < .005$). The imagery-based occupation, on the other hand, produced a more guided, longer, and more convoluted path than did the exercise condition, probably because the goal was more vague in that condition.

Sietsema, Nelson, Mulder, Mervau-Scheidel, and White (1993) tested the effect of goal on overall active range of shoulder motion of 20 adults with brain injury. Each subject reached to a point 3 inches above the center of a table placed to require full forward reach. Each also reached the same distance to play a computer-controlled game of flashing lights and sounds. Overall active range of motion was significantly greater as a result of the game than simply reaching to the more vague target (t_{19} = 5.77, $p < .001$).

At least in terms of motor responses, then, purpose does appear to organize behavior. Of course, much more study is required to verify this finding.

Meaningfulness in Occupation-as-Means

Whereas a meaningful occupation has purposefulness, strictly speaking, a purposeful activity may or may not be meaningful. Sharrott (1983) stated that the purpose of an action gives that action meaning. He may have been using *purpose* to denote the reason that a person does something, or the motive, rather than the goal of the action. I think that confounding these terms will impede research. The purpose is the goal, the expected end result. The meaning is the value that accomplishment of that goal has for the person. I have an anecdotal example of the separation between the two concepts. Some years back, my father had a right cerebrovascular accident with resultant hemi-inattention. The occupational therapist gave him parquetry blocks to do. There were two purposes. One was the goal of the activity—to place all the blocks on the diagram. He understood the goal and tried to do what he was told. However, it had no meaning to him; he viewed this activity as a children's game and found it degrading. The therapeutic purpose, of course, was to improve his hemi-inattention. That purpose had no meaning to him either; he did not think he had hemi-inattention and did not get the connection between the child's game and the therapeutic goal.

What do we mean by *meaningful* and how does that quality of occupation-as-means affect behavioral responses? Meaning related to occupation-as-means may relate to basic values held by the person—similar to the way meaning is derived for occupation-as-end. However, meaning is probably generated from a less profound source when it applies to particular, circumscribed, time-limited activities used to promote some performance component. The meaningful aspect of occupation-as-means may be the emotional value that an interesting and creative experience offers the patient (Ayres, 1958). Or meaningfulness may stem from familiarity with the occupation, or its power to arouse positive associations, or the likelihood that completion of it will elicit approval from others who are respected and admired (Cynkin & Robinson, 1990), or its potential to contribute to recovery.

Although we often count on meaningfulness to emanate from the activity, there is no inherent meaningfulness quality in a particular occupation. Meaningfulness is individual. Bruner (1990) said that "action is interpretable only by reference to what the actor says he or she is up to" (p. 20). In therapy, meaningfulness is developed through an exchange between the therapist and the person to construct the meaning of the activity within the context of culture, life experiences, disability (Fleming, 1990; Kielhofner, 1992), and present needs.

Research Related to Meaningfulness of Occupation-as-Means

The importance of meaningfulness to us as therapists is that we believe that it motivates. What evidence is there that meaning motivates behavior?

Meaningfulness has been operationalized in occupational therapy studies in one of three ways. One is to offer a choice, another is to provide a product, and the third is to enhance the context. The response, motivation, has been operationalized as the number of repetitions or length of time engaged in the occupation or as the effort expended.

Choice

Bakshi, Bhambhani, and Madill (1991) studied 20 female college students who chose their most preferred and least preferred activity from eight offered activities. They completed each under conditions of purpose and nonpurpose, defined respectively as working on a product or not. There were no differences in number of repetitions performed between the preferred and non-preferred occupation. Differences between product and no-product conditions were not significant due to high variability (see Table 16.1). On the other hand, LaMore and Nelson (1993), in a more controlled study, did find a significant increase in repetitions ($Z = 2.9, p < .01$) when 22 adult

Table 16.1. Mean Number of Repetitions as a Result of Preference and Purpose in Assigned Tasks

	Task Assigned	
Purpose	Preferred	Nonpreferred
Yes	63	63
No	83	84

Note. Based on Bakshi, R., Bhambhani, Y., & Madill, H. (1991). The effects of task preference on performance during purposeful and nonpurposeful activities. *American Journal of Occupational Therapy, 45,* 912–916.

subjects with mental disabilities were given a limited choice of which ceramic object to paint as compared with when they were told to paint a particular one.

Product

Thibodeaux and Ludwig (1988) tested whether performance time and heart rate (effort) would be significantly different when 15 occupational therapy students sanded a cutting board that they could keep as compared with when they sanded wood for no reason. Although the subjects reported enjoying the product-oriented activity significantly more and they worked longer at it, there was too much intersubject variability to detect significant differences between conditions (see Table 16.2).

Enhanced Context

Riccio, Nelson, and Bush (1990) studied the effects of enhanced context. They tested the effect of imagery-based activity and exercise on the number of repetitions of 27 elderly nursing home residents when they reached up to pretend to pick apples and reached down to pretend to pick up coins versus when they simply reached up or down for exercise. There was a significant difference between the two conditions for the up direction ($Z = 2.25, p = .012$), indicating that pretending to pick apples was more motivating than exercise. The outcome for reaching down was in the same direction, but nonsignificant ($Z = 1.60, p = .055$), possibly because of a confounding effect of fatigue.

Lang, Nelson, and Bush (1992) tested the responses of 15 elderly nursing home residents under three conditions: materials-based activity, imagery-based activity, and exercise. In the materials-based condition, subjects actually kicked a red balloon. In the imagery-based condition, they pretended to kick

Table 16.2. Effects of Product-Oriented and Nonproduct-Oriented Activities

	Product	
Measures	Yes (Cutting Board)	No (Wood)
Preference	4.8	3.4*
Increased heart rate	13	17
Performance time	172	148

*$p = .001$.

Note. Based on Thibodeaux, C. S., & Ludwig, F. M. (1988). Intrinsic motivation in product-oriented and nonproduct-oriented activities. *American Journal of Occupational Therapy, 42,* 169–175.

a described balloon. In the exercise condition, they kicked as demonstrated. The number of repetitions associated with really kicking the balloon (54) was significantly greater ($F_{2,28}$ = 6.62, p = .004) than those associated with imagining kicking the balloon (26) or kicking for exercise (18). This study was later replicated by DeKuiper, Nelson, and White (1993) on 28 elderly nursing home residents. Materials-based occupation produced significantly more repetitions than imagery-based occupation or rote exercise ($F_{2,54}$ = 12.1, p < .001). In this study they also measured effort in terms of distance the foot was raised and speed of kick. There were no significant differences among the various contextual conditions for these variables (see Table 16.3).

A number of other researchers (Bloch, Smith, & Nelson, 1989; Kircher, 1984; Miller & Nelson, 1987; Steinbeck, 1986; Yoder, Nelson, & Smith, 1989) all demonstrated significantly greater numbers of repetitions or duration for what they termed purposeful versus nonpurposeful activity. The differences in the activities were actually differences in meaning in terms of context, not differences in purpose—the motoric purpose was the same: jump up and down or jump rope, stir dough for exercise or stir dough that will be made into cookies that the subjects could smell baking, squeeze a bulb to keep a ping-pong ball suspended in air or squeeze the same bulb for exercise. Some demonstrated significantly greater effort (heart rate) expended for the enhanced condition, but this was not a consistent finding (Bloch et al., 1989; Kircher, 1984; Steinbeck, 1986).

Meaningfulness, as operationalized by enhanced context, and possibly by choice, appears to motivate continued performance. However, more definitive research is needed. Additionally, basic research on what makes occupation-as-means meaningful and how best to operationalize this in both research and practice is needed.

Practice and Research

As occupational therapists we want our patients to achieve role competence. We use occupation-as-end and occupation-as-means now to achieve that. We need to document the successes of our current practices, but we also need to reconsider some of our practices. For example, practice based on

an ascending hierarchical model has emphasized remediation of occupational components because it is assumed that lower-level skills and abilities are prerequisite to higher-level functioning. Although this assumption makes logical sense—persons who cannot lift their arms certainly cannot comb their hair in the usual way—practice has sometimes emphasized treatment to increase strength and other capacities and abilities to the exclusion of teaching functional skills. However, a thorough review of the literature on stroke rehabilitation (Wagenaar & Meijer, 1991a, 1991b) indicated that gains in component functions are small and do not automatically result in improved functional performance. When the results of several correlational studies were averaged together, the average correlation between motor impairment and ADL was .56 and between perceptual impairment and ADL was .58 (Trombly, 1995b). By squaring the r, the amount of variance of ADL accounted for by motor impairment was 31 percent (see Figure 16.6). Therefore, 69 percent of variance associated with ADL derives from other factors. Even if motor impairment were 100 percent remediated, would the patient be able to do ADL without specific training and adaptation? Studies are needed that compare skills training at the level of occupation-as-end with subskills training using occupation-as-means to effectively and efficiently achieve occupational functioning (Rogers, 1982).

How the purposefulness and meaningfulness aspects of both levels of occupation contribute to the therapeutic effect need explication to guide practice. We need to study in more detail how purposefulness organizes behavior and meaningfulness motivates performance. The literature reviewed here is a beginning in this regard. Some of the studies reviewed indicated that the organization of motor behavior is different when the purposes or contexts are different, even if they are similar. This finding suggests that treatment in simulated contexts using simulated objects and simulated goals may not help a patient learn occupational performance for real life. Studies are needed to compare effectiveness of treatment with actual objects in natural contexts versus treatment with simulated objects in clinical settings. Follow-up studies of carryover of occupational performance from treatment center to home are also needed.

Those golden moments that we have all experienced as therapists probably came about when the patient succeeded in doing something that had great meaning to him or her. Sometimes we get complacent, though, and offer activities and occupations that we think ought to be meaningful to the person but are not really, or we offer a choice of activities from a selection in which none of the choices are meaningful. Much more attention needs to be applied to discovering the meaning of, or creating meaning for, therapeutic occupation. Methods to evaluate meaningfulness are needed both for research and practice. We need more well-controlled studies that test the effect of meaningfulness on perseverance and effort during therapy.

Table 16.3. Average Effects of Materials-Based Occupation, Imagery-Based Occupation, and Rote Exercise

Measures	Type of Occupation and Exercise		
	Materials-Based	Imagery-Based	Rote
Repetitions to fatigue	127**	51	75
Distance foot lifted (cm)	29	31	26
Speed (cm/sec)	71	71	67

**p < .001

Note. Based on DeKuiper, W. P., Nelson, D. L., & White, B. E. (1993). Materials-based occupation versus imagery-based occupation versus rote exercise: A replication and extension. *Occupational Therapy Journal of Research, 13,* 183–197.

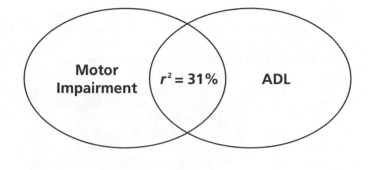

Figure 16.6. Pictorial description of r^2.

Conclusion

Occupational therapy was founded on the belief that engaging in occupation brought about mental and physical health. Over the years we have redefined health, for our purposes, as occupational performance having many levels of organization. In this context, occupation can be seen both as end and as means. In both dimensions, meaningfulness and purposefulness are key qualities. Purposefulness organizes and meaningfulness motivates. Purposeful occupation-as-end seems to organize time and a person's description of his life. Meaningful occupation-as-end motivates the person's participation in life. Purposeful occupation-as-means organizes behavioral responses, at least as far as motor responses are concerned. Meaningful occupation-as-means seems to motivate the person to persevere in his efforts long enough to achieve a therapeutic benefit. Research is needed to verify each of these hypotheses. I hope each occupational therapist will join me in taking responsibility to contribute to that effort.

Acknowledgments

Figures 1, 2, and 6, as well as all the slides in the original presentation, were prepared by Elizabeth (Boo) Murray, SCD, OTR, FAOTA, to whom I am very grateful. I further want to acknowledge the support and constructive critique of my colleagues in the Neurobehavioral Rehabilitation Research Center (NRRC), which is the American Occupational Therapy Association and American Occupational Therapy Foundation Center for Scholarship and Research at Boston University: Sharon Cermak, EdD, OTR, FAOTA; Wendy Coster, PhD, OTR, FAOTA; Anne Henderson, PhD, OTR, FAOTA; Karen Jacobs, EdD, OTR, FAOTA; Noomi Katz, PhD, OTR; Boo Murray, SCD, OTR, FAOTA; and Elsie Vergara, ScD, OTR, FAOTA.

References

Abler, R. R., & Fretz, B. R. (1988). Self-efficacy and competence in independent living among oldest old persons. *Journal of Gerontology: Social Sciences, 43,* S138–S143.

American Occupational Therapy Association. (1993). Position Paper—Purposeful activity. *American Journal of Occupational Therapy, 47,* 1081–1082.

American Occupational Therapy Association. (1994). Uniform terminology for occupational therapy—third edition. *American Journal of Occupational Therapy, 48,* 1047–1054.

Ayres, A. J. (1958). Basic concepts of clinical practice in physical disabilities. *American Journal of Occupational Therapy, 12,* 300–302, 311.

Bakshi, R., Bhambhani, Y., & Madill, H. (1991). The effects of task preference on performance during purposeful and nonpurposeful activities. *American Journal of Occupational Therapy, 45,* 912–916.

Bandura, A. (1977). Self-efficacy: Toward a unifying theory of behavior change. *Psychological Review, 84,* 191–215.

Barrows, M. (1917). Susan E. Tracy, R. N. *Maryland Psychiatric Quarterly, 6,* 57–62.

Bernstein, N. (1967). *The coordination and regulation of movements.* Elmsford, NY: Pergamon.

Bloch, M. W., Smith, D. A., & Nelson, D. L. (1989). Heart rate, activity, duration, and affect in added-purpose versus single-purpose jumping activities. *American Journal of Occupational Therapy, 43,* 25–30.

Bränholm, I. B., & Fugl-Meyer, A. R. (1992). Occupational role preferences and life satisfaction. *Occupational Therapy Journal of Research, 12,* 159–171.

Bruner, J. (1990). *Acts of meaning.* Cambridge, MA: Harvard University Press.

Cameron, R. G. (1917). An interview with Miss Susan Tracy. *Maryland Psychiatric Quarterly, 4,* 65–66.

Chiou, I. I. L., & Burnett, C. N. (1985). Values of activities of daily living: A survey of stroke patients and their home therapists. *Physical Therapy, 65,* 901–906.

Christiansen, C. (1991). Occupational therapy intervention for life performance (pp. 1–43). In C. Christiansen & C. Baum (Eds.), *Occupational therapy: Overcoming human performance deficits.* Thorofare, NJ: Slack.

Clark, F., Parham, D., Carlson, M. E., Frank, G., Jackson, J. Pierce, D., Wolfe, R. J., & Zemke, R. (1991). Occupational science: Academic innovation in the service of occupational therapy's future. *American Journal of Occupational Therapy, 45,* 300–310.

Cynkin, S., & Robinson, J. M. (1990). *Occupational therapy and activities health: Toward health through activities.* Boston: Little, Brown.

DeKuiper, W. P., Nelson, D. L., & White, B. E. (1993). Materials-based occupation versus imagery-based occupation versus rote exercise: A replication and extension. *Occupational Therapy Journal of Research, 13,* 183–197.

Dunton, W. R., Jr. (1914). Roundtable. *Maryland Psychiatric Quarterly, 4,* 20–32.

Editorial. (1929). Susan E. Tracy. *Occupational Therapy and Rehabilitation, 8,* 63–66.

Fleming, M. (1990). Untitled invited paper presented at the American Occupational Therapy Foundation planning meeting for the Occupation Symposium, Boston, MA.

Georgopoulos, A. P. (1986). On reaching. *Annual Review of Neurosciences, 9,* 147–170.

Haas, L. J. (1922). Crafts adaptable to occupational needs: Their relative importance. *Archives of Occupational Therapy, 1,* 443–455.

Haugen, J. B., & Mathiowetz, V. (1995). Contemporary task-oriented approach. In C. A. Trombly (Ed.), *Occupational therapy for physical dysfunction* (4th ed.) (pp. 510–528). Baltimore: Williams & Wilkins.

Hawking, S. W. (1988). *A brief history of time: From the big bang to black holes.* New York: Bantam.

Horak, F. B. (1991). Assumptions underlying motor control for neurologic rehabilitation. In M. Lister (Ed.), *Contemporary management of motor control problems. Proceedings of the II STEP Conference* (pp. 11–27). Alexandria, VA: Foundation for Physical Therapy.

Jeannerod, M. (1988). *The neural and behavioral organization of goal-directed movements.* Oxford: Clarendon.

Jebsen, R. H., Taylor, N., Trieschmann, R. B., Trotter, M., & Howard, L. A. (1969). An objective and standardized test of hand function. *Archives of Physical Medicine and Rehabilitation, 50,* 311–319.

Kamm, K., Thelen, E., & Jensen, J. L. (1990). A dynamical systems approach to motor development. *Physical Therapy, 70,* 763–775.

Kielhofner, G. (Ed.). (1985). *A Model of Human Occupation.* Baltimore: Williams & Wilkins.

Kielhofner, G. (1992). *Conceptual foundations of occupational therapy.* Philadelphia: F. A. Davis.

Kircher, M. A. (1984). Motivation as a factor of perceived exertion in purposeful versus nonpurposeful activity. *American Journal of Occupational Therapy, 38,* 165–170.

Lang, E. M., Nelson, D. L., & Bush, M. A. (1992). Comparison of performance in materials-based occupation, imagery-based occupation, and rote exercise in nursing home residents. *American Journal of Occupational Therapy, 46,* 607–611.

LaMore, K. L., & Nelson, D. L. (1993). The effects of options on performance of an art project in adults with mental disabilities. *American Journal of Occupational Therapy, 47,* 397–401.

Llorens, L. A. (1986). Activity analysis: Agreement among factors in a sensory processing model. *American Journal of Occupational Therapy, 40,* 103–110.

Llorens, L. A. (1993). Activity analysis: Agreement between participants and observers on perceived factors in occupation components. *Occupational Therapy Journal of Research, 13,* 198–211.

Lowney, M. E. P. (1930). The relationship between occupational therapy and rehabilitation. *Massachusetts Association for Occupational Therapy Bulletin, 4*(2).

Luria, A. R. (1973). *The working brain: An introduction to neuropsychology.* New York: Basic.

Mathiowetz, V. G. (1991). *Informational support and functional motor performance.* Unpublished doctoral dissertation, University of Minnesota.

Mathiowetz, V., & Haugen, J. B. (1994). Motor behavior research: Implications for therapeutic approaches to central nervous system dysfunction. *American Journal of Occupational Therapy, 48,* 733–745.

Mathiowetz, V., & Haugen, J. B. (1995). Evaluation of motor behavior: Traditional and contemporary views. In C. A. Trombly (Ed.), *Occupational therapy for physical dysfunction* (4th ed., pp. 157–186). Baltimore: Williams & Wilkins.

Marteniuk, R. G., MacKenzie, C. L., Jeannerod, M., Athenes, S., & Dugas, C. (1987). Constraints on human arm movement trajectories. *Canadian Journal of Psychology, 41,* 365–378.

McKinnon, A, L. (1992). Time use for self-care, productivity, and leisure among elderly Canadians. *Canadian Journal of Occupational Therapy, 59,* 102–110.

Meyer, A. (1977). The philosophy of occupational therapy. American Journal of Occupational Therapy, 31, 639–642. Reprinted from *Archives of Occupational Therapy, 1,* 1–10, 1922.

Miller, L., & Nelson, D. L. (1987). Dual-purpose activity versus single-purpose activity in terms of duration of task, exertion level, and affect. *Occupational Therapy in Mental Health, 1,* 55–67.

Morasso, P., & Zaccaria, R. (1986). Understanding human movement. *Experimental Brain Research, 15,* 145–157.

Neistadt, M. E., McAuley, D., Zecha, D., & Shannon, R. (1993). An analysis of a board game as a treatment activity. *American Journal of Occupational Therapy, 47,* 154–160.

Nelson, C. E., & Payton, 0. D. (1991). A system for involving patients in program planning. *American Journal of Occupational Therapy, 45,* 753–755.

Nelson, D. L. (1988). Occupation: Form and performance. *American Journal of Occupational Therapy, 42,* 633–641.

Nelson, D. L. (1990). Untitled invited paper presented at the American Occupational Therapy Foundation planning meeting for the Occupation Symposium, Boston, MA.

Nelson, W. L. (1983). Physical principles for economies of skilled movements. *Biological Cybernetics, 46,* 135–147.

Newell, K. M., & Corcos, D. M. (1993). Issues in variability and motor control. In K. M. Newell & D. M. Corcos (Eds.), *Variability and motor control* (pp. 1–12). Champaign, IL: Human Kinetics.

Parsons, S. E. (1917). Miss Tracy's work in general hospitals. *Maryland Psychiatric Quarterly, 6,* 63–64.

Purdum, H. D. (1911). The psycho-therapeutic value of occupation. *Maryland Psychiatric Quarterly, 1,* 35–36.

Riccio, C. M., Nelson, D. L., & Bush, M. A. (1990). Adding purpose to the repetitive exercise of elderly women through imagery. *American Journal of Occupational Therapy, 44,* 714–719.

Rogers, J. C. (1982). The spirit of independence: The evolution of a philosophy. *American Journal of Occupational Therapy, 36,* 709–715.

Sharrott, G. W. (1983). Occupational therapy's role in the client's creation and affirmation of meaning. In G. Kielhofner (Ed.), *Health through occupation: Theory and practice in occupational therapy.* Philadelphia: F. A. Davis.

Sietsema, J. M., Nelson, D. L., Mulder, R. M., Mervau-Scheidel, D., & White, B.E. (1993). The use of a game to promote arm reach in persons with traumatic brain injury. *American Journal of Occupational Therapy, 47,* 19–24.

Slagle, E. C. (1914). History of the development of occupation for the insane. *Maryland Psychiatric Quarterly, 4,* 14–20.

Smith, N. R., Kielhofner, G., & Watts, J. H. (1986). The relationships among volition, activity pattern, and life satisfaction in the elderly. *American Journal of Occupational Therapy, 40,* 278–283.

Steinbeck, T. M. (1986). Purposeful activity and performance. *American Journal of Occupational Therapy, 40,* 529–534.

Swaim, L. T. (1928). Does occupational work hasten recovery of the crippled? *Massachusetts Association of Occupational Therapy Bulletin, 2*(3).

Taylor, D. P. (1974). Treatment goals for quadriplegic and paraplegic patients. *American Journal of Occupational Therapy, 28,* 22–29.

Thibodeaux, C. S., & Ludwig, F. M. (1988). Intrinsic motivation in product-oriented and nonproduct-oriented activities. *American Journal of Occupational Therapy, 42,* 169–175.

Trombly, C. (1993). Anticipating the future: Assessment of occupational function. *American Journal of Occupational Therapy, 47,* 253–257.

Trombly, C. (Ed.). (1995a). *Occupational therapy for physical dysfunction* (4th ed.). Baltimore: Williams & Wilkins.

Trombly, C. A. (1995b). *Relationships between motor and perceptual performance components and activities of daily living.* Unpublished paper, Boston University.

Trombly, C. A., & Cole, J. M. (1979). Electromyographic study of four hand muscles during selected activities. *American Journal of Occupational Therapy, 33,* 440–449.

Tsai, P. L. (1994). *Activity analysis and activity selection among occupational therapists: A survey.* Unpublished master's thesis, Boston University, Boston.

Van der Weel, F. R., van der Meer, A. L. H., & Lee, D. N. (1991). Effect of task on movement control in cerebral palsy: Implications for assessment and therapy. *Developmental Medicine and Child Neurology, 33,* 419–426.

Wagenaar, R. C., & Meijer, O. G. (1991a). Effects of stroke rehabilitation (1): A critical review of the literature. *Journal of Rehabilitation Sciences, 4,* 61–73.

Wagenaar, R. C., & Meijer, O. G. (1991b). Effects of stroke rehabilitation (2): A critical review of the literature. *Journal of Rehabilitation Sciences, 4,* 97–109.

White, R. W. (1959). Motivation reconsidered: The concept of competence. *Psychological Review, 66,* 297–333.

Wu, C. Y. (1993). *The relationship between occupational form and occupational performance: A kinematic perspective.* Unpublished master's thesis, Boston University.

Wu, C. Y., Trombly, C. A., & Lin, K. C. (1994). The relationship between occupational form and occupational performance: A kinematic perspective. *American Journal of Occupational Therapy, 48,* 679–687.

Yerxa, E. J., & Baum, S. (1986). Engagement in daily occupations and life satisfaction among people with spinal cord injuries. *Occupational Therapy Journal of Research, 6,* 271–283.

Yerxa, E., & Locker, S. (1990). Quality of time use by adults with spinal cord injuries. *American Journal of Occupational Therapy, 44,* 318–326.

Yerxa, E. J., Clark, F., Frank, G., Jackson, J., Parham, D., Pierce, D., Stein, C., & Zemkè, R. (1990). An introduction to occupational science: A foundation for occupational therapy in the 21st century. *Occupational Therapy in Health Care, 6,* 1–32.

Yoder, R. M., Nelson, D. L., & Smith, D. A. (1989). Added purpose versus rote exercise in female nursing home residents. *American Journal of Occupational Therapy, 43,* 581–586.

PART III

Contextual Considerations for Engagement in Occupation and Participation

Introduction

A basic philosophical premise of occupational therapy is that a person and his or her occupations cannot be understood or worked with therapeutically without consideration of context. This premise was clearly evident in Part I in which the contextual aspects of occupational therapy were strongly emphasized by the founders of our profession and recently reaffirmed with the adoption of the *Occupational Therapy Practice Framework* (American Occupational Therapy Association [AOTA], 2002; reprinted as Appendix A in this volume). These contexts include the physical, social, cultural, spiritual, virtual, and temporal aspects of performance and service delivery. The influence of context on an individual's occupational performance and the occupational therapy process cannot be underestimated (AOTA, 2002).

As highlighted in the practice models provided in Part II, the meaningfulness and value of occupation cannot be understood without considering the contexts of occupational performance (Law, 2002). Assessing a person's ability to prepare a meal in a large, well-equipped, occupational therapy activities of daily living kitchen and providing intervention to teach meal preparation skills in this setting are totally irrelevant and virtually useless to the person whose only kitchen is a one-burner hotplate in a single-room occupancy hotel. As Cynkin (1995) stated, "The nature of everyday activities emerges only from the context in which they are embedded" (p. 13). Therefore, the occupational therapy practitioner must assess the individual's current and expected contexts throughout the occupational therapy process to ensure a comprehensive evaluation and a relevant plan of intervention (AOTA, 2002; Mosey, 1996).

This section has gathered literature that provide readers with the knowledge and skills needed to effectively assess the contexts of occupation and occupational therapy service delivery. Chapter 17 begins with a presentation of a comprehensive framework for considering the effect of context on human performance. Dunn, Brown, and McGuigan provide a broad, encompassing definition of context, emphasizing the importance of analyzing contextual features during occupational therapy evaluation and intervention. They review relevant literature from the social sciences and occupational therapy to identify pertinent environmental concepts and definitions, establishing a foundation for their Ecology of Human Performance (EHP) framework. This framework provides an organized structure for systematically considering the complexities of temporal, physical, social, and cultural contexts in occupational therapy practice. The authors describe context as a lens through which the individual views the world, with the interrelationships between the person and the contexts determining the tasks that are within the person's performance range. They propose and define five alternatives for therapeutic intervention that enable the occupational therapy practitioner to collaborate with the individual and the family to meet performance needs within the person's environmental contexts. Numerous case examples, illustrated schemata, and clear practical suggestions complete their discussion. The use of the EHP framework to thoroughly consider context can be invaluable to a practitioner, for it removes the limitations and potential dangers of evaluating performance and planning intervention out of context.

As noted in the EHP model and the *Practice Framework*, the cultural context is particularly important to consider throughout the occupational therapy process. Culture is external to the person and determines expectations, beliefs, and customs, but the individual also internalizes these factors (AOTA, 2002). Culture influences all aspects of occupation; that is, "what we do, how, when, where, for how long, and with whom we do it" (Cynkin, 1995, p. 151). Therefore, occupational therapy practitioners must have a thorough understanding of a person's cultural context to ensure the appropriateness of his or her evaluation and intervention. The next three chapters provide thoughtful analyses of the link between culture and occupation.

In Chapter 18, Schemm provides a comprehensive discussion of how culture influences the occupational therapy process and the outcome of treatment. A historical analysis of views about culture held by occupational therapy founders and theorists is presented. Levine defines culture and identifies components of culture, examining how they pertain to and affect occupational therapy clinical practice. The influence of culture on a person's perception of illness, health, and therapy and a person's belief in the meaning of his or her own life and activities are explored. Guidelines for considering cultural factors during evaluation and treatment are provided, along with a case study, highlighting the relevance of these factors to the ultimate outcome of occupational therapy.

Krefting, in Chapter 19, expands on Levine's exploration of culture, providing an in-depth analysis of the practical implications of culturally sensitive and culturally insensitive practice. She presents a multidimensional definition of culture, with emphasis placed on the individual level of culture and its effects on assessment and treatment. The importance of increasing awareness of one's own cultural orientation, values, and beliefs is highlighted. The costs of culturally insensitive therapy are analyzed, and strategies for enhancing cultural sensitivity are provided. Clinical examples from pediatric practice support these culturally sensitive principles, which are clearly relevant to all areas of occupational therapy practice.

Clearly, competent occupational therapy practitioners are aware of the need to address culture throughout the occupational therapy process. However, the authors of Chapter 20 propose that unclear definitions of culture provide little guidance to practitioners about how to recognize culture's effects in therapeutic encounters. They review diverse definitions of culture and examine the usefulness and limitations of description-based and rules-based approaches to defining culture. To counter these limits, Bonder, Martin, and Miracle adopt a third approach to examining culture. They put forth a pragmatic definition of culture as emergent in everyday interactions of individuals. This view

conceptualizes culture as a symbolic system that emerges through the interaction of individuals. They explore how this culture-emergent perspective requires a reconsideration of important characteristics of culture.

The conceptualization that culture is learned, localized, patterned, evaluative, and persistent is explored, with the authors concluding that these characteristics can change and adapt as a result of interaction. They propose that understanding culture as emerging from interaction, including the therapeutic relationship, has important implications for occupational therapy practitioners. Bonder, Martin, and Miracle analyze the influence of culture on occupation patterns and occupation choice, providing suggestions for occupational therapy practitioners to use to enhance therapeutic encounters. They emphasize that careful attention to the emergent nature of culture in each person, active curiosity about the cultural aspects of interactions, and self-reflection and self-evaluation of therapeutic interaction can enhance the occupational therapy process due to improved therapeutic collaboration. As Dickie (2004) reminds us, "attending to cultural moments, sensitivity to the possibility of difference, and awareness of the cultural in our own realities are strategies to help us achieve cultural competence in the moment" (p. 172).

One inherent component of culture that cannot be ignored in any occupational therapy practice is time. As Hall (1959) clearly explained in his landmark work on culture, "time is an element of culture which communicates as powerfully as language" (p. 140). The temporal context of occupation has a rich historical base in occupational therapy literature and practice, as evident in the founders' emphasis on the need for a temporal balance among work, self-care, play, and rest. The temporal context is still vitally important to occupational therapy evaluation and treatment as evident in the *Practice Framework's* exploration of performance patterns; therefore, the

next three chapters are presented to explore the temporal aspects of occupation and the nature of temporal adaptation.

In Chapter 21, Kielhofner's seminal exploration of temporal adaptation provides a comprehensive presentation of a conceptual framework for considering this concept in occupational therapy evaluation and intervention. Recognizing the value occupational therapy founders consistently placed on the temporal aspects of performance, Kielhofner calls for a renewed appreciation of this concept's influence on adaptation and dysfunction. He presents a review of the literature, describing characteristics of temporal adaptation and temporal dysfunction. A series of propositions about temporal adaptation are presented that can be used to develop strategies to evaluate temporal adaptation and treat temporal dysfunction in a socioculturally relevant manner. Two case examples demonstrate the application of this temporal adaptation framework to occupational therapy clinical practice.

A primary assumption underlying the occupational therapy process is that people's use of time as they participate in occupation is related to their overall quality of life and well-being. In Chapter 22, Farnworth asserts that time use, tempo, and temporality have been central to the profession since its founding, providing an overview of this philosophical heritage. However, Farnworth expresses concern that occupational therapy practitioners' understanding and use of these concepts have been fragmented and often invisible in actual practice. To help occupational therapy practitioners reclaim time as central to occupational therapy theory and practice, she presents a comprehensive review of the literature and recent research related to tempo, temporality, and time use. The relationship among these concepts and the presence and absence of health and well-being are strongly supported. Farnworth presents numerous societal and clinical scenarios to support her stance that tempo, temporality, and time use are strongly related to health outcomes. The expertise that occupational therapy practitioners can contribute to the well-being and quality of life of individuals and communities experiencing temporal dysfunction is highlighted. Farnworth concludes that, because society's recognition of our knowledge and skills in this area is nil, occupational therapy practitioners have a responsibility to explain, communicate, and research time use, tempo, and temporality because they are the essence of our profession.

As Farnworth noted, if occupational therapy practitioners do not investigate time use or establish their own expertise in this area, others will. The reality that research on time use is valued, meaningful, and relevant is strongly supported when one examines the temporal concept of flow and its related research. Chapter 23 by Emerson provides a comprehensive literature review on flow and occupation. She proposes that the shift in our profession's research to qualitative examinations of the subjective experiences of people engaged in occupation can greatly benefit from knowledge obtained through research on flow. This research conducted by Csikszentmihalyi and colleagues provides a wealth of information about the measurement of time spent in activity and the subjective experience of activity or pursuit. From this research, Csikszentmihalyi and colleagues developed a theory about the essence of intrinsic motivation, termed *flow*.

As Emerson reviews, flow is defined as a subjective psychological state, which occurs when one is completely immersed in an activity. She describes the characteristics of the flow experience and the positive outcomes of this experience, which has been viewed to be the highest level of well-being. The postulate that a match between environmental demands and a person's perception of his or her skills is needed to achieve flow is particularly relevant to

occupational therapy practitioners' knowledge and skills related to activity synthesis. Emerson reviews the continuum used to study flow, which contains the optimal state of flow, anxiety, boredom, and apathy. Flow activities and flow experiences across cultures, in adversity, and in everyday life are examined. The type of personality that is inclined to experience flow is explained. From this literature review, the relevance of flow theory to the philosophy and practice of occupational therapy is clearly evident. As Emerson notes, flow "names and frames" a phenomenon that is highly congruent with the core values and fundamental beliefs of our profession. She outlines eight principles for occupational therapy practitioners to use to help people engage in flow-inducing activities. Emerson concludes by posing several relevant research questions related to occupation and flow. She proposes that this is an appropriate time for the implementation of research that may support our profession's heritage and provide information that can enhance the occupational therapy process.

An important aspect of flow is that it is an intensely personal experience that is considered vital to growth. A context highly relevant to the occupational therapy process that is also intensely personal and often related to growth is the spiritual context. According to the *Practice Framework,* the spiritual context is internal to the individual; influences his or her personal beliefs, perceptions, and expectations; and inspires and motivates the individual, thereby influencing occupational therapy service delivery. This section's next two chapters explain important dimensions of spirituality and a person's inner life.

In Chapter 24, McColl presents her Muriel Driver Memorial Lecture, which explored spirituality, occupation, and disability. Her thought-provoking discussion is guided by the results of two spirituality studies and an extensive literature review. In this reflective work,

McColl examines definitions of spirituality, spirit, and transcendence and related themes from the occupational therapy literature. She then reinterprets these themes according to the definitions that she provides for spirituality, spirit, and transcendence. Her discussion of the essence of self, the power of will and intention, the connection among people, and the source of meaning raises many important issues and questions worthy of reflection. McColl also explores perspectives about the spiritual aspects of living with a disability and the ability to experience spirituality through occupation. The reality that the personal limitations of occupational therapy practitioners and practice-setting constraints restrict the embracement of spirituality in practice is honestly discussed.

While occupational therapy practitioners recognize the theoretical relevance of spirituality, McColl identifies a continuum of how spirituality is actually addressed in practice. She provides practical suggestions for assessment and intervention that can help expand the occupational therapy practitioner's role with respect to the spiritual realm. McColl's discussion of activities that are creative antecedents to spiritual experience is particularly noteworthy and provides practitioners with concrete ideas to increase the goodness-of-fit between our theoretical support of spirituality and our actual practices. Relevant quotes from her research studies support her interpretations and provide personal insights into the relationship among spirit, disability, and occupation.

Further reflections on the relationship between an individual's most personal characteristics and inner life are provided in Fine's 1990 Eleanor Clarke Slagle Lecture, which is presented in Chapter 25. In this inspiring work, Fine examines several concepts related to spirit as she answers the question "Who rises above adversity?" She explores remarkable examples of human adaptability and resilience in the face of extraordinary hardships and major adversity. Fine reflects on the reality that occupational therapy practitioners often work in a world of incredible trauma and stunning triumph. She examines factors that influence resilience, the relationship between these internal qualities and the external world, and the person's emerging capabilities to adapt to adversity. Several theories on stress and various perspectives on coping are provided. Fine's analysis of the social and personal meaning of trauma and resilience is interwoven with striking personal anecdotes and poetry from people who have experienced extraordinary trauma. Fine proposes that an increased appreciation of the power of a person's inner psychological life can strengthen the occupational therapy process. She reminds us that many people we work with will have their capacities for resilience threatened by an often unresponsive health care system and the constant challenges of living with chronic illness and disability. Therefore, occupational therapy practitioners must use our skills to provide timely and meaningful interventions to assist in the reintegration process and to transform adversity into possibilities, thereby facilitating the person's ability to attain an inner life that rises above adversity.

The process of becoming and living life as a self-actualized person is further analyzed by Rowles, who proposes that the essence of this process is a combination of knowing, doing, and being. In Chapter 26, Rowles analyzes the way in which the environment can become part of the person's being. Rowles explores people's immersion into culturally defined spatiotemporal environments. His analysis integrates concepts of physical space, time, and culture with the human processes of knowing, doing, and being. An emphasis on the understanding of the nature of "being in place" and methods for researching this vital process are provided through the discussion of the extensive enthnographic study conducted by Rowles. This study clearly substantiates the relevance of understanding individuals' immersion into their highly individualized life world (i.e., their "being in place"). Occupational therapy practitioners who are sensitive to the significance of the environment can identify interventions that are attuned to the individual's life world, whether that environment is a home of many years or a recent relocation. Rowles argues that increased attention and sensitivity to and concern for a person's "being in place" is a vital part of occupational therapy practice that is highly relevant to all people, whether they are living in a home environment or in a residential, institutional setting.

As Rowles reflected, an important aspect of "being" is "doing." We learn skills and develop a sense of accomplishment by engagement in occupations that vary across the life span. The next three chapters in this section explore developmental aspects of this personal context. In Chapter 27, Missiuna and Pollack explore the physical, social, personal, and environmental barriers that contribute to play deprivation in children with disabilities. They emphasize that self-initiated free-play experiences must be readily available to all children because play is the principle occupation that contributes to a child's normal growth and development. The nature, purpose, and benefits of play are highlighted, supporting the need for occupational therapy practitioners to help children with disabilities develop free-play skills. Missiuna and Pollock postulate that children with disabilities who are deprived of normal play opportunities develop secondary social, emotional, and psychological disabilities. These secondary disabilities hinder development and may limit potential for independence and adaptive functioning throughout the life span. They explore barriers to free play for children with disabilities, including restrictions set by caregivers and the physical, sensory, and personal limitations of the child.

Missiuna and Pollock advocate that occupational therapy practitioners assume an active role in developing and maintaining free play for the child with disabilities in many settings. Guidelines for comprehensively assessing developmental play levels; principles for collaborating with parents, teachers, and caregivers; and recommendations for a multitude of interventions are provided. The authors emphasize the need for occupational therapy practitioners to consider the child's developmental abilities, familial and peer relationships, adaptations of play materials, and environmental modifications. They conclude that the promotion and provision of active, self-initiated play in the home, school, and community will provide children with disabilities the developmental experiences needed to become productive members of society.

The need for occupational therapy practitioners to actively work with children with disabilities to develop their abilities for full social participation is strongly supported by Broillier, Shephard, and Markley's discussion of transitional planning for adolescents. While the developmental stage of adolescence is typically characterized by a great deal of decision-making and a large amount of personal growth, this normal transition can be further complicated when the adolescent has a disability. Therefore, there is a critical need to develop interventions for adolescents with disabilities designed to facilitate healthy transitions from adolescence to adulthood.

In Chapter 28, Broillier, Shepherd, and Markley address this vital need by discussing the use of individualized transition plans (ITPs) for students with disabilities. The development and implementation of an effective ITP can help students move successfully from a school setting into employment and community living. The authors describe the assessment and intervention process, focusing on functional activities within the home, school, community, recreational, and vocational environments. Standards for realistic, relevant goal setting, intervention principles, and service characteristics are provided. A strong emphasis is placed on developing those skills needed for safe, healthy, productive living and in fostering community integration and participation in adult activities. Their presentation is supported by a review of occupational therapy and special education literature on occupational performance, functional activities, and transitional planning. Federal initiatives and legislative mandates concerning vocational transition for youths with disabilities are also reviewed. The role of the ITP team in collaborating with the student and parents to develop and implement a comprehensive transition plan is discussed. Potential barriers to collaborative planning are explored, with suggestions to reduce these barriers and increase parental and student participation provided. The role of occupational therapy practitioners in adapting activities, modifying the environment, and providing technological aids to implement ITPs and develop adolescents' social, self-care, home management, work, school, and leisure skills to live and work within the community is clearly discussed.

The importance of achieving full community participation is further explored in Chapter 29 by Crist and Stoffel. In their discussion, they analyze the impact of the Americans with Disabilities Act (ADA) on the evaluation and enhancement of work environments for people with mental illness. Their comprehensive analysis integrates occupational therapy principles with literature on personal self-efficacy, employment readiness, and the ADA, and they provide a clear link between performance accomplishments and occupational therapy's focus on using purposeful activities and the "doing" process in intervention. ADA criteria for determining essential job functions, marginal job functions, and reasonable accommodations are clearly

identified. Implications for occupational therapy practice are discussed, including the development of advocacy and attitude training programs to reduce stigma and the provision of concrete assistance to employers seeking to provide reasonable accommodations to people with mental illness seeking preparation for successful employment. Although Crist's and Stoffel's main focus is on people with mental illness, the issues identified (particularly those regarding personal self-efficacy) are highly relevant to all people with disabilities in a work setting. The authors challenge occupational therapy practitioners to assume leadership positions and act as agents of change to assist people with disabilities in achieving efficacy and independence within their work environments.

In Chapter 30, Grady amplifies this challenge to create enabling environments in her 1994 Eleanor Clarke Slagle Lecture on building inclusive communities. She analyzes the nature and meaning of community and examines the relationships among individuals, their families, their culture, environmental contexts, and community. Foundations for building personal communities of choice are identified. The interaction among a person's past experience, present situation, future aspirations, and ability to choose are explored as they affect the relationship between the occupational therapy practitioner and the consumer of occupational therapy services. Grady discusses the challenge for practitioners in understanding each person's unique community and its culture, context, and foundation. She calls for occupational therapy practitioners to develop skills in analyzing environments and environmental interaction. Current ideas about the philosophy of inclusion, societal mandates, and legislative initiatives for inclusion, along with contrasting views about disability, are presented. Grady emphasizes the need to recognize disability as a dimension of diversity and not as a limiting handicap. She proposes four key values for

occupational therapy reflective of an interactive model of disability and supportive on inclusion and choice.

Grady also entreats occupational therapy practitioners to create opportunities for people with disabilities to develop their capacities within their chosen community environments. To achieve this goal, environmental barriers must be removed and supports and adaptations must be provided. Grady cautions that attitudinal and emotional barriers, supports, and adaptations must be considered along with the physical aspects of the environment. The removal of attitudinal barriers, the provision of emotional supports, and the development of physical adaptations can foster the person's ability to engage in meaningful activity within his or her natural environments. Grady also presents the spatiotemporal adaptation theory, which views development in children and ongoing functioning in adults as a transactional process between the individual and the environment. She describes a spiraling continuum of environments that promote inclusion, independence, interdependence, and successful adaptation. Interactive strategies for occupational therapy practitioners to use to build collaborative models of consumer-driven, community-based practice are presented with an emphasis on the therapeutic communication process.

This section's prior chapters on developmental considerations presented strong cases for interventions to achieve participation whether that participation is the play of a child or the work of the adult. However, as emphasized by Grady's discussion of inclusive community and highlighted in the *Practice Framework*, there often are political, social, and cultural barriers to the achievement of this outcome. Chapter 31 by Whiteford provides a thoughtful discussion about the effects of external restrictions on people. She proposes that, when these external factors are beyond the person's control and restrict the individual's ability to engage in occupations of meaning, the result is occupational deprivation. Whiteford defines occupational deprivation, emphasizing that deprivation does not result from limitations inherent within the person but rather from external forces. She analyzes the related phenomena of occupational disruption and dysfunction to clarify their differences from occupational deprivation. Whiteford explores the conceptual origins of occupational deprivation, noting that, while this is a relatively new term, the phenomenon itself has been present throughout world history. However, recent global trends such as advances in technology, the maldistribution of labor, the marginalization of people, and the experience of refugeeism are contributing to increased occupational deprivation. Whiteford reflects on the human costs of occupational deprivation and identifies ways that occupational therapy practitioners can address occupational deprivation. She suggests the adoption of a perspective that incorporates occupation with broader social, international, and cultural dimensions. Having a global viewpoint can help practitioners think and act in a manner that is congruent with our concerns for social and occupational justice. Most important, Whiteford presents a call to arms for occupational therapy practitioners to address occupational deprivation through social and political action.

The relevance of occupational deprivation and justice to occupational therapy is expanded on in Chapter 32 by Townsend and Wilcock. These authors explore the phenomena of occupational deprivation and propose that this is one of four types of occupational injustice that can be derived from their exploratory theory of occupational justice. Townsend and Wilcock examine the significance of these occupational injustices to occupational therapy and contend that the naming of these suggests four occupational rights: the right to experience meaning and enrichment in one's occupation, the right to participate in a range of occupations for health and social inclusion, the right to make choices and share decision-making power in daily life, and the right to receive equal privileges for diverse participation in occupations. Townsend's and Wilcock's reflections in their ongoing international dialogue about the relationship between occupation justice and client-centered practice provide a stellar example for occupational therapy practitioners seeking to work for justice. They accurately state that, because silence implies compliance with the status quo, practitioners should develop their own dialogue about occupational injustices to bring these issues to the forefront of our profession. They remind us that dialogue about occupational injustice is timely as occupational therapy practitioners around the world focus on providing best practices that synthesize and apply our knowledge, skills, and attitudes about occupation, enabling, and justice. In their treatise, Townsend and Wilcock present a persuasive argument that occupational therapy as a profession exists to address occupational injustice and that it is up to occupational therapy practitioners to make this proposal explicit to the world. They describe specific actions occupational therapy clinicians, managers, educators, policymakers, and researchers can take to support client-centered activism for occupational justice to ensure that all individuals attain and maintain their rights to occupation.

The concept that humans have an inalienable right to occupation is further explored by Wilcock, who developed a theory of the human need for occupation. This theory proposes that occupation is not just the purpose of human function but an integral component of each human being's relationship with the world. Wilcock explores this biological need to do and proposes that needs have a three-way role in maintaining the health and stability of the person. She relates these three functions to occupation, explaining how engagement in purposeful occupation contributes to the survival of the species. She argues that occupation fulfills basic human needs essential for survival and develops biological, social, and cultural capacities of the person, enabling the person to grow and adapt to environmental changes and challenges. Occupation also provides the mechanism for people to interpret socially and to form the foundation for community. She contends that occupation is the means by which humans demonstrate their value to their society and the world. Wilcock expresses concern that the centrality of occupation to the human experience is being threatened by sociocultural, economic, and political forces and that the occupational needs of people have became obscured by the increased complexities of a technological world.

Wilcock's reflections on the negative impact of technology on the fundamental need for occupation are important for readers to carefully consider. The *Practice Framework* has identified the virtual context as relevant to the occupational therapy process, and our society has largely enculturated us to view the use of technology as a positive development for people with disabilities. While there are undeniable recognizable benefits to technology, such as the use of electronic aids to daily living to master the environment, readers should carefully reflect on the full implementation of the definition of the virtual context. As defined in the *Practice Framework,* the virtual context is "the environment in which communication occurs by means of airways, computers, and *an absence of physical contact*" (italics added) (AOTA, 2002, p. 623). Because our profession's core philosophy supports the view that occupation is a fundamental human need, what is the impact on the person's health and spirit when physical contact is removed? Will our society's increased emphasis on technology further isolate people with disabilities?

Yerxa further examines the relationship among occupation, health, and spirit and explores post–industrial societal forces that are endangering human's occupational being in Chapter 33. She describes her view of health as the possession of a repertoire of skills that enable individuals to achieve desired goals in their chosen environments, not as the absence of pathology. Adopting this perspective means that health is possible for all people, including those with chronic illnesses and disabilities. Yerxa reviews the literature from occupational therapy and other disciplines to highlight the key influences of occupations on health. These influences include interests, satisfaction in everyday doing, balance, the latent consequences of work, and transcendence. Yerxa continues her exploration of the literature by focusing on research about the "hardy" personality and mortality. Yerxa concludes that both theory and research support a relationship among occupation, survival, health, and well-being. She challenges occupational therapy practitioners to create environments that enable meaningful occupation and provide all people with "just-right challenges" to achieve participation in life.

The fact that context influences participation has been strongly supported by all of the authors in this part. However, the reality that there exist significant contextual constraints to this participation cannot be ignored (Cottrell, 2003; Law, 2002). Therefore, occupational therapy practitioners must advocate for the development of community-based services, for this is the environment in which engagement in "real occupation" takes place. This advocacy is critical in today's political environment and health care delivery system that is emphasizing community-based care, yet limiting resources. As hospital lengths of stay decrease, individuals are being discharged with a multitude of limitations affecting their ability to participate in their environment in a need-satisfying manner. As a result, hospital-based occupational therapy practitioners must immediately evaluate the home and community environment to ensure that occupational therapy intervention is relevant to the person's discharge goals. Home-care and community-based practitioners must develop the necessary supports and provide the required adaptations and modifications to ensure the person's safe, active participation in his or her contexts. School-based practitioners must expand their vision beyond the classroom to view the broader environmental contexts of children with disabilities. This view is particularly critical as students "age out" of educational systems and sadly find few opportunities to participate fully within their community environment (Bremer, Kachal, & Schoeller, 2003).

All occupational therapy practitioners have an ethical responsibility to advocate for sociopolitical change supportive of full participation and for the allocation of adequate resources to enable people with disabilities to live in environments of choice (Williams, 2004). Current evaluations and interventions are rendered meaningless if people with disabilities are not participating members of their communities. A sociopolitical system that devalues people with disabilities by providing insufficient resources will force full participation to remain an elusive goal supported by empty rhetoric rather than becoming an achievable reality. As recognized in the *Practice Framework*, politics and legislation directly affects access to resources, limiting the power of occupation. Part 6 of this text explores these issues further. I believe that we all share a collective responsibility to use our occupational therapy knowledge and skills to fight for political actions and legislative initiatives that support and finance participation. The reality is that major societal change will be required to enable people with disabilities to affirm their fundamental right to participate in life (Williams, 2004).

Questions to Consider

1. Analyze your current living environment (e.g., your home and community). What are the physical, social, cultural, personal, spiritual, virtual, and temporal contexts of your occupations? What contextual characteristics are supportive of your occupational performance? What are the contextual barriers or constraints that limit your occupational performance?

2. Would the contextual supports identified above facilitate the achievement of occupational justice? Would the contextual barriers identified above result in occupational injustice? Are there incidences of occupational injustice in your local community (e.g., ADA noncompliant services and programs, inaccessible voting places, predominance of institutional-based care vs. community-based care)? How can occupational therapy practitioners act to end occupational injustices on a local level?

3. Imagine you acquired a serious, long-term disability. Describe your environment of choice. What environmental supports, adaptations, and modifications would be needed to maximize your occupational performance and ensure an acceptable quality of life? How would your use of time change? What occupations would be essential for you to engage in to achieve temporal adaptation and to fulfill your human need for occupation?

4. Have you ever experienced flow? What were the characteristics of the activity that resulted in flow? How can the concept of flow be incorporated into the occupational therapy process?

5. Pair up with a peer from a different cultural background. Discuss each culture's view of health, illness, treatment, and the therapeutic relationship. Identify your culture's

values, beliefs, and norms. How will these affect your role as an occupational therapy practitioner? What are potential biases of your cultural background that may affect your professional roles and tasks?

6. Has spirituality influenced your life? Has your resilience ever been challenged? What was the nature of these influences and challenges, and how might these experiences shape you as an occupational therapy practitioner? What is the relationship between spirituality and resilience? How can occupational therapy practitioners honor a person's spirituality and resilience throughout the occupational therapy process?

7. Visit several communities with different physical characteristics and a diversity of cultures. Identify existing supports and barriers for people with disabilities. Be certain to consider attitudinal supports and barriers, along with the physical characteristics. What recommendations would you make for additional supports, adaptations, and modifications to create communities of inclusion? What resources are available to support your recommendations?

References

American Occupational Therapy Association. (2002). Occupational therapy practice framework: Domain and process. *American Journal of Occupational Therapy, 56,* 609–639.

Bremer, C., Kachal, M., & Schoeller, K. (2003, April). *Research to Practice Brief: Self-determination—Supporting successful transition.* Retrieved on November 18, 2003, from http://www.ncset.org/publication/printresource.asp?id=962.

Cottrell, R. P. (2003, March 10). The Olmstead decision: Fulfilling the promise of ADA? Implications for occupational therapy. *OT Practice,* pp. 17–21.

Cynkin, S. (1995). Activities. In C. B. Royeen (Ed.), *The practice of the future: Putting occupation back into therapy* (Lesson 7). Bethesda, MD: American Occupational Therapy Association.

Dickie, V. (2004). Culture is tricky: A commentary on culture emergent in occupation. *American Journal of Occupational Therapy, 58,* 169–173.

Hall, E. (1959). The silent language. New York: Doubleday.

Law, M. (2002). Distinguished Scholar Lecture: Participation in the occupation of everyday life. *American Journal of Occupational Therapy, 56,* 640–649.

Mosey, A. (1996). *Psychosocial components of occupational therapy.* New York: Raven Press.

Williams, K. (2004, February 23). Advocacy: Step up to the plate. *Advance for Occupational Therapy Practitioners,* p. 10.

The Ecology of Human Performance: A Framework for Considering the Effect of Context

CHAPTER 17

Winnie Dunn, PhD, OTR, FAOTA
Catana Brown, MA, OTR
Ann McGuigan, PhD

A person does not exist in a vacuum; the physical environment as well as social, cultural, and temporal factors all influence behavior. Taken together, those factors that operate external to the person are identified as *context* for the purposes of this article. Each person's contextual experience is unique, although many elements are shared among persons.

Consider the unique way that adults talk to young children. They may change the tone of their voices, carefully select their words, bend down to make themselves smaller, or use gestures that animate the conversation. Adults make these adaptations because they recognize the importance of context when talking to young children, such as the level of the child's communication skills or how the child might feel about talking to a big person. Use of these adaptive strategies by an adult speaking at a work meeting would be considered inappropriate because the context of a work meeting dictates other communication methods. The same need for contextually selected behavior exists in many realms of daily life. A Catholic who attends services at a synagogue derives different meaning from the experience than does her Jewish friend. When a family eats at a fast-food restaurant, a different repertoire of behaviors may be sanctioned than if that same family went to a restaurant with menus at the table. Context influences behavior and performance in many ways; disciplines that address human behavior must consider the effect of these contextual features on target behaviors.

A recurring theme in the occupational therapy literature is the concept that environment (i.e., context) is a critical factor in human performance. Despite this emphasis, the potential contribution of contextual features in evaluation and intervention relative to performance components and performance areas has received little attention. For example, occupational therapy has many assessments that examine muscle strength, social skills, vestibular function, dressing, or use of leisure time. However, contextual features such as the physical qualities of an environment, the cultural background of the person, or the effect of friendships on performance are often missing from assessment tools typically used in occupational therapy. The Ecology of Human Performance (EHP) framework has been developed by the occupational therapy faculty members at the University of Kansas in response to the lack of consideration for the complexities of context. The framework provides a structure for thinking of context as a key variable in assessment and intervention planning, while elucidating the inherent dangers in examining performance out of context.

Ecology is concerned with the interrelationships of organisms and their environments. Occupational therapy is interested in the interrelationship of humans and their contexts and the effect of these relationships on performance; hence this framework is entitled the Ecology of Human Performance.

The EHP framework provides guidelines directed at including contextual features in occupational therapy research and practice (Mosey, 1992). It draws from occupational therapy and social science knowledge to contribute a complementary perspective of ecological principles. As a framework, it delineates and defines the relevant concepts and describes relationships among variables. It provides direction for the development of specific frames of reference concerned with context or the reexamination of existing frames of reference and their attention to context. The following literature review acknowledges the major contribution of others in the development of this framework and provides the groundwork for understanding the EHP.

Relevant Literature From Social Science

The EHP framework is founded on and synthesizes the work of scholars in several disciplines who have considered the interaction between person and environment. Much of the original work was conducted by environmental psychologists who examined the interrelationship of the physical environment and human behavior or experience. In environmental psychology, persons are considered to be interdependent with their immediate environment; the focus of research is on the interaction of the physical elements of a person's immediate environment with behavior (Holahan, 1986; Wicker, 1979).

Although the EHP framework shares this emphasis on examining the interdependent relationship between the person and the physical environment, it expands the concept of context–environment to include physical, temporal, social, and cultural elements. Employing a broader definition of environment allows researchers to make explicit those elements that have frequently been left implicit by the environmental psychologists. For example, Wicker (1979) described the effect of settings on behavior and detailed how behavior might be modified to be appropriate for a particular environment. Implicit in his analysis is the assumption of a shared concept of the external environment. The use of context in the EHP framework balances the emphasis on the external environment presented in environmental psychology and suggests that the researcher–practitioner consider what the environment means to the person.

Hart (1979) conceptualized the environment as an instrument of socialization. He presented the concept of environmental competence as the "knowledge, skill and confidence to use the environment to carry out one's own goals and to enrich one's experience" (p. 343). Like other environmental psychologists, he emphasized that the process of learning about self and the environment is interactional and he limited the concept of environment to the physical environment.

The idea that context and person are interactional is fundamental to the EHP. It is assumed that persons both affect and are affected by their context. Although the interactional relationship between person and environment is of primary importance to environmental psychologists, none has described this process as completely as Bruner (1989). He developed the concept of transactional contextualism as a process in which the person constructs the self in the context of the environment. For example, a child who grows up in a large family develops a different construction of self than a child who grows up without siblings.

Lawton's conceptualization of environment more closely resembles that of the EHP than do those of other environmental psychologists. He presented a broader concept of environment that includes the personal, suprapersonal, and social as well as the physical (Lawton, 1982). Applying Murray's (1938) concept of environmental press to the physical environment, Lawton (1982) developed an ecological model of aging that describes the dynamics of ecological change, competence, and environmental press in which a person's environment affects perceptions of competence. In this model, behavior is thought to be "a function of the competence of the individual and the environmental press of the situation" (p. 43).

Hall (1983) and Zerubavel (1981) have examined the concept of time as an aspect of environment. Both considered time as context. Hall portrayed time as a factor that is different when persons live it and when they consider it. He argued for a contextually bound, culturally idiosyncratic, realistic concept of time. Zerubavel asserted that time is a major parameter of environment and that the two must mesh to produce a meaningful gestalt. Csikszentmihalyi (1990) described "flow" experiences in which persons are so immersed in a selected task that they are unaware of the passage of time. These authors' discussions of time as context provide excellent examples of the importance of considering time to be a component of context.

Several issues have been raised by those who have considered the relationship of environment to behavior. Many authors have distinguished between the phenomenological and physical nature of the environment. The EHP recognizes the role played by both. Gibson (1986) discussed both these aspects in his consideration of the relation between ecological context and visual perception. He suggested that the environment is both physical and phenomenological in that persons perceive objects in the environment by the affordances they offer. The environment–context is meaningful to the person by what it offers or allows the person. The EHP framework incorporates this interpretive phenomenological perspective in its consideration of the relationship between the person and context.

Developmental psychologists have also examined the effect of environment on behavior. For the most part, they have emphasized social aspects of environment. Bronfenbrenner's (1979) ecological model for human development applied an ecological systems model to human development. It presented a system of social relationships that provided the context for child development. Bronfenbrenner also developed the concept of ecological validity, in which he argued that research was not valid unless it was grounded in context. The EHP framework might enable professionals to consider whether therapeutic intervention could be valid if it were not grounded in context.

Vygotsky (1978) also examined the contribution that social environment makes to development. Wertsch (1985) summarized Vygotsky's principles by describing how context could affect development in the theory of the zone of proximal development. For Vygotsky, the zone of proximal development was the distance between a child's actual development and a higher level of potential development. Vygotsky argued that intervention during periods of sensitivity might allow the child to develop to a higher level than might have otherwise occurred, that is, an alteration of the child's regular context could affect development.

The importance that the EHP framework places on context is consistent with the emphasis placed on ecology and context by Auerswald (1971). Auerswald's work on ecological epistemology was among the earliest applications of an ecological perspective to therapeutic intervention. He argued that the processing of information from a holistic ecological perspective should replace simpler linear cause-and-effect thinking in therapeutic intervention. He identified a keynote of this kind of ecological thought as the "concern with the context in which a phenomenon occurs" (1971, p. 263). His position was that contextual issues should be considered before any therapeutic intervention began.

Relevant Occupational Therapy Literature

The environmental psychologists have contributed to the thinking of many occupational therapists. Kiernat (1992) applied the Lawton-Nehamow ecological model in her discussion of the environment as a modality. Barris (1982) drew from the work of Wicker and Hall in her conceptualization of environmental interactions. Howe and Briggs (1982) described an ecological systems model for occupational therapy that included the theories of Auerswald, Bronfenbrenner, and Wicker, whereas Spencer (1991b) used the ideas of Hall and Lawton in her discussion of physical environment and performance.

The terms *environment* and *context* are used interchangeably in the present review, dependent on the word contained in the original work. Although the occupational therapy literature has most commonly used the term *environment*, more recent authors have used the term *context*. The latter term was chosen for the EHP framework because context encompasses more of the person's physical, social, and phenomenological experience.

The concept of environment in theoretical occupational therapy literature is typically explained from two positions. In one, the environment is described primarily as a tool employed by the therapist in the intervention process. For example, Llorens (1970) defined occupational therapy intervention as the provision of environments that assist persons whose developmental cycle has been disrupted. Fidler and Fidler (1978) (see Chapter 9) explained that persons develop skills and mastery through interaction with the human and nonhuman environment. She appreciated the individuality of this interaction and recognized the influence of social and cultural norms. King (1978) (see Chapter 10) described intervention as the use of the environment to elicit adaptive responses.

In the other position, the relationship of the environment and the person is characterized from the perspective of general systems theory. The application of general systems theory to occupational therapy has facilitated the understanding of person and environment interaction. Reilly (1962) (see Chapter 8) was the first to apply the constructs of general systems theory and to include the rules of hierarchy as organizing principles. The person and environment are therefore viewed as interdependent, interacting through a system of input, output, and feedback.

General systems theory and hierarchical structures provide a framework for the Model of Human Occupation (Kielhofner & Burke, 1980). The components of the environment are identified as objects, persons, and events that again interact with the person in an open system. Kielhofner and Burke included throughput as an element of the system that is made up of three hierarchically arranged subsystems: volition, habituation, and performance. Barris (1982) used the framework of the Model of Human Occupation to clarify environmental properties and their influence on the person.

Occupation science organizes the study of humans as occupational beings through the Model of Human Subsystems That Influence Occupation (Clark et al., 1991). This model, based on general systems theory, represents the person as six hierarchically arranged subsystems that interact with the environment in an open system.

Howe and Briggs (1982) developed the Ecological Systems Model, which uses general systems theory to portray interconnections of the person and the environment as concentric circles with the person at the center surrounded by environmental layers. They detailed the model's view of function and dysfunction, which considers both the person and the environmental context.

In defining occupation, Nelson (1988) described the dynamics of occupational form and occupational performance within the framework of a system. Occupational form was defined as "an objective set of circumstances, independent of and external to a person" (p. 633). Nelson emphasized that performance can only be understood in terms of the occupational form. Moreover, occupations are characterized as occurring at different levels.

Christiansen (1991) discussed the effect that general systems theory has had on organizing the complex concepts involved in occupational therapy. General systems theory has allowed these complexities to be understood while avoiding reductionistic views that oversimplify phenomena.

General systems theory is congruous with the EHP. However, the conceptualization of the EHP is distinguished by a nonlinear, dynamic perspective. Dynamic principles describe systems as multiply determined, complex, and self-organizing (Thelen, 1992). They eschew schemas and static programs and emphasize variability. Persons may tend toward certain modes, behaviors, or patterns; however, small changes in the person or context alter these tendencies. Persons self-organize by adapting to these changes. When persons are unable to successfully self-organize, the occupational therapist provides interventions that encompass the complex relationship of the person and his or her context. In dynamic systems, hierarchies can exist to suggest patterns but are not requisite parts of the system.

The EHP provides a framework for examining situations that occupational therapists encounter every day. For example, the framework illustrates why some people in the intermediate stages of Alzheimer's disease may be able to live in a home environment, whereas others may be more comfortable in a nursing facility (i.e., the supports available to enable the person to function safely at home may be available to the first person, but not to the second one). The framework also illustrates why not all persons require prevocational training before they can work competitively (i.e., the contextual supports and cues available in the actual work environment may enable the person to perform the work task more consistently than in simulated task performance, which does not contain these supports). The EHP deciphers the variance in disruption of daily life that persons experience with disability, illness, or stress from a contextual perspective.

Recently, context's significance has received more attention in the occupational therapy literature. Mosey (1992) included context as one of three categories in occupational therapy's domain of concern. She classified age and environment as the components of context that "provide the perspective from which performance components and occupational areas are viewed relative to the individual" (1992, p. 260). Schkade and Schultz (1992) described occupational adaptation as a frame of reference that gives equal importance to the environment and the person (see Chapter 11). Occupational adaptation is organized by a holistic, nonhierarchical approach; however, the linear perspective of occupational adaptation distinguishes it from the nonlinear view of the EHP framework.

Several authors have strongly advocated the inclusion of context in occupational therapy assessment. Dunn (1993) recommended using a contextual approach to assessment so that the assessment is relevant to the person and addresses the person's wants and needs. Kiernat (1990) stated that environment is a factor in disability and must be considered when assessing function. Fisher (1992) (see Chapter 11) advocated for the recognition of occupational therapy's unique perspective of function in the assessment process. She emphasized the importance of considering the meaningfulness of the measure and placing the assessment within context. Ethnographic methods have been proposed as a means of including context

in occupational therapy assessment (Spencer, Krefting, & Mattingly, 1993). Proponents of ethnography have suggested that these methods can present a more realistic analysis of the person relative to the expectations within a setting.

The current literature has also discussed the application of contextual elements. Spencer (1991a) studied the relationship of social and cultural factors to independent living alternatives. Barney (1991) identified culture as a basic contextual determinant when providing services to older adults in need of assisted living.

In summary, although the occupational therapy literature has consistently included environment as a salient feature of performance, no author has proposed a framework for systematic consideration of environment–context. It is imperative that occupational therapy begin to directly address the features of context; this knowledge will broaden perspectives on successful intervention possibilities.

The EHP Framework

The EHP was developed to provide a framework for investigating the relationship among important constructs in the practice of occupational therapy: person, context (temporal, physical, social, and cultural) [American Occupational Therapy Association, 1995], tasks, performance, and therapeutic intervention, to better understand the domain of human performance. The primary theoretical postulate fundamental to the EHP framework is that ecology, or the interaction between person and the environment, affects human behavior and performance, and that performance cannot be understood outside of context.

The person in this framework includes one's experiences and sensorimotor, cognitive, and psychosocial skills and abilities. The person is represented by a simple stick figure in the circle (see Figure 17.1). The circle surrounding the person represents the person's context (physical, temporal, social, and cultural features); the only way to see the person is to look through the context. In Figure 17.1, a wedge has been cut out of the context to make the person easier to view. The ellipse in the diagram is the cut edge, enabling the reader to see the person. In this model, it is impossible to see the person without first seeing the context.

The circles with the Ts inside represent the tasks that are available to persons. *Tasks* are defined as objective sets of behaviors necessary to accomplish a goal. Everyone has the opportunity or the possibility of performing myriad tasks. Persons use their skills and abilities to focus attention on specific tasks from these possibilities.

When persons use their skills and abilities to perform tasks, they use environmental cues and features to support performance. Figure 17.2 illustrates a typical person embedded in a context supporting regular behavior, who has a particular focus on a particular area of performance. For example, a person may notice that the red light is on at the street corner, indicating the need to stop. A person's contexts are

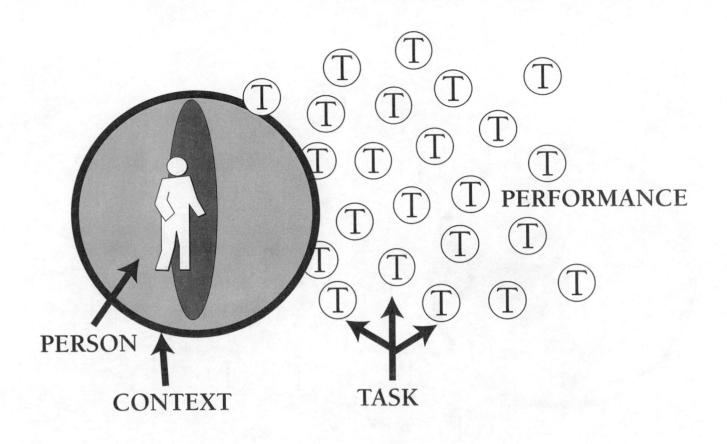

Figure 17.1. Schemata for the Ecology of Human Performance framework. Persons are embedded in their contexts. An infinite variety of tasks exists around every person. Performance results when the person interacts with context to engage in tasks.

continuously shifting; as contexts shift, the behaviors necessary to accomplish a goal also change.

When persons use their context to support performance, it is like using the lens within the eye to get a perspective on the world. As Figure 17.2 indicates, the contextual lens interacts with persons' skills and abilities to enable persons to perform certain tasks. The resulting scope of action is called the performance range (see Appendix). Persons view different potential tasks through their contextual filter, the accumulation of their experiences, and their perceptions about the physical, social, and cultural features of their current performance setting. One person might look toward being a downhill skier and another might look toward being a writer or a cook, but everyone looks through a context to derive meaning about needs or desires.

Occupational therapy also considers a person's life roles. Figure 17.3 illustrates how roles may be characterized in this model: it displays three roles (cook, mother, and wife) as a constellation of tasks; some of these roles overlap. Each person who has the roles of wife, cook, and mother includes a unique configuration of tasks in each role as a consequence of her skills and experiences and the demands of her context. For ex-

ample, if one person is a gourmet cook, she might have more tasks in the cook configuration than another person who uses a microwave oven to prepare meals or goes to restaurants.

The temporal context is also relevant to role characterization. For example, a child's role as cook might involve simpler recipes than an adult's. A person who has sustained an acute injury, such as a broken leg, may adapt the role of cook until it is possible to go out to restaurants again, whereas a person with a chronic disability, such as a head injury, may need to learn completely new cooking strategies. A person's configuration of the roles is based on the person's skills, abilities, context, and desires.

A person may have more limited skills and abilities but be embedded in a regular context that typically supports performance. This person may have the same possible cues and supports available in the context as that of the person in Figure 17.2, but the performance range is narrower because this person does not notice all the cues and supports. When a person has a more limited set of skills and abilities, then the person may either derive less meaning from the context or may not have the personal resources to support performance (see Figure 17.4). This person may not have the nec-

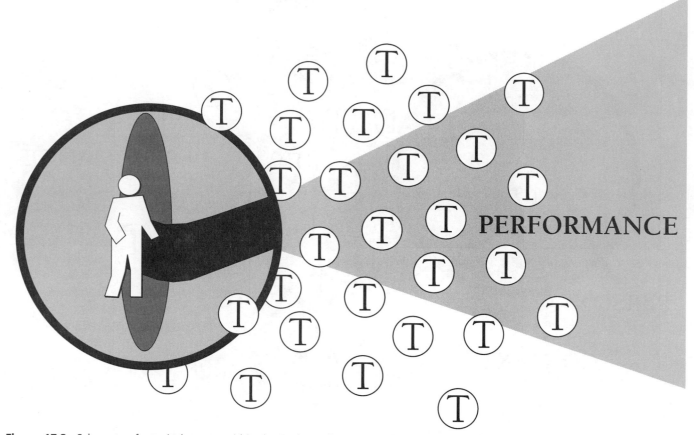

Figure 17.2. Schemata of a typical person within the Ecology of Human Performance framework. Persons use their skills and abilities to look through the context at the tasks they need or want to do. They derive meaning from this process. Performance range is the configuration of tasks that the persons execute.

essary physical capacities (e.g., a person who is blind may not be able to drive), may not pick up the cues the context provides (e.g., a child may fail to recognize that another child is trying the engage him or her in play), or may not know how to take advantage of contextual features (e.g., a person may stand in a full-service lane at the grocery store with only four items when an express lane is available). Each condition may result in a more limited performance range. The tasks that are possible are limited because the person is not able to use the resources that might be available to support performance in the context.

For example, if a person is learning to ski, all of the contextual features are available to support skiing but the person initially lacks the skills to perform the skiing behaviors and so has a more limited performance range. An adult with developmental disabilities may need transportation to work. The bus system is available in the context; all the features are there to allow persons to use the bus to get to work, but the person may not have the skills necessary to use those features to an advantage, so the performance range is limited. A child may have attentional deficits and limited social skills. Although the context for this child has the same cues that it has for every other child at school, the child who has poor

social skill development may not be sensitive to these cues. When the teacher frowns, this child may not understand its meaning, may not notice, or may misinterpret the frown and thus may behave in a way that is viewed as inappropriate for the context of the school day. Consequently, the performance range is limited by the inability to take advantage of the cues or by the irrelevance of the cues to the person. When a person has limited skills and abilities, these limitations can be compounded by inability to use contextual features to an advantage in support of performance.

Sometimes, there is a more limited contextual environment available to the person, but the person possesses typical skills and abilities (see Figure 17.5). For example, a gourmet cook may have extensive cooking skills, but in a kitchen with only a toaster oven, that cook has limited ability to demonstrate those skills and abilities. A skillful downhill skier has a difficult time demonstrating those skills in the tropics; the person must travel to a more contextually relevant location.

Persons with disabilities sometimes have limited skills and abilities and are also in an impoverished context (e.g., a person with severe mental illness who is also homeless). They do not have a context that provides them with the salient cues and the objects or events that are relevant to them to support

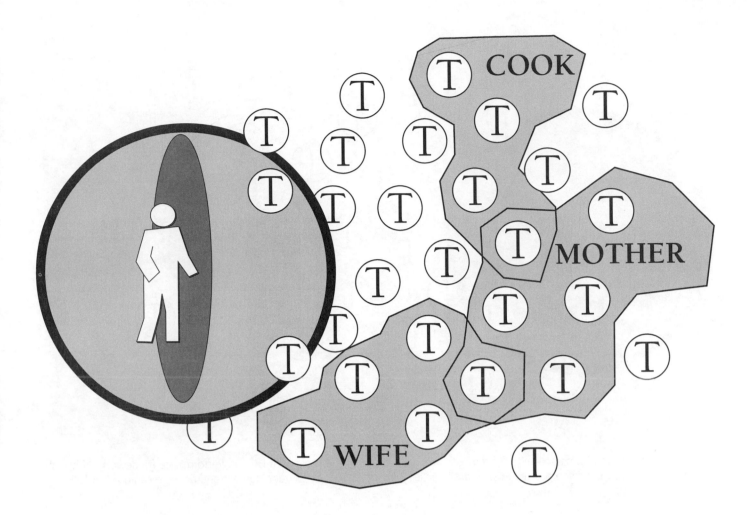

Figure 17.3. Illustration of roles in the Ecology of Human Performance framework. Life roles are a constellation of tasks. Persons have many roles; some tasks fall into more than one role. These role configurations are unique for each person.

performance. Performance of daily life tasks, work, or leisure activities in this situation becomes even more complex.

Therapeutic Intervention Within the EHP

Occupational therapy is most effective when it is imbedded in real life. If occupational therapists evaluate individual performance without considering the context of the performance, there is a great risk of interpreting the behavior inappropriately. Misinterpretation can lead to inappropriate choices about therapeutic intervention. For example, consider an occupational therapist working with a young woman and her daughter, who was physically ready to feed herself. The woman resisted the occupational therapist's repeated suggestions to use more independent eating strategies. Upon completing a home visit, the occupational therapist discovered that the mother only knew how to interact with her daughter during mealtime. At other times, the child sat on the floor with toys, but with no direction or interaction. The home visit made it clear to the occupational therapist that the mother was reluctant to give up her only time of interaction with her daughter.

This new insight helped the occupational therapist redirect therapeutic efforts so that the mother and child could play together in a manner that was satisfying to both. By not considering context, this occupational therapist would have put this mother in the difficult situation of having to compromise her relationship with her daughter by following the therapist's suggestions. Additionally, by not considering context, the therapist would have taken the risk that the child would not make progress because the mother might not have followed her suggestions.

A naturalistic study by deVries and Delespaul (1989) examined context and the experiences of persons with schizophrenia. They concluded that knowledge of context provided a new clinical tool. In one example, a man with schizophrenia was having severe problems with hypertensive illness. Clinical investigation to determine the cause of his high blood pressure was puzzling. An analysis of this man's context revealed that he worked as a dishwasher and became extremely anxious when he had to sort silverware during the lunch rush. The clinician was able to use this contextual

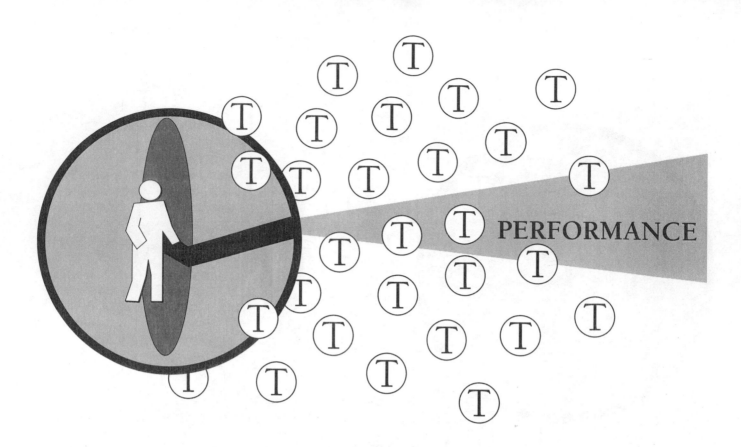

Figure 17.4. Schemata of a person with limited skills and abilities within the Ecology of Human Performance framework. Although context is still useful, the person has fewer skills and abilities with which to look through context and derive meaning. This lack limits the person's performance range.

information to convince the employer to change the employee's work tasks. Consequently, the man's blood pressure decreased to near normal.

Relationships among the EHP framework and the variety of interventions available to the occupational therapist are shown in Figure 17.6. Within this framework, therapeutic intervention is a collaboration among the person, the family, and the occupational therapist directed at meeting performance needs. Figure 17.6 displays five alternatives for therapeutic intervention; the Appendix contains definitions of each therapeutic intervention.

Establish or Restore

The first therapeutic intervention alternative is to establish or restore (remediate) the person's skills and abilities. In this category, the occupational therapist identifies the person's skills and the barriers to performance and designs interventions that improve the person's skills and abilities. The occupational therapist, person, and family might be concerned with reestablishing the person's role in the family, and so might work on coping skills or physical endurance to enable the person to perform tasks related to the family role. Restorative approaches are common options chosen by therapists, particularly within the medical model, which considers what is wrong

with the person and sets a plan to correct the problem. This approach is adapted, especially with young children, to include establishing needed skills for function. For example, a therapist might work on the muscle tone of a child with Down syndrome so that the child can move about to play with friends. Adults use these approaches within their own lives when they learn a new skill or when they work to restore a lost function (e.g., increasing range of motion in a joint after removing a cast).

Even when the focus of intervention is on skill development, context is still important. For example, Abreu and Hinojosa (1992) suggested that predictable environments provide the feedback necessary to correct motor behaviors. Toglia (1992) explained that an understanding of the interactions of person, task, and environment is essential to effective cognitive rehabilitation strategies.

Alter

The second therapeutic intervention alternative is to alter the actual context in which persons perform. This intervention emphasizes selecting a context that enables the person to perform with current skills and abilities. The person can be placed in a different setting that more closely matches his or her current skills and abilities, rather than changing the

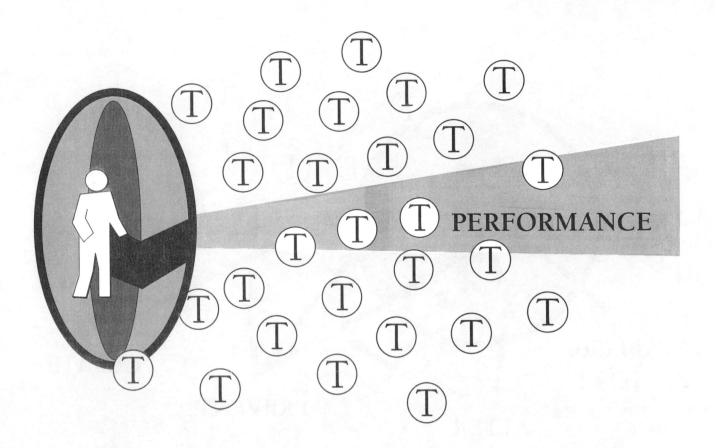

Figure 17.5. Schemata of a limited context within the Ecology of Human Performance framework. The person has adequate skills and abilities, but the context does not provide resources needed to perform. In this situation, performance range is limited.

Create a completely different context...etc. + task...etc.

present setting to accommodate the person's needs. The occupational therapist would consider the person's skills, abilities, and difficulties and find a context that was compatible with this performance profile. The important feature of the alter intervention is that the therapist does not set out to correct the person or the environment; instead, the therapist is looking for the best match between the person and current contextual features available. Allen (1992) acknowledged the lack of direction for occupational therapists working with persons beyond the acute phase of illness who must live with functional limitations. Her frame of reference provides guidelines for making the best fit for persons with cognitive disabilities and available contexts.

Fairweather (1980) used the alter strategy in his Lodge Society, a community program for persons with severe mental illness. He was concerned that persons who were able to succeed in jobs at the hospital were unsuccessful at work in the community because of the intolerance for behavior that was viewed as deviant. One strategy was to create janitorial crews that worked at times and in settings where their contact with others was limited.

Another example involves a person who has low assertiveness ability and needs to buy a car. Although the therapist could work on assertiveness skill development or visit the car dealer to offer some adaptations to the process to facilitate the person's purchase, an alternative that uses the alter intervention option would be for the therapist to suggest that the person buy a car at a dealership that employs the no-haggling approach. Some manufacturers market their sales strategy as one that minimizes the need for assertiveness because there is one price for their cars and no negotiating is necessary. The therapist does not have to change the context and the person can succeed with current skills to purchase the car.

Adapt

The occupational therapist can also adapt the contextual features and task demands to support performance in context. When therapists adapt, they design a more supportive context for the person's performance. Therapists might enhance some contextual features to provide cues and reduce other features to minimize distractibility and make the task more possible for the person. When children are distractible, therapists suggest shorter assignments for their seat work in class. When an adult with severe disabilities needs to manage the home environment, the therapist might select an environmental control unit. Therapists adjust desk and table configurations to meet individual needs. They might change a desk's height to match the person's postural support needs or might find a lower table

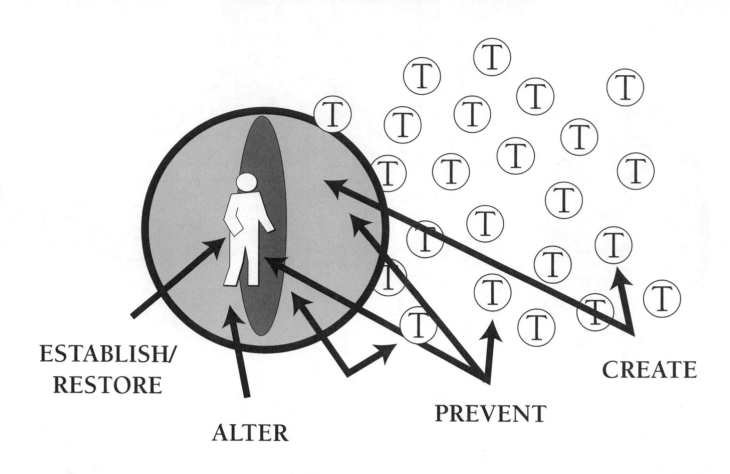

ESTABLISH/RESTORE

ALTER

PREVENT

CREATE

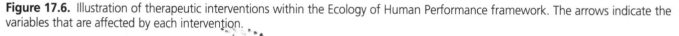

Figure 17.6. Illustration of therapeutic interventions within the Ecology of Human Performance framework. The arrows indicate the variables that are affected by each intervention.

in the dining area for someone whose ethnic background suggests preference for a lower eating surface. Many persons use stick-on notes to help them remember things they need to do. Persons whose vision is failing may purchase hard-cover novels because they have huger print than paperbacks. Buning and Hanzlik (1993) reported a single-subject study in which the person's context was considered in technological adaptations. In this case, computer technologies were used so that a doctoral student with severe visual impairments could complete her dissertation.

Prevent

The fourth therapeutic intervention option is to prevent the occurrence or evolution of maladaptive performance in context. Sometimes, therapists can predict that certain negative outcomes are likely unless intervention is provided. Therapists can create interventions to change the course of events by addressing person, context, and task variables to enable functional performance to emerge. This view is supported by Coulter (1992) who proposed that prevention efforts in mental retardation must take an ecological approach that focuses on the interaction between persons and their environment. Department managers employ a prevention approach when they provide an orientation for

newly hired employees; managers do not wait until the employee faces a problem to instruct them in proper procedures. Runners who stretch before running are employing a prevention approach. Occupational therapists teach persons with spinal cord injuries how to adjust their position frequently to prevent contractures and decubitus ulcers. Therapists also provide lifting classes in industrial settings to prevent work injuries. Therapists can construct a map of community services for a person with severe mental illness who is moving to a new apartment area to prevent him or her from feeling socially isolated. Prevention approaches anticipate possible and likely problems and change the course of activities to increase positive outcomes. Prevention approaches are good options for persons with long-term conditions that lead to secondary problems; the temporal context is relevant to these person's outcomes.

Create

The fifth therapeutic intervention option is creating circumstances that promote more adaptable or complex performance in context. This therapeutic intervention does not assume that a disability is present or that a disability has the potential to interfere with performance. The person or family seeking assistance may see the problem from a functional performance standpoint, not from a disability standpoint. The therapist participates by providing expertise to enrich contextual and task experiences that will enhance performance. Circumstances that do not presume disability are constructed; this is what distinguishes the create intervention from the prevent intervention, which addresses precluding the occurrence of a problem that is likely to arise. Early intervention programs are common examples of community-based programs that have an enriching philosophy; therapists use their expertise to plan age-appropriate tasks that embellish the young children's development. Therapists might also participate in the development of living communities for elders that provide varied and stimulating activities. These community settings do not presume their consumers have disabilities. They are designed to make the best possible use of environment to enhance living and development. For example, a large building complex may have many signs to lead visitors and workers to correct locations efficiently, not because there are presumed disabilities, but because signs make the environment easier for everyone. When adults play an icebreaker game at the beginning of a party they are creating an enriched environment for socialization.

Occupational therapists have many therapeutic choices with each person they serve, and at each point along the therapeutic relationship. Therapists often employ several intervention approaches either simultaneously or across time. Table 17.1 shows two examples of how an occupational therapist might deal with a person and family who need occupational therapy services from all of these approaches. When occupational therapists include context in the total perspective, it creates possibilities; when persons are viewed out of context, viable options are lost.

Directions for Future Work

The EHP proposes the relationships among the key variables of person, context, tasks, and performance. Within the domain of concern of occupational therapy, context is only relevant as it relates to human performance.

Mosey (1981) indicated that a frame of reference must describe postulates that allow application to practice and offer specific guidance for intervention. Scholars will therefore need to refine these constructs by assessing their adequacy and answering practice-oriented questions. Several lines of study provide important initial information that will refine current frames of reference that affect occupational therapy, develop new frames of reference, and create new assessment and intervention strategies.

Several questions emerge as fundamental to the investigation of basic relationships proposed in this framework. A primary question is: How do we capture contextual features objectively, and how do we then decide which features are salient for particular performance situations? We must also determine how a contextual feature becomes relevant for a particular person. There are many more contextual features

Table 17.1. Case Examples Applying the Ecology of Human Performance framework

Area Addressed	Strategy Employed/Information
CASE 1	
Background	M is 15 months old; he has two older siblings and both of his parents living in his home. He has very low muscle tone and a developmental delay and his family wants him to play and socialize.
Establish/Restore	The therapist decides to work on M's eye contact and vocalizing as ways for the family to know that M is paying attention to them.
Alter	The therapist suggests that the family enroll M in a part-time day care program so he can have the stimulation of the other children playing as a way to learn play skills.
Adapt	The therapist talks to the family about moving the toys closer, having the siblings move closer when they play with M. The therapist works with the siblings to help them learn how to change their voice tone so that M can pay attention easier.
Prevent	The therapist decides to work on functional communication strategies to prevent M's frustration at socializing. The therapist works with the family to pick some simple gestures and sounds that everyone recognizes as communication signals from M, so he can get some basic needs met.
Create	The therapist and parents discuss the usefulness of getting together with other families from the church that have similar aged children for a family gathering. This will be a positive socialization experience for all members, and involve M in a typical socialization opportunity.
CASE 2	
Background	Ms. T is a 75-year-old who has had a right hemisphere stroke. She lives with her son and daughter-in-law and two grandchildren.
Establish/Restore	The therapist decides to work on functional range of motion for reaching and stepping.
Alter	The therapist and Ms. T discuss her need to socialize and Ms. T expresses concern over her usual socializing in the quilting club, which expects a certain level of performance. The therapist suggests Sunday school as a place to socialize that doesn't require the fine motor control.
Adapt	The therapist brings clamps to help her with her stitching so that she could still do some stitching. The therapist brings her a stocking darner and velcro to attach to key items in the bathroom when she expressed desire to dress and complete personal hygiene.
Prevent	The therapist helps Ms. T to establish a daily routine to prevent joint, muscle, and skin breakdowns.
Create	The therapist helps her plan regular times to play with her grandchildren as part of the family routine.

available to persons in a particular context than are noticed or used by a person for successful performance. In particular performance situations, we need to determine which contextual features support or create barriers to performance. Are there particular contextual features that contribute to a person's resilience?

Occupational therapy assessment strategies also need to consider context. It will be important to determine whether standardized functional assessments are valid for capturing what is actually known about the person's performance in the natural context. For example, does the dressing item on a standardized test rate the person the same way that a therapist would rate the person if watching the person's morning dressing routine? This information will enable occupational therapists to construct initial data about persons so that planning can be individualized and relevant to their needs. It will also be important to create new, contextually relevant assessments in the future.

There are also questions that need to be answered about the proposed therapeutic interventions. For example, which interventions are the best choices for which performance problems? What is the effect of the proposed therapeutic interventions on performance outcomes? What is the difference in functional outcomes when therapeutic interventions occur in natural and contrived contexts? It is not likely that all the intervention options described here will be equally useful for all performance problems. Therefore, it will be important to test the relationships among particular performance problems and various intervention options.

The tendency to take ideas created through professional dialogue in the literature and regard them as certainty is tempting; in fact, in dialogue this is easy to do. Ideas must be tested, and it seems only fitting that ideas proposed about context be evaluated in that setting. As knowledge and understanding grow about the role of context in human performance, these initial proposals will need adaptation, a suitable outcome for a set of ideas about ecological relationships.

Appendix 17.A
Ecology of Human Performance: Definitions
Person
An individual with a unique configuration of abilities, experiences, and sensorimotor, cognitive, and psychosocial skills.

A. Persons are unique and complex and therefore precise predictability about their performance is impossible.
B. The meaning a person attaches to task and contextual variables strongly influences performance.

Task
An objective set of behaviors necessary to accomplish a goal.

A. An infinite variety of tasks exists around every person.
B. Constellations of tasks form a person's roles.

Performance
Both the process and the result of the person interacting with context to engage in tasks.

A. The performance range is determined by the interaction between the person and the context.
B. Performance in natural contexts is different from performance in contrived contexts (ecological validity, Bronfenbrenner, 1979).

Context (adapted from *Uniform Terminology for Occupational Therapy, 3rd edition*):
Temporal Aspects (Note: although temporal aspects are determined by the person, they become contextual due to the social and cultural meaning attached to the temporal features)

1. Chronological: person's age.
2. Developmental: stage or phase of maturation.
3. Life cycle: place in important life phases, such as career cycle, parenting cycle, educational process.
4. Health status: place in continuum of disability, such as acuteness of injury, chronicity of disability, or terminal nature of illness.
5. Period: the measurable span of time during which a task exists or continues.

Environment
1. Physical: nonhuman aspects of context (includes the natural terrain, buildings, furniture, objects, tools, and devices).
2. Social: availability and expectations of important persons, such as spouses, friends, and caregivers (also includes larger social groups that are influential in establishing norms, role expectations, and social routines).
3. Cultural: customs, beliefs, activity patterns, behavior standards, and expectations accepted by the society of which the person is a member (includes political aspects such as laws that shape access to resources and affirm personal rights; also includes opportunities for education, employment, and economic support).

Therapeutic Intervention
A collaboration between the person/family and the occupational therapist directed at meeting performance needs.

• Therapeutic interventions in occupational therapy are multifaceted and can be designed to accomplish any or all of the following.
• *Establish/restore* a person's abilities to perform in context. Therapeutic intervention can establish or restore a

person's abilities to perform in context. This emphasis is on identifying a person's skills and barriers to performance, and designing interventions that improve the person's skills and experiences.

- *Alter* actual context in which people perform. Therapeutic interventions can alter the context within which the person performs. This intervention emphasizes selecting a context that enables the person to perform with current skills and abilities. This can include placing the person in a different setting that more closely matches current skills and abilities, rather than changing the present setting to accommodate needs.

- *Adapt* contextual features and task demands so they support performance in context. Therapeutic interventions can adapt contextual features and task demands so they are more supportive to the person's performance. In this intervention, the therapist changes aspects of context and/or tasks so performance is more likely. This can include enhancing some features to provide cues, or reducing other features to reduce distractibility.

- *Prevent* the occurrence or evolution of malpractice performance in context. Therapeutic interventions can prevent the occurrence or evolution of barriers to performance in context. Sometimes, therapists can predict that certain negative outcomes are likely without intervention to change the course of events. Therapists can create intervention to change the course of events. Therapists can create interventions that address person, context, and task variables to change the course, thus enabling functional performance to emerge.

- *Create* circumstances that promote more adaptable/complex performance in context. Therapeutic interventions can create circumstances which promote more adaptable performance in context. This therapeutic intervention does not assume a disability is present or has the potential to interfere with performance. This therapeutic choice focuses on providing enriched contextual and task experiences that will enhance performance.

References

Abreu, B.C., & Hinojosa, J. (1992). The process approach for cognitive–perceptual and postural control dysfunction for adults with brain injuries. In N. Katz (Ed.), *Cognitive rehabilitation: Models for intervention in occupational therapy* (pp. 167–194). Stoneham, MA: Andover Medical.

Allen, D. K. (1992). *Occupational therapy treatment goals for the physically and cognitively disabled.* Rockville, MD: American Occupational Therapy Association.

American Occupational Therapy Association. (1995). Uniform terminology for occupational therapy—third edition. *American Journal of Occupational Therapy.*

Auerswald, E. H. (1971). Families, change, and the ecological perspective. *Family Process, 10,* 263–280.

Barney, K. F. (1991). From Ellis island to assisted living: Meeting the needs of older adults from diverse cultures. *American Journal of Occupational Therapy, 45,* 486–593.

Barris, R. (1982). Environmental interactions: An extension of the model of occupation. *American Journal of Occupational Therapy, 36,* 637–644.

Bronfenbrenner, U. (1979). *The ecology of human development.* Cambridge, MA: Harvard University Press.

Bruner J. *(1989). Acts of meaning.* Cambridge, MA: Harvard University Press.

Buning, M. E., & Hanzlik, J. R. (1993). Adaptive computer use for a person with visual impairment. *American Journal of Occupational Therapy, 47,* 998–1007.

Christiansen, C. (1991). Occupational therapy: Intervention for life performance. In C. Christiansen & C. Baum (Eds.), *Occupational therapy: Overcoming human performance deficits* (pp. 3–44). New York: McGraw-Hill.

Clark, F. A., Parham, D., Carlson, M. E., Frank, G., Jackson, J., Pierce, D., Wolfe, R. J., & Zemke, R. (1991). Occupational science: Academic innovation in the service of occupational therapy's future. *American Journal of Occupational Therapy, 45,* 300–310.

Coulter, D. L. (1992). An ecology of prevention for the future. *Mental Retardation, 30,* 363–369.

Csikszentmihalyi, M. (1990). *Flow: The psychology of optimal experience.* New York: Harper Perennial.

deVries, M. W., & Delespaul, P. A. E. G. (1989). Time, context, and subjective experiences in schizophrenia. *Schizophrenia Bulletin, 15,* 233–244.

Dunn, W. (1993). The Issue Is—Measurement of function: Actions for the future. *American Journal of Occupational Therapy, 47,* 357–359.

Fairweather, G. W., (1980). The prototype lodge society: Instituting group process principles. *New Directions for Mental Health Services, 7,* 13–32.

Fidler, G. S., & Fidler, F. W. (1978). Doing and becoming: Purposeful action and self actualization. *American Journal of Occupational Therapy, 32,* 305–310. Reprinted as Chapter 9.

Fisher, A. (1992). Functional measure, Part 1: What is function, what should we measure, and how should we measure it? *American Journal of Occupational Therapy, 46,* 183–185.

Gibson, J. J. (1986). *An ecological approach to visual perception,* Hilldale, NJ: Erlbaum.

Hall, E. T. (1983). *The dance of life.* New York: Doubleday.

Hart, R. (1979). *Children's experience of place.* New York: Irvington.

Holahan, C. J. (1986). Environmental psychology. *Annual Review of Psychology, 37,* 381–407.

Howe, M. C., & Briggs, A. K. (1982). Ecological systems model for occupational therapy. *American Journal of Occupational Therapy, 36,* 322–327.

Kielhofner, G., & Burke, J. P. (1980). A model of human occupation, Part 1. Conceptual framework and content. *American Journal of Occupational Therapy, 34,* 572–581.

Kiernat, J. M. (1990). Considering the environment. In C. B. Royeen (Ed.), *AOTA Self Study Series: Assessing function* (Lesson 6). Rockville, MD: American Occupational Therapy Association.

Kiernat, J. M. (1992). Environment: The hidden modality. *Journal of Physical and Occupational Therapy in Geriatrics, 21,* 3–12.

King, L. J. (1978). Toward a science of adaptive responses. *American Journal of Occupational Therapy, 32,* 429–437. Reprinted as Chapter 10.

Lawton, M. P. (1982). Competence, environmental press, and the adaptation of older people. In M. P. Lawton, P. G. Windley, & T. O. Byerts (Eds.), *Aging and the environment* (pp. 33–59). New York: Springer.

Llorens, L. A. (1970). Facilitating growth and development: The promise of occupational therapy. *American Journal of Occupational Therapy, 24,* 93–101.

Mosey, A. C. (1981). *Occupational therapy: Configuration of a profession.* New York: Raven.

Mosey, A. C. (1992). *Applied scientific inquiry in the health professions: An epistemological orientation.* Rockville: American Occupational Therapy Association.

Murray, H. A. (1938). *Explorations in personality.* New York: Oxford.

Nelson, D. L. (1988). Occupation: Form and performance. *American Journal of Occupational Therapy, 42,* 633–641.

Reilly, M. (1962). Occupational therapy can be one of the great ideas of 20th century medicine. *American Journal of Occupational Therapy, 16,* 1–9. Reprinted as Chapter 8.

Schkade, J. K., & Schultz, S. (1992). Occupational adaptation: Toward a holistic approach for contemporary practice, Part 1. *American Journal of Occupational Therapy, 46,* 829–837. Reprinted as Chapter 11.

Spencer, J. C. (1991a). An ethnographic study of independent living alternatives. *American Journal of Occupational Therapy, 45,* 243–251.

Spencer, J. C. (1991b). The physical environment and performance. In C. Christiansen & C. Baum (Eds.), *Occupational therapy: Overcoming human performance deficits* (pp. 125–140). New York: Slack.

Spencer, J., Krefting, L., & Mattingly, C. (1993). Incorporation of ethnographic methods in occupational therapy assessment. *American Journal of Occupational Therapy, 47,* 303–309.

Thelen, E. (1992). Development as a dynamic system. *Current Directions in Psychological Science, 1,* 189–193.

Toglia, J. P. (1992). A dynamical approach to cognitive rehabilitation. In N. Katz (Ed), *Cognitive rehabilitation: Models for intervention in occupational therapy* (pp. 104–143). Stoneham, MA: Andover Medical.

Wicker, A. W. (1979). *An introduction to ecological psychology.* Cambridge, MA: Cambridge University Press.

Wertsch, J. V. (1985). *Vygotsky and the social formation of mind.* Cambridge, MA: Harvard University Press.

Vygotsky, L. S. (1978). *Mind in society: The development of higher psychological processes.* Cambridge, MA: Harvard University Press.

Zerubavel, E. (1981). *Hidden rhythms: Schedules and calendars in social life.* Berkeley: University of California Press.

Culture: A Factor Influencing the Outcomes of Occupational Therapy

Ruth Levine Schemm,
EdD, OTR/L, FAOTA

Overview

People can accomplish seemingly impossible goals if invested in the outcome; on the other hand, few people are interested in activities that have no personal meaning. This paper will explore one of the factors that can make therapy more meaningful to our patients. The concept is a complex pattern of living, which is called *culture*. As therapists, we search for activities that will stimulate and interest our patients as well as promote functional abilities. This is no easy task because few of our patients come from the same culture group that we do. This paper will define culture, review the importance of culture in occupational therapy practice, and describe how cultural beliefs and values affect assessment and treatment in occupational therapy.

This chapter was previously published, under the name of Ruth Ellen Levine, jointly in *Sociocultural Implications in Treatment Planning in Occupational Therapy* (The Haworth Press, Inc., 1987) and in *Occupational Therapy in Health Care, 4*(1), 3–16. Copyright © 1987, The Haworth Press, Inc.

Let us begin with a treatment vignette that offers an introduction to the concept of culture.

Case Study

Mrs. W., a 57-year-old, attractive, upper-middle-class, urban housewife with Guillian-Barre syndrome, was hospitalized and transferred to a rehabilitation center and then to home care. Mrs. W. occupied a first-floor bedroom suite in the newly purchased home of one of her daughters. The family reasoned that Mrs. W. could interact with family members, walk short distances, and join the family for meals. The physical therapist felt that Mrs. W. was almost ready to return to her own home if it were adapted to accommodate her needs. Mrs. W. lived in a newly constructed three-story townhouse in center city. Although the OTR felt that referral to occupational therapy was perhaps too late for best results, she decided to visit the patient anyway.

On the day of the scheduled evaluation visit, the OTR was admitted into the gracious house by the maid because the daughter was conferring with an interior decorator. The OTR was led to the first-floor bedroom where Mrs. W. was propped up in bed while a full-time attendant fussed over her sheets and cleared her breakfast dishes. Mrs. W. ignored the therapist and continued her conversation with the attendant. After a few minutes, Mrs. W. briefly acknowledged the OTR and spent the next 15 minutes describing her symptoms as if the OTR was an unwanted, inexperienced newcomer. Mrs. W. praised "her" physical therapist and attributed her progress to his guidance and skill. The occupational therapist tried to guide their conversation toward the patient's previous interests and activities and her present views on self-care and independence, but Mrs. W. switched the conversation back to the physical therapist.

The OTR decided to define her role and the type of equipment that might improve Mrs. W.'s functional abilities. This seemed to make Mrs. W. act more defensively. The OTR tried to ameliorate her discomfort by pointing out useful safety rails and tub seats in an equipment catalog. Mrs. W. grew even more negative and told the OTR that she did not need adaptive equipment. The OTR soon realized that something was wrong with the interview but could not fathom why it was going so poorly. Mrs. W. became more upset as the therapist tried to win her approval by switching the topic to the other services offered by an occupational therapist, including work simplification and analysis of architectural barriers. Unfortunately, this topic also proved difficult, and Mrs. W.

interrupted the OTR and told her that the physical therapist said that she was making excellent progress. The OTR tried to explain that she was impressed with Mrs. W.'s efforts, but this praise did not impress Mrs. W.

The OTR decided there was nothing else to do so she concluded the evaluation by telling Mrs. W. that she would close the case because Mrs. W. had no interest in adaptive equipment. Mrs. W. said she hoped that she would never see the occupational therapist again and told the OTR that she planned to report her to the physical therapist.

Later, the physical therapist called the OTR to find out what had gone wrong with the evaluation. He reported that Mrs. W. was angry and upset and claimed that the OTR insisted that she would need "handicapped" equipment for the rest of her life. The OTR was both hurt and confused and wondered what she had done to infuriate Mrs. W. After all, she was doing exactly what she had been taught in her training for home health care.

The negative outcome of this evaluation visit affected all of the team members—patient, caretakers, physical therapist, nurse, and the occupational therapist. Each person was interpreting events from their own perspective. The meaning of the communication was, in part, determined by the person's values, interests, goals, roles, and habits. Each person's culture became a filter or screen that either passed information through or blocked it. The vignette demonstrates that even though the therapist's professional manner was similar to that prescribed during her professional training, the patient interpreted the visit as an attempt to jinx her hard-won progress. In retrospect, the OTR may have realized that two different opinions about the value of adaptive equipment started the tangled communication. Within a short time, the OTR could not extricate herself from the negative meaning that "handicapped" things had for Mrs. W. The therapist moved her treatment agenda too quickly without hearing what the patient was really saying. Mrs. W. was frightened by her diagnosis and did not want to see, touch, own, or talk about anything that implied that she might not regain her independence. In Mrs. W.'s culture outward appearances were of vital importance, people who used adaptive equipment were handicapped, and the thought that other people might regard her as disabled was more stressful than being dependent on an attendant.

Historical Overview

Occupational therapy founders first considered culture as an important aspect of treatment planning because of their belief in the interrelationship between mind and body. If an activity generated a patient's interests it could also promote functional independence. In the first occupations training course, Tracy identified activities that matched the patient's lifestyle,[1] and Dunton agreed and emphasized the need to stimulate the patient's interests by prescribing activities based on personal and cultural values.[2] Hall and Buck claimed that "brain workers should be given work that was largely physical and those

who worked with their hands, must have simpler, more primitive tasks."[3] Although the consideration of culture was not fully developed, the Founders searched for different ways to elicit a patient's interest through the use of novel experiences. In 1925 a committee of the American Occupational Therapy Association defined occupational therapy and formulated 15 principles, one-third of which emphasized the importance of considering the patient's interests and needs.[4] Thus, the early literature of the profession is filled with examples of attempts to consider the patient's culture during treatment.

As medical care became more scientific in the 1930s and 1940s, therapists began to concentrate more on the patient's pathology than on residual strengths; thus, decreasing their initial commitment to linking the patient's goals, interests and values, habits, and roles with the activity process. At the same time, many therapists were arts-and-crafts teachers who were committed to a philosophy that tended to encourage patients to refine their craft skills and produce an attractive end-product. It was believed that the quality product would enhance self-confidence. Other therapists concentrated on the benefits that occurred during the *doing* part of the activity process. Thus, ideological differences grew between the therapists and the diversionists.[5] Another factor that compromised initial consideration of culture during the Depression years was the scarcity of funds. Therapists had to treat large numbers of patients and market and sell patient projects in order to replenish department supply budgets. The patients' interests were subordinated to the department needs because some projects were more cost efficient than others.

The emphasis on arts and crafts with little concentration on the therapeutic use of activities may have prompted Eleanor Clarke Slagle to tell the 1930 graduating class at Sheppard and Enoch Pratt Hospital that "handicrafts are not enough" because " . . . the patient is being more and more considered in relation to his domestic and community life."[6]

Culture was as important in early practice as it must be today, because occupational therapy deals with goal-directed activities which are part and parcel of everyday life. Recently, modern therapists are rediscovering the importance of early beliefs that emphasized the interaction of mind and body during treatment. Theorists Mosey,[7] Fidler and Fidler (see Chapter 9),[8] Llorens,[9] Reilly,[10] Keilhofner and Burke,[11,12] Barris,[13] Nuse-Clark,[14] and Yerxa[15] all address the influence of culture in treatment. Using basic concepts from our past, present-day theorists still emphasize the importance of the patient's motivation, interests, goals, interests, values, habits, time-orientation, roles, caretaker network, and use of the nonhuman environment. All of these concepts are part of a person's culture.

Defining Culture

Culture has been described as a "blueprint" for human behavior, influencing individual thoughts, actions, and collectively influencing a particular society.[16] Culture can be viewed as a multifaceted influence which is learned by direct and indirect daily experiences based on what people do (cultural behavior), say (speech messages), make, and use (cultural artifacts). In short, a child learns a life pattern of beliefs and values which shape the way that he or she believes, thinks, perceives, feels, and behaves.[17] Culture is a way of life that encompasses kinetic or overt behavior, psychological expressions, and the material products of labor or industry. The major cultural transmission agents are behavioral and material elements simply because psychological states are not transferable.[18]

Kinetic or overt behaviors, the first elements of culture, are evident in actions performed by an individual and include body motions, speech patterns, distance selected during communication with others, and use of products and tools. People use their bodies in unique ways to indicate agreement, acceptance, rejection, discomfort, and other reactions.

Speech patterns are also culturally determined; rate of speech, expression and emphasis, pronunciation, and choice of words are part of a person's culture. Even the distance preferred between people during different activities is also culturally determined.[19] Tool use, as part of one's behavior, is another factor indigenous to one's culture: some people use handtools exclusively, others rely on sophisticated gadgets and technology, some others prefer to use only their hands in doing tasks. In examining culture one must also consider how people employ objects and other artifacts. For example, consider a patient who uses the same hammer over and over and seems to derive pleasure from completing a task by using this object which almost seems like a nonhuman friend. In contrast, another patient may be careless with tools and abuse them without giving it a second thought. Still another patient may regard the use of tools with disdain because handmade objects can be purchased and "time is money."

Psychological aspects, the second elements of one's culture, include knowledge, attitudes, and values that are shared by members of a given cultural group. These factors cannot be readily observed because they take place in a person's mind. Psychological factors are therefore more difficult for an observer to assess and observe. Although these factors are subjective they still deserve some of our attention because people exhibit different reactions to events in their daily lives. On the other hand, measurement of psychological factors is not precise and individual reactions may be inconsistent and variable even under the same circumstances. For example, if you introduce yourself to a patient using your first name only some people may feel right at home, welcome your informality, and respond with warmth and humor. On the other hand, another person may find it annoying but tolerable and respond stiffly to requests for additional information. We can speculate that the first patient equates the informality with a type of relationship where the therapist and he are equal partners. The second patient may feel that she has just met the therapist, and the use of first names indicates a forced familiarity that makes the patient feel guarded. Thus we see that the same event can

take on different meaning for each participant depending on one's cultural background.

The last element associated with culture, the "material products of labor or industry," are the objects and artifacts that comprise *the non-human environment.* This category includes signs, symbols, objects, tasks, roles, and social organizations used to create products in the environment. Consider the work produced by a given group of people, the way that ideas are transformed into reality, and the type of organization that is needed to produce the goods and services. Members of a group teach their children how to participate in their culture through a complex system of rewards and punishments which are conveyed through thoughts, actions, social beliefs, attitudes, communication patterns, perceptions, time orientation, and ways of handling animals, plants, and objects. In effect, a child is exposed to a pattern of beliefs, attitudes, perceptions, meanings, and emotions based on personal experiences in a particular setting.[20]

Culture imposes a conditioning variable that is internalized in the human psyche and not easily forgotten.[21] Values, interests, goals, habits, roles, time orientation, communication patterns, the ways in which one uses symbols and artifacts, selects nonhuman objects—all are well ingrained as one grows, making change difficult. In fact, Likroeber compared culture to the great coral reefs built by polyps. The polyps die, but their secretions leave a permanent record of their former life.[22] Thus, culture establishes a filter through which individuals interpret daily events. At the same time, one's group establishes patterns that become "commonly defined meanings and sanctioned behaviors favored by the group."[23] Individuals are never free of the group influence—sometimes subtle and sometimes more specialized—to meet individual physical and psychological needs.[24]

The Relevance of Culture in Occupational Therapy

Culture is a central component of occupational therapy because people judge the quality of their therapy through a filter which is comprised, in part, of past learning and emotions and which is based on three levels of beliefs: (1) the patient's perception of illness and health, (2) the patient's perception of therapy, and (3) the patient's belief in the meaning of his own life and activities. These factors overlap and are not discrete.

Illness is not the same to all individuals. Sociologists have long identified significant differences in the ways that members of specific cultures decide to seek health care, care for themselves, use family caretaker networks, take medication and follow prescribed remedies, participate in a healthful daily regime, assist other ill family members, and endure pain and suffering.[25,26,27,28,29,30] Occupational therapists cannot assume that people all react to the stress of illness, traumatic events, or other life disruptions in the same way. "Illness behavior" refers to the ways in which symptoms may be differently perceived, evaluated, and acted (or not acted) upon by different kinds of persons.[31] The behavior varies with a person's socioeconomic class, education level, community cohesiveness, and ethnic origin. The higher the social status of a population, the better educated and informed they will be about signs and symptoms of illness.[32]

Being "ill" certainly is not the same to everyone. Some people are not ill until they are incapable of performing daily roles, others are ill as soon as they note a slight change in their body, still others are ill only if the illness is labeled by the medical establishment and therefore given "official" sanction. Therapists must consider the issue of illness behavior in rehabilitation because of diverse reactions such as a patient who does not want to participate in therapy because he is "ill" and therefore is not *capable* of participation. This type of behavior was described in a case study depicting the progress of an elderly Italian–American, with a left hemiparesis, who maintained that he could not dress or toilet himself until his arm "got well." This response is logical if you understand the culture of the first-generation Southern Italian.[33,34]

Another question to consider is how well patients understand their treatment programs. Occupational therapy can only be perceived as meaningful and deserving of the patient's interest and cooperation if it is relevant to patients and their caretakers. Treatment is valued only if patients believe that they have been helped by it. If not, services are judged as irrelevant and inconsequential. Chances are that therapists who are capable of attending to the patient's cultural values by selecting relevant treatment activities are also able to convince the patient that therapy is important. Yet, it is difficult to tap into the interests of patients who have experienced a traumatic illness, accident, or event which has drained their energies and made adaptation seem overwhelming and taxing. Sharrott maintained that occupational therapists "play a profound role in creation, affirmation and experience of meaning" because therapy provides opportunities for patients to redefine their previous experiences in light of their present abilities and needs.[35] Effective therapy alters the patient's perception of meaningful existence by offering concrete feedback on daily performance in activities that are important in a patient's life roles. Unlike other treatment, occupational therapy mirrors the painful limitations wrought by traumatic incident, aging, development, or deprivation. But therapy sessions can alter the patient's perception of life by providing immediate evidence on what the patient *CAN* do rather than what is lost.[36]

Another factor frequently overlooked when designing therapy programs is the patient's beliefs and values regarding the nonhuman environment. Barris discussed the importance of the treatment environment because it should provide "adequate but not overbearing stimulation."[37] Patients will express culturally determined values about their environment, and these ideas should be respected. For example, some patients prefer to do their therapy activities alone and refuse to participate in a group project, whereas other patients like to be involved in the social interactions that evolve during work on a collective project. Relevance, or the link between therapy and the patient's reality, should become part of initial treatment planning because the therapist is responsible for developing a strong link between the patient's interests and the goals of the occupational therapy program. This is not to say that it is easy to develop therapy that is compatible with the patient's goals, values, and interests. These three factors—the patient's perception of illness and health, the patient's perception of therapy, and the patient's belief in the meaning of life and activities—are all considered in a successful therapy program.

Factors to Consider During Evaluation and Treatment

This section will use information presented in the earlier case study to demonstrate how the OTR could have improved her assessment if cultural factors had been considered during the evaluation visit.

Conceptual Framework

One way to systematically include culture in one's daily treatment is to select a conceptual framework or model that includes culture. Although many occupational therapy theories and models mention culture, the Model of Human Occupation[38,39] includes a conceptual structure that integrates data about the patient's values, goals, interests, personal causation, habits, and roles into occupational therapy.

Background

The next step is to observe and investigate the lifestyle of cultural group members. Consider the largest number of ethnic group members in your patient load and find out where group members live. Try to do a small-scale, informal ethnographic study by exploring a local store, restaurant, recreational center, or religious sanctuary.[40] During your visit use your clinical skills to observe the human and non-human environment and the way that group members interact. Consider the values that are conveyed through all of these cues.

For instance, if the OTR had visited Mrs. W.'s neighborhood, she would have found a row of exclusive townhouses in a village within center city. The colonial-style, three-story, brick houses have narrow stairways and small rooms—in no way a barrier-free environment. Each house faced an attractive courtyard with a few trees and benches in the center. Garages were hidden underground and could only be accessed by an enclosed walkway. The houses were situated near a cluster of exclusive stores where one could buy things like gourmet take-out food, imported wine, custom made tiles, designer clothing, or hand-made lampshades.

This upper-middle-class neighborhood conveyed an air of cosmopolitan homogeneity. Although the OTR could not assume that Mrs. W. shared all of her neighbors' values, she could still learn something about her patient's lifestyle. It is not realistic to visit every patient's neighborhood; nonetheless, one can choose the largest group among one's patients and gather some background information about them. This data is as important as looking up medication side-effects and unfamiliar medical diagnoses.

Reading offers another source of information. Research on particular cultural groups appears in sociological, anthropological, and historical journals. Books also depict life in a particular culture. For instance, Chute's novel about the pain, humiliation, and rage of a poverty-stricken New England family[41] offers insight into rural deprivation. Factual accounts are also useful, such as the story told by Wideman, a Black-American Rhodes scholar and English professor, who searches for an answer to why his brother, who was raised by the same parents in the same environment as the author is presently serving a life sentence for murder.[42] Television and film documentaries that portray family and community life are helpful in understanding different lifestyles. In short, the OTR should gather as much information as possible about a patient's cultural group before the evaluation visit.

Using the case-study as an example, the OTR did not adequately prepare for the evaluation visit. The nurse and the physical therapist could have been used as informants so the OTR could be introduced to the patient's lifestyle. The OTR tried to control the interview by taking charge and asking questions. Mrs. W. valued competition and outward appearances; moreover, it was important for her to act like the family matriarch. Thus, the OTR became a rival. During the first 15 minutes of the interview, the OTR could have satisfied Mrs. W.'s need for attention by listening to her description of her progress and offering support for her efforts. At the same time, the OTR could have thoroughly observed the environment.

Evaluation

The initial evaluation is a crucial time to establish trust and gather cues from the human and the non-human environment. There are a number of evaluation tools that can be used to direct these observations. Use a guide to begin your search for an effective instrument. The Kielhofner text *The Model of Human Occupation*[43] includes an overview of assessment tools or *Asher's Annotated Index of Occupational Therapy Evaluation Tools*[44] which includes profiles on 87 occupational therapy instruments, as well as information on where to find the tool.

Because no instrument is perfect, consider elements of the patient's lifestyle by observing values concerning life, death, health, productivity, work, family relations, human nature, time, meaningful activities, and religion. Be alert to ethnic myths and taboos which will impede care if misunderstood by the therapist. Use data gathered from the evaluation tools you use to refine your ideas about treatment. For example, Mrs. W. may have responded better if the OTR had explored one of her

interests and then used the activity to observe Mrs. W.'s functional abilities.

Specific tools which could have been used in conjunction with other ADL, cognitive, perceptual, or motor evaluations are the Occupational Role History,[45,46] a semi-structured interview on occupational choice, work experience, and leisure satisfaction, or The Occupational Questionnaire[47] which collects data on the patient's use of time in daily activities and how that relates to the patient's values, interests, and personal causation. Two other useful tools are The Role Checklist, which assesses productive adult life-roles by indicating the individual's perceptions of past, present, and future roles[48] and the Time Battery for gathering qualitative and quantitative data on temporal adaptation and use of time.[49] The OTR should have selected a tool which seemed to provide appropriate ideas for treatment planning.

Even if the OTR had used better interviewing skills, completed an ADL Evaluation, and administered an instrument such as the Occupational Questionnaire, she would still need to compare this data with cues from the environment. Thus, the OTR's observation skills are fundamental to evaluation and treatment planning because patients may not always mean what they say. Examine the "extent to which the patient's beliefs, values, and customs are congruent with a trifold set of standards: from the patient's culture or ethnic group, from the therapist's own culture, and from the setting in which the treatment takes place.[50] Consider the extent that the patient is "like all other humans, like some other humans, and like no other humans."[51] Take time to identify and label similarities and differences between the patient's culture and the therapist's. This will help to separate personal bias and needs from those of the patient. For example, not all patients want to be independent in self-care. Some want to direct their energies toward other activities and view assistance as a trade-off. This was certainly true for Mrs. W.

A final consideration is the setting in which treatment takes place. Is the therapist a guest in the patient's home or is the patient a visitor in the hospital? The answer to those questions will determine roles and relationships. Treatment must be appropriate for the setting. For example, the institution is not always the best place to teach cooking and toileting skills because the information must be retaught once the patient returns home. On the other hand, the home setting is not suitable for constructing complex equipment and hand splints.

Summary

This paper has explored the importance of culture in occupational therapy. Occupational therapy founders emphasized the need to consider the patient's interests in treatment. Today, we again realize that treatment must be meaningful to patients. Thus, cultural factors must be considered in evaluation and treatment. This is no easy task because we are all entrenched in our own value systems. However, although there are many differences among cultural groups, there are also many similarities. Occupations can serve as a "common light among cultures."[52]

N.B. Throughout this paper the author has used the term "patient" to refer to the recipient of treatment. The term "client" was eschewed because it did not reflect people who were receiving medical services.

References

1. Tracy, SE: *Studies in invalid occupations.* Boston: Whitcomb and Barrows. 1912.
2. Dunton, WR: *Occupational Therapy: A manual for nurses.* Philadelphia: WB Saunders Co. 1918.
3. Hall, H and Buck, MMC: *Handicrafts for the Handicapped.* New York: Moffatt, Yard and Company. 1916, p. xii.
4. American Occupational Therapy Association Committee. An outline of lectures in Occupational Therapy to medical students and physicians. *Occupational Therapy and Rehabilitation. 5,* 1925, p. 278.
5. Doane, JC: Presidential address delivered at AOTA annual meeting. Toronto, Canada, September 28–30, 1931. Reprinted as *Occupational Therapy and Rehabilitation, 10,* 1931, p. 365.
6. Slagle, EC: Address to Graduates, Sheppard and Enoch Pratt Hospital, Towson, Maryland, June 28, 1930. *Occupational Therapy and Rehabilitation, 9* 1930, p. 275.
7. Mosey, AC: *Occupational Therapy: Configuration of a Profession.* New York: Raven Press. 1981, p. 78.
8. Fidler, GS and Fidler, JW: Doing and becoming: the Occupational Therapy experience. In Kielhofner, G, *Health through occupation.* Philadelphia: FA Davis Company. 1983, p. 267–280. Reprinted as Chapter 9.
9. Llorens, LA: *Application of a developmental theory for health and rehabilitation.* American Occupational Therapy Association. 1976.
10. Reilly, M: The modernization of Occupational Therapy. *Amer J Occup Ther 25,* 1971, p. 243–246.
11. Keilhofner, G and Burke, JP: Components and determinants of human occupation. In Kielhofner, G (Editor): *A model of human occupation: theory and application.* Baltimore, Maryland: Williams and Wilkins. 1985, p. 12–36.
12. Kielhofner, G and Burke, JP: A model of human occupation, Part I. Conceptual Framework and content. *Amer J Occup Ther 34,* 1980, pp. 572–581.
13. Barris, R: Environmental interactions: an extension of the model of occupation. *Amer J Occup Ther 36,* 1982, pp 637–644 .
14. Nuse-Clark, P: Human development through occupation: A philosophy and conceptual model for practice, part 2. *Amer J Occup Ther 33,* 1979, pp. 577–585.
15. Yerxa, E: Audicious values: the energy source for occupational therapy practice. In Kielhofner, G. (Editor) *Health through occupation.* Philadelphia: FA Davis. 1983, pp. 149–162.
16. Leininger, M: *Transcultural nursing: concepts, theories, and practices.* New York: John Wiley and Sons. 1978, p. 80.
17. Spradley, JP, McDurdy, DW (Editors): *Conformity and conflict.* Boston: Little, Brown. 1980, p. 2.
18. Linton, R. *The cultural background of personality.* New York: Appleton-Century-Crofts, Inc. 1945, p. 38.
19. Hall, ET: *The hidden dimension.* Garden City, New York: Anchor Books. 1969.
20. Laudin, H: *Victims of culture.* Columbus, Ohio: Charles E. Merrill Pub. Co. 1973.
21. Opler, M: *Culture and social psychiatry.* New York: Atherton Press. 1967, p. 14.
22. Likroeber, Al: quoted in Laudin, op. cit. p. 4.
23. Ibid. p. 184.
24. Ibid. p. 189.
25. Mechanic, D: Response factors in illness: the study of illness behavior. In Jaco, EG. (Editor): *Patients, physicians and illness.* New York: The Free Press. 1972, pp. 128–141.
26. Leininger, op. cit.
27. Saunders, L: *Cultural difference and medical care.* New York: Russell Sage Foundation. 1954.
28. Scott, CS: Health and healing practices among five ethnic groups in Miami, Florida. *Public Health Reports. 89* 1974, pp. 524–32.
29. Suchman, EA: Social patterns of illness and medical care. *Journal of health and human behavior. 6,* 1965, pp. 2–16.
30. Wolff, BB and Langley, S: Cultural factors and the response to pain. A review, In Weisenberg, M (Editor): *Pain: clinical and experimental perspectives.* Saint Louis: The CV Mosby Co. 1975, pp. 141–143.
31. Mechanic, D. Religion, religiosity, and illness behavior. *Human organization. 22,* 1963, p. 202.
32. Suchman, EA: Sociomedical variations among ethic groups. *American Journal of Sociology. 70* 1964–5, pp. 319–331.
33. Lopreato, J: *Italian Americans.* New York: Random House, 1970.
34. Levine, RE: The cultural aspects of home care delivery. *Amer J Occup Ther 38,* 1984, pp. 736–737.
35. Sharrott, G: Occupational therapy's role in the client's creation and affirmation of meaning. In Kielhofner, G: *Health through occupation.* Philadelphia: FA Davis. 1983, p. 215.
36. Rogers, JC: The spirit of independence: the evolution of a philosophy. *Amer J Occup Ther 36,* 1982 pp. 709–715.
37. Barris, op. cit.
38. Kielhofner and Burke, op. cit.
39. Kielhofner, G. op. cit.
40. Merrill, SC: Qualitative methods in occupational therapy research: an application. *The occupational therapy journal of research. 5* 1985, pp. 209–222.
41. Chute, C: *The Beans of Egypt, Maine.* New York: Ticknor & Fields, 1985.
42. Wideman, JE: *Brothers and keepers.* New York: Penguin Books. 1984.
43. Kielhofner, op. cit.
44. Asher, IE: *Annotated index of Occupational Therapy evaluation tools.* Thomas Jefferson University, Department of Occupational Therapy, 1985.
45. Moorehead, L: The occupational history. *Amer J Occup Ther 23,* 1969, pp. 329–334.
46. Florey, LL & Michelman, SM: Occupational role history: a screening tool for psychiatric occupational therapy. *Amer J Occup Ther 36,* 1982 pp. 301–308.
47. Riopel, N & Kielhofner, G: *Occupational questionnaire.* In Asher, op. cit. p. 57.
48. Oakley, F: *The role checklist.* In Asher. op. cit. p. 58.
49. Larrington, G: *Time Battery.* In Asher. op. cit. p. 59.
50. Tripp-Reimer, T., Brink, PJ, Saunders, JM: Cultural assessment: content and process. *Nursing Outlook. 32,* p. 81.
51. Kluckholn, C: quoted in Brill, NI: *Working with people: the helping process.* Philadelphia: JB Lippincott, 1976, p. 19.
52. Malinowski, B: *Argonauts of the western pacific.* New York: EP Dutton and Co., Inc., 1961. p. 25.

The Culture Concept in the Everyday Practice of Occupational and Physical Therapy

CHAPTER 19

Laura Krefting, PhD

Although the concept of culture is a central tenet in the social sciences, it is only recently that its relevance to the provision of health care has been widely acknowledged. The purpose of this article is to present a concept of culture that has application in everyday practice, to describe the hazards of avoiding culturally sensitive practice, and to present some ways to facilitate the use of the culture concept in clinical practice.

This chapter was previously published in *Meaning of Culture in Pediatric Rehabilitation and Health Care,* The Haworth Press, (1991), 1–16.

The Culture Concept

In anthropology, where culture is a central theoretical concept, entire books have been devoted to its definition, suggesting the richness and complexity of the concept (see for a discussion Geertz, 1973;[1] Keesing, 1981;[2] Kroeber & Kluckholn, 1963[3]). In fact, after decades of debate anthropologists have not agreed on a single definition. There are, however, certain commonalities among the definitions which provide a basis for understanding the concept. Most agree that it is a system of learned patterns of behavior.[4] The idea that culture is learned rather than inherited biologically is important. Learning occurs through the socialization process—it is transmitted to the young of the group by other group members. Another commonality in definitions of culture is that it is shared by other members of a group rather than being the property of an individual. Finally, in many definitions, culture includes the concept of providing the individual and the group with effective mechanisms for interacting both with others and with the surrounding environment. In this way culture can be seen as adaptive. A shorter capsular definition of culture refers to culture as a blueprint or organizing framework to guide daily behavior.

An important aspect of culture is that the influence of culture on behavior is not always conscious. Hall calls it the silent language and describes cultural traditions and convention as largely subconscious.[5] He argues that most people do not recognize the effect of culture on themselves, yet behavior is rigidly influenced by it. For example, some cultural groups have a less rigid definition of "appointment time" than do most Western-trained therapists. The client that arrives 4 hours late, in the company of a friend who has brought his two children along for an assessment as well, can present problems to the therapist.

Those who use culture in practical ways, as advocate, often adopt a multidimensional definition of culture. Figure 19.1 depicts the different dimensions of culture as concentric circles. In the preceding definitions, culture refers to common patterns held by larger groups, e.g., states or nations. This outer regional circle is the one most often seen in cross-cultural studies. It focuses on visible, commonly held patterns; an example would be a comparison of mental health patterns in Ireland and the United States. I chose that particular cross-cultural example from the book *Saints, Scholars, and Schizophrenics* by Scheper-Hughes.[6] In this study she describes the dynamics behind the mental health patterns in Ireland and associates them with land tenure and customs related to family role. She focuses in particular on the custom of the youngest son staying on the small farm with aging parents while siblings emigrate to North America. The study illustrates that the life of these youngest "caretaker sons" is one that is conducive to the development of schizophrenia. In this example, types of industry, natural resources, and geographic diversity within the culture are pertinent factors. It is at this level that comparisons of health service delivery models are often made, e.g., comparing the more nationalized systems of Britain and Canada to that of the American health-care system. The regional level also includes the popular definition of groups, such as the Navaho or Inuit culture. Within these cultures, however, there is also variation.

In considering culture at a *community* level, smaller and more refined commonalities among people are noted. For example, there might be similarity in type of housing, ethnicity, and economic background among Caucasian middle-class suburbanites, particularly if compared to individuals in an inner-city core. Similarities in health care practices might be seen at the community level in how frequently and for what reasons community members see family physicians.

Even within these communities, cultures differ, as can be seen by comparing two neighboring families in the same community. Factors that might differ at the family level of

culture include family power structure, style and frequency of worship, and ways that stress are demonstrated. Potential differences are apparent when comparing the family reaction to the birth of a neonate with severe physical disability in a family which has lived in the area for 10 years and has experience with the health-care services to reactions in a family which has recently emigrated from a Latin American country and for whom the knowledge of appropriate services and how to access them is a major difficulty.

Finally, culture can be defined in terms of the individual, i.e., each person can be considered to have an *individual* culture. Although culture is a shared phenomenon, sharing is seen in the context of transmission and socialization. Moreover, individuals learn culture from a number of different people and places so that, in fact, each person's contact with and interpretation of the culture is unique. For instance, siblings brought up in the same home culture might differ in terms of food preference, coping style, and degree of interaction with peer group.

In looking at the different definitions of culture and the heterogeneity of cultural groups, it is important to consider the assimilation of cultures. Assimilation refers to the process whereby people of one culture lose their culturally unique characteristics and become more like those of the dominant culture.[7] Assimilation is the term often used in describing how well immigrants adapted to their new country. The degree of

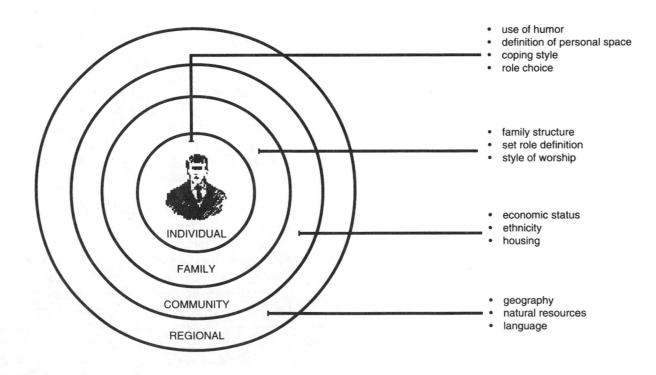

Figure 19.1. Cultural influence at different levels.

Note: From Krefting, L. H., & Krefting, D. V. (1991). Cultural influences on performance. In Christiansen, C. & Baum, C. (Eds). *Occupational Therapy: Overcoming Human Performance Deficits.* Thorofare, NJ: Slack Incorporated, p. 103.

assimilation depends on such factors as length of residence in new country or region, residential area, language spoken at home and fluency in the new language or dialect, and amount of contact with country of origin. Variety among groups, even of recent immigrants, can be noted. Differing characteristics include whether they belong to official cultural organizations (such as the Korean Students' Sports Club or a children's language training group), their clothing style, food preference, and involvement with others of the same cultural group. This dilution of stronger cultural characteristics prevents therapists from making broad generalizations about how members of certain groups will behave.

Further complicating the issue of cultural identity is the fact that some individuals are bicultural. These are individuals who may adapt to the dominant culture in one role in life, e.g., at work, yet retain their own cultural values and customs at home.[8] This can also be seen at the family level in which one family member, usually the wife or grandmother who stays at home with young children, retains more of the original cultural characteristics than the primary wage earner, who has more contact with the new cultural group through work. Intergenerational comparisons also illustrate the process of assimilation. For example, in some groups elders are the authority because they are the repositories of knowledge (where knowledge was passed orally). This changes when they emigrate to a new country or region with a different culture. In this new setting the young may become powerful because they more quickly learn the knowledge that helps them adapt to the new culture through attending school or work and through peer contact.

To summarize, the concept of culture can be understood on multiple levels. Each individual is a product of the integration of multiple levels of culture and can be seen to have a unique cultural identity. It is at this level that the definition of culture is of most use to physical and occupational therapists.

What Culture Is Not

One way to help clarify the complex definition of culture is to describe what it is not. A common misinterpretation of culture is that it is the same as ethnicity. Ethnicity is that part of one's identify derived from membership, usually through birth, in a racial, religious, national, or linguistic group or subgroup.[9] Ethnicity is an important component of culture but the terms are not synonymous. For example, two patients may come from the same neighborhood and share a strong Hispanic-American background but can differ in other cultural factors such as religion, family structure, ways of expressing pain or discomfort, and experience with the medical system. The broader concept of culture can be noted when considering the best approach to the families of two disabled children of Pakistani background: one a family of seven on social assistance whose members have had minimal contact with the formal medical system and another family of three in which one parent works in a hospital and the other is involved in community politics.

Unfortunately, the most common way that culture has been addressed in the occupational and physical therapy literature is to equate it with ethnicity or race. In this approach writers attempt to provide background information on certain "cultural groups." For example, McCormack discussed characteristic health beliefs and practices of Hispanics, Indo-Chinese, and African-Americans,[10] and Blakeney[8] used Appalachian peoples as a case example of the importance of addressing the values of a subculture.

As Litterst observes, such a narrow definition of culture neglects potential variation within groups.[11] Such articles imply a homogeneity among group members and can, if not carefully written, perpetuate stereotypes. Such anecdotal information provides a sort of practical definition of ethnic groups; without a cultural assessment at the individual level, therapists can easily develop preconceived ideas about how groups of people will manage their illness or disability.

Nor is culture synonymous with a geographic region. Culture can be misrepresented in this way in articles such as "Rehabilitation in India" or "Lower Limb Prosthetics in Irian Jaya." This geographic definition often describes a small slice of the disability experience (children with upper limb amputations) or of professional services (mental health occupational therapy) in a particular country while making the assumption that these experiences or services are homogeneous throughout a country. Such cultural analyses (I use that term loosely) often result from what is known as "windscreen" medical anthropology in which only brief contact has been made with a small segment of the health care system.

A third way that the culture concept has been misrepresented is in limiting its relevance only to immigrant health. Clearly, immigrant health highlights the importance of cultural diversity. Changing immigration laws and refugee policies, as well as increased mobility within regions of North America, have created a situation in which it is quite feasible for a therapist to work with people from nearly every cultural group in the world.[12,13] The area of immigrant health also reveals new types of illnesses or disabilities or ones that are no longer common in North America, e.g., post-typhoid paralysis, polio, and nutritional-related disabilities such as blindness due to vitamin A deficiency. New arrivals to a culture are also at risk for stress-related disorders or complications because they often suffer social, economic, and cultural dislocation.[14] These factors result in an increased visibility of immigrants in the rehabilitation system.

Although I have emphasized the importance of immigrant health issues, I must stress that culture in health care is much more than that. The idea of culturally sensitive treatment should not come to mind only when a therapist hears an unfamiliar accent or sees a note on the patient history indicating that the person in the treatment room is a recent immigrant. It should come to mind *every time* the therapist enters that treatment room.

In relation to what culture is not, it is important to realize that no specific rules exist for working with members of any particular cultural group. Thus you will not find the definitive article on working with the first generation Ethiopian patient. As Baptiste notes, a shopping list of cultural traits is not the answer for developing a culturally sensitive practice.[15] In fact, this is a challenge for clinical social scientists who are called in to consult about patients whose cultural background is different from that of the majority of the rehabilitation team. An example from my personal experience is a patient from Asia whose mother had moved into the hospital room, was sleeping on rugs by her daughter's bed, and, in following her religious traditions, was ensuring that her daughter was awake for all five calls to prayer. Because there are no set rules that help you interpret particular cultures, it is critical to understand the basic components of culture and then assess the cultural identity of each patient.

Cultural Pespectives in Therapy

Culture is often considered from the perspective of the patient/client and the family members. In any therapeutic relationship, however, the culture of both the patient and the therapist must be considered. Not only do the cultural factors influencing the patient's behavior need to be identified but their interaction with the cultural background of the therapist is important.[16]

It is not surprising that therapists who are typically from white middle-class backgrounds and possess the inherent values, mores, and expectations of those experiences[17] can be in conflict with patients. A potential dilemma might arise in the case of the therapist brought up as a rugged individualist who is fiercely independent in interaction with a parent who never leaves the disabled child's side, helping him or her with every activity. This sort of cultural blindness is a good example of ethnocentricity, in which unfamiliar cultures are judged or defined in terms of the health professional's own, with the sense that the professional's culture is superior.

Therapists, then, must try to understand the background of the patient and to identify how their personal values and biases may interfere with assessment and treatment. At the same time therapists must recognize the nature of their own background and how it influences the therapeutic situation. In this way, both partners in the therapeutic relationship can arrive at a common understanding of the problem areas, their priority in treatment, and means of intervention.

The Cost of Culturally Insensitive Therapy

What is the cost of dismissing cultural factors in everyday practice of providing health care? First, rapport will be difficult to establish thereby decreasing the patient's trust in the therapist. Poor rapport can develop into major communication problems. The situation in which different perspectives regarding the preferred outcome of treatment exist but are not communicated is an illustration. Such a situation might be one in which a child is determined to attend a regular school, one parent supports special education, and the other a nontraditional Montessori type of education, and the therapist prefers an educational program in a school–hospital setting. Such communication problems can result in noncompliance and patient dissatisfaction with treatment.

One of the keys to cultural sensitivity is understanding that culture affects illness behavior. Illness behaviors are the ways in which people respond to bodily indication and conditions that they come to view as abnormal.[18] It is the way in which people monitor their health, define and interpret symptoms, take remedial action, and use sources of available help. One of the major factors in illness behavior is whether patients and families adhere to various treatment regimes. Understanding the patient's culture helps the professional to influence health behavior in positive ways—whether that means following a schedule of home exercises or wearing a protective helmet.

Moreover, by ignoring cultural factors, the behavior of therapists can be affected. They can be left with feelings of helplessness, frustration, and anger because of differences in perception with patients and/or families. Most therapists have probably experienced the frustration of either trying to dissuade parents from "doing for" their child with a disability or, on the other hand, to persuade parents to carry out home therapy programs.

In addition to the frustrations experienced by therapists and patients, family members can also be affected by cultural problems, becoming antagonists rather than facilitators in the treatment process. In the field of pediatrics, in which parents are key members of the rehabilitation team, their satisfaction with the therapeutic relationship is critical.

To summarize, recognizing the role of culture in assessment and treatment can improve rapport and communication and increase compliance and perceived satisfaction with treatment, thereby creating treatment that is effective, efficient, and economical.

Culturally Sensitive Practice

The health-care professions have responded to the issue of providing service in a multicultural society in a number of ways.[19] One approach focuses on language barriers and involves recruitment of translators for key linguistic groups. This approach is superficial because it reduces the culture concept to the issue of language differences. A second approach is to provide limited awareness training for staff members. This might include bringing in a speaker on multicultural communication or having a staff member of a different cultural background discuss cultural barriers s/he has encountered in the medical system. A third approach is to recruit bicultural health care professionals or at least ones with a different ethnic background. (I call this the "United Nations in one rehabilitation department" strategy.) Again, this reduces culture to ethnic background or skin color and does not really address cultural diversity.

The fourth approach is to develop culturally sensitive assessment and intervention strategies that can be used by any therapist with any patient or family member regardless of the individual cultural background. The remainder of the paper will address a number of strategies that can be used to develop cultural sensitivity in occupational and physical therapy programs. An approach that is particularly useful in introducing cultural sensitivity is to involve a medical anthropologist or sociologist on a consultation basis, for example in weekly rounds in which cultural issues are discussed. This brings immediate relevance to the issues of multiculturalism and daily practice. Cultural sensitivity can also be encouraged by modifying the physical features of an occupational or physical therapy department. Multicultural prompts in orientation boards that include a number of religious and ethnic festivals (for example, the Duvali—the Indian Festival of Lights) might be used. Morse's article describing a nontraditional community program based in the Jewish cultural context illustrates the ways that cultural beliefs can be incorporated into a life-skill program for those with developmental delay.[16] Examples of activities integrating principles of the Jewish faith included preparation of Bar and Bat Mitzvahs, holiday cooking classes, and joining with other Jewish cultural groups.

A critical step in providing culturally sensitive service is to assess the cultural validity of standardized assessment instruments. The composition of the sample used to establish norms is one aspect to be evaluated. A perusal of most rehabilitation test norms will show that they are based on urban middle- and upper-middle class subjects. Another factor in cultural validity is the relevance of the evaluation tools and tasks to children of different cultural backgrounds. The following situation illustrates how research efforts were frustrated because of poor cultural validity of an instrument. A team of experienced researchers was conducting a study of developmental delay in a northern Canadian community. Although the particular test had excellent psychometric properties, the common tasks children were expected to do were impossible to do in a harsh northern climate where, for example, riding tricycles on the pavement was impossible both because of the lack of pavement and of money to purchase tricycles.

Cultural relevance of diagnostic tests are particularly important when scores are used to determine whether a child is "normal" or in some way delayed and requires special services. A remarkable article by Edgerton describes how an individual labelled as "brain damaged" as a child spent his youth receiving special services for persons with developmental delay.[20] When retested at the age of 17 years, he was found to be of normal intelligence.

One of the ways of approaching the cultural validity of assessments is to compare the test scores of children of different cultural backgrounds. An example of this approach is a recent Master's thesis studying the Miller Assessment for Preschoolers (MAP). Hohl noted that Mexican-American children in Texas scored significantly lower on the verbal index of the MAP when compared to normative data, emphasizing the potential for cultural differences among groups.[21]

An initial evaluation can be modified in several ways to ensure that culturally relevant data are gathered. The degree to which therapists, children, and their families agree that a disability exists is one area to assess. The identification of a specific physical or mental impairment as "illness" or "disability" varies from one culture to another as well as among social classes or ethnic groups within a single culture. For example, variation in the definition of disability by social class is seen in the middle-class American view of asthma, stuttering, and learning disabilities as handicaps requiring treatment; other cultural groups view them as personal characteristics not directly related to health at all.[22] The labeling of these conditions as "disabilities" by the therapist, when the patient and/or family does not believe there is a problem, can lead to nonadherence to treatment as well as frustration of all concerned.

A second question to include in a culturally sensitive intake evaluation is "what caused the illness?" This relates not to pathophysiology but to social or supernatural causes of an illness or disability. The influence of beliefs about "why my child" or "why now" are clearly illustrated in the disability detection program with which I am associated in Indonesia. Figure 19.2 illustrates the kinds of beliefs that are attributed to the birth of an infant with cleft palate—all of the causes are related to behavior of the parents. Knowledge of such information would clearly help a therapist to understand parents who were reluctant to bring a child to a screening clinic or for treatment.

A third type of question to include in an initial evaluation is related to patterns of help-seeking. Patterns of help-seeking are the culturally distinct ways in which people go about finding help at particular times in their illness. Help-seeking refers both to the range of alternatives open to an individual and how and why choices are made among various alternatives.[23] Therapists usually think of help-seeking in terms of the professional health care network such as physicians, sports medicine clinicians, and rehabilitation counselors. However, people seek help from a variety of nonmedical sources such as family and friends, naturopaths, faith healers, and acupuncturists.[24] Clinicians should not assume that health care professionals are the only alterative used by the patient.

Three studies illustrate the concept of help-seeking by describing different approaches to family caregiving for children with chronic illness. Anderson reports on caregiving patterns for chronically ill children in a Chinese-Canadian context.[25] She notes that immigrant families are often not able to integrate the ideological structures behind the Western health care system and that this may be reflected in nonadherence. A lack of understanding about "normalization" by immigrant families

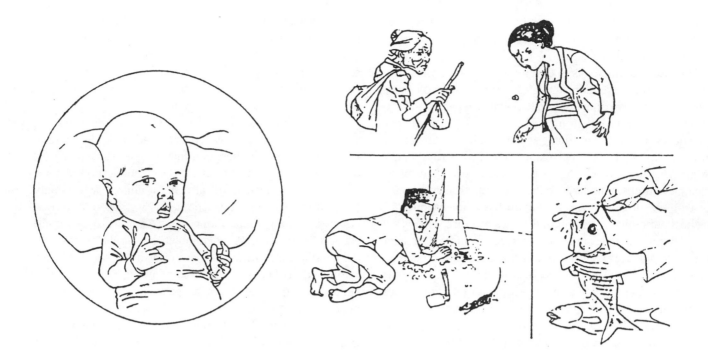

Figure 19.2. Cultural understanding of the cause of cleft palate. (Used with permission of Dr. Soeharso, Community Based Rehabilitation Centre, Surakarta, Indonesia).

was evident in a tendency to discontinue the exercise program or medication at the least bit of discomfort shown by the children. The family members' goal was the "happiness and contentment" of children rather than normalization procedures advocated in Western medicine.

An article by Oremland describes an ethnographic approach to studying work dynamics in family care of hemophilic children.[26] The division of labor surrounding family caregiving is clearly sensitive to cultural variation; in this study the central role that siblings play in caregiving is described. A third study describes "parental entrepreneurship"—activism among parents of children with a disability to promote better systems of professional caregiving.[27]

The concept of help-seeking has a number of practical implications for assessment and intervention. First, the history of help-seeking (including the perceived importance and success of each alternative) should be a part of any comprehensive assessment. Eliciting the child's and family's feelings about the use of informal sectors is often difficult because they may be reluctant to disclose "unmedical" or unsophisticated sources of help despite the fact that they have used them. One of the ways to facilitate communication is to convey an accepting attitude about the range of alternatives, perhaps by introducing the topic with a comment about the number of people you see in therapy who use nonmedical options.

It is important to consider therapeutic networks in which two or more options from different sectors are used simultaneously because occupational and physical therapy assessment and intervention might conflict with other alternatives.

An example is the situation in which an herbalist is advocating fasting and meditation for a chronic respiratory condition and the therapist is encouraging moderate exercise and postural drainage. Such a situation may create tension or anxiety for the child and family and may cause them to disregard the therapist's treatment choice. One approach is for therapists to try to incorporate non-traditional sources of help in his or her therapeutic program, for instance in preceding the therapy treatment sessions with relaxation or creative visualization.

The suggestions mentioned represent only a small number of examples of how therapists can begin to develop more culturally sensitive treatment approaches. They are meant to illustrate how the rather vague culture concept can be incorporated into daily practice.

Conclusions

Culture is a complex concept that is of central importance to the provision of effective services for infants and children who are disabled and to their families. I have argued that therapists must consider the cultural identity of the individual and avoid cultural "rule books" that assume all people of a particular ethnic or racial background are similar in health beliefs and practices. It is also important for therapists to evaluate their own cultural values and beliefs and to be aware of how these influence practice. A reconceptualization of all aspects of assessment and treatment is needed if the multicultural nature of today's society is to be acknowledged in the rehabilitation field. This article presents some ways to begin this process.

References

1. Geertz, C. (1973). *The interpretation of cultures.* New York: Basic Books.
2. Keesing, R. (1981). Theories of cultures. In R Casson (ed): *Language, Culture and Cognition.* New York: MacMillan.
3. Kroeber, A. L. & Kluckholn, C. (1963). *Culture: a Critical Review.* New York: Vintage Books.
4. Low, S. M. (1984). The cultural basis of health, illness, and disease. *Social Work in Health Care, 9,* 13–23.
5. Hall, E. (1959). *The Silent Language.* New York: Doubleday.
6. Scheper-Hughes, N. (1979). *Saints, Scholars, and Schizophrenics.* Berkeley: University of California Press.
7. Shawski, K. A. (1987). Ethnic/racial considerations in occupational therapy. *Occupational Therapy in Health Care, 4,* 37–49.
8. Blakeney A. B. (1987). Appalachian values: Implications for occupational therapists. *Occupational Therapy in Health Care, 4,* 57–72.
9. Hartog, J. & Hartog, E. E. (1983). Cultural aspects of health and illness behaviors in hospitals. *Western Journal of Medicine, 139,* 910–916.
10. McCormack, G.L. (1987). Culture and communication in the treatment planning for occupational therapy with minority patients. *Occupational Therapy in Health Care, 4,* 17–36.
11. Litterst, T. A. E. (1985). A reappraisal of anthropological fieldwork methods and concept of culture in occupational therapy research. *American Journal of Occupational Therapy, 39,* 602–604.
12. Dyck, I. (1989). The immigrant client: Issues in developing culturally sensitive practice. *Canadian Journal of Occupational Therapy, 56,* 248–255.
13. Health and Welfare Canada (1986). *Review of the Literature on Migrant Mental Health.* Ottawa: Department of National Health and Welfare.
14. Clarke, M. M. (1983). Cultural context of medical practice. *Western Journal of Medicine. 139,* 806–810.
15. Baptiste, S. (1988). Chronic pain, activity, and culture. *Canadian Journal of Occupational Therapy, 55,* 179–184.
16. Morse, A. (1987). A cultural intervention model for developmentally delayed adults: An expanded role for occupational therapy. *Occupational Therapy in Health Care, 4,* 103–113.
17. Robinson, L. (1987). Patient compliance in occupational therapy home health programs: Sociocultural considerations. *Occupational Therapy in Health Care, 4,* 127–137.
18. Mechanic, D. (1986). The concept of illness behavior: Culture, situation, and personal predisposition. *Psychological Medicine, 16,* 1–7.
19. Cuellar, I. & Arnold, B. R. (1988). Cultural considerations and rehabilitation of disabled Mexican Americans. *Journal of Rehabilitation,* 35–41.
20. Edgerton, R. B. (1986). A case of delabeling: Some practical and theoretical implications. In L. Langness & H. Levine (Eds). *Culture and Retardation* pp 101–126. Norwell, MA: Kluwer Academic Press.
21. Hohl, M. R. (1990). *The Performance of Mexican–American Children in Texas on the Miller Assessment for Pre-schoolers.* Unpublished master's thesis. Chapel Hill, NC, University of North Carolina at Chapel Hill.
22. Gliedman, J. & Roth, W. (1980). *The Unexpected Minority: Handicapped Children in America.* New York: Harcourt Brace Jovanovich.
23. Helman, C. (1984). *Culture, Health and Illness.* Bristol: John Wright and Sons.
24. Kleinman, A. (1980). *Patients and Healers in the Context of Culture.* Berkeley: University of California Press, pp 104–118.
25. Anderson, J. (1986). Ethnicity and illness experience: Ideological structures and the health care delivery system. *Social Science and Medicine, 22,* 1277–1283.
26. Oremland, E. K. (1988). Work dynamics in family care of hemophiliac children. *Social Science and Medicine, 26,* 467–475.
27. Darling, R. (1988). Parental entrepreneurship: A consumerist response to professional dominance. *Journal of Social Issues, 44,* 141–158.

Culture Emergent in Occupation

CHAPTER 20

BETTE R. BONDER, PhD, OTR/L, FAOTA
LAURA MARTIN, PhD
ANDREW W. MIRACLE, PhD

Culture influences occupation as well as perceptions of health, illness, and disability. Therapists are aware of the need to address culture in interventions. However, definitions of culture can be unclear, providing little guidance to therapists about how to recognize its effects in therapeutic encounters. A pragmatic definition of culture as emergent in everyday interactions of individuals encourages reconsideration of the main elements of culture, that it is learned, shared, patterned, evaluative, and persistent but changeable. Understanding of culture as emergent in interaction, including therapeutic intervention, suggests three important characteristics that therapists can cultivate to enhance clinical encounters: careful attention, active curiosity, and self-reflection and evaluation.

Introduction

Occupational therapists have long acknowledged that culture is an important aspect of occupation and of perceptions of health, disability, and illness. The founders of the profession emphasized that therapeutic activities should be prescribed based on the individual's personal and cultural values (Dunton, 1918). This recognition has led to many calls for cultural competence in the clinic (Barney, 1991; Dillard et al., 1992; Mirkopoulos & Evert, 1994; Wittman & Velde, 2002), a call now incorporated into standards for education of new therapists (American Occupational Therapy Association [AOTA], 1999). It is fair to say that "few occupational therapists are unaware of the importance of considering culture in the provision of occupational therapy services" (Fitzgerald, Mullavey-O'Byrne, & Clemson, 1997, p. 1).

Before cultural factors can be addressed in care, therapists must have a clear understanding of what culture is. Anthropologists, who have a primary focus on defining and describing culture, have throughout their history debated the definition of the term and still have not reached consensus (Kuper, 1999). It is therefore not surprising that therapists likewise are somewhat unclear about exactly what the construct means. Too often, race and ethnicity are used as representations of culture. For example, in their book on cultural competency, Wells and Black (2000) discuss what it is that "White American health practitioners" (p. 138) must be aware of in their practice, suggesting that White Americans constitute a single cultural group and that race is a central characteristic of cultural group identity. The equation of race or ethnicity with culture leaves therapists to puzzle about whether culture is something that applies only to those who look different from themselves or speak a different language (Pope-Davis, Prieto, Whitaker, & Pope-Davis, 1993). Because effective therapeutic interventions address cultural factors as a way to enhance quality of life and optimal performance (Barney, 1991; Dyck & Forwell, 1997), this confusion about what constitutes culture has a potentially damaging impact on client care.

Defining Culture

In the occupational therapy literature, an array of definitions of culture can be found. One definition is "a state of manners, taste, and intellectual development at a time or place. It is the ideas, customs, arts, etc. of a given people at a given time" (Baptiste, 1988, p. 180). At approximately the same time,

Levine (1987 [see Chapter 18]) described culture as "a 'blueprint' for human behavior, influencing individual thoughts, actions and collectively influencing a particular society" (p. 7). Krefting and Krefting (1991 [see Chapter 19]) called it "a filter or veil through which people perceive life's experiences" (p. 108). Christiansen and Baum (1997) define culture as referring to the "values, beliefs, customs and behaviors that are passed on from one generation to the next" (p. 61). Still another definition labels culture "an abstract concept that refers to learned and shared patterns of perceiving and adapting to the world" (Fitzgerald et al., 1997, p. 1).

Anthropologists have also developed multiple definitions for culture. Since it was first created by Edward B. Tylor (1871) and other late 19th-century scholars, use of the term has evolved. Not surprisingly, changes in usage have reflected the changed understandings of what it means to be human that have been in vogue at various times.

By the mid-20th century, the burgeoning influence of individual psychology began to affect scholarly approaches to culture. Sapir (1924/1949) and Wallace (1961) noted that the foundations for cultural traits resided in the minds of specific individuals; that is, while patterns of thinking and behavior might be widely shared across a society, the locus of culture is within individuals. Wallace's theory of mazeway as the mechanism for cultural change was explicit in this regard. For Wallace, culture change begins when a single individual incorporates a new element (e.g., through invention or borrowing) or when someone synthesizes traditional elements in a new configuration. If such innovation is perceived as useful, then additional individuals in the cultural group may adopt it and thus widespread change may be underway.

Geertz (1973) describes culture as "webs of meaning" in which people live. Kuper (1999) indicates that "in its most general sense, culture is simply a way of talking about collective identities" (p. 3). Holland, Lachicotte, Skinner, and Cain (1998) suggest that culture can be conceived in several different ways: as defining and determining individual human needs; as a superficial labeling of deep-seated needs; or as a formation of motivation during development. There has been considerable debate in anthropological circles about whether culture refers to behavior, or to the artistic expression of emotion, that is, culture in the sense of the arts and literature (Kuper, 1999).

Today, anthropologists (e.g., Reyna, 2002) work to explain the relationship between the biological and the cultural. Noting the work of anthropologists such as D'Andrade (1999) and Dressler and Bindon (2000), Handwerker (2002) concludes that a "theory of culture as cognitive elements and structure now dominates ethnographic research" (p. 119). Moreover, there is a growing recognition by psychologists (e.g., Hermans & Kempen, 1998; Pepitone, 2000) that the "discipline can no longer assume an acultural or unicultural stance" (Segall, Lonner, & Berry, 1998, p. 1101). And, sociologists (e.g., Cerulo, 2001) have begun to consider culture and cognition, especially in the context of race and ethnicity.

All of these conceptualizations carry some common themes related to individuals' actions, and their attributions of meaning and value to those actions. Two main strategies have typically been employed to create the necessary specificity in defining culture.

A Descriptive Approach

One strategy for elaborating on definitions of culture has been an approach characterized by a detailed description of particular groups through "the set of characteristics that an observer might record in studying the collective life of a human group" (Kuper, 1999, p. 24). This descriptive approach is exemplified in the thorough accounts by early ethnographers of New World indigenous groups, or by such works as Eliot's (1948) list of English cultural traits. Such descriptions involve a systematic identification of the particular characteristics and material goods of a given society. A full description of all the technological, economic, political, kinship, and religious characteristics of a people, together with the details of their socialization practices, rituals, and value systems, has been assumed to provide a description of the culture of that people. Providing a list of the major traits, patterns of behavior, and material objects the people produce or use is believed to offer a good approximation of a particular cultural group at a given moment in time. Examples of this kind of description are now widely available at Web sites focused on diversity, or on culture and health (for an example, see Cross-Cultural Health Care Program, www.xculture.org/resource/library/index/cfm).

Producing these descriptions is a demanding task. It is impossible to describe every relevant cultural fact about a given people. Even if the task itself were manageable, such a list can tell us nothing of the choices a single member of the group has made within the range of possibilities each culture provides. This approach assumes that by describing what seem (to the describer) to be the significant traits of a culture, outsiders can gain an appreciation of what life is like, at least superficially, for the people involved. Most of the time, though, descriptive approach products simply summarize cultures with just a few key values or characteristics. The ethnographies that abound in anthropology are excellent examples of the descriptive approach (cf., Hendrickson, 1995), but require constant updating as cultural circumstances change (Hendrickson, 1996).

Such summaries can be useful. They provide snapshots of particular groups at particular points in time, and a general sense of the important values and behaviors of the group. They provide for the observer, or the therapist, a starting point from which further exploration of the values of the specific individual within the culture can begin. But they are inevitably superficial. The potential exists to create stereotypes, or to replace one stereotype with another, rather than to reach a genuine understanding of the culture as represented by its individuals. This strategy also inevitably results in a limitation of scope. As an example, Hendrickson (1995) focused her attention specifically on weaving, providing much less information about other aspects of life in the Guatemala highlands, the lives of men, for instance, or the activities of women in villages where weaving was not typical.

A Rules Approach

Another strategy for enhancing cultural understanding focuses on the rules for belief and behavior. This approach assumes culture serves as a cognitive model of reality for each of the group's members. For example, Skinner (1989) provides a list of rules for the behavior of young girls in Naudada, a Hindu community in central Nepal. The list indicates what good daughters and good wives do. On the list is a rule indicating that good wives die before their husbands. Knowing this rule, that it is unseemly to outlive one's husband, helps the outsider understand why the term *Radi* (widow) is a pejorative term in that culture. Thus, understanding a culture means knowing how the people living in that culture view reality, how they make distinctions among categories of things, and how they generally make decisions about right courses of action (Schneider, 1976). Of course, in taking this approach it is necessary to know (and to describe for others) most of the things that exist in the world of those people. In this sense, the rules approach subsumes the descriptive one, but adds a list of the rules by which the culture determines meaning, molds behavior, and incorporates new information.

Taking the approach of listing rules can be quite helpful in providing a starting place for interaction. Many guides to cultural competence for health-care providers emphasize this strategy, indicating, for example, what the rules are for interaction between genders, how to address someone from a particular cultural group, or whether or not to make direct eye contact (Galanti, 1997; Wells & Black, 2000). Knowing the rules can provide the therapist with a starting point for asking appropriate questions about the preferences of the individual.

However, like descriptive accounts, rules studies are always incomplete because not everything can be included. Nor can it ever be known with certainty that the model provided by such an approach really describes reality as understood by all the people in a society or even by most of them. By imposing a static model of culture, this method also fails to accommodate the ranges of variability or the combinations of cultural influences experienced by most individuals, especially those living in culturally heterogenous communities.

In spite of the consistent association between action and meaning and the many examples of rules-based and description-based accounts, definitions of culture remain relatively vague from the occupational therapist's point of view. They fail to provide guidance regarding precisely how culture relates to occupation, and, therefore, how therapists might address culture in assessing clients and designing meaningful and relevant interventions. We believe that too often therapists fail to recognize that everyone in an encounter has culture (in fact, identifies with more than one culture, as will be discussed below), and that the cultural experiences of every participant in an encounter affect the nature of the interaction (cf., Bonder, Martin, & Miracle, 2002). It is equally easy to dismiss as "not really cultures" the regional differences (e.g., Appalachian) and other factors (e.g., sexual orientation, bicultural identities) that individual clients may self-describe as components of their cultural identities. For purposes of creating interventions, therapists need a pragmatic definition that can guide the kinds of questions they ask, their interpretation of responses, and their design of treatment.

The Model of Culture Emergent

A third approach to culture, the one we adopt here, is based on a pragmatic definition of culture as emergent in the everyday interactions of individuals (Bonder et al., 2002). It has been developed to elaborate on and reconceptualize factors found in traditional definitions of culture. This definition emphasizes both group patterns and individual variation to explain the multiple influences experienced by people who live and work in culturally diverse settings, and to allow for the interactive effects of noncultural influences from biological and psychological aspects of the person. Rather than attempt to define and delineate specific cultural groups, this approach suggests that the way any individual behaves is based on the array of influences, both those general to the group and those unique to her or his development. This idea is based on a conceptualization of culture as a *symbolic system that emerges through the interaction of individuals.*

Culture emergent suggests that the symbolic aspects of culture and cultural identity emerge in interaction and are displayed primarily through talk and through action. Both language and action are symbols (Holland et al., 1998; Kuper, 1999; Tedlock & Mannheim, 1995) that result from cultural learning and convey the values of the group. Talk and action are "processed through the filter of interpretation. Actions are artifacts, signs that are intended to convey meaning" (Kuper, p. 105). This symbolic language is public, thus, by extension the values of the culture are public (Kuper), and talk and action are conditioned by transient circumstances as well as by traditional patterns of behavior (Sherzer, 1987; Urban, 1991). Krefting (1991) (see Chapter 19) notes that "although culture is a shared phenomenon, sharing is seen in the context of transmission and socialization. Moreover, individuals learn culture from a number of different people and places, so each person's contact with and interpretation of the culture is unique" (p. 5).

Not only is culture uniquely expressed by the individual; its expression also changes constantly, based on new experiences and the influence of those experiences on perceptions. In these ways, "Culture is contested, temporal, and emergent" (Clifford, 1986, p. 19). Tedlock and Mannheim (1995) suggest that cultures emerge and are revised continuously in the interaction among individuals within the group through both dialog and action.

The theoretical framework of *culture emergent* takes into account the interactions of individuals and cultural development as well as the process of change in culture over time (Tedlock & Mannheim, 1995). Thus, the focus is away from cultural group–cultural mind-set and toward individuals making choices within culturally supported boundaries. The idea of culture emergent assumes that cultural patterns are dynamic and collectively negotiated by individuals through multiple interactions. The culture emergent approach views culture itself as having evolved from application of the social, problem-solving, task orientation of human beings. We assume that some cultural belief structures and behavior patterns are laid down in early childhood through learning and experience within the family and community, but we also assume that those structures and patterns are continually reevaluated. One only has to reflect on the differences between the values and behaviors demonstrated by his or her parents, perhaps on the issue of cultural diversity itself, and those represented by his or her peers and profession to see that even patterns learned very early in life are susceptible to modification over time and experience.

This approach also conceptualizes culture as a cognitive model of reality, a model that is based on the cumulative learning experiences of the individual. However, this model is not a unitary one shared by everyone in society, but a differentiated one located in individuals. And, because all individuals have had different experiences in life, personal models always vary at least slightly, even among individuals who live in similar environments and have shared many similar experiences. Inevitably, some elements of culture may be shared with one set of individuals, while other elements may be shared with other sets. Moreover, because individuals continue to have new experiences throughout life, the model reflects the fact that culture adapts and changes, sometimes dramatically though often slowly, through the actions of individuals. Culture emergent presupposes the individual—not the group—as the key cultural actor, and encourages careful examination of both the group and the individual. Within this framework, we highlight five important characteristics of culture, emphasizing the ways in which the concept of culture emergent affects traditional conceptualizations of culture.

Culture Is Learned

Most definitions suggest that culture is learned. It is transmitted from one generation to another through the process of enculturation, the acquisition of cultural knowledge that allows one to function as a member of a particular group. The learned aspect of culture sets it apart from the biological (Kuper, 1999). It is not inherited, but must be transmitted from individual to individual. Observation and discourse are the primary means of cultural transmission. One learns culture through interaction with others, listening, observing, and assessing those interactions.

Enculturation, the acquisition of culture, occurs both through purposeful instruction and through modeling and observation. One learns the culture of a profession like occupational therapy in part through direct teaching in the course of the professional education experience. Faculty teach not only the facts required to plan and provide intervention, but also the value system of the profession, through, for example, explication of the professional code of ethics, the mind-set that supports client-based care, or the importance of evidence-based practice. This initial learning may require organization around specific rules taught by others (Holland et al., 1998).

In addition to this purposefully taught information, specific individuals such as occupational therapy students acquire information from experience, interaction, and the evaluative responses of others. This kind of learning enables the learner to form a gestalt that directs action in new situations (Holland et al., 1998). Observing and modeling more experienced therapists during fieldwork and the early years of practice is a mechanism for learning about and practicing particular kinds of professional behavior. Both the intentional teaching and the less formal modeling serve to enculturate students to the professional culture.

Culture emergent suggests that because culture is learned, it must be presumed that the learning process is ongoing, and that new behaviors, beliefs, and values emerge as individuals acquire new information and experience. Further, because culture is learned, it also is shared with those from whom it is learned and those to whom it is taught. Each interaction with another individual provides an opportunity for learning culture and for reinforcing elements already acquired. This interactive sharing and mutual reinforcement has the effect of binding the individual to others and to the group. It is the mechanism by which group identities are formed.

Culture Is Localized

Culture is created and expressed through discrete interactions with specific individuals in particular locations. It is from such interactions that one draws meaningful elements that will be shared with some but not all individuals within society. Thus, culture is situated in personally meaningful locales. It is from such interactions, in the immediate surroundings, that individuals learn meaningful elements that will be shared with some, even most, of the other persons within the group. Rosaldo (1999) suggests that "all knowledge is local" (p. 31). Even in an era of mass electronic communication around the world, information is processed based on local values, mores, and norms (Abu-Lughod, 1999; Kuper, 1999).

Professional settings offer a kind of well-defined environment for the emergence of localized knowledge. For example, knowing how the occupational therapy clinic is set up, or how the supplies are classified, or how patient visits are prioritized is largely learned from experience or observation in a particular setting. The specifics of such knowledge need not be shared with others in different parts of the organization or with therapists in other clinics, although in general every occupational therapy practitioner will need to have similar information, regardless of work setting.

However, interactions in multiple social settings also provide multiple contexts for learning culture. Thus, the concept of culture emergent suggests that every individual embodies multiple cultural components, some based on ethnicity, race, or country of origin, and others based on life experience in other contexts such as professional, geographic, religious, social, or family settings. Everyone is a bundle of cultural threads, and social context influences individual choices about displaying one or another of them. In every interaction, only part of an individual's identity is being exhibited, making all understanding about that identity incomplete (cf., Holland et al., 1998).

This localization of culture is part of what makes it meaningful. Meaning is assigned to any particular cultural factor based in part on the perspective of the individual. Perspectives can be communicated and shared with others, and can be broadened through experience and training. Nevertheless, at any given moment, each individual is responding to a particular view of an interaction, a view that our model terms *vantage*. Like the position adopted by Bakhtin (1981) and drawing directly from Hill and MacLaurey (1995), this notion suggests that at another moment, a similar interaction may carry different interpretations because of a change of *vantage*. Vantage effects are clearly evident, for example, in the differing interpretations of a client's behavior from the perspective of a physician and a therapist. Similarly, asking someone "how are you" in a clinical setting carries a very different connotation than asking the same question in a social situation.

Culture Is Patterned

Patterning is essential for social behavior and for the development and maintenance of societies (Fitzgerald et al., 1997). It is essential that individuals develop patterns for behavior, because patterns help minimize ambiguity and relieve us from having to renegotiate each interaction from scratch (cf., Holland et al., 1998). Patterns emerge from the repetition of specific samples of behavior and talk. Repeated patterns establish the normal and customary expectations that structure interactions.

Culture is patterned in two senses. First, it is patterned in that the components of culture are integrated, reflecting generalizable patterns within which individual actions have meaning. Culture emergent theory suggests a second form of patterning, that is, culture is patterned in the repetitive behaviors of individuals, which become so ingrained that they seem like empirical reality. Through ritual, daily routine, and habitual behaviors, individuals express their cultural identities and affiliations, as well as their individual

preferences and characteristics (cf., Holland et al., 1998). For example, a woman dressing in India will have a different routine for donning her sari than a woman donning her pantsuit in the United States. Such routinized behaviors serve not only to structure daily life, but also to help shape an evaluative system for assessing one's own and others' behaviors. Both women must also make somewhat less routinized decisions while dressing, including determinations about the level of formality in dress that is required by a particular situation and personal preferences about style and color. These decisions reflect a degree of individual self-expression, even though the ranges in both cases are bound by culturally governed matters of availability, convention, and values. In general, we assume that the process of repetition leads to ritualization (i.e., assignment of symbolic meaning). Ritualized and routinized behavior leads to a shaping of the individual's "reality." From there it is only a short step to being the "right thing."

Culture Is Evaluative

Values are embedded in culture and are reflected in individual behavioral decisions and choices (Kuper, 1999). Values reflect the underlying organization of shared structures that facilitate social interaction. Society would not be possible without a significant level of shared values. Socialization within families and communities is one means of acquiring values. Ideally, there is considerable consensus about values within a society or a group, because commonality of evaluative perception is one of the factors that helps hold individuals together in social institutions. It is doubtful, though, that there is ever total agreement on values, even in small groups. Different cultures, different groups within a society, or different individuals within a group may agree or disagree on how to evaluate items or ideas.

Perhaps the most salient example of this difference in evaluation is one that is mentioned repeatedly in the occupational therapy literature. Occupational therapy is based on a set of values that holds independence to be an essential goal for individual well-being (Kinebanian & Stomph, 1992). However, in a number of cultures, independence is much less highly valued, with interdependence, or, in situations of illness or disability, dependence, being both expected and accepted (cf., Jang, 1995). Kinebanian and Stomph (1992) give the example of a Hindu man with hemiplegia who, although able to accomplish many tasks for himself, declined to do so, indicating that he was waiting for God to improve his physical status.

The idea of culture emergent emphasizes that individuals are shaped by their culture. However, it also emphasizes that socialization is not the same for all members of a given group. Individuals are continuously evaluating the applicability and relative weight of values in terms of personal relevance. Sometimes, contradictory values may exist, and decisions about which one to acknowledge are contingent on context. Spencer, Krefting, and Mattingly (1993) report that when one of the researchers was introduced as an occupational therapist, patients with traumatic brain injury identified their problems as double vision, instability in walking, and difficulty swallowing. When the same researcher was introduced as an anthropologist, patients identified their problems as loneliness, financial difficulties, and unhappiness about being labeled as retarded. In this case, patients' expectations about the culture of the researcher, either in terms of what they thought was expected of them or in terms of what they thought the researcher could help them with, imposed a screen in terms of what they identified as problematic. Gender, age, innate skills, and social position are among the variables affecting an individual's socialization experiences (Holland et al., 1998). These factors in turn affect the acquisition of values.

One's values, the concepts of what is desirable or abhorrent, change over the life course. Children, adolescents, young adults, middle-aged individuals, and elderly individuals may have differing value orientations as a result not only of differing needs and personal experience, but also because of what their interaction with the cultures around them has taught them. This variation is reflected in, and reflects, another important characteristic of culture emergent. While elements of culture are persistent, culture is also constantly evolving.

Culture Has Continuity With Change

Generally, culture is more or less stable through time. This consistency is an important characteristic of culture, essential if it is indeed to provide the values and beliefs that guide or pattern behavior. However, cultures are far from static (Sewell, 1999). They are constantly evolving (Sahlins & Service, 1960), and would, in fact, disappear if they did not. This is not to suggest that cultural difference is disappearing. Even in the face of global communication, differences persist, perhaps even sharpening (Clifford, 1986). This ability of cultures to incorporate new ideas, to borrow from other cultures, to assimilate new information, is a strength that enables cultures to persist.

One source of cultural change is the introduction of new technologies. As part of our research on the meaning of occupation for weavers in the highlands of Guatemala (Bonder & Martin, 2001), we found that weavers in small villages in the Guatemala highlands have begun to use the Internet to market their textiles as a way to maintain a traditional art that might otherwise disappear. By opening new markets selling on the Internet, they increased the revenue generated by this age-old activity, thereby sustaining themselves as well as the tradition.

Similarly, the cultural knowledge of an individual changes over the life course as new objects, situations, and interactions are encountered (Tedlock & Mannheim, 1995). The theory of culture emergent is particularly focused on this element of culture. Individual experiences serve to shape a unique person.

However, across a society, many individuals may experience forces for change almost simultaneously and respond in similar ways. The progress of digital technology in the United States and elsewhere offers us many examples of such forces for change and their relationships not only to life activities (e.g., job tasks) but to identity (e.g., technophobes versus technophiles) and values (e.g., role of Internet in discussions of plagiarism and reevaluations of intellectual property rights). Within larger cultural groups, smaller groups change at their own pace, often in response to trends elsewhere in the system. So, for example, demographic changes at a societal level produce organization change at an institutional level (cf., Martin & Bonder, 2003). The concept of emergence helps explain why this is so and helps manage it.

Usually, cultural groups are continuous over time. Except in cases of wholesale extermination through contact-induced disease or forcible conquest, cultural change seldom means replacement, especially for individuals. Though new cultural components are added to an individual's knowledge base, pre-existing components are not excised. For example, old ideas about technology may be supplanted. They cease to exist only when they are no longer learned by a new generation. Occupational therapists rarely work with their clients on shoeing horses or making soap or using typewriters. However, these used to be common cultural skills, and are still viable among some groups.

Culture changes in two ways. First, at the societal level, the collective patterns may change when many individuals alter their behavior over a short period of time, as a result of changes in the external context. For example, when environmental circumstances change, or when one group comes in contact with another on a widespread basis, cultural change is nearly inevitable and often invisible (Kuper, 1999). Second, the cultural knowledge of an individual continues to change over the life course as the person encounters new elements in the personal environment and incorporates them into life and interactions.

Implications for Practice

The idea of culture emergent has consequences for therapeutic intervention in occupational therapy as well as in other health-care encounters. It suggests a particular view of culture that has the potential to guide therapists' interactions.

Culture and Occupation

Culture is an important influence on occupational patterns, and occupational choices reflect cultural beliefs. A client's choice of activity level, engagement in particular occupations, and perceptions about the value of particular occupational outcomes are all influenced by his or her cultural beliefs. Kluckhohn and Strodtbeck (1961) suggest that every culture has a conception of human activity that conveys values that may be expressed through orientations on "being," "being-in-becoming," or "doing." In Western culture, the "being" orientation is somewhat devalued (Rowles, 1991) (see Chapter 26), while other cultures value that orientation more highly than the Western orientation toward "doing" (Jang, 1995). Some Far Eastern cultures emphasize harmony with nature, acceptance of fate, and personal reflection as being more central than active doing of occupations. If the therapist values the Western "doing" culture, there may be a conflict with a client who values a "being" perspective more highly.

Examples of cultural influences on occupation are ubiquitous. For instance, gender roles in some cultures are rigidly defined, such that women and men may have relatively restricted choice of productive (work) roles. In our observations in Maya communities in the highlands of Guatemala, women typically look after the home, weave using backstrap looms, and provide child care. Men work in the fields or take jobs in town. Women rarely run for public office or hold leadership positions in the church. However, individual personality and personal experience definitely influence these roles. Some women become influential in village politics through activities with women's weaving cooperatives, or through church activities linked to their husbands' roles in the church (Bonder, 2001). As educational opportunities, political activism, and social support for expanded women's roles increase, individual women will exercise new choices, and, over time, may alter the description of "typical" Maya women's work (Bonder & Martin, 2001).

Cultural constructions of occupation also influence the experience of disability. When disability interferes with accomplishment of occupations strongly linked to cultural values, life-satisfaction can be compromised. We spoke with a Maya woman who could no longer weave because of arthritis and who felt a great sense of personal loss. However, for her, modifying the activity was not acceptable because of the rigidity of her definition of its structure in her culture. The idea of sitting on a chair instead of the floor was not consistent with her view of how weaving occurred, even though in other villages nearby, weavers had all begun to sit on low stools. Alternatively, another Maya woman whose disability interfered with her weaving was able to substitute other activities that promoted a sense of self-worth for her (Bonder, 2001).

In clinical encounters, therapists must carefully explore the cultural construction of specific occupations and occupational patterns. Without such exploration, a process that characterizes the critical thinking that is vital to effective practice (Wittman & Velde, 2002), important aspects of occupation will be overlooked. In exploring culture, however, it is vital to recognize the emergent nature of culture in the individual. Knowledge of cultural facts is useful only as a means of generating preliminary hypotheses that must be tested for the specific client. It is also essential to recall that the therapist, too, has culture. The values and beliefs that accompany that culture also influence the interaction and must be given careful attention. It is not possible for the therapist to be an entirely objective observer of a situation (Bakhtin, cited in Willeman, 1994).

Framing Encounters

Sue (2000) suggests that effective intercultural clinical interaction has three primary characteristics. The first of these is *scientific-mindedness*. Sue refers here to the recognition that clinical encounters are based on forming hypotheses based on prior knowledge, with the expectation that these hypotheses must be tested in the specific encounter. Experience with individuals from a particular culture may well lead to a set of assumptions about all individuals from that culture. However, as Mattingly (1998) notes, therapists who carry those assumptions into intervention without examining their applicability to the specific client may well fail in their efforts. One must also cultivate what Sue has labeled *dynamic sizing skills*. The clinician must recognize when cultural generalizations apply to a particular situation and when individual factors predominate. In order to do so effectively, the clinician needs at least some *culture-specific expertise*, knowledge about the general characteristics of cultural groups.

Thus, therapeutic encounters become something of a dance between the individual and the cultural. The therapist must recognize the limitations of cultural generalities, but, at the same time, possess a fund of knowledge from which to begin. As an example, a therapist planning treatment for a Maya immigrant woman who has had a stroke will find it helpful to know that in Maya culture women do the cooking, and that typical meals include vegetables, beans, and tortillas. Tortillas are the staff of life for Mayans, carrying much ritual, mythological, and symbolic content. It is also helpful to know that the tortillas are made through a process involving soaking of the corn, grinding it into meal, mixing the dough, shaping it by clapping the dough between the hands, and cooking on a stone over a flame. However, if the Maya woman is a second- or third-generation resident of the United States, she may make her tortillas using purchased cornmeal, on a griddle over an electric burner, and may even shape the tortillas using a tortilla press. In fact, she might prefer to serve peanut butter and jelly sandwiches made with purchased white bread. Different movements and procedures are required for the different kinds of cooking, and treatment must be molded accordingly.

Intervention Strategies

Understanding of culture as emergent in intervention suggests three important characteristics that therapists can cultivate to enhance clinical encounters. The first of these is attending carefully to the interactional moment (Tedlock & Mannheim, 1995). Because culture emerges in interaction, each interaction is a new situation. Previous information about specific cultures, about the diagnosis of the client, and about other relevant factors must be understood in the context of the immediate situation. Therefore, attention to word choice, facial expression, body posture, voice tone, gestures, and other clues to the feelings and attitudes of the individual can be identified only through careful attention. The symbols that convey information about a culture are public and observable (Sewell, 1999), assuming one is attending carefully.

Active curiosity about the meaning of these clues is the second characteristic that therapists can bring to clinical encounters. It is impossible to know all there is to know about every labeled cultural group, Hispanics, for example, or Blacks. And as we have established, even knowing those facts would not provide adequate information in a particular encounter. Asking questions to help interpret observations can provide vital information to assist in understanding of the individual and framing of intervention.

Finally, therapists can engage in self-reflection and evaluation of interactions in order to improve subsequent encounters (Rosaldo, 1999). It is impossible always to notice the important clues, to ask the right questions, and to draw the right inferences. Nor are therapists neutral observers (Kuper, 1999). Reflection about choices made in one encounter can assist therapists to improve the next interaction. Their own culture, like that of their clients, is unavoidable (Greenfield, 2000), emergent in their clinical encounters, and, thus, subject to change. Self-reflection and evaluation can ensure that the change enhances future therapeutic interactions.

Conclusions

It is well-established that culture affects occupation and that occupational therapists must acknowledge its impact on daily life and on intervention strategies. Failure to do so can prevent establishment of rapport, decrease trust, and lead to communication difficulties, all of which can reduce effectiveness of intervention (Krefting, 1991) (see Chapter 19). However, culture is difficult to define and even more difficult to quantify. Efforts to group people on the basis of a set of cultural facts, as is done in much diversity training practice, are unlikely to be effective because these efforts fail to recognize the subtle but profound interplay of personal, experiential, and cultural factors in individual lives. Further, this approach fails to take into account the constant change that is part of individual lives.

The task of cultural understanding "involves observing what occurs between people in the intersubjective realm. These exchanges take place in the clear light of public interactions, they do not entail the mysteries of empathy or require extraordinary capacities for going inside people's heads or, worse, their souls" (Rosaldo, 1999, p. 30). Rather, the therapist, like a good ethnographer, "constructs data in a dialogue with informants, who are themselves interpreters" (Kuper, 1999, p. 214). Incorporation of the concept of culture emergent, that is, a definition of culture as a part of identity that emerges in individual interactional moments in specific locales, has the potential to enable clinicians to enhance clinical care by acknowledging the profound impact of culture, the unique nature of each individual, and the strategies that can lead to enhanced understanding and therapeutic collaboration.

References

Abu-Lughod, L. (1999). The interpretation of culture(s) after television. In S. B. Ortner (Ed.), *The fate of "culture": Geertz and beyond* (pp. 110–135). Berkeley, CA: University of California Press.

American Occupational Therapy Association. (1999). *Standards for accreditation of an occupational therapy education program*. Rockville, MD: Author.

Bakhtin, M. M. (1981). *The dialogic imagination: Four essays by M. M. Bakhtin*. In M. E. Holquist (Ed.). (C. Emerson & M. Holquist, Trans.). Austin, TX: University of Texas Press.

Baptiste, S. (1988). Murial Driver Memorial Lecture: Chronic pain, activity, and culture. *Canadian Journal of Occupational Therapy, 55*, 179–184.

Barney, K. F. (1991). From Ellis Island to assisted living: Meeting the needs of older adults from diverse cultures. *American Journal of Occupational Therapy, 45*, 586–593.

Bonder, B. R. (2001). Culture and occupation: A comparison of weaving in two traditions. *Canadian Journal of Occupational Therapy, 68*, 310–319.

Bonder, B. R., & Martin, L. (2001, November). *The meaning of weaving for Maya women in the Guatemala Highlands*. Paper presented at the Midwest Association for Latin American Studies, Cleveland, OH.

Bonder, B. R., Martin, L., & Miracle, A. W. (2002). *Culture in clinical care*. Thorofare, NJ: Slack.

Cerulo, K. A. (Ed.). (2001). *Culture in mind: Toward a sociology of culture*. New York: Routledge.

Christiansen, C., & Baum, C. (1997). Person–environment occupational performance: A conceptual model for practice. In C. Christiansen & C. Baum (Eds.), *Occupational therapy: Enabling function and well-being* (2nd ed., pp. 47–70). Thorofare, NJ: Slack.

Clifford, J. (1986). Introduction. In J. Clifford & G. E. Marcus (Eds.), *Writing culture: The poetics and politics of ethnography* (pp. 1–21). Berkeley, CA: University of California Press.

Cross-Cultural Health Care Program. (1996). CCHCP Library. Retrieved June 5, 2002, from http://www.xculture.org/resources/library/index.cfm

D'Andrade, R. (1999). Comment. *Current Anthropology, 40*(Suppl.), S16–S17.

Dillard, M., Andonian, L., Flores, O., Lai, L., MacRae, A., & Shakir, M. (1992). Culturally competent occupational therapy in a diversely populated mental health setting. *American Journal of Occupational Therapy, 46*, 721–726.

Dressler, W. W., & Bindon, J. R. (2000). The health consequences of cultural consonance. *American Anthropologist, 102*, 244–260.

Dunton, W. R. (1918). *Occupational therapy: A manual for nurses*. Philadelphia: Saunders.

Dyck, I., & Forwell, S. (1997). Occupational therapy student's first year fieldwork experience: Discovering the complexity of culture. *Canadian Journal of Occupational Therapy, 64*, 185–196.

Eliot, T. S. (1948). *Notes toward the definition of culture*. London: Faber & Faber.

Fitzgerald, M. H., Mullavey-O'Byrne, C., & Clemson, L. (1997). Cultural issues from practice. *Australian Occupational Therapy Journal, 44*, 1–21.

Galanti, G. (1997). *Caring for patients from different cultures* (2nd ed.). Philadelphia: University of Pennsylvania Press.

Geertz, C. (1973). *The interpretation of cultures*. New York: Basic Books.

Greenfield, P. M. (2000). What psychology can do for anthropology, or why anthropology took postmodernism on the chin. *American Anthropologist, 102*, 564–576.

Handwerker, W. P. (2002). The construct validity of cultures: Cultural diversity, culture theory, and a method for ethnography. *American Anthropologist, 104*, 106–122.

Hendrickson, C. (1995). *Weaving identities: Construction of dress and self in a Highland Guatemala town.* Austin, TX: University of Texas Press.

Hendrickson, C. (1996). Women, weaving, and education in Maya revitalization. In E. F. Fischer & R. M. Brown (Eds.), *Maya cultural activism in Guatemala* (pp. 156–164). Austin, TX: University of Texas Press.

Hermans, H. J. M., & Kempen, H. J. G. (1998). Moving cultures: The perilous problems of cultural dichotomies in a globalizing society. *American Psychologist, 53*, 1111–1120.

Hill, J. H., & MacLaurey, R. E. (1995). The terror of Montezuma: Aztec history, vantage theory, and the category of "person." In J. R. Taylor & R. MacLaurey (Eds.), *Language and the cognitive construal of the world. Trends in linguistics, studies, and monographs, 82* (pp. 277–329). Berlin, Germany: Mouton de Gruyter.

Holland, D., Lachicotte, W., Skinner, D., & Cain, C. (1998). *Identity and agency in cultural worlds.* Cambridge, MA: Harvard University Press.

Jang, Y. (1995). Chinese culture and occupational therapy. *British Journal of Occupational Therapy, 58*, 103–106.

Kinebanian, A., & Stomph, M. (1992). Cross-cultural occupational therapy: A critical reflection. *American Journal of Occupational Therapy, 46*, 751–757.

Kluckhohn, F. R., & Strodtbeck, F. L. (1961). *Variations in value orientations.* Evanston, IL: Row, Peterson, & Co.

Krefting, L. H. (1991). The culture concept in the everyday practice of occupational and physical therapy. *Occupational and Physical Therapy in Pediatrics, 11*(4), 1–16. Reprinted as Chapter 19.

Krefting, L. H., & Krefting, D. V. (1991). Cultural influences on performance. In C. Christiansen & C. Baum (Eds.), *Occupational therapy: Overcoming human performance deficits* (pp. 102–122). Thorofare, NJ: Slack.

Kuper, A. (1999). *Culture: The anthropologists' account.* Cambridge, MA: Harvard University Press.

Levine, R. E. (1987). Culture: A factor influencing the outcomes of occupational therapy. *Occupational Therapy in Health Care, 4*, 3–15. Reprinted as Chapter 18.

Martin, L., & Bonder, B. (2003). Achieving organizational change within the context of cultural competence. *Journal of Social Work in Long Term Care, 2*(1/2), 81–94.

Mattingly, C. (1998). *Healing dramas and clinical plots: The narrative structure of experience.* Cambridge, MA: Cambridge University Press.

Mirkopoulos, C., & Evert, M. M. (1994). Nationally speaking: Cultural connections: A challenge unmet. *American Journal of Occupational Therapy, 48*, 583–585.

Pepitone, A. (2000). A social psychology perspective on the study of culture: An eye on the road to interdisciplinarianism. *Cross-Cultural Research, 34*, 233–249.

Pope-Davis, D. B., Prieto, L. R., Whitaker, C. M., & Pope-Davis, S. A. (1993). Exploring multicultural competencies of occupational therapists: Implications for education and training. *American Journal of Occupational Therapy, 47*, 838–844.

Reyna, S. (2002). *Connections: Mind, brain and culture in social anthropology.* New York: Routledge.

Rosaldo, R. I. (1999). A note on the cultural essayist. In S. B. Ortner (Ed.), *The fate of "culture": Geertz and beyond* (pp. 30–34). Berkeley, CA: University of California Press.

Rowles, G. D. (1991). Beyond performance: Being in place as a component of occupational therapy. *American Journal of Occupational Therapy, 45*, 265–271. Reprinted as Chapter 26.

Sapir, E. (1924/1949). Culture, genuine and spurious. In D. Mandelbaum (Ed.), *Selected writings of Edward Sapir.* Berkeley, CA: University of California Press.

Sahlins, M., & Service, E. R. (Eds.). (1960). *Evolution and culture.* Ann Arbor, MI: University of Michigan Press.

Schneider, D. M. (1976). Notes toward a theory of culture. In K. Basso & H. Selby (Eds.), *Meaning in anthropology.* Albuquerque, NM: University of New Mexico Press.

Segall, M. H., Lonner, W. J., & Berry, J. W. (1998). Cross-cultural psychology as a scholarly discipline: On the flowering of culture in behavioral research. *American Psychologist, 53*, 1101–1110.

Sewell, W. H. (1999). Geertz, cultural systems, and history: From synchrony to transformation. In S. B. Ortner (Ed.), *The fate of "culture": Geertz and beyond* (pp. 35–55). Berkeley, CA: University of California Press.

Sherzer, J. A. (1987). Discourse-centered approach to language and culture. *American Anthropologist, 89*, 295–309.

Skinner, D. (1989). The socialization of gender identity: Observations from Nepal. In J. Valsiner (Ed.), *Child development in cultural context* (pp. 181–192). Toronto, Ontario, Canada: Hogrefe & Huber.

Spencer, J., Krefting, L., & Mattingly, C. (1993). Incorporation of ethnographic methods in occupational therapy assessment. *American Journal of Occupational Therapy, 47*, 303–309.

Sue, S. (2000, June). The provision of effective mental health treatment by service providers. National Institutes of Health Conference "Toward Higher Levels of Analysis: Progress and Promise in Research on Social and Cultural Dimensions of Health." Bethesda, MD.

Tedlock, D., & Mannheim, B. (1995). Introduction. In D. Tedlock & B. Mannheim (Eds.), *The dialogic emergence of culture* (pp. 1–32). Urbana, IL: University of Illinois Press.

Tylor, E. B. (1871). *Primitive society.* London: J. Murray.

Urban, G. A. (1991). *Discourse-centered approach to culture: Native South American myths and rituals.* Austin, TX: University of Texas Press.

Wallace, A. F. C. (1961). *Culture and personality.* New York: Random House.

Wells, S. A., & Black, R. M. (2000). *Cultural competency for health professionals.* Bethesda, MD: American Occupational Therapy Association.

Willeman, P. (1994). *Looks and frictions: Essays in cultural studies and film theory.* Bloomington, IN: University of Indiana Press.

Wittman, P., & Velde, B. P. (2002). The issue is: Attaining cultural competence, critical thinking, and intellectual development: A challenge for occupational therapists. *American Journal of Occupational Therapy, 56*, 454–456.

Temporal Adaptation: A Conceptual Framework for Occupational Therapy

CHAPTER 21

GARY KIELHOFNER, DRPH, OTR, FAOTA

In 1922, Adolf Meyer proposed a philosophy of practice for the newly formed profession of occupational therapy (see Chapter 2). He maintained that the key to successful application of occupational therapy would lie in an awakening to: "... a full meaning of time as the biggest wonder and asset of our lives and the valuation of opportunity and performance as the greatest measure of time...." (1)

Eleanor Clarke Slagle pioneered the application of Meyer's proposal that occupational therapy should view patients within the context of time through the unfolding of their daily lives. She implemented a program of "habit training" based on the principle that the normal use of time in a purposeful daily routine would exert an organizing force on even the most regressed, unmedicated mentally ill patients (2). Slagle intuitively recognized habit as a critical regulator of man's use of time and consequently as a significant component of his adaptation.

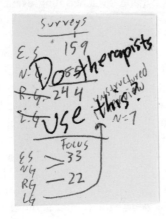

From Meyer and Slagle the profession received the proposition that in the richness of man's daily routines and his purposeful use of time, there was both health-maintaining and health-regenerating potential. Further, the way in which disabled individuals used and organized their time in daily life was revealed as a measure of their adaptiveness. Health was revealed in how patients functioned on a day-by-day, hour-by-hour basis. The temporal dimension in human adaptation was installed as a legitimate concern for occupational therapists. This temporal perspective gave to occupational therapy a special caretaker position for patients' activities of daily living.

However, occupational therapy practice has subsequently evolved away from a concern for patients' temporal functioning (3). The full appreciation of the meaning of time, which Meyer so strongly advocated, never came to pass in occupational therapy. Consequently, the broad humanistic theme of activities of daily living suffered a substantial loss of content. Presently, the concept of activities of daily living conveys little more than a checklist for self-care (4).

At a time when occupational therapy must face the reality of its "derailment," as Shannon suggests in his paper, it is imperative that the profession scrutinize its underpinnings and carefully examine its philosophy and practice for critical concepts that have been lost. The task that lies before the profession is to reclaim and revitalize those elements which made occupational therapy such a viable and energizing idea for the founders and early leaders of the profession.

The theme of temporal adaptation is a valuable scheme for practice and should be reintroduced to occupational therapy. Therefore, this paper first provides support for temporal functioning as a useful conceptual base from which human adaptation and dysfunction of the disabled can be better understood. Second, it proposes a temporal conceptual framework that serves as a background from which to generate evaluations and interventions.

The Temporal Dimension in Adaptation

The elderly person whose abundant leisure has become painful monotony, the physically disabled person whose self-care has been expanded into a long and tedious procedure, the psychiatric patient whose personal helplessness makes the future an unwelcome burden, and the mentally subnormal person for whom the string of events in time seems a jumble ... each represent a special difficulty in temporal adaptation. Although occupational therapists are thoroughly acquainted with such temporal problems, the systematic application of clinical intervention aimed at temporal dysfunction is not formally or consistently part of the clinician's treatment. In order to reintroduce temporal adaptation to clinical practice, this section provides a general, theoretical overview. *Temporal adaptation* serves in this paper as a descriptive term for integration of an entire spectrum of activities, the organization of which supports health on an ongoing daily life basis. *Temporal dysfunction* will refer to problems that arise in this daily life organization. Temporal adaptation and dysfunction represent descriptive terms for talking about complex daily activity from the specific but universal dimension of time.

Time is the inescapable boundary for human existence and activity. Hall describes it as the "unconscious determinant or frame upon which everything else is built," (5) and Henry states that for man time is a universal dimension, guiding and structuring his experience and his activity (6). Human adaptation is inextricably bound up in the conscious experience of time. Man's conscious placement in time is a function of the capacity to symbolize internally that which is perceived externally (7). Each man bears a complex symbolic model or image of himself located in time (8). His initial awareness of time results from the experience of change in the self and the environment (9). The model or image of external temporal reality is generated and continuously reorganized through the accumulated experience of changing events.

Armed with temporal consciousness, man is a supreme actor in time. Not only is he aware of changing events, but he is likewise conscious of the fact that he can have some effect on that course of events. The perception of the self as a cause comes from experiencing the results of one's own actions in time (10). Man's awareness of time, the awareness of his causative ability, and its potential for consequences are interrelated phenomena. The human condition is transformed by the awareness of the individual that he or she has acted, is acting, and will continue to act. Man's awareness of time makes possible this continuity of experience that transforms the nature of his adaptation. In John Dewey's words:

> Man differs from the lower animals because he preserves his past experiences . . . . With the animals, an experience perishes as it happens and each new doing or suffering stands alone. But man lives in a world where each occurrence is charged with echoes and reminiscences of what has gone before, where each event is a reminder of other things. Hence he lives not, like the beasts of the field, in a world of merely physical things, but in a world of signs and symbols. (11)

Although overt experiences occur as disconnected and episodic events, the inner symbolic experience is an uninterrupted flow in which past and future are orienting reference points for human adaptation. Man draws upon his past experiences as an information source for future action. He projects himself into the future, planning events, and setting goals that may not be realized for days, months, or even years. Through imagination, he can test alternative courses of action and contemplate their consequences (7). Once placed consciously in time, the human organism adapts through purposeful action. Man adapts through awareness of his own agenthood and placement in time that makes possible the conscious planning of action. Action and time are concomitant components of the human experience linked to purpose through hindsight and foresight.

The Conceptual Framework

The concepts of temporal adaptation can be put into operation through a conceptual framework designed to generate strategies of evaluation and treatment in occupational therapy. A preliminary framework was constructed as a series of propositions about temporal adaptation. The first four concern external factors and learning that influence temporal experience and activity. Propositions five and six concern the internal organization of temporal behavior. The seventh proposition concerns pathologies or dysfunctions of time.

Proposition 1: Each person bears a temporal frame of reference that is culturally constituted. Individuals carry an image of their placement in time that is a unique product of their culture (12). Their temporal frame of reference is maintained and transmitted within the culture in the form of norms and values and contains the basic notion and valuation of time (13).

In American society the notion of time is that of a straight line or path extending into the future. Time is experienced as a "supersensible medium or container, as a stream of infinitely extended warp upon which the woof of human happenings is woven …." (14) It is sectioned off and takes on the nature of enclosed or finite space, the segments of which are to be filled with activity (12, 13). This notion of time is exhibited in the American habit of scheduling events. Random behavior that lacks a pattern of organization is not functional in the mainstream of American society (6). The American culture values time as a commodity; it can be bought, sold, saved, or wasted (13). This sense of time is captured in the phrase *time is money* and, understandably, wasting time has a strong negative connotation in the culture.

Although the orderly, punctual life of Americans is not an innate feature of human existence, it is largely considered a fact of nature. This notion and valuation of time is the framework of the culture that sets boundaries for competent action in daily life. In order to adapt to the society the individual must to some degree internalize and order behavior according to the culture's temporal frame of reference.

Proposition 2: A unique temporal frame of reference is accumulated through learning and socializing experiences that begin in childhood. Although the basic ability to perceive time is a cognitive developmental phenomenon, the particular culture frame of reference is a product of socialization (6). The transmission of the temporal frame of reference has been classified by Hall into three levels of socialization or learning: technical, informal, and formal (13).

The technical learning of time occurs in a didactic framework, as when a child is taught to tell time and to comprehend the division of seconds, minutes, and hours. Informal time is learned through imitation of role models and the learning comprises activities and mannerisms that are so much a part of daily life that they are performed almost unconsciously. An example of informal time is knowing that being 5 minutes late for an appointment is acceptable, whereas 20 minutes is not. Formal learning is taught by precept and admonition, and concerns traditions and values transmitted through the expectations and prohibitions of each culture. As an example, the prohibition of wasting time is passed on in American culture as an important value.

From this teaching, modeling, precept, and admonition, children's socialization is accomplished through the internalization of a complex temporal frame of reference. It is within the family that children first learn to organize time under this framework toward fulfillment of a social role. The role of children or siblings within the family bears with it a whole set of activities ordered in time. Learning to be on time for meals, to do chores when assigned, to habitually care for themselves, and to periodically clean their rooms are all part of the complex schema children must incorporate. Learning temporal organization, which occurs within the family, generalizes to other roles children must take on later. Children not only know a particular set of behaviors ordered in time, but more importantly, also learn to organize activity in time.

In addition to learning how and when to behave, children learn a complex set of temporal expectations; Toffler gives the following poignant description.

From infancy on the child learns, for example, that when Daddy:

> … leaves for work in the morning, it means that he will not return for many hours…. The child soon learns that "mealtime" is neither a one-minute nor a five-hour affair, but that it ordinarily lasts from fifteen minutes to an hour. He learns that going to a movie lasts two to four hours, but that a visit with the pediatrician seldom lasts more than one. He learns that the school day ordinarily lasts six hours. He learns that a relationship with a teacher ordinarily extends over a school year, but that his relationship with his grandparents is supposed to be of much longer duration. Indeed some relationships are supposed to last a lifetime. (15)

Where the household temporal patterns are chaotic, children's learning of the temporal frame of reference may be maladaptive (6). Consequently, competent participation in the culture may be hindered as they falter in organizing tune to respond to other successive social institutions, such as school and the job setting.

Proposition 3: There is a natural temporal order to daily living organized around the life–space activities of self-maintenance, work, and play. Adolph Meyer pointed out that there is a natural rhythm in the organization of daily life around life spaces (1) (see Chapter 2). These life spaces are assigned to activities that represent a social order, determining appropriate times for role behavior. Reilly conceptualized daily living as divided into life spaces of existence, subsistence, and discretionary time (16). Existence is that time spent for eating, sleeping, personal hygiene, and other aspects of self-maintenance; subsistence is the life space devoted to working for an income; and discretionary time is that life space reserved for recreation and leisure. Recreation and leisure comprise dual aspects of play in adult life. Recreation is the period of time when man is made ready for the next cycle of work through relaxation. Leisure is earned time made possible by the satisfying performance of work.

Health consists of the proper balance of the life spaces that is both satisfying to individuals and appropriate for their roles within society. Balance refers to more than just so much work, play, and rest. Rather, balance recognizes an interdependence of these life spaces and their relationship to both internal values, interests, and goals, and external demands of the environment. It is the interrelated balance of self-maintenance, work, and play that comprises health.

While homeostasis is used to describe the biological health of the organism, a broader concept of balance in daily life describes the conditions for psychosocial health of the human organism. Occupational therapists are in a position to make critical statements about the health of their patients from both interrelated dimensions of homeostasis and balance. Far from being limited to the idea of self-care, activities of daily living refer to man's total state of health, which depends on both biological and psychosocial factors.

Proposition 4: Society requires its members to organize their use of time according to ascribed social roles. While cultural norms and values provide a contextual framework for man's use of time, his individual daily pattern must be organized around his occupational roles (17). Heard expands on this theme of role behavior in her paper. The sum total of man's activity within his life spaces has been referred to as occupational behavior (18). Life spaces are filled according to the occupational roles to which they are assigned. Within the daily routine, an individual's life spaces may be divided among several occupational roles such as the father, worker, and community volunteer. Adaptation requires individuals to use their time in a manner that supports their roles. The student must organize time for attendance at classes and homework, the worker for the job schedule, and the retiree for effective and satisfying use of leisure time.

The organization of time around one's roles is not a static skill. Occupational roles change and overlap; each individual passes through a succession of roles in a lifetime (19). Taking on a new role requires a new strategy for organizing one's time. When role change is abruptly forced upon an individual through an incurred disability, developing new temporal skills is a critical factor in adapting to the disability.

Proposition 5: An individual's use of time is a function of internalized values, interests, and goals. Values are commitments to action that organize an individual's use of time by establishing an internal order of what comes first and how much time will be allotted to various activities (20). An individual's values set priorities of actions, and their consequences create a personal valence that is ultimately translated into a lifestyle. Values serve an important function in the choice an individual makes to take on various roles. Although values reflect more serious commitments, interests also guide the commitment process. They are states of readiness for choices and action (21). Interests sustain action and serve thereby to maintain commitments over time. Like values, interests prioritize activities and lend organization to temporal behavior.

Goals represent strategies toward the fulfillment of values and interests. Values and interests yield automatic goal-setting and consequent adjustment and organization of daily patterns of time use. This process occurs at various levels of awareness and is necessary for ordering daily life. The individual who has no goals or has difficulty setting goals cannot organize daily life to use existing skills effectively and will, consequently, feel frustrated or helpless (22, 23). Further, an individual must be able to identify and execute appropriate actions for goal-attainment. Problems arise when an individual cannot identify and carry out in proper sequence those activities that lead to successful goal achievement (23, 24). Robinson expands this notion, sequencing action in time, in her paper on rules.

Proposition 6: Habits are the basic structures by which daily behavior is ordered in time and psychosocial health is maintained. While habits are traditionally thought of in terms of vices and virtues, they extend a more subtle and profound influence on daily temporal functioning. All that is familiar, routine, and predictable in daily life bears a relationship to habit. Without habit structure, an individual's daily life would be a chaotic series of disjointed events.

Habits are instantaneous, automatic choices of action made throughout the day (3). Although organized into unconscious routines, they are the products of once conscious choices made until they become automatic (3). Habits reflect actions related to values and interests cemented over time in daily patterns. Further, habits provide a crucial service to adaptation by organizing temporal behavior to meet societal requirements for competence. Consequently, habits perform an important role in assuring that skills are used in an adaptive manner. Skills must not only be present, but also organized into a daily routine.

Proposition 7: Temporal dysfunction may exist in relationship to categories of pathology. Temporal dysfunction may occur as an integral part of some mental illness or as a consequence of imposed physical disability.

When viewing individuals from the perspective of temporal adaptation, it becomes obvious that strategies for intervention cannot begin and end with the physical, mental, or emotional pathology. Each may be integrally related to a broader and often more difficult set of problems in the person's temporal adaptation.

Persons who are so disoriented in time that they cannot give the day, month, or year are readily suspected of being afflicted with dementia, senility, or some psychotic disorder (12). Actual distortions of the perception of time have been shown to occur in some cases of mental illness (9). Further, when individuals cannot organize their time toward fulfillment of their social roles, they may become candidates for psychiatric care (24). Disorganization of time is associated with the subjective sense of helplessness and incompetence seen in mental illness.

Disorganization of temporal adaptation may also be identified in the reaction of an individual to residual physical disabilities. Maintaining a pace of life comparable to individuals without disability may be impossible for some persons whose motor performance is dysfunctional. The impact of sudden disability often imposes tremendous distortions of daily life spaces by increasing the amount of time required for routine activities. Further, where one or more roles change or end as a result of acquired physical disability, the individual may be unable to find new meaningful activities and roles to fill the life–spaces formerly occupied by old ones.

Implementation

Propositions were formulated as a guiding framework for incorporating temporal adaptation into clinical evaluation and treatment. The clinician may use the framework for integrating clinical data with points raised in the propositions. The framework gives the clinician another dimension for viewing patient problems and for generating and interpreting data. It thereby serves as a basis for developing new treatment strategies. Three principles should be adhered to in applying the conceptual framework to evaluation. First, data should be collected on several variables contained in the propositions. Relevant data include the patient's values, interests, goals, balance of play and work, habit structure, and temporal frame of reference. Second, the evaluation should take into consideration internal constraints on time as revealed in the nature of the patient's physical, mental, or emotional disability. Third, the evaluation should also consider the external factors influencing time use: the patient's roles, family expectations, cultural background, and the demands of time and physical space that affect the patient's daily living.

Treatment intervention will be based on the particular pattern of temporal dysfunction revealed by the evaluation. As data is interrelated and considered in light of the conceptual framework, dysfunctional patterns should become evident. For example, one patient's chaotic day may be a reflection of a lack of ability to prioritize interests and to set goals. Without the ability to set priorities and goals, the patient cannot generate habits for a normal, satisfactory daily routine. By using the conceptual framework of temporal adaptation, the clinician should be able to formulate a more comprehensive treatment plan.

Case Examples

Two case histories, together with examples of clinical interventions that follow the principles above, are presented to serve as examples of how the temporal adaptation framework can be applied. Treatments described speak only to the temporal framework and assume the inclusion of other traditional occupational therapy interventions.

Case H.B.

H.B. is a 24-year-old, single male psychiatric patient. When admitted to the hospital, his presenting problems included depression and chronic repeated failures in work settings. H.B. graduated from college with a degree in music with plans to re-enter college for graduate study in musicology. He not only has definite skills as a musician but has also demonstrated a strong commitment by voluntarily organizing a teenage choir in a local church.

However, H.B. has not managed during the last 3 years to hold down a steady job and save enough money to re enter college. His recent occupational history includes such jobs as working in an electrical shop repairing fans, driving a school bus, and doing maintenance work in apartment complexes. H.B. was fired from each of these jobs because of his inability to concentrate on the work. He found the jobs uninteresting and had difficulty applying himself. He attempted to save money toward college, but used up his savings during periods of unemployment between jobs.

H.B. describes his daily life as highly variable and without routine. He has been unable to maintain any schedule and often finds himself late for work and appointments. Further, social activities have taken up a large part of his schedule so that he is negligent in doing many basic self-maintenance tasks. His housekeeping recently became so disorganized that he was evicted from his apartment. H.B. perceives his daily life as chaotic and complains that "there is so little time with so much to do, that I often get stuck on things and never get around to what I set out to do." He feels helpless and depressed because he is not close to his goal of re-entering college and does not feel he is progressing toward it. At this point

his response to this subjective state is to become inactive. He is without a job and recently does not even pursue his interests in music on a leisure basis.

When considered in light of the conceptual framework, H.B.'s temporal dysfunction can be outlined as follows. H.B. has internalized values and goals. He considers further education important and realistically has chosen an area of study within his capacities. His temporal dysfunction lies in the areas of: (a) identifying and pursuing reasonable short-term objectives that will bring him closer to his overall goal; (b) maintaining a satisfying daily schedule that would balance activities of work, play, and self-maintenance; and (c) organizing his time around present necessary role of being a worker. The temporal dysfunction that has eroded his competence in several areas augments his feelings of depression and helplessness.

Recommendations for treatment should include: 1. assisting H.B. in identifying how his present worker role will lead to the eventual goal of re–entering college and developing a strategy that balances his interest in music with the necessity of working on a daily basis; 2. practice in formulating a basic, balanced daily routine and adhering to it consistently; and 3. making beginning steps toward his overall goal, by gathering information on graduate programs in music, their requirements, and possible scholarships. By subdividing each of these goals into subroutines such as finding a new job or ways of pursuing his interest in music on a leisure basis, he may be able to overcome the vicious cycle of daily life incompetence, helplessness, and depression. Treatment would occur in graded steps toward the eventual reconstruction of daily living skills.

Case T.J.

T.J. is a 17-year-old male who sustained a spinal cord injury in an automobile accident. Five months after the injury, T.J., a paraplegic, remains depressed and withdrawn. When approached about his depressed state, T.J. responds that his life plans have been destroyed. Prior to his injury he was an excellent athlete with a promise of an athletic scholarship to a university.

Beyond his college training, T.J. had hoped to become a high school coach. Further, T.J. points out that he is now forced to spend days in bed or a wheelchair, whereas formerly he was active in a variety of intramural and varsity sports. He describes the present as boring and sees little prospect for change in the future. Also, data from his family points out that T.J.'s former positive self-image revolved around his physical appearance and athletic prowess; he now views himself as an invalid.

In T.J.'s case it should be noted that: (a) his former values and interests focused on activities he can no longer engage in or he must learn to participate in with some modifications; (b) his self-image and prospects for the future revolved around skills and capacities no longer intact; (c) his former daily routine revolved around his athletic role. In summary, those values and habits that formerly maintained a satisfying daily routine and those skills and goals which made the future desirable are no longer intact.

T.J.'s treatment under the framework of temporal adaptation would focus on the following sequence of treatment strategies: 1. reconstruction of the self-image through successful experiences in areas related to his past interests; 2. exploration of new activities to develop interests (in the clinic and his own community); 3. reconstruction of his daily routine, which will have to accommodate different life spaces—such as the expanded space necessary for self-care and personal hygiene; and 4. refocusing on his career goals so that a viable and acceptable objective could at least be tentatively pursued.

Conclusion

Temporal adaptation was identified as an early theme in occupational therapy that has been dropped out of clinical practice. The concept of temporal adaptation was reintroduced and formulated in a preliminary framework for clinical intervention. Temporal adaptation serves as a conceptual schema to broaden the clinician's current perspective and repertoire of skills and, as such, does not replace traditional therapeutic efforts but expands them into a more comprehensive framework. Temporal adaptation is a rich conceptual schema for occupational therapy because it speaks to a class of dysfunction found in the entire range of patients seen by occupational therapists.

Acknowledgment

This article is based in part upon material submitted in partial fulfillment of the requirements for the Master of Arts Degree, University of Southern California, Los Angeles. Partial financial support for this study was provided by the Division of Allied Health Manpower, Department of Health, Education and Welfare.

References

1. Meyer A: The philosophy of occupational therapy. *Arch Occup Ther 1*:1–10, 1922, p 9 Reprinted as Chapter 2.
2. Slagle EC: Training aides for mental patients. *Arch Occup Ther 1*:11–16, 1922.
3. Kielhofner GW: The evolution of knowledge in occupational therapy — understanding adaptation of the chronically disabled. Master's Thesis. Department of Occupational Therapy, University of Southern California, Los Angeles, 1973.
4. Reilly M: The modernization of occupational therapy. *Am J Occup Ther 25*:243–247, 1971.
5. Hall ET: The paradox of culture. In *In the Name of Life*, Bernard Landis and Edward S. Tauber, Editors, New York: Holt, Rinehart, and Winston, 1971, p 226.
6. Henry J: *Pathways to Madness*, New York: Vintage Books, Random House, 1971.
7. White R: Strategies of adaptation: an attempt at systematic description. In *Coping and Adaptation*, George Coelho, David Hamburg, and John E. Adams, Editors. New York: Basic Books, 1974.
8. Boulding K: *The Image*, Ann Arbor: University of Michigan Press, 1961.
9. Larrington G: An exploratory study of the temporal aspects of adaptive functioning. Master's Thesis. Department of Occupational Therapy, University of Southern California, Los Angeles, California, 1970.
10. DeCharms R.: *Personal Causation*, New York: Academic Press, 1968.
11. Dewey J: *Reconstruction in Philosophy*, New York: H. Holt and Company, 1920, p 36.
12. Hallowell I: *Culture and Experience*, New York: Schocken Books, 1955, p 217.
13. Hall ET: *The Silent Language*, Greenwich: Fawcett Publications, Inc., 1959.
14. Parkhurst HH: The cult of chronology. In *Essays in Honor of John Dewey*, New York: H. Holt and Company, 1929, p 23.
15. Toffler A: *Future Shock*, New York: Random House, 1970, p 360.
16. Reilly M: A psychiatric occupational therapy program as a teaching model. *Am J Occup Ther, 20*:2–10, 1966.
17. Newcomb T: *Social Psychology*, New York: Henry Holt and Company, 1959.
18. Matsutsuyu J: Occupational behavior a perspective on work and play. *Am J Occup Ther 25*:291–293,1971.
19. Arensenian J: Life cycle factors in mental illness. *Ment Hyg 52*:19–30, 1968.
20. Kluckhohn C: Values and value orientations in the theory of action: an exploration in definition and classification: In *Toward a General Theory of Action*, T. Parsons and E. Shils, Editors. Cambridge: Harvard University Press, 1951.
21. Matsutsuyu J: The interest checklist. *Am J Occup Ther 23*: 323–326, 1969.
22. Lakein A: *How to Get Control of Your Time and Your Life*, New York: The Signet, The New American Library, Inc., 1974.
23. Kiev A: *A Strategy of Daily Living*, New York: The Free Press, 1973.
24. Black MM: The evolution of social roles—a perspective on fantasy. Master's Thesis. Department of Occupational Therapy, University of Southern California, Los Angeles, 1973.

Time Use, Tempo, and Temporality: Occupational Therapy's Core Business or Someone Else's Business

2003 Sylvia Docker Lecture

LOUISE FARNWORTH,
BAPPSC, DIPCRIM, MA, PHD

I am deeply humbled and honored to present the 19th Sylvia Docker lecture. That I am here today has less to do with me than the fact that for many years now, I have been inspired by exceptional practitioners and the wisdom of a community of occupational therapy scholars, local, national, and international. These people strive selflessly in their pursuit of excellence and maintain exemplary professional standards. To these people I give thanks and dedicate this lecture.

My interest in time use began during my work in the prison environment in the late 1970s, a place where doing time was a fact of life. Nearly every day one of the inmates mutilated himself. The environment created occupational risk factors that would now be named occupational deprivation, occupational imbalance, and occupational alienation (Wilcock, 1998). The prison was a rich learning environment, although at many times, it was a disturbing one.

Throughout the 1980s, Linda King, a former lecturer at the Lincoln Institute, introduced me to concepts of the relationship among time, action, and health. She had a reputation for providing many pages of lecture notes to students. She did this because she believed that occupational therapists required great knowledge and skill to be able to exploit the characteristics of occupation to achieve health in the therapeutic environment. My belief is that we still have much to exploit. I argue here that it is the lack of attention to foundation knowledge on which rests the profession's core of knowledge that has made, and continues to make, occupational therapy vulnerable.

Knowledge is a fundamental element in the definition and operation of a profession (Higgs & Titchen, 1995). Wood (1996) contends that occupational therapy must assert itself as the rightful authority to be the sole keepers of its own practice and knowledge. This paper today, "Time use, tempo, and temporality," will be used as one illustration of knowledge that to date has not been rightfully asserted as occupational therapy's, even though it was central to our philosophical heritage at the profession's inception.

Wood (1996) argued that a strong, autonomous profession that distinguishes occupational therapists from other professionals, and enables occupational therapy practices to be translated into the future, should require graduates to leave educational environments with a complexity of knowledge. Wood suggested that knowing how, the knowledge that evolves through experience, does not require the knower be able to articulate, or possess, underlying theorems. In other words, you may know how, but not why or what if. This knowledge precedes the theory, that is, the ideas that have been the foundation for models of practice such as Sensory Integration (Ayres, 1979) and the Model of Human Occupation (Kielhofner, 1985, 1995, 2002). The danger is, that while knowing how is essential to practice, unless practitioners consciously understand what they know and, as a result, can explain, communicate, and investigate such knowledge, the knowing that, we will fail to achieve strong, autonomous, professional status. However, as suggested by Polanyi (as cited in Rogers, 1983), "... all knowledge is uncertain, involves risk, and is grasped and comprehended only through the deep, personal commitment of a disciplined search" (Rogers, 1983, p. 278). The topic of my paper does indeed require such professional and personal commitment. Would you expect anything less of someone who calls themself a professional?

Let me take you on a brief time trip through occupational therapy. Adolph Meyer (1922/1977) in his 1922 address to Occupational Therapists espoused the temporal dimension in human adaptation to disability as a legitimate concern for occupational therapy (see Chapter 2). He suggested that, "a full meaning of time ... and the valuation of opportunity and performance as the greatest measure of time, should be central to a philosophy of occupational therapy" (p. 642). He advocated not only that purposeful use of time had the potential to be both health maintaining and health regenerating, but also that the way in which individuals with a disablity used and organized their time in daily life was a measure of their adaptiveness. Such principles were applied in the newly developed occupational therapy in USA (Slagle, 1922), Scandinavia (Jonsson, 1998), and England (Wilcock, 1999) through the 1920s through to the beginning of World War II.

In relation to Australia, Sylvia Docker traveled to England in 1934 to learn how to become an occupational therapist (Anderson & Bell, 1988). She brought knowledge of occupational therapy to establish a fledgling profession in Australia. Although the profession was by that time well established in many countries, the knowledge base supporting this profession was still largely a mystery. Philosophical principles such as that espoused by Meyer were not subjected to further investigation in occupational therapy research, and practices using these principles declined. In Australia, as in other countries, research focused on demonstrating the effectiveness of specific techniques based on the exciting new developments in medical sciences, to gain professional recognition. Shortages of equipment, facilities, and personnel were of more immediate concern (Docker, 1959). What little has changed! Even in her 1975 Sylvia Docker lecture, Janet Sloan (1976) suggested that "there was nothing academically contrived about Australian pioneer occupational therapists in their approach [to practice]" (p. 7).

Kielhofner (1977) (see Chapter 21) revitalized Meyer's philosophies in a seminal paper on temporal adaptation. He described temporal adaptation as the integration of a spectrum of activities, the organization of which supports health on a daily basis. In this paper, Kielhofner outlined several propositions supporting the notion that temporal functioning was a useful conceptual base from which human adaptation and dysfunction could be better understood stating that, "action and time are concomitant components of the human experience" (p. 237). Kielhofner proposed that, because temporal adaptation was inclusive of all aspects of human dysfunction, unlike some other frames of reference at the time, it was not only suitable, but could unify all areas of occupational therapy practice. He suggested that a temporal conceptual framework could also facilitate the development of evaluations and interventions. His ideas, along with the ideas of several other colleagues were subsequently incorporated into a conceptual model of practice for occupational thera-

pists, A Model of Human Occupation (Kielhofner, 1985). In particular, the principles of temporal adaptation are embodied, though not clearly defined, in the concept of habituation (Kielhofner, 2002).

In summary, occupational therapy has a long, although fragmented association with the use of time as central to our philosophical underpinning. However, have we built on this association; should we do so, or is it really someone else's business? I am going to use the concepts of tempo, temporality, and time use to illustrate how I believe that time is at the heart of occupational therapy theory and practice. I ask you to reflect about how such knowledge may facilitate your distinctiveness as an occupational therapist and, through doing so, how it could further enable you to claim your rightful authority as sole keeper of your practice.

Tempo

> If the past is over, and the future has not yet come, all that exists is now; so how long does now last?
>
> St Augustine of Hippo (AD 354–430)

Tempo concerns not only the biological make-up of every individual, but also reflects how our values are translated occupationally. It therefore should be central to occupational therapy practice for individuals who experience challenges related to tempo. On this basis, we also should be at the forefront of public health developments on the consequences of desynchronization.

By tempo, I mean the pace of life, or time pressure. Tempo is intimately connected to our biological rhythms, described by Fraser (1987) as the characteristic patterns of recurring behavior. Tempo represents a flow of energy in time, and in relation to the environment. It is assumed that when rhythms are in synchrony, energy flows more effortlessly, and feelings are enhanced in the way described by Csikszentmihalyi & Csikszentmihalyi (1988) as flow. Biologically, for every individual, time felt, such as feeling rushed, is interpreted by the older regions of the brain and hence by the hidden levels of the mind. Time understood, or knowing the day or the hour, is interpreted by the newer regions of the brain, and hence by the easily accessible levels of the mind (Fraser). In this way, tempo is both beyond one level of awareness as well as being readily accessible at another.

Living systems are distinguished from non-living systems by our synchronization of a multitude of internal clocks—or circadian rhythms. For example, in the mouse, at least 60 internal rhythms have been identified in the functions of the hypothalamus, pituitary, and adrenal glands, in the chemical composition of bone marrow, and blood (Fraser, 1987). Conversely, measurable time has not always existed. Up until the 18th century, people could not be synchronized unless they were physically together (Fraser). Some used water towers, hour-glasses, sundials, or even the movement of birds.

The precursor of the modern clock was invented in approximately 1330, when the hour became the modern standard hour. It was not until 1764 that John Harrison was to build a marine chronometer that did not lose time (Sobel, 1998).

The sleep-wake cycle is the most obvious rhythm (Horne, 1988). Not only are we subject to rhythms across the day, but also the month (e.g. menstrual cycle) and yearly cycles, such as food selection habits attuned to seasonal climatic changes. There are also rhythms necessary to maintain life demonstrated by individuals in their local cultural and social context. To survive, it is necessary that the multitude of internal clocks be kept cycling in mutual dependence. When they are not properly maintained in synchrony, illness results; and a total lack of internal coordination leads to death.

While jet lag is the most obvious form of desynchronization, other examples of this can be seen in how shift workers manage or do not manage, changing shifts (Costa, 1996), or even at the level of whether a person is a morning or an evening person. As someone who does not function well in the morning, I dread the day when some bright young therapist comes to assess my functional capacities early in the morning, the consequences of which may lead to unreliable assessment results. Yet how often do we think about such timing of assessments in practice?

Not only does tempo impact on individuals, but it impacts on whole societies too. Several occupational scientists (Clark, 1997; Primeau, 1996; Wilcock, 1998; Yerxa, 1998 [see Chapter 34]) have discussed how the increased pace of life in industrialized societies, because of our restricted biological capacities, has resulted in detrimental health consequences. Clark suggested that, not only has this increased pace had an impact on individuals, but also, it potentially impacts on our humanity. She used Kundera's novel on *Slowness* to describe the 'secret bond between slowness and memory, between speed and forgetting' (Clark, 1997, p. 89). Kundera described how a man is walking down the street. At a certain moment, he tries to recall something, but the recollection escapes him. Automatically he slows down. Conversely, a person who wants to forget something unpleasant 'starts unconsciously to speed up his pace as if he were trying to distance himself from something still too close to him in time. That is, the degree of slowness is directly proportional to the intensity of meaning; the degree of speed is directly proportional to the intensity of forgetting' (p. 89).

Clark (1997) surmised that the increased pace of life in industrialized nations may not only produce stress and consequent ill health, but also robs people of a satisfying and meaningful life. She suggested that, 'it is not sufficient to simply participate in occupations; the occupational being must also be able to remember and understand them within the framework of an unfolding life story' (p. 89). Living organisms use valued occupations to meet biological needs, yet humans are increasingly driven by cultural priorities of money and power (Schor,

1991). Consequently, value is dominated by materialism that has little to do with meeting our biological needs.

In relationship to our own tempo and health as professionals, Young (1988) made a study of senior executives in Britain who were under extreme time pressure, subjecting themselves to an 8-day week, or a 30-hour day; always trying to do too much. They were continually harassed. When any said "I have no time" it was non-sensical. Young explained that, 'He had, or rather should have, the same amount of time as anyone else, instead of being permanently out of breath as he jogged past the stations in his calendar' (pp. 217–218). Claiming to have no time, according to Young, was a means of asserting status, measured by panting.

Time-use studies of the general population suggest that the average person's actual use of time has changed little in the last 40 years (Bittman, 2000). What has happened is that some people are working longer hours than ever before in our history, while others are disenfranchised from the labor market for reasons of disability, lack of available work, or appropriate skills and so on. Neither situation is likely to support health in the longer term. One might suggest that the scenario discussed by Young (1988) is in fact the reality not only of senior executives but of many professionals, which has little to do with asserting status. As such, you can see how tempo falls into our ambit as a public health issue.

Let me discuss one clinical application of knowledge on tempo. Sturgess (2003) has suggested that naturally occurring childhood play, such as climbing trees and jumping puddles, is being replaced by organized, active learning opportunities such as music lessons and competitive sports. That is, time is so precious that to use it fully, childhood play is one means to gain competitive advantage through enhahced learning opportunities. She claims, 'In this context, play is sometimes viewed as wasted time in which children dream and are aimless. They are seen to squander time that could be more usefully dedicated to active learning' (p. 106).

Part of this change is related to the political and social need to care for children economically in ostensibly 'safe and nurturing' environments while their parents are at work, fulfilling their time-use obligations as financial providers (Cunningham, 2003, as cited in Sturgess, 2003). As both parents increasingly spend more time in paid employment (Bittman, 2000), there is less time for engaging with children in naturally occurring play, or even building play into household chores such as gardening or cooking (Primeau, 1998) that now may be outsourced to a paid worker.

According to Sturgess (2003), children have less opportunity than was available even 10 years ago to challenge themselves with extending their ability to master physical feats purely for fun, such as walking along a length of fence. If children have fewer opportunities to experience a variety of sensory inputs, and are restricted because of fewer opportunities to play in natural environments with unsophisticated or "found" play materials, this impacts on the range of play skills achieved. The strength of play style created will be more limited. Play context, opportunity, stimulus, environment, and self-choice are the ingredients of healthy play opportunities that lead to healthy participation in occupations as adults. Sturgess suggested because occupational therapists have expertise on healthy growth and development through childhood play, we are ideally positioned to advocate for humanity, by arguing to keep time and space for childrens' impromptu, or improvised play, as well as structured play-related occupations.

In summary, tempo is internal and integral to healthy individuals and communities. Occupational therapists have expertise in the biological and occupational consequences of desynchronization for the individual, as well as the health consequences for societies. Such knowledge translates into our day-to-day clinical practice. Arguably, such expertise is not perceived as our domain at the public health level; however, it should be. At the very least, we can make a difference when we express our views in the media such as letters to the print media or on talk-back radio. If we do not, we relegate our wisdom as redundant, for others to claim as theirs.

Temporality

The future may never arrive whereas the past is gone forever—some of it has occurred and is not, while some is going to be and is not yet.

Aristotle (384–322 BC)

Whereas tempo is an internal, integral experience of time, temporality is a subjective perception of time. Temporality concerns the temporal character of occupation that is imbued with meaning in relation to one's sense of past, present, and future. All animals experience tempo, but only humans perceive temporality. As suggested by Young (1988), neither the future nor the past exist, but there is the present of past things (memory), the present of present things (direct perception), and the present of future things (expectations). That is, the past and future cannot be perceived except from inside the present. We do not wholly reinvent ourselves in each new present.

Rituals are a linking of past, present, and future (do Rozario, 1994; Hocking, Wright-St. Clair, & Bunrayong, 2002; Rosaldo, 1989; Turner, 1988). For example, an individual's activities at the wailing wall in Jerusalem are full of meaning only when we know that they represent religious rituals that link orthodox Jews to past and future generations of Jews, and that the wall, as the center of activities, has come to represent the tradition and the people who celebrate it. Rituals are recurrent events that can contain both continuity and change. People also bring such rituals with them to therapy, no matter how big or small, and these may impact on therapy.

People and groups differ in real and meaningful ways with respect to their time perspectives, and when they interact, conflicts often arise. Hall (1983) suggested that a future time perspective is the basic formulation for construal of events in what he calls American-European culture. That is, time is held as having value, and people who are perceived to waste it may offend those who see it as having value. The puritan work ethic has become the bureaucrat time ethic.

However, in some Nations of Aboriginal people in Australia, such as traditional Wiradjuri, there is no word for time as an abstract concept. Instead, according to Yalmambirra (2000), time is defined as 'a space in which something happened or did not happen, a space in which something continues but a space in which something has stopped' (p. 133). A future time perspective may have no relevancy in this context. However, it can produce behavior associated with health risks, and also extreme individualistic, and potentially antisocial patterns of behavior.

People who are centered in the present time perspective, such as was shown by Suto and Prank (1994) in a study of people with schizophrenia, may be perceived to lack ambition and feel apathetic about the future, not only for themselves, but for others. What is important is that there are different perspectives, and both have their place. The danger is, even when viewed within its own natural cultural context, as occupational therapists, our values on time use have the potential to impact on our valuation of what is meaningful for another individual.

To illustrate such time valuation in a clinical context, I borrow from the work of Seymour (2002), who focused on the relationship between disability and time. According to Seymour, many people we see in the occupational therapy context experience incidents that have become immortalized in time. For a person with a head injury, this may be the fatal moment of driving too fast, or for a person with schizophrenia who attributes their problems as starting with that shot of electricity in a workplace accident, or the person who survives the consequences of a heroin overdose. If the injury can be attributed to reckless or blameworthy behavior, the irresponsibility becomes suspended in time. The body becomes a constant reminder of individual carelessness or failure, and the moral judgements of others, impact, not only the potential success of intervention, but also one's future identity. In this way, Seymour suggested that time and the body become a constant reminder of the past.

Seymour (2002) also discussed ruptured time. Recently, I was listening to a young woman talk about the impact of having had a stroke. One day, she was working as an executive; the next she was attached to life support systems, but stressed about how she was going to finish the report that was due next week. Seymour explained: "Serious illness and disability disrupt the critical time-body relationship upon which our lives are based" (p. 138). Words from health professionals such as "unchangeable, impossible, indicate the impending foreclosure of previous plans and expectations. It is only when the people can reconceptualize their condition in relation to its temporal implications that meaning is given to the therapeutic experience" (p. 139). The danger for occupational therapists is, without this understanding, the person may be described as unmotivated or hostile, and may have difficulty moving on, that is, making progress in reconstructing a life and identity.

This leads naturally to *Reclaimed time* in which a serious disruption in life's prospects and expectations can offer people an opportunity to remake themselves, in a sense, to reclaim time that has passed. Contemporary films such as *A Beautiful Mind,* which portrays the life of John Forbes Nash Jr., a mathematical genius who needed to find a new way of life following the onset of a psychotic illness, serve to illustrate reclaimed time. The opportunity to review one's life, for some may now mean that they make the most of every moment in a lifestyle that previously has been taken for granted.

A final concept borrowed from Seymour (2002) is consumed time. Living with a disability is a time-consuming lifestyle. In talking about her son who had cerebral palsy, a mother described how it took 18 months of planning to achieve the family's goal of getting him into a mainstream school. First there was locating a school that would accept her son. Then, she needed to locate funding required to equip the school to meet the environmental demands required by a child with a disability. These demands impacted on her ability to resume her own professional life, let alone to engage in the normal day-to-day activities that provide healthy outcomes for a caretaker of someone with a disability. A day is still 24 hours, a week, just 7 days. Time for a person, or a caretaker of someone with a disability (Bittman & Thomson, 2000), becomes a scarce commodity that must be managed to achieve satisfaction in life's activities, or even just for life to proceed.

Temporality is not just an abstract concept for philosophical debate. It is a part of every person, therapist, and client. How big a part, and what part it may play in a client's illness and their therapy is our work. Understanding our client's concept of temporality helps complete the picture and is central in understanding the meaningfulness and purposefulness of the current occupations of our clients, without which, client-centered practice is compromised (Law, 1998).

Time Use

The final topic of this paper is time use, the area of social science that focuses on what we do with our time and why. This area of study is the most familiar to us as occupational therapists. It is conceptually uncomplicated, seemingly quite objective, and simple in application. But here again, familiarity has perhaps bred contempt and some of its value and many of its opportunities are being overlooked, to the detriment of the client and the profession.

As all human actions are located in time, including past, present, and future; time use is a commonality of the human condition. Time-use surveys in Western industrialized countries provide substantial data that indicate that employed adults have a relatively equal distribution of work, recre-

ational, and rest occupations (Australian Bureau of Statistics (ABS), 1998; Castles, 1993; Robinson & Godbey, 1999; Statistics Canada, 1995; Sturgis & Lynn, 1998). Because these surveys provide data about the time use of populations, they allow social scientists to compare people across cultures (Robinson, Andreyenkov, & Patrushev, 1988), age, lifestyle, and gender (Singleton & Harvey, 1995; Zuranek, 1998; Zuranek & Mannell, 1993) and thus, assess social change. For occupational therapists, analyzing how people allocate their time to activities, places, and interactions, by using the International Classification of Function terminology (ICF) (World Health Organization, 2001), allows us to understand the impact of disability on their participation in activities. Thus, comparison of patterns of time use of people with a disability with that of the population as a whole, can suggest where their activity participation is restricted or constrained; the disabling consequences of illness (de Vries, 1997). Time use is also an indicator of quality of life (Harvey, 1993). Nevertheless, studying a person's time use has not been central to occupational therapy practice.

In general, time-use studies of people with disabilities suggest that disability has a negative impact on time use in terms of the frequency of activities participated in, higher unemployment, and altered time allocation compared with the general population. This is important because people with disabilities also have been shown to experience less satisfaction with their performance of activities; so they do less and they enjoy less. Some studies have compared the time use of clinical and non-clinical populations. To illustrate, I will describe such studies with the elderly, spinal cord injury, and with mentally ill populations.

The study by Moss and Lawton (1982) of time use of older people found that those who were more functionally independent spent more time away from home and in obligatory tasks, such as housework, cooking, and shopping, than those receiving formal care. Those who were more impaired had a higher level of inactivity. Subsequent studies (Lawton, Moss, & Duhamel, 1995; Moss, Lawton, Kleban, & Duhamel, 1993) of severely impaired elders who were still living in the community but waiting for nursing home accommodation, indicated similar results with by far the greatest proportion of the day being spent in passive activities of resting, and listening to television or radio. While these data indicate a paucity of stimulating occupations for the elderly, they also indicate the potential opportunities for occupational therapy in facilitating caregivers to enrich their occupational opportunities.

In relationship to people with a spinal cord injury, Yenca and Locker (1990) used age and sex-matched adults' population-based time budgets to compare the quality of time use of community-based adults with spinal cord injuries with a non-disabled group. The participants with spinal cord injuries had a higher rate of unemployment and more daily free time than did their non-disabled counterparts. Similarly, Pentland,

Harvey, and Walker (1998) also studied the relationships between time use and health and well-being in 312 men with spinal cord injury. They found that men with spinal cord injury spent 39 percent more time on personal care, 20 percent more time in leisure, and 40 percent less time in productivity than men without spinal cord injury.

Studies of the time use and experience of time use of people with a mental illness, both living in the community and in institutions, consistently indicate lives dominated by solitary and passive leisure occupations (de Vries, 1997; MacGlip, 1991; Suto & Frank, 1994; Weeder, 1986). For example, the studies by Delespaul et al. (Delespaul, 1995; Delespaul & de Vries, 1987) in the Netherlands, suggested people with mental illness spend significantly more time doing nothing compared with a control group selected from census data. Similarly, Hayes and Halford (1996) compared the time use of men with schizophrenia, with employed and long-term unemployed men by using the 1987 Australian Bureau of Statistics data. They found that unemployed men and those with schizophrenia participated in more passive leisure (e.g. watching television) than the employed group, while those with schizophrenia participated in less social life, less active leisure, and slept more than the other two groups. Thus, this study suggested the time-use impact of experiencing a clinical disorder is similar to, but goes beyond that of, being unemployed. It also suggests that long-term unemployment is in itself, a disabling condition.

Harvey, Shimitras, and Fossey (2002) analyzed time-use data from over 200 people with schizophrenia involved in the epidemiological study by Harvey (1996) in London. Their finding matched the previous examples, but went further. Based on a logistic regression analysis of their data, Harvey et al. found those with longer illnesses were significantly less likely to be participating in productive occupations such as paid or unpaid work. Neither sex, social opportunities at home, nor negative symptoms predicted participation in productive occupations. Passive leisure participation was only predicted by social opportunities in the home; those who were living alone were significantly more likely to be participating in passive leisure. No significant illness-related or socio-demographic predictors of participation in active leisure or social occupations were found.

Based on these two analyses, Harvey et al. (2002) concluded that efforts to assist people with schizophrenia with impoverished lifestyles might focus on enabling them to participate in naturally occurring occupations that foster their social inclusion with peers in the community. Furthermore, they suggested that people with schizophrenia who are most likely to need assistance to pursue more active lifestyles are those with lengthier illness, and those living alone. Thus, people's social opportunities as well as their disability may impact on their successful pursuit of healthier lifestyles.

In summary, this clinically based research indicates that studying people's use of time can indicate their overall adaptation to the requirements of daily life. Each study points to problematic time use. Although the specific issue is different, each study suggests, and importantly, could be used to justify the need for the specialist knowledge and skills of occupational therapists.

Hayes (2000) argued that research should be the basis for clinical interventions in evidence-based occupational therapy practice. She called for the profession to provide research-based evidence for established initiatives in clinical practice, rather than expending limited research resources on developing novel and diverse interventions. It follows then that our expertise on understanding the relevance of time use as a major indicator of a person's quality of life, is one significant contribution occupational therapists can make in the health arena. However, consistent with the views of Hayes, we need to research this area more fully, to further develop and rigorously justify our clinical interventions based on time use. To do this, we will require trustworthy methodological procedures.

Methodologies for Studying Time Use

Time-use studies have used a variety of methodologies. One of the most common methodologies is time diaries. For example, the ABS has completed three large national time-use surveys since 1987 using time diaries (Australian Bureau of Statistics, 1987, 1998; Castles, 1993). The time diary requires the participant to complete a log or diary of the sequence and duration of activities engaged in, typically for 24 hours. All activities are recorded including the start and the finish time in addition to other information such as where, who with, and for whom the activity was done. A time diary places people engaged in their daily activities within their natural temporal context. An inventory is used to categorise time use that emphasizes the duration of occupations as the basis for comparing behaviors among subpopulations. For example, the 1997 Australian Bureau of Statistics Time-Use Diary included categories of: personal care, employment, childcare, education, and domestic-related activities; recreation and leisure activities; purchasing goods and services; and social and community interaction.

Comparable data sets of categories, or units of analysis or time have been developed internationally so that peoples' use of time from several nations can be compared (Harvey & Pentland, 1999). Because time diaries provide such rich population data on peoples' time use, they are of use for comparisons among people with activity participation restrictions. Confidentialized forms of these data are available for use by social scientists with an interest in analyzing the national time-use data for their own research purposes and could be made use of by occupational therapists (Bridge, Farnworth, & Fossey, 2002).

Two other clinical instruments designed to gather time-use information use a diary configuration: the Occupational Questionnaire (Smith, Kielhofner, & Watts, 1986) and the

National Institutes of Health (NIH) Activity Record (Gerber & Furst, 1992). The NIH Activity Record was developed for use with persons who have a physical disability and asks additional questions pertaining to pain, fatigue, and so on. Hence, it provides detailed information about how a disability influences performance of everyday activities. In this way, the activity record could be modified to elucidate other information such as perceived satisfaction, experience of well-being, and so on; issues that are of interest to clinicians.

Beeper methodologies such as Experience Sampling Method (ESM), is a methodology that makes use of a spot sampling strategy while avoiding the problems associated with the intrusive observer (Csikszentmihalyi & Csikszentmihalyi, 1988; Farnworth, Mosstert, Harrison, & Worrell, 1996). The data collected includes the person's time use in addition to their experience of engagement in occupation, which is placed within a physical and social context. A person is beeped at random times to alert him or her to fill out a form. The methodology lends itself to smaller scale studies, while the time-use data gathered is comparable with data collected by time-use diaries (Robinson, 1985). However, its uses are not restricted to research questions on time use (Kennedy, 1998; Toth-Fejel, Toth-Fejel, & Hedricks, 1998). In my study (Farnworth, 1998a, 1998b) using ESM and interviewing to investigate the time use and subjective experiences of young offenders, I found that 78 percent of their time was spent engaging in passive leisure and self-care occupations, but the dominant experience was that of boredom, particularly while engaged in these occupations. This understanding of the potentially negative health outcomes of engaging in such occupations could be addressed; a finding that may not be advocated on the basis of time-use findings alone.

Qualitative methodologies such as interviews can provide rich time-use data. Direct observation is potentially more accurate than interviews, but it is expensive and because of the intrusiveness of the observer, it may alter the participants' behavior. Nikitin and Farnworth (2001), for this reason, used a combination of data collection methods: time-use diaries, participant observation, and the Occupational Performance History Interview II (OPHI-II). The OPHI-II was designed to gather essential data on a person's occupational life history (Kielhofner et al., 1998). The semistructured interview is premised on the idea that current occupations are a consequence of life experiences and environmental influences. It includes questions about how people use time currently, and how that may differ from previous use of time.

Therefore, we have ABS and other international general population studies and a variety of time-use study methodologies that suit a number of applications. That is, we have diagnostic tools to further our understanding of the relationship between time use and a person's health and well-being. Not only that, but focusing on how a person uses his or her time immediately orients the occupational therapist to occupation-based practices. Because studying time use is about the occupations engaged in by the person, time use is about intact occupations, not component parts (Law, Baum, & Baptiste, 2002; McLaughlin Gray, 1998 [see Chapter 15]; Pierce, 2003). It is also about occupations across the day, not just the time in therapy. For example, a therapist may see a child daily for individual therapy. Knowing that this child spends 5 hours each day in a variety of individual therapies may alert the therapist to incorporate additional occupations to meet the needs of the child, such as outdoor and social occupations, which are appropriate for the developmental age of the child.

Time use is a constant that we can measure. It therefore provides a basis for comparison between those who are able to engage in a healthy range of occupations of their own choosing versus those who do not have such choices. For example, a therapist may find that a person wants to rest in bed all day, everyday. In being client centered (Law, 1998), the therapist may support this client's occupational choice. However, using time-use data based on healthy individuals for support, or reference to data that suggests a loss of skills through the lack of use (Farnworth, 2000), may lead the therapist to challenge clients about healthy occupations in which they could engage.

Another advantage of using time-use data is that it is a way of communicating our area of expertise. Cusick (2001) cautioned occupational therapists in using profession-specific language if we are to communicate effectively both outside and inside the profession. She suggested that: 'we need to look at the language of the world and see what terms suit us without too much tampering' (p. 107). Naming and framing the occupations of clients of occupational therapy as passive leisure or self-care can be easily explained. These concepts also are readily linked to the universal language of ICF (Hasselkus, 2000; McLaughlin Gray, 2001). Time-use findings become a significant marketing strategy for occupational therapy, which has the potential to enhance our visibility as a profession, precisely because people engage in occupation throughout their day; people relate to having too much or too little time to do what they want, and the implications that this may have on their health.

Time Use as a Health Outcome

Understanding a person's use of time also is a measurement of health outcome. One must not ignore the benefits of larger scale epidemiological studies on the time usage of people with disabilities, which can be used to support the development of public health policies such as that advocated by Wilcock (1998). Fisher (1999) suggested that instruments such as the RAND 36-item Health Status Survey (Hays, Sherbourne, & Mazel, 1993; Ware & Sherbourne, 1992), which are used to measure changes in sociability and general well-being among people experiencing various health problems, are attempting to make a generalized assessment of how people use their time. Several questions on the shorter versions of the SF36, such as the depression, anxiety, and sociability scale (DAS) (Coxon et al., as cited in Fisher) assess a person's sociability. These questions assume that a change in health status may also accompany a change in the proportion of time respondents spend alone, or with other people. Additionally, many of the activities about which people are asked to comment in SF36, such as participating in bathing and dressing, have long been categories of activities people are specifically asked about in time diaries. Fisher believed that the SF36 differs from existing time diary research interests only in asking specifically about the ability to perform activities rather than a person's engagement in the activity. She suggested that, because of this, time diaries allow the possibility of improving the quality of generalised health outcome research in three ways:

1. *Detecting chances in behavior associated with both the benefits and side-effects of treatments in relation to other activities.* Diaries facilitate the measurement of progressive change in behavior measured through use of time, prior to, during, and after intervention.
2. *More precisely measuring sociability, fatigue, and behavior related to the way people use their time.* The time diary measures how much time people spend with others, what they do, and where they do these activities. Whilt one may spend time talking with friends on the telephone, another may go to meet with these people. Both are social activities but the physical setting and activity engagement level is quite different. These differences may have different health benefits for the individual.
3. *Offering more precise cost-benefit analyses of the treatments for funding agencies.* Fisher (1999) suggested that time diaries can be applied to valuing the effects of health intervention. If, for example, a person with a severe mental illness was receiving therapy from an occupational therapist to re-engage in social and productive activities, such as working voluntarily at the local recycling outlet and becoming a consumer advocate, time diary data could provide quantitative data to support the costs versus the societal gains, for this person's new activities.

Finally, as proposed by Fisher (1999), because time diaries are a relatively innocuous form of assessment, and not costly to administer, using diaries to study a person's use of time produces results that are directly meaningful to the lived experience of people who complete them. Given occupational therapists' quest for suitable outcome measures that detect changes attributable to occupational therapy, in addition to maintaining authenticity, time diaries have many advantages.

Conclusion

In conclusion, the World Health Organization has focused attention on activity and participation with the development of the ICF which recognises that restrictions in participation in activities is a measure of disability. I believe that studying a person's time use can provide a rich insight into disability from an occupational perspective. Although occupational therapy, since its inception, has had a core interest in time use as an indicator of health and well-being, and there is much evidence on time use available internationally from population-based studies, we are yet to fully exploit the potential of such interests to validate our practice.

I have discussed several studies concerned with the tempo, temporality, and time use of people with a disability and methodological strategies for understanding further a person's use of time. Such knowledge and methods, if used, enhance our rightful authority to be the sole keepers of practices incorporating such ideas. However, to be able to do this, we need to know how to do it, and we need to explain, communicate, and investigate such knowledge further. The advantages for us professionally are enormous. We live in an increasingly temporally challenged society, not just for people with a disability. The development of policy that supports fair, and equitable, access of all people to a range of occupations that lead to or maintain health and well-being requires such expertise. As indicated in this paper, time use, tempo, and temporality are the essence of occupational therapy's business. If we don't pursue such knowledge, others will, and we risk becoming marginalized from what originated as our autonomous, professional authority, something that distinguished us from other professionals.

References

Anderson, B. & Bell, J. (1988). *Occupational therapy: Its place in Australia's history.* Victoria: N.S.W. Association of Occupational Therapists.

Australian Bureau of Statistics. (1987). *Information paper: Time use pilot survey, Sydney, May–June 1987* (Vol. Cat. No. 4111.1). Canberra: Australian Bureau of Statistics.

Australian Bureau of Statistics. (1998). *1997 Time use survey* (No. Cat. No. 4153.0). Canberra: Australian Bureau of Statistics.

Ayres, J. (1979). *Sensory integration and the child.* Los Angeles: Western Psychological Services.

Bittman, M. (2000). Now it's 2000: Trends in doing and being in the new millennium. *Journal of Occupational Science, 7,* 108–117.

Bittman, M. & Thomson, C. (2000). Invisible support: Determinants of time spent informal care. In: J. Warburton & M. Oppenheimer (Eds), *Volunteers and volunteering* (pp. 98–112). Annadale: The Federation Press.

Bridge, K., Farnworth, L., & Fossey, E. (2002). *Mining population surveys: Potential sources of activity participation knowledge for practice.* Paper presented at the World Federation of Occupational Therapists Congress 13th World Congress, Stockholm, June 23–28.

Castles, I. (1993). *How Australians use their time* (No. ABS Cat. No. 4153.0). Canberra: Australian Bureau of Statistics.

Clark, F. (1997). Reflections of the human as an occupational being: Biological tempo, biological need, tempo, and temporality. *Journal of Occupational Science: Australia, 4,* 86–92.

Costa, G. (1996). The impact of shift and night work on health. *Applied Ergonomics, 37,* 9–16.

Csikszentmihalyi, M. & Csikszentmihalyi, I. (1988). *Optimal experience: Psychological studies of flow in consciousness.* Cambridge: Cambridge University Press.

Cusick, A. (2001). The 2001 Sylvia Docker Lecture: EBPOT2000: Australian occupational therapy, evidence-based practice, and the 21st century. *Australian Journal of Occupational Therapy, 48,* 102–117.

de Vries, M. W. (1997). Recontextualizing psychiatry: Toward ecologically valid mental health research. *Transcultural Psychiatry, 34,* 185–218.

Delespaul, P. (1995). *Assessing schizophrenia in daily life: The experience sampling method.* Maastricht: IPSER.

Delespaul, P. & de Vries, M. (1987). The daily life of ambulatory chronic mental patients. *The Journal of Nervous and Mental Disease, 175* (9), 537–544.

Docker, S. (1959). Development of occupational therapy in Australia. *Bulletin: Australian Association of Occupational Therapists, 6,* 2–8.

do Rozario, L. (1994). Ritual, meaning, and transcendence: The role of occupation in modern life. *Journal of Occupational Science: Australia, 1,* 46–53.

Farnworth, L. (1998a). Doing, being, and boredom. *Journal of Occupational Science, 5,* 140–146.

Farnworth, L. (1998b). Time use and subjective experience of occupations of young male and female legal offenders. Unpublished doctoral Dissertation. Los Angeles: University of Southern California.

Farnworth, L. (2000). Time use and leisure occupations of young offenders. *American Journal of Occupational Therapy, 54,* 315–325.

Farnworth, L., Mostert, E. & Harrison, S., Worrell, D. (1996). The Experience sampling method: Its potential use in occupational therapy research. *Occupational Therapy International, 3,* 1–17.

Fisher, K. (1999). *Potential applications of time use data for measuring health outcomes.* Retrieved 20 April, 2002, from http://www.iser.essex.ac.uk/activities/iatur/.

Fraser, J. (1987). *Time, the familiar stranger.* Amherst: University of Massachusetts Press.

Gerber, L. & Furst, G. (1992). Validation of the NIH Activity Record: a quantitative measure of life activities. *Arthritis Care and Research, 5,* 81–86.

Hall, E. (1983). *The dance of life: The other dimension of time.* New York: Anchor Books.

Harvey, A. (1993). Quality of life and the use of time theory and measurement. *Journal of Occupational Science: Australia, 1,* 27–29.

Harvey, C. (1996). The Camden Schizophrenia Surveys. I: The psychiatric, behavioral, and social characteristics of the severely mentally ill in an Inner London health district. *British Journal of Psychiatry, 168,* 410–417.

Harvey, A. & Pentland, W. (1999). Time use research. In: W. Pentland, A. Harvey, M. P. Lawton, & M. A. McColl (Eds), *Time use research in the social sciences* (pp. 3–19.) New York: Kluwer Academic.

Harvey, C., Shimitras, L., & Fossey, E. (2002). Time use of people with schizophrenia living in the community: Participation in activities and rehabilitation implications. *Schizophrenia Research Supplement, 53,* 239.

Hasselkus, B. (2000). From the desk of the editor — Reaching consensus. *American Journal of Occupational Therapy, 54,* 127–128.

Hayes, R. (2000). Evidence-based occupational therapy needs strategically targeted quality research now. *Australian Journal of Occupational Therapy, 47,* 186–190.

Hayes, R. & Halford, K. (1996). Time use of unemployed and employed single male schizophrenia subjects. *Schizophrenia Bulletin, 22,* 659–669.

Hays, R., Sherbourne, C. D., & Mazel, R. (1993). The RAND 36-Item Health Survey 1.0. *Health Economy, 2,* 217–227.

Higgs, J. & Titchen, A. (1995). Propositional, professional, and personal knowledge in clinical reasoning. In: J. Higgs & M. Jones (Eds), *Clinical reasoning in the health professions* (pp. 129–146). Oxford: Butterworth-Heinemann.

Hocking, C., Wright-St. Clair, V., & Bunrayong, W. (2002). The meaning of cooking and recipe work for older Thai and New Zealand women. *Journal of Occupational Science, 9,* 117–127.

Horne, J. (1988). *Why we sleep — The functions of sleep in humans and other mammals.* Oxford: Oxford University Press.

Jonsson, H. (1998). Emst Westerlund — A Swedish doctor of occupation. *Occupational Therapy International, 5,* 155–171.

Kennedy, B. L. (1998). *Feeling and doing: Health and mind-body-context interactions during daily occupations of women with HIV/AIDS.* Unpublished PhD dissertation. Los Angeles, CA: University of Southern California,

Kielhofner, G. (Ed.) (1985). *A model of human occupation: Theory and application.* Baltimore: Williams & Wilkins.

Kielhofner, G. (1977). Temporal adaptation: A conceptual framework for occupational therapy. *American Journal of Occupational Therapy, 31,* 235–247. Reprinted as Chapter 21.

Kielhofner, G. (1995). *A model of human occupation: Theory and Application* (2nd edn). Baltimore: Williams & Wilkins.

Kielhofner, G. (2002). *A model of human occupation: Theory and application* (3rd edn). Baltimore: Lippincott Williams & Wilkins.

Kielhofner, G., Mallinson, T., Crawford, C., Nowllk, M., Rigby, M., Henry, A., et al. (1998). A User's manual for the OPHI-II: *The occupational performance history interview* (Version 2.0 ed). Chicago: Model of Human Occupation Clearinghouse.

Law, M. (Ed.) (1998). *Client-centered occupational therapy.* Thorofare, NJ: Slack, Inc.

Law, M., Baum, C., & Baptiste, S. (2002). *Occupation-based practice: Fostering performance and participation.* Thorofare, NJ: Slack, Inc.

Lawton, M. P., Moss, M., & Duhamel, L. (1995). Quality of life among elderly care receivers. *Journal of Applied Gerontology, 14,* 150–171.

MacGlip, D. (1991). A quality of life study of discharged long-term psychiatric patients. *Journal of Advanced Nursing, 16,* 1206–1215.

McLaughlin Gray, J. (1998). Putting occupation into practice: Occupation as ends, occupation as means. *American Journal of Occupational* Therapy, 52, 354–364. Reprinted as Chapter 15.

McLaughlin Gray, J. (2001). Discussion of the ICIDH–2 in relation to occupational therapy and occupational science. *Scandinavian Journal of Occupational Therapy, 8,* 19–30.

Meyer, A. (1922/1977). The philosophy of occupational therapy. *American Journal of Occupational Therapy, 31,* 639–642. Reprinted as Chapter 2.

Moss, M. & Lawton, M. (1982). The time budgets of older people: a window on four lifestyles. *Journal of Gerontology, 37,* 115–123.

Moss, M., Lawton, M. P., Kleban, M., & Duhamel, L. (1993). Time budgets of caregiving of impaired elders before and after institutionalization. *Journal of Gerontology: Social Sciences, 4S,* S102–l11.

Nikitin, L. & Farnworth, L. (2001). Time use and occupational history of a forensic psychiatric population. Unpublished manuscript. La Trobe University, Melbourne.

Pentland, W., Harvey, A., & Walker, J. (1998). Time use, time pressure, personal stress, mental health, and life satisfaction from a life cycle perspective. *Journal of Occupational Science, 5,* 14–25.

Pierce, D. (2003). *Occupation by design: Building therapeutic power.* Philadelphia: FA Davis.

Primeau, L. (1996). Work and leisure: Transcending the dichotomy. *American Journal of Occupational Therapy, 50,* 569–577.

Primeau, L. (1998). Orchestration of work and play within families. *American Journal of Occupational Therapy, 52,* 188–195.

Robinson, J. (1985). The validity and reliability of diaries versus alternative time use measures. In: F. Juster and F. Stafford (Eds), *Time, goods, and well-being* (pp. 33–62). Ann Arbor: Survey Research Center. Institute for Social Research, University of Michigan.

Robinson, J., Andreyenkov, V., & Patrushev, V. (1988). *The rhythm of everyday life: How Soviet and American citizens use time.* San Francisco: Westview Press.

Robinson, J. & Godbey, G. (1999). *Time for life: The surprising ways Americans use their time* (2nd ed.). University Park, PA: State University Press.

Time Use, Tempo, and Temporality

Rogers, J. (1983). *Freedom to learn from the 80s.* Ohio: Charles E. Merriil.

Rosaldo, R. (1989). *Culture and truth: The remaking of social analysis.* Boston, MA: Beacon Press.

Schor, J. (1991). *The overworked American: The unexpected decline of leisure.* New York: Basic Books.

Seymour, W. (2002). Time and the body: Re-embodying time in disability. *Journal of Occupational Science, 9,* 135–142.

Singleton, J. & Harvey, A. (1995). Stages of lifecycle and time spent in activities. *Journal of Occupational Science: Australia, 2,* 3–12.

Slagle, E. (1922). Training aides for mental patients. *Archives of Occupational Therapy, 1,* 11–17.

Sloan, J. (1976). Sylvia Docker lecture 1975: After the pioneers. *Australian Occupational Therapy Journal, 23,* 7–19.

Smith, N., Kielhofner, G., & Watts, J. (1986). The relationship among volition, activity pattern, and life satisfaction in the elderly. *American Journal of Occupational Therapy, 40,* 278–283.

Sobel, D. (1998). *Longitude.* London: Fourth Estate.

Statistics Canada. (1995). *The 1992 General Social Survey: Cycle 7. Time Use.* Ottawa: Statistics Canada.

Sturgess, J. (2003). Viewpoint: A model describing play as a child-chosen activity: Is this still valid in contemporary Australia? *Australian Occupational Therapy Journal, 50,* 104–108.

Sturgis, P. & Lynn, P. (1998). *The 1997 UK pilot of the Eurostat time use survey* (No. Government Statistical Service Methodology Series 1). London: Office for National Statistics.

Suto, M. & Frank, G. (1994). Future time perspective and daily occupations of persons with chronic schizophrenia in a board and care home. *American Journal of Occupational Therapy, 48,* 7–18.

Toth-Fejel, G. E., Toth-Fejel, G. F., & Hedricks, C. (1998). Occupation-centered practice in hand rehabilitation using the experience sampling method. *American Journal of Occupational Therapy, 52,* 381–385.

Turner, V. W. (1988). *The anthropology of performance.* New York: PAJ Publications.

Ware, J. E. & Sherbourne, C. D. (1992). The MOS 36-Item Short Form Health Survey (SF–36): I. *Medical Care, 30,* 473–481.

Weeder, T. (1986). Comparison of temporal patterns and meaningfulness of daily activities of schizophrenic and normal adults. *Occupational Therapy in Mental Health, 6,* 27–45.

Wilcock, A. (1998). *An occupational perspective of health.* Thorofare, NJ: Slack Inc.

Wilcock, A. (1999). 1999 Sylvia Docker Lecture: Creating self and shaping the world. *Australian Occupational Therapy Journal, 46,* 77–88.

Wood, W. (1996). Legitimizing occupational therapy's knowledge. *American Journal of Occupational Therapy, 50,* 626–634.

World Health Organization. (2001). *International classification of functioning, disability, and health, ICF.* Geneva: World Health Organization.

Yalmambirra. (2000). Black time ...white time: My time ... Your time. *Journal of Occupational Science, 7,* 133–137.

Yema, E. (1998). Health and the human spirit for occupation. *American Journal of Occupational Therapy, 52,* 412–418. Reprinted as Chapter 34.

Yerxa, E. & Locker, S. (1990). Quality of time use by adults with spinal cord injuries. *American Journal of Occupational Therapy, 44,* 318–326.

Young, M. (1988). *The metronomic society: Natural rhythms and human timetables.* Cambridge. MA: Harvard University Press.

Zuranek, J. (1998). Time use, time pressure, personal stress, mental health, and life satisfaction from a life cycle perspective. *Journal of Occupational Science, 5,* 26–39.

Zuranek, J. & Manneli, R. (1993). Gender variations in the weekly rhythms of daily behavior and experiences. *Occupational Science: Australia, 1,* 25–37.

Flow and Occupation: A Review of the Literature

HEATHER EMERSON, MSc, OT(C)

For the past 75 years occupational therapists have claimed an interest in occupation and its impact on human beings (Weimer, 1979). We have identified conditions of occupational engagement that seem to influence the quality and outcome of these experiences. Only during the past 15 years, however, have we begun to focus our research on the subjective experiences of people engaged in occupation in their natural settings (Kielhofner, 1981; Kremer, Nelson, & Duncombe, 1984; Johnson & Yerxa, 1989). The literature on flow theory by Csikszentmihalyi has also been addressing the subjective experiences of persons engaged in occupation. Studies on flow can provide occupational therapy and occupational science with data on subjective occupational experience and the personal and activity properties that relate to it. In addition, this literature offers theoretical and methodological considerations for future research on occupation. The purpose of this paper is to introduce the construct of flow to occupational therapists who may not be familiar with this body of literature and to offer some principles for the application of this knowledge to clinical practice.

This chapter was previously published in the *Canadian Journal of Occupational Therapy, 65,* 37–44. Copyright © 1998, CAOT Publications ACE (Canadian Association of Occupational Therapists). Reprinted with permission.

Occupation

Occupation refers to "the active or 'doing' process of a person engaged in goal-directed, intrinsically gratifying, and culturally appropriate activity" (Evans, 1987, p. 627). Occupational therapists have long recognized that occupation has a role in integrating the mind and body (Breines, 1984; Cynkin & Robinson, 1999), maintaining psychic order (Meyer, 1922/1982 [see Chapter 2]), motivating the individual (Kielhofner, 1992; Meyer, 1922/1982), and promoting a sense of worth and competence (Fidler & Fidler, 1978 [see Chapter 9]); (Yerxa, 1980). Other benefits of occupational engagement identified in the literature include its ability to influence time perception (Meyer, 1922/1982), (Yerxa et al., 1990); reconnect the individual with his or her natural environment (Yerxa, 1980); and focus attention on a clear goal and away from one's self or one's worries (Friedland, 1988; Levine, 1987 [see Chapter 3]).

What is it about occupation or activity that promotes feelings of competence and well-being? The literature suggests that the answer pertains to the interplay between an individual and an activity, yet the nature of this relationship is not clearly understood (Breines, 1984; Meyer, 1922/1982 [see Chapter 3]).

An American Occupational Therapy Association Position Paper (1993) on purposeful activity discussed properties of activities that influence one's sense of competence and well-being. Beneficial aspects of activity that were recognized include their adaptability in that they can be graded to match the individual's abilities, structured to direct attention toward a goal rather than to the process, and altered to provide direct objective feedback on performance.

Breines (1984) viewed the process of bringing a person's attention beyond choice into "automaticity," where actions are elicited without conscious awareness, as a benefit of occupation. Others have claimed that the success of outcomes is an important aspect of occupation (Baum, 1985; Fidler & Fidler, 1978 [see Chapter 9]). Yerxa (1980) recognized the importance of choice and self-initiation. Fundamental to occupational therapy's philosophy are the beliefs that humans have an innate need to explore and master the environment, and that an important reward of occupation is in the process of doing (Kielhofner, 1992; Reilly, 1960).

These reflections can be found in the philosophical writings of occupational therapy. They are grounded in the opinions, experience, and observations of occupational therapists. Until recently, occupational therapists have focused their research on properties and responses to activity identified by clinicians. However, during the past 15 years occupational therapists have begun to study the subjective experiences of individuals while they are engaged in activity (Kielhofner, 1981; Kremer, Nelson, & Duncombe, 1984; Johnson & Yerxa, 1989; Laliberte, 1993; Merrill, 1985; Park, 1995; Steinmetz, 1995). They have begun to look outside the clinic at how people experience occupation in their daily lives (Keilhofner, 1981, 1982). Yerxa and colleagues reflected this focus when they wrote "To fully understand occupation it is necessary to comprehend the experience of engagement in it" (1990, p. 9). The shift toward an appreciation for subjective occupational experiences has been influenced by many factors. These factors include increased knowledge of qualitative research methods, increased interest in occupational science, and the recognition that the profession has much to learn from other disciplines besides medicine (Yerxa et al., 1990).

Subjective Occupational Experience

One source from which occupational therapists can learn about the subjective experience of activity and its measurement is the literature on flow by Csikszentmihalyi and his colleagues (Carlson & Clark, 1991). Csikszentmihalyi (1990, 1992) has spent three decades examining the question "What makes some action patterns worth pursuing for their own sake, even without any rational compensation?" He examined literature on intrinsic motivation by such authors as Hebb, Maslow, McClelland, Harlow, Bem, and DeCharms (Csikszentmihalyi, 1975). Through interviews, diaries, time logs, questionnaires, ethnography, and a technique he devised called "experience sampling method" (ESM), he collected data about the subjective experience of people engaged in activities and occupations in their natural settings during their everyday lives (Csikszentmihalyi, 1975). The ESM uses beeper technology to randomly signal participants several times a day to prompt them to fill out a form describing their most recent activity, its context, and their subjective experience at the time. Through these studies he developed a theory about a source of intrinsic motivation called "flow." This theory articulates and explores many beliefs about occupation that are fundamental to the philosophy of occupational therapy.

Flow

Flow is a subjective psychological state that occurs when one is totally involved in an activity (Csikszentmihalyi, 1975). It is "the state in which people are so involved in an activity that nothing else seems to matter; the experience itself is so enjoyable that people will do it even at great cost, for the sheer sake of doing it" (1990, p. 4).

The flow experience is characterized by the ability to concentrate on the activity, a sense of control over one's actions, and a clear sense of purpose or goals (Csikszentmihalyi, 1975,

1988a). During flow there is a removal from awareness of one's worries, a loss of self-consciousness, and a distorted sense of time (Csikszentmihalyi, 1990). Other conditions connected with flow include a choice of participation, a sense that the outcome of the activity is under one's control and is meaningful, immediate clear feedback, a merging of awareness with activity, and a sense that the activity is rewarding in and of itself (Csikszentmihalyi, 1975, 1990).

When a person is in flow, a positive affective state, high motivation, high cognitive efficiency, and high activation are experienced. This activation involves arousal, alertness, energy, and interest (Csikszentmihalyi & Larson, 1987; Csikszentmihalyi & Mei-Ha Wong, 1991). Flow involves an active use of skills which causes "enjoyment" and growth, in contrast to the more passive construct of "pleasure," which does not require effort and is based on genetically programmed drives for survival of the species, such as eating and sexual behavior (Massimini, Csikszentmihalyi, & Delle Fave, 1988).

Csikszentmihalyi believed that the unfocused mind is in a state of chaos, "entropy," and that psychic order, "negentropy," is achieved by learning to control consciousness through the focusing of one's energy, attention, and skills on the goals offered through engagement in challenging activities (Csikszentmihalyi, 1988b). Flow is sometimes called "optimal experience" or "autotelic enjoyment" and is considered by some to be the highest level of well-being (Csikszentmihalyi & Mel-Ha Wong, 1991).

The Flow Channel

A match between an individual's perceptions of his or her skills and of the environmental demands has been identified as a prerequisite to this type of optimal experience (Csikszentmihalyi, 1975, 1988b, 1988c; Massimini et al., 1988). Educators on flow believe that to sustain a combination of interest, enjoyment, and motivation, the dimensions of perceived skill and perceived challenge must be matched and considered above average for that individual (Csikszentmihalyi, 1988b). This balance between high skills and high challenges is referred to as "the flow channel" (Csikszentmihalyi & Csikszentmihalyi, 1988, p. 261).

In models of flow, this optimal state is contrasted with states of anxiety, boredom, and apathy (Csikszentmihalyi, 1975; Massimini, Csikszentmihalyi, & Carli, 1987). When environmental demands are perceived by the individual as exceeding his or her capacity, anxiety states are apt to occur (Csikszentmihalyi & Larson, 1984). When the demands of the environment do not tax the individual's perceived skills, boredom or apathy may occur (Csikszentmihalyi & Larson, 1984; Massimini et al., 1987). Csikszentmihalyi and Larson (1984) claim that, to remain in the flow channel with an activity, the person must believe that the demands are increasing as his or her skills improve.

ESM studies have measured time in flow using the high skill/high challenge criterion. There is variance in the amount of time spent in flow from person to person. Some studies use the four-channel model (anxiety, apathy, flow, and boredom) while others use eight or 16 channels. Using the four-channel model, LeFevre studied 107 adults who volunteered from five Chicago companies (1988). On average, they spent 33 percent of work time in flow, 34 percent in apathy; while leisure time was spent 19 percent in flow channel, and 42 percent in apathy (LeFevre, 1988). LeFevre found that managers had more flow at work than did blue collar workers, but that the opposite was true of leisure time. Wells' (1988) four-channel study of working mothers found that time in flow ranged from 4 to 40 percent and averaged 23 percent. Occupational therapy practitioners in physical rehabilitation settings spent about 23 percent of their work time in flow, and a surprising 44 percent of work time in the anxiety channel of this model (Jacobs, 1994).

An eight-channel model has also been used in some ESM studies (Csikszentmihalyi & Mei-Ha Wong, 1991). In addition to the states of flow, boredom, apathy, and anxiety, these studies measured time in the intermediate states of arousal, control, relaxation, and worry (Massimini, Carli, & Cikszentmihalyi, 1988). Because a person's time is divided among eight, rather than four channels, the proportion of time in each channel is expected to be less than on studies using four-channel models. Studies using this model found that adolescents in Milan spent an average of 19 percent of their time in flow, while adolescents in Chicago spent 16 percent of their time in flow (Carli, Delle Fave, & Massimini, 1988; Massimini et al., 1988).

Flow Activities

Activities that bring about flow are called "autotelic activities" after the Latin *auto* meaning *self* and *teleos* meaning *goals* (Csikszentmihalyi, 1975). Csikszentmihalyi said of autotelic activities, "the most basic requirement is to provide a clear set of challenges" and the most basic challenge is that of "the unknown, which leads to discovery, exploration, and problem-solving" (1975, p. 30). Although these activities differ from person to person, they have some properties in common (Csikszentmihalyi, 1975, 1988b, 1990). They provide opportunities for action that match the person's skills. There are clear goals with adequate means for reaching them. Clear consistent feedback on performance is provided. The stimulus field is limited to decrease distraction. The activity is viewed by the person as having surmountable goals and outcomes that he or she can influence.

Often autotelic activities involve competition, rules, and risks. These activities are not necessarily virtuous or instrumental (Csikszentmihalyi & Larson, 1984). A youth who lacks prosocial skills may find flow in antisocial activities such as stealing. Sometimes flow activities are addictive in that they are so intriguing or appealing that the individual

may neglect or fail to find enjoyment in other aspects of life (Csikszentmihalyi, 1975).

Autotelic activities occur in leisure, self-care, and work contexts. Examples include playing chess, rock climbing, ocean cruising, yoga, painting, performing surgery, playing with one's child, and doing sports (Csikszentmihalyi, 1975, 1988b, 1990; Jackson, 1994).

Flow Experience Across Cultures

The potential for flow is felt to be both universal and individualized. It exists across a variety of cultures, ages, and social classes (Carlson & Clark, 1991; Csikszentmihalyi & Larson, 1984; Massimini et al., 1988). Sato (1988) wrote about a collective of "group flow" experienced by Japanese youths on motorcycle runs. Delle Fave and Massimini (1988) studied flow in alpine villages in northern Italy and found that, while members of the traditional culture experienced flow through farm work, the modern generation experienced flow primarily in leisure contexts. Han (1988) found that life satisfaction for Korean immigrants was more closely tied to flow for women than men and suspected that women were more sensitive to the affective effects of flow. There have been studies of flow among Italian cave explorers, drug addicts, students from Bangkok, Navajo college students, white collar workers, dancers, and blind nuns (Csikszentmihalyi & Csikszentmihalyi, 1988; Massimini et al., 1988).

Flow theory has been applied in retrospect to some trends documented in history. Researchers who have reviewed historical documents and anthropological writings have found evidence to suggest that flow experiences may have occurred among pygmies, Shuswap Indians, fourth-century Japanese shrine builders, natives of New Guinea, Mayan ball players, Indian Brahmins, Athenian citizens, Chinese intellectuals, and violent warriors of the ancient Turkish and Tartar cultures (Csikszentmihalyi, 1990). It was hypothesized that the Jesuit order of St. Ignatius of Loyala in the 1500s attracted young missionaries because of the complex system of graded challenges that provided flow opportunities (Csikszentmihalyi, I., 1988).

The types of activities that promote flow differ based on gender, a finding that may relate to differing opportunities for skill development (Csikszentmihalyi, 1975). It seems that as age and socioeconomic status increase, people are more inclined to enjoy activity engagement for its own sake. The characteristics of flow are the same in all cultures, but the contexts and opportunities differ. Flow can be found in cultures where there are goals, rules, and challenges matched to the skills of the population (Csikszentmihalyi, 1990). Csikszentmihalyi viewed flow as a higher-level need, essential for happiness, but not necessarily for survival of an individual. Flow seems to only occur, and take precedence, in cultures and times where basic survival and safety needs are not threatened (Csikszentmihalyi, 1990).

The Autotelic Personality

There are differences from person to person in the inclination to experience flow (Adlai-Gail, 1994; Csikszentmihalyi & Mei-Ha Wong, 1991; Massimini et al., 1988). In LeFevre's (1988) sample of 107 workers, 40 percent seemed content to spend their time in the apathy channel, while another 40 percent sought situations that placed a higher demand on their skills. Studies of students have suggested that for some, the desire to avoid anxiety-provoking situations is stronger than the desire to face challenges (Carli et al., 1988; Nakamura, 1988).

People who seek out flow opportunities have "autotelic personalities" (Csikszentmihalyi, 1988b). They welcome opportunities for action and are most content when involved in a challenging activity (Logan, 1988). These individuals seem to have reduced cortical activity when focused on tasks inducing the flow state (Hamilton Halcomb & Csikszentmihalyi, 1975). Kimiecik and Stein (1992) discovered that athletes with autotelic personalities were more task-oriented and less ego-oriented than those without autotelic traits. Although just about everyone has the potential for flow, individuals who are self-centered or self-conscious seem less inclined to experience flow (Csikszentmihalyi, 1988b, 1990; Logan, 1988). When people focus their thoughts on themselves, there is less energy left to devote to their activities. Csikszentmihalyi suggested that individuals with stimulus over-inclusion problems, such as schizophrenia and attention deficit disorder, lacked the ability to focus adequately on a task to experience flow (1990).

Some researchers claim that differences in the predisposition to flow are inherent (Csikszentmihalyi, 1993). The cause of these genetic differences is unclear but may relate to differences in ability to focus attention. In addition, certain conditions in a family seem to influence the child's development of "autotelic personality." These conditions may include choices; clarity of feedback; and a focus on activity, trust, and manageable challenges (Rathunde, 1988).

Flow in Adversity

Differences in the ability to achieve flow may account for differences in the ability to cope with conditions of chronic stress among people (Csikszentmihalyi, 1990; Logan, 1988). Massimini et al. (1988) studied flow among persons with visual and physical disabilities and persons who have survived extremely tragic human conditions. His team concluded that it was the ability to experience flow in everyday life that accounted for differences in the capacity to cope effectively in the face of adverse or disastrous conditions. Individuals who were able to cope most effectively transformed seemingly hopeless conditions into a series of manageable challenges with clear goals. They could report positive experiences in striving to meet these goals. They were able to find flow experiences in everyday living. When faced with adversity they followed a sequence of actions where they would scan the environment, set a goal, monitor progress, and increase the level of difficulty as they achieved success (Logan, 1988).

Flow in Everyday Life

Flow experiences can occur in everyday life when individuals engage in activities that match their skills with task demands. Flow is best seen on a continuum, rather than as an all-or-nothing phenomenon (Csikszentmihalyi, 1975). It is a subjective state that varies in intensity, depth, and strength of purpose. How often flow states occur for an individual depends on how flow is defined by the researcher (Csikszentmihalyi, 1992).

Graef (1975a) used the term "microflow activities" for trivial, sometimes automatic behavior patterns that require less skill but are intrinsically rewarding, enjoyable, and may facilitate involvement with more structured activities. He suggested that people need to involve themselves in seemingly unnecessary activities that provide activation, structure, and goals to cope with gaps in daily routine. Examples of microflow activities include doodling, jokes, foot-tapping, word games, and other noninstrumental activities.

Individuals who have been deprived of flow or microflow activities experience negative effects (Graef, 1975b). Following a 48-hour flow-deprivation experiment, college students reported feeling dull and unreasonable (Graef, 1975b). Some individuals were disorganized and had a sense of no longer being actively in control of the environment. Graef pointed out similarities between the disorganized state brought on by flow deprivation and the cognitive disorganization reported by individuals with acute schizophrenia. He suggested that microflow activities help make reality manageable and that there may be a relationship between flow and psychopathology (1975b).

While microflow falls at one end of the flow continuum, intense memorable flow experiences that are difficult to interrupt fall at the opposite end. These "deep flow" or "macroflow" experiences share features with Maslow's "peak experience" and other spiritual experiences (Csikszentmihalyi, 1975). In deep flow there is a sense of transcendence and harmony with one's surroundings. The literature has reported such experiences during rock climbing, chess, and figure skating (Csikszentmihalyi, 1975; Jackson, 1992).

Significance of Flow

The flow experience is considered vital to adaptation and growth, while constant involvement with low challenge environments leads to regression and disorganization (Logan, 1988; Massimini et al., 1987). Research has related flow to happiness, self-esteem, work productivity, role satisfaction, and satisfaction with life (Carlson & Clark, 1991; Csikszentmihalyi, 1988b, 1990, 1993; Han, 1988; Jacobs, 1994; Kipper, 1992; Logan, 1988; Massimini et al., 1988). Applications of flow theory have influenced the design of school curriculums, museums, homes for the aged, work sites, leisure products, and rehabilitation programs for juvenile delinquents (Csikszentmihalyi, 1990).

Massimini and colleagues (1987) have suggested that monitoring the experience of flow in everyday contexts could provide information applicable to psychiatric rehabilitation. They noted emotional atrophy among people with psychiatric diseases. They hypothesized that if flow theory applies to this population, then the prescription for psychiatric patients would include involvement in activities that are challenging, but do not overwhelm the individual's skills. These comments echo the sentiments of Meyer, one of the early founders of occupational therapy:

> Thus, with our patients we naturally begin with a natural simple regime of pleasurable ease, the creation of an orderly rhythm in the atmosphere....We naturally heed also the other factors—the personal interests and personal fitness....To get the pleasure and pride of achievement and use of one's hands and muscles, the feeling of worthwhileness of a little effort and of a well fitted use of time is the basic remedy for the blase tedium that characterizes the indifference or hopeless depression that stands in the way of rallying thwarted personalities. (1921/1982, p. 84)

Limitations of Flow Research

When Csikszentmihalyi (1975) first began to identify elements of flow, his intention was to eventually operationalize flow with a standardized assessment, for fear its essence might be lost (1992). Researchers have differed in their opinions about whether all elements associated with flow must be present, and whether some of these are more important to the identification of flow than others (Kimiecik & Stein, 1992). While in some studies researchers have defined flow by the performer's account of the subjective experience (Csikszentmihalyi, 1975; Sato, 1988), in others flow is operationalized by the perceived presence of certain conditions, such as a balance between challenges and skills (Carli et al., 1988; Csikszentmihalyi, 1975; LeFevre, 1988; Massimini et al., 1988).

Another limitation of flow studies is that, although flow falls somewhere on the continuum between microflow and macroflow, different researchers have used different boundaries along this continuum (Csikszentmihalyi, 1992). In addition, while some researchers have used the four-channel model to study time in flow (Wells, 1988), others have used eight channel, and 16 channel models (Carli et al., 1988; Massimini et al., 1988). Therefore, cross comparisons among experience-sampling studies require caution. Also, Wernick (1992) found that the channels used in flow studies were not sufficient to encompass all of the diverse subjective experiences of work.

Because data collection is disruptive to flow experience, descriptions are based on retrospective recall. There are very few critiques of flow in the literature. The study of flow is less than 25 years old, and much of what is written is philosophical and exploratory, without empirical evidence to support it.

Flow and the Occupational Therapy Literature

The occupational therapy literature contains some references to this construct. Howe and Schwartzberg (1988) include flow in a list of considerations for running a group, and Jacobs (1994) studied job satisfaction and flow among occupational therapy practitioners at work in physical rehabilitation settings. Jackson (1989) referred to flow studies in describing considerations for designing an independent living skills program for adolescents. In her Muriel Driver Lecture, Law (1991) discussed the connection between flow and occupational satisfaction. Flow is seen as relevant to occupational science (Primeau, Clark, & Pierce, 1990; Yerxa et al., 1990). The ESM was described by Carlson and Clark (1991) as an innovative method for naturalistic research. Finally, do Rozario (1994) discussed flow in terms of changing societies and the belief that deep flow and spiritual experiences came more naturally through occupation in traditional societies than in modern technological societies. Although flow has been discussed as a useful construct, it has not been well examined in the occupational therapy literature.

Relevance of Flow to Occupational Therapy

The study of flow is important to occupational therapists because it "names and frames" a phenomenon consistent with the fundamental beliefs of the occupational therapy profession (Carlson & Clark, 1991; Schon, 1982; Yerxa et al., 1990). Naming and framing permit discussion and study of a phenomenon. The autotelic, or intrinsically motivating, nature of this experience is congruent with the conviction that activity is rewarding in itself and that "occupation gives meaning to life" (Polatajko, 1992, p. 1923). The philosophy underlying occupational therapy includes the belief that the experience of becoming absorbed in a "just-right challenge" is therapeutic and influential to one's overall sense of well-being (Yerxa et al., 1990). If occupational therapists can understand more about the properties and conditions of the flow experience, they can help in the client's discovery of occupations that are intrinsically motivating and that promote this sense of well-being and meaning.

The following principles, extracted from the literature on flow, may be useful to occupational therapy practitioners in helping clients engage in activities that may induce flow:

1. The client's own perception of his or her capabilities, and of the challenges inherent in the task, must be appreciated by the occupational therapy practitioner as indicators of the complexity which may provide the "just-right challenge."

2. The occupational therapy practitioner may solicit descriptions of experiences that the client found enjoyable in the past. Exploration and analysis of these accounts may clarify whether the constructs of enjoyment and flow are synonymous, and uncover information about the conditions that induce enjoyment and/or flow for the client.

3. The client should have a clear sense of the goals of the task and feel in control of these requirements. The practitioner should ensure that the requirements of the task are clear to the client and that the client is able to set his or her own standards for success.

4. The outcomes must be meaningful to the client. The practitioner may explore the client's values, needs, and interests for cues about what challenges may be meaningful to the individual.

5. Consistent feedback on performance of tasks must be available. The client must be able to see the connection between his or her performance and outcomes of these actions.

6. The practitioner must continually observe the client for signs of boredom or anxiety and adjust task demands to increase or decrease the level of challenge perceived by the client.

7. To induce flow, the client must have opportunities to focus deeply on the task. Thus, the environment may need to be adapted to eliminate other demands on his or her energy and attention.

8. The potential for flow varies from person to person, and for each person it varies across time. The practitioner should keep in mind that the individual may have more pressing concerns, for example, needs related to safety, security, and avoidance of anxiety.

Areas for Future Research

In 1960 Reilly said, "For us, in occupational therapy, the most fundamental area for research is, and probably will always be, the nature and meaning of activity" (p. 208). Several questions are crucial to the understanding of flow and its place in occupational science and occupational therapy: Can everybody experience flow? Is flow experienced differently by certain groups of people than by others? What conditions promote and inhibit flow for our clients? How do flow experiences affect rehabilitation outcomes? How do flow experiences affect health and well-being among persons with disabilities? Do people who frequently experience flow differ in occupational adaptation from those who do not? Are people with stimulus inclusion problems really unable to experience flow? If so, what are the consequences of genuine, long-term flow deprivation?

Given occupational therapy's concern for the impact of occupation on human beings, and the availability of innovative techniques for naturalistic data collection, the time is right for us to explore these questions. The answers may provide support for the philosophical foundation of our profession and lead us in directions that can improve the subjective occupational experience of our clients.

Acknowledgments

The author is indebted to Dr. Joanne Valiant Cook, Associate Professor in the School of Occupational Therapy at the University of Western Ontario, for her editorial and content suggestions for this paper.

References

Adlai-Gail, W. (1994). Exploring the autotelic personality (competence). DAI-B 55/4, p. 1684. [CD-ROM]. Abstract from: ProQuest File: Dissertation Abstracts Item: AAC 9425350.

American Occupational Therapy Association. (1993). Position paper: Purposeful activity. *American Journal of Occupational Therapy, 47,* 1081–1082.

Baum, C. (1985). Growth, renewal, and challenge: An important era for occupational therapy. *American Journal of Occupational Therapy, 39,* 778–784.

Breines, E. (1984). The Issue Is: An attempt to define purposeful activity. *American Journal of Occupational Therapy, 38,* 543–544.

Carli, M., Delle Fave, A., & Massimini, F. (1988). The quality of experience in the flow channels: Comparison of Italian and U.S. students. In M. Csikszentmihalyi & I. Csikszentmihalyi (Eds.), *Optimal experience: Psychological studies of flow in consciousness* (pp. 288–306). Cambridge, UK: Cambridge University Press.

Carlson, M., & Clark, F. (1991). The search for useful methodologies in occupational science. *American Journal of Occupational Therapy, 49,* 235–241.

Csikszentmihalyi, I. (1988). Flow in historical context: The case of the Jesuits. In M. Csikszentmihalyi & I. Csikszentmihalyi (Eds.), *Optimal experience: Psychological studies of flow in consciousness* (pp. 232–247). Cambridge, UK: Cambridge University Press.

Csikszentmihalyi, M. (Ed.). (1975). *Beyond boredom and anxiety: The experience of play in work and games.* San Francisco, CA: Jossey-Bass.

Csikszentmihalyi, M. (1988a). The flow experience and its significance for human psychology. In M. Csikszentmihalyi & I. Csikszentmihalyi (Eds.), *Optimal experience: Psychological studies of flow in consciousness* (p. 15–35). Cambridge, UK: Cambridge University Press.

Csikszentmihalyi, M. (1988b). Introduction. In M. Csikszentmihalyi & I. Csikszentmihalyi (Eds.), *Optimal experience: Psychological studies of flow in consciousness* (pp. 3–14). Cambridge, UK: Cambridge University Press.

Csikszentmihalyi, M. (1988c). The future of flow. In M. Csikszentmihalyi & I. Csikszentmihalyi (Eds.), *Optimal experience: Psychological studies of flow in consciousness* (pp. 364–383). Cambridge, UK: Cambridge University Press.

Csikszentmihalyi, M. (1990). *Flow: The psychology of optimal experience.* New York: Harper & Row.

Csikszentmihalyi, M. (1992). A response to the Kimiecik & Stein and Jackson Papers. *Journal of Applied Sport Psychology, 4,* 181–183.

Csikszentmihalyi, M. (1993). Activity and happiness: Toward a science of occupation. *Australian Journal of Occupational Science, 1*(1), 38–42.

Csikszentmihalyi, M., & Csikszentmihalyi, I. (1988). Introduction to part IV. In M. Csikszentmihalyi & I. Csikszentmihalyi (Eds.), *Optimal experience: Psychological studies of flow in consciousness* (pp. 251–265). Cambridge, UK: Cambridge University Press.

Csikszentmihalyi, M., & Larson, R. (1984). *Being adolescent: Conflict and growth in the teenage years.* New York: Basic Books.

Csikszentmihalyi, M., & Larson, R. (1987). Validity and reliability of the experience-sampling method. *Journal of Nervous and Mental Disease, 1975,* 526–535.

Csikszentmihalyi, M., & Mei-Ha Wong, M. (1991). The situational and personal correlates of happiness: A cross-national comparison. In F. Strack, M. Argyle, & N. Schwartz (Eds.), *Subjective well-being* (pp. 193–212). Toronto, ON: Pergammon Press.

Cynkin, S., & Robinson, A. (1990). *Occupational therapy and activities health: Toward health through activities.* Boston, MA: Little, Brown.

Delle Fave, A., & Massimini, F. (1988). Modernization and the changing contexts of flow in work and leisure. In M. Csikszentmihalyi & I. Csikszentmihalyi (Eds.), *Optimal experience: Psychological studies of flow in consciousness* (pp. 193–213). Cambridge, UK: Cambridge University Press.

do Rozario, L. (1994). Ritual, meaning, and transcendence: The role of occupation in modern life. *Australian Journal of Occupational Science, 1,* 46–53.

Evans, K. (1987). Nationally speaking: Definition of occupation as the core concept of occupational therapy. *American Journal of Occupational Therapy, 41,* 627–628.

Fidler, G., & Fidler, J. (1978). Doing and becoming: Purposeful action and self-actualization. *American Journal of Occupational Therapy, 31,* 305–310. Reprinted as Chapter 9.

Graef, R. (1975a). Flow patterns in everyday life. In M. Csikszentmihalyi (Ed.), *Beyond boredom and anxiety: The experience of play in work and games* (pp. 140–160). San Francisco, CA: Jossey-Bass.

Graef, R. (1975b). Effects of flow deprivation. In M. Csikszentmihalyi (Ed.), *Beyond boredom and anxiety: The experience of play in work and games* (pp. 161–178). San Francisco, CA: Jossey-Bass.

Hamilton Halcomb, J., & Csikszentmihalyi, M. (1975). Enjoying work: Surgery. In M. Csikszentmihalyi (Ed.), *Beyond boredom and anxiety: The experience of play in work and games* (pp. 123–139). San Francisco, CA: Jossey-Bass.

Han, S. (1988). The relationship between life satisfaction and flow in elderly Korean immigrants. In M. Csikszentmihalyi & I. Csikszentmihalyi (Eds.), *Optimal experience: Psychological studies of flow in consciousness* (pp. 138–171). Cambridge, UK: Cambridge University Press.

Howe, M., & Schwartzberg, S. (1988). Structure and process in designing a functional group. *Occupational Therapy in Mental Health, 8*(3), 1–8.

Jackson, J. (1989). En route to adulthood: A high school transition program for adolescents with disabilities. *Occupational Therapy in Health Care, 6*(4), 33–51.

Jackson, S. (1992). Athletes in flow: A qualitative investigation of flow states in elite figure skaters. *Journal of Applied Sport Psychology, 4,* 161–180.

Jacobs, K. (1994). Flow and the occupational therapy practitioner. *American Journal of Occupational Therapy, 48,* 989–996.

Johnson, J., & Yerxa, E. (Eds.) (1989). *Occupational science: The foundation for new models of practice.* Binghamton, NY: Haworth Press.

Kielhofner, G. (1981). An ethnographic study of deinstitutionalized adults: Their community settings and daily experience. *Occupational Therapy Journal of Research, 1,* 135–141.

Kielhofner, G. (1982). Qualitative research: Part two: Methodological approaches and relevance to occupational therapy. *Occupational Therapy Journal of Research, 2,* 150–164.

Kielhofner, G. (1992). *Conceptual foundations of occupational therapy.* Philadelphia, PA: F.A. Davis.

Kimiecik, I., & Stein, G. (1992). Examining flow experiences in sports context: Conceptual issues and methodological concerns. *Journal of Applied Sport Psychology, 4,* 141–160.

Kipper, D. (1992). The dynamics of role satisfaction: A theoretical model. *Group Psychotherapy, Psychodrama, and Sociometry, 44,* 71–86.

Kremer, E., Nelson, D., & Duncombe, L. (1984). Effects of selected activities on affective meaning in psychiatric patients. *American Journal of Occupational Therapy, 38,* 522–528.

Laliberte, D. (1993). *An exploration into the meaning seniors attach to activity.* Unpublished master's thesis. London, ON: University of Western Ontario.

Law, M. (1991). Muriel Driver Lecture. The environment: A focus for occupational therapy. *Canadian Journal of Occupational Therapy, 58,* 171–179.

LeFevre, J. (1988). Flow and the quality of experience during work and leisure. In M. Csikszentmihalyi & I. Csikszentmihalyi (Eds.), *Optimal experience: Psychological studies of flow in consciousness* (pp. 307–318). Cambridge, UK: Cambridge University Press.

Levine, R. (1987). The influence of the arts-and-crafts movement on the professional status of occupational therapy. *American Journal of Occupational Therapy, 45,* 248–254. Reprinted as Chapter 3.

Logan, P. (1988). Flow in solitary ordeals. In M. Csikszentmihalyi & I. Csikszentmihalyi (Eds.). *Optimal experience: Psychological studies of flow in consciousness* (pp. 172–180). Cambridge, UK: Cambridge University Press.

Massimini, A., Carli, M., & Csikszentmihalyi, M. (1988). Systematic assessment of flow in daily experience. In M. Csikszentmihalyi & I. Csikszentmihalyi (Eds.), *Optimal experience: Psychological studies of flow in consciousness* (pp. 266–281). Cambridge, UK: Cambridge University Press.

Massimini, A., Csikszentmihalyi, M., & Carli, M. (1987). The monitoring of optimal experience, *Journal of Nervous and Mental Disease, 1975,* 545–549.

Massimini, F., Csikszentmihalyi, M., & Delle Fave, A. (1988). Flow and bio-cultural evolution. In M. Csikszentmihalyi & I. Csikszentmihalyi (Eds.), *Optimal experience: Psychological studies of flow in consciousness* (pp. 60–81). Cambridge, UK: Cambridge University Press.

Merrill, S. (1985). Qualitative methods in occupational therapy research: An application. *Occupational Therapy Journal of Research, 5,* 213–222.

Meyer, A. (1922/1982). Worth repeating: The philosophy of occupational therapy. *Occupational Therapy in Mental Health, 2,* 79–86. Reprinted as Chapter 2.

Nakamura, J. (1988). Optimal experience and the uses of talent. In M. Csikszentmihalyi & I. Csikszentmihalyi (Eds.), *Optimal experience: Psychological studies of flow in consciousness* (pp. 319–326). Cambridge, UK: Cambridge University Press.

Park, H. (1995). *Occupation, well-being, and women with rheumatoid arthritis.* Unpublished master's thesis. London, ON: University of Western Ontario.

Polatajko, H. (1992). Muriel Driver Lecture: Naming and framing occupational therapy: A lecture dedicated to the life of Nancy B. *Canadian Journal of Occupational Therapy, 59,* 189–192.

Primeau, L., Clark, F., & Pierce, D. (1989). Occupational therapy alone has looked upon occupation: Future applications of occupational science to pediatric occupational therapy. *Occupational Therapy in Health Care, 6,*(4), 19–32.

Rathunde, K. (1988). Optimal experience and the family context. In M. Csikszentmihalyi & I. Csikszentmihalyi (Eds.), *Optimal experience: Psychological studies of flow in consciousness* (pp. 342–363). Cambridge, UK: Cambridge University Press.

Reilly, M. (1960). Research potentiality of occupational therapy. *American Journal of Occupational Therapy, 14,* 206–209.

Sato, I. (1988). Bosozoku: Flow in Japanese motorcycle gangs. In M. Csikszentmihalyi & I. Csikszentmihalyi. (Eds.), *Optimal experience:*

Psychological studies of flow in consciousness (pp. 92–117). Cambridge, UK: Cambridge University Press.

Schon, D. (1982). *The reflective practitioner.* New York: Basic Books.

Steinmetz, H. (1995). *Occupational performance and life satisfaction among community-dwelling stroke clients: A pilot study.* Unpublished master's thesis. London, ON: University of Western Ontario.

Wells, A. (1988). Self-esteem and optimal experience. In M. Csikszentmihalyi & I. Csikszentmihalyi. (Eds.), *Optimal experience: Psychological studies of flow in consciousness* (pp. 327–341). Cambridge, UK: Cambridge University Press.

Wernick, R. (1990). Work: An analysis of subjective work experience utilizing Cikszentmihalyi's theory of play. [CD-ROM]. DAI-A 51/06, p. 2173, Dec. 1990. Abstract from ProQuest File: Dissertation Abstracts Item: AAC 9033369.

Wiemer, R. (1979). Traditional and nontraditional practice arenas. In American Occupational Therapy Association (Ed.), *Occupational therapy 2001* (pp. 43–53). Rockville, MD: author.

Yerxa, E. (1980). Occupational therapy's role in creating a future climate of caring. *American Journal of Occupational Therapy, 34,* 529–534.

Yerxa, E., Clark, F., Frank, G., Jackson, J., Parfiam, D., Pierce, D., Stein, C., & Zemke, R. (1990). An introduction to occupational science: A foundation for occupational therapy in the 21st century. In J. Johnson & E. Yerxa (Eds.), *Occupational science: The foundation for new models of practice.* Binghamton, NY: Haworth Press.

Spirit, Occupation, and Disability

MURIEL DRIVER MEMORIAL LECTURE

CHAPTER 24

MARY ANN McCOLL, PHD, OT(C)

As the topic for my Muriel Driver Memorial Lecture, I have chosen spirituality—a topic that has been much in the spotlight in recent years. A few years ago, in the process of collaborating in research on spirituality and disability with colleagues from theology, philosophy, and pastoral care, I began to take courses in theology as a means of obtaining some theoretical preparation for further work of this kind. But it was a personal story from a friend that confirmed my resolve to address this topic in my lecture. The story involved a group of old friends who got together for dinner once a month. About a year ago, one of the group revealed that she was ill and didn't know how much longer she would be able to join them for dinner. So they began meeting at her house instead and bringing dinner in. As the months passed, these evenings became understandably more difficult. Then one night, one of the friends asked if it would be alright if she said a prayer. After a number of sideways glances and much shuffling of feet, the group agreed that it would be alright. Then, according to my friend, something happened— everyone in the room knew it, but no one could adequately describe it later. I knew what the theological explanation would be: that by means of prayer, spirit was invoked. In other words, something mysterious and otherworldly was experienced as a function of "spirit." It occurred to me that this was a different spirit from the one we talk about in occupational therapy. It took me down a road of exploring this difference, and sharing with you what I have learned.

Specifically, the lecture will address three things:

1. How we have defined spirituality and related concepts in occupational therapy;
2. What we know about the spiritual aspects of living with a disability; and
3. What we are doing or might do in occupational therapy in the spiritual realm of practice.

To guide my discussion, I have consulted four bodies of information that I will try to bring together:

1. As part of a project funded by the Fetter Institute, we interviewed 16 people with recently acquired disabilities about spiritual issues that might have arisen for them since the onset of their disability (see Table 24.1). We spoke with 12 men and four women, with an average age of 40, and an average duration of disability of 23 months, all of whom had had a traumatic-onset disability (spinal cord injury or brain injury) and had been discharged from rehabilitation up to 2 years (McColl et al., 2000).
2. As an adjunct to that study, we collected information from 40 occupational therapists across the country about how spirituality was expressed in their practice. The sample was recruited randomly from the CAOT membership list and had an average of 9.5 years of experience working in occupational therapy. Of 112 initially approached by mail, 36 (32 percent) responded saying they did not want to participate, 31 (28 percent) did not respond, and five could not be located at the address we had. The study addressed the questions in Table 24.1.
3. The literature in occupational therapy and other health disciplines provides a contemporary snapshot of spirituality as it is conceptualized and discussed by occupational therapists.
4. Finally, there is a wealth of literature in theology on spirit and spirituality and a growing body on spirituality as it relates to health and disability.

Objective 1: Definitions

Spirituality

Before I go any further, I will address the definition of spirituality. To date, we have insisted on a secular definition of spirituality in occupational therapy (Canadian Association of Occupational Therapists, 1997; Townsend, DeLaat, Egan,

Table 24.1. Study Questions for Two Spirituality Studies

Disability Study Questions:
1. Would you describe yourself as a spiritual person?
2. Has your understanding of yourself changed since you acquired your disability?
3. Have your relationships with others changed since your disability?
4. Has your way of viewing the world changed since your disability?
5. Have your beliefs changed since the onset of your disability?
6. Have your religious practices changed?
7. Has your soul or spirit been affected by your disability?

Occupational Therapy Study Questions:
1. In your practice as an occupational therapist:
   - Do you see evidence of the spiritual aspect of your patients?
   - Have you seen people whose understanding of themselves has changed when they acquired a disability?
   - Have you seen people whose relationships with others have changed after the onset?
   - Have you seen people whose way of viewing the world had changed after the onset?
   - Have you seen people whose belief in a Supreme Being or higher power changed?
   - Have you seen people whose religious practices changed after the onset of a disability?
2. Do you feel adequately prepared to deal with these issues when they arise with your patients?

Thibeault, & Wright, 1999). This secularity is a reflection of a number of 20th-century trends that have had similar effects on most of the health professions (do Rozario, 1994; Falardeau, 1997; Kroeker, 1997; McSherry & Draper, 1998):

- Religion has been shifted from a public to a private focus (privatization);
- Science has displaced religion as the source of ultimate answers (rationalism);
- Confidence in human beings has surpassed confidence in a supreme being in many instances (humanism);
- The focus on individual rights has overtaken the focus on community responsibilities (individualism);
- Waves of immigration have created a heterogeneous, multiethnic North American society (pluralism); and
- We have become increasingly tolerant of differences, including religious differences (liberalism).

We can point to a number of indicators in occupational therapy of how current practice continues to be influenced by these trends, such as evidence-based practice, belief in the worth and value of all persons, client-centred practice, and a secular approach to spirituality.

However, secular can mean two things:

- To some it means not dependent on any particular faith tradition or religious belief; that is, not explicitly religious;
- To others, it means strictly of this world, observable, tangible, not sacred or mysterious (Kroeker, 1997).

I suggest that in occupational therapy, when we talk about a secular approach to spirituality, we mean to say the former. We mean for our definition of spirituality to be inclusive of all faiths and beliefs and inclusive even of those people who do not adhere to a particular faith tradition (Townsend et al., 1999; Urbanowski & Vargo, 1994). However, in an effort to preserve the liberal pluralism that marked the development of our profession over the past century, we may have gone too far. In our efforts to be inclusive on religious grounds, we appear to have ended up with a definition of spirituality that is evacuated of its mysterious, sacred, supernatural content (Collins, 1998; Howard & Howard, 1997; Vrkijan, 2000).

I'm going to ask you to proceed with me on the basis of a very simple definition of spirituality: Spirituality is "sensitivity to the presence of spirit." According to this definition, spirituality is a quality that human beings possess to a greater or lesser degree, that allows them to be aware of the presence of spirit (Toole-Mitchell, 1999). There are two things I like about this definition: it is simple and easy to carry around and, it distinguishes between spirituality, which is a quality of humans, and spirit, which I suggest is not. This brings us to two considerably thornier questions: What, then, is spirit? And how do we experience spirit?

Spirit

First, what is spirit? Colloquial uses of the term "spirit" are listed in Table 24.2 to illustrate the many different ideas that are associated with it. The dictionary listed no less than 20 definitions of spirit, but one that serves our purpose is the following: Spirit is "the force that animates the body of living things" (Emblen, 1992). The dictionary also offered an interesting insight based on etymology—that the word "spirit" derives from the Latin for breath (Emblem, 1992; Enquist, Short-DeGraff, Gliner, & Oltejenbruns, 1997). This derivation squares with what the theological literature says about spirit—that like breath, spirit is something:

- That is shared among humans, with other creatures, and with the natural world;
- That we use and pass on;
- That enters us and is transformed, but not diminished;
- That we become aware of only fleetingly in our day-to-day lives.

Whereas spirituality is a human characteristic, spirit is not. Spirit is something that exists independent of us and can be incorporated into our lives to a greater or lesser extent, depending on the extent to which we are able to experience it—that is, depending on the extent of our spirituality.

Transcendence

So how do we experience spirit? Many of the definitions found in the health science literature talk about the senses, the emotions, and the intellect as the vehicles through which we experience spirit. However, the theological literature offers another

Table 24.2. Colloquial Uses of the Term Spirit and Ideas Associated With Them

Colloquial Use	Related Ideas
• Keep your spirits up	• Energy
• She was a very spiritied child	• Will
• Triumph of the human spirit	• Resilience, unassailability, indomitability
• Have some team spirit	• Comraderie
• I'll be there in spirit	• Not constrained by time and space
• Entering the world of the spirit	• Mysterious
• The Holy Spirit or divine spirit	• Sacred
• His spirit was broken	• Humanity
• If the spirit moves you	• Motivation
• The spirit is willing, but the flesh is weak	• Embodied
• She was spirited away	• Secretive
• It's not in the spirit of our agreement	• Essential
• An ounce of spirits	• Alcohol-related
• Light a spirit lamp	• Alcohol-related

possibility. It suggests that we do not experience spirit through the usual human channels, but rather through transcendence; that is, an experience that goes beyond normal human experience (Christiansen, 1997; Reed, 1992; Ross, 1995; Thibeault, 1997; Thibodaux, 1998; Van Amburg, 1997). We may use the senses, the emotions—they may feel like wonder, fear, attraction, awe, mystery, uncanny coincidence. But in fact the experience itself defies expression. We have no language to describe the experience of transcendence. Instead we use symbols and metaphors as bridges between what we can know and understand, and what we cannot (McFague, 1982; Richards, 1997; Sontag, 1977).

Peloquin (1997) offers a metaphor that I found very helpful for understanding transcendence. She likens it to those mysterious Magic Eye puzzles on the back page of the weekend section of the paper, that you have to hold up to your face to be able to see into the third dimension of the picture. Like transcendence, the third dimension of the Magic Eye puzzle is not immediately obvious to the casual onlooker—the picture looks flat, two-dimensional. However, if you can shut down your normal focusing apparatus and learn to see in a new way, suddenly the third dimension or the depth of the picture becomes clear. But as soon as you try to actually look at it, using your normal focusing apparatus, it disappears again. The first few times you try it, it is difficult to see anything except the flat picture. However, if you do it every Saturday, it gets easier, until you can flip into the third dimension with only a few seconds of holding the paper up to your nose!

Transcendent experiences are like that too. I'm sure you are aware of times when you could "see into the third dimension" of a situation or experience, but as soon as you tried to study, analyze, or capture it, it was gone. You were aware that some-

thing unusual and mysterious had happened, but when you tried to describe it, simulate it, or repeat it, it was gone. Some theologians would say that those experiences were glimpses into the eternal, infinite, unknowable realm of spirit; that they connect us, even if only fleetingly, with the whole cosmos and perhaps also with a supreme being (Collins 1998; Toomey, 1999). Further they would say that spirituality is the human capacity to recognize those experiences when they happen, and, just like with the Magic Eye puzzles, it gets easier the more you do it.

Themes About Spirituality

The occupational therapy literature emphasizes at least four themes in talking about spirituality:

* That spirituality entails an innate knowledge of the essence of the self;
* That it is the source of our will, intention, self-determination;
* That it is responsible for the connection among people;
* That it invests our daily occupations with meaning. (CAOT, 1997; Egan & DeLaat, 1997; Enquist et al., 1997; Townsend et al., 1999).

I would like to try to reinterpret these ideas in light of the three definitions that I have offered for spirituality, spirit, and transcendence.

The Essence of the Self

The occupational therapy literature suggests that spirituality is the essence of the self (CAOT, 1997; Collins, 1998; Egan & DeLaat, 1994, 1997; Vrkljan, 2000). It entails a clear sense of who the self is, a strong positive identity or self-image, and a view of the self as an intact whole. The idea of an essence comes from Plato; it refers to the idea that there is a perfect image of every creature that is its essence, and throughout its life, it tries to discover and live up to this essence.

But what if we believed that the spirit was shared rather than possessed by the self, and that spirituality was about transcendence rather than introspection? Then spirituality would not be about the essence of the self but rather about the ability to transcend the self and to recognize the possibility of a power greater than the self (Bing, 1997; Lindsel 1996; Moyers, 1997; Thibeault, 1997). Several authors describe illness as a distortion of the importance of the self and an undue emphasis on how the world relates to the self (Moyers, 1997; Reed, 1992; Watkins, 1997). Spirituality on the other hand, allows the individual to perceive the self in the context of the grander scheme, in relation to the cosmos as a whole, and even perhaps as a reflection of a divine will (Bing, 1997; Watkins, 1997).

The Source of Will and Intention

A second theme that I discovered in the literature on spirituality in the health field was that spirituality was the source of our will, that it motivated and impelled us, that it was an internal drive (CAOT, 1997; Gutterman, 1990). These concepts strike me as dangerously close to psychological concepts, and in fact several authors cautioned against interpreting spirituality in this way for that very reason (Townsend et al., 1999; Urbanowski & Vargo, 1994).

However, if we agreed that spirit is not within the person, but instead is an energy that passes between people and the world, then we might see it as transformative and inspirational, rather than simply motivational. I suggest that spirit acts through us, rather than in us. That is not to say that our free will is compromised by spirit, but that our potential is enhanced by it.

Responsible for the Connection Among People

There are many references in the literature to the fact that spirit is the part of us that connects with other people (CAOT, 1997; Lindsey, 1996; Soeken & Carson, 1987). But what if spirit is not a part of us at all, but rather the force that dissolves the boundaries between the self and others, and helps us to realize that other people and other parts of the world are real? The late Iris Murdoch said that one of the hardest things for us to do is to realize that "something other than oneself is real" (1959, p. 51). In our day-to-day lives, we experience this realization only fleetingly, and like other transcendent experiences, the moment we try to objectify and analyze it, the experience is gone (Buber, 1970).

One of the ways that the spiritual connection among people is expressed is the quest to seek spiritual answers together, to express our spirituality communally, and to extend social justice and liberation to all (BarbWire Collective, 1997;

Egan & DeLaat, 1997; Horsburgh, 1997; Robinson, 1994; Townsend, 1997).

The Source of Meaning

Finally, the occupational therapy literature gives pride of place to the concept of meaning in discussions of spirituality (CAOT, 1997; Christiansen, 1997; Rose, 1999; Tryssenaar, Jones, & Lee, 1999); that is, specific cognitive interpretations of events or circumstances (Fife, 1994). Not only does spirituality invest activities with meaning, but also meaningful activities express spirituality. We distinguish between meaning IN life (or lower-order meaning), referring to specific activities and the meanings they carry, and the meaning OF life (or higher-order meaning), referring to the meaning of one's whole life (do Rozario, 1994; Smith, 1995; Urbanowski & Vargo, 1994).

However, if we speak specifically of the opportunity for transcendence in everyday activities, then we recognize that meaning is not a characteristic of specific activities. Rather meaning derives from the opportunity to see universal truths in specific activities, to obtain a view of the whole cosmos in relation to a particular daily pattern of life, and to see one's life as a whole in relation to the grander scheme of things (Thibodaux, 1998). Sir William Osler (in Bing, 1997) talked about "appreciation for the poetry of the commonplace," and I think this is what he meant—that commonplace activities and occupations can afford us a view of the presence of spirit that is beyond our senses, but within our spiritual capacity.

Spirituality and Disability

From the perspective of occupational therapy, there are at least two aspects of spirit in which we might be interested:

- Spirituality among people with disabilities, and
- Spirituality as it is experienced through occupation.

To date, the occupational therapy literature has focused primarily on the latter, and I will come back to this, but let me begin by assembling some ideas about spirituality and disability. First of all, why should we be interested in the spiritual aspect of life with a disability? For a number of reasons, disability evokes spiritual searching and reflection:

1. The sheer magnitude of the question about why this happened and why it happened to a particular individual defies simple, deterministic explanations (Droege, 1991). The disability and its implications are so pervasive and overwhelming that they impel individuals to seek meaning in spiritual terms; that is, to seek answers in the realm of the mysterious, the unknown, or the unexplainable (Fitcher, 1981; Narayanasamy, 1996; Toombs, 1995).
2. Often, disability brings individuals closer either to death itself or to the idea of death. Just as the proximity of death

in old age often raises existential questions (Berggren-Thomas & Griggs, 1995; Clark et al., 1996; Ross, 1995; Young, 1993), a disability may also act as a catalyst for the search to understand the finitude of life in terms of the infinite (Droege, 1991; Fitzgerald, 1997; Toombs, 1995; Young, 1984).

3. Disability may separate individuals from the capacities that previously permitted them to experience and express spirit (Bowers, 1987; Howard & Howard, 1997; Ross, 1995; Soeken & Carson, 1987; Vanier, 1998; Zola, 1982). It may thereby render them cut off from their previous sources of spiritual life. Even if the pursuit of spiritual development had not been a high priority prior to the onset of disability, its loss may be an impetus for a search for meaning.

4. Finally, it has been suggested that events like the onset of disability arouse doubts in our assumptions about the essential goodness of the world (BarbWire Collective, 1997; Fine, 1991 [see Chapter 25]; Frankl, 1984; Young, 1984). C.S. Lewis (1962), in his exploration of the meaning of pain, suggested that the existence of illness, disability, and death challenges our view that the world is an orderly, just, and good place. In order to restore meaning in the chaos of disability, individuals are often impelled to a re-examination of basic beliefs and a renewed search for meaning (Fitcher, 1981; Lewis, 1962; Tryssenaar et al., 1999; Yancey, 1990).

In our own research and that of others, we have seen evidence of the spiritual aspect of disability. Participants in our study said to us over and over again that they had "never really thought about the things we were asking them, but ..." and then proceeded to produce an extremely cogent and thoughtful response to even the most abstract questions.

They expressed:

- Appreciation for the people who had helped them and stuck by them;
- Hopes for the future, as well as fears about what they might face;
- Questions and thoughts about a divine presence, which some called God and others called by other names;
- Candid awareness of the presence and proximity of death (McColl et al., 2000; McColl et al., in press; Smith, 1999).

Referring to both our interviews with people with disabilities and to the literature, it seems that there are at least four ways in which individuals experience spirit when disability overtakes their world.

1. Disability as reminder of humanity:

One way that spirit was experienced by our participants in relation to their disability was as a reminder of their physical vulnerability and mortality (Barnard, 1995; Bogdan & Taylor, 1993; Eiesland, 1994; Soeken & Carson, 1987).

Many of the interviewees stated that as a result of their injury, they recognized that they were not invincible or immortal; they had a new understanding of their own humanity and mortality.

> "I have to understand that it has happened, and that I'm just a human being, and somewhere there is an end to me, somewhere down the line. So I feel I understand myself as humanity, as human, not being invincible."

> "The major thing is I'm not indestructible any more. Before, I would do things that any other person would call crazy, just to make people laugh, and not care about myself or whether I got hurt. I would just do it. Now I'm more cautious. I actually think before I do stuff."

2. Disability as mission:

Another possible perspective is the idea that the disability is accompanied by a special purpose or mission (Sanford, 1997). Most commonly, participants told us that the purpose of their lives had changed as a result of the injury. Often they did not yet know exactly what their new purpose was, but there was a sense that it would be revealed with time. Some participants stated that they did not have a purpose before their injury, but now did as a result of the disability:

> "I just believe I was saved for a purpose—to help somebody or to do something. There is actually a reason for me to be here. I'm not just a statistic—another brain injury file. I'm here for a purpose."

> "(A member of my community) says that my purpose in life now is to get better and to help others that have brain injuries. I need to go and talk to them, because I understand what they've been through."

3. Disability as punishment:

It is clear that some people experience spirit in the face of disability as a moral judgement on a life not properly lived (Droege, 1991; Low, 1997; Ohsberg, 1982; Selway & Ashman, 1998):

> "I take it as a punishment in a way, for a lot of things I've done wrong. I look at it as the way God has of repaying."

The implication of this view is that the disabled individual lives not only with the difficulties imposed by the disability, but also with some combination of confusion, guilt, and shame:

- Confusion about what they have done wrong to deserve such a punishment;
- Guilt for whatever wrong-doing they are being punished for, and
- Shame as a result of the evidence provided by the disability for all to see (Murphy, 1990).

4. Disability as a warning:

Another possible experience that our participants related was the understanding of the disability as a warning (Young, 1984). As the quotes illustrate, some felt that a mysterious, universal force was sending them a very personalized message to make a change:

> "Just as long as you live a normal life and do the right things, then life will be okay. But if you start to get off the track, that's when He steps in and makes a correction."

> "Something had to slow me down. Before my accident, I was in the fast lane. I was gung-ho to go somewhere, but I don't know where it was. Something had to come along to slow me down."

This message seems to have been received with a combination of chagrin and gratitude. Unlike the punishment theme just discussed, this message appears to have been greeted with an acknowledgement of its inevitability and appreciation for the care for which it provides evidence.

Spirituality and Occupation

Finally, how do we as professional occupational therapists deal with this issue of spirituality? The therapists we talked to offered a very consistent picture of their feelings about the spiritual aspect of therapy. They were consistent in their recognition of spirituality as an important aspect of occupation and of occupational therapy (Baptiste, 1997; CAOT, 1997; Enquist et al, 1997; Rose, 1999). They were aware of its position in the Canadian model (CAOT, 1997), and to a large extent unquestioning of the centrality of spirituality for human occupation:

> "Our own occupational performance model talks about spirituality as being the central core to being able to understand a person and enabling a person to participate in occupations in everyday life"

> "It's part of a therapist's overall perspective on things."

However that was in theory—in practice, the topic of spirituality invoked admissions of guilt, embarrassment, and ambivalence:

> "I find that when we get into those deeper issues, I sometimes feel like I've gone too far. I don't feel like I've got the experience or background to really delve into it as much as some people would like you to."

> "I'm probably not comfortable asking it, because I'm not asking about it. It's the same as asking people about their sexuality"

> "I never bring it up—I guess that makes me a bad OT, because I'm not using the CAOT formula."

> "It's kind of a hard thing to bring up. They might kind of wonder what this is all about, because there are a lot of

misconceptions around spirituality and religion, and they may think you are some kind of religious person .... So it almost seems like it's taboo."

The therapists who agreed to talk to us reported uniformly that they had not had adequate preparation in their occupational therapy education to allow them to feel comfortable talking about spirituality (Antolikova, 1999; Rose, 1999). They reported that their preparation was too brief; too vague; given by people without adequate credentials; and not sufficiently practical. They indicated that they needed more information about other religions, language, and terminology for talking about spirituality and basic ideas or tenets pertaining to spirituality:

> "It's always in the models—they mention it, so you are always thinking about it, but I can't think of anything offhand (that I learned in school)."

> "Personally and professionally, I don't think I have any expertise to offer them in that area."

> "I don't recall it ever really being addressed directly as to how you would look at that. It was one of those things that you were always supposed to consider, but then what...?"

However, in spite of this, both the therapists we talked to, and the literature reviewed, gave some practical and helpful ideas about what therapists were doing or could do in practice.

Assessment

As regards assessment, we asked therapists specifically about how spirituality came up in their practice, how they were aware of it, and how it was initially addressed. Their responses formed the continuum shown in Figure 24.1. There were some therapists who brought it up directly:

- They asked clients about their faith tradition and religious practices, usually from the perspective of whether or not the disability might inhibit their ability to worship or practice their faith (Bryant, 1993).
- Another direct approach involved asking people who they thought was in control, if there was a reason things happened the way they did, if the disability had a purpose for them or happened for a reason.
- Another direct approach had to do with the source of strength, where people derived their inner strength, what allowed them to go on from day to day in the face of their difficulties.

Other therapists reported that they brought spirituality up indirectly, by:

- "Giving permission" for clients to raise spiritual issues;
- Creating an environment that was conducive to spiritual discussions.

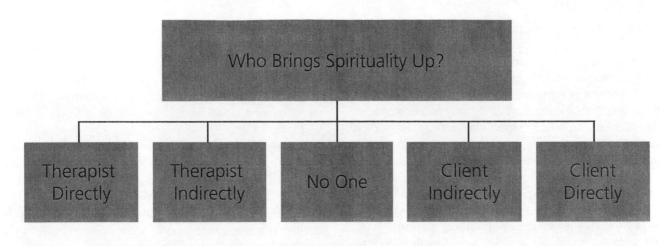

Figure 24.1. Continuum of addressing spirituality in occupational therapy practice.

In other cases, clients brought spirituality up directly:

- Most commonly, clients asked the "Why me?" type questions, as a signal that there were spiritual answers that they were searching for;
- Others expressed the idea that their faith had been challenged, that they were re-examining their basic beliefs and assumptions;
- Others referred specifically to a supreme being, questioning its benevolence or even its existence in the face of their own experience.

Therapists also reported that they felt some clients brought spiritual issues into the therapy relationship in an indirect manner:

- They made reference to religious participation;
- They exhibited religious or spiritual symbols, such as the wearing of a star, a cross, or a guardian angel, or the presence of religious artifacts in their room or home;
- They referred to death or near-death experiences.

In the middle of the continuum are those circumstances when no one discusses spirituality. Therapists offered the following reasons for this (Enquist et al., 1997; Russell, Sinclair, & Young, 1998; Tryssenaar et al., 1999):

- They don't know how to talk about it; don't have language for it other than religious language and aren't comfortable with that;
- They don't want to impose their own beliefs on anyone else;
- They don't know enough about other faiths besides their own to feel comfortable talking to people about their spirituality;
- They feel that spirituality is too personal to talk to clients about; some compared it with sexuality; others called it "taboo";

- They find it too emotional to talk to clients about spirituality—they end up crying or feeling frightened;
- They consider it a luxury that payers wouldn't be interested in; and that only gets addressed when there is a lot of time;
- They feel that the therapy milieu is inappropriate for discussions of this kind;
- They feel that their therapeutic relationships are not of sufficiently long duration to build the trust necessary for these discussions;
- They assume that their clients are incapable of these discussions because of cognitive or emotional disabilities.

Is there an ideal place for occupational therapists in Canada to be on this continuum, or is there some place on the continuum for which we should be striving? While we may not be ready yet to pronounce on this question, it may be helpful to discover that such a continuum exists, and that there is the possibility of understanding where one stands in relation to other therapists. If we were to decide we wanted to move from one position to another on the continuum of assessing spirituality (and I use the word assessment in its broadest possible context), it would involve other decisions about what information we wanted from clients about spiritual issues and what we were going to do with the information once we had it (Chapman, 1987; Enquist et al., 1997; Rose, 1999).

Intervention

What are therapists doing in practice in the realm of spirituality, and what are experts writing about in terms of occupational therapy practice that incorporates spirituality? There seems to be an assumption that what we want to be doing, or perhaps ought to be doing, is talking about spirituality with our clients. However, this is not how we deal with the other components of humans in occupational therapy. Let's use the example of the physical component of human beings. We do not typically engage our clients in discussions about their anatomy or physiology when we deal with the physical component of humans. We may draw on our knowledge of anatomy and physiology to understand and explain a problem with the physical aspect of some occupation. But we don't typically get into a technical discussion of the physical component. In fact, we don't particularly expect clients to know or even care about the problem at that level. And yet we know that it is important for us to understand the origins and insertions of particular muscles, and the levels and paths of their innervation. In most cases, it's enough that we understand those intricacies, because what we want from clients is for them to be able to DO something with their physical component.

Let me try to apply this analogy to spirituality. Perhaps what we want to happen in therapy is for clients to actually do something, or to have an experience that invokes spirit, that creates an opportunity for transcendence. But we get stuck, because we don't have any theoretical preparation that would compare:

- With our understanding of anatomy, physiology, kinesiology, medical sciences for the physical component;
- Or with our knowledge of psychology and psychiatry for the psychological component;
- Or with our background of sociology for the sociocultural component.

While we accept that we need theory from other disciplines to understand three of the components of human beings, for the one component that we have elevated to the central position of our guiding model, we have only our own upbringing and personal study to guide our professional role.

Therefore, the reluctance that therapists expressed to actually DO anything about spirituality may be well founded. It

may be based on their recognition of how potentially powerful spirituality is, and their realization that to do anything about it could be frightening, dangerous, and possibly professionally irresponsible (Kroeker, 1997). After all, if we did DO something or encouraged a client to DO something of a spiritual nature, and it backfired, how could we defend ourselves? (See Figure 24.2).

Let me suggest an alternative. We do know some things about spirituality and occupation. We know, for example, that spirit can be invoked spontaneously, or it can be induced (Cameron, 1992; Collins, 1998). We know that there are some activities that are more likely to invoke the presence of spirit. Activities that are antecedents to spiritual experience can be categorized as either existential, meditative, or creative. We have talked already about existential antecedents to spiritual experiences, specifically the disability itself. That leaves meditative and creative experiences.

Meditative experiences are direct methods of accessing spirit—including prayer, worship, meditation, and pastoral counseling. To further exploit the analogy with the physical component of human beings, the direct approach would be akin to asking a client to contract a particular muscle. It is something that we recognize is best left to another type of professional—in the example, a physical therapist; in the spiritual area, a religious or pastoral care professional (Christiansen, 1997; Smith, 1999).

The other way to invoke spirit is the indirect method, that is, the creative antecedents to spiritual experience. There are five that I encountered in my research and reading. Occupational therapists are using these methods, writing and talking about them, in a conscious or unconscious effort to involve the spiritual component of humans in the therapy process. They are using activities to invoke spirit in much the same way that they would use activities to involve the physical component in particular occupations.

1. Narrative

Perhaps the most widely discussed of the five ways of indirectly invoking spirit in occupational therapy is the use of narrative. Narratives have a number of features that make them attractive to occupational therapists, as several authors have outlined:

- They place the individual at the center of the process of therapy;
- They connect the client's past and present with the future;
- They give the client voice, power, control;
- They have a significant tolerance for paradox, contradiction, and complexity (Collins, 1998; Egan & Delaat, 1997; Frank, 1995; Fulford, 1999; Howard & Howard, 1997; Kirsch, 1996; Kleinman, 1988; McAdams, 1993).

However, none of these features is what makes narrative a potentially spiritual experience. After all, not every story is a

---

JUDGE:	Ms. OT, what training do you have to qualify you to undertake this sort of therapy involving spirituality with the plaintiff?
OT:	Why none, Your Honor, except for the fact that I'm a very spiritual person myself.
JUDGE:	And what evidence do you have to support the use of this form of therapy with clients like the plaintiff?
OT:	Why none, Your Honor, but surely you know yourself how meaningful occupation is in your daily life.
JUDGE:	And what would be considered a minimum standard of practice in your profession as regards to spirituality?
OT:	Why simply to do nothing, your Honor, but to know in my heart that spirituality is very important.

Figure 24.2. How would we defend ourselves?

spiritual story. The aspect of narrative that affords the possibility of transcendence is its potential to show one's personal story in relation to the story of the whole cosmos—in relation to other people, in relation to the natural world, and in relation to one's own belief in a supreme power. Therefore, for the narrative to succeed in being a spiritual or transcendent experience, the therapist may have to use his or her knowledge of spirituality to point out the mystery of every person's connection to the universal narrative (do Rozario, 1994).

2. Ritual

A second activity that the literature discusses in terms of spiritual experience is ritual. Ritual is a process that transforms an everyday activity into an activity with special meaning. It changes the activity from a mundane to a sacred one (Eliade, 1987). It emphasizes the symbolic significance of an activity, rather than the practical significance (do Rozario, 1994; Frank et al., 1997; Thibeault, 1997; Thibodaux, 1998). For example, one therapist told me of a client who had made a ritual of honoring the new self by burying something that had been a symbol of the predisability self. Burying a coffee can containing a piece of jewelry is not a sacred activity, but the ritual associated with it allowed the individual to transcend the ordinariness of the activity and to reach a new level of understanding of her place in her own life, in her relationships, and in the world.

3. Appreciation of nature

A third type of transcendent experience can occur in the presence of the natural world (Christiansen, 1997; McFague, 1997; Unruh, 1997). Numerous authors have written of the power of nature to invoke spirit; that is, to dissolve the boundaries between the self and the world, and to take one beyond a self-centered experience, and make one more aware of the mystery and connectedness of the world. Again, simply going to a national park may not do it, any more than setting up an activity in front of a client will make a particular occupation happen. It may require that the therapist facilitate the experience or create the possibility of a spiritual experience.

4. Creativity

A fourth type of experience that has the potential to invoke spirit is creative activity (Rose, 1999), or what Peloquin (1997) refers to as "making rather than doing" (p. 168). Creative activity affords an opportunity for unconstrained expression of spirit. According to Cameron (1992), creativity comes from a divine source. It is an individual's expression of universal truths and an attempt to communicate spirit in a universally accessible medium.

Occupational therapists talk about the experience of "flow" in relation to expressive or creative activities, meaning quite literally the experience of transcending the self, time, and place in the process of doing an activity (Collins, 1998; do

Rozario, 1994; Toomey, 1999). While neuropsychological explanations for this phenomenon are surely available, it is also possible that this is a transcendent or spiritual experience (Cousins, 1976).

5. Work

Finally, the balance of work and rest are activities that offer an opportunity for experiencing spirit. Several authors talk about a number of themes relating work and spirituality (Christiansen, 1997; Frank et al., 1997; Howard & Howard, 1997; Thibodaux, 1998):

- The opportunity for service and contribution through work;
- The dignity that is restored with work;
- The perspective of the self in relation to a universal mission;
- The rhythm and routines of work and rest, and the extent to which time is ordered and honored by these routines.

Conclusion

To this point, I have offered definitions of spirit, spirituality, and transcendence. In these definitions, I have emphasized:

- A distinction between spirituality and spirit; that is, a separation of person and spirit, and
- An affirmation of the mystery and other-worldliness that is the essence of spirit and of transcendent experiences of spirit.

Specifically, I have referred to how these definitions might make a difference in our views about spirituality as it relates to two central concepts in occupational therapy: disability and occupation.

We appear to be balanced in a precarious position as regards spirituality in occupational therapy. On the one hand, our profession, and particularly the Canadian arm of it, has achieved international recognition and admiration for incorporating the notion of spirituality in the occupational therapy model (Clark Green, 2000). On the other hand, occupational therapists from across the country tell us that almost 20 years later, spirituality is still not a comfortable fit for them; in fact, it is a source of distress and guilt.

Where are we to go with this? The options appear to be threefold.

1. We could stay where we are; that is, we could continue to talk about spirituality at some levels of the profession, but not at others; and we could continue to maintain a safe distance from the mysterious and supernatural aspects of spirituality;

2. We could become more expert and more involved with the concept of spirit as it plays a part in the lives of our clients. The primary implication for this option is educational; or

3. We could back off from our professional role in the area of spirituality, recognizing that we have neither the knowledge nor the expertise to play a meaningful role in this important part of peoples' lives.

Occupational therapy is an interesting example of the discussions that are currently taking place about the interface between science and religion (Autiero, 1992; Droege, 1997; Kevin & Wildes, 1992; Kroeker, 1997; McSherry & Draper, 1998). We can trace elements of our history to both camps, and now at the beginning of the 21st century, as we attempt to reconcile the two threads of our history, spirituality is at center stage in the discussion.

Acknowledgment

I gratefully acknowledge my friends and colleagues from the COPM group, who nominated me for the Muriel Driver Memorial Lectureship; my friend Nancy Pollock in particular, who spearheaded the nomination; the staff in the CAOT office, especially Geraldine Moore, for support in the preparation and delivery of the lecture; and the CAOT for conferring upon me this honor.

References

Antolikova, S. (1999). *Occupational therapy curriculum and spirituality.* Unpublished undergraduate thesis. University of Toronto, Toronto, ON.

Autiero, A. (1992). Dignity, solidarity, and sanctity of human life. In K.M. Wildes, F. Abel, & J.C. Harvey (Eds.), *Birth, suffering, and death: Catholic perspectives at the edges of life* (pp. 79–84). Dordrecht, Netherlands: Kluwer Academic.

Baptiste, S. (1997) Spiritually speaking.... *Canadian Journal of Occupational Therapy, 64,* 104–8.

BarbWire Collective. (1997). *Not all violins.* Toronto, ON: United Church Publishing House.

Barnard, D. (1995). Chronic illness and the dynamics of hoping. In S.K. Toombs, D. Barnard, & R.A. Carson (Eds.), *Chronic illness: From experience to policy.* Bloomington, IN: Indiana University Press,

Berggren-Thomas, P., & Griggs, M.J. (1995). Spirituality in aging: Spiritual need or spiritual journey? *Journal of Gerontological Nursing, 21,* 5–10.

Bing, R.K. (1997)."And teach agony to sing": An afternoon with Eleanor Clarke Slagle. *American Journal of Occupational Therapy, 51,* 220–227.

Bogdan, R., & Taylor, S.J. (1993). Relationships with severely disabled persons: The social construction of humanness. In M. Nagler (Ed.), *Perspectives on disability* (pp. 97–108). Palo Alto, CA: Health Markets Research.

Bowers, C.C. (1987). Spiritual dimensions of the rehabilitation journey. *Rehabilitation Nursing, 72,* 90–91.

Bryant, M.D. (1993). Religion and disability: Some notes on religious attitudes and views. In M. Nagier (Ed.), *Perspectives on disability* (pp. 91–95). Palo Alto, CA: Health Markets Research.

Buber, M. (1970). *I and thou.* New York: Scribners.

Cameron, J.A. (1992). *The artist's way.* New York: G.P. Putnam & Sons.

Canadian Association of Occupational Therapists. (1997). *Enabling occupation: An occupational therapy perspective.* Ottawa, ON: CAOT Publications ACE.

Chapman, L.S. (1987). Developing a useful perspective on spiritual health. *American Journal of Health Promotion, 1,* 31–39.

Christiansen, C. (1997). Acknowledging a spiritual dimension in occupational therapy practice. *American Journal of Occupational Therapy, 51,* 169–71.

Clark, F., Carlson, M., Zemke, R., Frank, G., Patterson, K., Ennevor, B.L., Rankin-Martinez, A., Hobson, I., Crandall, J., Mandel, D., & Lipson, L. (1996). Life domains and adaptive strategies of low-income well-older adults. *American Journal of Occupational Therapy, 50,* 99–128.

Clark Green, M. (2000 May/June). Editorial: The Canadian way. *Occupational Therapy Now, 2*(3), 3.

Collins, M. (1998). Occupational therapy and spirituality: Reflecting on quality of experience in therapeutic interactions. *British Journal of Occupational Therapy, 61,* 280–284.

Cousins, N. (1976). Anatomy of an illness. *New England Journal of Medicine, 295,* 1458–63.

do Rozario, L. (1994). Ritual, meaning, and transcendence: the role of occupation in modern life. *Journal of Occupational Science, 1,* 46.

Droege, T. (1991). *The faith factor in healing.* Philadelphia, PA: Trinity Press.

Egan, M., & DeLaat, D. (1997). The implicit spirituality of occupational therapy practice. *Canadian Journal of Occupational Therapy, 64,* 115–21.

Egan, M., & DeLaat, D. (1994). Considering spirituality in occupational therapy practice. *Canadian Journal of Occupational Therapy, 61,* 95–101.

Eiesland, N. (1994). *The disabled God: Toward a liberatory theology of disability.* Nashville, TN: Abingdon Press.

Eliade, M. (1987). *The sacred and the profane.* San Diego, CA: Harcourt Brace.

Emblen, J.D. (1992). Religion and spirituality defined according to current use in nursing literature. *Journal of Professional Nursing, 8,* 41–7.

Enquist, D.E., Short-DeCraff, M., Gliner, J., & Oltjenbruns, K. (1997). Occupational therapists' beliefs and practices with regard to spirituality and therapy. *American Journal of Occupational Therapy, 51,* 173–80.

Falardeau, M. (1997). Intervenir apres des personnes souffrant de depression en tenant compte de la dimension spirituelle. *Canadian Journal of Occupational Therapy, 64,* 127–137.

Fife, B. (1994). The concept of meaning in illness. *Social Science and Medicine, 38,* 309–16.

Fine, S.B. (1991). Resilience and human adaptability: Who rises above adversity? *American Journal of Occupational Therapy, 45,* 493–503. Reprinted as Chapter 25.

Fitcher, J.H. (1981). *Religion and pain: Spiritual dimensions of health care.* New York: Crossroads Publishing.

Fitzgerald, J. (1997). Reclaiming the whole: Self, spirit, and society. *Disability and Rehabilitation, 19,* 407–13.

Frank, A.W. (1995). *The wounded storyteller: Body, illness, and ethics.* Chicago, IL: University of Chicago Press.

Frank. G., Grenardo, C.S., Propper, S., Noguchi, F., Lipman, C., Maulhardt, B., & Weitze, L. (1997). Jewish spirituality through actions in time: Daily occupations of young orthodox Jewish couples in Los Angeles. *American Journal of Occupational Therapy, 51,* 199–206.

Frank, V. (1984). *Man's search for meaning.* New York: Washington Square Press.

Fulford, R. (1999). *The triumph of narrative.* Toronto, ON: Anansi Press.

Gutterman, L. (1990). A day treatment program for people with AIDS. *American Journal of Occupational Therapy, 44,* 234–237.

Horsburgh, M. (1997). Toward an inclusive spirituality: Wholeness, interdependence, and waiting. *Disability and Rehabilitation, 79,* 398–406.

Howard, B.S., & Howard, J.R. (1997). Occupation as spiritual activity. *American Journal of Occupational Therapy, 51,* 181–185.

Kevin, M., & Wildes, S.J. (1992). Finitude, religion, and medicine. The search for meaning in the post-modern world. In K.M. Wildes, F. Abel, & J.C. Harvey (Eds.), *Birth, suffering, and death: Catholic perspectives at the edges of life* (pp. 1–10). Dordrecht, Netherlands: Kluwer Academic.

Kirsh, B. (1996). A narrative approach to addressing spirituality in occupational therapy: Exploring personal meaning and purpose. *Canadian Journal of Occupational Therapy, 63,* 5–61.

Kleinman, A. (1988). *The illness narratives*. New York: Basic Books.

Kroeker, T. (1997). Spirituality and occupational therapy in a secular culture. *Canadian Journal of Occupational Therapy, 64*, 122–126.

Lewis, C.S. (1962). *The problem of pain*. New York: MacMillan.

Lindsey, E. (1996). Health within illness: Experiences of chronically ill/disabled people. *Journal of Advanced Nursing, 24*, 465–72.

Low, J.F. (1997). Religious orientation and pain management. *American Journal of Occupational Therapy, 51*, 215–219.

Mairs, N. (1990). *Carnal acts*. New York: HarperCollins.

McAdams, D. P. (1993). *The stories we live by*. New York: Guilford Press.

McColl, M.A., Bickenbach, J., Johnston, J., Nishihama, S., Schumaker, M., Smith, K., Smith, M., & Yeatland, B. (in press). Spiritual issues associated with traumatic-onset disability. *Disability and Rehabilitation*.

McColl, M.A., Bickenbach, J., Johnston, J., Nishihama, S., Schumaker, M., Smith, K., Smith, M., & Yealland, B. (2000). Changes in spirituality following disability. *Archives of Physical Medicine and Rehabilitation, 87*, 817–823.

McFague, S. (1982). *Metaphorical theology*. Minneapolis, MN: Fortress Press.

McFague, S. (1997). *Super, natural Christians*. Minneapolis, MN: Fortress Press.

McSherry, W., & Draper, P. (1998). The debates emerging from the literature surrounding the concept of spirituality as applied to nursing. *Journal of Advanced Nursing, 27*, 683–91.

Moyers, P. (1997). Occupational meaning and spirituality: The quest for sobriety. *American Journal of Occupational Therapy, 51*, 207–14.

Murdoch, I. (1959). The sublime and the good. *Chicago Review, 13*, 50–52.

Murpy, R. (1990). *The body silent*. New York: W.W. Norton.

Narayanasamy, A. (1996). Spiritual care of chronically ill patients. *British Journal of Nursing, 5*, 411–416.

Ohsberg, H.O. (1982). *The church and persons with handicaps*. Kitchener, ON: Herald Press.

Peloquin, S.M. (1997). The spiritual depth of occupation: Making worlds and making lives. *American Journal of Occupational Therapy, 51*, 167–168.

Reed, P. G. (1992). An emerging paradigm for the investigation of spirituality in nursing. *Research in Nursing and Health, 75*, 349–57.

Richards, E. (1997). A door to hope. In BarbWire Collective, *Not all violins*. Toronto, ON: United Church Publishing House.

Robinson, A. (1994). Spirituality and risk: Toward an understanding. *Holistic Nursing Practice, 8*.

Rose, A. (1999). Spirituality and palliative care: The attitudes of occupational therapists. *British Journal of Occupational Therapy, 62* 307–312.

Ross, L. (1995). The spiritual dimension: Its importance to patients' health, well-being, and quality of life, and its implications for nursing practice. *International Journal of Nursing Studies, 32*, 457–68.

Russell, M., Sinclair, H., & Young, H. (1998). Struggling with spirituality in the Canadian Model of Occupational Performance. *The National, 15*, 3.

Sanford, J.A. (1977). *Healing and wholeness*. New York: Paulist Press.

Selway, D., & Ashman, A.F. (1998). Disability, religion, and health. *Disability and Rehabilitation, 73*, 429–39.

Smith, D.W. (1995). Power and spirituality in polio survivors: A study based on Rogers' science. *Nursing Science Quarterly, 8*, 133–9.

Smith, M. (1999). *Growth through disability; strength through adversity: Spiritual healing with the post-rehabilitation person*. Unpublished master's thesis. Queen's Theological College, Kingston, ON.

Soeken, K.L., & Carson, V.J. (1987). Responding to the spiritual needs of the chronically ill. *Nursing Clinics of North America, 22*, 603–11.

Sontag, S. (1977). *Illness as metaphor*. Toronto, ON: McGraw-Hill-Ryerson Press.

Thibeault, R. (1997). A funeral for my father's mind: A therapist's attempt at grieving. *Canadian Journal of Occupational Therapy, 64*, 107–114.

Thibodaux, L.R. (1998). *Acknowledging the spiritual dimension of occupational therapy*. Paper presented at 12th International Congress of World Federation of Occupational Therapists. Montreal, Quebec.

Toole-Mitchell, K. (1999 June). Pentecost is more than a season. *United Church Observer*, p. 51.

Toombs, S.K. (1995). Sufficient unto the day: A life with MS. In S.K Toombs, O. Barnard, & R. A. Carson (Eds.), *Chronic illness: From experience to policy* (pp. 3–23). Bloomington, IN: Indiana University Press.

Toomey, M.A. (1999). The art of observation: Reflecting on a spiritual moment. *Canadian Journal of Occupational Therapy, 66*, 197–9.

Townsend, E. (1997). Inclusiveness: A community dimension of spirituality. *Canadian Journal of Occupational Therapy, 64*, 146–55.

Townsend, E., DeLaat, D., Egan, M., Thibeault, R., & Wright, W.A. (1999). *Spirituality in enabling occupation: A learner-centered workbook*. Ottawa, ON: CAOT Publications ACE.

Tryssenaar, J., Jones, E.J., & Lee, D. (1999). Occupational performance needs of a shelter population. *Canadian Journal of Occupational Therapy, 66*, 188–196.

Unruh, A. (1997). Spirituality and occupation: Garden musings and the Himalayan Blue Poppy. *Canadian Journal of Occupational Therapy, 64*, 156–160.

Urbanowski, R., & Vargo, J. (1994). Spirituality, daily practice, and the occupational performance model. *Canadian Journal of Occupational Therapy, 61*, 88–94.

Van Amburg, R. (1997). A Copernican revolution in clinical ethics: Engagement versus disengagement. *American Journal of Occupational Therapy, 57*, 186–90.

Vanier, J. (1998). *Becoming human*. Toronto, ON: Anansi Press.

Vrkijan, B.H. (2000 Mar/Apr). The role of spirituality in occupational therapy practice. *Occupational Therapy Now, 2*(2), 6–9.

Watkins, E. (1997). Essay on spirituality. *Journal of Substance Abuse Treatment, 14*, 581–583.

Yancey, P. (1990). *Where is God when it hurts?* Grand Rapids, MI: Zondervan Publishing House.

Young, C. (1993). Spirituality and the chronically ill Christian elderly. *Gerontological Nursing, 14*, 298–303.

Young, E.W.D. (1984). Spiritual health—An essential element in optimum health. *Journal of the American College of Health, 32*, 273–6.

Zola, I. (1982). *Missing pieces: A chronicle of living with a disability*. Philadelphia, PA: Temple University Press.

Resilience and Human Adaptability: Who Rises Above Adversity?

1990 Eleanor Clarke Slagle Lecture

CHAPTER 25

Susan B. Fine, MA, OTR, FAOTA

We work in a world of traumas and triumphs. Most of the persons we serve come to us out of necessity, struggling with the sequelae of disease and illness or the aftermath of natural or manmade disasters. We bring our expertise and compassion; they bring their bodies, minds, and compromised lives. Our worlds converge around a shared task: identifying and enhancing their capacities for daily living. We pursue problems of movement, perception, cognition, affect, and social capacity within the context of their roles and aspirations. Our contacts may be extensive, but often they are brief and only partially fulfilled. Our patients move on with varying degrees of functional ability—some with determination and buoyancy, others with little confidence that life is actually worth living. We remain, frequently knowing little about the factors that have influenced the outcome of our efforts, in spite of their compelling importance to our patients, our professional viability, and the health care system.

This Eleanor Clarke Slagle Lecture is a study of outcome— outcome that often defies the odds. It is a study of lives characterized by extraordinary hardships and remarkable abilities to move beyond them. It poses a core question: Who rises above adversity? It ventures beyond traditional concerns for pathology and vulnerability, beyond theoretical and statistical methods. In fact, its most valuable data come directly from the personal experiences of those confronted with chronic or terminal illness, physical and mental disabilities, abuse, impoverishment, the Holocaust, and other disasters. I have pursued many life narratives, not as a test of endurance in the face of human suffering (although it made for a more tearful year than most), not in search of heroes and heroines (although there were many), but in an effort to more fully understand factors that influence resilient responses. The voices of the resilient send a powerful message: Personal perceptions and responses to stressful life events are crucial elements of survival, recovery, and rehabilitation, transcending the reality of the situation or the interventions of others. The inner life (affective and cognitive processes and content) holds the potential for transforming traumas into varying degrees of triumph. Ironically, these same phenomena are often ignored in the clinical reasoning and practice of many health professions, including our own.

Consequently, this paper is intended to heighten the reader's appreciation of the powerful interaction among a person's inner psychological life, his or her relationship to the surrounding world, and his or her emerging functional capacities. It pursues these themes by first providing an overview of theoretical constructs about the human response to adversity. Second, it focuses on extreme life events and the personal and social meaning ascribed to them. Third, it addresses the phenomenon of resilience and the means by which persons in extreme situations have coped. Implications for occupational therapy practice are then considered.

Overcoming Adversity: A Human Condition

The experience of adversity and the drive to rise above it are themes that characterize the human condition. The inevitability of life's trials and tribulations and the struggles between good and evil are evident in religious traditions, myths, the arts, and everyday conversation. Although adversity is ultimately a personal experience, in the bigger scheme of things it is faceless and timeless. We have grown up with both the ascendance of Cinderella and the failure of Icarus.

We share such maxims as "It's always something" (Radner, 1989) or "You have to take the bad with the good." These universal themes attempt to guide us in matters of social order and disorder.

There is also professional literature devoted to understanding the human response to disruptions, the search for order and balance, and the consequences of prolonged imbalance. Although taxonomies and belief systems vary, a central theme, linked to Canon's (1939) work in biology and physics, identifies a recurring cycle of disruption and reintegration as a natural and necessary part of one's growing capacities to adapt to internal and external change (Flach, 1988). In today's lexicon we speak of risk, stress, coping, competency, crisis theory, and biopsychosocial models. The past has been marked by a more disparate array of assumptions.

The relationship of stress to disease has been the highest priority among clinicians since Hippocratic times. Attempts at developing broader, systematic constructs have emerged from a number of disciplines. Psychoanalysis has given us ego mechanisms of defense as a metaphor for mental processes that handle crises and threats. Freudian views emphasize a hierarchy of defenses that transform conflict-ridden impulses into more acceptable thoughts and actions. Ego psychology promotes reality-oriented, purposeful, conflict-free capacities (i.e., attention, perception, and memory) that are future-oriented and that render one capable of transforming situations rather than being transformed by them. In this formulation, adaptive functioning is seen as the relative use of coping capacities over defense mechanisms (Anthony & Cohler, 1987). The growth and cumulative effects of coping resources and skills over the life span are reflected in Erikson's (1963) classic development theories.

A behaviorist tradition also emerged with an early emphasis on the consequences of concrete problem solving. Today, as cognitive behaviorism, it is concerned with the cognitive components of coping skills and the Eriksonian belief that "successful coping promotes a sense of self-efficacy, which in turn, inspires more efforts at mastering difficult situations" (Moos & Schaefer, 1984, p. 6).

Endocrinologist Hans Selye (1978) assumed importance in the disruption–reintegration debate. Half a decade of work on stress and its hormonal and neurochemical correlates has had a great impact on professional and popular views of prevention and disease management. Selye's original emphasis on the singular importance of the stressful event itself has been mediated by a growing belief that the physical or psychological impact of any demand will vary depending on how we interpret the situation and how able we are to do something about it (Lazarus & Folkman, 1984).

Moos and Billings (1982) elaborated by organizing coping skills into three areas: appraisal-focused coping (i.e., efforts to understand and find meaning in a crisis), problem-focused coping (i.e., attempts to deal with the reality and consequences of the crisis and create a better situation), and emo-tion-focused coping (i.e., handling the feelings provoked by the crisis).

The cognitive appraisal process (how we interpret personal experiences) is central to a great deal of contemporary thought on coping. Stress itself has been defined as a "relationship between person and environment that is appraised by the person as taxing or exceeding his or resources and endangering his or her well being" (Lazurus & Folkman, 1984, p. 19). Although social psychology traditionally emphasizes the role of external stressors and cognitive strategies (i.e., logical analysis, mental preparation, cognitive redefinition, and avoidance or denial), internal phenomena must not be ignored. Personal theories of reality about oneself and one's world, developed over time and generally outside of awareness, serve as a filter through which we perceive, interpret, and respond to experiences (Janoff-Bulman & Timko, 1987). Disturbing thoughts and memories can also heavily influence the appraisal process (Houston, 1987).

The credibility of the cognitive appraisal paradigm is enhanced by the newly integrated discipline of psychoneuroimmunology, which is "the study of the intricate interaction of consciousness (psycho), brain and central nervous system (neuro), and the body's defense against external infection and aberrant cell division (immunology)" (Pelletier & Herzing, 1988, p. 29). The impact of personal mood and attitudes on the immune system has opened new doors for researchers and clinicians. Studies have found that one's immune system benefits from confronting traumatic memories, looking at life optimistically, and living at a mildly hectic pace (Goleman, 1989). This line of thought will no doubt continue to provide us with newer and different hypotheses about the law's disruption and reintegration.

For now, contemporary biopsychosocial formulations represent a robust model. Capacities to meet challenging demands and stand up to disruptions depend on inborn and acquired skills, the material and interpersonal resources in the environment, and the psychosocial capacities to handle anxieties that arise when one is performing various life tasks. Successful adaptation is dependent on the degree of fit among these factors. Although mastery is both developed and sustained by manageable challenges, challenges that are too demanding or too dangerous defeat resources for coping and reintegration (White, 1976).

And dangers there are! The law of disruption and reintegration does not promise, or always deliver, a rose garden. Life events continually test the durability of the balance we try to maintain.

Ordeals Beyond Our Control

There are life events that are experienced as traumatic because they are severe ordeals beyond our control. Under circumstances of predictable, moderate stress, persons call on conventional patterns and solve problems with characteristic resources and adaptive styles. But extreme situations and the stress accompanying them are not conventional. By their nature they are beyond the range of the predictable; previous experiences have not prepared us for them. How does one prepare for a spinal tumor, a brain injury, a schizophrenic episode, or a devastating earthquake? How does one comprehend Auschwitz or Dachau, where:

> Dreams used to come in the brutal nights,
> Dreams crowding and violent
> Dreamt with body and soul,
> Of going home, of eating, of telling our story.
> Until quickly and quietly, came
> The dawn reveille:
> *Wstawàch.*
> And the heart cracked in the breast. (Levi, 1965, p. xi)

Extreme experiences such as these are characterized by a lack of conventional social structure, a loss of anchor in reality, and a lack of ability to predict or anticipate outcomes (Torrance, 1965). Although we associate such phenomena with the high drama of hostage situations, prolonged combat, or concentration camps, they may also define the experience of persons whose lives are linked with ours on a daily basis, that is, our patients. Perhaps we ourselves have endured trauma or the sudden onset of a life-threatening illness:

> Being full of strength and vigor one moment and virtually helpless the next ... with all one's powers and faculties one moment and without them the next ... such a change, such a suddenness, is difficult to comprehend and the mind casts about for explanations. (Sacks, 1984, p. 21)

There are those, like Lifton (1988), who view man "as perpetual survivor ... of 'holocausts' large and small, personal and collective, that define much of existence" (p. 12). Although the Holocaust was a horrifying reality, as a metaphor it illuminates many other ordeals, helping us to understand and negotiate them. The vivid words and images of those with illness and disability also reveal the deeper meaning of their experiences—meaning that defines the nature of their adaptive task and shapes the quality of their reintegration.

The Personal and Social Meaning of Trauma

There are many reasons to perceive extreme life events as threatening. The most stressful dimensions appear to be those that challenge personal assumptions about oneself and the structure of the world one lives in. Much of this is linked with the phenomenon of control: the ability (or the perceived ability) to change, predict, understand, or accept environmental transactions within a meaningful context (Potocki & Everly, 1989). The sense of being in control and the desire for such control are believed to be crucial aspects of personality affecting physical and mental health as well as recovery potential.

The perception of self, with its elements of body image, identity, and self-worth, were dominant themes in every narrative I encountered, whether the trauma occurred in Vietnam, Theresienstadt, a hospital in London, or a city in Arizona. The pervasive threat to, or loss of, identity was as potent a force as—and sometimes more significant than—any real threat to life and limb. The tattooed number on the arm of a concentration camp inmate had its counterpart in the history number on a hospital ID bracelet. As startling as this analogy may seem, in the eyes of the "number" it may well mean humiliation, a lack of personal validation, and varying degrees of dehumanization. Just as prisoners of war are stripped of rank, role, and place in their reference group, victims of fires suffer losses of important nonhuman anchors for personal identity (Rosenfeld, 1989). Stroke victims, made captive by their disease and an impersonal hospital environment, lose the ability and opportunity to act on their own behalf.

In losing one's identity, one must replace it with another. How one chooses the new altered self is no small task. "Feelings of fear, vulnerability ... sadness over losses and weakness about not being able to control one's life or one's emotional reactions, contribute to feelings of defectiveness" (Marmar & Horowitz, 1988, p. 96). The impact of confinement, isolation, and perceptual distortions are described by neurologist Oliver Sacks following a near-death accident, serious leg injury, disturbing hospitalization, and role change from doctor to patient:

> I was physiologically, in imagination, and feeling ... a pygmy, a prisoner, a patient ... without the faintest awareness. How could one know one had shrunk, if one's frame of reference itself shrunk? (1984, p. 157)

Experiences that reflect a loss of self-control are often a central issue in psychiatric disorders as well. It is evident in schizophrenia, for example, when unpredictable symptoms turn "sparkles of light into demon eyes" (McGrath, 1984) or when a partially observing ego is "aware enough to recognize the dangers of not being able to control what I'm doing or thinking" (A patient, personal communication, October 1989).

Psychological stress, induced by threats of loss of self or failure, is also highly dependent on social values and the person's acceptance of the culture's definitions of what is valuable. Finding a new self or coming to terms with the only self one has ever known is reflected in the mirror others place before us. There is humiliation and pain generated:

> by a gait to embarrass, to make children laugh, a clumsy countering locomotion ... from only the most exacting; determined efforts to control. Inside my rolling head, behind my shocked, magnified eyeballs, my brain orders, with utmost precision, each awkward jerk of thigh, leg, foot. (Weaver, 1985, p. 43)

Jean Améry provides us with a powerful metaphor for thinking about a person's sense of his or her own body and place in the world when mastery and control of that body is violated through intentional political torture, abuse, or from the pain of illness and medical procedures.

> He who has suffered torture can no longer feel at ease in the world. Faith in humanity—cracked by the first slap across the face, then demolished by torture, can never be recovered. (Améry, 1986, p. xiii)

There are, of course, many forms of torture. The torture that physical illness may bestow need not be limited to bodily discomfort or pain, but "visits upon [people] a disease of social relations no less real than the paralysis of the body" (Murphy, 1987, p. 4). Anthropologist John Murphy viewed his spinal tumor, growing paralysis, and confinement as an assault on his identity and a disruption of ties with others. In depicting his illness as an extended field visit to an unfamiliar culture, he identified a primal scene of sociology—the social confrontation of persons with significant flaws, where someone looks or acts differently and we are uncertain as to what to say or where to look. This robs the encounter of cultural guidelines, leaving those involved uncertain about what to expect and what to do. For Murphy, "it has the potential for social calamity" (p. 87).

This calamity is also experienced as being in limbo. Sacks (1984) viewed this as a byproduct of his body agnosia and the empathic agnosia of his surgeon, who insisted that nothing was wrong. His disease and lack of a human foothold (i.e., adequate communication and validation) left Sacks with a sense of double nothingness, "Now doubly, I had no leg to stand on; unsupported, doubly" (p. 109). Kleinman (1988), in turn, characterized limbo, for those with chronic illness, as "the dangerous crossing of borders, the interminable waiting to exit and reenter normal everyday life ... the perpetual uncertain of whether one can return at all" (p. 181).

I heard this again and again: a common thread, a theme that plagued Holocaust survivors and Vietnam veterans as well as the physically and mentally disabled—the gulf between the self and others (family, friends, caregivers, society). Who will listen? Who will understand what we are experiencing? Who will believe where we have been and what we have endured? Who will validate us as we continue to deal with adversity and its imprints?

Resilience

For some, the imprints are so deeply etched that they succumb. Others endure under conditions that seem unsupportable to health. Redl's (1969) work with adolescents who have beaten the odds inspired the concept of *ego resilience*, that is, the capacity to withstand pathogenic pressure, the ability to recover rapidly from a temporary collapse even without outside help, and the strength to bounce back to normal or even supernormal levels of functioning. Demos (1989) suggested that, in its most developed state, such buoyancy requires "an active stance, persistence, the application of a variety of skills over a wide range of situations and probabilities ... [and] flexibility ... to know when to use what" (p. 5).

The formal study of resilience emerged in epidemiological studies on susceptibility to heart disease over 25 years ago. It is only within the last 15 years, however, that more rigorous efforts have been made to extricate it from a disease model and focus instead on "good psychosocial capacities such as competence, coping, creativity, and confidence (Anthony & Cohler, 1987, p. x). Although healthfulness remains a less-than-perfect body of knowledge, a variety of popular and scientific resources provide direction for the reader's ongoing investigation, including descriptions of personal experiences (Brown, 1990; Browne, Connors, & Stern, 1985; Cousins, 1979; Egendorf, 1986; Gill, 1988; Heller & Vogel, 1986; Miller, 1985; Minear, 1990; Nolan, 1987; Sheehan, 1982; Trillin, 1984), situational studies of combat (Elder & Clipp, 1988; Rahe & Genender, 1983), studies of disasters (Bolin & Trainer, 1978; Lifton & Olson, 1976) and illness (Cleveland, 1984; Cohen & Lazarus, 1973), studies of the invulnerable child (Anthony & Cohler, 1987; Dugan & Coles, 1989; Garmezy & Masten, 1986; Murphy & Moriarty, 1976), and longitudinal investigations of adaptation (Chess & Thomas, 1984; Vaillant, 1977; Werner & Smith, 1982).

Resilience has been chronicled in studies of famous men and women who were highly stressed and traumatized as children, among them, George Orwell, Charles Dickens, Anton Chekov, Kathe Kollowitz, Pablo Piccaso, and Buster Keaton (Goertzel & Goertzel, 1962; Miller, 1990; Shengold, 1989). Resilience, however, is evident in all walks of life. What is less clear is how persons manage to marshal the necessary resources. What enabled young Ryan White, confronted with two life-threatening illnesses, humiliation, and rejection, to become so articulate a spokesman for AIDS? What contributed to the brutalized Central Park jogger's remarkable recovery and recent promotion in her highly competitive investment banking firm? These are questions whose answers have as many nuances as there are people and ordeals, for resilience is not all of one piece.

Resilience is made operational by cognitive and behavioral coping skills and the recruitment of social support. Lazarus and Folkman (1984) suggested that such skills do not come all at once. Rather, they are acquired through a developmental process—a process of selecting from available alternatives and having persons reinforce the skills that are necessary to make coping possible. Studies of vulnerability and competence in children and adolescents have provided valuable insight into some aspects of this multifaceted and shifting phenomenon. Theoretical models of stress resistance view the relationship between stress and personal attributes from several perspectives: as compensation (personal attributes help to improve adjustment when stress diminishes competence), as protection (personal traits interact with stress in predicting adjustment), or as a challenge (stressors enhance competence) (Garmezy, 1983). Dispositional attributes of the child, family cohesion and warmth, and the use of external support systems by parents and children are mechanisms that buffer stress and promote resilient responses. Temperament, sex, intellectual ability, humor, empathy, social problem-solving skills, social expressiveness, and an inner locus of control have been found to influence adaptation under adverse conditions (Garmezy, 1985). These phenomena, however, show variability over time and at different developmental periods (Werner & Smith, 1982) and are influenced by changing demands of the environment. Coping, for children and adults alike, reflects trait-like and situation-specific elements (Kahana, Kahana, Harel, & Rosner, 1988).

Resilience is often measured behaviorally on the basis of the person's competence and success in meeting society's expectations despite great obstacles. Internal indexes (thoughts and feelings) are often ignored, despite evidence that impressive social competence may well be heavily correlated with depression and anxiety (Miller, 1990; Peck, 1987). Clinicians and researchers are alerted to attend to the distinctions and interactions between adaptive behavior and emotional status. Resilience needs to be examined and understood from both perspectives.

Resilient Perspectives

Truly functional coping behavior has been characterized as not only lessening the immediate impact of stress, but also as maintaining a sense of self-worth and unity with the past and an anticipated future (Dimsdale, 1974). It involves two distinct tasks: a response to the requirements of the situation and a response to the feelings about the situation. Author Nancy Mairs (1986), struggling with multiple sclerosis, chronic depression, and agoraphobia, explained the process:

> Each gesture ... carries a weight of uncertainty, demands significant attention: buttoning my shirt, changing a light bulb, walking down stairs. The minutiae of my life have had to assume dramatic proportions. If I could not ... delight in them, they would likely drown me in rage and self-pity.
>
> Yet I am unwilling to forgo the adventurous life; the difficulty of it, even the pain, the ... fear, and the sudden brief lift of spirit graces ... the pilgrimage. If I am to have it ... I must change the terms by which it is lived.... I refine adventure, make it smaller and smaller ... whether I am feeding fish flakes to my bettas ... lying wide-eyed in the dark battling yet another bout of depression, cooking a chicken ... [or] meeting a friend for lunch.... I am always having the adventures that are mine to have. (pp. 6–7)

Mairs accepted the challenge and altered her lifestyle in the face of unpredictable capacity while maintaining some semblance of control over her life through a commitment to scaled-down adventures. Even in the presence of many serious problems she demonstrated what Kobasa (1979) and colleagues have called *hardiness*. Hardiness is characterized by challenge, commitment, and control attributes. Challenge is expressed as a belief that change, rather than stability, is

normal in life and is an incentive for growth rather than a threat to security. Control is expressed by feeling and acting as if one is influential rather then helpless. Influence is operationalized through the use of imagination, knowledge, skill, and choice. Commitment is a tendency to involve oneself rather then feel alienated from situations; it involves a generalized sense of purpose that allows one to find events, things, and people meaningful and to approach situations rather than avoid them.

In extraordinarily stressful situations (the ones that diminish social structure, connections with reality, and a sense of predictability), opportunities to operationalize commitment, control, and challenge orientations are greatly compromised. Nonetheless, cognitive and behavioral coping mechanisms and efforts to recruit social support emerge and find expression in the most remarkable ways. The personal perspectives of the persons whose anecdotes follow are a tribute to the resourcefulness of the human mind and spirit. Their thoughts, feelings, and actions reflect the true character of resilience.

Hope and the Will to Overcome

Hope and the will to overcome are evident in the poignant poetry of children who found comfort and inspiration in the resilience of nature while confined in a Czechoslovakian camp in 1944:

> The sun has made a veil of gold
> So lovely that my body aches.
> Above, the heavens shriek with blue
> Convinced I've smiled by some mistake.
> The world's abloom and seems to smile.
> I want to fly but where, how high?
> If in barbed wire, things can bloom
> Why couldn't I? I will not die!
> (Anonymous, in *I Never Saw Another Butterfly*, 1978, p. 52)

Hope and the will to overcome emerge in others as a fierce, sometimes raging will to live, that is, "the burning desire to tell, to bear witness" (Gill, 1988, p. 59), "to testifying on behalf of all those whose shadows will be bound to mine forever" (Wiesel, 1990, p. 15), "to live not for oneself, but to lament those who died [in Hiroshima]" (Tamiki, 1990, p. 30).

Affiliation and the Recruitment of Social Support

Acquiring a sense of belonging to a social group or, for that matter, to all of life, is a powerful way to sustain oneself in the face of death or other extremes. It may manifest itself by turning one's attention inward to memories and images of loved ones, by participating in an organized underground movement, or by devising a tap code to communicate through cell walls to other Vietnam prisoners of war. It also emerges through the collaboration of a therapist and a severely mentally ill woman who is struggling against great odds to restore a semblance of autonomy and self-respect:

You believed in me ... were willing to take a chance on my being able to handle an apartment when my family felt it would be a waste of money. We had hopes; I didn't want to let you down and I haven't. (A patient, personal communication, 1989)

Finding Meaning and Purpose

The identification of purpose, or finding meaning in an ordeal, was described by Viktor Frankl (1984) as "the last of human freedoms"—choosing one's attitude in any given set of circumstances, having at least the power and the control over how you interpret and explain what happens to you. Individuals find meaning and purpose in many different ways. Some find it in an increased commitment to religion, a political ideal, or a social cause. Others find it by using intellect and creativity to combat devastating fear. Many concentration camp victims and prisoners of war played chess and built houses, nail by nail, in their mind's eye; one man prepared a full German–English dictionary on scraps of paper during his incarceration and published it after his release. Others claimed that even forced labor was sustaining.

Interestingly, despite confining, constraining situations with extremely limited resources, many sought to find meaning and retain interests, values, and skills through focused, self-regulating activity. "The prisoners who fared the best in the long run were those who ... could retain their personality system largely intact ... where previous interests, values and skills could to some extent be carried on" (Hamburg, Coelho, & Adams, 1974, p. 413). In situational studies of combat, illness, and the anticipated death of family members, Gal and Lazarus (1975) reported reductions in anxiety and feelings of helplessness even when activities did not provide actual control over the situation. In contrast, the vulnerable were described by Eitinger as those who "felt completely helpless and passive, and had lost their ability to retain some sort of self-activity" (Hamburg et al., 1974, p. 413). Our continuing efforts to understand the complex role of occupation in remediating illness and maintaining health may be greatly enhanced through studies of the spontaneous behavior of those in stressful situations.

The Capacity to Step Back

Frankl's (1984) disgust with his own trivial preoccupations with survival found him, in fantasy, lecturing on the psychology of concentration camps. Both he and his troubles became the object of a psychoscientific study undertaken by himself that later contributed to the development of a school of psychotherapy. Frankl demonstrated the capacity to step back and, in so doing, preserved a part of himself from extraordinary degradation, pain, and loss. Functioning somewhat like a solution to a figure–ground problem, this process provides one with the opportunity of ignoring aspects of the situation that are out of one's control. It may appear as a differential focus on the good, or it may be marked by a heightened capac-

ity for observation, that is, a period of exalted receptivity when details of events, faces, words, or sensations are retained (Levi, 1987). This is evident in the writings of Wiesel (1990), Cousins (1979), Heller and Vogel (1986), Brown (1990), and Nolan (1987). None perceived themselves to be victims or survivors, but rather, witnesses to their own experience.

There Is More to Oneself Than Current Circumstance Suggests

The discovery of the new or real self is artfully reflected in Frank's (1988) study of embodiment—the experience and meaning of disability in American culture. She described a young woman born with quadrilateral limb deficiencies who stressed her assets instead of her deficits—her womanly figure (like Venus de Milo's) and her ability to write better with her stumps than with her artificial arms. Interestingly, her rehabilitation team viewed her refusal to use prosthetics as poor adaptation.

Dugan and Coles (1989), in turn, described a 6-year-old Black girl who was initiating school desegregation in New Orleans in the face of mobs, violence, and threats to her life. She hoped she would "get through one day and then another," and if she did, "it will be because there is more to me than I ever realized" (p. xiv).

Novel Applications of Problem-Solving Strategies

Coping involves creative and reflective behavior (White, 1976). Resilience is manifest in the ability to turn a familiar way of solving problems into a novel application, one that may save a life. When Sacks (1984) sustained his injury while mountain climbing alone, he was at great risk for dying of exposure. He reported that there came to his aid a kinetic melody, rhythm, and motor music. "Now, so to speak, I was musicked along" (p. 30). Remembrances of the Volga Boatmen's Song gave him the strength and rhythm to "row" himself along the ground for many hours until he found help.

Transforming Dross Into Gold

Vaillant's (1977) longitudinal study of the life and coping strategies of a group of Harvard graduates documented the way in which the mature ego mechanisms of altruism, humor, suppression, and sublimation function to transform disturbances into adaptive behavior, thus turning "dross into gold" (p. 16). This is, in part, the way the speechless, palsied Irish poet Christopher Nolan (1987) found his mellifluous voice:

> Fossilized for so long now, he was going to speak to anyone interested enough to listen.... Now he shared the same world as everyone else, he could choose how much to tell and craftily decide how much to hold back. His voice would be his written word. (p. 98)

The same mechanisms allowed comedian Buster Keaton to devote his life to making others laugh, while unable to laugh spontaneously himself (Miller, 1990). Long before Norman

Cousins found health and fame in laughter and neuroscience linked it to our immune systems, humor was acknowledged to be one of the truly elegant defenses in the human repertoire (Lefcourt & Martin, 1986). "Like hope, humor permits one to bear and yet to focus upon what may be too terrible to be borne" (Vaillant, 1977, p. 386). This is precisely what ailing critic Anatole Broyard (1990) did when he quipped, "What a critically ill person needs above all is to be understood. Dying is a misunderstanding you have to get straightened out before you go" (p. 29).

Resilience is not a miraculous rescue. It can be a mere thread that wrestles itself to the surface of an otherwise despairing existence. It is reflected in the struggle of a 50-year-old chronically mentally ill woman who sustains her sense of altruism despite unrelenting suspiciousness, fear, and rigid thought processes. She is an ardent giver of small gifts, of greeting cards weeks before the actual event, and of postage stamps she hopes will acquire great value for the recipient's future grandchildren. The dignity and control she experiences in giving to others when she herself is in such great need allows her more comfort than she might otherwise have. It buffers her from the painful realization of how isolated and vulnerable she really is.

Hamburg et al. (1974) summarized the essence of survival under extreme duress by underscoring the importance of the maintenance of self-esteem, a sense of human dignity, a sense of group belonging, and a feeling of being useful to others.

How Durable Is Resilience?

Resilient responses to ordeals have phase-specific attributes. In the acute phase, energy is directed at minimizing the impact of the stress and stressor. In the reorganization phase, a new reality is faced and accepted in part or in whole. And then there is the rest of one's life. How durable is resilience? We know it is neither a single act nor a constant state. How and under what circumstances does it emerge, shift, or fail the person? Camus (as cited by Maquet, 1958) described its emergence: "In the depth of winter I finally learned that within me there lay an invincible summer." In contrast, Monette (1988) experienced its decline: "I used up all my optimism keeping my friend alive. Now that he's gone, the cup of my health is neither half full nor half empty. Just half " (p. 2).

The suicides of Primo Levi and Bruno Bettelheim prompt similar questions. Why did Levi, successful chemist and award-winning author who recorded his Holocaust experiences because there "were things that imperiously demanded to be told" (1987, p. 9), choose to die? Did cancer and the ill health of his mother chip away at the mission he had set for himself? Did a history of exemplary behavioral competence distract from the depression and anxiety that often accompanies it? Did a major depression go untreated? What about Bettelheim? His essays bore witness to Nazi atrocities; his provocative style challenged a world he saw as too passive and naive. He enacted solutions to some of humanity's problems by developing therapeutic environments for severely disturbed children. Did retirement, physical ailments, or the loss of a familiar social network limit his ability to play out a meaningful life story? Did his resilience run out? Or was this last sorrowful act a measure of his need to be in control, exercising his own will, his way, while he could? He spoke prospectively of these issues in the introduction to *The Uses of Enchantment: The Meaning and Importance of Fairy Tales* (1977):

> If we hope to live not just from moment to moment, but in true consciousness of our existence, then our greatest need and most difficult achievement is to find meaning in our lives.... Many have lost the will to live, and have stopped trying, because such meaning has evaded them. An understanding of the meaning of one's life is not suddenly acquired at a particular age, not even when one has reached chronological maturity. (p. 3)

These anecdotes demonstrate the changing and highly personal nature of resilience, often attained at the cost of some degree of spontaneity and flexibility. This and the interplay among such factors as age, general health status, and changing roles and relationships may conspire to diminish the once raging will to live in some, while allowing others to continue to find meaning and commitment in changing life circumstances. Resilience appears to be less an enduring characteristic and more a process determined by the impact of particular life experiences on particular conceptions of one's own life history (Cohler, 1987), leading one, once again, to conclude that it is not so much what happens to people but how they interpret and explain it that makes a difference.

Integrating Personal Meaning, Behavior, and Reality: Implications for Practice

Who rises above adversity? Perhaps it is sufficient to say that human capacities can shrink, hibernate, and flourish under circumstances of extreme stress; the influence of personal perspective; and the people, places, and things in the environment. The lives I sampled in the course of this study heightened my appreciation for the richness of the coping process and the difficulties many face with the unrelenting demands of their illness and the oft-times unresponsive health-care system. Even a resilient outcome does not represent a simple linear trajectory. It often requires the empathic attention and skillful assistance of those, like us, who are empowered by training and, I hope, by inclination.

Ordeals Provide a Window of Opportunity

Physical and emotional disruptions, the circumstances that bring us and our consumers together, provide a window of opportunity. Timely and meaningful interventions can have a significant impact on the reintegration process. These interventions may involve us in multiple tasks, such as helping persons find meaning in their crises, helping them handle feelings provoked by their situation, helping them with the reality and consequences of their condition, and fostering the functional skills and behaviors that they will need to fulfill their potential. Unfortunately, individual needs and capacities do not necessarily run on the same time standard as that of third-party payers. Potential for resilience may be noted and nurtured, but not necessarily birthed in 6 inpatient days or 12 annual reimbursed outpatient visits. Illness, and certainly disability, is an ongoing process in which personal problems may constantly emerge to undermine technical control, social order, and individual mastery (Kleinman, 1988). The conflicts that arise among individual needs, professional values, and the system's priorities pose real challenges to those who need access before the window of opportunity is shut. We must examine our own role in perpetuating this dilemma. We must re-evaluate and, in some instances, reframe, short- and long-term practice models. Additionally, we must educate colleagues, administrators, and insurers to the personal and financial impact of psychosocial factors on recovery and rehabilitation outcome in all areas of specialization.

Many Factors Influence Individual Response to Ordeals

Many intervening variables affect patients' major life changes on the one hand and illness outcome on the other. The good news is that those who rise above adversity do not belong to an exclusive club. It is not a closed system. However, some people are their own best facilitators, while others need help. Neither group should face its ordeals at the hands of caregivers and environments that induce more stress by diminishing humanistic contacts and links with reality, by neglecting the person's need to predict or anticipate outcomes, or by ignoring the inner elements of coping and competency behaviors. It is troubling to note how well many of our treatment centers fulfill the criteria for extremely stressful, negative life events.

The variability of resilience may come as bad news for some, because it does not permit a simple recipe for treatment. Instead, we must commit ourselves to understanding the complexities of personality, coping capacities, and environmental influences and use them to identify goals, interventions, and environments that are meaningful to a given person under a given set of circumstances.

Transforming Adversity Into Possibilities

Murphy (1987) reminded us that "there is a need for order in all humans that impels us to search for systematic coherence in both nature and society, and when we can find none, to invent it" (p. 33). Thoughts, feelings, and actions, influenced by neurobiology and environment, are the means by which our patients attempt to invent coherence and order that is acceptable to themselves and the outside world (White, 1976). The experiences documented in the present paper are testimony to how innovative and powerful human thoughts, feelings, and actions can be.

These capacities are also our most elegant professional tools for transforming adversity into possibilities, when we take the time to conceive of them as such. As always, Sacks (1984) captured the essence of this phenomenon best:

> Rehabilitation involves action; acts ... [and] must be centered on the character of acts—and how to call them forth, when they have come apart, disintegrated, been "lost"—or "forgotten." (p. 182)

Calling forth the character of acts involves the therapist's understanding and using the patient's thoughts and feelings, collaborating with him or her, establishing trust, and reaching for the personal context that is partner to external reality and individual potentials for functional behavior.

Professional Entreaties

How well do we call forth the character of acts? I believe that as a group we are far more effective at defining reality and assessing and promoting performance then we are at assessing and making use of patients' views of themselves and their situation. Although our clinical prowess has grown greatly, we are too often committed only to present manifest performance. These snapshot approaches to capacity fail to reflect the unique adaptive style and potential of each person. If we are to enhance outcome, we must integrate the patients' experience of their condition and their pre-existing patterns of self-regulating activity with our concerns and strategies for functional mobilization.

Kleinman (1988) proposed the use of clinical mini-ethnographic methods for acquiring a better picture, much like an anthropologist does in assessing a different culture. The ethnographer draws on knowledge of the context to make sense of behavior, allowing herself to sample the subject's experience. Occupational therapists are ethnographers of sorts. We have unique access to information about activities of everyday living and what it is like to live with an illness or disability. We need only to acknowledge and actualize it. But do we? Do we draw out the patient's perception of his or her situation? Or do we focus only on those aspects of function we can see, palpate, or measure?

Practice has changed dramatically over the past 30 years, as much a product of outgrowth and development as it is a measure of new knowledge and shifts in the health-care system. We certainly have not been idle. It is therefore no surprise that we find ourselves pursuing the future with such vigor that we sometimes fail to look back to see if we have left something of value behind. I believe we are at great risk of leaving in our wake some of the most central and precious components of our practice—how people think and feel about themselves and the world in which they live. Evidence suggests that we may have already reframed the rehabilitation process to fit today's economy rather than to fit today's patients.

Our connections to the deeper personal experiences of our patients seem to be unduly mediated by professional objectivity, our personal reluctance to hear, and a narrow view of what belongs to a given area of specialization. Fleming (1989) identified the presence of practice dichotomies concerning the relative importance of the patient's personal phenomenological status and how best to relate to him or her. Although some therapists appear to use such information and their relationship in treatment, their ambivalence about acknowledging it relegates it to an underground practice and reflects troublesome conflicts in values. We must remind ourselves that psychosocial phenomena belong to everyone, irrespective of their diagnosis and health status. Practice that separates feelings from function and psychosocial from physical perpetuates disorder rather than fostering reintegration.

The profession's current efforts to examine the actuality of clinical reasoning shows great promise for rescuing the person inside our patients and for allowing us to acknowledge the credibility of this element of clinical activity. Similarly, the study of resilient persons provides us with important opportunities to share their experience, rethink our beliefs about occupational therapy's domain of concern, and enrich the emerging science of occupation. Like the subjects of this paper, "each of us maintains a personal theory of reality, a coherent set of assumptions developed over time about ourselves and our world that organizes our experiences and understanding and directs our behavior" (Janoff-Bulman & Timko, 1987, p. 136). I believe that our responsiveness to the inner lives of others can add perspective to our professional assumptions and enhance our understanding of human performance capacity. In so doing, we will find ourselves far better able to help our patients refine their adventures, find meaning and purpose in their ordeals, discover there is more to themselves than current circumstance suggests, and transform the dross of their adversity into the gold of their accomplishments.

Epilogue

This is a work in progress. My purpose has been to examine the relevance of resilience to our practice. However, one person's efforts to orchestrate the chorus of resilient voices cannot do them justice. I urge the reader to explore this literature as well. It is likely to stimulate extraordinary personal and professional awakening. Moreover, it merits our collective thought and action, because the efforts of many are needed to give meaning to the hardships our patients endure and the difference occupational therapy can make.

Acknowledgments

I dedicate this lecture to three resilient women whose adaptive style and commitment to challenge have greatly enriched my personal and professional life: my mother, Elsie Babbitt; my mentor and friend, Gail Fidler; and my daughter, Deborah Fine. All three not only see the cup as half full, but strive to keep it overflowing for themselves and others.

References

Améry, J. (1986). *At the mind's limits: Contemplations by a survivor on Auschwitz and its realities.* New York: Schocken.

Anthony, E. J., & Cohler, B. J. (Eds.). (1987). *The invulnerable child.* New York: Guilford.

Bettelheim, B. (1977). *The uses of enchantment: The meaning and importance of fairy tales.* New York: Knopf.

Bolin, R., & Trainer, P. (1978). Modes of family recovery following disaster: A cross national study. In E. L. Quarantelli (Ed.), *Disaster theory and research* (pp. 233–247). London: Sage.

Brown, C. (1990). *Down all the days.* London: Mandarin.

Browne, S. E., Connors, D., & Stern, N. (1985). *With the power of each breath: A disabled women's anthology.* San Francisco: Cleis.

Broyard, A. (1990, April 1). Good books about being sick. *New York Times Book Review,* p. 1, 28–30.

Cannon, W. (1939). *The wisdom of the body.* New York: Norton.

Chess, S., & Thomas, A. (1984). *Origins and evolution of behavior disorders: From infancy to early adult life.* New York: Brunner/Mazel.

Cleveland, M. (1984). Family adaptation to traumatic spinal cord injury: Response to crisis. In R. H. Moos (Ed.), *Coping with physical illness* (pp. 159–171). New York: Plenum.

Cohen, F., & Lazarus, R. S. (1973). Active coping processes, coping dispositions, and recovery from surgery. *Psychosomatic Medicine, 35,* 375–389.

Cohler, B. J. (1987). Adversity, resilience, and the study of lives. In E. J. Anthony & B. J. Cohler (Eds.), *The invulnerable child* (pp. 363–424). New York: Guilford.

Cousins, N. (1979). *Anatomy of an illness.* New York; Bantam.

Demos, E. V. (1989). Resiliency in infancy. In T. F. Dugan & R. Coles (Eds.), *The child in our times: Studies in the development of resiliency* (pp. 3–22). New York: Brunner/Mazel.

Dimsdale, J. E. (1974). The coping behavior of Nazi concentration camp survivors. *American Journal of Psychiatry, 131,* 792–797.

Dugan, T. F., & Coles, R. (1989). *The child in our times: Studies in the development of resiliency.* New York: Brunner/Mazel.

Egendorf, A. (1989). *Healing from the war: Trauma and transformation after Vietnam.* Boston: Shambala.

Elder, G. H. Jr., & Clipp, E. C. (1988). Combat experience, comradeship, and psychological health. In J. P. Wilson, Z. Harel, & B. Kahana (Eds), *Human adaptation to extreme stress from the Holocaust to Vietnam* (pp. 131–154). New York: Plenum.

Erikson, E. (1963). *Childhood and society.* New York: Norton.

Flach, F. (1988). *Resilience: Discovering a new strength at times of stress.* New York: Fawcett Columbine.

Fleming, M. (1989). The therapist with the three-track mind. In *The AOTA Practice Symposium guide 1989* (pp. 70–73). Rockville, MD: American Occupational Therapy Association.

Frank, C. (1988). On embodiment: A case study of congenital limb deficiency in American culture. In M. Fine & A. Asch (Eds.), *Women with disabilities* (pp. 41–71). Philadelphia: Temple University Press.

Frankl, V. E. (1984). *Man's search for meaning.* New York: Washington Square Press.

Gal, R., & Lazarus, R. S. (1975, December). The role of activity in anticipating and confronting stressful situations. *Journal of Human Stress, 1,* 4–20.

Garmezy, N. (1983). Stressors of childhood. In N. Garmezy & M. Rutter (Eds.). *Stress, coping and development in children* (pp. 43–84). New York: McGraw-Hill.

Garmezy, N. (1985). Stress-resistant children: The search for protective factors. In J. E. Stevenson (Ed.), *Recent research in developmental psychopathology* (pp. 213–233). Elmsford, NY: Pergamon.

Garmezy, N., & Masten, A. S. (1986). Stress, competence, and resilience: Common frontiers for therapist and psychopathologist. *Behavior Therapy, 17,* 500–521.

Gill, A. (1988). *The journey back from hell: An oral history—Conversations with concentration camp survivors.* New York: Morrow.

Goertzel, V., & Goertzel, M. G. (1962). *Cradles of eminence.* Boston: Little, Brown.

Goleman, D. (1989, April 20). Researchers find optimism helps body's defense system. *New York Times,* p. B15.

Hamburg, D. A., Coelho, G. V., & Adams, J. E. (1974). Coping and adaptation: Steps toward a synthesis of biological and social perspectives. In G. V. Coelho, D.A. Hamburg, & J. E. Adams (Eds.), *Coping and adaptation* (pp. 403–440). New York: Basic.

Heller, J., & Vogel, S. (1986). *No laughing matter.* New York: Avon.

Houston, B. K. (1987). Stress and coping. In C. R. Snyder & C. E. Ford (Eds.), *Coping with negative life events* (pp. 373–399). New York: Plenum.

I never saw another butterfly: Children's drawings and poems from Terezin Concentration Camp, 1942–1944 (1978). New York: Schocken Books.

Janoff-Bulman, R., & Timko, C. (1987). Coping with traumatic events, The role of denial in light of people's assumptive worlds. In C. R. Snyder & S. E. Ford (Eds.), *Coping with negative life events* (pp. 135–155). New York: Plenum.

Kahana, E., Kahana, B., Harel, Z., & Rosner, T. (1988). Coping with extreme trauma. In J. P. Wilson, Z. Harel, & B. Kahana (Eds.), *Human adaptation to extreme stress: From the Holocaust to Vietnam* (pp. 55–76). New York: Plenum.

Kleinman, A. (1988). *The illness narratives: Suffering, healing, and the human condition.* New York: Basic.

Kobasa, S C. (1979). Stressful life events, personality, and health: An inquiry into hardiness. *Journal of Personality and Social Psychology, 37,* 1–11.

Lazarus, R. S., & Folkman, S. (1984). *Stress, appraisal, and coping.* New York: Springer.

Lefcourt, H. M., & Martin, R. A. (1986). *Humor and life stress: Antidote to adversity.* New York: Springer-Verlag.

Levi, P. (1965). *The reawakening.* New York: Collier.

Levi, P. (1987). *Moments of reprieve.* New York: Penguin.

Lifton, R. J. (1988). Understanding the traumatized self. Imagery, symbolization, and transformation. In J. P. Wilson, Z. Harel, & B. Kahana (Eds.), *Human adaptation to extreme stress: From the Holocaust to Vietnam* (pp. 7–31). New York: Plenum.

Lifton, R. J., & Olson, E. (1976). The human meaning of total disaster. *Psychiatry, 39,* 1–17.

Mairs, N. (1986). *Plaintext: Deciphering a woman's life.* New York: Perennial Library.

Maquet, A. (1958). *Albert Camus. The invincible summer.* New York: Braziller.

Marmar, E. R., & Horowitz, M. J. (1988). Post-traumatic stress disorder. In J. P. Wilson, Z. Harel, & D. Kahana (Eds.), *Human adaptation to extreme stress: From the Holocaust to Vietnam* (pp. 81–103). New York: Plenum.

McGrath, M. (1984). First-person accounts: Where did I go? *Schizophrenia Bulletin, 10,* 638–640.

Miller, A. (1990). *The untouched key: Tracing childhood trauma in creativity and destructiveness.* New York: Doubleday.

Miller, V. (Ed.). (1985). *Despite this flesh: The disabled, stories and poems.* Austin, TX: University of Texas Press.

Minear, R. H. (Ed.). (1990). *Hiroshima: Three witnesses.* Princeton, NJ: Princeton University Press.

Monette, P. (1988). *Borrowed time: An AIDS memoir.* New York: Avon.

Moos, R., & Billings, A. (1982). Conceptualizing and measuring coping resources and processes. In L. Goldberger & S. Breznitz (Eds.), *Handbook of stress: Theoretical and clinical aspects* (pp. 212–220). New York: Macmillan.

Moos, R. H., & Schaefer, J. A. (1984). The crisis of physical illness: An overview and conceptual approach. In R. H. Moos (Ed.), *Coping with physical illness* (pp. 8–25). New York: Plenum.

Murphy, L. B., & Moriarty, A. (1976). *Vulnerability, coping, and growth: From infancy to adolescence.* New Haven, CT: Yale University Press.

Murphy, R. F. (1987). *The body silent.* New York: Henry Holt.

Nolan, C. (1987). *Under the eye of the clock.* New York: Dell.

Peck, E. C. (1987). The traits of true invulnerability and posttraumatic stress in psychoanalyzed men of action. In E. J. Anthony & B. J. Kohler (Eds.), *The invulnerable child* (pp. 315–360). New York: Guilford.

Pelletier, K. R., & Herzing, D. L. (1988). Psychoneuroimmunology: Toward a mind-body model: A critical review. *Advances, 5,* 27–56.

Potocki, E. R., & Everly, G. S. Jr. (1989). Control and the human stress response. In G. S. Everly, Jr. (Ed.), *A clinical guide to the treatment of the human stress response* (pp. 119–136). New York: Plenum.

Radner, G. (1989). *It's always something.* New York: Simon & Schuster.

Rahe, R. H., & Genender, E. (1983). Adaptation to and recovery from captivity stress. *Military Medicine, 148,* 577–585.

Redl, F. (1969). Adolescents—Just how do they react? In G. Caplan & S. Lebovici (Eds.), *Adolescence: Psychosocial perspectives* (pp. 79–90). New York: Basic.

Rosenfeld, M. S. (1989). Occupational disruption and adaptation: A study of house fire victims. *American Journal of Occupational Therapy, 43,* 89–96.

Sacks, O. (1984). *A leg to stand on.* New York: Harper & Row.

Selye, H. (1978). *The stress of life* (2nd ed.). New York: McGraw-Hill.

Sheehan, S. (1982). *Is there no place on earth for me?* New York: Vintage.

Shengold, L. (1989). *The effects of childhood abuse and deprivation.* New Haven, CT: Yale University Press.

Tamiki, H. (1990). Summer flowers. In R. H. Minear (Ed.), *Hiroshima* (pp. 19–114). Princeton NJ: Princeton University Press.

Torrance, E. P. (1965). *Constructive behavior: Stress, personality, and mental health.* Belmont, CA: Wadsworth.

Trillin, A. S. (1984). Of dragons and garden peas: A cancer patient talks to doctors. In R. H. Moos (Ed.), *Coping with physical illness* (pp. 131–138). New York: Plenum.

Vaillant, G. E. (1977). *Adaptation to life.* Boston: Little, Brown.

Weaver, G. (1985). Finch the spastic speaks. In V. Miller (Ed.), *Despite this flesh: The disabled in stories and poems* (pp. 35–45). Austin, TX: University of Texas Press.

Werner, E. E., & Smith, R. S. (1982). *Vulnerable but invincible: A study of resilient children.* New York: McGraw-Hill.

White, R. W. (1976). Strategies of adaptation: An attempt at systematic description. In R. H. Moos (Ed.), *Human adaptation: Coping with life crises* (pp. 17–32). Lexington, MA: Heath.

Wiesel, E. (1990). *From the kingdom of memory: Reminiscences.* New York: Summit.

CHAPTER 26

Beyond Performance: Being in Place as a Component of Occupational Therapy

GRAHAM D. ROWLES, PHD

The essence of becoming and remaining human is a combination of *knowing, doing,* and *being* (Knos, 1977). An accumulation of information results in our knowing everything from how to brush our teeth through how to prepare a salad to more complex tasks such as servicing an automobile. Knowing also involves expertise acquired through practice, as we apply learned skills in activities of self-care, work, and play. We learn and achieve a sense of accomplishment by doing (Fidler & Fidler, 1978) (see Chapter 9). Finally, to live as a fully self-actualizing person involves the process of being, of simply experiencing life and the environment around us, frequently in an accepting, noninstrumental way. Being, in this sense, involves the realms of meaning, value, and intentionality that imbue our lives with a richness and diversity that transcends what we know and what we do (Maslow, 1966). Appreciation of the beauty and fragrance of a rose, the meaning of a home as distinguished from the house where one resides, the warmth of a lifelong relationship with a friend, one's sense of self, and one's perspective on the meaning of existence all fall within this rubric.

In recent decades, occupational therapy has tended to emphasize knowing and doing as focal concerns. The purpose of this article is to suggest that occupational therapists may significantly enhance their contribution to improving the quality of life by more explicitly incorporating within everyday practice and research an increased concern with understanding *being in place,* which is one important aspect of their clients' being. Such a reorientation may be especially useful in working with and understanding elderly people and other less mobile populations for whom the environment may have come to assume particular significance.

An expanded, more experientially grounded focus would seem to be timely in view of several trends in occupational therapy. These trends include (a) a growing concern with differentiating occupational therapy from a purely medical model (Kielhofner & Burke, 1977; Mosey, 1974, 1980; Reilly, 1969; Rogers, 1982); (b) increased interest in promulgating basic research; (c) the quest for a dominant research paradigm and for theory, a science of human occupation (Christiansen, 1981; Kielhofner & Nicol, 1989; Llorens, 1984); and (d) a rediscovered concern with the evolution of a holistic perspective on human occupation that places emphasis on the role of the environment as an influence on capacity for functional independence (Barris, 1986; Kiernat, 1982, 1987).

In developing this perspective, I focus on three themes: the need for increased emphasis on the nature of being in place; some methodological implications of adopting such an expanded philosophy in terms of the need for naturalistic and qualitative research; and illustrations, drawn from my own research as a social geographer and gerontologist, of the kind of basic insights that can emerge from such a perspective.

Adding Being to Knowing and Doing

Emphasis in occupational therapy on knowing and doing as cornerstones of practice and research is the outcome of a philosophy premised on maximizing individual competence and autonomy in activities of daily living. Such a perspective involves a number of limiting assumptions about individual needs and the nature of well-being that are deeply embedded in western industrial and postindustrial culture. First, this perspective places an emphasis on performance and productivity as life goals (for a notable exception, see Reilly, 1974). Often this translates into a therapeutic focus on instrumental relationships and activities rather than on interpersonal and socioemotional aspects of identity—the belief that people's sense

This chapter was previously published in the *American Journal of Occupational Therapy, 45,* 265–271. Copyright © 1991, American Occupational Therapy Association.

of worth and fulfillment arises from what they do or how they perform rather than from who they are and who they have been. A second implicit assumption is an underestimation of persons' ability to respond creatively to incapacity and to compensate without occupational therapy intervention for particular dysfunctions through life-style adjustments, psychological accommodation, or enhancement of other domains of their lives. Third is a pervasive assumption that an orientation toward knowing and doing is invariant over the life span—in short, that there are no developmental changes in the degree to which people are or wish to be passive and contemplative rather than active and productive. For example, children at play characteristically spend lots of time "hanging around" with their peers. They engage in seemingly nonproductive activities that generate the familiar response of "Nothing!" to the "What are you doing?" of an inquisitive adult. At the other end of the life cycle, people who are growing older may have an increasing propensity for reminiscence, life review, and more reflective modes of being in the world (Butler, 1963; Coleman, 1986).

Finally, there is an underestimation of the role of a person's environment as a source of identity and well-being. In this article, environment is viewed as far more than the physical or social setting. Environment is the *lifeworld*—the culturally defined spatiotemporal setting or horizon of everyday life (Buttimer, 1976). This phenomenological perspective embraces physical, social, cultural, and historical dimensions of an environment of lived experience. Thus, the lifeworld not only includes the person's current setting but also has a space–time depth that is uniquely experienced within the framework of personal history. Being in place expresses immersion within such a lifeworld.

Increased understanding of clients' being in place can be achieved by exploration of the meanings, values, and intentionalities that underlie their experience of particular environments. Through this process, it will be possible to develop insights that both contribute to theory and enhance practice. Such an endeavor has significant epistemological implications.

Implications for Epistemology

There is a need for basic research on normative populations that explores the nature of being in place. How do healthy people experience their lives in different environmental contexts? Clearly, in an increasingly multidisciplinary world, much can be learned from insights developed in other disciplines. Such borrowing needs to be complemented by original research with an explicitly occupational therapy focus that probes the underlying meanings, values, and intentionalities associated with adaptations healthy people normally make in the way they use their homes and conduct activities of self-care, work, and play as they pass through various phases of their lives (King, 1978) (see Chapter 10). Basic research is also necessary on the way in which people cope experientially with illness and reduced competence in different environments, both with and without occupational therapy intervention.

To develop such insight, it is important to nurture growing acceptance within occupational therapy of the value of qualitative research (Kielhofner, 1982a, 1982b; Merrill, 1985; Philips & Pierson, 1982; Schmid, 1981). A major feature of such research is an imperative to study people's experience in naturalistic context outside the laboratory. As Barris, Kielhofner, Levine, and Neville (1985) noted,

> Because persons both shape and are shaped by their environments, occupational function and dysfunction reflect the individual's history of environmental interactions. As a result, no attempt to understand a person's behavior will ever be complete without some understanding (or assessment) of the environments from which the person came and the behavior patterns that were encouraged by these environments. (p. 60)

Implicit within this observation is an acknowledgment that each person's response to a situation is uniquely conditioned by personal history and temporal context. A person's handling of recovery from a stroke may be as dependent on previous patterns of response to personal crises or the prevalent values of his or her age cohort as upon physical and occupational therapy regimens (Kaufman, 1988). Finally, qualitative research focuses on the phenomenological world of the individual to reveal experience as he or she actually understands it rather than as externally interpreted. Such research delves into the experiential meaning of having a stroke and the way this meaning impinges on the path to recovery and the effectiveness of interventions.

What does this mean in practical terms? There are now many sources of information on both philosophies and methodologies of qualitative research (Bogdan & Taylor, 1975; Kielhofner, 1982a, 1982b; Lofland & Lofland, 1984; Miles & Huberman, 1984; Reinharz & Rowles, 1988; Spradley, 1979; Van Maanan, 1983–1989). Although this information will not be reviewed in detail, several underlying themes are worth highlighting.

The quest for depth of insight frequently necessitates the use of limited numbers of subjects selected through purposive or theoretical sampling procedures (Glaser & Strauss, 1967). Emphasis is placed on the establishment of strong interpersonal relationships with these subjects. In developing such relationships, the researcher endeavors to be open to the sociocultural and environmental context and to develop a sense of empathy and mutual trust that will enable the subject to reveal dimensions of experience that might otherwise remain taken for granted and unexpressed (Von Eckartsberg, 1971). This process often entails a lengthy investment of time by the research participants (researcher and subject) in developing a shared language. By developing such a lexicon, the researcher is able to assume the role of translator of the subject's experience.

Significant contamination of the research situation can result from such intimate and potentially intense involvement by the researcher. In qualitative research, however, this is not a problem, because the focus of inquiry is descriptive and oriented toward the development of hypotheses and the generation of original insight. Such insight arises through inductive generalization from case studies. In contrast with traditional experimental and survey research, the criteria for verification are intuitive: They rely on the degree to which the researcher can authentically convey the essence of the research experience, rather than on measures of statistical significance. The presentation of qualitative findings becomes a crucial determinant of their usefulness. Presentation is characteristically detailed and descriptive. It relies on the researcher's ability to write, not only in a way that evokes the nuances of the research situation, but also in a manner that effectively conveys the environmental context and the process involved in arriving at conclusions—the natural history of the project.

Having provided the outlines of a methodology for exploring people's being in place, a study of elderly people living in a rural Appalachian environment will be used to illustrate the value of such an approach in occupational therapy.

The Colton Study

In the spring of 1978, I began a 3-year ethnographic study of 15 elderly residents of Colton,[1] a community of approximately 400 people (Rowles, 1980, 1981, 1983a, 1983b, 1983c). The subjects, 11 women and 4 men, ranged in age from 62 to 91 at the outset of the study. Most were lifelong residents of Colton or its vicinity.

Close interpersonal relationships were developed with each participant to explore their involvement with the places of their lives. Particular emphasis was placed on attempting to reveal their relationship with the Colton environment. This involved learning about their daily activity patterns, identifying social networks, assessing perceptions of local space, and trying to reveal the phenomenological meaning of the setting that had been their home for so many years. In addition to observation and both unstructured and semistructured tape-recorded interviews, data gathering included time–space activity diaries, mental mapping procedures, aerial photography of the space around each participant's residence, social network measures, and a variety of morale and life-satisfaction scales. The overall objective was to develop a comprehensive understanding of each participant's lifeworld and the role of being in place in conditioning their experience of growing old.

Analysis involved both ongoing interpretation during interactions with the participants and inductive sorting of material following the fieldwork. Descriptive case studies were developed on each person. In addition, the dossiers compiled on each of the participants were carefully reviewed in a search for common themes. A clear image of what it is like to live and grow old in Colton gradually emerged through this process. Three themes in particular carry implications for occupational therapy.

The Rhythm and Routine of Taken-for-Granted Behavior

Each participant inhabited a highly individualistic lifeworld characterized by distinctive patterns of daily activity, a unique set of social relationships, and a highly personalized emotional affinity with the Colton environment. Early in the research, it became apparent that there were a number of shared underlying motifs that characterized elderly Colton residents' being in place. One of these was the way daily behavior had become highly routinized and taken for granted. There are two aspects of this phenomenon.

First is the concept of body awareness, an implicit sensitivity to the physical context that allows the person to effectively negotiate space on a preconscious level. This phenomenon, originally identified by French phenomenologists and elaborated by Seamon (1979), involves the way the repetition of actions within a familiar environment may allow a person to transcend sensory capabilities. For example, typing proficiency developed by practice enables us to produce a memorandum on our personal computers without having to identify each letter; our fingers seem to know where to place themselves. We climb the stairs many times in our residences without being conscious of the number of steps involved. When driving on the freeway, we may suddenly become aware that we have traveled 20 miles while daydreaming and yet have not driven off the pavement. In each case the body's "automatic pilot," or learned awareness of the context, has guided our actions. This phenomenon is clearly manifested in the lives of the Colton elderly. Walter, 82 years of age when my research began, had lived with his 81-year-old wife, Beatrice, in the same house for more than 57 years. He did not have to think about the location of the throw rugs or about the camber on the porch steps that made them particularly treacherous following a rainstorm. Intimate familiarity with the layout of his home had served him well as he had grown increasingly constrained by failing vision. Beatrice's use of this environment was also facilitated by her body awareness of the placement of furniture. The configuration of furniture had gradually evolved over the years in a manner that provided places for her to hold on should she experience one of the dizzy spells to which she had become prone. Body awareness may become particularly adaptive in old age. It may compensate for sensory decrements and allow elderly people to continue functioning effectively in residences that might otherwise preclude independent living. Such familiarity may be a factor in the strong attachment

---

[1]Pseudonyms are employed for all persons and locations referred to in this account.

to home and reluctance to leave displayed by many elderly people (O'Bryant, 1983).

Body awareness of the larger environment beyond the residence may contribute to the rhythm and routine that characterizes elderly Colton residents' everyday use of space within the community. Every morning, shortly before 10:00 a.m., Walter takes a leisurely 400-yard stroll down the hill from his house to the trailer that serves as the post office to "pick up the mail." He traces exactly the same path each day. Several male age peers from different locations within Colton embark on the same trip at about the same time. Of course, there is often no mail to be collected, but that is not the point. Rather, picking up the mail provides a rationale for an informal gathering of the elderly men of the community at the bench outside the Colton Store, which is located adjacent to the post office. The men generally linger throughout the morning. They watch the passing traffic, converse with patrons of the store, and discuss events of the day. Then, around lunchtime, the group disperses and Walter wends his way home again. There is also a spatiotemporal rhythm to the way in which the elderly women of Colton use community space. Their activity patterns tend to be focused on the Senior Center during the noontime hour when lunch is served. Indeed, most elderly Colton residents exhibit highly regular and routinized activity patterns focused on a limited number of behavior settings (Barker, 1968; Barker & Barker, 1961). Considered together, this regular interaction of diverse activity patterns reveals an ongoing "place ballet" (Seamon & Nordin, 1981). The spatiotemporal consistency of this place ballet may be highly adaptive. It provides a sense of security, because deviation from the regular pattern (e.g., the failure of Walter to appear at the bench outside the Colton Store) is characteristically noted and investigated.

Recognition of taken-for-granted and routinized behavior as a component of normative adaptation is not new (King, 1978; Meyer, 1922) (see Chapters 10 and 2, respectively), but it is a theme that merits re-emphasis in occupational therapy. To what extent is it possible to enrich practice through exploring interventions that build on these aspects of being in place? Recognizing the importance of taken-for-granted behavior also suggests that individual functioning—the freedom and confidence to participate in the environment beyond the home—may be closely related to the sociocultural ambience (accepted rules and norms of behavior) of the community environment. It becomes important to study not only actual behavior but also the underlying premises that condition such behavior—premises that include community expectations with respect to the assumption of mutual responsibility for the welfare of the vulnerable.

The Surveillance Zone

A second theme concerns the importance of certain zones of space as components of many elderly people's being in place. There is now a large and growing literature on the meaning and significance of home (Altman & Werner, 1985; Rybczyn-ski, 1987). Most occupational therapists are at least implicitly aware of the significance of this space to many of their clients. Only a few, I suspect, are equally cognizant of the significance of space immediately beyond the threshold. In Colton, the surveillance zone (space within the visual field of home) assumed increasing importance in many elderly persons' lives as they grew older (Rowles, 1981). For some, particularly the homebound, this space became the arena of their lives—space that could be viewed from the window or from the porch. Several of the study participants spent many hours each day watching events as they transpired on the street below. In some cases this involved the development of unspoken relationships with those who passed by. In turn, this was the zone of space in which they were watched by concerned neighbors. Some of the participants had developed a system of signals whereby they would open their shades or switch on the porch light at prearranged times each day. They gained a sense of security from the knowledge that they would be checked on should they fail to follow this procedure.

The surveillance zone often becomes the focus of both practical and social support relationships among neighbors. Some of the participants engaged in a process of setting up for surveillance. They would position a favorite chair by the window and place their telephone, television remote control, sewing, lunch tray, and other needed items within arm's reach. The significance of the surveillance zone is illustrated by 68-year-old Peggy, who perceived herself as virtually housebound. Following the death of her husband, she had the window by which she spent much of her time replaced with a larger picture window affording a better view.

The surveillance zone view from the window may have therapeutic value not only for elderly people but also for those who are sick (Ulrich, 1984). Occupational therapists may significantly enrich their clients' lives by showing increased sensitivity to the potential of this space. This might be accomplished by facilitating the process of setting up for surveillance, recommending the removal, where feasible, of obstacles to vision (e.g., trees or high sills), and engaging in efforts to enhance communication with neighbors within the visual field.

Environment as a Component of Self

One of the most important findings from the research was that for many of Colton's older residents, particularly persons 75 and older, the environment had become almost literally a part of the self (Rowles, 1983c). Over many decades of residence, the environment had developed a time-depth as it accumulated layer upon layer of meaning. Participants in the study had known the setting in a variety of different contexts. They had known it in childhood as a bustling and vibrant railroad and coal town of more than 800 residents. They could visualize the excitement of the annual Oyster Day when one of the local businessmen would arrange for oysters to be brought in from Baltimore and the whole community would celebrate an unofficial holiday. They could recall the first kiss of adolescence, stolen by the pond in Raccoon Hollow, a favorite teenage haunt. They had also known this place during the hard times of the Great Depression. They remembered the day in 1931 when the bank closed its doors; they remembered the stores that had gone out of business, the abandonment of homes, and the departure of the young in search of employment in cities beyond Appalachia. Indeed, over the years, they had accumulated memories of incidents and events within a series of different Coltons that had evolved during their lifetimes.

For each person the reservoir of memories was unique. It represented a collage of incident places, that is, locations where particular events transpired, that are grounded in personal history and suffused with emotional significance. Each participant was able to vicariously immerse himself or herself within the places of the past and in so doing was able to transcend the bounds of both physical competence and the contemporary environment. Acknowledging this ability enables us to understand how the environment, particularly for those who have lived in the same setting for many years, may become a repository of meaning, a part of the self that is inextricably linked to self-identity.

Such fusion with the environment is well illustrated by the way many older people, and young ones too, manipulate their physical setting in a way that transforms it into an expression of who they are and have been. For example, Walter had assembled a working set of railroad lights and signals in his front yard. The trains no longer stopped in Colton, but these memorabilia served not only to remind him of the focus of his working life as a railroader but also presented a statement of his enduring identity to all who passed by.

Similar insight can be gleaned from the environment that Dan, a burly 86-year-old former coal miner, had created for himself. Dan shared a home with one of his daughters and her husband; it was located on a hillside overlooking the center of Colton. During our early meetings, I met with Dan in his bedroom or in the living room of the house. His sparsely decorated room contained many of the artifacts one might expect to find in the home of a rugged person who had enjoyed hunting. There was a gun rack on the wall and photographs recording successful fishing exploits. During our initial conversations, Dan would sometimes refer to his "rooms." I assumed that he was referring to his bedroom. One day, after I had come to know him a little better, he decided to show me the rooms. There were two of them, interconnected and located on the second floor of the house. As we entered, I was surprised to be confronted with a blaze of color. The walls were covered with decorated china plates and the tables, cabinets, and shelves were crammed with neatly arranged vases, china dolls, and ceramic and glass ornaments. When Dan was in his early 30s his wife had died, leaving him alone to raise five children. He had been obliged to adopt a more conventionally feminine role. In the process,

he had begun to accumulate the artifacts, and gradually his interest had evolved to the point where he would search out such items at yard sales and local fairs. His rooms both reflected and symbolized an important aspect of an unusual life experience that had become a part of his identity and a source of feelings of accomplishment in his old age.

By attempting to reveal and become sensitive to the spatiotemporal meaning and significance of the environment to their clients, occupational therapists may be able to identify intervention strategies more attuned to the experiential worlds of those they seek to serve. Such sensitivity may be especially important in dealing with people who have resided for many years in the same setting or who recently relocated from such a familiar environment. From a pragmatic perspective, developing deeper understanding of being in place will necessitate research. In-depth qualitative studies may be valuable in developing a clearer understanding of why some people respond positively to specific occupational therapy interventions and conscientiously follow recommendations but others seem resistant to efforts to assist them (Merrill, 1985). Such research may suggest ways in which environmental manipulation may be used to substitute or compensate for losses and to foster a continued sense of self-identity. This may be an important complement to more traditional skill- and competence-building interventions. Finally, research into the existential meaning of environment to clients may contribute significantly to the development of more sophisticated theory in occupational therapy.

Conclusion

In developing my thesis, I am not suggesting that knowing, doing, and being are discrete and mutually exclusive components of human occupation. They are intimately interrelated. Indeed, implicit within the illustrations from Colton are elements of knowing and doing. Physical routines of moving around within the environment, the process of scanning the surveillance zone, and accumulating artifacts to reinforce a sense of identity are all active components of occupying place. They undergird the person's experience of being in place and are prerequisite to it.

My argument is that widely accepted and internalized tenets of contemporary occupational therapy philosophy may be compromising and limiting the potential of the field. Emphasis on performance, as manifested by knowing and doing, has tended to relegate the notion of being (as a component of well-being and a fulfilling life) to an ancillary role. One outcome of this has been inadequate consideration, at least until recently, of the role of the person's experienced spatiotemporal environment in conditioning his or her response to dysfunctions and to the intervention strategies designed to remedy them.

More explicit incorporation of concern for understanding the person's being in place will enrich occupational therapy research and practice in several domains. First, it becomes possible by employing naturalistic and qualitative methodologies to more directly incorporate within emergent theory, consideration of the influence of the environmental context as a component of the meanings, values, and intentionalities with which clients imbue their occupation (be it self-care, work, or play).

Revelation of the nature of being in place in all of its space–time complexity in both normative and therapeutic situations facilitates discovery of ways in which compensatory strengths may be manifest in both the person and his or her environmental context (Rogers, 1982). Such strengths may emanate from dimensions of human experience that are neither productivity nor performance driven. They may arise through the identity-reinforcing potential of reminiscence, through vicarious immersion in spatially or temporally displaced environments, or through other noninstrumental aspects of being in place that are part of the context in which occupational therapy is practiced.

Finally, concern with an exploration of the nature of being in place offers the potential for improved understanding of the way in which many people function as their own occupational therapists or as therapists for their peers. They may accomplish this by developing an invariant daily routine in their use of the environment, by increasing the size of a picture window, or by surrounding themselves with artifacts and memorabilia that provide a constant reminder of their enduring identity— who they are and who they have been. Such simple and frequently taken-for-granted facets of being in place may assume great importance in persons' striving for continuing independence and autonomy as they accommodate to changing abilities and personal circumstances.

In making these observations, I am not suggesting that occupational therapy should turn away from other aspects of its mission—for example, from concern for increasing a person's range of motion, or for enhancing a person's ability to cope with or overcome physical or sensory losses. Rather, I am reinforcing recent arguments for a return to the more holistic perspective that characterized the origins of occupational therapy in the early part of this century as the field evolved out of a Moral Treatment tradition (Kielhofner & Nicol, 1989). I am advocating that efforts to enhance performance be framed within the broader context of increased sensitivity to and concern for clients' being in place. It is these sometimes subtle components of a person's lifeworld that may continue to sustain him or her as a fully self-actualizing human being in spite of the circumstances that have necessitated occupational therapy intervention.

Acknowledgment

I thank Gary Kielhofner, DrPH, OTR, of the University of Illinois at Chicago for his helpful comments on an earlier version of this article.

References

Altman, I., & Werner, C. M. (Eds.). (1985). *Home environments*. New York: Plenum.

Barker, R. G. (1968). *Ecological psychology*. Stanford: Stanford University Press.

Barker, R. G., & Barker, L. S. (1961). The psychological ecology of old people in Midwest, Kansas, and Yoredale, Yorkshire. *Journal of Gerontology, 61*, 231–239.

Barris, R. (1986). Activity: The interface between person and environment. *Physical and Occupational Therapy in Geriatrics, 5*, 39–49.

Barris, R., Kielhofner, G., Levine, R. E., & Neville, A. M. (1985). Occupation as interaction with the environment. In G. Kielhofner (Ed.), *A Model of Human Occupation: Theory and application* (pp. 42–62). Baltimore: Williams & Wilkins.

Bogdan, R., & Taylor, S. J. (1975). *Introduction to qualitative research methods. New York:* Wiley Interscience.

Butler, R. N. (1963). The life review: An interpretation of reminiscence in the aged. *Psychiatry, 26*, 65–76.

Buttimer, A. (1976). Grasping the dynamism of lifeworld. *Annals of the Association of American Geographers, 66*, 277–292.

Christiansen, C. H. (1981). Editorial: Toward resolution of crisis: Research requisites in occupational therapy. *Occupational Therapy Journal of Research, 1*, 115–124.

Coleman, P. G. (1986). *Aging and reminiscence processes: Social and clinical implications*. New York: Wiley.

Fidler, G. S., & Fidler, J. W. (1978). Doing and becoming: Purposeful action and self-actualization. *American Journal of Occupational Therapy, 32*, 305–310. Reprinted as Chapter 19.

Glaser, B. G., & Strauss, A. (1967). *The discovery of grounded theory: Strategies for qualitative research*. New York: Aldine.

Kaufman, S. R. (1988). Stroke rehabilitation and the negotiation of identity. In S. Reinharz & G. D. Rowles (Eds.), *Qualitative gerontology*. New York: Springer.

Kielhofner, G. (1982a). Qualitative research: Part One—Paradigmatic grounds and issues of reliability and validity. *Occupational Therapy Journal of Research, 2*, 67–79.

Kielhofner, G. (1982b). Qualitative research: Part Two—Methodological approaches and relevance to occupational therapy. *Occupational Therapy Journal of Research, 2*, 150–164.

Kielhofner, G., & Burke, J. P. (1977). Occupational therapy after 60 years: An account of changing identity and knowledge. *American Journal of Occupational Therapy, 31*, 675–689.

Kielhofner, G., & Nicol, M. (1989). The model of human occupation: A developing conceptual tool for clinicians. *British Journal of Occupational Therapy, 52*, 210–214.

Kiernat, J. M. (1982). Environment: The hidden modality. *Physical and Occupational Therapy in Geriatrics, 2*, 3–12.

Kiernat, J. M. (1987). Promoting independence and autonomy through environmental approaches. *Topics in Geriatric Rehabilitation, 3*, 1–6.

King, L. J. (1978). 1978 Eleanor Clarke Slagle Lecture: Toward a science of adaptive responses. *American Journal of Occupational Therapy, 32*, 429–437. Reprinted as Chapter 10.

Knos, D. S. (1977). On learning. In M. Sarris (Ed.), *New perspectives on geographic education: Putting theory into practice.* (pp. 1–11). Dubuque, IA: Kendall/Hunt.

Llorens, L. A. (1984). Theoretical conceptualizations of occupational therapy: 1960–1982. *Occupational Therapy in Mental Health, 4*(2), 1–14.

Lofland, J., & Lofland, L. (1984). *Analyzing social settings. A guide to qualitative observation and analysis*. Belmont, CA: Wadsworth.

Maslow, A. (1966). *The psychology of science: A reconnaissance*. Chicago: Henry Regnery.

Merrill, S. C. (1985). Qualitative methods in occupational therapy research: An application. *Occupational Therapy Journal of Research, 5,* 209–222,

Meyer, A. (1922). The philosophy of occupation therapy. *Archives of Occupational Therapy, 1,* 1–10. Reprinted as Chapter 2.

Miles, M. B., & Huberman, A. M. (1984). *Qualitative data analysis*. Beverly Hills, CA: Sage.

Mosey, A. C. (1974). An alternative: The biopsychosocial model. *American Journal of Occupational Therapy, 28,* 137–140.

Mosey, A. C. (1980). A model for occupational therapy. *Occupational Therapy in Mental Health, 1*(1), 11–31.

O'Bryant, S. L. (1983). The subjective value of "home" to older homeowners. *Journal of Housing for the Elderly, 1,* 29–43.

Philips, B. U., & Pierson, W. P. (1982). Commentary: Qualitative research in occupational therapy. *Occupational Therapy Journal of Research, 2,* 165–170.

Reilly M. (1969). The educational process. *American Journal of Occupational Therapy, 23,* 299–307.

Reilly, M. (Ed.). (1974). *Play as exploratory learning*. Beverly Hills, CA: Sage.

Reinharz, S., & Rowles, G. D. (Eds.). (1988). *Qualitative gerontology*. New York: Springer.

Rogers, J. C. (1982). Order and disorder in medicine and occupational therapy. *American Journal of Occupational Therapy, 36,* 29–35.

Rowles, G. D. (1980). Growing old "inside": Aging and attachment to place in an Appalachian community. In N. Datan & N. Lohmann (Eds.), *Transitions of aging* (pp. 153–170). New York: Academic Press.

Rowles, G. D. (1981). The surveillance zone as meaningful space for the aged. *Gerontologist, 23,* 304–311.

Rowles, G. D. (1983a). Between worlds: A relocation dilemma for the Appalachian elderly. *International Journal of Aging and Human Development, 17,* 301–314.

Rowles, G. D. (1983b). Geographical dimensions of social support in rural Appalachia. In G. D. Rowles & R. J. Ohta (Eds.), *Aging and milieu: Environmental perspectives on growing old* (pp. 111–130). New York: Academic Press.

Rowles, G. D. (1983c). Place and personal identity in old age: Observations from Appalachia. *Journal of Environmental Psychology, 3,* 299–313.

Rybczynski, W. (1987). Home: A short history of an idea. London: Penguin.

Schmid, H. (1981). Qualitative research and occupational therapy. *American Journal of Occupational Therapy, 35,* 105–106.

Seamon, D. (1979). *A geography of the lifeworld: Movement, rest and encounter*. New York: St. Martin's.

Seamon, D., & Nordin, C. (1981). Marketplace as place ballet: A Swedish example. *Landscape 24,* 35–41.

Spradley, J. (1979). *The ethnographic interview*. New York: Holt, Rinehart & Winston.

Ulrich, R. (1984). View through a window may influence recovery from surgery. *Science, 224,* 420–421.

Van Maanan, J (Ed.). (1983–1989). *Qualitative methodology*. Beverly Hills, CA: Sage.

Von Eckartsberg, R. (1971). On experiential methodology. In A. Georgi, W. F. Fischer, & R. Von Eckartsberg (Eds.), *Duquesne studies in phenomenological psychology*. (Vol.1, pp. 66–79). Pittsburgh, PA: Duquesne University Press/Humanities Press.

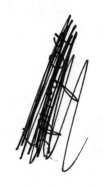

Play Deprivation in Children With Physical Disabilities: The Role of the Occupational Therapist in Preventing Secondary Disability

CHERYL MISSIUNA, MSc, OT(C)
NANCY POLLOCK, MSc, OT(C)

Self-initiated free play experiences are vital for the normal growth and development of all children. In this chapter, children with physical disabilities who are deprived of normal play opportunities are viewed as having a second disability that hinders their potential for independent behavior and performance. Physical, social, personal, and environmental barriers that may limit the play experiences of children with physical disabilities are delineated. Studies of the interactions of these children during play are discussed, and a case is made for the promotion of active, free play in the home, the school, and the community. As facilitators of this process, occupational therapists must consider a variety of factors, including the unique capabilities of the child, the influence of parent–child and peer relationships, the role of other caregiving adults, the adaptation of toys and materials, and the impact of the environment and setting.

Occupational therapists are unique in their emphasis on productive activity. A primary productive activity for young children is play (Bundy, 1989). In therapy, we frequently use play activities to achieve treatment objectives such as fine motor skill development, postural control, and concept development. This widely accepted use of toys and playful activity can be contrasted with another less evident function of play: the value of free play for its own sake. Rast (1986) noted, "Play and therapy almost appear to be mutually exclusive. A child's play is an intrinsically motivating activity done voluntarily and for its own sake; therapy proceeds according to the therapist's plan to achieve definite treatment objectives" (p. 30). If we consider play to be the primary productive activity for children, then the development of play skills becomes, in itself, an important goal for therapeutic intervention. Play acts as an antecedent for work and adult recreation and also serves to develop competence. We need to concern ourselves with play skills and also with the child's playfulness and motivation to engage in play.

In this paper, literature is used to demonstrate the purpose and benefit of free play experiences and to outline some of the barriers to free play that may be encountered by children with physical disabilities. The role of occupational therapists working with parents in preventing play deprivation and secondary disability is explored.

What Is Play?

Play is a complex, multifaceted behavior that is relatively easy to observe and describe but difficult to define theoretically (Rubin, Fein, & Vandenberg, 1983). Two characteristics that would be considered by most to be essential to the construct of play are that it be intrinsically motivated and that it be pleasurable (Ellis, 1973; Lindquist, Mack, & Parham, 1982; Mack, Lindquist, & Parham, 1982). In an occupational behavior framework, play is considered to be the primary activity of the child, a prerequisite to competence in occupational roles later in life (Reilly, 1974). Play has an exploratory component that is engaged in for its own sake and a competency component that results from an inner drive to master the environment (Reilly, 1974). Work and play are viewed along a developmental continuum, with play continuing to serve an adaptive function in adulthood (Kielhofner & Barris, 1984; Matsutsuyu, 1971). Sheridan (1975) elaborated on this work-play distinction by defining play as "eager engagement in pleasurable, physical or mental effort to obtain emotional satisfaction" (p. 5). Work, in contrast, is defined as "voluntary engagement in disciplined physical or mental effort to obtain material benefit" (p. 5).

The benefits of play are well-established (Ayres, 1981; Ellis, 1973; Erikson, 1963; Garvey, 1977; Gralewicz, 1973; Kielhofner & Barris, 1984; McHale & Olley, 1982; Piaget, 1951, 1952; Reilly, 1974; Vandenberg & Kielhofner, 1982). During play, children have the opportunity to discover what effect they can have on objects and people in their environment and to develop and test social and occupational roles. As children move around and explore their world, they receive information through their senses, gain knowledge about the nature and properties of objects, and develop rules about their own location in time and space (Robinson, 1977). The skills that are developed during play permit children to interact with and respond to the demands of their environment (Anderson, Hinojosa, & Strauch, 1987). This, in turn, leads to perceptual, conceptual, intellectual, and language development and, it has been argued, to the eventual integration of cognitive abilities (Levitt, 1975; Weininger, 1979, 1980, 1988; Weininger & Fitzgerald, 1988).

Occupational therapists working within sensory integrative, neurodevelopmental, occupational behavior, and developmental perspectives have recognized the sensorimotor, social, and constructive benefits of play and have justified its wide use in therapy as a treatment modality (Anderson et al., 1987). It is important for us, as therapists, to examine whether or not the benefits that may be attributed to the playful use of activity can be equated to the definition of play as a pleasurable activity that is emotionally satisfying. The distinction between the two forms of play can be highlighted by referring to the latter form as free play. In contrast to planned therapy sessions that are designed to produce specific responses through play, free play is spontaneous, intrinsically motivated, and self-regulated and requires the expressive personal involvement of the child (Calder, 1980; Garvey, 1977; Gunn, 1975; Yawkey, Dank, & Glossenger, 1986).

Primary and Secondary Forms of Play Deprivation

The designation, children with physical disabilities, is used in this paper to refer to children with sensory impairments, multiple handicaps, or limitations in voluntary movement or mobility. The impact of any of these disabilities can range from mild to severe in the degree to which the disability interferes with the child's ability to function independently. A child with mild cerebral palsy may have poor hand function, limiting his or her ability to manipulate a toy as desired; a child with a more severe impairment may be unable even to communicate his or her interest in a toy. Regardless of the individual circumstances, Mogford (1977) has proposed that the ability of children with physical disabilities to "explore, interact with, and master their environment is impaired with

a consequent distortion or deprivation of normal childhood experiences" (p. 171).

The deprivation described by Mogford can be considered from two perspectives. First, a physical disability often implies an absence of, or deficiency in, sensory and motor information being received by the child. A child will inevitably be deprived of the play experiences that cannot be made available to him or her due to the disabling condition. For example, a child with a visual impairment will not be able to experience directly the effect of play with lights or colors, nor will a child with a hearing impairment have the opportunity to play with voices and musical sounds. Alternative forms of play can be substituted, but this primary form of deprivation will remain unchanged.

Second, the occupational therapist is concerned with the secondary disabilities that may arise as an indirect result of play deprivation. Children with physical disabilities are often more dependent on their caregivers and other people than are nondisabled children (Rubin et al., 1983). Brown and Gordon (1987), in a study of the activity patterns of children with physical disabilities, found that disabled children spent more time in self-care and passive activities in their own homes than did nondisabled children. The child who is unable to experience normal childhood play because of a physical disability may encounter secondary social, emotional, and psychological disabilities. Examples of this form of play deprivation are children with visual impairments who are not permitted to climb monkey bars because they might fall, children with hearing impairments who are not allowed to play outside because they might not hear a car, and children in wheelchairs who are unable to cross the street to get to a park.

Free play provides a forum for children to explore their own capacities, to experiment with objects, to make decisions, to understand cause-and-effect relationships, to learn, to persist, and to understand consequences. This type of play also fosters creativity and allows a child to develop social skills when the play involves peers. Cotton (1984) suggested that, in addition to developing competence through play, the child also learns to cope with anxiety, frustration, and failure.

If children with physical disabilities are deprived of the opportunity to regularly engage in free play, it seems plausible that particular types of secondary disabilities are likely to result. Increased dependence on others, decreased motivation, lack of assertiveness, poorly developed social skills in unstructured situations, and lowered self-esteem are a few of the difficulties that may be experienced by children with disabilities (Clarke, Riach, & Cheyne, 1977/1982; Levitt & Cohen, 1977; Mogford, 1977; Philip & Duckworth, 1982). These secondary disabilities have an impact not only on the child's play and development, but also on later functioning in the school setting, the community, and the workplace. It is in the prevention of secondary disabilities that the role of the occupational therapist becomes important.

Barriers to Free Play

Play deprivation, primary and secondary, may occur as a result of many different forms of barriers. For children with physical disabilities, the areas that have been addressed most frequently in the literature are limitations imposed by caregivers, physical and personal limitations of the child, environmental barriers, and social barriers.

Limitations Imposed by Caregivers

Children need the freedom to initiate and engage actively in activities, the chance to make decisions and take risks, and the opportunity to master their physical selves or to accomplish a task they have chosen (Diamond, 1981). Well-meaning parents and teachers frequently overprotect children who have disabilities and may not permit their participation in normal activities (Calder, 1980; Hewett, Newson, & Newson, 1970; Philip & Duckworth, 1982; Williams & Matesi, 1988). Whether due to fear of injury, pity, compassion, or lack of knowledge about a child's abilities, adults may intervene too quickly and may unnecessarily limit the child's opportunity to play (Diamond, 1981; Levitt, 1975). In addition, concern for the child's physical development and progress may lead caregivers to fail to appreciate his or her need for play, with the result that free time may be used for therapy or for catching up on schoolwork (Calder, 1980; Mogford, 1977).

Physical and Personal Limitations of the Child

The natural exploration of the environment observed even in infancy in nondisabled children may not be possible for the child with a physical disability. Lack of mobility, limited communication, difficulty with reach and grasp, and impaired sensory responses may all interfere with the child's ability to play with toys or household objects. Children with physical disabilities may not be provided with chances to engage in nonstructured forms of play, such as launching an assault on the kitchen cupboards, bouncing on the bed, roughhousing, and participating actively in the neighborhood, at the park, and on the playground (Levitt, 1975; Russell, 1978). Csikszentmihalyi (1975) stressed the importance of matching a person's skills to the challenges of the environment. In the case of the child with a physical disability, environmental challenges often exceed the child's skills, leading to anxiety and frustration.

In addition to the apparent physical and sensory limitations, a number of authors have suggested that there may be factors within the child that limit participation in play. Limited intrinsic motivation (Levitt & Cohen, 1977; Mogford, 1977), lack of drive and decreased concentration (Salomon, 1983; Sheridan, 1975), and withdrawal due to lack of skill or frustration (Calder, 1980) have all been proposed as problems that may be inherent in the disabled child. It is not possible to state with certainty whether these problems originate within the child or arise secondarily due to a lack of opportunity for participation in self-initiated play activities.

Environmental Barriers

Barriers imposed by the physical environment (e.g., steps, narrow doorways) may severely limit the disabled child's opportunities for free play. These barriers may be present in the home as well as in the community (e.g., schools, recreational facilities, and playgrounds). The physical structure of toys, materials, and equipment may limit children's ability to express themselves and to explore objects (Rubin et al., 1983). Changes within the child's home environment may have been made to suit the child's individual needs; however, in the authors' experience, these modifications are rarely extended to the broader community environment. For the most part, buildings and playgrounds have been constructed to meet the needs of the young person without physical disabilities. A safe environment that allows opportunity for freedom of movement and that is filled with familiar play materials is considered to be optimal for free play (Knox, 1989). How often is this type of environment available for the child with physical disabilities?

Social Barriers

Interaction With Peers

Most normal free-play experiences center around interaction with peers. Parten (1932), in the now-familiar hierarchy of social interaction during play, described the increasingly complex stages of play ranging from parallel play to cooperation among players to achieve a common goal. Through these increasingly sophisticated interactions, the child learns societal norms and rules of behavior, is given the chance to experiment with different roles (e.g., leader, organizer), and models the social behaviors of other children. Children with physical disabilities are often limited in their interactions with other players due to both physical limitations and exclusion by their peer group. With decreased opportunities for interaction during the early years, the child with a disability may have a limited repertoire of social skills, which further increases his or her isolation. To illustrate this point, consider the presence of a child with physical disabilities in a mainstreamed kindergarten program. The child may not know how to initiate play with another child or how to join a group of children already playing at an activity center. It is no wonder that studies have repeatedly demonstrated that children with physical disabilities have poorly developed social skills (Clarke et al., 1977/1982; Philip & Duckworth, 1982).

Interaction With Parents

The lack of playfulness present in many parental interactions is another potential area of social deprivation during play (Kogan, Tyler, & Turner, 1974; Oster, 1984). Therapists may ask parents to become the child's teacher-therapist in the home environment. Although consistency and carryover of treatment ideas and approaches are beneficial to achieve therapy objectives, the question of the cost to the parent-child relationship must be raised. The interaction of a parent functioning as a therapist can be very different from normal parent-child interaction, and professionals have recently begun to question the effect of this interaction on the social development of the child with a disability (Rogers, 1988). It has further been proposed that the role of home therapist may produce an emotional conflict for the nurturing, accepting parent (Foster, Berger, & McLean, 1981). If parents are asked to follow a regimen established by a therapist, then their unique role and interaction with the child may be diminished (Kaiser & Hayden, 1984).

A number of studies performed in recent years have addressed this issue through an examination of the play of mothers with children who have physical disabilities. In contrast to nondisabled children, results suggest that mothers of disabled children perceive play and teaching situations as similar (Oster, 1984); show more negative affect and perceive the play situation as unrewarding (Kogan, 1980; Kogan et al., 1974); and are more directive and controlling (Brooks-Gunn & Lewis, 1982a, 1982b; Crawley & Spiker, 1983; Cunningham & Barkley, 1979; Hanzlik, 1989; Hanzlik & Stevenson, 1986; Oster, 1984). Many parents have expressed concern about the "one good hour" that they may have with their child: Their desire to simply cuddle and play with the child is rapidly extinguished when they recall the necessity to perform a home program (Kaiser, 1982). Similarly, several adults with cerebral palsy reported to Kibele (1989) that therapy had a negative effect on their relationships with their mothers. The demands of home programs limited their leisure time and, in some cases, led to the impression that they were disappointing their parents, particularly when skill development did not improve. It is essential for a parent to have positive interactions with his or her child, yet it is also important for the child's development to be stimulated whenever possible. Free play, not disguised therapy, may achieve similar objectives with less stress on the family.

Overcoming Barriers to Play: The Role of the Occupational Therapist

Occupational therapists may be in an ideal position to develop and maximize the free play opportunities of the child with physical disabilities in many settings. As professionals who are concerned with the child's development in the areas of self-care, productivity, and leisure, occupational therapists have the opportunity to work with the child in the home, in a treatment facility, or in a wide variety of community settings. Awareness of the barriers that the child frequently encounters and an understanding of the child's capabilities may facilitate the consultative process.

Assessment

Naturalistic observation and appraisal of a child's developmental play level is as essential to an occupational therapy assessment as evaluation of other activities of daily living. The play history, the types of play engaged in (e.g., active, exploratory, imitative, constructive, dramatic), the stage of play (e.g., solitary, independent, parallel, associative), and the developmental progression of object play (e.g., functional, relational, symbolic, combinatory) may all receive consideration. (Good reviews of these areas can be found in Behnke & Fetkovich, 1984; Florey, 1981; Kielhofner & Barris, 1984; Sheridan, 1975; and Sparling, Walker, & Singdahlsen, 1984.) Other important parts of a complete assessment are the frequency of play times, the variety of toys available, the physical location, and the opportunities for social interaction with peers and caregivers during these times.

Intervention

Providing opportunities for free play. Children with physical disabilities often have much less time available for play than do their nondisabled peers, in part due to the time spent in therapeutic programs (Brown & Gordon, 1987). If play is believed to be an important component of the child's life, then time must be built in to allow for free play experiences in the classroom, the therapeutic setting, the home, and the community.

In any play situation, a child needs to have the opportunity to choose, to explore, to create, and to respond to change if the result is truly to be called free play. Consideration can be given to the play space, recognizing the child's need for both personal play space and free ranging space in contact with other people (Stout, 1988). Whenever possible, caregiving adults can be encouraged by the therapist to let the child explore and interact independently. Numerous studies have indicated that adults working with physically disabled children tend to intervene too quickly, with the result that the children become highly dependent on this intervention during play (Federlein, 1979; Field, 1980; Field, Roseman, de Stefano, & Koewler, 1982; Levitt, 1975).

Consultation with parents. The therapist's expectations of, and recommendations to, the parent in the home environment must be thoughtfully considered. Parental participation in a child's play is not only positive but may be essential for children with more severe impairments. Many parents view this play time, however, as a time to "learn to use materials and to learn to use them correctly" (Oster, 1984, p. 156). To maximize play opportunities, parents may first need to be convinced of the importance of free play to the total health and development of the child. Understanding the educational value of play as well as the sequence of development that occurs in play may help parents view play as more than a pastime. Henderson and Bryan (1984) have suggested that parents must believe that self-direction is important and must trust their child's ability to learn from his or her own play experiences. The parent-child relationship is reciprocal, and parental expectations and beliefs will have an impact on the quality of the play. In addition, some of the apparent benefits of play—increased motivation, improved self-concept, and more active participation—may be viewed negatively by parents. For example, children who were previously satisfied with the vicarious experiences provided by television may become more demanding in their desire to have an active play life. In these instances, increasing the involvement of siblings or peers at home or in a play setting may be beneficial.

Consultation with teachers and caregivers. When therapists talk to teachers or caregivers about play and make recommendations for toys and play activities, the specific barriers that may limit the child's play in that setting must be addressed. The limitations imposed by caregivers are usually grounded in a genuine concern for the safety and welfare of the child. It is important for the therapist to acknowledge these concerns and to discuss with caregivers or teachers the extent to which their fears are realistic. Suggestions can be provided regarding the child's optimal positions for play and the extent to which he or she may need assistance. The child's capabilities, not limitations, should be stressed for two reasons: First, a child can demonstrate unique abilities and be remarkably creative when motivated to move or perform an activity, and second, a child needs to be enjoyed as a child, not as a child with a disability. Free play periods may offer this opportunity.

Integrated preschool and school settings offer ideal opportunities for peer interactions. Both the therapist and the caregiver should maximize the child's opportunities to be involved with his or her peers, without interfering with the spontaneity of these situations. Children with physical disabilities may need assistance with mobility, positioning, and access to playthings and equipment in order to allow them to participate to their maximum potential; however, dependence on the presence of an adult should be discouraged. The child may need some instructions on how to enter a play group, but this skill can also be learned from peer models. The role of the adult is to structure the environment, both physically and socially, and then allow play to happen.

Recommendations about playthings. The toys and activities that are made available for the child will influence both the type and quality of play. Sensitivity must be shown to social, emotional, physical, and educational needs and also to the interests of the child. A toy that is suitable for one child may be extremely unsuitable for another because of differences in temperament, motivation, and previous life experiences. To maximize the play experience, careful consideration must be given to the child's current developmental level. Toys of intermediate novelty are usually optimal: A toy should have an element of familiarity to the child but be sufficiently novel to induce exploration. Gradual pacing of activities will encourage the child to experiment and take risks but will ensure that the resulting information can be integrated into knowledge acquired previously. For example, familiarity with pouring water from cups into the bathtub might lead to the introduction of a funnel, a sieve, or a can with holes punched in it. The same items carried to the sandbox will produce entirely new results for the child. As a guideline for the development of intrinsic motivation, Ellis (1973) proposed that activities should be paced to the next developmental level, possess sufficient complexity to require investigation, be manipulable and responsive, and pose questions to be pondered by the child.

Advances in technology and computer applications have opened up a new world of play for even the most severely disabled child. Langley (1990) provided a thorough review of many toys that are suitable for children with physical disabilities. More traditional toys and materials, however, may still require modification by the occupational therapist (Lemire, 1988). The size, shape, weight, and consistency of materials may need to be adapted to suit the individual child (Anderson et al., 1987). A toy library may be helpful, allowing parents to borrow the more expensive electronic toys or to test adapted toys on a trial basis. Equipment modifications (e.g., an adapted playground, foot straps and back rests for a tricycle) may also serve to make an out-of-bounds activity accessible to the child. The "toys" that normal children discover in cupboards, basements, and backyards (e.g., pots and pans, insects, cardboard boxes, sticks) must not be overlooked for the child with a disability. As Diamond (1981), a physically disabled adult, pointed out, spitting 3 feet away and playing in the mud are also accomplishments for the child.

Summary

Free play has been proposed in this paper as a vitalizing element in the development of the whole child. The experiences derived from childhood play include exploration, mastery, decision-making, achievement, increased motivation, and competency—qualities that will eventually help children to develop occupational roles and to become more productive members of society (Bundy, 1989). Children—already restricted by physical limitations—who are not given adequate opportunities to engage in free play may be acquiring secondary disabilities, including diminished motivation, imagination, and creativity; poorly developed social skills; and increased dependence. The occupational therapist may be able to prevent some of these secondary problems by enhancing free play opportunities for the child who has a physical disability.

Acknowledgments

The development of this paper was supported in part by scholarships awarded to the first author by the Easter Seal Research Institute and the Social Sciences and Humanities Research Council of Canada.

References

Anderson, J., Hinojosa, J., & Strauch, C. (1987). Integrating play in neurodevelopmental treatment. *American Journal of Occupational Therapy, 41,* 421–426.

Ayres, A. J. (1981). *Sensory integration and the child.* Los Angeles: Western Psychological Services.

Behnke, C. J., & Fetkovich, M. M. (1984). Examining the reliability and validity of The Play History. *American Journal of Occupational Therapy, 38,* 94–100.

Brooks-Gunn, J., & Lewis, M. (1982a). Affective exchanges between normal and handicapped infants and their mothers. In T. Field & A. Fogel (Eds.), *Emotion and early interaction* (pp. 161–188). Hillsdale, NJ: Erlbaum.

Brooks-Gunn, J., & Lewis, M. (1982b). Development of play behavior in handicapped and normal infants. *Topics in Early Childhood Special Education, 2*(3), 14–27.

Brown, M., & Gordon, W. A. (1987). Impact of impairment on activity patterns of children. *Archives of Physical Medicine and Rehabilitation, 68,* 828–832.

Bundy, A. (1989, November). Play: The occupation of childhood. Workshop presented to the Occupational Therapy Play Research Group, Hamilton, Ontario.

Calder, J. E. (1980). Learn to play–Play to learn. In J. K. Atkinson (Ed.), *Too late at eight. Prevention and intervention, young children's learning difficulties* (pp. 163–188). Brisbane, Australia: Fred & Eleanor Schonell Educational Research Centre.

Clarke, M. M., Riach, J., & Cheyne, W. M. (1982). Handicapped children and pre-school education [Report to Warnock Committee on Special Education, University of Strathclyde]. Cited in M. Philip & D. Duckworth (Eds.), *Children with disabilities and their families.* Windsor, England: NFER-Nelson. Original report published 1977.

Cotton, N. (1984). Childhood play as an analog to adult capacity to work. *Child Psychiatry and Human Development, 14,* 135–144.

Crawley, S. B., & Spiker, D. (1983). Mother-child interactions involving two-year-olds with Down syndrome: A look at individual differences. *Child Development, 54,* 1312–1323.

Csikszentmihalyi, M. (1975). Play and intrinsic rewards. *Humanistic Psychology, 15,* 41–63.

Cunningham, C. E., & Barkley, R. A. (1979). The interactions of normal and hyperactive children with their mothers in free play and structured tasks. *Child Development, 50,* 217–224.

Diamond, S. (1981). Growing up with parents of a handicapped child: A handicapped person's perspective. In J. L. Paul (Ed.), *Understanding and working with parents of children with special needs* (pp. 23–50). New York: Holt, Rinehart & Winston.

Ellis, M. J. (1973). *Why people play.* Englewood Cliffs, NJ: Prentice-Hall.

Erikson, E. (1963). *Childhood and society.* New York: Norton.

Federlein, A. C. (1979, April). *A study of play behavior and interactions of preschool handicapped children in mainstreamed and segregated settings.* Paper presented at the annual meeting of the Council for Exceptional Children, Dallas, TX.

Field, T. (1980). Self, teacher, toy, and peer-directed behaviors of handicapped preschool children. In T. Field, S. Goldberg, D. Stein, & A. Sostek (Eds.), *High-risk infants and children: Adult and peer interactions* (pp. 313–360). New York: Academic Press.

Field, T., Roseman, S., de Stefano, L. J., & Koewler, J. (1982). The play of handicapped preschool children with handicapped and nonhandicapped peers in integrated and nonintegrated settings. *Topics in Early Childhood Special Education, 2*(3), 28–38.

Florey, L. L. (1981). Studies of play: Implications for growth, development, and for clinical practice. *American Journal of Occupational Therapy, 35,* 519–524.

Foster, M., Berger, M., & McLean, M. (1981). Rethinking a good idea: A reassessment of parent involvement. *Topics in Early Childhood Special Education, 1*(3), 55–65.

Garvey, C. (1977). *Play.* Cambridge, MA: Harvard University Press.

Gralewicz, A. (1973). Play deprivation in multihandicapped children. *American Journal of Occupational Therapy, 27,* 7072.

Gunn, S. L. (1975). Play as occupation: Implications for the handicapped. *American Journal of Occupational Therapy, 29,* 222–225.

Hanzlik, J. (1989). The effect of intervention on the free play experience for mothers and their infants with developmental delay and cerebral palsy. *Physical and Occupational Therapy in Pediatrics, 2*(2), 33–51.

Hanzlik, J., & Stevenson, M. (1986). Mother-infant interaction in families with infants who are mentally retarded, mentally retarded with cerebral palsy, or nonretarded. *American Journal of Mental Deficiency, 77,* 492–497.

Henderson, G., & Bryan, W. V. (1984). *Psychosocial aspects of disability.* Springfield, IL: Charles C Thomas.

Hewett, S., Newson, J., & Newson, E. (1970). *The family and the handicapped child.* Chicago: Aldine Publishing.

Kaiser, C. E. (1982). *Young and special.* Baltimore: University Park Press.

Kaiser, C. E., & Hayden, A. H. (1984). Clinical research and policy issues in parenting severely handicapped infants. In J. Blacher (Ed.), *Severely handicapped young children and their families* (pp. 275–317). Orlando: Academic Press.

Kibele, A. (1989). Occupational therapy's role in improving the quality of life for persons with cerebral palsy. *American Journal of Occupational Therapy, 43,* 371–377.

Kielhofner, G., & Barris, R. (1984). Collecting data on play: A critique of available methods. *Occupational Therapy Journal of Research, 4,* 150–180.

Knox, S. (1989, April). *The power of play as therapeutic media.* Paper presented at the 69th Annual Conference of the American Occupational Therapy Association, Baltimore, MD.

Kogan, K. L. (1980). Interaction systems between preschool handicapped or developmentally delayed children and their parents. In T. Field, S. Goldberg, D. Stein, & A. Sostek (Eds.), *High-risk infants and children: Adult and peer interactions* (pp. 227–247). New York: Academic Press.

Kogan, K. L., Tyler, N., & Turner, P. (1974). The process of interpersonal adaptation between mothers and their cerebral palsied children. *Developmental Medicine and Child Neurology, 16,* 518–527.

Langley, M. B. (1990). A developmental approach to the use of toys for facilitation of environmental control. *Physical and Occupational Therapy in Pediatrics, 10*(2), 69–91,

Lemire, E. (1988). Toy adaptations in pediatrics. *Occupational Therapy in Health Care, 5,* 87–93.

Levitt, E., & Cohen, S. (1977). Parents as teachers: A rationale for involving parents in the education of their young handicapped children. In L. G. Katz (Ed.), *Current topics in early childhood education* (Vol. 1, pp. 165–178). Norwood, NJ: Ablex.

Levitt, S. (1975). A study of the gross-motor skills of cerebral palsied children in an adventure playground for handicapped children. *Child: Care, Health and Development, 1,* 2943.

Lindquist, J. E., Mack, W., & Parham, L. D. (1982). A synthesis of occupational behavior and sensory integration concepts in theory and practice, part 2: Clinical applications. *American Journal of Occupational Therapy, 36,* 433–437.

Mack, W., Lindquist, J. E., & Parham, L. D. (1982). A synthesis of occupational behavior and sensory integration concepts in theory and practice, part 1. Theoretical foundations. *American Journal of Occupational Therapy, 36,* 365–374.

Matsutsuyu, J. (1971). Occupational behavior A perspective on work and play. *American Journal of Occupational Therapy, 25,* 291–294.

McHale, S. M., & Olley, J. G. (1982). Using play to facilitate the social development of handicapped children. *Topics in Early Childhood Special Education, 2*(3), 76–86.

Mogford, K. (1977). The play of handicapped children. In B. Tizard & D. Harvey (Eds.), Biology of play (pp. 170–184).London: Spastics International.

Oster, K (1984). *Physical disabilities in children: An exploratory study in mother and child interactions.* Unpublished doctoral dissertation, University of Toronto.

Parten, M. B. (1932). Social participation among preschool children. *Journal of Abnormal Psychology, 27,* 243–269.

Philip, M., & Duckworth, D. (1982). *Children with disabilities and their families.* Windsor, England: NFER-Nelson.

Piaget, J. (1951). *Play, dreams and imitation in childhood.* New York: Norton.

Piaget, J. (1952). *The origins of intelligence in children.* New York: Norton.

Rast, M. (1986). Play and therapy, play or therapy? In The American Occupational Therapy Association, Inc., *Play. A skill for life* [Monograph] (pp. 29–4 1). Rockville, MD: American Occupational Therapy Association.

Reilly, M. (1974). *Play as exploratory learning.* Beverly Hills, CA: Sage.

Robinson, A. L. (1977). Play: The arena for acquisition of rules for competent behavior. *American Journal of Occupational Therapy, 31,* 248–253.

Rogers, S. J. (1988). Characteristics of social interactions between mothers and their disabled infants: A review. *Child: Care, Health, and Development, 14,* 301–317.

Rubin, K. H., Fein, G. G., & Vandenberg, B. (1983). Play. In P. H. Mussen & E. M. Hetherington (Eds.), *Handbook of child psychology* (Vol. 4, pp. 693–774). New York: Wiley.

Russell, P. (1978). *The wheelchair child.* London: Souvenir Press.

Salomon, M. K. (1983). Play therapy with the physically handicapped. In C. E. Schaeffer & K. J. O'Connor (Eds.), *Handbook of play therapy* (pp. 455–469). New York: Wiley.

Sheridan, M. D. (1975). The importance of spontaneous play in the fundamental learning of handicapped children. *Child: Care, Health and Development, 1,* 3–17.

Sparling, J. W., Walker, D. F., & Singdahlsen, J. (1984). Play techniques with neurologically impaired preschoolers. *American Journal of Occupational Therapy, 38,* 603–612.

Stout, J. (1988). Planning playgrounds for children with disabilities. *American Journal of Occupational Therapy, 42,* 653–657.

Vandenberg, B., & Kielhofner, G. (1982). Play in evolution, culture, and individual adaptation: Implications for therapy. *American Journal of Occupational Therapy, 36,* 20–28.

Weininger, 0. (1979). *Play and education: The basic tool for early childhood learning.* Springfield, IL: Charles C Thomas.

Weininger, 0. (1980). The learning potential of play. *Canadian Journal of Early Childhood Education, 1,* 21–28.

Weininger, 0. (1988). "What if" and "as if": Imagination and pretend play in early childhood. In K. Egan & D. Nadaner (Eds.), *Imagination and education* (pp. 141–149). New York: Teachers College Press.

Weininger, O., & Fitzgerald, D. (1988). Symbolic play and interhemispheric integration: Some thoughts on a neuropsychological model of play. *Journal of Research and Development in Education, 21*(4), 23–40.

Williams, S. E., & Matesi, D. V. (1988). Therapeutic intervention with an adapted toy. *American Journal of Occupational Therapy, 42,* 673–676.

Yawkey, T. D., Dank, H. L., & Glossenger, F. L. (1986). *Playing. Inside and out.* Lancaster, PA: Technomic Publishing.

Transition From School to Community Living

CHAPTER 28

CHESTINA BROLLIER, PhD, OTR, FAOTA

JAYNE SHEPHERD, MS, OTR

KERRI FLICK MARKLEY, MS, OTR

The education and services for children with disabilities have improved since the Education of All Handicapped Children Act of 1975 (Public Law 94–142) (U.S. Department of Education, Office of Special Education and Rehabilitative Services, 1991). Yet between 50 percent and 75 percent of persons with disabilities remain unemployed (Harris, 1986; Hasazi, Gordon, & Roe, 1985; Wehman, 1992a). Nearly the same percentage of the 250,000 to 300,000 students with disabilities who have left the public schools each year had no jobs or independent living arrangements (Wehman, 1992a). These statistics suggest that transition planning for special education students deserves the attention of professionals such as school-based occupational therapists. *Transition planning* is the process by which a student is prepared to leave the school setting and enter into employment and community living (Wehman, 1992a). A literature search on this topic revealed little occupational therapy coverage.

Because the emphasis in transition programs is on functional daily life skills, occupational therapists' knowledge of activities of daily living, work, and leisure is applicable. The literature review, our clinical experiences, and research have led us to question whether some school system occupational therapists may be underemphasizing occupational performance areas while overemphasizing a developmental approach and sensorimotor occupational performance components (Barber, McInerney, & Struck, 1993; Spencer & Sample, 1993). This paper synthesizes some key issues for the transition process by reviewing occupational therapy and special education literature on functional activities and transition planning. The following key issues for the transition process are highlighted: federal initiatives, team efforts, parental involvement, assessment, goal setting, service characteristics, and roles for occupational therapy.

Federal Initiatives

The Office of Special Education and Rehabilitative Services (OSERS) has made vocational transition for students who have moderate to severe disabilities a national priority (Will, 1984). OSERS calls for the availability of services necessary for transition from school to work for all persons with disabilities and for a goal of sustained employment.

Additionally, the federal government has passed numerous laws concerning transition. The Education of the Handicapped Act Amendments of 1983 (Public Law 98–199) and 1986 (Public Law 99–457) mandated secondary education and transition services for youth with disabilities between the ages of 12 and 22 and authorized funding for research on the transition process. The Carl D. Perkins Vocational Education Act of 1984 (Public Law 98–524) provided funding for vocational education and legislated that students and their parents be made aware of vocational opportunities in the school one year before services are provided, or by the time the student reaches the ninth grade. The 1986 amendments to this act (Public Law 99–506) funded supported employment services in all states (Wehman, Moon, Everson, Wood, & Barcus, 1988). The Carl D. Perkins Vocational and Applied Technology Education Act of 1990 (Public Law 101–392) guaranteed full vocational education for youth with disabilities (National Information Center for Children and Youth with Disabilities [NICHCY], 1991).

In 1990, Congress passed the Education of the Handicapped Act Amendments of 1990 (Public Law 101–476), called the Individuals with Disabilities Education Act (IDEA). This law includes transition services and assistive technology as new definitions of special education services that must be included in a student's individualized education program (IEP) (NICHCY, 1991).

The Individualized Transition Planning Team

An individualized transition planning (ITP) team is essential to establishing a comprehensive transition plan (Giangreco, 1992; Rainforth, York, & MacDonald, 1992). The team may include special educators, occupational therapists, physical therapists, speech and language pathologists, representatives from adult service agencies, a vocational rehabilitation counselor, parents, the student, and, often, an employer. With this many team members, collaboration among agencies is essential to avoid duplication of services (Wehman, 1992a).

IDEA requires formal transition planning as part of the IEP process for all 16-year-old special education students (and those at a younger age, if considered appropriate) (Code of Federal Regulations, 1992). For many students with moderate to severe disabilities, transition planning and community living experiences are needed in the elementary and middle school years even if a formal ITP team has not been developed (Spencer & Sample, 1993).

Parental Involvement

A key issue in transition planning is active involvement by parents. First, they have the legal right to be involved in the education of their children. Second, they know their children better than anyone and are a significant source of information regarding skills needed by the student (Bates, Renzaglia, & Wehman, 1981; Wehman, 1992a). Third, after completing mandatory education, the former student and his or her family are responsible for carrying out the goals of an ITP. If they are not invested in these future plans, the targeted outcomes for transition may fail.

Studies on parental involvement in ITP development (Karge, Patton, & de la Garza, 1992) and IEP conferences (Vaughn, Bos, Harrell, & Lasky, 1988) found that parents took a passive role. Vacc and colleagues (1985) had similar results. They found that academic and social functioning were the most discussed IEP topics; topics receiving relatively little attention included planning for parental involvement, learning about student preferences and future environments, and integration of the student into real life settings. These confirmed those of Lynch and Stein's (1982) study, in which only 18 percent of 400 parents of students with disabilities reported participating in the development of the IEP. Additionally, Lynch and Stein found that parents of 13- to 14-year-old students participated significantly less in IEP meetings than parents of younger students. This study warrants current replication because transition planning for teenagers is legally required.

Parental input may be affected by several obstacles: logistical problems (lack of transportation, lack of child care, and inconvenient times), communication problems (language barriers and misunderstanding of terminology), inferiority feelings, and uncertainty about their child's disability (Lynch & Stein, 1982; Turnbull & Turnbull, 1990). Parents may resist transition planning due to concerns about their child's safety or about the questionable potential for success. They may worry about the attitudes of others, the school district's commitment to this programming, and the quality of the program (Hanline & Halvorsen, 1989). Parents also may have difficulty accepting the change in therapy programming from remediating medical problems to developing life skills; they may have difficulty thinking about the future and seeing their children in more adult roles (Turnbull & Turnbull, 1990). Therefore, transition planning may be an emotional event for families that influences their level of participation in the ITP.

There are several ways to reduce the barriers to parental participation in ITP meetings. Parents can be given a choice about when and where to meet. They, along with their child, can help select the specific professionals to be involved in the ITP process (Turnbull & Turnbull, 1990). Depending on their wishes and abilities, they can be given a list of possible topics to prepare for discussion at the ITP meeting. A few sample topics are living arrangements, jobs, guardianship, social security benefits, sexuality, fitness, and medical access (Sample, Spencer, & Bean, 1990). Besides preparation time, parents can be given information on what services are currently available and about the need for changes in service provision. Respect for cultural preference and open communication can promote effective working relationships among all team members, including the parents.

Functional, Environmentally Referenced Assessments

Before the ITP meeting, each member of the team uses functional, environmentally referenced assessments to determine the student's current levels of functioning relative to the previous year's IEP goals (Spencer & Sample, 1993). Dividing duties, the team evaluates the student's performance at home, in school, in the community, during recreation, and during temporary job placements (Brown et al., 1991; Spencer, Murphy, Bean, & Schelly, 1991). Functional performance, environmental demands and expectations, performance gaps, and support or training needs are noted (Spencer & Sample, 1993). Parents, teachers, and other key people are also interviewed for their input.

To determine which activities to assess within various environments, team members ask, "If the student does not learn this activity, will someone else have to do it for him or her?" (Brown et al., 1986; LaVesser & Shealey, 1986). If the answer is yes, the activity is functional and should be evaluated. For example, the ability to use a toilet is a functional skill and may be evaluated in multiple environments (e.g., school, a restaurant, a work site, a movie theater). Additional activities considered for the evaluation are those the student and parents prefer, those that reflect his or her culture, and those that influence safety or health (Brown et al., 1991; NICHCY, 1990).

After completion of the functional, environmentally referenced assessments, a discrepancy analysis is performed. This analysis determines what part of a desired skill the student can perform, what specific aspect of a skill is difficult for the student and why, and whether assistive technology could help this student.

Compared to functional, environmentally referenced assessments, standardized developmental tests often used in school system occupational therapy practice may have several shortcomings in transition programming for students with severe disabilities. Many of these assessments test isolated skills that may not be used in a student's home, community, or work (Rainforth & York, 1987), and they do not provide clear information on the student's and parent's priorities. Furthermore, because students with severe disabilities do not necessarily develop skills in the "normal" sequence (Orelove & Sobsey, 1991), an emphasis on performance components may not be appropriate. Additionally, developmental tests often lack information about a student's learning style (Falvey, 1986; Lehr, 1989).

Goal Setting

After completing the evaluation, the ITP team discusses long-term transition goals. These focus on the student's desired lifestyle after the school years in terms of domestic or home life, ability to function out in the community, and leisure and vocational activities (Spencer & Sample, 1993). The student's current levels of functioning and needs influence the IEP goals. Each annual goal addresses some need related to a long-term goal.

There are six areas to examine when setting goals: (a) preference, (b) number of environments in which the skills are used, (c) number of occurrences, (d) social significance, (e) probability of skill acquisition, and (f) safety and health issues (Brown et al., 1986; Meyer, Peck, & Brown, 1991). Preference refers to the judgments of all team members, especially those of parents and students. Each person comes to the ITP meeting with opinions about what skills are most important.

Determining the number of environments in which a skill is to be used is important in prioritizing goals. For example, many special education students have been taught to sort cubes or cones by color, a prereadiness activity not usually required in many environments. In contrast, matching clothes by color is a skill used in dressing at home or in doing laundry at home or at a work placement (Brown et al., 1986; Wehman et al., 1988; Wehman, 1992a).

The more a skill is practiced throughout life, the more likely it is that the skill will be learned and used (Billingsley, 1986; Brown et al., 1986). For example, washing dishes or loading a dishwasher may only be used in a home or vocational setting, but they are skills used several times a day for years. Therefore, these skills often will be of high priority.

Social significance refers to how a skill affects the social acceptance of the student. According to Brown and associates (1986), failing to teach the student some skills may hinder peer acceptance. For example, although a student may be instructed in ordering food from a restaurant, if he or she acts out by yelling or throwing food, he or she is less likely to be accepted by peers. However, teaching a 16-year-old how to operate an age-appropriate device, such as a switch to a radio rather than one connected to a infant's toy, may influence social acceptance by peers. Even the choice of equipment or assistive devices the student will need has social significance. For example, children and teens may reject a deltoid sling because of its appearance even though it can make eating easier.

Probability of skill acquisition is another area to be appraised when setting goals. Is the development of a skill worth the time and effort of instruction? (Brown et al., 1986; Wehman, 1992a). For example, independence in dressing may not be an appropriate goal for many students with severe physical disabilities.

When distinguishing which skills or activities are important for the student to acquire, the team must emphasize those that will assist the student in learning safety measures and that promote healthful living (Brown et al., 1986; Wehman et al., 1988; Wehman, 1992a). Because students with disabilities have typically been taught in sheltered environments, they may not have experience in dealing with environmental obstacles or potential dangers (e.g., stairs, toilets without railings, street crossing, cooking).

Service Characteristics

Each annual ITP goal is accompanied by a list that identifies who will be responsible for goal attainment, who will provide consultation, what adaptations or supports are needed by the student, when the goal is to be achieved, and what environments will be used for training (Spencer & Sample, 1993). Several team members may be responsible for different aspects of the same goal. The student's responsibilities are also delineated (Ward, 1992).

A number of authors (Brown et al., 1991; Chandler, 1992; Sailor et al., 1986; Wehman, 1992a) have successfully implemented a functional life skills curriculum. Such curricula use the classroom in a regular public school or an integrated private school; nonclassroom areas such as the cafeteria, library, hallways, and playground; community areas such as parks, restaurants, work environments, and residential settings; and other age-appropriate community environments or areas in which to teach life skills. These curricula require careful planning for the needs of each student and increased time for community-based instruction as the student gets older. Students from 12 to 16 years old may spend as much as 75 percent of their time out of school in community-centered instruction (Brown et al., 1991; Sailor et al., 1986). The work force for community training programs can be provided by occupational therapy personnel, teachers, teachers' aides, physical therapists, speech and language pathologists, and parents and volunteers (Giangreco, York, & Rainforth, 1989). One adult to three students is the recommended ratio for effective community training and integration (Hutchins & Talarico, 1985). Examples of functional assessment and intervention activities that may be used in a life–skills curriculum are shown in Table 28.1.

Intervention Principles

There are several key principles of intervention for effective transition services. These are:

- Teach at natural times, using naturally occurring cues, reinforcers, and consequences.
- Teach in natural environments.
- Use real materials.
- Teach all day and across environments to promote generalization.
- Use partial participation (What part of a task can the student do?).
- Keep student data to determine effectiveness of intervention.
- Integrate student with nondisabled peers.
- Use functional activities.

Intervention concentrates on specific skills that help to integrate the student into the community and ensure participation in adult activities (Bellamy & Wilcox, 1982; Brown et al., 1991; Spencer, 1989; Wehman, 1992b).

Roles for Occupational Therapy

IDEA mandates that transition services address work, education, independent living, and community participation. These domains are synonymous with the occupational performance areas delineated by the American Occupational Therapy Association's (AOTA) *Uniform Terminology* (AOTA, 1989). Occupational therapists in transition programs can address these performance areas by providing direct or indirect therapy, consultation, and monitoring while offering services in school and community environments (Dunn, 1991; Giangreco, 1986; Giangrceco, Edelman, & Dennis, 1991; Niehues, Bundy, Mattingly, & Lawlor, 1991).

Occupational therapy transition services concentrate on functional life skills programming. In Table 28.2, functional activities are contrasted with fewer functional activity choices and simulations that may not be generalized to natural environments. Occupational therapists use the tasks of everyday living to help students develop the self-care, home management, work, school, and leisure skills necessary to live and work in their community.

Occupational therapists can structure the physical environment to facilitate the learning of functional life skills. This process may lead to task or environmental modifications and the use of technological assistive devices (TADs). The physical environment may be modified to promote accessibility, work simplification, appropriate positioning of the student, the effective level of sensory stimulation, or combinations of the above.

Environmental modification often involves the use of technological assistive devices. Speech pathologists and occupational therapists frequently are the primary ITP members with expertise in assistive technology (Spencer & Sample, 1993) and often recommend equipment for students to become more integrated within their environments (Bain, 1989). Besides assessing and recommending TADs, the therapist can be responsible for instructing the student, parent, or teacher in proper use and maintenance of the equipment (Trefler, 1987).

A variety of technological aids are available to assist students with severe disabilities, including augmentative communication devices, computers, telephones, power wheelchairs, environmental control units, and adaptive aids (Mann & Lane, 1991; Vanderheiden, 1987). The same criteria used for selecting transition goals (listed above) help in prioritizing which technological aids to use.

One technological aid frequently used is the computer. Computer games are used to help improve visual perceptual skills. However, these games may not be adequate for an older student who has severe disabilities because the skills may not transfer to doing schoolwork or a job placement even though they may provide appropriate recreation. For example, skills learned in using the Muppet Learning Keys[1] do not transfer easily to those needed for word processing skills because the letter configuration on the Muppet Learning Keys keyboard is not similar to other computer keyboards found in work and home environments. With team input, the occupational therapist can carefully select the hardware, software, and peripherals to increase the student's functional outcomes in multiple environments (e.g., postschool training, employment, and home management).

Occupational therapists can also structure the temporal environment while teaching functional life skills. This allows students to work at peak performance times. Temporal cues may aid a student's performance. For example, watches or clocks with alarms can be placed in the environment to cue students to begin, change, or end tasks. Or students may be taught when to perform a job or a self-care task according to the time of day when it is needed.

Structuring the social environment can facilitate the development of interpersonal and social skills likely to prove beneficial across many domains of adult life (NICHCY, 1993). This social structuring may include positioning the student with peers or role models who support appropriate behaviors and

---

[1]Manufactured by Sunburst Communications, 39 Washington Avenue, Pleasantville, NY 10570.

Table 28.1. Examples of Functional Assessment and Intervention Activities for Life-Skill Programs

Student	Domestic	Community	Leisure	Vocational
TB, 10 years old, autistic-like behaviors, considered to be at trainable mentally retarded level	Picking up toys, washing dishes, making beds, dressing, grooming, eating skills, toileting skills, sorting clothes, emptying trash (lives at home with parents)	Eating meals in a restaurant, using restroom in a local restaurant, putting trash into container, giving the clerk money for an item he wants to purchase, recognizing and reading pedestrian safety signs, participating in local scout troop, going to neighbor's house for lunch	Climbing on swing set, playing simple board games, playing tag with neighbors, tumbling activities, running, playing kickball, riding bicycles, playing with age-appropriate toys	Cleaning the room at the end of the day, working on a task for designated period (15–30 min), wiping table after meals, following 2- to 4-step oral instructions, taking messages to people
JS, 17 years old, post-brain injury, right hemiplegia with behavioral problems; ambulates with a walker	Sweeping and dusting at place of residence, cooking simple meals (bowl of cereal, sandwich), operating simple machines (microwave, TV, stereo, tape recorder), putting the groceries away, caring for personal hygiene, dressing independently Ready to leave parents and live within a group residence	Using bus system to get around community; getting in and out of community stores and restaurants; negotiating steps, curbs, and revolving doorways; simple comparative shopping; using community health facilities (physician, pharmacist); interacting courteously with public	Watching college basketball, playing card games, listening to and recording music, going to movies with friends, playing video games	Performing janitorial duties at local store, food stocking duties at grocery store, inventory and reshelving videos at video store, ticket-taking duties at local movie theater

Adapted with permission from Wehman, P., Moon, M. S., Everson, J. M., Wood, W., & Barcus, J. M. (1988). *Transition from school to work: New challenges for youth with severe disabilities.* Baltimore: Brookes.

assisting students in determining the appropriate time and place for socialization. Besides structuring the environment, knowledge of psychosocial performance components (AOTA, 1989) helps occupational therapists teach skills such as stress management, time management, and self-management techniques. For example, if a student is having difficulty behaving in socially appropriate ways, ITP objectives may include learning appropriate greetings; knowing differences among strangers, friends, and employers and how each should be treated; or developing conversational skills appropriate for job or social settings.

When modifying environments, task analysis and adaptation can be the basis for teaching functional skills. Task analysis identifies not only all the steps necessary for successful performance of a task, but also the intellectual, psychosocial, perceptual, and motor skills required. Information gained from the analysis of a task is placed into a step-by-step learning sequence. The transition team often relies on the occupational therapist to adapt the activity, or the learning sequence (Spencer & Sample, 1993). Physical and verbal cuing, cue cards, or photo reminders can be used to prompt the learning of complex tasks. For example, a teenage student with mental retardation who is unable to follow verbal three-step directions may be taught feminine hygiene skills through photo cue cards and an adaptive aid.

Roles for occupational therapy in transition programming are multifaceted. Occupational therapists not only teach functional daily living skills, but also help structure the physical, temporal, and social environments. Through task analysis and adaptation, therapists help modify the student's skills to meet environmental demands.

Conclusion

Transition programming for a student with moderate to severe disabilities involves an appropriate life-centered, functional school-based program, formalized plans involving the parents and the entire array of community agencies that are responsible for providing services, and multiple quality options for gainful employment or meaningful postschool training and appropriate community living arrangements. School-based occupational therapists have much to offer the transition process when they concentrate on real-life functional activities.

Table 28.2. Contrasting Activity Choices for Students With Severe Disabilities

Community Living Functional Activities	Less Functional Activities
Sorting silverware	Working with pegs and patterns
Setting table	Working with block designs
Clipping coupons	Cutting predrawn shapes
Dressing and undressing self for gym and outdoors	Using activities of daily living (ADL) button, lacing, and zipper boards
Using money to purchase items in cafeteria, school store, fast-food restaurant, drugstore	Practicing simulated shopping with play money
Using real washer and dryer at home, laundromat, or in work setting	Using simulated washing machine
Applying telephone skills, making real business and social calls	Practicing telephone skills by talking to occupational therapist
Completing application for desired part-time job	Using simulated copies of job application
Finding a specific classified advertisement or telephone number	Using figure–ground worksheets (e.g., "circle all the *E*s")
Practicing specific social skills with peers without disabilities and non-staff adults	Practicing social skills training with a special needs group
Using computers to do school assignments, write letters, etc.	Playing computer games or using visual–perceptual training programs
Practicing wheelchair mobility in school, home, and community environment	Practicing wheelchair mobility only in school or classroom environments

Acknowledgments

This paper is based in part on a faculty-designed research project conducted by the third author while a professional master's-degree student in occupational therapy at Virginia Commonwealth University. Presentations on this topic have been given at the 1991 Great Southern Occupational Therapy Conference and the 72nd Annual Conference of the American Occupational Therapy Association Conference, Houston, Texas, March 1992.

We thank the following organizations for their participation in the ongoing transition project, of which this paper is a part: The Richmond Cerebral Palsy Center, The Chesterfield County Public Schools, and The Virginia Commonwealth University Rehabilitation Research and Training Center.

References

American Occupational Therapy Association. (1989). Uniform terminology for occupational therapy—Second edition. *American Journal of Occupational Therapy, 43,* 808–815.

Bain, B. (1989). Assessment of clients for technological assistive devices. In *Technology review '89: Perspectives on occupational therapy practice* (pp. 55–59). Rockville, MD: American Occupational Therapy Association.

Barber, M., McInerney, C., & Struck, M. (1993, June). Training for independence: Transition from school to work. *Work Programs Special Interest Section Newsletter,* pp. 1–2.

Bates, P., Renzaglia, A., & Wehman, P. (1981, April). Characteristics of an appropriate education for the severely and profoundly handicapped. *Education and Training of the Mentally Retarded, 16,* 142–148.

Bellamy, G. T., & Wilcox, B. (1982). Secondary education for severely handicapped students: Guidelines for quality services. In K. P. Lynch, W. E. Kiernan, & J. A. Stark, *Prevocational and vocational education for special needs youth: A blueprint for the 1980's* (pp. 65–80). Baltimore: Brookes.

Billingsley, F. (1986). Where are the generalized outcomes? An examination of instructional objectives. In H. Powell (Ed.), *PILOT: Project for independent living in occupational therapy* (pp. 96–103). Rockville, MD: American Occupational Therapy Association.

Brown, L., Falvey, M., Vincent, L., Kaye, N., Johnson, F., Ferrara–Parrish, P., & Gruenewald, L. (1986). Strategies for generating comprehensive, longitudinal and chronological age-appropriate individualized education programs for adolescent and young adult severely handicapped students. In H. Powell (Ed.), *PILOT: Project for independent living in occupational therapy* (pp. 104–115). Rockville, MD: American Occupational Therapy Association.

Brown, L., Schwarz, P., Udvari–Solner, A., Kampschroer, E., Johnson, F., Jorgensen, J., & Gruenewald, L. (1991). How much time should students with severe intellectual disabilities spend in regular education classrooms and elsewhere? *Journal of the Association for Persons with Severe Handicaps, 16,* 39–47.

Carl D. Perkins Vocational Education Act of 1984 (Public Law 98–524).

Carl D. Perkins Vocational Education Act Amendments (Public Law 99–506). (1986).

Carl D. Perkins Vocational and Applied Technology Education Act of 1990 (Public Law 101–392).

Chandler, B. (1992). How to design and implement classroom programming. In C. Royeen (Ed.), American Occupational Therapy Association Self-Study Series, *Classroom applications for school-based practice.* Rockville, MD: AOTA.

Code of Federal Regulations 300–301 (1992, October). Final Regulations; Correction: Assistance to states for the education of children with disabilities program and preschool grants for children with disabilities. *Federal Register, 57*(208).

Education of All Handicapped Children Act (Public Law 94–142). (1975).

Education of the Handicapped Act Amendments of 1983 (Public Law 98–199).

Education of the Handicapped Act Amendments of 1986 (Public Law 99–457), 20 U.S.C., § 1400.

Dunn, W. (Ed.). (1991). *Pediatric occupational therapy: Facilitating effective service provision.* Thorofare, NJ: Slack.

Falvey, M. (1986). *Community-based curriculum: Instructional strategies for students with severe handicaps.* Baltimore: Brookes.

Giangreco, M. F. (1986). Delivery of therapeutic services in special education programs for learners with severe handicaps. *Physical and Occupational Therapy in Pediatrics, 6*(2), 5–15.

Giangreco, M. F. (1992, February). *Integrating related services in the education of students with disabilities.* Symposium on using the transdisciplinary approach to related services in classrooms, Williamsburg, Virginia.

Giangreco, M., Edelman, S., & Dennis, R. (1991). Common professional practices that interfere with the integrated delivery of services. *Remedial and Special Education, 12*(2), 16–24.

Giangreco, M., York, R., & Rainforth, B. (1989). Providing related services to learners with severe handicaps in educational settings: Pursuing the least restrictive option. *Pediatric Physical Therapy, 1*(2), 55–63.

Hanline, M., & Halvorsen, A. (1989). Parent perceptions of the integration transition process: Overcoming artificial barriers. *Exceptional Children, 55,* 487–492.

Harris, L. (1986). *International Center for the Disabled survey of disabled Americans. Bringing disabled Americans into the mainstream: A nationwide survey of 1,000 disabled people.* New York: International Center for the Disabled.

Hasazi, S., Gordon, L., & Roe, C. (1985). Factors associated with the employment status of handicapped youth exiting high school from 1973–1983. *Exceptional Children, 51,* 455–469.

Hutchins, M., & Talarico, D. (1985). Administrative considerations in providing community integrated training programs. In P. McCarthy, J. Everson, M. S. Moon, & M. Barcus (Eds.), *School-to-work transition for youth with severe disabilities.* Project Transition into Employment, Rehabilitation Research & Training Center, School of Education, Virginia Commonwealth University, Richmond, Virginia.

Individuals With Disabilities Education Act (Public Law 101–476). (1990).

Karge, B. D., Patton, P. L., & de la Garza, B. (1992). Transition services for youth with mild disabilities: Do they exist, are they needed? *Career Development for Exceptional Individuals, 15,* 47–68.

LaVesser, P., & Shealey, S. (1986). The occupational therapy process. In H. Powell (Ed.), *PILOT: Project for independent living in occupational therapy* (pp. 87–95). Rockville, MD: American Occupational Therapy Association.

Lehr, D. (1989). Educational programming for young children with the most severe disabilities. In F. Brown & D. Lehr (Eds.), *Persons with profound disabilities: Issues and practices* (pp. 213–237). Baltimore: Brookes.

Lynch, E. W., & Stein, R. (1982). Perspectives on parent participation in special education. *Exceptional Education Quarterly, 3*(2), 56–63.

Mann, W. C., & Lane, J. P. (1991). *Assistive technology for persons with disabilities: The role of occupational therapy.* Rockville, MD: American Occupational Therapy Association.

Meyer, L., Peck, C., & Brown, L. (1991). *Critical issues in the lives of people with severe disabilities.* Baltimore: Brookes.

National Information Center for Children and Youth with Disabilities. (1990, December). Transition summary. *NICHCY, 6,* 1–13.

National Information Center for Children and Youth with Disabilities. (1991). The education of children and youth with special needs: What do the laws say? *NICHCY, 1*(1), 1–11.

National Information Center for Children and Youth with Disabilities. (1993, March). Transition summary. *NICHCY, 3*(1), 1–20.

Niehues, A., Bundy, A., Mattingly, C., & Lawlor, M. (1991). Making a difference: Occupational therapy in the public schools. *Occupational Therapy Journal of Research, 11,* 195–211.

Orelove, F., & Sobsey, D. (1991). *Educating children with multiple disabilities: A transdisciplinary approach* (pp. 231–258). Baltimore: Brookes.

Rainforth, B., & York, J. (1987). Integrating related services in community instruction. *Journal of the Association for Persons with Severe Handicaps, 12,* 190–198.

Rainforth, B., York, J., & MacDonald, C. (1992). *Collaborative teams for students with severe disabilities: Integrating therapy and educational services.* Baltimore: Brookes.

Sailor, W., Halvorsen, A., Anderson, J., Goetz, L., Gee, K., Doering, K., & Hunt, P. (1986). Community intensive instruction. In R. Homer, L. Meyer, & B. Fredericks (Eds.), *Education of learners with severe handicaps* (pp. 251–288). Baltimore: Brookes.

Sample, P., Spencer, K., & Bean, G. (1990). *Transition planning: Creating a positive future for students with disabilities.* Fort Collins, CO: Office of Transition Services, Department of Occupational Therapy, Colorado State University.

Spencer, K. (1989). The transition from school to adult life. In S. Hertfelder, & C. Gwin (Eds.), *Work in progress: Occupational therapy in work programs* (pp. 157–179). Rockville, MD: American Occupational Therapy Association.

Spencer, K., Murphy, M., Bean, G., & Schelly, C. (1991). Vocational needs assessment: A functional, community-referenced approach. In K. Spencer (Ed.), *From school to adult life: The role of occupational therapy in the transition process* (pp. 185–213). Fort Collins, CO: Department of Occupational Therapy, Colorado State University.

Spencer, K., & Sample, P. (1993). Transition planning and services. In C. Royeen (Ed.), *Classroom applications for school-based practice* (pp. 6–48). Rockville, MD: American Occupational Therapy Association.

Trefler, E. (1987). Technology applications. *American Journal of Occupational Therapy, 41,* 697–700.

Turnbull, A., & Turnbull, R. (1990). *Families, professionals, and exceptionality: A special partnership.* Columbus: Merrill.

U.S. Department of Education, Office of Special Education and Rehabilitative Services. (1991). *Thirteenth annual report to Congress on the implementation of the Education of the Handicapped Act.* Washington, DC: U.S. Government Printing Office.

Vacc, N. A., Vallecorsa, A. L., Parker, A., Bonner, S., Lester, C., Richardson, S., & Yates, C. (1985). Parents and educators' participation in IEP conferences. *Education and Treatment of Children, 8*(2), 153–162.

Vanderheiden, G. (1987). Service delivery mechanisms in rehabilitation technology. *American Journal of Occupational Therapy, 41,* 703–710.

Vaughn, S., Bos, C., Harrell, J., & Lasky, B. (1988). Parent participation in the initial placement/IEP conference 10 years after mandated involvement. *Journal of Learning Disabilities, 21*(2), 82–89.

Ward, M. J. (1992). Introduction to secondary special education and transition issues. In F. R. Rusch, L. DeStefano, J. Chadsey-Rusch, L. A. Phelps, & E. Szymanshi (Eds.), *Transition from school to adult life: Models, linkages, and policy* (pp. 387–389). Sycamore, IL: Sycamore.

Wehman, P. (1992a). *Life beyond the classroom: Transition strategies for young people with disabilities.* Baltimore: Brookes.

Wehman, P. (1992b, Summer). Transition from school to adulthood for young people with disabilities. *Rehabilitation Research and Training Center Newsletter,* p. 1.

Wehman, P., Moon, M. S., Everson, J. M., Wood, W., & Barcus, J. M. (1988). *Transition from school to work: New challenges for youth with severe disabilities.* Baltimore: Brookes.

Will, M. C. (1984). *OSERS programming for the transition of youth with disabilities: Bridges from school to working life.* Washington, DC: Office of Special Education and Rehabilitative Service, U.S. Department of Education.

The Americans With Disabilities Act of 1990 and Employees With Mental Impairments: Personal Efficacy and the Environment

CHAPTER 29

PATRICIA A. H. CRIST, PHD, FAOTA
VIRGINIA C. STOFFEL, MS, OTR

Paid employment carries both practical and symbolic significance, because work results in compensation for basic needs, provides resources for community participation and giving, and is a symbol of full citizenship (Mancuso, 1990; Rhodes, Ramsing, & Bellamy, 1988). Productive work is highly valued in our society and is often the focal point around which self-care, leisure, and rest pursuits are selected and planned; it is one of the two determinants of our socioeconomic status. Unfortunately, many qualified Americans who have a mental disability may have been denied employment because of their mental health problems. Fortunately, we now have Title I of the Americans With Disabilities Act of 1990 (ADA) (Public Law 101-336), which mandates that qualified persons with physical or mental impairments not be excluded from employment and work activities because of disability.

This chapter was previously published in the *American Journal of Occupational Therapy, 46,* 434–443. Copyright © 1992, American Occupational Therapy Association.

When President Bush signed the ADA on July 26, 1990, he referred to the law as the new "Declaration of Independence" for 43 million Americans with disabilities (Staff, 1990). Occupational therapy philosophy, values, and rehabilitation goals are supported by the ADA, and our professionals can serve a central role in the implementation of this legislation. Recently, Townsend (1991) discussed a vision for the profession's future:

> I do not believe that it is enough to treat our patients in the confines of our hospitals and clinics without regard to factors outside that realm that influence their right to life and happiness.... As we look beyond our clinics out into the larger world and make our presence felt in a broad and meaningful way, we become instruments of change for our patients and the greater society. Occupational therapy is grounded in the respect for, search for, and achievement of maximum human potential for all of those we serve. (p. 873)

The ADA provides a mechanism for occupational therapists to be the "instruments of change" in helping persons with mental health impairments realize their potential as employees and productive citizens. Because the environment influences job performance and personal competence (Christiansen, 1991), occupational therapists can adapt individual job skills or the work site or both.

The purpose of this paper is to describe the role of occupational therapy in implementing the ADA to enhance the employment of persons with mental health problems. To achieve this goal, aspects of the ADA necessitating special attention for psychosocial disabilities are reviewed, and the influence of personal competence (self-efficacy) and the environment on performance are discussed. For the purposes of this paper, the job environment consists of four environmental components:

1. Employer and co-worker attitudes toward persons with mental health impairments.
2. Definition of essential job functions related to mental health.
3. Reasonable accommodations for employment skills associated with dysfunctional employee behavior resulting from mental impairments.
4. Access to employee functions.

Each of these components is necessary to fully comply with the ADA for employment processes (Lotito & Pimental, 1990).

The ADA and Mental Health

Under the ADA, mental or psychological disorders include mental retardation, organic brain syndrome, emotional or mental illness, and specific learning disabilities (National Mental Health Association, 1990). Excluded conditions include current illegal use of alcohol or drugs, homosexuality and bisexuality, sexual behavior disorders not resulting from physical impairments, compulsive gambling, kleptomania, and pyromania. Human immunodeficiency virus, AIDS, and other communicable diseases are protected under the ADA.

Persons disabled by drug addiction or alcoholism are covered under the law as long as the person is not currently abusing drugs or alcohol. Persons entitled to protection in the workplace are those who are (a) former users who have successfully completed a supervised rehabilitation program and no longer use illegal substances, (b) participants in a supervised drug rehabilitation program who no longer use illegal substances, and (c) persons using alcohol or drugs who are erroneously regarded as engaging in illegal drug use (i.e., using a drug that is illegal unless prescribed by a physician) (ADA, Title 1, § 104).

Legal drug use is that which occurs under the care of a licensed health care professional. A person who is currently abusing drugs is protected against discrimination under the ADA only if the present disability is not related to the illegal drug use. Protection is only for the defined disability and is not concurrent with drug- or alcohol-related disability problems. Employers may require a drug-free workplace and hold illegal drug users and alcoholics to the same performance standards as other employees, as established pursuant to the Drug-Free Workplace Act of 1988 (National Mental Health Association, 1990; Watson, 1990). Drug testing to identify illegal drugs during preemployment screenings is permitted, as are employment decisions made solely on drug test results. Termination and disciplinary actions can be taken, and no reasonable accommodations are required under the ADA for active drug and alcohol users.

Employers are not required to offer mental health coverage as part of their insurance benefits. An employer could not use the ADA to justify not employing a qualified applicant because the employer's current insurance plan does not cover the person's disability or because the cost of insurance benefits to the employer may increase. This is true for both health and liability insurance. Reasonable accommodation does not require that the employer provide alcohol or drug rehabilitation. A person with a drug addiction cannot be denied health and rehabilitation services if he or she was otherwise entitled to such coverage under the employer's medical plan.

The ADA protects persons with mental impairments from discrimination and supports inclusion in employment (Title 1) as well as access to public accommodations and services (Title III) that enhance employability and employees' rights. For successful engagement in productive work roles, a person with mental health problems must experience personal competence or self-efficacy in performing employment-related tasks.

Personal Self-Efficacy and Employment Readiness

To be successfully employed, one must view oneself as employable. Employability is a match among work-related skill, one's judgments regarding work abilities, and the job itself. According to the ADA, skills required to perform a job are delineated in the job description and referred to as *essential job functions*. Work skill is the ability to do work tasks. However, one's judgment regarding one's ability to work may be an even more important contributor to employability than work skills themselves.

Bandura (1977) described this judgment about one's skills or competence as *self-efficacy*. Efficacy allows a person to competently engage with the environment using multiple subskills and to execute courses of action required to deal with situations. Bandura stated that perceived self-efficacy influences a person's choice of activities and environmental settings, the effort expended, and persistence. Through research, he demonstrated that perceived self-efficacy is a better predictor of subsequent behavior than are performance skills (Bandura, 1982). Success as an employee is the result of perceived self-efficacy. Because persons with mental impairments often have low self-esteem, Bandura's theory can be used to develop strategies for persons with mental health problems to acquire self-efficacy. The self-efficacy will then allow them to perform the essential functions of a job, with or without accommodation, as addressed in the ADA.

Bandura's (1977) theory is based on the assumption that psychological procedures create and strengthen expectations of personal efficacy. In this model, two personal efficacy expectations are differentiated—efficacy expectations and outcome expectations:

> An efficacy expectation is the conviction that one can successfully execute the behavior required to produce the outcomes. An outcome expectation is defined as the person's estimate that a given behavior will lead to certain outcomes. Individuals can believe that a particular course of action will produce certain outcomes, but if they entertain serious doubts about whether they can perform the necessary activities, such information does not influence their behavior. Expectations of personal mastery affect both initiation and persistence of coping behavior. (Bandura, 1977, p. 193)

For persons with mental impairments to successfully engage in employment, both components of self-efficacy need to be developed, reinforced, and maintained to achieve the desired outcome, which is appropriate work behaviors. Persons with mental impairments are unlikely to report self-efficacy beliefs. Despite possessing the skills to perform the essential functions of a job, a person will not succeed if he or she has poor self-efficacy beliefs. Thus, development of positive work-related self-efficacy judgments is critical for employability. Occupational therapists can assist with the development of positive self-efficacy beliefs. Employability of persons with mental health problems can be enhanced through an understanding of the criteria used to judge employability. Therapists can then implement activities that enhance the employee's self-efficacy.

Bandura (1977, 1986) identified four sources of judgements about one's self-efficacy and, ultimately, the ability to perform: (a) emotional arousal, (b) verbal or social persuasion, (c) vicarious experience, and (d) performance accomplishments. These are hierarchically ordered from least influential to most influential in the development and maintenance of competency behavior.

As stated by Bandura (1977), *emotional arousal* is a source of physiological information used to judge anxiety and vulnerability to stress. Experience with stressful situations enables the development of coping skills and competency to deal effectively with fearful situations. *Verbal persuasion* involves leading people to believe that they can cope successfully with what has overwhelmed them in the past. Verbal persuasion can contribute to the successes achieved through performance, because people can be socially persuaded that they possess the capabilities to master difficult situations. *Social persuasion*, without arrangements for conditions to facilitate effective performance, will most likely lead to failures that discredit the persuaders and further undermine self-efficacy. *Vicarious experience* involves seeing others perform difficult activities without adverse consequences. This experience can generate expectations of the observers that they too will improve if they persist in their efforts. Vicarious experience relies on inferences from social comparison used to model another person's behavior. Modeled behavior with clear outcomes conveys efficacy information. Observing another's performance, which results in repeated successes with evident consequences, enhances the observer's efficacy expectations. *Performance accomplishments*, the most influential and enduring sense of personal efficacy, involve personal mastery experiences. Successes raise mastery expectations; failures lower them. Mishaps that occur early in the course of events erode self-efficacy beliefs more than later failures during the development of self-efficacy. Repeated success lessens the negative effect of occasional failures, which in themselves can reinforce self-efficacy if failures are overcome. Performance exposure with a model present conveys powerful efficacy information, because verbal persuasion, vicarious experiences, and performance accomplishments are available to develop self-efficacy judgments. Opportunities to translate personal behavioral conceptions into appropriate successful actions and to make

corrective refinements toward the perfection of skills are essential to the development of self-efficacy.

Psychological self-efficacy is probably acquired through more than one type of efficacy experience. Efficacy results from capability, which is the result of cognitive, social, and behavioral skill organization; but capability is only as good as its execution (Bandura, 1982). Once established, enhanced self-efficacy will generalize to other performance.

Bandura's (1977, 1982) self-efficacy model and occupational therapy are mutually supportive. Occupational therapists value all four types of efficacy experiences, and Bandura's emphasis on the importance of performance accomplishments is consistent with our focus on the doing process in treatment using purposeful activity. The importance of selected functional activities is to provide actual performance experience, the preferred facilitator for self-efficacy beliefs. Simulation, modeling, observation, and repeated movement exercises are only preliminary or underpinning experiences to the development of self-efficacy through actual performance. In occupational therapy, the value of actually performing the functional activity combined with using the three other forms of efficacy experiences is underscored.

Occupational therapists in mental health are aware of the importance of the emerging trend called *supported and transitional employment* in providing work-related efficacy expectations in their clients. Supported and transitional employment approaches assume that all people can do meaningful, productive work in competitive employment settings, if it is what people choose to do and if they are given necessary supports or accommodation appropriate for the setting (Anthony & Blanch, 1987). ADA outcomes will include the increased use of supported or transitional employment and opportunities to engage in regular work roles with reasonable accommodations. An example follows:

A 51-year-old woman with mental retardation who had never gone to school or worked lived at home with her 92-year-old mother until her mother's increasing age required both of them to move to a nursing home together. The head nurse at the nursing home requested that this woman engage in more productive work than that offered by the activity specialist. Both the client and her mother did not believe that she was employable.

Initial observation by the occupational therapist during a 3 hour trial in the workshop revealed that the client was able to do the essential job functions for several tasks in the sheltered workshop with minimal support from a female staff member. However, when a male supervisor or male co-worker addressed her or stood nearby, she became angry, hostile, and unable to keep working. The issue of tolerance for the opposite sex was considered to be a marginal job function.

The treatment plan, which was also a reasonable accommodation for a marginal job function, was simply to place the client in a work room with other women only. As expected, her work skills developed. Modeling by peers and the therapist, verbal persuasion by the therapist and others, and practice facilitated the development of her self-efficacy as a worker.

The outcome of the treatment plan was to have this client successfully employed in nearby industry. The treatment program incorporated the behavioral approach of desensitization, so that she would be able to work alongside men and talk with them without it disrupting her work. This would be less isolating for the client in the workplace. A second alternative, if not successful, was to seek reasonable accommodation in the workplace.

A person's perceived self-efficacy influences choice and structures needs for specific types of support and transition. Frequently, persons with mental health problems are not able to accurately report their job abilities. However, coupling one of the self-efficacy approaches with a person's job expectations may reveal the person's true abilities and decrease the influence of negative or limiting perceived expectations. The following case exemplifies the importance of self-efficacy experiences:

In the television show "L.A. Law," the character named Benny has developmental disabilities and started working at the law firm by helping with mail delivery, performing relatively simple filing, and making deliveries. His view of his own skills was narrow, based on living in a loving home environment with his mother, who provided for all of Benny's needs but not for the development of work attitudes or behaviors. The work environment was new to him. As Benny's strengths were reinforced by performance experiences and accommodation, he got clear, strong, powerful feedback from his supervisors and other personnel as to the importance of the service he provided. His confidence in his skills increased to the point where when accused of losing a file, he would respond with "No, I know exactly where that file is," and would produce it. He demonstrated mastery and accompanying self-efficacy and participated in employee activities and work-related social events.

Important aspects of the work environments described in the above examples were the employers' positive attitude regarding each person's employability, accurate definitions of essential job functions, appropriate accommodations for both marginal and essential job functions, and full access to employee privileges. Each of these aspects is described below.

Attitudes Toward Mental Impairment

The ADA does not require a person to disclose a disability. Information regarding an identified disability must remain confidential, except in employment situations where supervisors and managers need to be informed regarding restrictions or accommodations. The greatest challenge for persons with mental impairments may be the decision to disclose a mental health impairment to a potential employer. On the one hand, disclosure can provide protection under the law; on the other hand, many psychosocial disabilities are invisible or just considered eccentric behaviors, making disclosure of mental impairment a matter of individual choice. The decision to report a mental impairment can be difficult because of the stigma associated with mental health problems:

The stigma associated with mental illness often results in attitudinal barriers that hinder a person's ability to work or enjoy life. Concerns by employers regarding productivity, safety, insurance, ability, attendance, and acceptance by co-workers and customers have been identified as common barriers that frequently result in the exclusion of persons who have sought mental health care from the work force. (National Mental Health Association, 1990, p. 7)

A person cannot be rejected from a job because of stereotypes, stigma, myths, or fear associated with mental illness. Stigma and stereotypic expectations regarding the ability of persons with mental impairments to be suitable employees are often founded in bias and a lack of knowledge by both the public and employers (Combs & Omvig, 1986; Howard, 1975). Just as with attitudes about race, culture, and sex, assumptions and attitudes toward any minority group not only define our perceptions, but also direct our actions toward the group (Lotito & Pimental, 1990). Hartlage and Roland (1971) reported that employers viewed persons with mental health problems as less desirable employees and as having behavioral problems that lead to poor work abilities. Such negative attitudes are a serious impediment to the successful employment of many persons with psychiatric disabilities. These persons are being deprived of the opportunity to restore their mental health through engagement in productive work roles (Howard, 1975). These attitudes and perceptions are counterproductive to the intent of the ADA and are cause for action.

Persons with psychosocial disabilities can be educated to become self-advocates. Ultimately, the decision to disclose information about one's mental impairment is the employee's. Advocacy training may allow the person to disclose this information in order to assist with beneficial accommodations instead of continuing negative patterns of behavior, which might limit or prevent full participation in work roles. Personal advocacy training should begin before the need for job accommodation arises. Self-advocates are able to share concerns regarding their mental impairments with employers and suggest beneficial accommodations.

The reduction of stigma associated with mental illness will also require the education of people in the workplace and the community regarding appropriate attitudes and behaviors toward persons with mental impairments. Common strategies to use in assisting with attitude change include personnel training for managers and supervisors, advocacy training for staff and persons with mental health problems, visibility of successful employees with mental health impairments, employee counseling and consultation, and modeling of normal interactions among co-workers. Occupational therapists can provide information, encouragement, counseling, and suggestions to employers and co-workers regarding employment of persons with mental health problems. Training sessions that focus on capabilities, understanding, and acceptance of the employee with a mental impairment can help create a work environment where reasonable accommodation is understood and the employee is able to work more effectively.

Occupational therapists might use the following format for employer and co-worker training. This information could be included for self-advocacy training also.

1. Self-assessment of common myths and expectations regarding mental impairments.
2. Group discussion of self-assessment and information to dispel myths.
3. Information regarding mental impairments.
4. Discussion of the ADA regarding employment.
5. Presentation of successful employees with mental impairments either through personal testimony or audiovisual resources.
6. Identification of workers' behaviors and related reasonable accommodations needed by persons with mental impairments.
7. Protection of confidential information and civil rights during pre-employment interviewing and employment.

When this general foundation is in place in co-workers, employment practices can be reviewed and accommodations designed to meet the specific individualized needs of the employee with mental impairments.

The individual qualified for a job is not required to prove that the employer's concerns regarding the influence of mental impairment on job performance are invalid. Under the ADA, a person's employability is established through assessment of his or her fitness for duty using the essential functions of a job.

Essential Job Functions

Every job in society, regardless of skill level and perceived efficacy, can be described in great detail (Lotito & Pimental, 1990). The ADA stipulates that job functions can be divided into two categories: essential and marginal. These two categories become the basis for the job description, pre-employment screening, medical examination, and employment processes. The focus during these activities is on the person's abilities, not the disability. Job descriptions guide the other processes, because they provide a clear explanation of each job, its performance expectations, and its relation to other jobs.

The employer determines what needs to be done, what each job will look like, how jobs interrelate, and the employee qualifications needed in each job. The ADA mandates that hiring and employment policies not discriminate against qualified employees on the basis of their disability. These job descriptions must differentiate between essential and marginal performance requirements.

Essential job functions are work tasks that are critical, fundamental, indispensable, required, and necessary. A person who, through reasonable accommodation, can demonstrate the ability to perform essential job functions is considered to be qualified for the job. *Marginal job functions* are work tasks that are nonessential, peripheral, extra, or incidental; they cannot be used to disqualify an otherwise qualified person with mental health impairment. All marginal job functions require reasonable accommodation. The following is an example of mental impairment that requires accommodation of marginal, not essential, job functions:

A worker with a history of depression is employed as a cashier in a fast-food restaurant. Essential job functions include taking accurate orders, handling money, and providing change to customers with accuracy and in a timely manner. Marginal functions included smiling at each customer and making positive, energetic statements to customers when greeting them. The worker found that after 2 hours at the counter, he was unable to maintain accuracy and speed in the essential job functions as well as fulfill the marginal job functions. The worker's self-esteem was affected, and he consulted with an occupational therapist. The therapist recognized this situation as contributing to low self-efficacy and discussed with the worker how to adapt the situation. Following a supervisory session between the worker and supervisor, reasonable accommodations were made by scheduling the worker for half an hour at the counter followed by 45 minutes of cleanup duties, a break, and then a repeat of that schedule. The worker was coached by the therapist to alert the supervisor to fatigue and to an increase in his negative thoughts that might precede a potential negative interaction with a customer. The supervisor also provided the worker with verbal praise at half hour intervals throughout the work shift.

The accommodations in the case above qualify as reasonable accommodations under the ADA.

Occupational therapists are familiar with job analysis in work settings that have physical, emotional, cognitive, or social requirements. A job analysis is unique to each work environment and job description. Occupational therapists can use their skills in job analysis to assist employers with defining job descriptions and potential reasonable accommodations. An important task will be defining essential job functions related to emotional and psychosocial performance and differentiating the essential ones from the marginal. In the process of developing job descriptions, therapists can identify attitudes needing to be changed.

In the following situation, Bowman (1991) demonstrated that mental or emotional health can be identified as an essential job function:

An occupational therapy position is available in a psychiatric treatment program that is behaviorally oriented. The therapist working in the program is expected to model appropriate social behavior. A new therapist is hired who has an emotional problem resulting in her exhibiting irrational, inappropriate social behavior when she is in stressful situations. The occupational therapist is terminated and files suit against the manager and facility for discrimination. The evidence used to determine if the [therapist] has been discriminated against is the job description. If the job description did not include "modeling appropriate social behavior" as an essential job function, the manager could not claim it was essential. Unwritten assumptions about what a job requires no longer apply. The performance skills required must be outlined in the job description, which must be shown to the applicant. (p. 2)

In this situation, two critical parts were present that are necessary under the ADA. First, the modeling of appropriate social behavior was defined as an essential function in the job description for this position, and, second, there was no suitable, reasonable accommodation that could substitute for this essential job requirement.

Reasonable Accommodation

There is pressing need for widespread education regarding reasonable accommodations within the mental health field (Mancuso, 1990). Reasonable accommodations reduce the gap between a worker's capabilities and job demands. In planning for employment, one must examine both elements. Occupational therapists can assist both the employee and employer with this planning, as demonstrated below:

A computer programmer with a mental disability and related problems with fatigue was seen by an occupational therapist during outpatient sessions. Assessment revealed that the fatigue increased in relation to the amount of stress associated with programming responsibilities and with the client's sleeping patterns. Recently, she had been working overtime for 2 weeks to solve problems in a new inventory system. She reported that the increased hours disrupted her normal sleep cycle and that previously discussed adaptations were not helping. An adaptation was planned to prevent this fatigue.

She requested from her supervisor 3 days of sick leave to work with her physician and to get the necessary rest to get back into a normal awake-sleep cycle. She informed the supervisor of the employer's policy for employees to use paid sick time to see their physician. The supervisor agreed to her sick leave. The supervisor will use two other programmers to solve any computer problems that occur during the client's 3-day absence. Upon her return, both parties agreed to discuss other job accommodations to prevent this level of fatigue from occurring in the future.

A person is qualified for accommodation whether the disability is a condition that exists prior to employment or develops during employment, as indicated in the following example:

An employee recovering from alcohol dependence (i.e., he has not had a drink for 1 1/2 months) has been a sales and delivery person for 3 years with a company that sells and distributes snack products. Of the 100 customers in the employee's sales territory, seven are liquor stores or taverns that the employee used to frequent. He reported to his occupational therapist how stressful it was to continue to serve these accounts.

The employee was a participant in an employer-sponsored alcohol rehabilitation program. The employer wanted the employee to return to work as soon as possible and asked for a planning meeting. The occupational therapist from the rehabilitation program was asked to assist in the decisionmaking process, and the problems with the assigned territory were discussed. A reasonable accommodation involved transferring these accounts to another salesperson in a nearby territory. In exchange, this employee would service appropriate accounts from the nearby territory. Thus, the employee was able to return to work sooner than expected, and the employer was able to continue business.

Accommodation must also reflect limitations that are static or changing. For example, job accommodation for people with personality disorder behaviors may need to be implemented only once and are predictable, whereas for people with bipolar disorders, accommodation may need to vary depending on the current behavior pattern.

Reasonable accommodation may include (a) making existing employment facilities accessible to and usable by persons with disabilities; (b) job restructuring; (c) part-time or modified work schedules; (d) reassignment to a vacant position; (e) acquisition or modification of equipment or devices; (f) appropriate adjustment or modification of examinations, training materials, or policies; and (g) provision of qualified readers or interpreters and other similar accommodations for persons with disabilities [ADA, Title I, § 101.9.(A)]. Reasonable accommodation for persons with mental disabilities might include the following:

- Part-time or flexible work schedules to allow for medical appointments.
- Provision of unpaid leave days.
- Redelegating assignments.
- Exchanging assignments with another employee.
- Reassignment to a vacant position if this would prevent the employee from being unemployed or the employer from losing a valuable employee. (National Mental Health Association, 1990, p. 13)

Under the ADA, reasonable accommodation is expected of the employer; it is usual or typical and not an exception, as seen in the following situation.

A job is open for a purchasing clerk in a large, open work space that has 16 purchasing clerks. A person with an anxiety disorder is able to meet all the essential job functions for the clerk position except that she has difficulty concentrating on multiple tasks. The occupational therapist reviewed the situation and made suggestions.

Reasonable accommodations included placing the employee's desk within a three-sided portable wall system to decrease general office distractions and developing an in-out work basket system outside this immediate work area to decrease interruptions. Follow-up by the occupational therapist indicated that these accommodations supported satisfactory work behaviors.

These two accommodations are not exceptional because they are also appropriate for a nondisabled employee with poor concentration on the job (e.g., the office socializer). Implied is the fact that persons with disabilities cannot be disqualified because of their inability to perform nonessential, or marginal, functions of the job and that reasonable accommodation be made to help such persons meet legitimate criteria (National Mental Health Association, 1990). As of July 1, 1992, employers will have to defend discrimination charges related to their standards, selection criteria, tests, and refusal to accommodate in employment-related decisions (ADA, Title I, § 107).

According to the ADA, employers who interview a potential employee or consider an employee's continued employment are not allowed to focus on what a person cannot do or on the diagnosis itself. They must focus instead on essential job functions and the capability of the person in question to perform the job tasks. An occupational therapist could assist the employer in making plans to address potential problems, such as in the following scenario:

A certified public accountant for a medium-sized business, whose condition is diagnosed as bipolar affective disorder, appears agitated at tax time and highly sensitive to the supervisor's questions about the time line for submitting tax documents. Instead of confronting the worker and requesting immediate documentation, the employer along with the occupational therapist could plan a reasonable accommodation that would entail asking the worker to meet the supervisor the next day with a time line and to be prepared to identify the need for additional help or personnel. Additionally, at the meeting, the supervisor could offer the employee support for his diligent efforts. The supervisor could also encourage the employee to take time to see a physician to make sure his medications are conducive to his work responsibilities. These actions demonstrate positive regard for the employee's work and facilitate the employee's performance and self-efficacy beliefs.

Occupational therapists can help the employer and employee identify desired work behaviors and plan reasonable accommodations to facilitate essential work behaviors. Psychiatric disabilities present functional limitations that recur and require adaptation during employment. Mancuso (1990) identified these limitations as (a) duration of concentration, (b) screening out environmental stimuli, (c) maintaining stamina throughout the workday, (d) managing time pressures and deadlines, (e) initiating interpersonal contact, (f) focusing on multiple tasks simultaneously, (g) responding to negative feedback, and (h) physical and emotional side effects of psychotropic medications. (See the Appendix of this chapter for an expanded list and reasonable accommodations for work-related behaviors associated with mental impairment.) This list may be useful for employers who, in good faith, want to employ persons with mental impairments, for occupational therapists who will oversee the work site, and for persons with mental health problems to identify potentially beneficial accommodations that allow them to successfully engage in work. The selection of accommodation must reflect the person's functional abilities, his or her self-efficacy, and the work environment. For example, if a person cannot do word processing for more than 90 minutes, then the accommodation may be to require a 10-minute break every 90 minutes, and the software package itself could notify the employee when it is time for a break.

Not providing reasonable accommodations to a qualified person with a disability is prohibited discrimination, unless the change would be unreasonably burdensome. The legal term for this employer burden is *undue hardship*. Undue hardship is an action requiring significant difficulty or expense when considered in light of the nature and cost of the accommodation needed and the overall operational, financial, and personnel resources of the facility. Accommodation is required unless it creates a significant difficulty or expense. Employers must provide evidence to support their undue hardship decisions when denying employment to a qualified individual with a mental impairment. If there is more than one way for an employer to provide accommodation, he or she may choose the easiest one to implement or the least expensive. The following example describes a potential undue hardship:

An aging day-care worker has shown signs of cognitive deterioration, forgetfulness, and shortened concentration. The day-care center meets the strict state-mandated standards for number of personnel assigned to care for the various age groups. The employee continues to be a warm, gentle person who wants to maintain her full-time job and denies any cognitive problems. Because she has developed such a good, long-standing relationship with the children and their parents, the supervisor consulted with an occupational therapist and decided to add part-time workers to assist the day-care worker in her assigned room.

The agency suffered a significant financial loss due to the increased personnel costs of providing for the safety of the children and the worker. During the consultation, the supervisor said that this increased financial outlay could not be continued. The worker was aware of the change in her abilities and agreed to resign her position. Knowing that the worker enjoys children, the therapist helped her find a church-based nursery to volunteer her services.

In this case, the employer could claim undue hardship as long as access to adequate financial resources to cover the financial loss were not available. For example, a small, privately owned day-care center could claim undue hardship, whereas a facility owned by a large corporate entity would need to prove undue hardship based on total corporate assets.

Two related important factors influence decisions regarding reasonable accommodation for persons with mental impairment under this law—direct threat and fitness for duty. If direct threat or fitness for duty are used in employment decisions, either must be shown to be job related and consistent with business necessity. Mental illness is hard to define, and the stability of an emotionally disturbed person is difficult to assess and predict (Strasser, 1991). Strasser said that not only should a person be able to perform a job, but the person should perform it safely and, in doing so, not endanger himself or herself, his or her co-workers, or society.

Essential job functions regarding safety should be included in the job description, and occupational therapists, physicians, and job interviewers should be instructed to assess for this ability. According to Section 103 of Title 1, employers may write and screen for job qualifications that exclude persons with mental health conditions from consideration if they pose a significant safety risk for other employees (Verville, 1990). A person with a history of aggressive, violent behavior in the work environment, for example, could be excluded from jobs where the behavior could create an unsafe working environment. The following example reviews such an instance:

A slaughterer from a local meat-packing company was hospitalized because he had been swinging meat cleavers at fellow workers, saying he was going to kill them. Clearly, this behavior is life threatening. The employer with a carefully constructed job description could justify excluding this person from this job and show that the company was not violating the employee's civil rights by not providing reasonable accommodation. The occupational therapist could inform the worker and employer of their rights and return-to-work expectations.

Direct threat is defined in the law as a significant risk to health or safety of others that cannot be eliminated by reasonable accommodation. Direct threat can be used as a qualification standard when screening a person for a specific job. Regarding mental illness, this section of the law ensures that decisions pertaining to a person's qualifications for a job are based on current, objective evaluation rather than on misconceptions and stereotypes (National Mental Health Association, 1990). To disqualify a person for a job, an employer must obtain objective evidence that an applicant or employee has

recently that threatened injury or has committed overt, threatening, or harmful acts. The specific risk and behavior posed by the disability must be identified. The perceived threat of harmful actions in the future is not a factor. The following case exemplifies the direct-threat issue:

In the process of interviewing a person for hire as a bank clerk, the manager discovered that the applicant had been treated for cocaine addiction 2 years earlier. The applicant openly talked about his recovery and his current involvement in support groups. The manager's previous experience with cocaine addicts was negative and assumed that this employee could not be trusted with cash, would try to steal money for cocaine, or might have cocaine-addicted friends who would use the applicant to rob the bank in the future. The employer is considering not hiring him to work at the bank.

In the above example, the employer would be in conflict with the ADA, because these conclusions had no objective basis or no current behavioral indicators related to this employee's ability to perform the essential job functions; they were based on misconceptions or stereotypes. An occupational therapist who offered seminars for employers regarding cocaine addiction and rehabilitation could increase this employer's understanding and maybe his acceptance of addiction.

A second qualification standard related to direct threat is fitness for duty, which also requires individualized, objective assessment. In the ADA, *fitness for duty* is defined as the degree of risk justifying disqualification that demonstrates reasonable probability of serious or substantial harm. The likelihood, seriousness, and imminence of injury are factors that one would consider in determining the legality of exclusion. The recurrence of a clinical condition could be used to estimate this standard for each person in a specific job. Both individual factors and job-related factors should be considered (Maffeo, 1990). Additionally, established scientific bases for determining risk may contribute to fitness-for-duty decisions. For example, Maffeo (1990) stated that an employer who is concerned about an applicant who has threatened suicide in the past must assess (a) both the applicant and the requirements of the job, with attention to the applicant's current and past mental health problems; (b) the published data on suicide risk, general nature, and specific hazards in the target job; and (c) adequacy of the applicant's performance at previous jobs. The final decision must be based on information from objective data about known risk factors and possible accommodations to permit essential and marginal job functions.

Employers are reminded that concerns regarding direct threat and fitness for duty cannot circumvent the prohibition against pre-employment inquiries into a person's disability (ADA, 1990). This includes generalized requests or inquiries related to medical records, mental health history, or mental disability under the guise of wanting to ascertain the possibility of direct threat posed by the applicant. Instead, employers must focus on the ability of the applicant or employee to perform the essential functions of a job with or without reasonable accommodation.

Access to Employee Functions

Employees with mental health disabilities are entitled to attend any function provided to any other employee. Any public accommodation or service provided to other employees must be accessible to them as well. Employees cannot be excluded from annual office retreats, use of the corporate condominium, or business trips, as shown in the example below:

> The company holiday party for employees and their families has been announced and the personnel department is taking reservations. An employee who has a 14-year-old daughter with mental disabilities made her reservation. Personnel is aware that this daughter has been known to be loud and distracting in her speech, and they are concerned about her behavior being disruptive and inappropriate in the restaurant's elegant setting. The company is considering asking this employee not to bring her daughter.

Under ADA protection, the company cannot make such a request. The employee's right to equal access for her family to join in the employer's holiday party is protected by Title III.

Employers must ensure that employees have access to employment-related activities that may occur off the job site. For example, a business with a staff of 75 employees offers supported employment for 12 mentally retarded persons. A bowling league is being set up for interested employees, and seven of the supported employees wish to join the bowling league. Under the ADA, it is discriminatory not to offer the persons with mental disabilities access to the integrated bowling league.

Clearly, Titles I and III work in concert with each other when addressing access to employment-related activities, whether these activities are at the work site or are related to employer-sponsored activities.

Implications for Occupational Therapy

The focus on employment and reasonable accommodations for clients with mental disabilities focuses more on abstract psychosocial components of employment, including interpersonal behaviors and personal beliefs, and less on assistive technology. Occupational therapists can help persons with mental disabilities become a part of the work force by doing the following:

- Providing attitude and advocacy training for persons with disabilities as well as for employers and co-workers.
- Preparing persons with mental impairments to be successful employees through training programs to promote self-efficacy as a worker.

- Collaborating with employers who want to employ persons with mental impairments by helping them to identify the essential functions of jobs and determine reasonable accommodations for persons with mental disabilities.

If employment is a goal of any mental health rehabilitation program, then occupational therapists should plan meaningful treatment activities that simulate work and provide opportunity to acquire self-efficacy as a worker. Bandura's (1977, 1982) model, which is consistent with occupational therapy philosophy, provides a mechanism for returning clients to work roles. This model also has implications for keeping persons with mental impairments on the job. Thus, the self-efficacy model provides a mechanism to ensure successful employability within the guidelines of the ADA.

Occupational therapists in mental health will see numerous related roles emerge as the ADA is implemented, including those of advocate, educator, designer, provider of reasonable accommodations, and, perhaps, liaison between employers and employees with disabilities. We hope that implementing the suggestions made in this paper will direct ADA-related decisions about those with mental disabilities toward access and participation in life roles, especially the most meaningful role—that of worker—for persons with mental impairments (Gonzalez & Gordon, 1990). Occupational therapists can facilitate the process of integrating Americans with mental disabilities into the mainstream of life and be instrumental in providing leadership to assist in the full implementation of this new civil rights legislation. As agents of both personal and environmental change, we as occupational therapists can demonstrate application of our knowledge in a timely way to help persons with mental disabilities attain their employment rights and support this declaration of independence.

References

Americans With Disabilities Act of 1990 (Public Law 101–336), 42 U.S.C. § 12101.

Anthony W. A., & Blanch, A. (1987). Supported employment for persons who are psychiatrically disabled: An historical and conceptual perspective. *Psychosocial Rehabilitation, 11*(2), 5–23.

Bandura, A. (1977). Self-efficacy: Toward a unifying theory of behavioral change. *Psychological Review, 84,* 191–215.

Bandura, A. (1982). Self-efficacy mechanism in human agency. *American Psychologist, 37,* 122–147.

Bandura, A. (1986). Fearful expectations and avoidance actions as coeffects of perceived self-efficacy. *American Psychologist, 41,* 1389–1391.

Bowman, O. J. (1991, September). Managers to play an important role in implementing the Americans With Disabilities Act. *Administration and Management Special Interest Section Newsletter,* pp. 1–2.

Christiansen, C. (1991). Occupational therapy: Intervention for life performance. In C. Christiansen & C. Baum (Eds.), *Occupational therapy: Overcoming human performance deficits* (pp. 2–43). Thorofare, NJ: Slack.

Combs, I. H., & Omvig, C. P. (1986). Accommodation of disabled people into employment: Perceptions of employers. *Journal of Rehabilitation, 52,* 42–45.

Gonzalez, E. G., & Gordon, D. M. (1990). Americans With Disabilities Act: The crumbling of another wall. *Archives of Physical Medicine and Rehabilitation, 71,* 951.

Hartlage, L., & Roland, P. (1971). Attitudes of employers toward different types of handicapped workers. *Journal of Applied Rehabilitation Counseling, 2,* 115–120.

Howard, G. (1975). The ex-mental patient as an employee: An on-the-job evaluation. *American Journal of Orthopsychiatry, 45,* 479–483.

Lotito, M. J., & Pimental, R. (1990). *The American With Disabilities Act: Making the ADA work for you.* Northridge, CA: Milt Wright.

Maffeo, P. A. (1990). Making non-discriminatory fitness-for-duty decisions about persons with disabilities under the Rehabilitation Act and the Americans With Disabilities Act. *American Journal of Law and Medicine, 14,* 279–326.

Mancuso, L. L. (1990). Reasonable accommodation for workers with psychiatric disabilities. *Psychosocial Rehabilitation Journal, 14,* 3–19.

National Mental Health Association. (1990). *ADA. Americans With Disabilities Act of 1990 (Public Law 101-336): Legislative summary series.* Alexandria, VA: Author.

Rhodes, L. E., Ramsing, K. D., & Bellamy, G. T. (1988). Business participation in supported employment. In G. T. Bellamy, L. E. Rhodes, D. M. Mank, & J. M. Albin (Eds.), *Supported employment: A community implementation guide* (pp. 247–261). Baltimore: Brookes.

Staff. (1990, July-August). Americans With Disabilities Act signing: "Declaration of Independence" for 43 million. *Quality of Care,* pp. 8–9.

Strasser, A.L. (1991). Americans With Disabilities Act raises ethical considerations for physicians. *Occupational Health and Safety, 60*(2), 26.

Townsend, B. (1991). Nationally Speaking—Beyond our clinics: A vision for the future. *American Journal of Occupational Therapy, 45,* 871–873.

Verville, R. E. (1990). The Americans With Disabilities Act: An analysis. *Archives of Physical Medicine and Rehabilitation, 71,* 1010–1013.

Watson, P. G. (1990). The Americans With Disabilities Act: More rights for people with disabilities. *Rehabilitation Nursing, 15,* 325–328.

Appendix. 29.A. Reasonable Accommodations for Recurrent Functional Problems Among Persons With Psychiatric Disorders

Personal Self-Efficacy

Reinforce or coach appropriate behaviors.

Test for job skills on the job and avoid self-report of abilities.

Place in job where there is a model to follow or imitate.

Teach self-advocacy skills.

Provide successful job experiences. Use positive feedback.

Begin with close supervision and then cut back slowly as skills are maintained.

Maintain similarity or consistency in work tasks.

Encourage positive self-talk and eliminate negative self-talk.

Duration of Concentration[a]

Put each work request in writing and leave in "to-do" box to avoid interruptions.

Provide ongoing consultation, mediation, problem solving, and conflict resolution.

Provide good working conditions, such as adequate light, smoke-free environment, and reduced noise.

Provide directive commands on a regular basis.

Screening Out Environmental Stimuli[a]

Place in a separate office.

Provide opaque room dividers between workstations.

Allow person to work after hours or when others are not around.

Ensure that workstation facilitates work production and organization.

Maintaining Stamina Throughout the Workday[a]

Provide additional breaks or shortened workday.

Allow an extended day to allow for breaks or rest periods.

Avoid work during lunch, such as answering the phone; buy an answering machine instead.

Distribute tasks throughout the day according to energy level.

Job share with another employee.

Develop work simplification techniques, such as collect all copying to be done at one time or use a wheeled cart to move supplies.

Have a liberal leave policy for health problems, flexible hours, and back-up coverage.

Individualize work agreements.

Verify employees' efficacy regarding their ability to sustain effort or persist with a task.

Teach on-the-job relaxation and stress-reduction techniques.

Appendix. 29.A. Reasonable Accommodations for Recurrent Functional Problems Among Persons With Psychiatric Disorders (Continued)

Managing time pressure and deadlines[a]

Maintain structure through a daily time and task schedule using hourly goals.

Provide positive reinforcement when tasks are completed within the expected time lines.

Arrange a separate work area to reduce noise and interruptions.

Screen out unnecessary business.

Initiating interpersonal contact[a]

Purposely plan orientation to meet and work alongside co-workers.

Allow sufficient time to make good, unhurried contacts.

Make contacts during work, break, and even lunch times, adjusting the conversation to the situation.

When standing, instead of facing each other, try standing at a 90-degree angle to each other.

Allow the person to work at home.

Have an advocate to advise and support the person.

Communicate honestly.

Plan supervision times and maintain them.

Develop tolerance for and helpful responses to unusual behaviors.

Provide awareness and advocacy training for all workers.

Focusing on multiple tasks simultaneously[a]

Eliminate the number of simultaneous tasks.

Redistribute tasks among employees with the same responsibilities, so each can do more of one type of job task than a lot of different tasks.

Establish priorities for task completion.

Arrange for all work tasks to be put in writing with due dates or times.

Responding to negative feedback[a]

Have employee prepare own work appraisal to compare with supervisor's.

Work together to establish methods employee can use to change negative behavior.

Provide positive reinforcement for observed behavioral change.

Provide on-site crisis intervention and counseling services to develop self-esteem, provide emotional support, and promote comfort with accommodations.

Establish guidelines for feedback.

Symptoms secondary to prescribed psychotropic medications[a]

Provide release time to see psychiatrist or primary physician.

Encourage employee to work with physician to establish a time schedule to take medications that are conducive to work responsibilities.

Provide release time or changes in job tasks that match condition.

[a]From Mancuso (1990).

Building Inclusive Community: A Challenge for Occupational Therapy

1994 ELEANOR CLARKE SLAGLE LECTURE

ANN P. GRADY, MA, OTR, FAOTA

Preparation of the Eleanor Clarke Slagle Lecture promotes reflection on the values and philosophy of occupational therapy. I chose the topic *Building Inclusive Community: A Challenge for Occupational Therapy* because it provided me with an opportunity to explore my own values and the values of the profession regarding inclusion of all persons into the community they choose and into the world community at large. The topic particularly led me to review my own work in adaptation theory developed with Elnora Gilfoyle (Gilfoyle, Grady, & Moore, 1990) in light of changes occurring or being promoted in society regarding opportunities for inclusion of all persons in all aspects of living.

Ideas about inclusion; the meaning of community; the relationship between environment and community; the interaction among a person's past experience, present situation, and future hopes and dreams and its effect on the relationship that develops between an occupational therapist and a person seeking therapy services all became focal points for exploring our role in building inclusive community. The result has been some expansion of our understanding of the environment category of the spatiotemporal adaptation theory and exploration of the relationship between environment and community. In addition, exploring the concepts of the theory led to consideration of its relevance for enhancing our ability to plan with consumers of service who are creating or returning to their own community. Focal points for exploring the challenges related to building inclusive community include:

- An understanding of the meaning of community building within a person's own environment and according to his or her choices.
- A review of current ideas about the nature of disability in relation to both philosophy and mandates for inclusion.
- An expansion of ideas about the role of environment in a person's adaptation to community living.
- A consideration of strategies for promoting choice and inclusion.

For as far back in time as we know, human beings have gathered together to share in daily living and use some form of symbols as means for communicating with each other, hence the building of community (Dance & Larson, 1972). To this day, we share meaning in our communities through symbols composed of pictures, words spoken in our own culturally determined language, and gestures or nonverbal expressions of our thoughts or feelings. Native Americans in the southwestern regions of our country choose to tell the stories of their community living and beliefs through petroglyphs, or rock art (Patterson–Rudolph, 1993). One expert in petroglyphs compared attempts at identifying subject matter and its significance to cloud watching in that no two people will interpret what they see in the same way. Petroglyphs were apparently not intended to represent words of a language as we know it, but instead were meant to convey more general concepts or global ideas about the society, such as ideas about religion, medicine, governance, art, war, and peace. An artist's rendition of petroglyphs titled "Circle of Friends" (see Figure 30.1) is chosen to represent

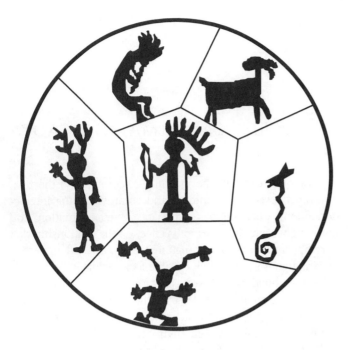

Figure 30.1. Circle of Friends petroglyph. Original metal sculpture by Kevin Smith, Golden, Colorado. Appears with permission of Kevin Smith.

ideas about community and inclusion that are central to the themes of this article. In rock art, spirals, concentric circles, and other geometric shapes are interpreted to be universal symbols used to convey conceptual ideas (Patterson, 1992). There are dozens of possible interpretations connected to each figure in the circle because rock art is interpreted not only according to the individual symbols present, but also by the figures that are combined in a panel, just like words in spoken language. For me, the Circle of Friends represents the encompassing nature of a community, whether it is the community that each of us constructs for ourselves or the larger environment in which we discover ourselves. The circle represents the wholeness of a community, and the figures relate to diversity that can exist within the community. Just as the circle is considered a symbol of inclusion and wholeness, the extension of the circle as a spiral is well known as a symbol of growth and continuity. Spirals frequently appear as symbols of continuity in Native American culture (Patterson, 1992). The spiral reflects evolution and renewal with growth emanating from continuous learning and new challenges. The spiral and its embedded circles will be used in this article to represent change and continuity.

Why is the idea of building inclusive community important to us as people and as occupational therapists? The idea is both profound and simple. Simply, we believe that people belong together regardless of real or perceived differences. All persons have the right to choose where they wish to live, work, learn, and play and with whom they wish to spend time. On a deeper level, we believe that people belong to-

gether *because* of differences. There is a richness that characterizes a community constructed with appreciation for both differences and similarities among its members. The idea is not new, but as Winston Churchill said, "Men [and women] stumble over the truth from time to time, but most pick themselves up and hurry off as if nothing had happened" (McWilliams, 1994, p. 413).

The Nature of Community and Choice

Community provides a context for actualizing individual potential and experiencing oneness with others (McLaughlin & Davidson, 1985). The human condition yearns for a greater sense of connectedness, expressed as a need to reach out, deeply touch others, and throw off the pain and loneliness of separation. The term *community* encompasses *communication* and *unity*. Yankelovitch said that the community evokes in the individual the feeling that "here is where I belong—these are my people, I care for them, they care for me, I am part of them, I know what they expect from me and I from them, they share my concerns. I know this place, I am on familiar ground, I am at home" (1981, p. 224).

There are established communities such as towns, neighborhoods, schools, and workplaces, and there are personal communities we create for ourselves, which include family, friends, acquaintances, how and where we spend our time formally or informally, and the relationships we build over time. Our personal communities do not necessarily depend on specific location or specific time, although they are often embedded in established communities. Building inclusive community refers to both the larger, more formal community context and the smaller, informal community that a person identifies as a personal community. Ideas about diversity and inclusion in community in this article apply to all people, but we as occupational therapists have particular concerns for assuring choice in community living for persons with disabilities and chronic health problems, as well as persons for whom disability and health issues can be prevented.

Personal community building begins at the center of the circle, where the person is embedded in family and close relationships (see Figure 30.2). Networks of informal support develop in the center of a personal community. Relationships grow because persons choose to be connected. The unique culture of personal community is created from family experience. Values are established; heritage, myths, and traditions are communicated. The foundation for building personal community is established within the family:

> We all come from families. Families are big, small, extended, nuclear, multigenerational, with one parent, two parents, and grandparents. We live under one roof or many. A family can be as temporary as a few weeks, as permanent as forever. We become part of a family by birth, adoption, marriage, or from a desire for mutual support. Families are dynamic and are cultures unto themselves, with different values and unique ways of realizing dreams. Our families

create neighborhoods, communities, states, and nations. (Shelton & Stepanek, 1994, p. 6)

For both children and adults, family provides a personal culture of embeddedness. Each person creates a community of family culture in the broadest sense of the concept of community. Like all cultures, each culture we create within our community is based on our values and may differ substantially from another's uniquely consummated community. However the family is constituted, whether we judge it adequate or not according to our value system, a person is embedded in his or her family and that is our starting place for inclusion. *A challenge for occupational therapy practitioners is understanding each person's unique community, including its culture and the context in which it was formed.*

The concept of community is broadened to include relations with acquaintances, coworkers, and schoolmates as well as locations like neighborhoods, workplace, and town. The community circle includes both formal and informal sources of support. The environment provides the context in which communities are formed. It is composed of persons, objects, and space—all of which can be combined for personal or formal community building. The environment generally provides formal support to persons in community. Community is not a static structure in the environment, but an ongoing process of interaction among persons, objects, and space. Community provides familiarity with daily interactions that reduces the uncertainty experienced in new and challenging situations and creates a sense of belonging.

A sense of belonging in a community provides the comfort and security needed to explore and use one's gifts. According to Maslow's hierarchy, belonging is an important component in the development of self-esteem. Building blocks to self-esteem include a sense of safety in one's immediate community, a sense of self-acceptance, identity, affiliation with others, and a sense of competence and mission. In some instances, we seem to expect children and adults with disabilities to demonstrate a sense of self-esteem before they can be included in a typical classroom or work or living environment forgetting that belonging to a typical community is the means by which a person develops a sense of self (Kunc, 1994). *One of the challenges we often face is resolution of the conflict we have over the need for persons with disabilities to prove themselves capable before they are included in typical communities of their choice rather than creating opportunities for them to develop their capacities in their community with appropriate supports.*

Choice is a valued dimension of our community life. Choice means having alternatives from which to make a selection. As occupational therapists, we recognize the importance of choice in every person's pursuit of self-actualization, particularly as he or she fulfills occupational roles of daily living, work, school, and play and leisure. Choice in occupational therapy has traditionally meant that the person seeking services takes an active part in planning and

carrying out a therapy program. Yerxa (1966) maintained that one of the most important roles an occupational therapist plays is providing choice in selection of therapeutic activities, interaction with the activities, and, most important, establishment of objectives for a therapy program. Exercising choice in a therapeutic environment provides opportunities to explore capabilities and options for life outside the therapy setting. Making choices is another way of exploring personal values about daily living, relationships, roles, and the physical, psychological, social, and spiritual communities in which living needs to occur to pursue self-actualization. Making choices in therapy is only a prelude to the choices people need to make regarding their life in the community. How will I make a living? Where will I live? Where will my child go to school? What supports will I need to live fully in the community of my choice? *A challenge for occupational therapy practitioners is fostering choice that reflects their consumers' priorities for living and accomplishing occupational tasks, even if there are differences among them regarding values or perceptions of expertise.* Schön (1983) wrote that the interactive practitioner realizes that he or she is not the only one in the situation to have relevant and important knowledge. The consumer interacts by joining with a service provider to make sense of the situation and, by doing so, gains a sense of increased involvement and action—or choice.

Being part of a community provides opportunities for lifelong development. Persons with disabilities and their family members have a right to pursue and participate in all levels of their community, whether it is one they have known well or one they wish to build to accommodate new circumstances and fulfill new or old dreams. Each person creates a community of his or her own culture in the broadest sense of the concept. Like all cultures, each culture we create within our community is based in our values and may differ substantially from another's uniquely consummated community.

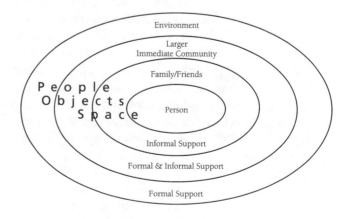

Figure 30.2. Personal community building.

Creating community opens doors to new cultural vistas with opportunities to cooperate with each other and participate in community activities. Inclusion in a community also means an end to loneliness and helplessness and the beginning of empowerment to fulfill dreams (McLaughlin & Davidson, 1985). Building inclusive communities with all persons provides opportunities for members of the community to experience different relationships. Each of us has the capacity for creating inclusive community through our work with individuals as well as our ability to influence society and its established institutions.

The Nature of Disability and Inclusion

A new sociopolitical environment is developing in which persons with disabilities are taking or creating social and political actions on their own behalf. Changing perceptions of disability and the histories of the civil rights movement in the 1960s and the women's rights movement in the 1970s resulted in substantial legislative action for disability rights. In his book *No Pity*, Shapiro (1993) chronicled the course of the disability rights movement in the United States. Shapiro stated that persons with disabilities insist simply on common respect and the opportunity to build bonds to their community as fully accepted participants in everyday life. In the past, disability was usually viewed as a medical problem with the expectation that, to be accepted, persons with disabilities needed to be as much like persons without disabilities as possible without regard for their own uniqueness. Now, persons with disabilities are thinking differently about themselves. Many no longer think of their physical or mental differences as a source of shame or something to overcome in order to be like others or inspire others. In *Flying Without Wings*, Beisser, who contracted polio as an adult, said "When I stopped struggling, working to change, and found means of accepting what I had already become, I discovered that changed me. Rather than feeling disabled and inadequate, I felt whole again" (1989, p. 169). Beisser views disability as a difference among people. Considering disability as a difference is in itself neutral and changes the way persons with disabilities view themselves and are viewed by others. For example, in the village of Chilmark on Martha's Vineyard Island in Massachusetts, more than half the residents in the 1800s were genetically deaf (Groce, 1985). All the people in the village were fluent in sign language. It has been reported that spoken and sign language were used simultaneously or, if a person who was deaf joined a speaking group, group members immediately started to use sign as well as speech. Deafness was not a disability in Chilmark. Disability is a dimension of diversity not unlike ethnic background, color, religious, or gender differences (Shapiro, 1993). Differences do not necessarily equal limitations, but rather create opportunities for meaningful interaction (J. Snow, personal communication, 1994) as long as people are living together naturally.

Just as perceptions of disability are changing, so are the reasons that disability was so often seen as a limitation. The difference within the person is no longer viewed as the main problem; instead, the environment that cannot accommodate the person is considered responsible for society's failure to include persons with disabilities in the mainstream. Social considerations have led to a shift from the traditional medical view of disability to an interactional model that accounts for the relationship between person and environment. Gill (1987) summarized this shift in perspective as follows:

> According to the medical view, disability is considered a deficit or abnormality. In an interactional model, disability is a difference.
>
> In the medical view, being disabled is perceived as negative. In an interactional model, being disabled is in itself neutral.
>
> Medicine views disability as residing in the individual. In an interactional model, disability is derived from problems encountered during interaction between the individual and their environment.
>
> In medicine, the remedy for disability-related problems is cure or normalization of the individual. In an interactional model, the remedy for disability-related problems is a change in the environmental interaction.
>
> Finally, the medical view identifies the agent of remedy as the professional. An interactional model has proposed that the agent of remedy may be the individual, an advocate, or anyone who affects the arrangements between the individual and society.

The last interactional category in Gill's summary can have a significant effect on the roles for occupational therapists. The shift from a medical perspective to an environmental framework is not difficult for us to understand. Occupational therapists have always recognized that disability was not an illness that could be cured by medicine. *The challenge for us is to promote the interactive model for practice regardless of the venue of our practice. A concurrent challenge is to increase support for more practice venues in the community where engagement in real occupation takes place.*

Change in perception of disability has fostered the disability rights movement and legislative action. The disability rights movement has focused on the rights of persons with disabilities to be included in society according to the choices they make for themselves and their families. The rights movement could also be called an *inclusion* movement. Inclusion in community means that all persons regardless of differences participate in natural environments for living, learning, playing, working, resting, and recreating. For persons with disabilities, participation may be with specific support from others or with adaptations to the environment. According to Gill (1987), inclusion means removal of barriers to power, which results in a greater number of alternatives or choices.

Shapiro (1993) identified the 1960s as the beginning of the disability independent living movement started by Ed Roberts and other students at the University of California–Berkeley. The movement spread to include action in Washington, DC, that initiated funding for independent living. Groups of parents of children with disabilities began to form around the country at about the same time, primarily to provide support to other parents in the same situations. The groups were often connected to existing organizations like United Cerebral Palsy or the Easter Seal Society. Later, parent organizations would emerge as independent, social change groups.

The 1970s saw adoption of Section 504 of the Rehabilitation Act (Public Law 93–112) prohibiting discrimination on the basis of disability. But Section 504 was not implemented for nearly 5 years after its adoption and was implemented only after a group led by Roberts and others staged a sit-in at Department of Health, Education, and Welfare office in San Francisco. Besides succeeding in obtaining regulations for Section 504, the event in San Francisco created an awareness that linked groups of adults around the country in a civil rights movement. Also in the 1970s, Public Law 94–142 was adopted as the Education for All Handicapped Children Act (1975), mandating public education in the least restrictive environment for children with disabilities who were 5 years of age and older.

In the 1980s, support was provided for that act through the establishment of statewide parent information and advocacy centers in every state. The legislation was expanded to include infants and toddlers with passage of the Education of the Handicapped Act Amendments of 1986 (Public Law 99–457). With this expanded legislation for education came the components of family-centered care, or respect for a family's central role as decision maker for a child, or support for an adult, which is now considered best practice across the life span. Public Law 94–142 and Public Law 99–457 were combined and expanded in reauthorization as the Individuals With Disabilities Education Act of 1990 (IDEA) (Public Law 101–476). Meanwhile, the Technology-Related Assistance for Individuals With Disabilities Act (Public Law 100–407) (1988) began the process of changing policy and availability of assistive technology for persons with disabilities in all states. The legislative decade of the 1980s culminated with the Americans With Disabilities Act of 1990 (ADA) (Public Law 101–336). ADA encompasses ideology from all previous legislation by ensuring that the barriers to inclusion be eliminated for persons with disabilities. Although far-reaching disability rights legislation was officially adopted in the 1980s, we are still struggling with implementation of all the laws in the 1990s.

The disability rights movement and legislation has focused primarily on removing physical and legal barriers to inclusion. Legislative mandates serve the purpose of forcing inclusion. The spirit of inclusion only comes with attitude change supported by community preparation and relationship building. In a midwestern city, 9-year-old Amy, who has cerebral palsy, visited Santa Claus last year and had only one wish for Christmas—just one day in school when the kids did not tease her about her cerebral palsy. Clearly, Amy was present in school with her typical peers, and being there is a start. But she is not truly included because a community that accepts her for who she is has not been created. She needed a school community that gave her a sense of familiarity, caring, and belonging. She needed relationships that she could depend upon for support ("Disabled Girl Asks Santa," 1993). In another city, 14-year-old Kevin, who has Down's syndrome, has been with typical peers from the beginning of his school career. His inclusion has focused on preparation and relationship building that included Kevin along with the teachers and children in the building. When asked what it would be like if he was not included in typical school, he replied that he'd feel sad. "I like to be in school with my friends— I learn from them and they learn from me" (Kevin, personal communication, February 1993).

Inclusion is about relationships. Judith Snow, a consumer advocate in Canada, has said that the only real disability is having no relationships (personal communication, January 1994). Inclusion means participation. Inclusion in school is only the prelude to inclusion in life. Participation may require support not only in the traditional sense of personal assistance and adaptations, but also in terms of preparing the persons in the community to welcome differences into their community and help develop natural support systems. A challenge for occupational therapy is development of programs that prepare persons and their families for life in the community while working to prepare the community and persons in it to welcome the gifts of diversity. If we espouse the interactive model of disability, we can affect the arrangements between the individual and society and make unique contributions to the interactive model of change. We can assist with remediation of the person's physical or psychological problem to the extent that the manifestations of the problem can be changed. We can participate in modification of the person's environment so that it can accommodate the needs. We can assist with building community with the person or family in order to create a place for belonging that includes both the formal and informal sources of support. We can continue to promote inclusion as a value through our sociopolitical systems.

Building inclusive community sometimes requires change in value-based practices. The spiral (see Figure 30.3) serves as a model to illustrate that when we recognize differences in values, we may experience conflicts within ourselves or with others. If we cannot move beyond the downward spiral between values and differences, we will not be able to move beyond conflict. But if we move upward to change our perspective to

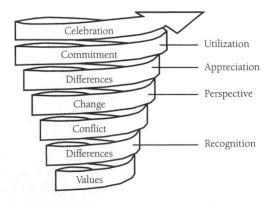

Figure 30.3. Celebrating diversity: Individual and society.

one of appreciating differences, we can make a commitment to using differences in ways that productively build community. The spiral begins with a small, defined center focusing on personal values about differences. These values were established with past experience. As the spiral moves upward and widens, new experiences are included. The person uses past experience to respond to new situations. The response may be use of past behavior or of a new behavior that will modify old behaviors. For example, Bobbie wants to live alone in an apartment, but he cannot tie his shoes, button his shirt, prepare meals very well, or use the telephone to summon help. If your values about independence mean a person can only choose between doing everything alone or living in a segregated community, then Bobbie's proposal is different, causes conflict, and probably elicits a negative response. If you stay in a downward spiral of conflict between values and differences, you will continue to respond negatively to full inclusion for persons who cannot perform all tasks independently. But if you take an interactive view of disability, your perspective changes. You appreciate that Bobbie's disability resides in the community that cannot accommodate his differences. A change in perspective leads to modification of old behavior by new responses. A commitment to using rather than rejecting differences creates new possibilities for removing the barriers to inclusion. *The challenge for individual occupational therapists and the profession is making a commitment to inclusion in community for all persons with disabilities and chronic health problems.* The following values are proposed for occupational therapy:

- Every person has a right to be an integrated member of a community of choice.
- Every person has a right to active participation in decision making for self and family
- Every person has a right to information and options as part of decision making.
- Every person has a right to choice of services delivered in natural environments in order to maximize success in occupational roles.

The Nature of Adaptation and Environment

To explore means for occupational therapists to meet the challenges of building inclusive community. I would like to turn to the spatiotemporal adaptation theory developed with my colleague Elnora Gilfoyle. The theory was developed when we were both involved in pediatric practice and education. During those years, pediatric occupational therapy and other disciplines focused knowledge development and research on typical child development as a means for designing programs for children who were not developing typically. Although the spatiotemporal adaptation theory articulated the importance of interaction between the child and the environment, it emphasized ways in which therapists could influence the child's development rather than ways in which the environment could be prepared to accommodate the child's function. In light of the shift from medical to interactive approach to disability, it seems appropriate to reexamine the categories of the theory, especially the environmental category of the model. The original categories in the theory included *movement, environment, adaptation, and spiraling continuum of development* (Gilfoyle et al., 1990).

In the theory, both development in children and ongoing functioning of adults is seen as a transactional process between a person and the environment; for example, movement provides a means for action and the environment presents a reason to act. The person influences and is influenced by the environment through a process of adaptation. According to Kegan, "adaptation is not just a process of coping or adjusting to events (of the environment) as they are, but an active process of increasingly organizing the relationship of self to the environment" (1982, p. 113). The relationship is transactional because persons organize themselves around events of the environment while simultaneously organizing environmental events to meet their needs (Yerxa, 1992). Adaptation as a category of the theory is viewed as an ongoing process of change in behavior. The spiral again provides the model for the adaptation process (see Figure 30.4). Throughout the life span, a person uses past experience, including values established in early life, to adapt to current situations and prepare for future adaptations. Through adaptation, more complex behaviors evolve to respond to more extensive demands from the environment. If the demands of the current or future situations exceed the ability to adapt, the person may recall past behavior to respond until environmental events can be reorganized to elicit a higher-level response. With adaptation as a process for organizing one's self and environment, interaction between person and environment sets up a system of relationships.

Environment as a category in the adaptation theory is all-inclusive. Environment represents the complete setting or surrounding in which a person lives, including self, other persons, objects, space, and relationships among all components in the environment (see Figure 30.2). According to Winnicott, a "good enough" (1965, p. 67) environment meets and challenges a person's need to grow and develop by adapting to stimulation from continually changing situations. Yerxa (1994) (see Chapter 57) noted that persons need just the right challenge to make an adaptive response. Daloz said that:

> how readily we grow—indeed whether we grow at all—has a great deal to do with the nature of the world in which we transact our lives' business. To understand human development, we must understand the environment's part, how it confirms us, contradicts us and provides continuity (1986, p. 68).

Environment–person relationships (see Figure 30.5) are conceptualized on a spiraling continuum from a *holding environment,* which promotes inclusion, to a *facilitating environment,* which promotes independence, to a *challenging environment,* which increases independence, to an *interactive environment,* which fosters interdependence. The holding environment begins in infancy and provides support through physical and psychological holding. Winnicott maintained that the holding environment is the context in which early development takes place. The infant experience can influence a lifetime. Kegan referred to holding as the "culture of embeddedness" (1982, p. 115), which means an environment that is for growth as well as for accumulating history and mythology. In the holding environment, the infant begins to acquire a culture based on values and traditions communicated during this phase. According to Kegan, there is no single holding environment in early life, but a succession of holding environments, a life history of embeddedness. Holding environments are psychosocial environments that hold us and let go of us. If the infant's experience is satisfactory, it becomes a reference point whenever holding or support is needed later in life. The holding environment promotes a sense of inclusion or belonging, which usually precedes movement away from sources of support and is vital for all persons' development of independence.

The facilitating environment motivates a person to move beyond a familiar setting and on to new challenges and independence. It provides just enough support for moving, literally or figuratively, into new situations.

The challenging environment focuses on separating the person from embeddedness in order to develop and test potential. Just the right amount of challenge is needed if the person is to make an adaptive response to the situation. Increased independence evolves from successful adaptation to challenges.

Finally, the interactive environment promotes interplay between person and environment by combining a sense of self with an appreciation for relationships with others. Interactive environment supports interdependence. Winnicott stated that independence is never absolute. The healthy person does not become isolated, but relates to the environment in such a way that person and environment can be considered interdependent. The different functions of environment and the spiraling sequence of relating to environment can be useful for helping

persons identify the environment they need to seek or create for their own health and well-being.

The role of the therapist is construction of Winnicott's "good enough" environment, depending on the person's adaptation needs (Letts et al., 1994). A new parent of a child with significant health problems may need a supportive holding environment to learn the special care that will be given at home. A teenager with a spinal cord injury may seek a facilitating environment when he decides to go to college. He may begin assembling the sources for assistance and adaptations he will need to live independently as well as the advocacy skills he will need to act on his own behalf. A woman recovering from a head injury may have regained considerable function in a rehabilitation setting, but may be fearful of being back in her community. She will need challenge to regain her independence but with enough support and facilitation to ensure pro-

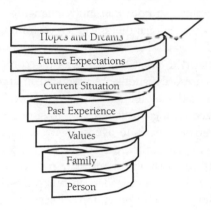

Figure 30.4. The person in life span.

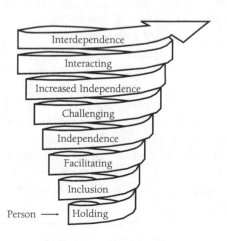

Figure 30.5. Environment–person relationships.

gressively successful adaptation. She may want to reconstruct the life she led before the accident, or she may construct a new community and need resources for her new life. An infant may literally require a supportive environment to learn sensorimotor skills or speech or to focus on learning through play. For all of us, gaining and maintaining a balanced interaction between self and environment is a work in progress. We often need to challenge ourselves if we wish to move ahead. Or we seek facilitation for new situations, or support in difficult times. A challenge for occupational therapy practitioners is development of skill in analyzing environments and helping consumers to identify the type of environmental milieu that will facilitate their adaptation process.

Interactive Strategies for Choice and Inclusion

The promise of occupational therapy lies in our ability to continuously combine the mandates put forth in the early tenets of our discipline with our constantly changing practice environments. Occupational therapy emerged from both community and medical models of practice although our philosophy is more related to what we know as the community-based model because occupations are practiced in community settings. For decades we tended to practice more in institutions or specialized settings, usually trying to simulate real-life settings to prepare persons to live in their community. Some of our more visionary colleagues set the course toward a future that focused on community consultation models of service delivery. The founders and leaders in our profession have fostered the importance of providing services in a person's own setting and according to the person's own choices and priorities for gaining or regaining specific skills for living. Our philosophy from the beginning of our profession has included the value of choice, relevance, and active participation through engagement in meaningful occupations. Occupation provides a context for organizing one's self and one's environment, thus promoting the transactional process of adaptation within a community setting (Engelhardt, 1977; Gilfoyle et al., 1990; Grady, 1992; Meyer, 1922 [see Chapter 2]; Schwartz, 1992; Yerxa, 1966). Therapy programs are designed to prevent or remediate the effects of disability or health issues and promote independent living in the community through occupations such as self-care and daily care of others, ability to play independently or with other children, ability to learn as a child and engage in lifelong learning as an adult, ability to be engaged in meaningful work to make a living or for one's own satisfaction or both, ability to balance work and recreation, and ability to blend all occupational activity with rest. Although models for community service delivery have been promoted from within the profession, external mandates for change have also influenced expansion of our practice environments. The voices heard from our consumers, our colleagues, legislation at state and national levels, and rapidly changing payment systems direct us toward service delivery that focuses on consumers'

priorities for goals and naturally occurring venues for activities. The new directions in practice allow us to combine our past experience and founders' mandates with the current realities of practice in ways that lead us to realize the future hopes and dreams of our consumers, ourselves as individuals, and the profession as a whole.

To build collaborative models of consumer-driven, community-based practice, we need to focus on a communication process that helps us understand other persons' unique culture and priorities for life occupations as well as meaning associated with past experiences, current situations, and hopes for the future. Recent developments in the field support a focus on communication that enhances a shift from medically focused to interactive models of practice in which the therapist serves as an agent of remedy to affect the arrangements between the individual and society. The use of narrative for storytelling has increased our understanding of a person's past and present experience. Reflective practice and clinical reasoning support our ability to gain insight into the interactive roles that can unfold between a therapist and a person seeking services. Ethnographic approaches to research have in general heightened our knowledge of persons living in their own environments (Clark, 1993; Mattingly & Fleming, 1994; Schön, 1983; Yerxa, 1994 [see Chapter 57]).

Therapist–consumer collaborative practice models mean that communication among the therapist, the person seeking services, the family members, and the close community members is critical. From the beginning, it is the relationships we build that are critical to our ability to collaborate effectively. Listening, talking, reflecting, informing, and demonstrating are all part of the ways we establish relationships. Human beings are uniquely constituted for giving and receiving information, making and sharing meaning. We have the capacity to use intrapersonal communication skills to explore the meaning of our own values and experiences, and interpersonal communication skills to link with another person's values and experiences. *Intrapersonal communication* refers to the creating, functioning, and evaluating of symbolic processes that operate within us. Such activities as thinking, reflecting, solving some problems, and talking with oneself are part of our unique intrapersonal communication system (Dance & Larson, 1972). Intrapersonal communication is active within us whenever meaning is attached to an internally or externally generated source of stimulation. Meaning associated with past events and current situations is deeply embedded in the intrapersonal system of both the persons seeking services and the service provider. Interpersonal communication serves to link us through verbal and nonverbal expression so that we can more explicitly share information and meaning. Through interpersonal communication, we can tell our stories; explore the meaning of relationships, events, and circumstances; reflect on similarities, differences, strengths, and challenges; and develop plans for working together toward future goals. Kegan said, "If you want to understand another person in

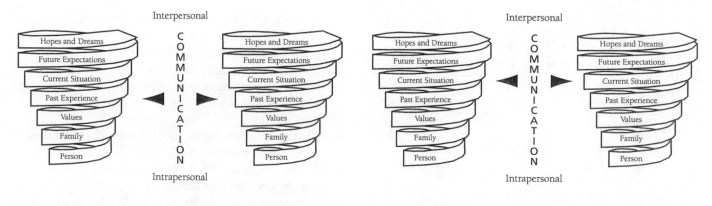

Figure 30.6. Linking past experiences.

Figure 30.8. Linking current information.

some fundamental way, you must know where the person is in his or her evolution. You need to understand his or her underlying structure for making meaning" (1982, p. 113). The context in which we as therapists seek and receive the information shared by persons seeking services can enhance our communication and collaborative planning. A communication model of collaboration can be illustrated by the spiraling model of person in life span (see Figure 30.4). If we place spirals side by side and let one spiral represent the consultant therapist and the other represent a person seeking services, we can visualize the communication sequences that occur. Communication moves from intrapersonal reflection to interpersonal linking through listening and speaking (see Figure 30.6). A closer look at the circle representing past experience provides details that can be shared about the meaning embedded in values and culture of childhood, family, and personal community (see Figure 30.7). We can discuss past experiences in terms of activities and relationships with family and close friends, with personal community, and with the larger environment. Exploring the past provides insight into the values that have directed past choices and the types of environments that the person has experienced. Discussing the current situation (see Figures 30.8 and 30.9) in the same context allows the therapist to understand the extent and meaning of the change that has occurred in the person's life as well as the priorities and

types of environments that need to be foremost in planning together. The persons can glean considerable information about the therapist's perspective on the current situation on the basis of past experience. The interpersonal linking increases understanding and promotes collaborative goal setting between person and therapist. As much as we have moved toward collaboration in family-centered and person-centered planning, we are still sometimes heard to say that we are having difficulty with a person receiving services accepting the goals we have set for their therapy. Interactive strategies mean that persons receiving services set the goals and therapists collaborate to design programs with them that will help address the goals. Information shared and the meaning it holds for both consumer and therapist provide the basis for collaboratively planning the future (see Figures 30.10 and 30.11). According to Schön (1983), there is gratification and anxiety for the reflective, interactive practitioner in becoming an active participant in a process of shared inquiry. For a therapist or consumer who wishes to move from traditional to reflective communication, there is the task of reshaping expectations for the relationship. But if we are to be agents of remedy in the arrangements between a person and the environment, we need to be able to share with and receive comprehensive information from the persons who are seeking choices for inclusion in their community.

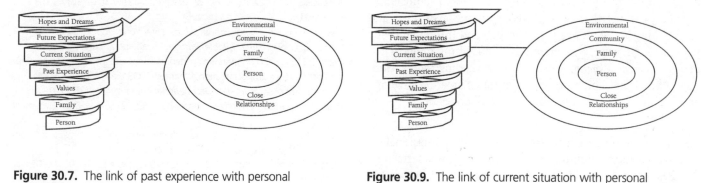

Figure 30.7. The link of past experience with personal community.

Figure 30.9. The link of current situation with personal community.

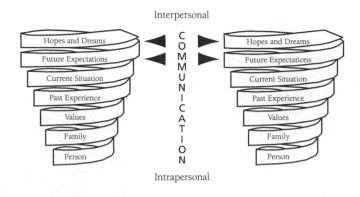

Figure 30.10. Exploring future possibilities.

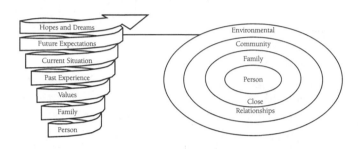

Figure 30.11. The link of hopes, dreams, and future expectations with personal community.

Summary

We have had an opportunity to focus on the challenges and opportunities for building inclusive community with the persons with whom we work in occupational therapy. We have gained understanding about the meaning of community and choice, reviewed current ideas about the nature of disability and mandates for inclusion, expanded ideas about environment and adaptation, considered strategies for promoting choice and inclusion, and related these concepts to the philosophy of occupational therapy. I had the extraordinary opportunity to explore my own values, past experience, current situation, and hopes for the future and I am forever changed by the experience. As Emily Brontë reflected, "I've dreamt in my life—dreams that have stayed with me ever after, and changed my ideas: they've gone through and through me, like wine through water, and altered the color of my mind" (cited in *The Quotable Woman*, 1991, p. 185). Leading the development of inclusive community is right for occupational therapy and we all have it in us to do it. The challenges before us are as follows:

1. Understanding each person's unique community, including its culture and the context in which it was formed.
2. Resolving the conflict we have over the need for persons with disabilities to prove themselves capable before being included in typical communities of choice rather than creating opportunities for developing capabilities in the community with appropriate supports.
3. Fostering choice that reflects a person's priorities for living and accomplishing occupational tasks, even when there are differences regarding values or perceptions of expertise.
4. Promoting the interactive model for practice, regardless of the venue of practice.
5. Increasing support for more practice venues in the community where engagement in real occupation takes place.
6. Developing programs that prepare people and their families for life in the community while working to prepare the community to welcome the gifts of diversity.
7. Making a commitment to inclusion in community for all persons.
8. Developing skill in analyzing environments and helping people identify the type of environmental milieu that will facilitate their adaptation process.

Acknowledgments

I thank Ellie Gilfoyle for leading the Eleanor Clarke Slagle nomination process and for a lifetime of creative collaboration; my colleagues who supported the nomination and by doing so offered focus for the topic; Lou Shannon for ongoing support and inspiration; my colleagues at The Children's Hospital for their support; Anita Wagner, Jackie Brand, and all the other parents who enlightened me with their perspectives and changed the course of my professional life; Betty Yerxa, whose philosophy and writings have influenced my thinking for many years; and my family, who is in the center of my personal community. I also thank Carol Wassell from Instructional Services at Colorado State University for creating beautiful slides for the presentation and graphics for this article and Diane Brians for drawing the Circle of Friends.

This lectureship is dedicated to my parents, the late Marion and James Grady, with deep love and appreciation for the strong focus on family and community that they lived and instilled in their children.

References

Americans With Disabilities Act of 1990 (Public Law 101–336) 42 U.S.C. § 12101.

Beisser, A. (1989). *Flying without wings.* New York: Doubleday.

Brontë, E. (1991). *The quotable woman.* Philadelphia: Running Press.

Clark, F. (1993). Occupation embedded in a real life: Interweaving occupational science and occupational therapy. 1993 Eleanor Clarke Slagle Lecture. *American Journal of Occupational Therapy, 47,* 1067–1078.

Daloz, L. (1986). *Effective mentoring and teaching.* San Francisco: Jossey–Bass.

Dance, F., & Larson, C. (1972). *Speech communication: Concepts and behavior.* New York: Holt, Rhinehart, & Winston.

Disabled girl asks Santa to end teasing. (1993, December 14). *The Denver Post,* p. 1.

Education for All Handicapped Children Act of 1975 (Public Law 94–142).

Education of the Handicapped Act Amendments of 1986 (Public Law 99–457).

Engelhardt, H. (1977). Defining occupational therapy: The meaning of therapy and the virtues of occupation. *American Journal of Occupational Therapy, 31,* 666–672.

Gilfoyle, E., Grady A., & Moore, J. (1990). *Children adapt* (2nd ed.). Thorofare, NJ: Slack.

Gill, C. (19877). A new social perspective on disability and its implication for rehabilitation. *Occupational Therapy in Health Care, 7,* 1.

Grady A. (1992). Nationally Speaking—Occupation as vision. *American Journal of Occupational Therapy, 46,* 1062–1065.

Groce, N. (1985). *Everyone here spoke sign language: Hereditary deafness on Martha's Vineyard.* Cambridge. MA: Harvard University Press.

Individuals With Disabilities Education Act of 1990 (Public Law 101–476).

Kegan, R. (1982). *The evolving self.* Cambridge, MA: Harvard University Press.

Kunc, N. (1994). *The other side of therapy.* Port Alberni, BC: Axis Consultation and Training.

Letts, L., Law, M., Rigby, P., Cooper, B., Stewart, D., & Strong, S. (1994). Person–environment assessments in occupational therapy. *American Journal of Occupational Therapy, 48,* 608–618.

Mattingly, C., & Fleming, M. (1994). *Clinical reasoning: Forms of inquiry in a therapeutic practice.* Philadelphia: F. A. Davis.

Meyer, A. (1922). The philosophy of occupation therapy. *Archives of Occupational Therapy, 1,* 1. Reprinted as Chapter 2.

McLaughlin, C., & Davidson, G. (1985). *Builders of the dawn.* Summertown, TN: Book Publishing.

McWilliams, P. (1994). *Do it again!* Los Angeles. Prelude.

Patterson, A. (1992). *Rock art symbols of the greater Southwest.* Boulder, CO: Johnson.

Patterson–Rudolph, C. (1993). *Petroglyphs and Pueblo myths of the Rio Grande* (2nd ed.). Albuquerque, NM: Avanyu.

Rehabilitation Act of 1973 (Public Law 93–112), 29 U.S.C. § 794.

Schön, D. (1983). *The reflective practitioner.* New York: Basic.

Schwartz, K. (1992). Occupational therapy and education: A shared vision. *American Journal of Occupational Therapy, 46,* 12–18.

Shapiro, J. (1993). *No pity.* New York: Times.

Shelton, T., & Stepanek, J. (1994). *Family-centered care for children needing specialized health and developmental services.* Bethesda, MD: Association for the Care of Children's Health.

Technology-Related Assistance for individuals With Disabilities Act (Public Law 100–407) (1988).

Winnicott, D. (1965). *The maturational processes and the facilitating environment.* New York: International Universities Press.

Yankelovitch, D. (1981). *New rules.* New York: Random House.

Yerxa, E. (1966). Eleanor Clarke Slagle Lecture—Authentic occupational therapy. *American Journal of Occupational Therapy, 21,* 1–9.

Yerxa, E. (1992). Some implications of occupational therapy's history for its epistemology, values, and relation to medicine. *American Journal of Occupational Therapy, 46,* 79–83.

Yerxa, E. (1994). Dreams, dilemmas, and decisions for occupational therapy practice in a new millennium: An American perspective. *American Journal of Occupational Therapy, 48,* 586–589. Reprinted as Chapter 57.

Occupational Deprivation: Global Challenge in the New Millennium

CHAPTER 31

GAIL WHITEFORD, BAppSc, MHSc, PHD

Occupational deprivation is, in essence, a state in which a person or group of people is unable to do what is necessary and meaningful in their lives due to external restrictions. It is a state in which the opportunity to perform those occupations that have social, cultural, and personal relevance is rendered difficult if not impossible. It is a reality for numerous people living around the globe today.

To highlight that occupational deprivation is a real and pressing phenomenon affecting the lives of many individuals, consider the situation of Trkulja Ljubica. She is a refugee living in Belgrade and reflects here on her former life:

> I remember my violets that remained blooming in the window of my kitchen. And all the flowers too. My violets flourished in various colors: blue, pink, white. I watched them there, one next to the other as if in conversation, not knowing that I would go from there and that my hand would not nourish them any more. Oh God, where is the end of this hell, when will I have violets and other flowers in my flat again? I always think how my violets dried up and died, dropping their gorgeous flowers. (Ljubica, 1996, p. 6)

Ljubica's story is part of a compelling collection of narrative accounts of the experience of refugeeism. This is the experience of being forcibly removed from home, family, and community, of being disenfranchised and of being unable to engage in the everyday occupations of life such as growing violets. In other words, it is preclusion from those everyday occupations that bring meaning and coherence to existence.

This is an experience that is difficult for many of us to imagine as we orchestrate the numerous occupations that compete for time on a daily basis. Most of us have the freedom and opportunity to make choices about what we will, or will not, do today based on personal preference and individual or social need. The lives of Bosnian women like Ljubica, as well as the numerous refugees around the world in Rwanda, Kosovo and, more recently, East Timor, stand in sharp contrast. Their lives speak of trauma, upheaval, dislocation, and occupational deprivation. While their situation is extreme, they are, however, not alone. Globally, groups of people that (arguably) include ethnic, cultural, and religious minority groups; prisoners; chronically unemployed people; political prisoners; child laborers; and women exist in the context of restricted occupational choice and diminished occupational opportunities.

In this article, definitions of occupational deprivation are presented and explored alongside the related phenomena of occupational disruption and dysfunction. Populations susceptible to the experience of occupational deprivation are identified, as are the impacts of occupational deprivation and the

This chapter was previously published in the *British Journal of Occupational Therapy, 63*(5), 200–204. © Copyright 2000, British Association of Occupational Therapists, College of Occupational Therapists. Reprinted with permission.

social, political, and economic contexts in which it occurs. Narrative accounts from individuals are included to highlight their realities. In conclusion, some ideas as to how occupational therapists can address occupational deprivation as part of their orientation toward social and occupational justice are posited for consideration.

Defining and Clarifying: What Is Occupational Deprivation?

Wilcock (1998) originally defined *occupational deprivation* as being characterized by "the influence of an external circumstance that keeps a person from acquiring, using, or enjoying something" (p. 145). Based on this original definition of Wilcock and on focused inquiry into the phenomenon, the author's definition of occupational deprivation is:

> A state of preclusion from engagement in occupations of necessity and/or meaning due to factors that stand outside the immediate control of the individual.

The intention of the latter is to highlight the occupational and meaning dimensions within the definition so as to bring to the foreground their importance and relevance both to occupational therapy (Christiansen et al. 1999) and to occupational science (Zemke and Clark, 1996).

The important concept tacit to both these definitions, however, is that occupational deprivation as a term implies that *someone or something external to the individual is doing the depriving.* This concept is of central importance in understanding occupational deprivation. The state of deprivation arises not as a result of limitations inherent within the individual, but due to forces outside his or her control. The forces and conditions that may cause such deprivation are complex and are discussed more fully below.

Occupational Disruption

There are two other occupational terms that, while sounding similar, describe quite different phenomena. These are occupational disruption and occupational dysfunction. Occupational disruption is a state that is usually temporary or transient rather than prolonged. Occupational disruption occurs when a person's normal pattern of occupational engagement is disrupted due to significant life events (such as having a baby), environmental changes (such as moving house or location), becoming ill, or sustaining an injury from which full recovery is expected. The most important thing to remember about occupational disruption is that it is a *temporary state and one that, given supportive conditions, resolves itself.* Occupational deprivation differs in that it usually occurs over time and in a context in which there is an absence of supporting conditions. More often, the forces that create a state of occupational deprivation, such as civil conflict leading to refugeeism or the economic constraints necessitating a redundancy, are experienced as hostile.

Occupational Dysfunction

Occupational dysfunction differs from occupational disruption in several key respects. Rather than conceptualizing it as a discrete phenomenon, it can be viewed more usefully either as a byproduct of nonresolved occupational disruption, as a result of specific occupational performance deficits, or as arising from a prolonged state of occupational deprivation. It is a phenomenon that is "nested in a complex of factors all of which reflect and contribute to sustaining the performance, patterns of behavior, identities, choices and so on, that reflect a life in trouble" (Kielhofner, 1995, p. 156). Occupational dysfunction arising from a state of occupational deprivation may be characterized by atrophy of some of the innate human capacities for occupation (Wilcock, 1993). (See Chapter 33.)

Understanding and Identifying Occupational Deprivation

As may be evident, occupational deprivation is a relatively new term for a phenomenon that has arguably existed in human society for some time. The histories of human societies are characterized by groups of people subordinating others to themselves and depriving them of liberty (Toch, 1977) and, hence, occupational freedom. In today's world, occupational deprivation still results from such direct social and cultural exclusions, but may also exist as a byproduct of institutional policies, technological advancements, economic models, and political systems (Wilcock, 1998).

The Impact of Technology

If the impact of technology in particular is considered, it is evident that whole communities of people previously involved in both primary and manufacturing industries have been disenfranchised by mass unemployment due to new technologies in the workplace. As Tomlinson (1999) pointed out, technology never solves problems or creates better societies; rather, it serves to highlight social inequalities and political conflicts. That this is very much the case with the growing numbers of technology-driven redundancies is evident in the "ghosting" of the blue-collar worker (Toulmin, 1995). In an excellent analysis of the complex technological, economic, and market-driven forces that have an impact on unemployment, Jones (1998) suggested that the twin phenomena of high levels of unemployment and high levels of participation occur because:

> ...males who were traditionally in work are now out of it and females who were traditionally out are now in. This phenomenon illustrates the development of a dual labor market and is broadly characteristic of most OECD countries. However, this is of no consolation to the unemployed, especially unskilled and semiskilled workers. (p. 129)

Maldistributed Labor

As indicated, economic conditions coupled with the new fiscal rationalism in many Western countries seem to be shaping occupational trends of concern. Of note is the paradoxical rise of chronic unemployment alongside overemployment; in other words, fewer people are doing more while lots of people are doing less. Bittman and Rice (1999) cited the Geneva-based International Labour Organization (ILO) which suggested that the new flexibility demanded of modern employees about when and for how long they worked resulted in a maldistribution of working hours. Such a maldistribution, they argued, generated still more unemployment as well as increasingly precarious employment, and had "the overall impact of reducing the bargaining capacity of organized labor" (p. 1).

Such an increasing trend toward maldistributed labor reflects an increasing polarization of working hours, creating a scenario of two distinct groups in society: those with too much to do and those with too little. Those in the latter category, that is, those deprived of opportunities to engage in the occupation of paid employment, have the time in which potentially to engage in other occupational pursuits but have little available financial resources with which to do so. This is problematic in a modern context because, as Lobo (1999) suggested, leisure has become commodified to the extent that it requires significant discretionary income. Increasingly, as he pointed out, you need money to be a leisure participant in Western society. This situation, that is, one in which people are already marginalized through lack of paid employment, lack of discretionary income and, subsequently, diminished opportunities to engage in leisure occupations, can over time evolve into a scenario of occupational deprivation.

Marginalization

Besides unemployed people, underemployed people and those living in poverty, Wilcock (1998) included prisoners of war, prison inmates, minority groups (particularly indigenous peoples), and women in her list of people who are most vulnerable to occupational deprivation. This list reflects a collection of those individuals and groups who have traditionally had little or no legitimate "voice" in mainstream society. Voice and representation reflect levels of participation in mainstream forms of cultural production (Giroux, 1996). If you are occupationally deprived, such legitimate participation is difficult if not impossible. When this is the case, engagement in nonlegitimated occupations, such as vandalism and participation in occupational groups like gangs (Snyder et al. 1998), may become a seemingly attractive alternative.

Certainly, from an occupational perspective, such participation represents an understandable response. However, while there exist some perceived individual benefits in terms of identity construction and structured time use,

engagement in such occupations is also potentially dangerous. Involvement has the potential for serious and negative consequences that represent a "downward spiraling trend" (Snyder et al. 1998, p. 134) at both personal and social levels. Antisocial activity, gang participation, and marginal group identity are modern and largely urban phenomena and certainly beyond the scope of full exploration in this article. However, if framed as essentially occupational phenomena, that is, as byproducts of sustained, socially constructed occupational deprivation, they warrant further inquiry as a matter of some urgency.

The Experience of Refugeeism

Refugees, as suggested above, are another group within society that are potentially at risk of becoming occupationally deprived. The experience of refugeeism is profound and life changing, leading to potentially serious and pervasive problems (Faderman, 1998). While the temporary accommodation (which in some instances becomes long term) of refugee camps may be experienced as a holding space affording few normative occupational opportunities, the country of resettlement can prove as hostile to full occupational participation. To highlight this point, it is worth considering a case illustration. Boua Xa Moua (1998) is an Hmong refugee who resettled in the USA. His story is compelling in that his dream of a new life in relative security sours as he finds himself isolated and occupationally restricted. He feels robbed of his previous legitimated social roles and describes his sense of being unable to "do" in the confusing and restricting world of contemporary urban USA:

> Life in America is very tough ... I can't do anything, I would rather go back if I had the choice. I have been here so long but I have not learned how to speak English or how to read and write ... whenever you want to go anywhere, all the time, you have to wait for someone. I mean if they don't come you can't go where you want because you don't know how to go ... Like I said, if I would have a choice, I would have remained in Laos, or if I could. I would like to go back now. It's much nicer and peaceful back home. Here everything feels too lonely. Everything is too much. I always find myself lost in this world. (Boua Xa Moua, 1998, p. 101)

This account suggests that resettlement in another country does not necessarily predicate a successful outcome for refugees. Societal structures, economic and language barriers, as well as cultural and religious differences, can prevent community integration and occupational participation (Wilcock, 1998). Even when financial status is secure through employment, the deprivation from occupations of meaning can have a devastating and long-term impact. As Boua Xa Moua (1998) reflected, there is little left but to wish for the place in which a meaningful occupational identity existed: home.

The Human Costs of Occupational Deprivation

A decade ago, Yerxa (1989) stated that "Occupation is not just something nice to do, rather, it is wired into the human" and that "Individuals are most true to their humanity when engaged in occupation" (p. 7). What happens, then, when people are deprived of this apparently innate feature of existence, of something so central to our humanity, as Yerxa put it? What are the consequences, both personal and social, of occupational deprivation?

There are few answers in the literature because, currently, there is a lack of existing research dealing with the negative consequences of occupational deprivation. This, in turn, is due to the fact that occupational deprivation (like numerous emergent occupational concepts) has been relatively recently framed as such within the occupational therapy profession. In order best to understand it, as well as other occupational phenomena and their respective relationships to health and well-being, focused inquiry using a range of methodological strategies is required in the near future (Law et al., 1998). In the absence of an in-depth research base to draw upon, the following reflections on the impacts of occupational deprivation are based upon the author's experience of undertaking an occupational needs assessment of a special assessment unit in a high-security prison (Whiteford, 1995, 1997).

Lack of Meaningful Time Use

One of the most problematic dimensions associated with the direct experience of occupational deprivation is time use. Consistent with the study by Christiansen et al. (1999) pointing to the positive relationship between time spent engaging in meaningful occupation and perceived well-being, lack of time spent engaged in meaningful occupations in the prison setting appeared detrimental to health and well-being. The dynamic relationship among time use, sense of efficacy, and identity seemed, in the penal context, to be compromised by prolonged occupational deprivation.

Evidence of this came from the inmates' narratives. Many of those interviewed had experienced repeated psychotic breakdowns due to gross disturbances in orientation: they were unable to "locate" themselves in time. With few occupations (except eating) to provide structure and punctuate the day, and with little variation in time-use patterns between days of the week and months of the year, they reported feeling "adrift" in an undifferentiated sea of time. Many comments reflected a sense of hopelessness born of a deteriorating sense of efficacy because, where there is little or no perceived control over occupational choices, "there is no sense of efficacy" (Kielhofner, 1995, p. 45).

The prisoners' descriptions reflected these themes and varied from "Time is long and it passes slowly" to "The days go fast but time is slow" and "Time is nothingness." Additionally, they commented that increased occupational opportunities

had the potential to "Keep my mind occupied and diverted from thoughts that make me crazy," "Give me an opportunity to bring a picture of something I have in my head to life," "Give me a chance to change my behavior," and "To let out anger and frustration" (Whiteford, 1997, p. 129).

Maladaptive Responses

Not surprisingly, sleep was reported by the inmates as a predominant response to their occupationally deprived state. Sleep, however, was not the only maladaptive response; the prison unit also had a high rate of suicide and suicide attempts. While acknowledging the multiplicity of factors that may have contributed to it, this disturbing feature of life in the unit was discerned by the author to be, at least in part, due to pervasive occupational deprivation. Clearly, this is an area requiring further investigation.

Barrier to Community Reintegration

The major concern with respect to these inmates is that, for them, the experience of occupational deprivation appeared to be a significant barrier to successful community reintegration. They had, to varying degrees, adapted to the occupationally barren environment, reflected in the inmate comment "I've spent most of my life in institutions so the bars don't bother me" (Whiteford, 1997). With severely restricted occupational role repertoires and diminished capacities for structuring and using time effectively, the inmates faced the challenge of living successful occupational lives in the communities to which they would ultimately return. Prolonged occupational deprivation very probably diminishes the likelihood of adaptive responses to new environments, a scenario that could be remediated through the conscious creation of "occupationally enriched" (Molineux & Whiteford, 1999) prison environments.

Wider Impact of Occupational Deprivation

While these observations have been drawn from interactions with a population of occupationally deprived prisoners, it can be argued that diminished opportunities to engage in occupations of meaning for any individual or group of people may potentially have similar results. After all, what we do in life is inextricable from the meaning we ascribe to it (Hasselkus, 1997). Atrophied occupational capacities (Wilcock, 1995), diminished self-efficacy beliefs, and truncated identity constructions may all be byproducts of this dehumanizing phenomenon. Understanding just what impact this has on individuals, families, communities, and societies is a central challenge in the new millennium and worthy of immediate attention.

Future Challenges

The cogent question, then, is how should occupational therapists address occupational deprivation? There are three dimensions to how this can be done.

Adopting an Occupational Perspective

First, it requires occupational therapists to make a conceptual shift to an occupational perspective: to view the world through occupational eyes, seeing phenomena that have previously been viewed from other perspectives (for example, medical, psychological, and social) as essentially occupational phenomena (Townsend, 1999). An occupational perspective is a requisite to considering the occupational needs of people as individuals and within society separately from consideration of how these can be met through the provision of therapeutic interventions. Such a perspective will serve to centralize the role of occupational therapists in being the key agents in the future to address challenging occupational phenomena. Although it has been suggested that there is a "renaissance" of occupation in occupational therapy (Whiteford et al., 2000), it still seems that a gap exists as to how occupation is incorporated into practice. This is an issue when, as Wood (1998) suggested, other professional groups are embracing occupation as pivotal to their interventions.

Acting at a Broader Social and Cultural Level

Second, occupational therapists need to think and act at a broader social and cultural level. Armed with an occupational perspective of society, there is a need to invest more energy into influencing social and institutional structures and policies, which preclude people from full occupational participation. In doing this, the profession comes closer to realizing occupational therapy's social vision (Townsend, 1993).

Embracing Occupational Justice

Third, occupational therapists need to embrace the concept of "occupational justice": to mobilize resources with the aim of creating occupationally "just" societies, societies based on people and their need, and indeed right, to do. Occupational justice is concerned with "economic, political and social force that create equitable opportunity and the means to choose, organize and perform occupations that people find useful or meaningful in their environment" (Townsend, 1999, p. 154). Dignity, as created through the opportunity to interact with the world in a meaningful way through living diverse occupational lives, not just those focused on material gain (Fromm, 1998), will be a central feature of an occupationally just future. Embracing the principles of equity, justice, diversity, and ecological sustainability will be central to the process of achieving this. In the excellent critique of a range of health promotion models presented by Wilcock (1998), that of "social justice" appears to provide the best blueprint for action in addressing occupational deprivation. The model is described as promoting:

> ... social and economic change to increase individual, community and political awareness, resources and equitable opportunities for health ... participatory analysis of occupational disadvantage, underlying occupational determinants, and uncovering occupational injustice ... social

action for change of occupational policies toward occupational equity and justice [including] social and political lobbying. (p. 230)

Such action and activism represent a big, but necessary, brief for occupational therapy in the years ahead: the face of the new millennium is, to a greater or lesser extent, up to occupational therapists. This is because, as futurist Dator (paper given at the International Futures Conference, Auckland, 1992) suggested some time ago, we won't get the future we necessarily want, but we will get the future we deserve. It is a challenging prospect.

Summary

This article has explored occupational deprivation as a potentially challenging phenomenon in the new millennium. It has considered some definitions of the term and their origins and has explored some related occupational phenomena. The article has considered briefly the conditions that contribute to occupational deprivation and the individuals and groups most vulnerable to it. A consideration of the human and social cost of occupational deprivation preceded a call to arms for occupational therapists to address, through social and political action, this challenging problem now and in the future.

References

Bittman M, Rice J (1999) Are working hours becoming more unsociable? *Australian Social Policy Research Center Newsletter, 74*, 1–5.

Boua Xa Moua (1998) Boua Xa Moua's story. In: L Faderman, ed. *I begin my life all over: the Hmong and the American immigrant experience.* Boston: Beacon Press.

Christiansen C, Backman C, Little B, Nguyen A (1999) Occupations and well-being: a study of personal projects. *American Journal of Occupational Therapy, 53*(1), 91–99.

Faderman L (1998) *I begin my life all over the Hmong and the American immigrant experience.* Boston: Beacon Press.

Fromm E (1998) *Between having and being.* New York: Continuum.

Giroux H (1996) *Living dangerously: multiculturalism and the politics of difference.* New York: Peter Lang.

Hasselkus B (1997) Meaning and occupation. In: C Christiansen, C Baum, eds. *Occupational therapy: enabling function and wellbeing.* Thorofare, NJ: Slack, 362–77.

Jones B (1998) Redefining work: setting directions for the future. *Journal of Occupational Science, 5*(3), 127–32.

Kielhofner G (1995) *A model of human occupation.* 2nd ed. Baltimore: Williams & Wilkins.

Law M, Steinwender S, Leclair L (1998) Occupation, health, and well-being. *Canadian Journal of Occupational Therapy, 65*(2), 81–91.

Lobo F (1999) The leisure and work of young people: a review. *Journal of Occupational Science, 6*(3), 27–33.

Ljubica T (1996) Violets. In: R Zarkovic, ed., *I remember: writings of Bosnian women.* San Francisco: Aunt Lute Books.

Moiineux M, Whiteford G (1999) Prisons: from occupational deprivation to occupational enrichment. *Journal of Occupational Science, 6*(3), 124–39.

Snyder C, Clark F, Masunaka-Noriega M, Young B (1998) Los Angeles street kids: new occupations for life programme. *Journal of Occupational Science, 5*(3), 133–39.

Toch H (1997) *Living in prison: the ecology of survival.* New York: MacMiilan.

Tomlinson J (1999) *Globalization and culture.* Cambridge: Polity.

Townsend E (1993) Occupational therapy's social vision. *Canadian Journal of Occupational Therapy, 60*(4), 167–83.

Townsend E (1999) Enabling occupation in the 21st century: making good intentions a reality. *Australian Occupational Therapy Journal, 46*(4), 147–59.

Toulmin S (1995) Occupation, employment, and human welfare. *Journal of Occupational Science: Australia, 2*(2), 48–58.

Whiteford G (1995)A concrete void: occupational deprivation and the special needs inmate, *Journal of Occupational Science: Australia, 2*(2), 80–81.

Whiteford G (1997) Occupational deprivation and incarceration. *Journal of Occupational Science: Australia, 4*(3), 126–30.

Whiteford G, Townsend E, Hocking C (2000) Reflections on a renaissance of occupation. *Canadian Journal of Occupational Therapy, 67*(1), 61–69.

Wilcock A (1993) A theory of the human need for occupation. *Journal of Occupational Science: Australia, 1*(1) 17–24. Reprinted as Chapter 33.

Wilcock A (1995) The occupational brain: a theory of human nature. *Journal of Occupational Science: Australia, 2*(2), 68–73.

Wilcock A (1998) *An occupational perspective of health.* Thorofare, NJ: Slack.

Wood W (1998) It is jump time for occupational therapy. *American Journal of Occupational Therapy, 52*(6) 403–11.

Yerxa E (1989) An introduction to occupational science: a foundation for occupational therapy in the 21st century. In: J Johnson, E Yerxa, eds. *Occupational science: the foundations for new models of practice.* New York: Haworth.

Zemke R, Clark F (1996) *Occupational science: the evolving discipline.* Philadelphia: FA Davis.

Occupational Justice and Client-Centered Practice: A Dialogue in Progress

CHAPTER 32

ELIZABETH TOWNSEND, FCAOT

ANN A. WILCOCK, PHD, REGOT(SA)

This paper reports our ongoing, international dialogue about the relationship among occupation, justice, and client-centered practice. We will discuss two foundations informing the dialogue, four exploratory cases of occupational injustice, implications for occupational therapy's client-centered practice, and concluding reflections. The question that frames our discussion is how do occupational therapists work for justice? Dialogue on this question seems timely as occupational therapists around the world articulate what distinguishes this numerically small, rather invisible profession and its contributions to individuals, populations, and societies.

Foundations of the Dialogue

When we first met in 1997 in South Australia, we discovered a strong synergy of ideas about justice, occupation, and the convergence of those interests in what we began to describe as occupational justice. In sharing our visions of an occupationally just world, we are raising questions about how individuals and populations could flourish as equal citizens in daily lives comprised of health-building occupations (Townsend & Wilcock, 2004; Wilcock & Townsend, 2000).

Occupational therapists already understand that participation in occupations is the means or medium of occupational therapy, and ideally is also the ends or outcomes (Gray, 1998 [see Chapter 15]; Rebeiro, 1998). History tells us that visions are what propel people to reach beyond what is. John Locke's (Locke, 1690) Essay Concerning Humane Understanding and Southwood Smith's social reforms in the British Industrial Era (Guy, 1996) remind us of the power inherent in articulating and critiquing beliefs, principles, and reasoning. With awareness of the power of visions to spur action, we are pursuing a dialogue about what could be possible if societies utilize participation in the daily life occupations of a community, including but not limited to work, as both a means and a benchmark to advance occupational justice for individuals and populations.

With World War II as an early life marker, we both grew up in white, middle-class families of British culture. Wilcock moved as an occupational therapist from Britain to Australia to see the world and challenge her ideas in urban and rural communities. With her British cultural background, Townsend left Toronto to see the world and challenge her ideas by working in East Africa then in Prairie, Ontario, and Atlantic communities in rural and urban Canada. On the one hand, we express Western concerns for individual meaning, fulfillment, choice, identity, and autonomy, as well as for citizen participation, empowerment, and civil society. On the other hand, we recognize that daily life, including occupational therapy as a profession, is embedded in a complex environment of power relations. We value cultural differences and Eastern concerns for belonging in community, understanding that communities shape individuals and groups while individuals and groups shape their communities. While optimistically seeking to understand how occupation produces health, well-being, and justice, our critiques attempt to identify forces that produce alienation, deprivation, marginalization, and imbalance. Over the 5 years since 1997, we have been exploring justice from

Table 32.1. Two Foundations to Explore Occupational Justice

Knowledge Foundations	Concerns for Justice	Example of Occupational Injustice
1. Occupation Humans are occupational beings. Their existence depends on enablement of diverse opportunities and resources for participation in culturally defined and health-building occupations (Wilcock, 1993, 1998).	Denial of universal access to opportunities and/or resources to participate in culturally defined, health-building occupations is unjust.	Occupational alienation Occupational deprivation Occupational imbalance
2. Client-centered practice Enabling of social inclusion is a justice-oriented, client-centered practice to create diverse opportunities and resources for people to participate in culturally defined, health-building occupations (Townsend, 1993, 1998).	Lack of enabling, client-centered practices restricts the opportunities and/or resources required for diverse people to participate in the occupations of a society.	Occupational deprivation Occupational marginalization Occupational imbalance

the perspective of two complementary knowledge foundations: occupation and client-centered practice (see Table 32.1).

Wilcock's research, using a history of ideas methodology (Wilcock, 1998, 2001), has generated historical, analytic knowledge about humans as occupational beings and an occupational perspective of health. She found that people in each historical era have implicitly or explicitly employed occupation as the mechanism to survive and promote health and well-being. Underlying occupational determinants, such as the type of economy, social structure, and belief system, shape health. Wilcock reasoned that because occupations are central to human existence, injustices occur when, for example, populations experience occupational alienation or deprivation.

Townsend's research, using an institutional ethnography methodology (Townsend, 1998; Townsend, Ripley, & Langille, 2003), has generated social, analytic knowledge about occupational therapy's social vision of client-centered approaches for enabling empowerment through occupations. She found that occupational therapists may enable some people to flourish, but professional dominance, standardized treatment and documentation, market-driven economies, insurance, laws, and political conditions can overrule our good intentions. Townsend reasoned that injustices occur when client-centred, empowerment approaches are overruled to the extent that populations are occupationally underdeveloped or marginalized.

Language of the Dialogue

Occupational therapy is not alone in its interest in justice, nor even in occupation. Many research and practice fields have an interest in everyday life, participation, occupation, and justice, expressed in diverse ways, examples being found in adult education, community development, community psychology, law, and social work. There are many theories about how social, political, legal, and economic practices determine possibilities and limits for promoting justice and civil society. Survivors of potentially disabling conditions, such as Galipeault, Gidden, Little, Moore, and Sherr Klein (Townsend, 2003a) all highlight their fundamental need to participate in various occupations as empowered citizens.

What, then, distinguishes this profession and its contributions to individuals, populations, and societies? We perceive that occupational therapists' best practices offer a unique synthesis and application of knowledge, skills, and attitudes about three interconnected pillars of knowledge: occupation, enabling, and justice. To distinguish occupational therapists' interests in justice, we use the language of *occupation* to describe participation in various aspects of daily life. We use the language of enabling to describe therapy that uses participatory, empowerment-oriented approaches, what occupational therapists have named client-centered practice. And we use the language of justice to talk about determinants and forms of occupational well-being and social inclusion that take differences in people and contexts into account.

Use of the term occupation to encompass all participation in daily life is as problematic in English as it is in other languages. Popular, research, and government references to occupation in English focus narrowly on work (Jarman, 2003), or aggressively on the military occupation of territory. As occupational scientists and therapists, we make strategic, political use of the term occupation to bring issues of participation in daily life to visible, public attention. We ally ourselves with those who use the term "enabling" to encompass culturally variable processes that invite active client participation in the decision-making and priorities of therapy as well as in daily life occupations—despite the tensions of going against the grain in hierarchically organized systems (Byrne, 1999; Deegan, 1997; Polatajko, 2001; Townsend et al., 2003). Whereas concerns for social justice have raised issues about equality, we want to bring to public awareness the injustices that persist when participation in occupations is barred, confined, restricted, segregated, prohibited, undeveloped, disrupted, alienated, marginalized, exploited, excluded, or otherwise restricted.

It seems that societies tolerate an occupational apartheid (Kronenberg & Simo Algado, 2003). Occupational apartheid may describe situations where occupations are classified, paid, valued, and enhance life for some, while in the same places and times occupations are taken for granted, exploited,

Table 32.2. Word Associations: Occupation, Justice, and Occupational Justice[1]

Occupation	Justice	Occupational Justice
• Doing	• Equality	• Enablement of fairness and equal opportunity (possibly with different resources)
• Action	• Fairness	
• Being	• Opportunity	• No discrimination based on ability, age, or other factors
• Everyday life	• Resources	
• Work	• Shared power	• Social commitment to universal design and accessibility
• Leisure	• Empowerment for all	
• Parenting	• Rights	• Enabling everyone to flourish to their greatest potential individually or as members of communities
• Performance	• Responsibilities	
• Participation	• Social network	
• Meaningful doing	• Politics	
• Engagement	• Regulations	
• Meditation	• Doing the right thing	
• More than activity	• Ethics	
• Not a technique/task	• Moral principles	
• Vocation	• Civil society	
• Census classification	• Citizen participation	

[1] Words and phrases from workshop discussions between 1999 and 2002.

and trivialized for others (Townsend, 2003b). It seems that occupational therapists innately know that everyday injustices are right in front of our eyes (H. Fujimoto, personal communication, July 2003). We assert that justice is an implicit, invisible foundation of occupational therapy's occupation-focused, client-centered practice (Townsend, 1993; Wilcock, 1993).

Methods

To draw others into our dialogue on occupational justice, our starting point was to review the literature and to organize workshops. We wanted to generate open discussion and critique, without confining participants to questions on a survey or other impersonal research tool.

Occupational Justice Workshops

Workshops and presentations on occupational justice in Australia, Britain, Canada, Portugal, Sweden, and the United States were the first initiatives to draw others into the dialogue. Participants to date have been occupational scientists and therapists, plus a few from sociology, urban and rural planning, social work, and nursing. Their words and phrases illustrate a range of responses to the questions What is occupation? What is justice? and What is occupational justice? (see Table 32.2) Typical comments to date have been:

- This concept feels like a good fit with occupational therapy.
- What is the difference from social justice? Do we need another concept?
- Occupational justice is interesting, but I can't see what I can do about it in my practice.
- There's already too much emphasis on theory [in occupational therapy] and new graduates have less and less skill to actually practice.

- Until the concepts are clearer, there is nothing new in this idea of occupational justice.
- I want to know more about this concept—it makes sense to my practice [as an occupational therapist].
- At last there is a name for something I have felt was behind my occupational therapy practice.

Literature Review

We will highlight references that we find particularly helpful in supporting or challenging our thinking on occupational justice. To understand the breadth of occupation and the relationships among occupation, health, and justice, we honor the contributions of Americans Mary Reilly (1962) (see Chapter 8) and Elizabeth Yerxa (1967, 1979, 1993) in particular who reminded us that occupation is our domain of interest as occupational therapists. Contemporary authors include Karen Rebeiro (2001) in Canada who is drawing in the voices of mental health consumers' experiences of marginalized participation in occupations. Borell and colleagues (2001) in Sweden are building a body of research that illuminates how older adults experience their occupations, becoming diminished in scope and highly controlled by caregivers. Forces that support and limit the occupational development of children with disabilities have been identified in Sweden and the United States (Hemmingsson & Borell, 2002; Royeen, Duncan, Crabree, Richards, & Clark, 2000).

In looking beyond individual experiences of occupation, from his professional and academic perspective that bridges Western (Canadian) and Eastern (Japanese) epistemologies, Iwama (1999, 2003) has asked if we are listening to understand the cultural context of occupations. Fujimoto (H. Fujimoto, personal communication, July 2003) echoes this call to cultural relevance in her formulation of occupational justice for children who are ventilator-dependent. Whiteford (2000) (see Chapter 31) contributes a global, structural perspective on contexts that produce occupational deprivation as a form of injustice, using examples that range from refugee and aboriginal contexts, to the occupational contexts of prisoners, women, and those who are geographically isolated in the Australian outback.

Outside more than inside occupational therapy, the concept of enabling has been repeatedly emphasized. Dunst and his colleagues (Dunst, Trivette, & Deal, 1988) in social work and Noyes (2000) in nursing have described enabling as a participatory, empowerment-oriented process. Enabling is also a policy and legal concept used to describe how regulations undermine or enable social inclusion in community health, building, design, and legislation (Rosenau, 1994). In the Ottawa Charter for Health Promotion, the World Health Organization (1986) recommended enabling, advocating, and mediating as three necessary approaches for promoting health for all. McKnight (1989) articulated links among enabling, empowerment, and health. Labonte (1989) affirmed that enabling the empowerment of poor people in inner cities promotes health when they form new action communities, for instance to grow their own food.

The broad view of occupation that occupational scientists and therapists use expresses a critical, social perspective on occupations. We have drawn insights on occupations, enabling, and justice particularly from Elizabeth Casson, a physician and founder of occupational therapy in Britain (Wilcock, 2002), from Adolf Meyer (1922) (see Chapter 2), a psychiatrist who contributed to the founding of occupational therapy in the United States, and from Goldwin Howland (Howland, 1944), a Canadian physician whose vision advanced occupational therapy in this country following World War I. Dorothy Smith's (1987, 1990a, 1990b) sociology for women has been helpful in theorizing and tracing the interconnectedness of governance, from policies to media images, embedded in the everyday world. She described how power relations are formed and perpetuated invisibly and often unconsciously through a multiplicity of work processes, similar to our broad view of occupations.

To develop an understanding of justice, we have been guided by both general writings, as well as research on particular instances of injustice. Justice is an ethical, moral, and civic concept (Adelson, 1995; Bores, 2000; Rawls, 1975; Young, 1990) which is applied in various ways to particular circumstances. Underlying Western conceptions of justice may be beliefs about individual autonomy, or what constitutes scientific knowledge (Heitman, 2000). For instance, the notion of individual rights is based on the Enlightenment view of individual agency and moral capacity (Ignatieff, 2000). Whereas Irani (1995), Grammenos (2003), and Zanetti (2001) have emphasized that justice may be viewed outside Western thinking not as a matter of equal distribution of rights or goods, but as matters of trust and loyalty versus exploitation and betrayal. Because justice is culturally bound, ideas, beliefs, principles, and reasoning about civic governance and state regulation tend to establish justice within particular social and institutional frameworks (Armstrong, 2000; McKay, 2000; Metz, 2000).

In specific jurisdictions, such as correctional services, the North American concept of restorative justice has developed to consider debates about the long-term impact on crime rates of rehabilitation or punishment approaches with prisoners (Pogge, 2000). From a consumer perspective, justice related to mental illness is construed as a matter of empowerment (Deegan, 1997). In North American health services, the concept of distributive justice has been used to assess the equality of distribution of particular medical services across various populations (Cookson & Dolan, 2000; Daniels, Kennedy, & Kawachi, 1999; Emanuel, 2000). Principles of justice have been used to guide rationing and spending cuts in health services (Cookson & Dolan, 2000). These views of justice present health as a commodity that can be modified by rationing and distribution.

Two influential sources in developing our occupational perspective of justice have been Iris Morton Young (1990) and Vicki Schultz (2000), researchers in American law. Young challenges the distributive paradigm of justice based on

Table 32.3. An Exploratory Theory of Occupational Justice[2]

Ideas about occupational justice	Reasoning about occupational determinants, forms, and outcomes
• People are occupational as well as social beings • Humans' occupational needs differ with each person • Differing forms of enablement address a variety of occupational needs, strengths, and potentials	• Occupational experiences and environments are determined by economic, policy, cultural, and other determinants • Media, parenting, education, and employment are examples of occupations that shape and are shaped by other occupations • Potential outcomes of occupational injustice are, for example, occupational alienation or occupational marginalization

Beliefs and principles about occupational justice	Occupational justice versus social justice
• Humans participate in occupations as autonomous yet interdependent agents in their societal context • Health depends on participation in health-building occupations • Empowerment depends on enabling choice and control in occupational participation	Emphasis in occupational justice on: • Participation in all daily occupations • Differences in occupational participation • Enablement of differences in occupational participation

[2]Townsend & Wilcock, 2003.

sameness and individual rights by proposing that "issues of decision-making power and procedures, division of labor, and culture" (p. 15) require a paradigm based on enablement of opportunities that respond to differences across social groups. Only in examining power as a social relation rather than as a commodity for distribution, Young argues, can we understand how taken for granted injustices persist—injustices that oppress everyday life for women, persons with disabilities, persons of color, and immigrants. Writing in the Columbia Law Review, Schultz provides a feminist critique of work that has applicability for other populations who are denied fair opportunities or rewards for their work. She envisions a "social order in which work is consistent with egalitarian conceptions of citizenship and care" (p. 1886). To her, work can be structured negatively or positively: "if people's lives can be constrained in negative ways by their conception of their occupational roles, they can also be reshaped along more empowering lines by changing work or the way it is structured or understood" (p. 1891).

Exploratory Theory of Occupational Justice

A brief overview of an exploratory theory of occupational justice (Townsend & Wilcock, 2003) summarizes our own beliefs, principles, ideas, and reasoning to date, as highlighted in Table 32.3. We believe that people are occupational as well as social beings. We recognize that, individually or as members of particular communities, we have differing occupational needs, strengths, and potential which require differing forms of enablement to flourish. With an acknowledged Western view of individual autonomy exerted within an environment or context, we support the principle that occupations are the practical means through which humans exert citizen empowerment, choice, and control. It seems that various forms of participation—doing, being, or becoming through occupations—are essential in promoting health, well-being, and social inclusion in various cultural, economic, institutional, social, and political contexts. Occupational determinants, forms, and outcomes, such as unemployment and poverty, create or limit possibilities for occupational justice. Occupational justice appears to complement and extend understandings of social justice. An occupational perspective, we believe, sparks new perspectives and insights on injustices particularly related to participation in occupations.

Cases of Occupational Injustice

We propose four cases (see Table 32.4) which emerged when we discussed occupational justice together and with workshop participants. The four cases imply the possibility of extending concepts of social justice by defining occupational rights:
- To experience occupation as meaningful and enriching;
- To develop through participation in occupations for health and social inclusion;
- To exert individual or population autonomy through choice in occupations;

Table 32.4. Proposed Occupational Rights

Right to experience occupation as meaningful and enriching
Occupational injustice: occupational alienation

Right to develop through participation in occupations for health and social inclusion
Occupational injustice: occupational deprivation

Right to exert individual or population autonomy through choice in occupations
Occupational injustice: occupational marginalization

Right to benefit from fair privileges for diverse participation in occupations
Occupational injustice: occupational imbalance

*Injustices noted are examples only. They are not categorically limited consequences of restricted rights.

- To benefit from fair privileges for diverse participation in occupations socially excluded from full citizenship without participation in the typical range of occupations of a community.

Occupational Alienation

The case described as occupational alienation focuses on the right of populations as well as individuals to experience meaningful, enriching occupations, contrasted against experiences of alienation. Whereas social justice might address freedom to choose where and how to live, from an occupational perspective, the underlying concern is whether choices are available for all populations to experience meaning and enrichment as they participate in occupations. Occupational alienation is named here as a social condition of injustice, not a psychological state.

With awareness of the complex and problematic notions of meaning and enrichment, we associate occupational alienation with prolonged experiences of disconnectedness, isolation, emptiness, lack of a sense of identity, a limited or confined expression of spirit, or a sense of meaninglessness. Such experiences may occur whether or not people are busy or wealthy. Occupational alienation may be a community or population experience of spiritual emptiness or lack of positive identity. Experiences of meaning and enrichment, enjoyment, health, identity, and quality of life within chosen places and routines appear to be derived from participation in one's occupations (Barnes, 2000; Blair, 2000; Christiansen, 1999 [see Chapter 42]; Hasselkus, 2002; Nygård & Borell, 1998; Primeau, 1996; Tindale, 1999; Vrkljan, 2001). Lack of opportunities or resources to enable occupational meaning and enrichment, then, is viewed as unjust.

Prime examples of occupational alienation occur when people are physically removed from their own cultural occupations through slavery, refugee confinement, or industrial policies that require them to work in demeaning jobs that pay them low wages, possibly great distances from their home or loved ones. Persons with physical or mental disabilities or persons who live in homes for seniors may experience occupational alienation if they are required to participate in occupations that they find meaningless. If the only choices offer no meaningful or enriching occupational experiences for some, then these people may experience occupational alienation, even through others may find the same choices meaningful or enriching. Sheltered workshops for adults with disabilities, senior activity centers, and workfare programs for people without paid employment may carry a managerial and professional vision of meaningful occupation. Yet the actual experience for some may be demeaning, soulless, tiresome, coercive participation in occupations they find meaningless. The concept of occupational alienation may help us to understand the tragedies of aboriginal and other peoples who are denied opportunities and resources to experience meaningful cultural rituals and language. Occupational alienation may offer insights on the desperation of people who are displaced from their homes and communities through mass relocation or war. Consideration of occupational alienation might explain the apparently soulless behavior of people who are institutionalized for long periods without meaningful, enriching participation in occupations.

The right not to be occupationally alienated speaks to the importance of what Fearing and Clark (Fearing & Clark, 2000) have described as occupational dreams. With attention to the dreams of populations or communities as well as individuals, the case of occupational alienation makes visible and conscious the social conditions required for humans to develop through participation in the range of daily life occupations that are typical of a community.

Occupational Deprivation

Whiteford (2003) defines occupational deprivation as "a state of prolonged preclusion from engagement in occupations of necessity and/or meaning due to factors that stand outside the control of the individual" (p. 222). Whiteford's cases of occupational deprivation consider geographic isolation, unsatisfactory conditions of employment (underemployment, unemployment, and overemployment), incarceration, sex-role stereotyping, refugeeism, and disability (pp. 223–239). She distinguishes the prolonged nature of occupational deprivation from temporary occupational disruptions related to injuries, or moving to a new home.

In North America and other jurisdictions, the right to work may be a fundamental value and concept associated with social justice. Yet we know that life is more than work, and work does not necessarily promote health and social inclusion. As knowledge about the impact of daily life expands, it is becoming clear that humans need to do more than work. Humans need the right to develop through participation in occupations for health and social inclusion. Of particular concern in naming occupational deprivation as a form of injustice are those who are confined or otherwise limited from participating in work. Occupational deprivation may also arise when populations have limited choice in occupations because of their isolated location, their ability, or other circumstances.

One of Whiteford's (2003) examples of occupational deprivation is geographic isolation. She describes the daily lives of aboriginal women who live in remote Australian communities with too little companionship and opportunity to flourish. The concept of occupational deprivation might be useful for explaining the losses to children with a disability if they cannot participate in the natural school and play opportunities available around their home. Given the normative expectations of ability and competence, people who are old or living with a disability may also be socially excluded from participation in transportation, health care, recreation, shopping, farming, mining, fishing, industry, business, public service, or other occupations typical of their communities.

The case of occupational deprivation recognizes that the right to work is not sufficient to capture what people need and want to do to flourish from birth to death. One might say that being deprived of occupations is the ultimate punishment. Those who work or live in prisons, locked forensic mental health hospital wards, or refugee camps know the power of occupational deprivation—we call it isolation. When we want to control or punish others, we deprive them of something to do. The argument that occupational deprivation is a matter of justice is that participation in the range of occupations is the day-to-day means through which we exercise health, citizenship, and social inclusion. We are denied these opportunities when deprived of occupations.

Occupational Marginalization

Advocates for social justice have fought for the universal right to vote, a right that enables individuals to exert their macro decision-making power to determine political leadership and exercise citizenship. From an occupational perspective, marginalization may occur despite people having the macro-decision right to vote. Occupational marginalization speaks to the need for humans to exert micro, everyday choices and decision-making power as we participate in occupations. Occupational marginalization may not be overt discrimination to bar certain groups, for instance, from paid occupations or recreation.

Rather, occupational marginalization operates invisibly, a major force of injustice being normative standardization of expectations about how, when, and where people "should" participate. Humans need to participate in and make choices about their occupations for physical, mental, and spiritual health (Frank & Engelke, 2001; Wilcock, 1998). People also need to exert self-determination and decision-making capacities in what they do (Sprague & Hayes, 2000). In its support for the International Classification of Function (ICF), the World Health Organization (1980, 2001) has defined participation restrictions as a matter of citizenship and justice as well as health. Yet managerial systems persist in seeking efficiencies through standardization efficiencies that control time, places, policies, laws, and funding (Stein, 2001; Wells, 1990), potentially overruling the empowerment approaches of client-centered practice.

In their discussion of sociological and geographic perspectives on the environment, O'Brien, Dyck, Caron, and Mortenson (2002) remind us that "spaces may be socially constructed around ideas of normalcy and ablement and therefore create environments which are exclusionary for people with disabilities by restricting their physical access or social opportunities" (p. 231). To date, people who are chronically sick or disabled remain stigmatized and excluded from mainstream life (Dewolfe, 2002). Occupational marginalization may occur, for instance, when people with disabilities are excluded from employment opportunities and have few expectations that employment is even possible (Nagle, Cook, & Polatajko, 2002). A common image that the body is an absent presence, not a determinant of life, may result in social policy that overlooks physical differences (Twigg, 2002). In other words, regulatory policies, built environments, funding, and laws, more than bodily impairment, may undermine opportunities for client-centered practice (Campbell, 2002).

The case of occupational marginalization emerged with recognition that humans, individually and as populations, need to exert micro, everyday choices and decision-making power as we participate in occupations. Moreover, we need choices related to participation in a wide range of occupations. The argument is that choice and control in what we do to participate in occupations is the basis of our empowerment as humans, and empowerment is a determinant of health for individuals and populations.

Occupational Imbalance

Occupational imbalance is used as a population-based term to identify populations that do not share in the labor and benefits of economic production. The right to equal privileges and pay for equal work is a cornerstone of social justice principles. An occupational perspective, oriented to meaning, enrichment, health, social inclusion, choice, and everyday decision-making raises questions about the right to fair privileges as the just rewards for diverse participation in the occupations of a family, community, or nation.

Occupational imbalance can be described as a form of occupational apartheid if one recognizes three major occupational classes: unoccupied, underoccupied, and overoccupied. Underemployed people are at risk for ill health because they are less likely to experience sufficient mental, physical, and social exercise that provides meaning and enrichment in their lives. Overemployed people are also at risk for ill health because they are too busy to look after themselves, their families, or their communities. Therefore, unemployment is not only an economic status; it is a matter of injustice. People without paid employment may be unoccupied, if historical and present circumstances leave them in an environment where there is very little to do. Or unemployment may release

people from paid occupations but leave them underoccupied, without opportunities to participate in occupations through which they can derive meaning and empowerment. It is important to recognize that unemployment may also result in overoccupation. Those who are unemployed may experience ill health because they become overoccupied with survival through multiple paid and unpaid occupations. While occupational imbalance may ring with concerns born of a Western work ethic, this case speaks to being occupied too much or too little to experience meaning and empowerment. Occupational imbalances relate to market rewards for work, as well as to the need for a range of occupations that promote health-giving routines and social inclusion.

Occupational segregation associated with gender, disability, race, or other forms of difference are actually forms of occupational imbalance, possibly also occupational alienation, occupational deprivation, occupational marginalization, or possibly occupational apartheid (Kronenberg & Simo Algado, 2003). To examine occupational imbalances in a community, we could identify conditions where occupations are classified, paid, valued, and enhance life for some, while in the same places and times occupations are taken for granted, exploited, and trivialized for others (Townsend, 2003b).

There are huge dilemmas in addressing occupational imbalances, because we are not only referring to having too little or too much to do, but also to the privileges and benefits associated with occupations. An imbalanced division of labor may be associated with imbalanced economic conditions. There may be economic and class gaps between those who are highly rewarded for their occupations, and those who receive few benefits for their participation in occupations. Therefore, an analysis of occupational imbalance needs to target the typical values and institutionalized practices of paying less for homemaking, child care, and physical labor than for intellectual or managerial occupations. The existence of welfare systems is an acceptance that some social groups are disadvantaged because they cannot survive without economic assistance in their participation in occupations. One is left asking, Would occupational justice be advanced by having a system of guaranteed wages, or a communal system of resource sharing, regardless of differences in daily life participation? What Would an economy look like if societies calculated an economic value for the participation of children, persons with disabilities, seniors, and others whose occupations are not currently counted in economic calculations?

Implications for Occupational Therapy's Client-Centered Practice

Why is this discussion relevant to occupational therapy practice, beyond being a topic of interest? Our response is that occupational therapy exists as a profession to address occupational injustices. We believe this because occupational therapists' primary populations of concern are those who are vulnerable to injustices because their participation in occupations

Table 32.5. Working for Occupational Justice Through Client-Centered Practice

Occupational therapy clinicians and practitioners with individual clients	• Consider client participation in occupations and what occupations are used in therapy • Examine policy support for client participation in all decision-making re: all aspects of services • Seek practice opportunities with groups, communities, and populations as well as with individuals
Occupational therapy educators	• Consider visibility of occupation, enabling approaches, and justice in curriculum • Incorporate student projects with occupational justice theme • Enable students to critically appraise power, economic, cultural, social, and political issues that impact equity and occupational justice
Occupational therapy managers	• Consider how policies on time use, service types, travel costs, and other data support and capture client-centered approaches targeting occupational justice rights
Occupational therapy researchers	• Employ qualitative methods with participants to explore experiences of occupational justice/injustice • Employ quantitative methods with participants to measure occupational participation, etc. • Employ critical theories/methods, e.g., critical ethnography, PAR (participatory, action research), liberation, and emancipatory approaches with participants to analyze and change social structures and policies

is restricted by injury, chronic illness, disability of various types, mental illness, incarceration, old age, or other circumstances. Moreover, occupational therapists' values, beliefs, and practical approaches advocate that we work as professionals in client-centered, just ways with persons who are active agents in therapy and their own lives. The most explicit link to occupational justice can be found in our goals and objectives to collaborate with clients to promote social inclusion, using various enabling methods that emphasize client decision-making about their participation in occupations (Townsend, 1993). The broad implication is that, in health, community services, employment support, housing, school, transportation, corrections, higher education, private business, and other systems worldwide, occupational therapists can choose to either advocate consciously with others for justice, or comply with occupational injustices through silence and inaction. Given occupational therapists' populations of concern, professional values, beliefs, and client-centered intentions, and focus on social inclusion, occupational justice is an implicit issue, whether or not we choose to make it explicit.

However, we know that occupational therapists' good intentions may be overruled by policies and funding priorities which are not yet organized to support client-centered practice (Sumsio & Smyth, 2000; Townsend, 1998; Wilkins, Pollock, Rochon, & Law, 2001). Occupational therapists' and others' enabling, client-centered approaches go against the grain of professionals' traditional, hierarchical decision-making about those who are dependent on their services (Cervaro & Wilson, 1999; Townsend, 2003a). Moreover, today's corporate efficiency models emphasize standardization over attention to justice (Stein, 2001).

In light of these difficulties, what actions can occupational therapists take? First, occupational therapy clinicians, educators, managers, policy makers, or researchers who want to make justice more explicit can extend the dialogue summarized here by developing a personal and professional self-critique and a social critique. The implication is to develop critical, reflexive rather than technical, prescriptive practice (Falardeau & José Durand, 2002; Stern, Restall, & Ripat, 2000). We advocate dialogues and research that combine critical analysis of the everyday lives of our populations of concern, the systems in which we work, and our profession, with hope and visions of possible futures. Dialogues could consider how to use client-centered approaches more explicitly in order to counter professionals' traditional, structured dominance and authority (Campbell, Copeland, & Tate, 1998; Griffin, 2001). Dialogues could also brainstorm cases as a way of developing greater cultural competence to address clients' diversity in the areas, settings, and populations that we encounter (Whiteford & St. Clair, 2002).

Second, with critical reflection, occupational therapists can brainstorm possible actions, examples being the actions suggested in Table 32.5. As difficult as it sounds, those focused on working with individuals might collectively make time away, through professional development in-service sessions or retreats, from the pressing demands of individualized caseloads. The profession might develop strategies for change if we learn what limits us in the use of simulated and real occupations as therapy in health and other systems. Justice might be more consciously incorporated in occupational therapy curricula by educators. And justice could be made explicit in student projects in academic or fieldwork settings, encouraging students to learn to critically appraise the power relations that control clients' and occupational therapists' opportunities. Because management and research occupational therapists are positioned to gather and use data, these occupational therapists can develop critiques of policies on time use, service types, travel costs, and other issues to determine what supports and limits client-centered practice. Researchers might employ qualitative, critical, and/or quantitative methods to develop guidelines for evidence-based practice that would make occupation, enabling, and justice more explicit and known to others. Historical research could be taken to provide the facts and analysis about this profession's grounding in moral treatment and the therapeutic use of occupation with those who live with various restrictions in daily life (Friedland, 2001).

Third, the profession might engage with our communities. Taking a client-centered, action-research approach to matters of justice (Figure 32.1) could crystallize debate around apparent occupational injustices that occupational therapists confront every day. Looking beyond an individual's local family or work environment, as a profession we could record and talk publicly about social determinants of health (the economy, national priorities and policies, and societal values) and how these impact the individuals and groups with whom occupational therapists work. Occupational therapists can contribute to society by using our knowledge pillars (occupation, enabling, justice) to address health and social inclusion.

Examples of potential contributions would be to educate the public on the therapeutic power of occupation (Pierce, 2001) (see Chapter 63). We could use a sociological and geographic analysis of the environment (O'Brien et al., 2002) as a basis for enabling changes in the social and physical environment while involving those who tend to be socially excluded as participants (Dunn, 2000; Fazio, 2001). Use of participatory evaluation tools, such as the Canadian Occupational Performance Measure, can remind us to attend closely to clients' goals and to involve clients in designing interventions (Wressle, Eeg-Olofsson, Marcusson, & Henriksson, 2002). Client-centered evaluation of community-based services would enable us to partner with clients to determine the relevance and impacts of our practice on people's lives (Hebert, Thibeault, Landry, Boisvenu, & Laporte, 2000). Explicit justice-oriented work would involve us in more alliances with consumers who are advocating for greater empowerment in and beyond health services (Deegan, 1997; Sherr Klein, 1997). Qualitative inquiry (Hammell, 2002) would open up insights on clients' own perceptions of their involvement and decision-making in occupational therapy services. Evaluation studies that include client perceptions of occupational therapy services and outcomes would help to identify issues that may not be visible from a professional perspective (McKinnon, 2000). Action toward justice for and with persons with a disability should motivate and empower (them) to make appropriate, constructive responses. Actions consistent with occupational justice would develop community awareness through community groups, the Internet, and the media and provide role play or other opportunities for clients to practice the skills for becoming their own advocates. An international

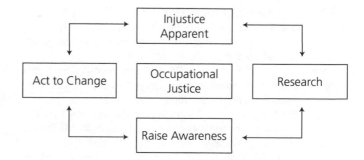

Figure 32.1. Client-centered activism for occupational justice.

perspective would enable occupational therapists to take into account diverse Western and Eastern cultural constructions of occupation, enabling, and justice.

Reflections and Conclusions

This paper has highlighted an ongoing dialogue about occupational justice both to record it and to draw others into a widening circle of inquiry. We posed the question Do occupational therapists work for justice? Our answer is that occupational therapists may work for justice. We recognize that some occupational therapists are more interested in the methods and techniques of practice than in activism. Moreover, we cannot always see where injustices lie from our own position of power and privilege, even when that power is limited as it is for occupational therapists. Occupational therapists may be caught in our own experiences of occupational injustice as we struggle to keep up with workloads, let alone consider idealistic notions of justice. With acknowledgement of the struggle, we view the work of enabling occupational justice as congruent with worldwide activism. Dialogue about occupational justice seems timely as occupational therapists around the world articulate what distinguishes this numerically small, rather invisible profession and its contributions to individuals, populations, and societies.

References

Adelson, H. L. (1995). The origins of a concept of social justice. In K. D. Irani & M. Silver (Eds.), *Social justice in the ancient world* (pp. 25–38). Westport, CT: Greenwood Press.

Armstrong, H. (2000). Reflections on the difficulty of creating and sustaining equiable communicative forums. *Canadian Journal for Studies in Adult Education, 14*, 67–85.

Barnes, C. (2000). A working social model? Disability, work, and disability politics in the 21st century. *Critical Social Policy, 20*, 441–457.

Blair, S. E. (2000). The centrality of occupation during life transitions. *British Journal of Occupational Therapy, 63*, 231–237.

Borell, L., Lilja, M., Sviden, G. A., & Sadlo, G. (2001). Occupations and signs of reduced hope: An explorative study of older adults with functional impairments. *American Journal of Occupational Therapy, 55*, 311–316.

Bores, A. (2000). A comparison between the ethics of justice and the ethics of care. *Journal of Advanced Nursing, 32*, 1071–1075.

Byrne, C. (1999). Facilitating empowerment groups: Dismantling professional boundaries. *Issues in Mental Health Nursing, 21,* 55–71.

Campbell, J. (2002). Valuing diversity: The disability agenda—We've only just begun. *Disability and Society, 17,* 471–478.

Campbell, M., Copeland, B., & Tate, B. (1998). Taking the standpoint of people with disabilities in research: Experiences with participation. *Canadian Journal of Rehabilitation, 12,* 95–304.

Cervaro, R. M., & Wilson, A. L. (1999). Beyond learner-centred practice: Adult education, power, and society. *Canadian Journal for the Study of Adult Education, 13,* 27–38.

Christiansen, C. (1999). Defining lives: Occupation as identity: An essay on competence, coherence, and the creation of meaning. *American Journal of Occupational Therapy, 53,* 547–558. Reprinted as Chapter 42.

Cookson, R., & Dolan, P. (2000). Principles of justice in healthcare rationing. *Journal of Medical Ethics, 26,* 323–379.

Daniels, N., Kennedy, B. P., & Kawachi, I. (1999). Why justice is good for our health: The social determinants of health inequalities. *Daedalus, 128,* 215–251.

Deegan, P. (1997). Recovery and empowerment for people with psychiatric disabilities. *Social Work in Health Care, 25,* 11–24.

DeWolfe, P. (2002). Private tragedy in social context? Reflections on disability, illness, and suffering. *Disability and Society, 17,* 255–267.

Dunn, W. (2000). *Best practice occupational therapy: In community service with children and families.* Thorofare, NJ: Slack.

Dunst, C., Trivette, C., & Deal, A. (1988). *Enabling and empowering families: Principles and guidelines for practice.* Cambridge, MA: Brookline Books.

Emanuel, E. J. (2000). Justice and managed care: Four principles for the just allocation of health care resources. *Hastings Center Report, 30,* 8–16.

Falardeau, M., & José Durand, M. (2002). Negotiation-centered versus client-centered: Which approach should be used? *Canadian Journal of Occupational Therapy, 69,* 135–142.

Fazio, L. (2001). *Developing occupation-centered programs for the community.* Upper Saddle River, NJ: Prentice-Hall.

Fearing, V., & Clark, J. (2000). *Individuals in context: A practical guide to client-centered practice.* Thorofare, NJ: Slack.

Frank, L., & Engelke, P. (2001). The built environment and human activity patterns: Exploring the impacts of urban form on public health. *Journal of Planning Literature, 16,* 202–218.

Friedland, J. (2001). Knowing from whence we came: Reflecting on return-to-work and interpersonal relationships. *Canadian Journal of Occupational Therapy, 68,* 266–271.

Grammenos, S. (2003). *Illness, disability, and social inclusion.* Brussels: Centre for European Social and Economic Policy.

Gray, J. M. (1998). Putting occupation into practice: Occupation as ends, occupation as means. *American Journal of Occupational Therapy, 32,* 354–364. Reprinted as Chapter 15.

Griffin, S. (2001). Occupational therapists and the concept of power: A review of the literature. *Australian Occupational Therapy Journal, 48,* 24–34.

Guy, J. R. (1996). *Comparison of the art of the possible: Dr. Southwood Smith as social reformer and public health pioneer.* Cambridgeshire: Octavia Hill Society.

Hammell, K. W. (2002). Informing, client-centered practice through qualitative inquiry: Evaluating the duality of qualitative research. *British Journal of Occupational Therapy, 65,* 175–194.

Hasselkus, B. R. (2002). *The meaning of everyday occupation.* Thorofare, NJ: Slack.

Hebert, M., Thibeault, R., Landry A., Boisvenu, M., & Laporte, D. (2000). Introducing an evaluation of community-based occupational therapy services: A client-centered practice. *Canadian Journal of Occupational Therapy, 67,* 146–154.

Heitman, E. (2000). Ethical values in the education of biomedical researchers. *The Hastings Center Report, 30,* S40–S44.

Hemmingsson, H., & Borell, L. (2002). Environmental barriers in mainstream schools. *Child Care, Health, and Development, 25,* 57–63.

Howland, G. W. (1944). Occupational therapy across Canada. *Canadian Geographical Journal, 28,* 32–40.

Ignatieff, M. (2000). *The rights revolution.* Toronto, ON: House of Anansi.

Irani, K. D. (1995). The idea of social justice in the ancient world. In K. D. Irani & M. Silver (Eds.), *Social justice in the ancient world* (pp. 3–8). Westport, CT: Greenwood Press.

Iwama, M. (1999). Are you listening? Cross-cultural perspectives on client-centered occupational therapy practice: A view from Japan. *Occupational Therapy Now, 1,* 4–6.

Iwama, M. (2003). Toward culturally relevant epistemologies in occupational therapy. *American Journal of Occupational Therapy, 57,* 582–588.

Jarman, J. (2003). What is occupation: Interdisciplinary perspectives on defining and classifying human activity. In E. Townsend (Ed.), *Introduction to occupation: The art and science of living* (pp. 47–62). Upper Saddle River, NJ: Prentice-Hall.

Kronenberg, E., & Simo Algado, S. (2003). *The political nature of occupational therapy.* University of Linkoping, Linkoping, SW.

Labonte, R. (1989). Community empowerment: The need for political analysis. *Canadian Journal of Public Health, 80,* 87–88.

Locke, J. (1690). *An essay concerning humane understanding.* London: T. Basset.

McKay, S. (2000). Gender justice and reconciliation. *Women's Studies International Forum, 23,* 561–570.

McKinnon, A. L. (2000). Client values and satisfaction with occupational therapy. *Scandinavian Journal of Occupational Therapy, 7,* 99–106.

McKnight, J. L. (1989). Health and empowerment. *Canadian Journal of Occupational Public Health, 76* (Supplement 1), 37–38.

Metz, T. (2000). Arbitrariness, justice, and respect. *Social Theory and Practice, 26,* 24–45.

Meyer, A. (1922). The philosophy of occupational therapy. *Archives of Occupational Therapy, 1,* 1–10. Reprinted as Chapter 2.

Nagle, S., Cook, T. V., & Polatajko, H. (2002). I'm doing as much as I can: Occupational choices of persons with a severe and persistent mental illness. *Journal of Occupational Science, 9,* 71–82.

Noyes, J. (2000). Enabling young ventilator-dependent people to express their views and experiences of their care in hospital. *Journal of Advanced Nursing, 31,* 1206–1215.

Nygård, L., & Borell, L. (1998). A life-world of alternating meaning: Expressions of the illness experience of dementia in everyday life over three years. *Occupational Therapy Journal of Research, 18,* 109–136.

O'Brien, P., Dyck, I., Caron, S., & Mortenson, P. (2002). Environmental analysis: Insights from sociological and geographic perspectives. *Canadian Journal of Occupational Therapy, 69,* 229–238.

Pierce, D. (2001). Occupation by design: Dimensions, therapeutic power, and creative process. *American Journal of Occupational Therapy, 55,* 249–259. Reprinted as Chapter 63.

Pogge, T. W. (2000). On the site of distributive justice: Reflections on Cohen and Murphy. *Philosophy and Public Affairs, 29,* 137–169.

Polatajko, H. (2001). The evolution of our occupational perspective: The journey from diversion through therapeutic use to enablement. *Canadian Journal of Occupational Therapy, 68,* 203–207.

Primeau, L. A. (1996). Running as an occupation: Multiple meanings and purposes. In R. Z. F. Clark (Ed.), *Occupational science: The evolving discipline* (pp. 275–286). Philadelphia: F.A. Davis.

Rawls, J. (1975). A Kantian conception of equality. *The Cambridge Review,* 94–99.

Rebeiro, K. (1998). Occupation-as-means to mental health: A review of the literature and a call for research. *Canadian Journal of Occupational Therapy, 65,* 12–19.

Rebeiro, K. (2001). Enabling occupation: The importance of an affirming environment. *Canadian Journal of Occupational Therapy, 68,* 80–89.

Reilly, M. (1962). Occupational therapy can be one of the great ideas of 20th century medicine. *American Journal of Occupational Therapy, 16,* 1–9. Reprinted as Chapter 8.

Rosenau, P. V. (1994). Health politics meet post-modernism: Its meaning and implications for community health organizing. *Journal of Health Politics, Policy and Law, 19,* 303–333.

Royeen, C., Duncan, M., Crabree, J., Richards, J., & Clark, G. F. (2000). Effects of billing Medicaid for occupational therapy services in the schools: A pilot study. *American Journal of Occupational Therapy, 54,* 429–433.

Schultz, V. (2000). Life's work. *Columbia Law Review, 100*(7), 1981–1964.

Sherr Klein, B. (1997). Foreword in *Enabling occupation: An occupational therapy perspective* (pp. vii–x). Ottawa, ON: CAOT Publications ACE.

Smith, D. (1987). *The everyday world as problematic: A feminist sociology.* Toronto, ON: University of Toronto Press.

Smith, D. (1990a). *The conceptual practices of power: A feminist sociology of knowledge.* Toronto, ON: University of Toronto Press.

Smith, D. (1990b). *Texts, facts, and femininity: Exploring the relations of ruling.* New York: Routledge.

Sprague, J., & Hayes, J. (2000). Self-determination and empowerment: A feminist standpoint analysis of talk about disability. *American Journal of Community Psychology, 28,* 671–695.

Stein, J. G. (2001). *The cult of efficiency.* Toronto, ON: House of Anansi.

Stern, M., Restall, G., & Ripat, J. (2000). The use of self-reflection to improve client-centered practice. In V. G. Fearing & J. Clark (Eds.), *Individuals in context* (pp. 145–158). Thorofare, NJ: Slack.

Sumsion, T., & Smyth, G. (2000). Barriers to client-centredness and their resolution. *Canadian Journal of Occupational Therapy, 67,* 15–21.

Tindale, J. (1999). Variance in the meaning of time by family cycle, period, social context, and ethnicity. In W. E. Pentland, A. S. Harvey, M. P. Lawton, & M. A. McColl (Eds.), *Time use research in the social sciences* (p. 155). New York: Kulwer Academic/Plenum Publishers.

Townsend, E. (1993). Muriel Driver Lecture: Occupational therapy's social vision. *Canadian Journal of Occupational Therapy, 60,* 174–184.

Townsend, E. (1998). *Good intentions overruled: A critique of empowerment in the routine organization of mental health services.* Toronto, ON: University of Toronto Press.

Townsend, E. (2003a). Power and justice in enabling occupation. *Canadian Journal of Occupational Therapy, 70,* 74–87.

Townsend, E. (2003b). Occupational justice: Ethical, moral, and civic principles for an inclusive world. Keynote presentation at the Annual Conference of the European Network of Occupational Therapy Educators, Czech Republic, Prague, October.

Townsend, E., Ripley, D., & Langille, L. (2003). Professional tensions in client-centered practice. *American Journal of Occupational Therapy, 57,* 17–28.

Townsend, E., & Wilcock, A. A. (2004). Occupational justice. In C. Christiansen & E. Townsend (Eds.), *An introduction to occupation: The art and science of living* (pp. 243–273). Upper Saddle River, NJ: Prentice Hall.

Twigg, J. (2002). The body of social policy: Mapping a territory. *Journal of Social Policy, 31,* 421–439.

Vrkljan, B. (2001). Meaning of occupational engagement in life-threatening illness: A qualitative pilot project. *Canadian Journal of Occupational Therapy, 68,* 237–246.

Wells, L. (1990). Responsiveness and accountability in long-term care: Strategies for policy development and empowerment. *Canadian Journal of Public Health, 81,* 382–385.

Whiteford, G. (2000). Occupational deprivation: Global challenge in the new millennium. *British Journal of Occupational Therapy, 64,* 200–210. Reprinted as Chapter 31.

Whiteford, G. (2003). When people cannot participate: Occupational deprivation. In C. Christiansen & E. Townsend (Eds.), *An introduction to occupation: The art and science of living* (pp. 221–242). Upper Saddle River, NJ: Prentice Hall.

Whiteford, G., & St. Clair, V. W. (2002). Being prepared for diversity: In practice: Occupational therapy students' perceptions of valuable intercultural learning experiences. *British Journal of Occupational Therapy, 65,* 129–137.

Wilcock, A. A. (1993). A theory of the human need for occupation. *Journal of Occupational Science: Australia, 1,* 17–24. Reprinted as Chapter 33.

Wilcock, A. A. (1998). *An occupational perspective of health.* Thorofare, NJ: Slack.

Wilcock, A. A. (2001). *Occupation for health: A journey from self-health to prescription* (Vol. I). London: British Association and College of Occupational Therapists.

Wilcock, A. A. (2002). *A journey from prescription to self-health* (Vol. 2). London: British Association and College of Occupational Therapists.

Wilcock, A. A., & Townsend, E. (2000). Occupational justice: Occupational terminology interactive dialogue. *Journal of Occupational Science, 7,* 84–86.

Wilkins, S., Pollock, N., Rochon, S., & Law, M. (2001). Implementing client-centered practice: Why is it so difficult to do? *Canadian Journal of Occupational Therapy, 68,* 70–79.

World Health Organization. (1980). *International classification of impairments, disabilities, and handicaps: A manual of classification relating to the consequences of disease.* Geneva: Author.

World Health Organization. (1986). *Ottawa charter for health promotion: An international conference on health promotion,* retrieved March, 2003 from the Health Canada web site: www.hc-sc.gc.ca/hppb/phdd/docs/charter.

World Health Organization. (2001). *International classification of functioning, disability, and health (ICF).* Geneva: World Health Organization.

Wressle, E., Eeg-Olofsson, A., Marcusson, J., & Henriksson, C. (2002). Improved client participation in the rehabilitation process using a client-centered goal formation structure. *Journal of Rehabilitation Medicine, 34,* 5–11.

Yerxa, E. J. (1967). 1966 Eleanor Clarke Slagle Lecture: Authentic occupational therapy. *American Journal of Occupational Therapy, 21,* 1–9.

Yerxa, E. J. (1979). *The philosophical base of occupational therapy: 2000 AD.* Rockville, MD: American Occupational Therapy Association.

Yerxa, E. J. (1993). Occupational science: A new source of power for participants in occupational therapy. *Occupational Science: Australia, 1,* 3–10.

Young, I. M. (1990). *Justice and the politics of difference.* Princeton, NJ: Princeton University Press.

Zanetti, V. (2001). Global justice: Is interventionalism desirable? *Metaphilosophy, 32,* 196–211.

A Theory of the Human Need for Occupation

CHAPTER 33

ANN WILCOCK, PHD, REG OT(SA)

"It is the unique blend of biology and culture that makes the species 'Homo sapiens' a truly unique kind of animal.... Humans are different, not so much for what we do ... but rather the fact that we can do more or less what we want."[1]

Occupation, that is, purposeful activity, is a central aspect of the human experience. In developing a theory of the human need for occupation, an exploration of occupational evolution as well as the biological and the sociocultural aspects of occupational behavior is necessary. This paper, which is based on a study of human occupational behavior throughout history, explores the proposition that, although in most instances the conception, expression, and execution of occupation is unique and motivated by sociocultural values and beliefs, the need to engage in purposeful occupation is innate and related to health and survival.

This chapter was previously published in *Occupational Science: Australia*, *1*(1), 17–24. Copyright © 1993, Occupational Science Australia. Reprinted with permission.

All animals appear to have some special characteristic which is paramount to their survival. This varies among and within species. For some it is speed, for others the ability to camouflage, and for yet others, highly developed visual or auditory capacities. Many animals possess qualities and characteristics once thought unique to humans, which is not surprising as all mammalian brains have neuronal circuitry and systems which enable then to receive, attend to, interpret, communicate with, and act upon information from the environment. In fact *"there is no strong evidence of unique brain–behavior relationships in any species within the class Mammalia."[2]* The difference among species is in the degree of capacities. Ethologist Konrad Lorenz contends that:

"Among humans" ... "perceptions of depth and direction, a central nervous representation of space, Gestalt perception and the capacity for abstraction, insight and learning, voluntary movement, curiosity and exploratory behavior" and "imitation" ... are more strongly developed than any of them is among an animal species, even if they represent for those animals a fulfilment of the most vital life-furthering functions."[3]

The difference between humans and the other mammals is manifest in the size of the human brain. It is 6.3 times larger than expected for mammals of the same body size[1], with the difference mainly attributable to an increase in association areas of the cortex. These are responsible for the mediation of cognitive processes such as the capacities noted by Lorenz, and complex communication, language, thinking, forward planning, problem solving, analysis, judgement, and adaptation. It is these highly developed cognitive capacities, along with consciousness, which are the special survival characteristics of humans, enabling them to adapt to and meet the challenge of many different environments and dangers.

These differences in degree of cognitive capacity are central to the occupational nature of humans who go beyond survival needs in their pursuit of occupation because they free them from the functional constraints of most animals, enabling them to use their apparently strong drive to engage in daily, new, or adventurous occupations. People are able to undertake activities with individuality of purpose; to think about the effects, conceptualize, and plan beforehand; and to reflect and mentally alter future behavior as a result of outcomes. Children, through play, the predominant occupation of the young, learn practical skills to enable them to survive, to interact with others, to choose future roles, in fact to develop according to their environment and cultural values. Occupation provides the mechanism for social interaction, and societal development and growth, forming the foundation stone of communal, local, and national identity, because not only do individuals engage in separate pursuits, they are able to plan and execute group activity to the extent of national government or to achieve international goals, for individual, mutual, and community purposes. As Marx suggests *"History is nothing but the activity of man pursuing his aims."*[5] Individuals dream and communities plan what they will "do" in the future. Such dreams and plans often predict potential accolades for what will be achieved, reflecting how occupations are the outward expression of culturally desired intellectual, moral, and physical attributes. Occupation is the mechanism by which individuals demonstrate the use of their capacities by achievements of value and worth to their society and the world. It is only by their activities that people can demonstrate what they are or what they hope to be. Occupational achievement usually results in self development and growth experiences, which Hegel and Marx described as *"labour as man's act of self creation."*[6]

Marx founded much of his philosophy on the idea that labor is the collective creative activity of mankind, in fact, is *"man's species nature."*[7] As people engage in occupation to master their environment and improve human opportunities, well-being, and survival, the physical and social environment is altered. The more sophisticated the occupation, the greater the change to the environment, which in turn causes further change to and development of people, and *"by thus acting on the external world and changing it, he at the same time changes his own nature."*[8] In the same vein, Braverman proposes that people are the special product of purposeful action, arguing that occupation which *"transcends mere instinctual activity is the force which created human kind and the force by which humankind created the world as we know it."*[9]

The idea that occupation is not just the object of human function but is an integrated part of each person's being in relationship with the world suggests the need to explore the biological purpose of the human need to "do." This need is so much a part of our being that we have, to this time, paid scant attention to its purpose, other than, in post-industrial societies, as an objective of living. In considering people as occupational beings it is implied that humans need to engage in occupation in order to flourish, and that as Selye observes, purposeful use of time is a biological necessity because *"our brain slips into chaos and confusion unless we constantly use it for work that seems worthwhile to us."*[10] Further, Sigerist argues that work is essential in maintaining health *"because it determines the chief rhythm of life, balances it, and gives meaning and significance. An organ that does not work atrophies, and the mind that does not work becomes dumb."*[11]

Biological Need

Because basic biological needs are now obscured by millions of years of acquired values, present day awareness may not reflect human needs which were, and probably still are, fundamental to healthy survival. In fact, the study of biological needs has been neglected of late either because, as Allport remarked on fashion in scientific inquiry, *"we never seem to solve our problems or exhaust our concepts; we only grow tired of them,"*[12] or because of a false dichotomy between disciplines concerned with the study of biology and sociology which mirrors the Cartesian division of mind and body. In the long-running nature-versus-nurture debate, the need to consider both is poorly recognized except perhaps by disciplines such as ethology, sociobiology, and occupational therapy.

Biological mechanisms aimed at ensuring survival are basic to all animals, and the proposition put by Omstein and Sobel in "The Healing Brain"[13] that *"the major role of the brain is to mind the body and maintain health"* appears more logical than some of the lofty purposes attributed to it by those seeking to differentiate humans from their animal heritage. The brain, they argue, by making *"countless adjustments"* is able to maintain stability between *"social worlds, our mental and emotional lives, and our internal physiology."* It is contended here that biological "needs" have an integral role in this process.

It was in the early 1930s that the "concept of need" as a *"central motivating variable"* made its debut into academic psychology, eventually replacing the notion of instinct, although unlike instinct it does not have a *"repertoire of inherited, unlearned action patterns."*[14] Many needs theorists of the time were influenced by physiological discoveries such as those pertaining to homeostasis, and the notions propounded about "drives" as persistent motivations, organic in origin, which *"arouse, sustain, and regulate human and animal behavior."* These were seen as distinct from external determinants of behavior such as *"social goals, interests, values, attitude and personality traits."*[15] Dashiell in "Fundamentals of Objective Psychology,"[16] for example, argues that

> *"The primary drives to persistent forms of animal and human conduct are tissue conditions within the organism giving rise to stimulations existing the organism to overt activity. A man's interest and desires may became ever so elaborate, refined, socialized, sublimated, idealistic; but the raze basis from which they are developed is found in the phenomena of living matter."*

Lorenz in examining *"the purposefulness of the anatomic characteristic as well the behavior patterns of every living creature"*[17] observes that humans do lack *"long, self-continued chains of innate behavior patterns"* but that they have more *"genuinely instinctive impulses than any other animal."*[18] It is such impulses which express biological needs. In the 1973 *Dictionary of Behavioral Science*, "Need" is described as:

> *"the condition of lacking, wanting or requiring something which if present would benefit the organism by facilitating behaviour or satisfying a tension."*

and also as

"a construct representing a force in the brain which directs and organises the individual's perception, thinking and action, so as to change an existing, unsatisfying situation."[19]

The view held here accepts and extends this concept, arguing that "needs" relate not only to correction of disequilibrium but to facilitating what is required for living organisms—plants, animals, or humans to fulfil potential and flourish.[20 21] With this view, biological needs are seen as inborn health agents which recognize the organism as a "whole in interaction with the environment" as part of an open system. They do not differentiate among physical, mental, or social issues in the way of modern society, or as does medicine, psychology or sociology, but work as part of *"a flow of processes"* within the biological hierarchy relating structures and function,[22] and are integral to the collaboration between biological rhythms and homeostasis as described by Campbell.[23]

Using a cybernetic—that is, a transfer of information and feedback model to assist understanding of the processes, it is proposed that needs have a three-way role in maintaining the stability and health of the organism (Figure 33.1). They serve to warn after a problem occurs, to protect and prevent potential disorder, and to prompt and reward use of capacities so that the organism will flourish and reach potential. To warn and protect, needs are experienced as a form of discomfort which calls for some kind of action to satisfy or assuage the need. Examples of these experiences are pain, fatigue, hunger, cold, fear, boredom, tension, depression, anxiety, anger, or loneliness. To prevent disorder and prompt use of capacities, needs are experienced in a positive sense, such as a need to spend extra energy, walk, explore, understand or make sense of, utilize ideas, express thoughts, talk, listen or look, spend time alone or with others, and so on. The third category of needs considered here to be integral to the healthy survival of individuals are those that reward use of capacities, such as the need for purpose, satisfaction, fulfillment and pleasure. Pleasure and happiness have been recognized as powerful human needs by many, such as, Aristotle 2,300 years ago, and current writers such as Argyle[24] and Csikszentmihalyi.[25] These three categories of needs are structured physiologically to provide both motivation and feedback.

Founded on these notions about biological needs and following an exploration of human occupation from early in evolution, a theoretical framework attributing a place for purposeful occupation in maintaining and enabling the health of individuals and survival of the species is proposed. Three major functions of occupation are identified. They are:

- To provide for immediate bodily needs of sustenance, self-care, and shelter;
- To develop skills, social structures, and technology, aimed at safety and superiority over predators and the environment;
- And to exercise personal capacities to enable maintenance and development of the organism.

It is assumed that occupational behaviors of early humans of the hunter–gatherer period reflect basic phylogenic needs of humans more closely than those of the present day because they would be less affected by culturally acquired knowledge, values, and behavior. Within hunter–gatherer societies the direct provision of daily requirements formed the foundation of occupational behaviour. This simple occupational structure did not obscure innate physiological needs, but catered for them to the extent that the environment was able to furnish these needs, and people were able to adapt to changes of habitat. Virey, French physician–philosopher in "L'Hygiene Philosophique,"[26] asserted that humans in a state of nature are endowed with an instinct for health which permits biological adaptation and which civilized humans have lost, and it has been observed *"that people living a culturally primitive life (with less medical care) are generally more physically perfect than those from afflluent societies."*[27] This view is supported by reports from explorers in their initial contacts with people of primitive cultures which suggest that they appeared both happy and healthy. For example, Captain James Cook recorded in his Journal, 1768–1771, that he found the natives of the Pacific Islands he visited happy, healthy, and full of vigor, and of the Australian aborigine he wrote *"they are far happier than we*

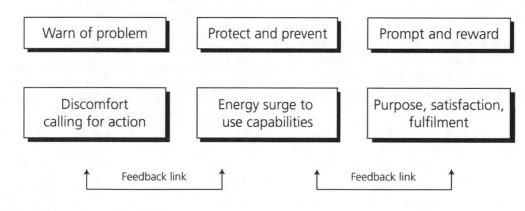

Figure 33.1. Needs: Three-way role in health.

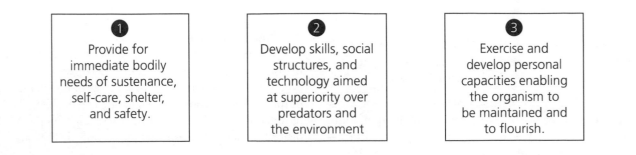

| **1** Provide for immediate bodily needs of sustenance, self-care, shelter, and safety. | **2** Develop skills, social structures, and technology aimed at superiority over predators and the environment | **3** Exercise and develop personal capacities enabling the organism to be maintained and to flourish. |

Figure 33.2. Occupation: Three major functions in species survival.

Europeans ... they live in tranquility ..." and "they think themselves provided with all the necessarys of Life, and that they have no Superfluities (sic)."[28] On the whole, health and well-being seem to have sat easily with the unequivocal lifestyle.

The occupational technology and social structures of this prolonged era aimed at safety and superiority over predators and the environment were in accord with the natural world and are generally considered not to have disturbed the environmental balance. The "overexploitation of natural resources" does not occur in the ecology of plants and animals, because human hunter–gatherer cultures "influence their biotope in a way no different from that of animal populations."[29] While some may argue this assertion, it is supported, on the whole, by observation of cultures such as that of the Australian aborigine which does not appear to have overexploited the environment, and "in full tribal life ... presented an excellent example of a society working in rhythm with its environment."[30]

From such simple beginnings social structures and technology have become dominant and self-perpetuating forces, with most people seeming to accept whatever eventuates as an inevitable and useful progression, to the extent they are seldom considered as having grown from basic human needs. In fact, the needs of people pale into insignificance beside the drive to create more and more sophisticated technology, and more regulated societies which are no longer in step with ecology. The exercise of personal capacities to enable maintenance and development of the organism is perhaps the most primary and least appreciated function of human occupation. The organism, and all its parts, have to be active in order to remain healthy. Maslow observed that:

"capacities clamor to be used, and cease their clamor only when they are well used. That is, capacities are also needs. Not only is it fun to use our capacities, but it is also necessary for growth. The unused skill or capacity or organ can become a disease centre or else atrophy or disappear."[31]

In other words, capacities need exercise to maintain homeostasis and health, and the expanded human brain with its capacity to think, surmise, problem solve, anticipate, and plan for the future imposes upon the need for activity, the need for purpose. For millions of years, basic survival provided the purpose for required activity. With changes to occupation and

purpose due to cultural evolution, particularly over the last 200 years, the balanced use of capacities is compromised, and ultimately long-term health and survival of the species may be under threat.

Sociocultural Factors

This may have come about because biological needs are not easy to distinguish from socioculturally acquired needs and wants, and neither are they omnipotent. They are subject to scrutiny of, and adaptation by, cognitive and intellectual capacities which are the most recent evolutionary processes of the human brain. These are primarily responsive to the sociocultural environment with a functional capacity to formulate acquired needs. Although acquired and biological needs work in partnership, acquired needs are able to override biological needs because of the hierarchical structure of the central nervous system. "In evolution, new structures of body and brain are often added on to existing ones," but are involved in the same functions. "A tension can exist between the old and the new. Such tensions are especially pronounced in ... humans [who are] equipped with a powerful cortex [which] can say 'no.'"[32]

However, it can be argued that the biological mechanism of needs has focused human energies toward developing sociocultural structures to meet those needs. Humans' intellectual, cognitive, and cultural capacity has enabled them through engagement in occupation, to satisfy, in large measure, the three categories of needs identified earlier. Because of this, and despite diverse challenges, humans, unlike other mammals, have been successful survivors—to the point of overpopulation. In post-industrial countries, action to satisfy or assuage discomfort, such as food production, the regulation of temperature, and measures to reduce pain, have reached a level of sophistication far beyond the simple methods used by all other animals living in natural habitats. To prevent disorder, humans have developed ways of using their capacities in adaptive, inventive, and exploratory fashions to the extent that they provide purpose, reward, and the pursuit of happiness.

The human brain's capacity to adapt to and indeed construct social environs different from those in which humans evolved appears to alter the significance of biological needs, so that "even phylogenetically evolved programs of ... behavior are adjusted to the presence of a culture."[33] This has led to "culture *itself*" creating "*norms of human behavior that, in a certain sense, can step in as substitutes for innate behavior programs.*"[34]

Humans' ability for sociocultural adaptation enables infants at a very early age to assimilate and retain information from the environment, before a conscious appreciation of meaning or significance is possible. This early absorption of observed behaviors enables ontogenic development to be in step with sociocultural expectations. Attitudes, as well as behavior are absorbed and adopted, and it is those formed before intellectual capacities are sufficiently advanced to allow for adequate understanding or refuting, that have the strongest, because "unconscious," hold on individuals. While this mechanism was central to early humans' healthy survival because it allowed essential learning to occur from birth and stimulated cognitive capacities to develop, in latter-day cultures, despite these benefits, what is absorbed may have little to do with health. Sociocultural survival as observed by infants is, in post-industrial societies, concerned, in large part, with material things. In addition, infants are encouraged to hide many physiological actions, such as yawning or scratching, because they are counter to sociocultural rules. In this way biological needs are gradually suppressed to the point where, in order to meet social expectations, they are not adequately recognized. It is from views such as this that sociologists developed one of the fundamental postulates of the modern discipline, that human actions are limited or determined by past and present environments, and that humans are the products and the victims of their society.[35]

In a continuous but accelerating process, occupation has increased in complexity and division along with sociocultural change. In large part changes to the sociocultural world can be traced to occupational technology and the human need to exercise intellectual capacities to meet challenges imposed by social and ecological environments. Purposeful use of time is an issue of great complexity which has been poorly recognized because it forms the substance of everyday life and is taken for granted."[36] As Primeau, Clark, and Pierce[37] describe, each day, people weave together their own particular multiplicity of occupations within the context of contemporary society, with its many stresses, pressures, regulations, and changing values. The gradual evolution of complex occupational structures in response to cultural forces has led to the present situation in which it is difficult to tease out the survival and health maintaining behaviors which were once dominant in human occupation and, on the whole, health and well-being seem to sit uneasily amid the rush and stresses of present-day occupational structures.

This raises the question of whether occupational structures, the social environment and political agendas which support these structures, provide people with opportunities for health-enhancing, balanced and stimulating use of physical, mental, and social capacities and whether the passion to continue developing technology, which is known to be to the detriment of the ecology, is also to the detriment of basic human needs.

John Maynard Keynes, the economist, in 1931 observed "*the struggle for subsistence, always has been hitherto the primary, most pressing problem of the human race....Thus we have been expressly evolved by nature.*" If this need is removed:

> "*mankind will be deprived of its traditional purpose....Thus for the first time since his creation man will be faced with his real, his permanent problem—how to use his freedom,... how to occupy the leisure, to live wisely and agreeably and well.... It is a fearful problem for the ordinary person, with no special talents, to occupy himself, especially if he no longer has roots in the soil or in the custom or in the beloved conventions of a traditional society.*"[38]

This suggests that if the human need to use cognitive capacities continues in the present direction without consideration of how basic biological needs for occupation can be met, health, well-being, and survival may well suffer. The human use of capacities has changed as occupation has changed and as technology builds upon technology. Human creativity has effectively changed "*manual work into machine work: machine work into paper work: paper work into electronic simulation of work, divorced progressively from any organic functions or human purposes, except those that further the power system.*"[39] This changed use of human energies and potentials via technology is primarily to meet production purposes rather than human needs. It is argued that the state of technology and the social structures which support it are not conducive to the maintenance of occupational balance for the majority of people, the result being boredom or burnout. Ironically, in part, boredom or burnout is caused by the drive for human creativity and cognitive capacity. In part it is also caused by the arbitrary dividing of occupation resulting from cultural evolutionary forces which makes it difficult to consider occupation from a holistic perspective. This impedes the conscious awareness of the need to balance mental, physical, and social occupations as integral aspects of health; to balance energy expenditure and rest; and social activity and solitude. Additionally, although affluent societies appear to have an abundance of occupational choices offering opportunity for the exercise and development of physical, mental, and social skills, the structures and values placed upon different aspects of occupation may well affect how successfully individuals access these opportunities. People may be restricted in their choice by many factors such as lack of time or material resources. They may be disadvantaged in comparison with early humans because they are not socialized into selecting occupations conducive to health. They may lack opportunity to provide for their own basic needs because changing occupational structures and technologies:

- Restrict freedom of action by ever-increasing rules and regulations,
- Replace ongoing human endeavor with technological labor-saving devices,

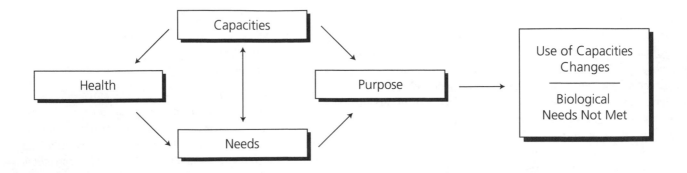

Figure 33.3. Capacities and needs are subjugated to external purpose.

- Reduce the availability of paid employment,
- Create an addictive way of life out of step with sustaining the ecology.

It is argued here that post-industrial societies have reached a stage in which the need to use human capacities is being overlooked. We are now creating a world in which what has been created by the capacities of humans appears more important than the balanced use of capacities. Use of capacities and needs are subjugated to external purpose which, for mankind in a natural state, was the motivation to use capacities. The purpose takes on a life form of its own and becomes a primary sociocultural need, such as the apparently overwhelming need at present for technology or money. The greater the need for the created rather than for the creating, the less health enhancing it becomes (Figure 33.3).

People need to make use of their capacities through engagement in individually motivating and ongoing occupations, and if they are able, or encouraged to pursue this need, they will, apart from supplying sustenance for survival and safety, enhance their health. As was possible prehistory, the total range of an individual's purposeful and fulfilling occupations can provide individuals with sufficient exercise to maintain homeostasis, to keep body parts and neuronal physiology and mental capacities functioning at peak efficiency, and enable maintenance and development of satisfying and stimulating social relationships. A range of occupations can provide balance among physical, mental, and social challenges and relaxation. This is part of the complex neural system aimed at maintenance of homeostasis, growth, and development because occupations act as a focus for integrating physical, mental, and social capacities.

Humans are occupational beings with a need to use time in a purposeful way. This need is innate and related to health and survival because it enables individuals to utilize their biological capacities and potential, and thereby flourish. Because of the adaptive capacity of the human brain the innate drive for purposeful occupation has been influenced over time by sociocultural forces and values which has added ever-increasing complexity to the relationship between biological needs and how people "spend their time."

This paper has proposed a theory of the primary functions of occupation and how they relate to health and survival, and it has proposed that sociocultural factors are deflecting occupation from its primary functions. It is desirable that following increased articulation and research into the possible consequences of the changes, political, social, and health policy can be influenced so that human rather than economic needs are central in future societies.

References

1. Leakey R, Lewin R. *People of the lake: man: his origins, nature, and future.* Penguin Books, 1978: 38–39.
2. Kolb B, Whishaw I Q. *Fundamentals of human neuropsychology.* 3rd ed. San Francisco: W H Freeman and Company, 1990: 106.
3. Lorenz K. *The waning of humaneness,* Munich: R Piper & Co Verlag, 1983. Translated USA: Little Brown and Company, 1987: 57–58.
4. Jerison H J. *Evolution of the brain and intelligence.* New York: Academic Press, 1973.
5. Marx K. The holy family. 1845: 125. In: Fischer E. *Marx in his own words.* London: Alien Lane The Penguin Press, 1970.
6. Marx K. Economic and philosophical manuscripts. 1843. In: Fischer E. *Marx in his own Words.* London: Alien Lane The Penguin Press, 1970: 31.
7. Marx K. Economic and philosophical Manuscripts. 1843. In: Fischer, E. *Marx in his own words.* London: Alien Lane The Penguin Press, 1970: 37.
8. Marx K. Capital 1.1867: 179–180. In Fischer E. *Marx in his own words.* London: Alien Lane The Penguin Press, 1970.
9. Braverman H. *Labor and monopoly capital: the deregulation of work in the twentieth century,* New York: Monthly Review Press, 1974.
10. Selye H, Monat A, Lazarus R S. *Stress and coping: an anthology.* 2nd ed. New York: Columbia University Press, 1985: 28.
11. Sigerist H E. *A history of medicine, Vol. 1,* primitive and archaic medicine. New York: Oxford University Press, 1955: 254–255.
12. Allport G W. The open system in personality theory. *Journal of abnormal and social psychology.* 1960, 61: 301–311.
13. Omstein R, Sobei D. *The healing brain: a radical new approach to health care.* London: MacMillan, 1988, p. 11–12.
14. Eysenck H S, Arnold W, Meili R. *Encyclopedia of psychology.* New York: Continuum Books The Seabury Press, 3979: 705–706.
15. Young P T. Drives. In: Sills D L, ed. *International encyclopedia of the social sciences.* The Macmillan Co & The Free Press. 1968: 275–276.
16. Dashiell J F. *Fundamentals of objective psychology.* Boston: Houghton Mifflin, 1928:233–234.
17. Lorenz K. *The waning of humaneness,* Munich: R Piper & Co Verlag, 1983. Translated USA: Little Brown and Company, 1987: 21.
18. Lorenz K. *Civilized man's eight deadly sins,* translated by M. Latzke. London: Methuen & Co Ltd, 1974: 3–5.
19. Wolman B, ed. *Dictionary of behavioral science.* New York: Van Nostand Reinold Co, 1973: 250.

20. Anscombe G E M. Modern moral philosophy. *Philosophy.* 1958: 33.

21. Watts E D. Human needs. In Kuper A, Kuper J, eds. *The social science encyclopedia.* London: Routledge, 1985.

22. Bertalanffy L von. *General systems theory.* New York: George Baziller. 1968. 27.

23. Campbell J. *Winston Churchill's afternoon nap.* London: Paladin, 1988: 79

24. Argyle M. *The psychology of happiness.* London: Methucn and Co Ltd, 1987.

25. Csikszentmihalyi M. *Flow: the psychology of optimal experience.* New York: Harper and Row, 1990.

26. Virey. *L'hygiene philosophique.* Paris: Crochard, 1828.

27. Stephenson W. *The ecological development of man.* Sydney: Angus and Robertson, 1972: 217.

28. Wharton W J L, ed. *Captain Cook's journal during his first voyage around the world made in HM Bark Endeavour, 1768–1777.* London: Eliot Stock, 1893: 323.

29. Lorenz K. *Civilized man's eight deadly sins,* translated by M. Latzke. London: Methuen & Co Ltd, 1974: 12–13.

30. King-Boyes M J E. *Patterns of aboriginal culture then and now.* Sydney: McGraw-Hill Book Company, 1977.

31. Maslow A H. *Toward a psychology of being.* 2nd ed. New York: D Van Nostrand Company, 1968.

32. Campbell J. *Winston Churchill's afternoon nap.* London: Paladin, 1988: 14.

33. Lorenz K. *The waning of humaneness.* Munich: R Piper & Co Verlag, 1983. Translated USA: Little Brown and Company, 1987: 124.

34. Lorenz K. *The waning of humaneness.* Munich: R Piper & Co Verlag, 1983. Translated USA: Little Brown and Company, 1987: 124.

35. Shils E. Sociology. 799–810. In Kuyper A, Kuyper J, eds. *The social science encyclopedia.* London & New York: Routledge, 1985: 805.

36. Cynkin S, Robinson A M. Occupational therapy and activities health: toward health through activities. Boston: Little Brown and Company, 1990.

37. Primeau L A, Clarke F, Pierce D. Occupational therapy alone has looked upon occupation: future applications of occupational science to pediatric occupational therapy. *Occupational therapy in health care.* New York: Haworth Press, 1989: 6 (4).

38. Keynes J M. Economic possibilities for our grandchildren. In *Essays in persuasion,* London: MacMillan, 1931.

39. Mufiiford L. *The condition of man.* London: Heinemann, 1944 and 1963.

Health and the Human Spirit for Occupation

CHAPTER 34

ELIZABETH J. YERXA, EdD, LHD (HON),
ScD (HON), OTR, FAOTA

Reilly's (1962) fundamental hypothesis "that man, through the use of his hands as energized by mind and will, can influence the state of his own health" (p. 2) proposes a significant relationship between engagement in activity, as dictated by the human spirit for occupation, and healthfulness (see Chapter 8). I shall explore that connection by describing my views of occupation and health, sharing some assumptions, reviewing relevant ideas from an array of disciplines, and drawing implications for occupational science and its application in occupational therapy.

This article is based on my continuous search for ideas from other disciplines, a synthesis of which may contribute to the scholarly foundations of occupational therapy (occupational science) and should therefore be seen as a work in progress.

Views of Occupation and Health

The human spirit for activity is actualized, in a healthy way, through engagement in occupation: self-initiated, self-directed activity that is productive for the person (even if the product is fun) and contributes to others. Occupations are organized into patterns or the "elemental routines that occupy people" (Beisser, 1989, p. 166). These activities of daily living (ADL) are categorized by our culture as play, work, rest, leisure, creative pursuits, and other ADL that enable us to adapt to environmental demands. Dewey's (1910) criteria for a child's occupation were that it be of interest, be intrinsically worthwhile (relevant personally and socially), awaken curiosity, and lead to development. Engagement in occupation enables humans to learn competency.

I shall view health, not as the absence of organ pathology, but as an encompassing, positive, dynamic state of "well-beingness," reflecting adaptability, a good quality of life, and satisfaction in one's own activities. Notice that this perspective of health does not exclude persons with disabilities. They may have irremediable impairments but still possess the potential to be healthy, for example, by developing and using skills to achieve their vital goals (Pörn, 1993).

What is the connection between engagement in occupation and health? This question is crucial for humankind in the new millennium, for the 21st century will certainly usher in an unprecedented "era of chronicity" due to advances in medicine's ability to preserve life. What is thought about how people, including those with chronic impairments, achieve healthfulness through the use of their hands, minds, and will?

Assumptions

I always urge my graduate students to make their assumptions explicit, so I have to follow my own advice:

1. I shall view people as complex, multileveled (biological, psychological, social, spiritual), open systems who interact with their environments (Kagan, 1996) by using occupation to make an adaptive response to its demands. Consequently, human beings cannot be reduced to a single level, say that of the motor system, and retain their richness or identity. Similarly, water cannot be reduced to hydrogen and oxygen and still be wet and drinkable.

This chapter was previously published in the American Journal of Occupational Therapy. 52, 412–418. Copyright © 1998, American Occupational Therapy Association.

2. The occupational therapy profession is founded on an optimistic view of human nature (Reilly, 1962). Occupational therapists discover a person's resources and emphasize what that person can or might be able to do instead of the person's incapacities; what's right instead of what's wrong. We are "search engines" for potential. Our profession is committed to improving life opportunities for all people, including those with so-called chronic impairments, a category that includes most of the persons we serve.

3. The postindustrial society is in danger of creating masses of throw-away people, a burgeoning underclass whose chronic impairments, homelessness, mental illness, and inadequate education and skills leave them outsiders in an increasingly technical, complex, and fast-paced society. In important respects, *most* of society, except for an elite superclass, may become an endangered species occupationally. As Beisser (1989) said when he lost the ability to work as a physician due to paralysis, "My place in the culture was gone" (p. 167). Similarly, for large segments of society, Rifkin (1995), an economist, predicted the "end of work." Work as we have known it may be replaced by a "technopoly" managed by an elite class who keeps the robots and computers operating, leaving millions without a job or a place in society. This endangerment to health and well-being is profound because our society lacks an agreed-upon, valued substitute for work. Because we often view work as an economic necessity rather than a biological, moral, and social imperative, we frequently fail to recognize the potential impact of unemployment and loss of occupational role on human health. The more than 70% of working-age persons with disabilities who are currently unemployed provides a window into the future (Bickenbach, 1993).

Relation of Engagement in Occupation to Health

Interests

Storr (1988), a British psychiatrist, proposed that our society has overvalued intimate relationships while paying too little attention to "work in solitude" as a source of health and happiness. Two opposing motives operate throughout life, one to bring us closer to people and another for autonomy. The second is as important as the first.

Creative persons classed among the world's great thinkers often lacked close personal ties. For example, Descartes, Newton, Kant, Nietzche, Kierkegaard, and Wittgenstein lived alone for most of their lives, finding their chief value in the "impersonal" (Storr, 1988). The impersonal includes *interest* in doing almost anything from breeding carrier pigeons to designing aircraft. Such interest contributes to the economy of human happiness by fulfilling the need for autonomy, leading to both adaptation and creativity.

Storr (1988) criticized psychiatry and the social sciences for overlooking the importance of pursuing interests to meaning, happiness, discovery, creative contribution, and the human search for some pattern that makes sense out of life. Such pursuits can be a matter of life and death. Acting on interests may prevent mental collapse and subsequent death for persons in states of extreme deprivation. The capacity to be alone while pursuing one's unique interests is a valuable health resource, fulfilling the need for autonomy and achieving personal integration through activity one believes is worth doing. Interests energize occupation.

Satisfaction in Everyday Doing

When I become discouraged by the high-tech, business-oriented, specialist trajectory of our culture, I read Adolph Meyer (1931/1957). He never fails to revitalize my enthusiastic respect for the idea of occupation. Meyer (1922/1977) (see Chapter 2) focused on the person's everyday doings and actual experiences as primary resources for health. Health was assessed by one's relative capacity for *satisfaction,* "doing and getting enough" in those cycles of activity and composure that mark the rhythms of life. Meyer's (1931/1957) formula for satisfaction included the components shown in Figure 34.1. His view of satisfaction and health suggests major concepts for investigation by occupational scientists. For example, *capacity* implies that people be viewed as individuals who have unique skills and resources; *opportunity* requires attention to environmental qualities such as novelty, affordances, attractors, and challenges that will stimulate activity; and *ambition* involves energizers of action such as interest, curiosity, will, desire, and personal perceptions of skills. In interaction, these contribute to satisfaction by influencing both performance (generating feedback) and mood (encompassing one's being).

Meyer (1931/1957) placed this dynamic relationship within a cultural context, showing that both other people's appreciation of what we do and our own expectations of ourselves contribute to satisfaction. The formula suggests that health may be influenced by discovering or developing new capacities, changing the environment, nurturing ambition, improving performance, and modifying mood, all in ways appreciated by one's culture and acceptable to oneself. Meyer (1922/1977) proposed that occupational therapists provide opportunities rather than prescriptions in the spirit of this formula (see Chapter 2).

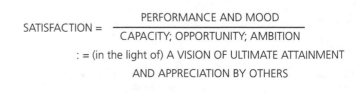

Figure 34.1. Formula for satisfaction (Meyer, 1931/1957, p. 81).

His formula applied to *all* people—physicians, psychiatric patients, and the public. Thus, health via satisfaction was possible for all, rather than requiring a special, separate track for those with psychopathology. Patients with mental illness were part of the mainstream of society, seeking the same satisfactions as anyone else, capable thereby of influencing their own health.

Meyer (1931/1957) saw potential everywhere; all people possessed assets and capacities: "A study and use of the assets, at the same time we attempt a direct correction of the ills, is the first important condition of a psychobiological therapy" (p. 157). But he was not blind to the challenge he posed: "To use the patient's assets is a more difficult problem than using something under our control" (p. 157). Capabilities discovered and nurtured could overcome psychiatric problems, which he viewed as problems of adaptation.

Meyer's (1931/1957) optimistic view of people emphasizing their resources, capabilities, habits, and skills that enable them to adapt to their environments with joy, satisfaction, and harmony places the spirit for occupation as central to human healthfulness. It is remarkable that his philosophy was applied in the early 1900s, long before the advent of psychotropic medications, because his patients must have exhibited severe symptoms rarely seen today. Yet he viewed even these persons as capable of healthy satisfaction through occupation.

Balance

Activity. Many theorists whose ideas are relevant to occupation and health propose the need for some sort of "healthy" balance. For example, Meyer (1922/1977) noted that people organize themselves in a kind of rhythm as they carry out their daily rounds of activity. To be healthy, people needed to be attuned to

> the larger rhythms of night and day, of sleep and waking hours, of hunger and its gratification and finally the big four—work and play and rest and sleep which our organism must be able to balance even under difficulty. (p. 641)

Meyer asserted that only by "actual doing" (p. 641) or performance could this balance be obtained. Consequently, all people needed to be provided with opportunities to work to achieve pleasure in their own achievement, and to learn a happy appreciation of time and the sacredness of the moment. This balance was learned through organizing one's own actions.

Pörn (1993), a contemporary philosopher, related health to people's ability to achieve their own goals through engagement in daily life activities and routines. He viewed people as acting subjects (not reacting objects). People, as actors, draw on three essentials: "a repertoire," an organized collection of abilities to act; an environment; and goals. Vital goals are personal objectives necessary for minimal happiness (p. 303). According to Pörn, health consists of achievement of a complex balance or equilibrium between people's environmental circumstances and the ability to realize their goals through a repertoire of abilities. Health is a kind of wholeness and general adaptedness that does not require freedom from pathology.

How could such healthfulness be assessed? We could look at the adequacy of one's repertoire (organized abilities to act), the appropriateness of one's environment (especially the opportunities it provides to exercise abilities), and the extent of realism in the person's goals in relation to both the environment and the repertoire.

How might health be fostered in a way that preserves and defends adaptation? This might be accomplished by addressing the repertoire (e.g., developing new skills for increased competence), the environment by its challenges, and the goals by helping the person alter his or her objectives. All three components need to be balanced for holistic care directed toward human agency.

Occupational therapists know this in their bones and hearts. In Sweden, they participated in research that validated Pörn's (1993) theory between persons with and without impairments. In this research, ability to achieve one's vital goals (via a repertoire of skills) was found to be more important to life satisfaction than degree of physical impairment among those with stroke (Bernspång, 1987).

Other theorists who have related balance to health include Csikszentmihalyi (1975), who posited the need for a balance between self-perceived skills and environmental demands, and Reilly (1962 [see Chapter 8], 1969, 1974), who related health to a balance between degree of environmental challenge and capacity for learning the skills, rules, and habits necessary to fulfill occupational role expectations. Offering a "just-right challenge" that enables an adaptive response promotes a crucial balance for health-promoting occupational therapy practice.

Information. Klapp (1986), a sociologist, proposed the need for another sort of balance concerning information and action. Today, health is threatened by the boredom that permeates postmodern life, creating a thick cloud over people's everyday experience. We feel trapped, satiated, habituated, and desensitized because we are bombarded by meaningless stimuli from the media, "noise" that requires no response. Listen to the monotonous, ever-urgent tones used by announcers and observe the sheer volume of noise created by the endless commercials and repetitious banality of the media. "Our ears are overwhelmed while we are denied a voice," Klapp observed (1986, p. 51). He defined information as "useful knowledge," contrasting it with "entropy" (p. 120), a tendency to randomness and confusion. When input does not arouse interest but continues relentlessly, people often escape into passivity or health-threatening "social placebos," such as alcohol, drugs, and other mood-altering addictions.

The desired balance that buffers boredom and contributes to health consists of "meaningful variety" that encourages learning and "meaningful redundancy," which is so familiar, reliable, and reassuring that it contributes to warm memories and a sense of community (Klapp, 1986, p. 118). (I think here of cultural rules and rituals.) People need to develop *skill* to respond to this overload of meaninglessness by learning to view their boredom as a signal for action. To be healthy, they need to be taught to create an individualized balance of meaningful variety and redundancy through discovering, developing, and acting on their own interests and by participating in the rules, habits, and rituals of their cultures.

Meyer's (1922/1977) vision of providing opportunities rather than prescriptions, contributing to performance and mood, offers occupation as an alternative to this health-threatening imbalance. Instead of escaping into unhealthy social placebos to alter their moods, people could learn to achieve their own balance of meaningful variety and meaningful ritual through engagement in activity worth doing (see Chapter 2).

Aristotle might have been right about the golden mean. Health as adaptation, satisfaction, and quality of life experience seems to require achievement of a desirable balance between environmental and personal attributes. Such a balance is highly individualized and is learned through opportunities to act on the environment as an agent. We need to learn much more about such healthy balances and how they might be fostered.

The Latent Consequences of Work

Recently a psychiatrist asked me, "Why is work so important to our patients? Why can't some other activity take its place?" Liebow's (1993) anthropological study of homeless women revealed their obsessive preoccupation with looking for and finding a job. Our own research with men who had spinal cord injuries found that they reserved the category of "work" almost exclusively for paid employment, even though they were engaged in many occupations that could have been called work (Yerxa & Baum, 1986). How is participation in the apparently significant occupation of work related to health as adaptation?

In technologically sophisticated societies, work is separated from other activities, such as leisure. Relationships that are largely based on work constitute a major source of societal structure and order (Argyle, 1987). Work appears to have a psychologically stabilizing effect on people. Leisure, to be satisfying in any important sense, needs to be viewed as the moral equivalent of work (Argyle, 1972) to fill its culturally significant role. People who are unemployed and have no organized leisure often become depressed, losing their sense of identify and purpose in life as well as their health.

Jahoda (1981) asked, why is work, as Marx observed, such a fundamental condition of human existence that people eat to work, not the other way around? She differentiated the "latent consequences" (p. 188) of work from its manifest outcome of earning a living. Latency meant the unintended but significant "by-products" of being employed (p. 188). Five latent consequences of employment seem relevant to health:

- Employment imposes a time structure on one's day.
- Employment implies regularly shared experiences and contacts with persons outside one's immediate family.
- Employment links persons to goals and purposes transcending their own.
- Employment defines important aspects of personal status and identity.
- Employment enforces activity, providing a predictable demand for action (Jahoda, 1981, p. 188).

Jahoda (1981) did not address the experience of "flow," that autotelic satisfaction in simply doing the work (Csikszentmihalyi, 1975), which is an important product for many people, nor did she discuss work's latent consequences for social units such as the family. However, her observations support the importance of work to health. Remove employment and you remove a person's strongest tie to reality (Freud, 1930), his or her place in the culture, threatening healthfulness. Work is supportive of health even under poor conditions. People may dislike their jobs, but they often dislike unemployment more (Argyle, 1987).

I still await the predicted utopia in which leisure becomes our major occupation. For leisure to be health promoting, it would have to convey the same latent consequences as work. Instead, the laboratory of unemployed persons with impairments and others who have lost their jobs due to corporate downsizing demonstrates the stubborn significance to health and quality of life of having work worth doing.

In many respects, the desire to engage in the occupation of work and its significance to human health and happiness are not fully appreciated until the opportunity to engage is taken away, whether by revolutionary social upheaval, as in today's postindustrial, increasingly automated society, or by the onset of impairment. Vash (1981), a woman who was severely paralyzed by polio as a teenager and later became a psychologist, put it this way: "The impact of disablement is largely contingent on the extent to which it interferes with what you are doing" (p. 15), not only the actual activities, but also the potential ones. Beisser (1989), who had been an ardent tennis player and medical student before he contracted polio, believed that "my place in the culture was gone" because he was no longer able to engage in the "elemental routines that occupy people" (pp. 166–167) and was disconnected from the familiar roles he had known in family, work, and sports. Yet the public, seeing Carolyn Vash and Arnold Beisser, would probably view inability to move as their most important characteristic, rendering them "disabled." Important though such impairment is, preoccupation with the loss of motor control blinds us to the significant loss of something important to do, the frustrated spirit for occupation, no longer served by their bodies, culture, or environment. Both of these articulate people believed that *this loss* was more important than their physical impairments. They echo Pörn's (1993) theory of health and Jahoda's (1981) latent consequences of work, revealing the connection between engagement in occupation and healthy adaptation.

Transcendence

The experiences of persons incarcerated under extreme conditions of deprivation and despair support the transcending effects of engagement in occupation that fosters survival and sanity (Storr, 1988). Frankl (1984), a psychiatrist who lived through Auschwitz, stated: "In the Nazi concentration camps, one could have witnessed that those who knew there was a task waiting for them to fulfill were most apt to survive" (p. 126). He reported that psychiatric investigations into Japanese, North Korean, and North Vietnamese prison camps reached the same conclusions.

The manuscript of Frankl's first book was confiscated when he was searched before incarceration. He felt this as a profound loss. His unfulfilled desire to rewrite the book not only helped him survive the rigors of camp life, but working on it, reconstructing the manuscript, and scribbling key words in shorthand on tiny scraps of paper, also enabled him to ward off attacks of delirium. Engagement in occupation, albeit mental, also enabled him to transcend his immediate disgust and despair. He visualized himself in a warm lecture room in front of an attractive audience. He was giving a lecture on the psychology of the concentration camp. By so doing, he rose above the suffering of the moment. Occupation enabled him to objectify and describe his oppressing situation from the "remote viewpoint of science" (Frankl, 1984, p. 95), transforming his emotions from despair into an interesting scientific study that he, himself, conducted.

Extreme environmental degradation reveals the potential transcending effects of occupation in stark clarity. People were more likely to survive such conditions when they had interests and tasks worth doing and were able to create transcending experiences that restored their sense of autonomy (Frankl, 1984).

Relevant Research on Occupation and Health

Hardy Personality

Kobasa (1982), an existentialist, believed that people construct a dynamic personality—"being in the world" (p. 6)—through their own actions. Because their life situations are always changing, they inevitably encounter stress. She asked, how do people confront unavoidable stresses and shape their lives successfully?

Her theory and research supported the idea of a "hardy personality" that resists stress and remains healthy. (In contrast to my definition, she defined health as lack of physical or psychiatric symptoms.) The three characteristics contributing to hardiness should interest occupational therapists:

- *Commitment*—"ability to believe in the value of who one is and what one is doing" (Kobasa, 1982, p. 6) involving oneself fully in life, including work, family, and social institutions. An overall sense of purpose, goals, and priorities acts as a buffer to stress.
- *Control*—"tendency to believe and act as *if* one can influence the course of events" (p. 7). Stress was viewed as a predictable consequence of one's own activity and subject to one's own direction.
- *Challenge*—a "belief that change rather than stability is the normative mode of life" (p. 7). Stress was viewed as an opportunity or incentive rather than as a threat. Hardy people search for new, interesting experiences and know where to turn for resources.

These three components contribute to "hardiness" or the ability to resist stress and maintain health. Kobasa hypothesized that when life is stressful, people with such hardiness would remain healthy. Her hypothesis was supported by research with male business executives, male general practice lawyers, and female medical outpatients in retrospective and prospective studies, using subjective and objective reports of illness indicators.

Kobasa's (1982) research connecting commitment, control, and challenge to hardiness in the face of stress supports the use of occupation as therapy to prepare people for engagement in the practical endeavors of everyday life. For if Meyer (1931/1957) was correct that people learn to achieve health in the doing, then such hardiness may be learned and developed through engagement in occupation. Gaining a sense of commitment in what one is doing, a sense of control over the course of events, and the seeking of challenges as a source of interest are products of one's adaptive responses to a "just-right" degree of challenge. In Kobasa's (1982) work, these products resisted the inevitable stressors of daily life and enabled people to maintain health. The most important piece missing from Kobasa's work is the *process* by which such characteristics are constructed by the person's actions in real life. I propose an important role for occupation.

Mortality

In today's world, engagement in some occupations is often trivialized, sometimes considered merely diversion. This view may reflect our ignorance of the contribution of engagement in occupation not only to health, but also to actual survival.

In an 11-year study of the long-term survival of persons with spinal cord injuries, Krause and Crewe (1991) compared the characteristics of those still alive with those known to have died. The researchers hypothesized that the survivors would have superior medical and psychosocial adjustment. "Medical adjustment" measured by nonroutine medical appointments and hospitalizations, was expected to be the *most important* predictor of survival. But neither recent medical history nor emotional adjustment predicted survival. Instead, strong support was found for a relationship between *activity level* and survival. Those who were more active, vocationally and socially, in participating in a round of daily occupations were more likely to have survived. Activity level was more important than medical history or a mediating emotional state. The authors, both psychologists, concluded that "counseling must go beyond facilitating emotional adjustment" (p. 84). Rather, people need to be taught the skills to participate in life, skills that might influence *survival* itself.

In another study (Wright, 1983), 100 patients with severe disabilities underwent rehabilitation in a hospital that encouraged their maximum participation. Patients designed their own schedules and solved problems as they arose. If a wheelchair needed repair, the patients worked out how to get it done. One year after discharge, these more "occupationally autonomous" patients not only showed a greater degree of sustained improvement in activities of daily living, but also a *lower mortality* rate than did the control group.

Both theory and research demonstrate that an environment that provides opportunities for active engagement in life contributes to health, well-being, independence, and survival. We need to take another look at the trivialization of occupation. What could be less trivial than survival?

Conclusions

An increasing body of knowledge from an array of disciplines supports Reilly's (1962) (see Chapter 8) great hypothesis. Humans can influence the state of their own health, provided that they are given the opportunity to develop the skills to do so. The human spirit for occupation, developed through eons of time in evolution, unfolding through development, and actualized through daily learning, needs to be nurtured to contribute to the health, quality of life, and survival of persons and society.

Occupational therapists and occupational scientists need to reaffirm that engagement in occupation, rather than being trivial, is an essential mediator of healthy adaptation and a vital source of joy and happiness in one's daily life. In the new millennium, the era of chronicity and the potential "end of work" as we have known it will pose particularly strenuous challenges: How can our profession help create an environment in which people have opportunities to engage in the "moral equivalent of work" and thus contribute to their own health? How can all people be provided with opportunities or "just-right challenges" to discover their interests and potential for something worth doing?

Occupational therapy could promote a new concept of health to replace the traditional view. Health, perceived as possession of a repertoire of skills enabling people to achieve their valued goals in their own environments, would then be possible for *all people,* including those with chronic impairments. A major objective would be to achieve "equality of capability" (Bickenbach, 1993). To do this, we need to learn much, much more about how human beings develop the adaptive skills, rules, and habits that enable competence as well as how occupational therapists might create a "just-right environmental challenge" to enable an adaptive response. Such "coaching" from occupational therapists could benefit all people who need to develop skills in order to survive, contribute, and achieve satisfaction in their daily life activities, whether or not they have impairments.

To serve humankind well requires that we discover much more knowledge about people as agents, in their own environments, engaged in daily occupations. We need to broaden our concept of ADL beyond self-care to include study of the daily routines that occupy people in real-life contexts. To learn what we need to know requires that we accept the challenge of becoming ardent students of life's daily activities, grappling courageously with the ambiguity and complexity of occupation, the occupational human, and the contexts in which occupation takes place. Only then will we fulfill our commitment to persons with chronic impairments and assure that our humanistic values are expressed in an occupational therapy practice that contributes to life opportunities and health for a new millennium.

Acknowledgments

A major portion of this article was presented as the Wilma West Lecture at the Ninth Occupational Science Symposium at the University of Southern California on April 12, 1996. It is respectfully dedicated to the memory of Wilma West, MA, OTR, FAOTA, who contributed so much of her spirit to occupational therapy.

References

Argyle, A. (1972). *The social psychology of work.* New York: Laplinger.

Argyle, M. (1987). *The psychology of happiness.* London: Methven.

Beisser, A. (1989). *Flying without wings: Personal reflections on being disabled.* New York: Doubleday.

Bernspång, B. (1987). *Consequences of stroke. Aspects of impairments disabilities and life satisfaction with special emphasis on perception and occupational therapy.* Unpublished medical dissertation, Umeå University, Umeå, Sweden.

Bickenbach, J. (1993). *Physical disability and social policy.* Toronto, Ontario: University of Toronto Press.

Csikszentmihalyi, M. (1975). *Beyond boredom and anxiety: The experience of play in work and games.* San Francisco: Jossey-Bass.

Dewey, J. (1910). *How we think.* Lexington, MA: Heath.

Frankl, V. (1984). *Man's search for meaning* (Rev. ed.). New York: Washington Square.

Freud, S. (1930). *Civilization and its discontents.* London: Hogarth.

Jahoda, M. (1981). Work, employment, and unemployment: Values, theories, and approaches in social research. *American Psychologist, 36,* 184–191.

Kagan, J. (1996, January 12). Point of view: The misleading abstractions of social scientists. *Chronicle of Higher Education, XLII,* p. A52.

Klapp, O. (1986). *Overload and boredom: Essays on the quality of life in the information society.* New York: Greenwood.

Kobasa, S. (1982). The hardy personality: Toward a social psychology of stress and health. In G. Sander & J. Sules (Eds.), *Social psychology of health and illness,* (pp. 3–32). Hillsdale, NJ: Erlbaum.

Krause, J. S., & Crewe, N. M. (1991). Prediction of long-term survival of persons with spinal cord injury: An 11-year prospective study. In M. Eisenberg & R. Glueckauf (Eds.), *Psychological aspects of disability* (pp. 76–84). New York: Springer.

Liebow, E. (1993). *Tell them who I am. The lives of homeless women.* New York: Penguin.

Meyer, A. (1957). *Psychobiology: A science of man.* Springfield, IL. Charles C. Thomas. Original work published 1931.

Meyer, A. (1977). The philosophy of occupation therapy. *American Journal of Occupational Therapy, 31,* 639–642. Original work published 1922. Reprinted as Chapter 2.

Pörn, I. (1993). Health and adaptedness. *Theoretical Medicine, 14,* 295–303.

Reilly, M. (1962). Occupational therapy can be one of the great ideas of 20th century medicine, 1961 Eleanor Clarke Slagle Lecture. *American Journal of Occupational Therapy, 16,* 1–9. Reprinted as Chapter 8.

Reilly, M. (1969). The educational process. *American Journal of Occupational Therapy, 23,* 299–307.

Reilly, M. (1974). *Play as exploratory learning.* Beverly Hills, CA: Sage.

Rifkin, J. (1995). *The end of work.* New York: Putnam.

Storr, A. (1988). *Solitude. A return to the self.* New York: Ballantine.

Vash, C. L. (1981). *The psychology of disability. Springer series on rehabilitation, 1.* New York: Springer.

Wright, B. (1983). *Physical disability: A psychosocial approach* (2nd ed.). New York: Harper & Row.

Yerxa, E. J., & Baum, S. (1986). Engagement in daily occupations and life satisfaction among people with spinal cord injuries. *Occupational Therapy Journal of Research, 6,* 271–283.

PART IV

The Therapeutic Relationship: Joining With the Person

Introduction

As Yerxa asserted in Chapter 34, our profession's humanistic values are needed to counter the hi-tech, business-oriented, specialist trajectory of our culture. The interrelationships among the therapist, the person, and occupation cannot be ignored. One cannot adequately understand the personal meaning of occupation if one has not developed a positive therapeutic relationship. The therapist may consider an occupation to be therapeutic and purposeful, yet the person may not be motivated to participate in its related activity (American Occupational Therapy Association [AOTA], 2002; Arnsten, 1990). As therapists, we do not apply activity, or "do" an activity "on" or "to" a person; rather, we do activity *with* a person, thereby facilitating a therapeutic relationship (Gilfoyle, 1980). A partnership and a mutual cooperation develop (Yerxa, 1980), enabling the therapist to use himself or herself therapeutically (Sachs & Labovitz, 1994). This partnership has historically and traditionally considered the art of occupational therapy practice (Gilfoyle, 1980; Mosey, 1996).

However, there are many forces that challenge our ability to practice this art. Shorter lengths of stay, reimbursement-driven practice, increased demands for productivity, and staff shortages are several of the trends that place pressure on occupational therapy practitioners to use mechanistic and technological techniques rather than humanistic and holistic approaches (Peloquin, 1994; Yerxa, 1980). Based on the realization of these challenges, the *Occupational Therapy Practice*

Framework places a strong emphasis on the use of a client-centered approach that facilitates the person's engagement in occupation. By its very nature, occupational engagement must be internally motivating, individually determined, and self-directed; therefore, the person's participation and a collaborative relationship are required (AOTA, 2002). It is hoped that the chapters in this part will provide a solid foundation for the recognition of the vital importance of forming therapeutic relationships, along with the necessary skills and tools for implementing this philosophy into practice. This appreciation and skill development is essential to keeping the art of practice in occupational therapy and for sustaining a client-centered approach.

Devereux begins this part with a thoughtful analysis of the caring relationship, which she presents as the basis for our profession's philosophy and practice. She emphasizes in Chapter 35 that the development of a caring relationship between the person and the practitioner reinforces the holistic approach of our field, enabling us to make a unique societal contribution by being a caring profession. Devereux explores the therapeutic relationship and discusses how to develop a caring relationship with individuals to assist them in reconnecting to occupations that are meaningful. Equally important is her analysis of how the practitioner can care for himself or herself to be able to enter into and maintain caring therapeutic relationships. She concludes with an exploration of how occupational therapy can maintain its caring focus in a complex and challenging health care system.

The benefits of forming therapeutic relationships are strongly identified by Devereaux. The efforts that must be made to deal with health care system constraints are clearly worthwhile. Her view that caring is an inherent part of the art of occupational therapy practice is strongly supported by the exploration of client-centered practice in Chapter 36. In this analysis, Law, Baptiste, and Mills define and discuss key concepts and issues related to the implementation of client-centered practice. The roots of the construct of client-centeredness are highlighted. Concepts of client-centered practice, including individual autonomy and choice, partnership, therapist and client responsibility, enablement, contextual congruence, accessibility, and respect for diversity, are examined from both a current collaborative perspective and the traditional therapist-directed perspective. These concepts provide a basis for the authors' definition of a client-centered practice and for the formation of key assumptions about this approach. Implications for occupational therapy practice and challenges to the implementation of a client-centered approach are realistically discussed. Two practice examples are used to illustrate client-centered concepts and assumptions and to raise consciousness about obstacles to the practice of client-centered occupational therapy. The authors review research about the efficacy of a client-centered approach in enhancing client satisfaction, increasing functional outcomes, and improving client participation in the occupational therapy process.

Law, Baptiste, and Mills conclude with a call for research on client-centered practices to increase our understanding of the effects of implementing approaches that promote the person's control of the occupational therapy process. The efficacy of client-centered practices based on a collaborative model versus therapist-directed practices based on a scientific model is analyzed in Mattingly's landmark study of the narrative clinical-reasoning process. The discussion of this research is presented in Chapter 37. Mattingly argues that a narrative model of reasoning is fundamental to the thinking of occupational therapy practitioners. Traditional scientific modes of reasoning are viewed as incongruent with the occupational therapy process because practitioners think with stories. This story thought process became evident during the American Occupational Therapy Association/ American Occupational Therapy Foundation's seminal clinical-reasoning study, which found that occupational therapy practitioners actively listen to the stories told to them by their clients and relate stories about the people they work with to others. Mattingly presents a compelling argument for the value of this storytelling process. Storytelling helps the practitioners understand an individual's uniquely personal experience of illness or disability. It also enables both practitioners and clients to make sense of this experience.

In addition to storytelling, Mattingly found that occupational therapy practitioners also create stories that allow the person to remake the story of his or her life now that it has been altered by an illness or disability experience. When occupational therapy practitioners create a prospective treatment story, they imagine the potentialities of the person's future. Mattingly terms this process "therapeutic emplotment," for this envisioned future guides the occupational therapy process. The power of narrative reasoning in helping practitioners make sense of the uniquely human experience of living with illness and disability and its effectiveness in helping us uncover different motiva-

tional possibilities to move people to act is strongly supported by a case example. The story of the development of the "NY Gang" is a stellar example of the power of client-centered practice based on narrative reasoning.

As Mattingly emphasized, a major aim of narrative reasoning is to ensure that the occupational therapy process proceeds in a manner that enables the person to successfully meet challenges and develop "increased confidence and commitment to take on challenges" as his or her story unfolds. This perceived self-efficacy contributes to the person's motivation to act and implement his or her story. As a result, the ability to engage in the occupational therapy process can be highly influenced by one's judgment of his or her capabilities. Simply put, a person is less likely to engage in an activity that is viewed as beyond his or her capacities. Therefore, occupational therapy practitioners must consider the person's perceived self-efficacy when planning and implementing occupational therapy intervention. Gage and Polatajko explore this construct of perceived self-efficacy in-depth in Chapter 38. They consider the effects of perceived self-efficacy on activity selection, engagement, and performance. Perceived self-efficacy's origin, history, definition, parameters, and relationship to self-esteem, behavior, treatment outcome, and psychological well-being are discussed in a comprehensive manner. A literature review highlights relevant research, and clinical examples support the impact of perceived self-efficacy on performance. Gage and Polatajko postulate that assessing and monitoring perceived self-efficacy and using activities that closely approximate community and similar real-life activities will result in better treatment outcomes and enhanced occupational performance. The benefits of considering perceived self-efficacy in occupational therapy assessment, treatment planning, and intervention implementation are clear. The authors challenge occupational therapy practitioners to identify and incorporate this construct into daily

practice. We can structure task experiences to be successful and provide a therapeutic relationship supportive of clients having a "real" voice about their treatment, thereby strengthening clients' perceived self-efficacy.

The need for occupational therapy practitioners to collaborate with those we work with and consider the uniqueness of each individual's experience is strongly supported in Chapter 39. In this thoughtful work, Gitlin, Corcoran, and Leinmiller-Eckhardt present an ethnographic framework for providing occupational therapy in the home—sensitive to the inner life of caregivers—enabling them to be active agents throughout the occupational therapy process. Their framework is founded on four key principles derived from ethnographic methodology. These include the identification of an informant, use of an insider approach, engagement in self-reflection, and interpretation of information. The authors clearly describe each of these terms and the principles that they reflect. Underlying strategies to use these principles are provided to foster an understanding of the personal meaning of caregiving and its unique provision in a family. Specific aspects of caregiving that can be viewed as problematic by family members are also explored. This enhanced understanding of the family perspective allows occupational therapy practitioners to develop services that reflect the unique individual needs of caregivers and that are congruent with and respectful of a family's values and belief system.

Gitlin, Corcoran, and Leinmiller-Eckhardt provide a series of excellent questions that are simple and straightforward, and yet the answers to these questions can provide a wealth of information about each family's unique caregiving experience and guide occupational therapy practitioners in the development and implementation of a family-centered plan. A case example clearly and realistically illustrates the ethnographic framework and the application of the provided questions to a home-based caregiving situation.

Although this example involves an older person, the use of these questions and the ethnographic framework is relevant to all caregiving experiences across the life span. Particularly relevant is this case's emphasis on the importance of using this framework to help identify and address potential ethical dilemmas. As the authors note, the caregiver (as the lay practitioner) has the decision control when there is a conflict in beliefs or priorities. They advocate that occupational therapy practitioners actively use reflexivity to continually examine their personal and professional values and beliefs and analyze how these interact with the family's values and beliefs to shape occupational therapy service delivery.

The power of beliefs to shape care and the client–therapist relationship is eloquently explored in Chapter 40 by Peloquin. She thoughtfully examines societal beliefs that shape the patient–therapist relationship and our ability to provide care. Peloquin explores the voices of people who have received occupational therapy services through the presentation of several stories that reflect caring practice and, unfortunately, numerous stories that reflect depersonalized practice. She examines three societal constructs that devalue caring and the formation of a therapeutic relationship. These constructs—an emphasis on the rationale fixing of the health care problem; over-reliance on methods and protocols; and a health care system driven by business, efficacy, and profit—are carefully analyzed by Peloquin and strongly substantiated by comprehensive narrative data. Her thoughtful and sensitive analysis of these societal constructs is invaluable to occupational therapy practitioners struggling to maintain a level of caring in the current health care delivery system, which is largely unsupportive of therapeutic caring.

The incongruence between occupational therapy, which values caring and person-directed interventions, and the medical model, which values scientific techniques and applied expertise, becomes glaring when one considers our society's emphasis on evidence-based practice. Many perceive that joining with the person to form a therapeutic relationship is not possible in an evidence-based practice environment. The view that evidence-based practice must only be objectively scientific (and not personally contextual) is strongly resisted in Chapter 41 by Lee and Mills. They contend that occupational therapy practitioners should not use definitions of evidence-based practice that have been put forth by experts in evidence-based medicine because these definitions identify research as the sole source of evidence. While Lee and Mills recognize the excellence of these definitions and the value of research, they argue that any definition of evidence-based practice used to guide occupational therapy practice must reflect the contextual nature of the occupational therapy process. As a result, the experiences, beliefs, values, and knowledge of the practitioner and client must be accepted as valuable sources of evidence and thereby included in the definition of evidence-based practice.

To support their assertion, the authors contrast the standardized procedures used in medicine with the highly contextual and dynamic nature of the occupational therapy process. Each discipline also views the role of the individual quite differently. Medicine places people receiving services in a passive-recipient role, while occupational therapy considers each person to be unique and equal in a collaborative therapeutic relationship. The implications of these differences are clear. Evidence-based practice in occupational therapy must recognize the variety of evidence brought by the person and practitioner to the clinical context. Lee and Mills review and critique classical views about methods of evidence, concluding that the methods of appraising belief can provide a unique classification for the different types of evidence that the therapeutic relationship brings to occupational therapy interventions. They provide thoughtful reflections on possible beliefs and perspectives of the person and practitioner that should be considered in evaluating the potential outcome of an occupational therapy intervention. They present an evidence matrix that summarizes the varieties of evidence methods and perspectives that should be considered during the occupational therapy process. An overview of the process of evidence-based clinical decision-making is provided in an illustration, with the authors emphasizing a dynamic approach to integrating evidence. Lee and Miller describe four strategies—intrusion, parsimony, consensual validation, and cross validation—that can be flexibly applied to a diversity of evidence, highlighting the continuous and often circular nature of evidence-based clinical decision-making.

While everyone may not agree with all of Lee's and Mill's assertions about evidence-based practice (see Chapter 60 for additional viewpoints on evidence-based practice as put forth in Holm's Eleanor Clarke Slagle Lecture), the issues that they raise about the core values and fundamental being of our profession in an evidence-based medical model context are worthy of much dialogue. Their emphasis on recognizing that all people bring their own uniqueness to the occupational therapy process, even when it is an evidence-based process, is a reality that cannot (and should not) be denied.

The importance of personal identity to the occupational therapy process is analyzed in great depth in Chapter 42. In this noteworthy Eleanor Clarke Slagle Lecture, Christiansen explores how people develop and express their personal identities. His thoughtful treatise asserts that occupation is the principal means through which each particular individual creates and maintains his or her own unique identity. Christiansen supports his assertion based on a review of theory and research from which he derived four key propositions about the human need to express a personal identity in a meaningful manner. These propositions—identity shapes and is shaped by interpersonal relationships, identity is linked to doing and these actions are interpreted in an interpersonal context, identity is a central component a person's life story and provides meaning for his or her everyday doings and life itself, and identity is essential for well-being and life satisfaction—are viewed as tentative due to the need for research on the construction and maintenance of identity.

However, Christiansen's discussion of each of these propositions provides useful reflections for occupational therapy practitioners to consider about identity throughout the occupational therapy process. His elaboration on the roots of identity—reflexive consciousness, interpersonal aspects of selfhood, and the agential aspects of the self—provide an additional framework for understanding the implications of identity for occupational therapy practice. The relationship among identity, people's life stories, how people make sense of these life stories, and how life experiences shape identities and create life meaning are explored. Christiansen proposes that identity is instrumental to social life because it gives the person a context that enables him or her to derive meaning from daily experiences and interpret his or her life story. He also proposes that identity provide a framework for goal-setting and motivation because the person can envision a future "possible self" that includes images in action. Christiansen further asserts that these thoughts of actions are influenced by social approval and competent performance, thereby shaping identity. Because engagement in occupations shapes identity, performance limitations, impairments, illnesses, participation restrictions, and disability can threaten the development of an identity based on competence. In addition, Christiansen contends that stigma and bodily disfigurement can hinder the development of identity because of the lack of social approval. Occupational therapy practitioners can help address the identity challenges faced by those we work with, enabling

them to maintain or reclaim an identity acceptable to self, based on occupational competence. Christiansen claims that the resulting identity will provide a sense of coherence and well-being for the person. What could be a better outcome for the occupational therapy process and the formation of a therapeutic relationship?

The health care system challenges identified by Devereux as beginning in the 1980s mushroomed in the 1990s. Our current era continues to present increased complexities. Therefore, occupational therapy practitioners must develop knowledge, skills, and attitudes for effectively dealing with these challenges (Fleming, 2001). It is hoped that the chapters in this section will provide a solid foundation for the recognition of the vital importance of forming therapeutic relationships, along with the necessary skills and tools for implementing this philosophy into practice. This appreciation and skill development is essential to keeping the art of practice in our profession and for sustaining a client-centered approach.

Questions to Consider

1. What are your personal values regarding caring? How does your culture view caring? How do these values influence your ability to formulate caring therapeutic relationships with others?
2. What are societal views of caring? What is the market value of caring? Does the fact that occupational therapy is a predominately female profession influence the profession's view of caring and society's view of the profession?
3. Given current health care system trends, how can occupational therapy practitioners maintain a focus on caring? How can practitioners create a humanizing environment in an often dehumanizing, medical-model health care system? How can you care for yourself in this demanding and evolving time in health care?

4. What are the potential external constraints on adopting a contextual definition of evidence-based practice? What are the benefits to our profession of broadening the definition of evidence-based practice to include beliefs, perspectives, and context? What are the potential ramifications of being considered less scientific in our evidence?
5. How can occupational therapy practitioners contribute to the formation and maintenance of a positive self-identity across the life span? How do practice-setting constraints, cultural values, and contextual issues (e.g., a school, the home, a skilled nursing facility) influence one's identity and the development of an identity based on occupational competence and social approval?

References

American Occupational Therapy Association. (2002). Occupational therapy practice framework: Domain and process. *American Journal of Occupational Therapy, 56,* 609–639. Reprinted as Appendix A.

Amsten, S. M. (1990). Intrinsic motivation. *American Journal of Occupational Therapy, 44,* 462–463.

Baum, G. M. (1980). Occupational therapists put care in the health-care system. *American Journal of Occupational Therapy, 34,* 505–516.

Gilfoyle, E. M. (1980). Caring: A philosophy of practice. *American Journal of Occupational Therapy, 34,* 517–521.

Fleming, V. (2001). Muriel Driver Memorial Lecture: Change: Creating our own reality. *Canadian Journal of Occupational Therapy, 68,* 208–215.

Mosey, A. C. (1996). *Psychosocial components of occupational therapy.* New York: Raven Press.

Peloquin, S. M. (1994). Occupational therapy as art and science: Should the older definition be reclaimed? *American Journal of Occupational Therapy, 48,* 1093–1096.

Sachs, O., & Labovitz, O. R. (1994). The caring occupational therapist: Scope of professional roles and boundaries. *American Journal of Occupational Therapy, 48,* 997–1005.

Yerxa, E. J. (1980). Occupational therapy's role in creating a future climate of caring. *American Journal of Occupational Therapy, 34,* 529–534.

Occupational Therapy's Challenge: The Caring Relationship

CHAPTER 35

ELIZABETH B. DEVEREAUX,
MSW, ACSW/L, OTR/L, FAOTA

Caring exists only in relation to something; caring simply does not exist alone or in a vacuum. Before caring can exist or be relevant, it must be in relation to a living organism, a thing, or a thought. The relationship object may be tangible or intangible, the person may be self or other, and the living organism may be animal or human.

Occupational therapists are concerned about caring. We talk about this concern and act on it. In this paper my initial focus is on developing a caring relationship with the patient; this is followed by a discussion of the need to care for self as an integral part of developing any caring relationship with another and of the elements of therapeutic relationships. Finally, our functioning as caring professionals within the context and constraints of today's health-care environment is explored.

Relationship With the Patient

We are all attracted to a health care profession because we are caring people. We value caring relationships, and the health-care arena provides the structure within which our natural feelings and skills can find expression. Of even greater importance is the fact that we chose occupational therapy as the profession within the total health-care field. Occupational therapy does not do to, or for, the patient, but it instead does with. Through our treatment, we facilitate the patient's doing for him- or herself. When we treat a patient, it is with the awareness of the person, first, and the person who may have problems, second (1, p. 787). All health-care practitioners recognize the pathology when they look at a patient; however, occupational therapists not only see the pathology and deal with it as a part of the treatment process, but we also recognize and focus on what is healthy about the individual. What is there to build on? What do we have to work with that can help this person learn, or relearn, the skills necessary to perform life tasks? We deal with the whole person, described by West (2) as "the mind-body-environment interrelationships activated through occupation." (p. 22) The concept of wholism is expressed eloquently in the report of the *Project to Identify the Philosophy of Occupational Therapy* (3).

> Embodiment or wholism is that perspective where mind and body are perceived as inextricably connected, integrated as one entity, in contrast to the dualistic perspective where mind and body are perceived as separate and hierarchically related entities (one entity superior to the other).... (p. 21)

To discuss a patient as "the kidney in room 319" or "the hand in the second treatment room" represents, to me, the height of dualism. Where and who are the people to whom these anatomic parts are vital? What right does anyone have to depersonalize them so? Ciardi (4) says, "If you don't really care, any reason is good enough." (p. 158) Menninger (5) and

Thomas (6) advised that physicians and health care providers should periodically become patients to experience, or reexperience, the patient role, to enhance sensitivity to what it's like to be a patient, and to see the effect of various provider behaviors on the patient's illness. Thomas said the following:

One of the hard things to teach, is what it feels like to be a patient ... (p. 222) being a patient is hard work ... (p. 223) The nearest thing to a personal education in illness is the grippe. It is almost all we have left in the way of on-the-job training.... (p. 221)

There is, of course, an emotional, or psychological, component to every physical illness. During the stress of illness, a person reverts to a dependent role, to the wish—the need—to be taken care of. The awareness of this wish sets up an inner struggle, a push–pull relationship, an ambivalence between dependence and independence. Not only do we want to be cared for, we also want to remain in control of (as much as possible) our lives and our relationships.

Patients sometimes resent both the need to be cared for and the people who fill the need. As caring professionals, it is our responsibility to know and understand the emotions of illness, to be sensitive to the many variations of these emotional manifestations in patient behavior, and to acknowledge this in empathic, yet therapeutic, responses as an integral part of our treatment. This is the essence of the holistic approach to treatment. Although we may know the complete history of the patient (e.g., employment, family, economic, interests, developmental, medical), if we do not in some way communicate to the patient our *understanding* of what his or her illness means to his or her life, our treatment reflects the dualistic mind–body dichotomy; thus, we are treating only "the kidney in room 319" or "the hand in the second treatment room." When patients know that we care enough to understand them as people, then we are contributing to their drive toward action (7), toward the reawakening of their drive for mastery of their environment. We then have helped patients to accept whatever level of dependency must be there for however long, and we have helped them reach for independence. This is an integral part of Reilly's (7) "nurturing of the spirit of man for action." (See Chapter 8.)

Several years ago a colleague and I were asked to consult with an occupational therapist working in a renal dialysis unit. This was the therapist's first job, and little about the role of occupational therapy treatment with renal dialysis patients had been published at that time. This pioneering therapist was questioning why she was there, her effectiveness, and whether she was actually "doing occupational therapy." She was particularly distressed about one patient, Charlotte (fictitious name), because Charlotte had been generally angry, hostile, and uncooperative, and was resistant to get involved in the discussion groups and other activities the therapist initiated. However, the therapist persisted in her attempts to engage

Charlotte, and eventually Charlotte's behavior changed a great deal; Charlotte was involved and pleasant, and she even seemed to enjoy the activities and talked with the therapist and the other patients. The therapist was pleased but puzzled with this change in Charlotte's behavior. My colleague and I talked with the therapist about issues such as when is help helpful, patient resistance, and the concept of each patient having his or her own timing. We then went to talk with Charlotte. Charlotte told us about her husband at home who was even more seriously ill than she. She was concerned that her dialysis treatment 3 days each week took her away from caring for him. She told us about their two sons: one who had died from the same type of kidney disease Charlotte had and the other who was recently diagnosed as having this same disease. Charlotte talked of her anger, her despair, her feeling of hopelessness and helplessness, her inability even to drive a car, and her dependency on others for the trips to the dialysis unit. Charlotte said that each time she came for treatment, it reinforced the losses in her life caused by the illness. [Let me point out two important points here: (a) that being compliant by coming to treatment can have a negative and a positive component for the patient, that this action (of coming for treatment) prevents the denial of the illness, and (b) that the use of occupation during the treatment period helps the patient avoid getting caught in the emotional flooding of feeling the losses resulting from the illness and then connecting them to all the losses in his or her life.] She said that everything was out of control in her life but that she kept coming to dialysis because she could not function without it. She said the therapist accepted her in spite of her anger; one day, Charlotte reluctantly started working on a needlepoint project offered to her by the therapist, and an amazing thing happened. Charlotte said, "As I got involved, suddenly, I realized that this little piece of needlepoint was the only place I had any control in my life, but that I did have control here! Then I started looking around to see what other little things I could control. I knew I could not control my illness or that of my son or husband, and I couldn't drive, but I could control my behavior and I could become a more pleasant person and I could try to get and give more pleasure out of my time here. And that's what occupational therapy has meant to me so far, and I'm still looking for other places for me to control."

The story of Charlotte introduces another situation: some patients are simply not very lovable. We therapists dread the next treatment session of these patients, and we feel guilty that we do not like them. These patients are often noncompliant with treatment but are constantly demanding, and we frequently feel the impulse to grab them by both shoulders and say, "Hold still while I help you!" The therapist's anger and resentment may result in his or her becoming noncompliant also, if he or she becomes noncaring. As contradictory as it may seem, some manipulative patients learn to be powerful within the context of the dependent patient role; they have few behaviors that permit dependence and cooperation, while maintaining a sense of independence and coping within the patient role. As in Charlotte's case, a patient's resistance is often stirred by the mixture of emotions surrounding the disruptions in his or her life caused by the illness, the feelings of fear, anger, powerlessness, and the despair of having no hope for the future. In this type of situation, it is generally possible for the therapist to get under or around the resistance by empathetically understanding and acknowledging what the patient is experiencing.

Patients have their own timing for change, and we can facilitate this change, not by pushing, but by being supportive while they become sensitive to and in touch with that timing. We need to acknowledge that we cannot care for every patient. We need to accept that we cannot turn our caring feelings on and off at will. It is sometimes possible to refer a patient that we dislike to another therapist who can feel more positively for the patient, but at times this possibility is not an option. Whatever the situation, our responsibility is to deliver the best professional care. This ". . . in itself, is a kind of caring." (8, p. 235)

The same colleague who participated in the renal dialysis consultation (B. Bennett) recently commented (in a discussion, March 1984) that she wondered if the importance of what we do lies in our awareness. In her view, occupational therapy allows for and promotes "connectedness." Our patients are human beings who have had some aspect of human functioning taken away from them. They have been deprived of the mechanisms for connectedness in some part of their relationships. Occupational therapy may invent connectedness where perhaps none existed or create opportunities for reconnecting the patient to other human beings and the environment. We reawaken the patient's capacity to care. Often the patients are unattached to people and institutions. Daily life activities are often the connectors among people; that is, the mechanisms of caring. Occupational therapists care by helping people disengage from despair and dysfunction and by helping them look forward, to see their loss as being able to be ameliorated through adaptation and occupation.

Occupational therapists are specialists in making caring happen. We know how to enrich all the transactions in the relationship with the patient. These become caring gestures. We augment the power of individuals to achieve their own objectives. In the same discussion mentioned earlier, Bennett continued that part of caring is knowing when to stop caring, to stop what she calls "emotional hemorrhaging"; walking the fine line between the two frequently becomes a balancing act. Finally, she added, when the structure of the treatment plan has been followed without the "spirit" of the plan, caring has been abandoned. (9) Caring implies quality of care and for us quality of life.

Occupational therapy is not the only caring profession. It demonstrates caring differently. To illustrate, a surgeon excised a malignant sarcoma from the hip joint of a middle-aged man and also removed about half the muscle tissue forming the buttocks on that side; the psychotherapist used family therapy to help the patient and his family deal with their fears of cancer, the changes in their lives, and the overwhelming feelings focused on his illness; the occupational therapist molded a special cushion allowing the patient to sit more comfortably while he drove a car and while he pursued his hobby of tinkering with cars. These "helpers" were all important to this patient, to his life, and to his quality of life. The occupational therapist's intervention was different in that it helped the patient reconnect to those occupations meaningful to him.

What is the market value of caring and who pays for it? Fromm (9) said, "... human energy and skill are without exchange value if there is no demand for them under existing market conditions." (9, pp. 70–71) In discussing employment settings for occupational therapists, Jantzen (10) said, "Caring for others and other altruistic motives seem to me rarely sufficient to generate dollars for salaries." (p. 72) The relationship between caring, *along with* the competence of the health care professional, and patient treatment compliance and its effect on malpractice litigation is well documented. Menninger (5) stated the following:

> ... more often than not, the breakdown has been in the "caring" aspect the physician–patient relationship—not in the quality of technical care and treatment provided ... Caring is an important aspect of health care quality. (p. 837)

He further advocated including an assessment of caring within the professional standards review.

So far, caring has not been a part of the professional standards review. I do not believe that it ever will be, because the quality of caring is difficult to measure. However, every patient knows whether or not it is present. The ability of the health professional to develop a caring relationship with patients falls within the art rather than the science of health care. I am convinced that a profession that consistently provides treatment giving patients a clear sense of having both their physical and psychological needs well tended and contributed to will not only survive, but will also experience an increase in the demand for their services. Occupational therapy is such a profession.

Relationships With Self

The emphasis so far has been on the patient and on the development of the caring relationship as an integral part of the treatment. The focus now shifts to another relationship: that which we have with ourselves. Is it a caring relationship?

> If I am not for myself, who will be?
> If I am for myself alone, what am I?
> If not now, when? (11, p. 237)

The meaning of these lines may be quite different for each person who hears them. Each individual's concept of self "... is composed of the thousands of perceptions varying in clarity, precision, and importance ..." gathered since birth (12). Our own perceptions screen every experience in our world and interpret that experience uniquely for each of us, thus constantly shaping our self-concept. "The most important single factor affecting behavior is the self-concept." (8, p. 39) What we do at every moment in our lives is a product of how we see ourselves and the situations we are in. While situations may change, the beliefs, values, and purposes we have about ourselves are ever-present factors in determining our behavior. "Freud defined the ego (or the self) as that part of the mind which is aware of reality, stores up experiences (in the memory), avoids excessively strong stimuli (through flight), deals with moderate stimuli (through adaptation), and causes changes in the external world to its own advantage (through activity)." (12, p. 86) The self is the star of every performance, the central figure in every act (8, p. 39). Therefore, we who are engaged in a helping profession need the broadest possible understanding of the nature, origins, and functions of the self-concept, not only for our own benefit but for that of our patients (8, pp. 6, 39).

The ability to develop caring relationships with others is in direct proportion to the ability to care for self. This caring for self is not an egocentric, narcissistic focus on self, but rather it is the sensitivity and knowledge of self that leads to personal growth. Just as Thomas (6) advocated a good case of the grippe to sensitize medical students to what it's like to be a patient (p. 222), I recommend that we occupational therapists perform an Activity Configuration on ourselves to gain a more objective view of how we use ourselves. How many "shoulds" have we grown up with that are no longer valid in our lives? Once when I was agonizing over whether or not to attend a meeting that I felt I "should" but did not really want to, a friend offered the perspective that "the world is not minimized by your lack of participation in it."

The process of helping others helps one's self: it is satisfying, therapeutic, and curative. There is an exhilaration in helping others that "is the result of something deeper than the power involved or the satisfaction of professional pride and a job well done." It is "the curative power of being human." The response of patients to genuine caring is enormous. It mobilizes "assets and self-curative resources on the part of a person being helped which too often he cannot tap on his own." Helping others increases our own self-esteem as we become aware of the strength and resources being mobilized for this effort and the power they activate in relationships (13, pp. 214–216).

Caring, for self and for others, "... orders other values around itself." (14, p. 51) A life that is ordered through caring has some telling features. It acquires a special kind of certain-ty, not a stewing need to feel certain and to seek guarantees. It is restful, yet dynamic, as opposed to static, giving security that retains vulnerability (14). "Such inclusive ordering requires giving up certain things and activities, and may thus be said to include an element of submission. But this submission, like the voluntary submission of the craftsman to his discipline and the requirements of his materials is basically liberating and affirming." (14, p. 53) Caring brings an order to our lives and relationships that frees our energy to be creative and productive, and provides parameters for our daily decisions. The energy thus freed, converted from negative to positive energy, has a direct effect on our productivity. Caring for self means choosing to attend to my needs first sometimes, not always second or third, because the less I give to me, the less I have to give to others.

We use relationships to define ourselves. As we look inward we see certain things about ourselves, but in the reflections from relationships we begin to see other facets of ourselves. Through relationships with our mothers, fathers, and others, we experience different levels of caring; our perceptions of that caring and how we use that information determine the kind of person we become. It is through this lifelong process that we learn to care for self and others. Our capacity to care and our ability to show we care are dependent on the kinds and quality of caring we receive. This is an ever-changing process for us, because once a word is spoken or an action has occurred, it becomes a part of our experience of the world. It is, in a psychic sense similar to the law of nature that for every action there is an equal and opposite reaction: we receive, we give; we give, we receive.

"One's actions are a part of one's existence" according to Pablo Casals (15). "... One feels it a duty to act, and whatever comes one does it—that's all—a very simple thing. I feel the capacity to care is the thing which gives life its deepest significance and meaning." (15, p. 156)

> If I am not for myself, who will be?
> If I am for myself alone, what am I?
> If not now, when? (11, p. 237)

The Elements of Therapeutic Relationships

It is self-evident that caring alone is not enough to establish an effective therapeutic relationship. Caring is the base; its presence enriches all other aspects of the relationship. The following are additional elements essential to the development of such a relationship:

1. *Competence.* We may be the most caring therapists in existence, but without the knowledge, skill, and ability to provide the needed treatment, we may develop only minimally therapeutic relationships. We have the responsibility to develop an ongoing continuing education program for ourselves. This personalized program should include studying the research being reported and

translating treatment efficacy into treatment effectiveness. It should include studying the literature of related fields and studying our own. Developing and maintaining competence is also a part of caring . . . for ourselves and for our patients.

2. *Belief in the dignity and worth of the individual.* This element is conveyed in mostly subtle ways. It involves believing in the integrity of the individual, including his or her need for mastery and control, which we must not violate, but preserve as important.

3. *Belief that each individual has the potential for change and growth.* The individual already has the capacity to adapt and grow. The occupational therapist provides a road map in a sense and facilitates the journey of adaptation through "occupation to improve health and performance." (16)

4. *Communication.* True communication involves listening, hearing the words and the feelings behind the words, making sensitive observations, and sending clear messages.

5. *Values.* Values are reflected in our beliefs. They are our standards for living, and provide stability and meaning in our lives and parameters for our behavior. Values are the foundations of our selectivity, for saying, "This is good, this I believe; that is not good, that is not the way I will go."

6. *Touch.* Rather than elaborating on the use of this powerful therapeutic element here, I urge you to read again Huss's 1976 Slagle Lecture (17, pp. 11–18).

7. *Sense of humor.* A judicious use of humor can do much to bypass resistance or defuse a tense situation. It can introduce perspective for both patient and therapist. And it promotes health. In the introduction to Cousins' book, Bernard Lown, Harvard professor of cardiology, quoted the famous 17th-century physician Thomas Sydenham: "The arrival of a good clown exercises more beneficial influence upon the health of a town than twenty asses laden with drugs." (18, p. 24)

These are some of the elements necessary to therapeutic relationships. Individual therapists can expand this list by adding important elements from their experience. Taken individually, these elements are splinter skills; used collectively, they enable and enhance the use of self as a therapeutic tool. These elements become a part of us and a part of the treatment process; and, rather than requiring extra time to include, most often they save time, because we and our patients are in synchrony, and our actions and reactions are mutually supportive of our goals.

These same elements are eminently transferable to our relationships with co-workers, whether lateral, hierarchical, or interdisciplinary. Before staff members can relate to patients in a humanistic way, they have to be dealt with that way. How difficult it is for staff members to create a humanizing environment for patients within a setting where staff are being dealt with in a dehumanizing manner. I have observed that it is difficult to increase or even maintain productivity in situations like this.

Relationships Within Today's Health-Care Environment

No discussion of relationships in health care today is complete without some mention of how these relationships are affected by the complexity of the health-care system. The push for productivity makes it necessary for us to cut costs of providing services and maintain larger caseloads. At the same time, we are being asked to increase documentation. All of these demands make it difficult for us to retain our motivation to develop relationships with our patients that go beyond a superficial level.

Additionally, we are experiencing the initial impact of the prospective payment system. Patients are leaving health facilities before their complete rehabilitation needs have been addressed. We are participating in a health-care system that, for the first time, views our service as a cost as opposed to something directed toward supporting human function. Our educational programs face enrollment problems and decreased federal funding. These are definitely challenging times.

Along with the thrust for increased productivity and accountability in the health-care arena, a new round of regulation has emerged. "Health care costs have been growing out of control and threaten to consume larger and larger shares of our national wealth. Even more perplexing is the fact that while we outspend other nations on health care we do not enjoy the best of health. We're clearly not getting our money's worth." (19, p. 6)

Not only is the federal government sending the message to the health-care system to do more, faster and better, with less, but also many states have enacted cost-containment legislation, and third-party payers are strictly following their criteria for reimbursement in the effort to control their risks. Now patients—the health-care consumers—are demanding more active participation in their own health care; that is, less dependence on and more accountability from their health-care providers. One of the fastest growing consumer groups is the 35,000-member People's Medical Society, which has been in existence for just 1 year but adds 1,000 members each week. This past January, the organization asked all the physicians of West Palm Beach to sign a 10-point Code of Practice, which would include fees posting, complete and open discussion of proposed treatment, and the physician's particular competency to perform that treatment. Charles Inlander, the organization's executive director, said that the Code of Practice "simply affirms basic patient rights. We're only asking doctors the same questions they ask their Mercedes dealer's service department—up-front costs, prognosis, and 'You can't go ahead and do anything until I give you my full approval.' The only difference is we're not asking for the parts back." (20, p. D-2)

The shifting relationships in today's health care environment are yet another phase of the action–reaction process that has its roots, at least in American medicine, in the beginning of this country. However, for our purposes, a few comments about the past decade will illustrate the pattern.

According to Starr (21), "Medicine, like many other American institutions, suffered a stunning loss of confidence in the 1970s!" (p. 379) Until then, the federal government had supported the beliefs that more medical services were needed and decisions regarding the delivery of these services should be made by the private medical sector. As costs continued to rise, but with no proportionate improvement in health care, government regulations and constraints increased as never before. This reaction was more than an economic one, because it included concern about the rights of patients, about the effectiveness of medical treatment, and about the moral values of medicine. Women, in particular, began to assume more responsibility for their own health, thereby diminishing the power, influence, and control of the medical profession (21, pp. 379, 380). It was no longer just a question of whether hospitalizations and surgery were necessary; rather, whether medical care made any difference in the health of the American people. "The nineteenth century doctrine of therapeutic nihilism—that existing drugs and therapies were useless—was revived in a new form. Now the net effectiveness of the medical system as a whole was [questioned]." (21, p. 408)

Starr's (21) comments indicate that the pendulum does swing—action, reaction—and that the "doctrine of therapeutic nihilism" (p. 408) appeared in both the 19th and 20th centuries, although in a different form the second time around. That pendulum will certainly swing again. While Starr's book focuses on the medical profession, we, as associates of that profession, must closely evaluate our capacity to address the effectiveness of our services and maintain the relationships that give us a position within the system itself. The turbulence within the health-care system today is but a reflection of the turbulence within society as it struggles to hold onto the old ways while also reaching to the new that are unknown. "One important characteristic to recognize is that if any one part of the system is changed, then all other parts within the system and any related system are changed as a result." (22, p. 800) Thus, the restructuring of society, from the changing profile of the labor force to the graying of America, affects the health care system. Those of us who are in the health care arena are scrambling to find our new place, to restore balance and security to our environment. In this competitive environment, it is important to do what we do well and maintain the relationships that will support our patients' needs, along with our own.

The greater the use of technology, the greater the depersonalization of the individual. Caring is the counterbalance:

the "high touch" human response to the introduction of "high tech." (23, p. 39) From its beginning, occupational therapy treatment has been inextricably involved with high touch. We have helped our patients to do, participate, work, and enjoy, despite their dysfunction. Baum (24) has stated that, "As a profession, occupational therapy harnesses will and gives the individual control through activity. That is human, that is care." (p. 515)

Summary

The constraints in today's health-care environment make it extremely difficult to do the job we've been trained to do. With the possible exception of continuing competency, the elements of a therapeutic relationship described earlier do not increase the cost of health care, do not require additional time in the treatment process, and give the patient a clear sense of having both his or her physical and psychological needs well tended and contributed to. As occupational therapists, we have superb skills for developing and tending caring relationships. Let us continue to use them well.

Acknowledgments

The author thanks Carolyn Baum, MA, OTR, FAOTA; Binni Bennett, MSW; and Wanda Ellis-Webb for their invaluable support and assistance.

References

1. Devereaux E: Community home health care—in the rural setting. In *Willard and Spackman's Occupational Therapy,* 6th edition, Hopkins and H Smith, Editors. Philadelphia: Lippincott, 1983, p. 787.
2. West W: A reaffirmed philosophy and practice of occupational therapy for the 1980s. *Am J Occup Ther 38*:22, 1984.
3. *Project to Identify the Philosophy of Occupational Therapy.* Rockville, MD: AOTA, Jan 1983, p. 21.
4. Ciardi J: In *Choose Life,* B Mandelbaum, Editor. New York: Random House, 1968, p. 158.
5. Menninger W: "Caring" as part of health care quality. *JAMA 234*:836–837, 1975.
6. Thomas L: *The Youngest Science: Notes of a Medicine-Watcher.* New York: Viking, 1983, pp. 220–223.
7. Reilly M: Occupational therapy can be one of the great ideas of 20th century medicine. *Am J Occup Ther 16*:1–9, 1962. Reprinted as Chapter 8.
8. Combs A, Avila D, Purkey W: *Helping Relationships: Basic Concept for the Helping Professions.* Boston; Allyn & Bacon, 1971, pp. 6, 39.
9. Fromm E: *The Art of Loving.* New York: Bantam Books, 1956, pp. 70–71.
10. Jantzen A: The current profile of occupational therapy and the future professional or vocational? In *Occupational Therapy: 2001 AD.* Rockville, MD: AOTA, 1978, p. 72.
11. Ethics of the fathers (chapt 1, verse 14). In *Choose Life,* B Mandelbaum, Editor. New York: Random House, 1968, p. 237.
12. Appelton W: *Fathers and Daughters.* New York: Doubleday, 1981, p. 86.
13. Rubin T: *Through My Own Eyes.* New York: Macmillan, 1982, pp. 214–216.
14. Mayeroff M: *On Caring.* New York: Perennial Library, Harper & Row, 1971.
15. Casals P: In *Choose Life,* B Mandelbaum, Editor. New York: Random House, 1968, p. 156.

16. Representative Assembly: Occupation as the common core of occupational therapy. In *Policies of the AOTA, Inc.* Rockville, MD: AOTA, 1979, #1.12.

17. Huss J: Touch with care or a caring touch? *Am J Occup Ther 31*:11–18, 1977.

18. Cousin: Introduction. In *The Healing Heart, Antidotes to Panic and Helplessness.* New York: Norton, 1983, p. 24.

19. Schneiderman L: The "Molting" of America's welfare system. In *NASW News.* Silver Spring, MD: National Association of Social Workers, Sept 1983, p. 6.

20. Peirce N: Citizen's group going after more medical accountability. In *The Herald Dispatch.* Huntington, WV: Gannett Feb 19, 1984, p. D-2.

21. Starr P: *The Social Transformation of American Medicine.* New York: Basic Books, 1982, pp. 379–380, 408.

22. Baum C, Devereaux E: A systems perspective—Conceptualizing and implementing occupational therapy in a complex environment. In *Willard and Spackman's Occupational Therapy,* 6th edition, Hopkins and Smith, Editors. Philadelphia: Lippincott, 1983, p. 800.

23. Naisbitt J: *Megatrends.* New York: Warner Books, 1982, p. 39.

24. Baum C: Occupational therapists put care in the health system. *Am J Occup Ther 34*:515, 1980.

CHAPTER 36

Client-Centered Practice: What Does It Mean and Does It Make a Difference?

MARY LAW, PHD, OT(C)
SUE BAPTISTE, MHSC, OT(C)
JENNIFER MILLS, BHSC, OT(C)

Occupational therapists in Canada were one of the first health professional groups to describe and endorse a model of client-centered practice (Canadian Association of Occupational Therapists & Department of National Health and Welfare, 1983). Throughout the development of a clear framework for the unique contribution of the discipline of occupational therapy in Canada, the concept of client-centeredness has been constant (CAOT, 1991; Law et al., 1990; Townsend, Brintnell, & Staisey, 1990). The development of a client-centered approach reflects changes wanted by consumers who desire more control in defining health issues as well as changes in how health is viewed. According to the Ottawa Charter for Health Promotion (World Health Organization, 1986), health is viewed as a "resource for living." The implications of these changes have led to increased emphasis on consumer rights and public participation in health issues.

Although the Guidelines for the Client-Centred Practice of Occupational Therapy have been widely distributed and used in Canada (Blain & Townsend, 1993), there has been little discussion about the concepts and issues inherent in client-centered practice. In fact, in researching the literature for this paper, a definition of client-centered practice—along with a description of its concepts and assumptions, was not found. Because of the lack of discussion about the meaning of client-centered practice, it is difficult for therapists to understand and implement these ideas in their practice.

The purpose of this paper is to define and discuss concepts and issues fundamental to client-centered practice. Concepts such as individual autonomy and choice, partnership, therapist and client responsibility, enablement, contextual congruence, accessibility, and respect for diversity will be examined. From these concepts, assumptions of client-centered practice emerge. The challenge of implementing the assumptions of client-centered practice on a day-to-day basis is illustrated through two occupational therapy practice examples. The paper concludes with a brief discussion of research evidence about the effectiveness of client-centered practice in enhancing client outcomes. The ideas raised in this paper should be of interest to occupational therapists in clinical practice, education, and research.

Client-Centeredness

The underpinnings of the construer of client-centeredness are found in original works of Carl Rogers just prior to World War II. Historically, the term *client-centered practice* first arose from Rogers in a book entitled *The Clinical Treatment of the Problem Child* (Rogers, 1939). Rogers recognized a number of key constructs of client-centeredness (1951). He emphasized the importance of cultural values, the dynamic nature of the therapist–client interaction, the need for a client to have an active role in approaching problems and concerns, and the need for openness and honesty within the clinical relationship (Rogers, 1951). The most important contributions of Rogers in articulating client-centered practice were the concept of listening and his discussion of the quality of therapist–client interactions. Growth of the client-centered movement continued into the mid-1960s with its main focus in utilization being within the discipline and practice of social work.

Though Rogers' interpretation of client-centered practice may be different from the occupational therapy interpretation, it is important to note from whence this term emerged. It was within the last two decades that the profession of occupational therapy in Canada articulated a congruence between the theoretical framework of occupational performance and the core value of client-centeredness (CAOT, 1991). In the development of these concepts for occupational therapy, the importance of the relationship between client and therapist reflects the contribution of Rogers' thinking. The initial version of the Guidelines for the Client-Centred Practice of Occupational Therapy (CAOT & DNHW, 1983) emphasized ideas about the worth of the individual and a holistic view of the individual. Ideas about client-centered practice have, however, evolved over time and now reflect the importance of client–therapist partnership, the rights of clients to make choices about occupations, the influence of a client's environment, and the need for intervention at a societal and policy level (Law, 1991; Polatajko, 1992; Townsend, 1993).

Concepts of Client-Centered Practice

There is increasing evidence that occupational therapists, as reflective practitioners, value a therapist–client relationship defined by trust, caring, and competence (Doble, 1988; Mattingly & Fleming, 1994; Peloquin, 1991). Client-centeredness is a philosophy of practice built on concepts that reflect changes in the attitudes and beliefs of clients and occupational therapists. There are a number of concepts which form the underpinnings of a client-centered approach.

Autonomy/Choice

It is recognized that each client is unique and brings that perspective to the occupational therapy experience (CAOT, 1991). Clients are experts about their occupational function. Only they can truly understand the experiences of their daily lives, express their needs, and make choices about their occupations. "The real experts on disability are the people who live with a disability" (Canadian Association of Independent Living Centers (CAILC), 1992, p. 58). Crabtree and Caron-Parker (1991) have suggested that Thomasma's freedoms—freedom from obstacles, to know one's options, to choose, to act, and to create new options—be the cornerstone of occupational therapy service.

Clients have the right to receive information to enable them to make decisions about occupational therapy services that will or will not effectively meet these needs. They expect that their opinions will be sought, their values will be respected, and that they will maintain their dignity and integrity throughout the therapy process (Polatajko, 1992). To enable this to occur, clients need to be provided with information in a format that is understandable and that will enable them to make decisions about their needs.

Partnership and Responsibility

Client-centered practice necessarily leads to a change in power so that clients have more say in defining the priorities of intervention and directing the intervention process (Kaplan, 1991;

Sumsion, 1993). In client-centered practice, the goal of the client–therapist relationship is an interdependent partnership to enable the solution of occupational performance issues and the achievement of client goals. Assessment and intervention reflect the client's visions and values, taking into account the roles that they have and the environments in which they live. In such a therapist–client relationship, power is defined as a process by which the client and the therapist achieve together what neither could achieve alone (Crabtree & Caron-Parker, 1991; Law, 1991).

With partnership comes responsibility. The responsibilities of the therapist and client, in this practice model, change from responsibilities as viewed within a medical model. Traditionally, therapists have taken an active role in the assessment and definition of occupational performance issues and the delineation of methods to resolve those concerns. In a client-centered practice, the client has a more active role in defining both the goals of intervention and the desired outcomes of intervention. The role of the therapist shifts to one of facilitator in working with the client to find the means to achieve those goals (Kaplan, 1991). Client and therapist become partners in the intervention process. Therapists' responsibilities include providing information which will enable client choice and utilizing their expertise to facilitate a broad range of solutions to occupational performance issues (Matheis-Kraft et al., 1990; Sokoly & Dokecki, 1992). Clients have a responsibility to be active participants in the therapy process, both in defining issues for therapy intervention and in facilitating the intervention process. Such a partnership leads to the therapist and client working together, questioning issues, trusting, and learning from each other throughout the therapy process.

Clients may choose to define problems or seek intervention which puts them at risk to themselves or at risk for failure. Therapists recognize that such risks are often valuable learning experiences, provided that the client is competent to understand the consequences of risks and the therapist is not supporting actions which are unethical, could lead to harm, or could be considered as malpractice. In client-centered practice, it is important that therapists discuss openly with clients if they believe that the course of action the clients are undertaking puts them at risk. There may be situations when a therapist is uncomfortable with a client's choice, more because of a difference in values than the fact that the client is not competent to make that choice. Therapists must clearly outline when they cannot support clients in pursuing an action plan.

Enablement

Occupational therapy practice in the past has focused largely on remediation of functional difficulties by facilitating change in individual performance components. A client-centered approach in which clients define the central issues for occupational therapy intervention supports a shift from a deficit model of intervention to an enablement model (Polatajko

1992). Within such a model, therapists work with clients to enable them to achieve occupational goals that they have set for themselves. The occupational therapy process can focus on prevention, remediation, development, or maintenance of occupational performance (CAOT, 1991). Achievement of these goals is facilitated through a variety of means, including changes in individual skills, changes in environments, and changes in occupations. All intervention alternatives are explored. In the therapy encounter, the process of providing services is important. There is a need for increased emphasis on the use of listening and emphasis on the use of language that is understood by clients and provision of information to facilitate client decision-making (Baxendale, 1993). Peloquin (1993) found that clients desire more than simply technical competence from therapists. Clients value the caring which is shown by therapists who truly listen and learn from their experiences.

Contextual Congruence

The importance of clients' roles, interests, environments, and culture are central to the occupational therapy process within client-centered practice. Occupational therapy assessment and intervention using a client-centered approach places importance on the individualization of assessment and intervention (Dunn, 1993; Law, 1991; Law, Baptiste, et al., 1994). Consideration of the context in which a client lives demands a flexibility in the approach of the therapist in all intervention situations (Dunn et al., 1994) (see Chapter 17. For example, the use of a set protocol of assessments and intervention for diagnostically defined types of clients is not supported within client-centered practice. Research about assessment has also indicated that results depend on the environment in which the assessment occurs (Park, Fisher, & Velozo, 1993). In practice, there may be situations where therapists use different levels of client-centeredness, depending on the nature of the intervention and the needs of the client. One of the most challenging dimensions of client-centered practice is "how to adjust consultation style to the needs of the moment" (Moorhead & Winefield, 1991, p. 345). It is also important to note that a client of occupational therapy may not always be an individual. Clients can include other family members or can be communities, private companies, or organizations.

Accessibility and Flexibility

In client-centered practice, services are provided to clients in a timely and accessible manner. Services are constructed to meet the needs of the client, rather than the client fitting into a service model. A client-centered approach to practice is flexible and dynamic, with an emphasis on learning and problem solving. •Therapists work to enable clients to access services with a minimum of bureaucratic red tape.• The successful client-centered therapist exhibits an openness and honesty within the client–therapist relationship. This includes the pro-

vision of a welcoming service with attention paid to such details as parking, waiting lists, information brochures, and ongoing therapy procedures.

Respect for Diversity

Intervention based on clients' visions and values demonstrates a respect for the diversity of values that clients hold. It is important for therapists to recognize their own values and not impose these values on clients. What may seem to be an irrational choice by a client is often exactly what is right for that person at that time, based on all the information they have about their lives and values (Kaplan, 1991). The strengths and resources that a client brings to an occupational therapy encounter are recognized and used to facilitate the achievement of occupational performance goals. The client-centered approach recognizes that differences in values and opinions will occur, but supports a mediation approach to the resolution of these conflicts.

Definition and Assumptions of Client-Centered Practice in Occupational Therapy

One of the difficulties in discussing client-centered practice in occupational therapy has been the lack of a definition of client-centered practice. Using the concepts discussed in the previous section, a definition of client-centered practice in occupational therapy was developed.•**Client-centered practice is an approach to providing occupational therapy, which embraces a philosophy of respect for, and partnership with, people receiving services. Client-centered practice recognizes the autonomy of individuals, the need for client choice in making decisions about occupational needs, the strengths clients bring to a therapy encounter, the benefits of client–therapist partnership, and the need to ensure that services are accessible and fit the context in which a client lives.**•"The goal of the [client] centered philosophy is to create a caring, dignified and empowering environment in which clients truly direct the course of their care and call upon their inner resources to speed the healing process" (Matheis-Kraft, George, Olinger, & York, 1990, p. 128).

From the concepts and definition of client-centered practice, assumptions about practice can be developed. These assumptions can be used to guide the structure and process of occupational therapy practice as well as research directed at exploring the effects of a client-centered practice philosophy. They include:

- Occupational therapists using a client-centered approach recognize that clients and families are all different and unique and they know themselves best (King, Rosenbaum, Law, King, & Evans, 1994).

- Optimal client outcomes occur when clients and therapists work in partnership throughout the therapy process and focus on the resolution of client-defined occupational performance issues.

- Provision of information to clients about their occupational function will enable them to make choices about what services they need and the desired outcome.
- Optimal client outcomes occurs when occupational therapy services consider the environment and roles important to each client.

Implications for Occupational Therapy Practice

The concepts and assumptions of client-centered practice raise a number of client–therapist partnership issues that must be addressed. These include 1) defining the nature of the presenting occupational issues; 2) discussing and deciding on the need for intervention and the desired outcome; and 3) deciding the focus of occupational therapy intervention. In addressing these issues, it is important for therapists to determine who the client is, to respect the client's value system and culture, to facilitate the client in setting occupational goals, to provide education and information to facilitate personal choices and problem solving, and to use their skills to help the client achieve their occupational performance goals.

Because client-centered practice suggests a particular philosophical approach, it is difficult to list specific implications for practice. The challenges of basing intervention on priorities and client choice, increasing client participation in program planning, allowing clients to succeed but also to risk and to fail, changing therapist roles to enable facilitation, and broadening the focus of intervention are all critical challenges to be met and resolved. These ideas may not mean changing one's clinical practice entirely, as occupational therapists have always supported a holistic approach to practice. However, client-centered practice needs to be more clearly articulated in our day-to-day clinical activities and in how we approach interactions with clients.

Differences between a more traditional and a client-centered approach begin from the initial contact. In a recent survey, Neistadt (1995) found that the majority of occupational therapists use very informal methods to determine client priorities. In client-centered practice, considerable thought should go into how an occupational therapy encounter begins. For example, key questions (listed below) could be used by therapists to analyze the nature of this aspect of practice.

- How much power does the client have at initial contact?
- How much time is spent discussing the client's values and goals?
- How much of the occupational therapy assessment focuses on performance components compared to occupational performance issues?
- How much of the assessment process uses standardized assessment procedures as compared to procedures tailored to the needs of the client?
- Is the client aware of the system within which they are receiving service?

- Is the occupational therapy intervention plan addressing the roles and environments that are relevant to the client?
- Are educational materials tailored to the relevant needs of the client?

The following examples illustrate some of the key concepts and assumptions of client-centered practice as used within two occupational therapy clinical encounters.

Example 1

Mr. S. was a 76-year-old man who was admitted to an acute inpatient medical floor because of severe dehydration. Mr. S. was found at home, unable to get out of bed, incontinent, and unable to manage any aspect of personal care. His spouse had a history of moderately advanced dementia, and did not pursue medical attention until there was severe physical deterioration Occupational therapy was requested because of his dependence in basic activities of daily living. In therapy, Mr. S.'s main objective was to get well enough to return home. The occupational therapist worked with the client to facilitate a return to independence in self-care skills. Eventually, he was able to perform all aspects of personal care independently. After this stage of successful rehabilitation, the client had many options and choices to make regarding discharge from the hospital. Psychological assessment found Mr. S. to be competent to make his own decisions. The occupational therapist provided information regarding the risks and consequences of returning to his previous living arrangement. With this knowledge, Mr. S. made an informed decision to return to a home environment that was placing him at a fairly high safety risk, with minimal community supports accepted by his wife.

This case study highlights the concepts of autonomy/personal choice, client responsibility for goal setting, and respect for diversity of the client. It is an example of a situation that involved a client making an apparently irrational choice, but a decision that was accepted as right for him at that time. The degree of client-centeredness evolved throughout the therapy process. As Mr. S.'s acute medical crisis stabilized, he was able to assume more control for directing his therapy goals and interventions.

Example 2

Mrs. R. was a 39-year-old woman diagnosed with fibromyalgia. The home care occupational therapist was requested to assist with management of daily activities. Initial assessment found that, Mrs. R. had severe pain in the arms, neck, back, and legs; stiffness limiting range of motion; chronic fatigue; and problems sleeping. In addition, other concerns included being a single mother of two young boys, geographic isolation, recent marriage separation, and financial difficulties.

To identify and prioritize problems and goals, the Canadian Occupational Performance Measure was administered (Law et al., 1994). The occupational performance problems identified were sleeping discomfort, preparing meals, use of toilet and bathing, playing with children, and pursuing meaningful roles outside the home. The process of setting occupational performance goals was challenging for Mrs. R., as she was quite focused on her individual physical problems. The use of the COPM, a client-centered assessment focusing on occupational performance areas, facilitated a shift in the therapy process from a deficit model to an enablement model of goal setting and intervention. The client-centered assessment process allowed subsequent intervention and education to be focussed on client priorities throughout the therapy process. This helped to ensure that these sessions were meaningful, and it allowed the client to assume responsibility for developing solutions which fit her lifestyle. Using the COPM also gave the client an indication of progress as the scores on the measure changed from 2.2 and 2.4 for performance and satisfaction to 5.2 and 4.9 after intervention.

Intervention involved providing education regarding the modification of her physical environment, implementing energy conservation and relaxation strategies, and counseling regarding a paced approach to resuming meaningful roles. By focusing on the potential functional outcomes, Mrs. R. was able to identify the need to implement changes in her lifestyle. For example, she decided that a scooter was acceptable because of the freedom it allowed for outings with her children. After this, the occupational therapist was able to provide her with practical methods of accessing a scooter for her regular use.

Central to this therapeutic process were the client-centered concepts of autonomy, personal control, partnership, responsibility, and enablement. The client-therapist relationship fostered skills in self-management for use by Mrs. R. in the present and for the future.

Challenges to Implementation

It must be recognized that working in a client-centered model of practice is challenging and complex. The therapist must be aware of obstacles that exist in the therapy process which may hinder the implementation of client-centered principles. Obstacles may arise from various sources, including the client, the therapist, and the organization.

Clients themselves may present barriers that alter the extent to which the therapy can be client-centered. For example, if a client does not have well-developed problem-solving skills, the therapist may have to be more directive than with other clients. As well, some clients may be reluctant to assume responsibility for their care. This creates an obvious challenge to the therapist, and challenges the therapist to act

as a mediator to ensure that these issues are discussed and to work for potential solutions.

The therapist may also be the source of some obstacles toward client-centered practice. The process of giving more power/control to the client threatens the traditional view of the therapist as expert, and may elicit feelings of discomfort. In addition, separating personal and professional values from client values can be a challenge, especially when the client is making a decision that appears to entail unnecessary risk. One must be careful that the client-centered approach is not used to absolve therapists or the system of responsibility for providing excellent quality of service. If a client chooses not to adhere to recommendations, it is easy to assume that it is because the client is noncompliant. This may be the case, but it is important for the therapist to reflect back on the process and identify any barriers which may have prevented adherence. For example, did the client understand the rationale for such recommendations, any risks from nonadherence to them, and any other options which were available?

The third source of barriers may be at the organization or systems level. For example, in a program setting dominated by the medical model, it may be difficult to implement some concepts of client-centered practice such as autonomy, responsibility, and enablement. It may also be difficult to determine who is the primary client: the referred person, family, school, insurance company, hospital, or industry.

The obstacles will vary depending on the clinical setting, and the personal characteristics of the client and therapist involved. This discussion has highlighted only a few examples that may occur. It is important to be aware of the potential barriers to client-centered practice, so that they can be foreseen, identified, and solutions created.

Does Client-Centered Practice Make a Difference?

While occupational therapists may be comfortable with and support the philosophy of client-centered practice, it is important to determine whether the concepts and values inherent in client-centered practice make a difference, both in the service provision process and in client outcomes. A review of the occupational therapy literature yielded very few studies examining the effect of client-centered practice, so the review was expanded to examine studies in other disciplines as well.

Research findings indicate that providing respectful and supportive services, an aspect of client-centered practice, leads to improved client satisfaction and adherence to health service programs (Greenfield, Kaplan, & Ware, 1985; Hall, Roter, & Katz, 1988; Wasserman, Inui, Barriatua, Carter, & Lippincott, 1984). In a review of the service process, King, King, and Rosenbaum (1994) found that there is evidence that respectful and supportive treatment, information exchange, and practices enabling client professional partnerships are all significantly associated with increased client satisfaction.

Provision of information to clients to enable client decision-making has been shown to lead to both improved functional outcome and improved client satisfaction. In studies involving clients with diabetes or peptic ulcer disease, Greenfield, Kaplan, and Ware (1985) evaluated the effect of providing client education. Clients were randomized into two groups, an experimental group which received a 20-minute educational intervention about how to read their medical charts and ask for pertinent information, and another group receiving a standard education program. Clients receiving the experimental intervention were more satisfied with their services and had improved functional outcomes one month later. Moxley-Haegert and Serbin (1983), in a clinical trial comparing parent education about developmental issues to parent education about general parenting or a control group, found that parents who received developmental education were more able, after one year, to identify key issues related to their child's development and had increased adherence to service program suggestions. As well, children of parents who had received developmental education had improved developmental outcomes after one year.

Development of a client–therapist partnership has been demonstrated to lead to increased client participation, increased client self-efficacy, and improved satisfaction with service (Dunst, Trivette, Boyd, & Brookfield, 1994; Greenfield, Kaplan, & Ware, 1985). An individualized flexible approach to occupational therapy intervention, where the client defines goals which then become the focus of intervention, has been shown to lead to improved occupational performance outcome and improved satisfaction (Law, Polatjko, et al., 1994; Sanford, Law, Swanson, & Guyatt, 1994).

Conclusion

Client-centered practice is an approach to therapy that supports a respectful partnership between therapists and clients. It is the philosophical basis for the national occupational therapy guidelines published by the Canadian Association of Occupational Therapists (CAOT, 1991). Although client-centered practice is evident throughout the history of occupational therapy, its significance and implications for practice are only recently being explored in the occupational therapy literature and research. More research to understand the effect of promoting personal control and enablement through a client-centered approach is needed. It is important that the meaning and application of client-centered practice continues to be developed. The term client-centered is popular in many areas of health service, but using the term does not necessarily translate into a truly client-centered practice. As health care policy becomes influenced more by consumers, it is an opportune time for occupational therapists to integrate the concepts of client-centered practice into program planning and intervention.

References

Abramson, J.S. (1990). Enhancing patient participation: Clinical strategies in the discharge planning process. *Social Work in Health Care, 14*, 53–71.

Baxendale, B. (1993, June). *Being a patient...becoming a person*. Paper presented at the Canadian Association of Occupational Therapists Conference, Regina, SK.

Blain, J., & Townsend, E. (1933). Occupational therapy guidelines for client-centered practice: Impact study findings. *Canadian Journal of Occupational Therapy, 60*, 271–285.

Canadian Association of Independent Living Centres. (1992). Research as an empowerment process for the Independent Living movement. *Abilities, Fall-winter*, 58–59.

Canadian Association of Occupational Therapists. (1991). *Occupational therapy guidelines for client-centered practice*. Toronto, ON: CAOT Publications ACE.

Canadian Association of Occupational Therapists & Department of National Health and Welfare. (1983). *Guidelines for the client-centered practice of occupational therapy* (H39–33/1983E). Ottawa, ON: Department of National Health and Welfare.

Crabtree, J.L., & Caron-Parker, L.M. (1991). Long-term care of the aged: Ethical dilemmas and solutions. *American Journal of Occupational Therapy, 45*, 607–612.

Doble, S. (1988). Intrinsic motivation and clinical practice: The key to understanding the unmotivated client. *Canadian Journal of Occupational Therapy, 55*, 75–60.

Dunn, W., Brown, C., & McGuigan, A. (1934). The ecology of human performance: A framework for considering the effect of context. *American Journal of Occupational Therapy, 48*, 595–607. Reprinted as Chapter 17.

Dunst, C.J., Trivette, C.M., Boyd, K., & Brookfield, J. (1994). Help-giving practices and the self-efficacy appraisals of parents. In C.J. Dunst, C.M. Trivette, & A.G. Deal (Eds.), *Supporting and strengthening families (Vol. 1): Methods, strategies and practices*. Cambridge, MA: Brookline Books.

Greenfield, S., Kaplan, S.H., & Ware, J.E. (1985). Expanding patient involvement in care: Effects on patient outcomes. *Annals of Internal Medicine, 102*, 520–528.

Hall, J.A., Poter, D.L., & Katz, N.R. (1988). Meta-analysis of correlates of provider behavior in medical encounters. *Medical Care, 26*, 657–675.

Kaplan, R.M. (1991). Health-related quality of life in patient decision-making. *Journal of Social Issues, 47*, 69–30.

King, G., Rosenbaum, P., Law, M., King, S., & Evans, J. (1994). *A framework for family-centered service*. Hamilton, ON: McMaster University, Neurodevelopmental Clinical Research Unit.

King, G., King, S., & Rosenbaum, P. (1994). *Interpersonal aspects of caregiving and client satisfaction, adherence, and stress: A review of the medical and rehabilitation literature*. Hamilton: McMaster University, ON, Neurodevelopmental Clinical Research Unit.

Law, M., Baptiste, S., McColl, M., Opzoomer, A., Polatajko, H., & Pollock, N. (1990). The Canadian Occupational Performance Measure: An outcome measurement protocol for occupational therapy. *Canadian Journal of Occupational Therapy, 57*, 82–87.

Law, M. (1991). The environment: A focus for occupational therapy. *Canadian Journal of Occupational Therapy, 58*, 171–179.

Law, M., Baptiste, S., Carswell, A., McColl, M.A., Polatajko, H., & Pollock, N. (1994). *Canadian Occupational Performance Measure Manual* (2nd edition). Toronto, ON: CAOT Publications: ACE.

Law, M., Polatajko, H., Pollock, N., Carswell, A., Baptiste, S., & McColl, M. (1994). The Canadian Occupational Performance Measure: Results of pilot testing. *Canadian Journal of Occupational Therapy, 61*, 191–197.

Matheis-Kraft, C., George, S., Olinger, M.J., & York, L. (1990). Patient-driven healthcare works. *Nursing Management, 21,* 124–128.

Mattingly, C., & Fleming, M.H. (1994). *Clinical reasoning: Forms of inquiry in a therapeutic process.* Phiiadelphia: F.A. Davis.

Moorhead. K., & Winefield, H. (1991). Teaching counseling skills to fourth-year medical students: A dilemma concerning goals. *Family Practice, 8,* 343–346.

Moxley-Haegert, L., & Serbin, L.A. (1983). Developmental education for parents of delayed infants: Effects on parental motivation and children's development. *Child Development, 54,* 1324–1331.

Neistadt, M.E. (1995). Methods of assessing clients' priorities: A survey of adult physical dysfunction settings. *American Journal of Occupational Therapy, 49,* 428–436.

Park, S., Fisher, A.C., & Velozo, C.A. (1993). Using the Assessment of Motor and Process Skills to compare performance between home and clinical settings. *American Journal of Occupational Therapy, 48,* 697–709.

Peloquin, S.M. (1991). Time as a commodity: Reflections and implications. *American Journal of Occupational Therapy, 45,* 147–154.

Polatajko, H. J. (1992). Naming and framing occupational therapy: A lecture dedicated to the life of Nancy B. *Canadian Journal of Occupational Therapy,* 59, 189–200.

Rogers, C. R. (1939). *The critical treatment of the problem child.* Boston: Houghton Mifflin.

Rogers. C. R. (1951). *Client-centered therapy.* Boston: Houghton Mifflin.

Sanford, J., Law, M., Swanson, L., & Guyatt. G. (1994). *Assessing clinically important change as an outcome of rehabilitation in older adults.* San Francisco: American Society on Aging Conference.

Sokoly, M.M., & Dokecki, P.R. (1992). Ethical perspectives on family-centered early intervention. *Infants and Young Children, 4,* 23–32.

Sumsion, T. (1999). Client-centered practice: The true impact. *Canadian Journal of Occupational Therapy, 60,* 6–8.

Townsend. E., Brintnell, S., & Staisey, N. (1990). Developing guidelines for client-centered occupational therapy practice. *Canadian Journal of Occupational Therapy, 57,* 69–76.

Wasserman, R.C., Inui, T.S., Barriatua, R.D., Carter, W.B., & Lippincott, P. (1984). Pediatric clinicians' support for parents makes a difference: An outcome-based analysis of clinician–parent interaction. *Pediatrics, 74,* 1047–1053.

World Health Organization. (1986). *Ottawa charter for health promotion.* Ottawa: World Health Organization.

The Narrative Nature of Clinical Reasoning

CHAPTER 37

CHERYL MATTINGLY, PhD

Many professions identify good thinking with a process that resembles the scientific method—an application in practice of empirically tested abstract knowledge (theories) and generalizable factual knowledge. Here reasoning involves the recognition of particular instances of behavior in terms of general laws that regulate the relationship between the cause and a caused state of affairs (see Mattingly, 1991, for a related discussion of this point). There are many debates within the philosophy of science about whether this model of objective knowledge characterizes even the hard sciences, such as physics (Kuhn, 1962; Putnam, 1979; Rorty, 1979). Also debated is whether the scientific method provides an appropriate model with which to characterize professional reasoning (Dreyfus & Dreyfus, 1986; Schön, 1983, 1987). I enter these debates in arguing that a narrative model of reasoning, as opposed to scientific reasoning in the traditional sense, is fundamental to the thinking of occupational therapists.

Book: Clinical Reasoning. Therapists = a 3 treat mind.

Therapists think with stories in two distinct, but equally important, ways—through storytelling and story creation. Storytelling constitutes an extremely important and underrated mode of discourse in occupational therapy. Recently, there has been a surge of interest in the health professions in eliciting stories from patients (Coles, 1989; Kleinman, 1988). It became clear in the course of the American Occupational Therapy Association/American Occupational Therapy Foundation Clinical Reasoning Study that therapists not only listen to the stories that their patients tell them, but also tell stories about their patients. Furthermore, an important part of this storytelling involves the therapist's understanding of the patient's way of dealing with disability and with puzzling about how to approach a problematic patient. The creation of clinical stories in clinical time is the second way in which occupational therapists use narrative in their reasoning process. I call such creation *therapeutic emplotment.*

Narrative Reasoning and Storytelling: Making Sense of the Illness Experience

What does it mean to say that occupational therapists think about their patients through the telling of stories and that this constitutes a primary form of thinking in their therapeutic practice? Jerome Bruner (1986, 1990), a psychologist noted for his studies of cognitive development, argued that humans think in two fundamentally different ways. He labeled the first type of thinking paradigmatic, that is, thinking through propositional argument, and the second, narrative, that is, thinking through storytelling. The difference between these two kinds of thinking involves how we make sense of and explain what we see. When we look at something and try to understand it through propositional argument, we are trying to take a particular and see it in general terms, as an instance of a general type. For example, when we see a patient with a set of symptoms, we may note that we are seeing a severe case of Parkinson's disease. According to Bruner, in linking the particular symptoms to a general disease category, we are thinking propositionally.

Conversely, when we are thinking narratively, we are trying to understand the particular case. Specifically, we are trying to understand a particular person's experience. Narrative thinking is our primary way of making sense of human experience. We do this primarily through an investigation of human motives (Burke, 1945; Gardner, 1982). We think narratively when we want to explain not whether someone has Parkinson's disease, but rather, why this patient's wife is so unwilling to have her husband be discharged home. The difference between these two modes of thinking in occupational therapy is illustrated by the way in which therapists use storytelling to talk about their cases over lunch or to present cases to colleagues in weekly departmental staff meetings.

At University Hospital in Boston, where the Clinical Reasoning Study took place, the therapists drew on two modes of talking to discuss patients. Case presentations consisted of two distinct parts: "chart talk" and storytelling. The first, chart talk, involved a familiar biomedical presentation. When speaking chart talk, therapists focused on the pathology in general. The items ordinarily addressed were (a) key symptoms; (b) major typical physical impairments and primary needs, especially activities of daily living needs; (c) assessment goals and other ways of rating a patient's extent of impairment; and (d) typical treatment modalities and strategies.

The second form of case presentation was through storytelling. Here the therapists shifted their focus from a discussion based on pathology to one based on the specific patients they had worked with and their experiences of disability. One example of such storytelling comes from a staff meeting in which an affiliating student was doing a presentation of a patient with Parkinson's disease. After discussing Parkinson's disease as a pathology, she turned to describe her problems with a specific patient with Parkinson's disease whom she was treating and how his wife was responding to her husband's disability. As part of her description of treating the patient, she recounted her interchanges with his wife. Here is part of the student's story:

> He [the patient] said that something would have to be changed because his bedroom was downstairs in the basement. His wife wanted to keep him downstairs but finally agreed that he could have a bedroom in the living room. He progressed rapidly, and after a week and a half he was smiling, becoming more social. His wife told me, "He does nothing at home." I don't know if she could hear what we were telling her. We said, "He is not just sitting around. Many times he simply can't do anything because of the disease." When the wife heard that he would be on medication and that this would improve his functioning, she said to him, "Good. There's a lot of chores around the house you can do." I don't know how much she heard of what we were telling her.

This story triggered a storytelling exchange in which others around the table offered their own experiences in treating patients with Parkinson's disease, emphasizing how the disease was experienced by the patient, the family, or

themselves rather than its general medical features. Nearly all of the speakers told stories that elaborated on themes raised by the initial story. What does this storytelling have to do with clinical reasoning? When the student told her story about the wife of the patient with Parkinson's disease, she identified a critical problem for clinical reasoning: What is she supposed to do with the patient's wife? How should she best treat this patient, given his wife's feelings? How does the wife really feel? What are this wife's denial and anger about? Or is the wife displaying something that is being mistaken for denial or anger? These are all narrative questions whose answers require a kind of clinical reasoning that is fundamentally narrative in form. To return to Bruner's (1986, 1990) distinction, when we think in propositional arguments, we try to transcend particulars and strive for abstraction (i.e., for truths that transcend any particular historical situation). But narrative is rooted in the particular. Whereas propositional arguments are concerned with understanding phenomena in terms of general causes, narratives are concerned with the likely connections among particular events. Bruner gave a simple example to illustrate the difference. The statement "if x, then y" belongs to propositional argument. An occupational therapist is relying on propositional reasoning when she says, "If you see these symptoms, then you probably have a case of Parkinson's disease." Such if–then statements are aimed at providing an abstract description of a causal relationship that holds up generally or, ideally, universally across concrete individual cases.

This genre of descriptive and explanatory statements can be contrasted with a very different mode of explanation. Bruner (1986) gave the following illustration, borrowed from E. M. Forster (1927). The statement, "The king died, and then the queen died" (pp. 11–12) is a narrative statement that not only concerns the particular, that is, some specific king and queen, but also, suggests causes that lead one to wonder about intentions. Did the queen die of grief? Was the queen murdered? We investigate the meaning of a narrative statement by trying out different motivational possibilities; we search for what guided the action that the statement reports. And human action, unlike a pathological process, is motivated. Narratives make sense of reality by linking the outward world of actions and events to the inner world of human intention and motivation. To ask in a narrative sense why something happened is to ask what motivated the actors to do what they did. In the philosophy of history, this mode of narrative explanation has been called "explanation by reason" (Dray, 1971, 1980). In a story, a person's actions are accounted for—or explained—by their placement in some specific historical context that shows how and why they were begun, what other actions unfolded as a result, and how they evolved over time. So when we hear about a particular patient with Parkinson's disease whose wife complains that he does not do enough housework and we want to explain what is going on, we start asking the narrative questions enumerated earlier.

In moving between chart talk and storytelling, therapists present the clinical problem in different ways. The shift in presentation from an abstract discussion of Parkinson's disease to a story of a patient with Parkinson's disease who has an uncooperative wife involves much more than a move from the general to the concrete or from the objective to the subjective.

In chart talk, the focus is on a disease. The disease is the main character. But in storytelling, it is the patient's situation or experience with the disease that is the central clinical problem. The therapist might ask, What is the best way to treat the patient with Parkinson's disease who is going home to this particular wife? The severity and nature of the patient's dysfunctions are still important, but they are only one part of the picture that the therapist has to put together with the unique features of one patient's situation.

Therapists often speak of expert practice as involving the ability to "put it all together" for a particular patient. I suggest that what they mean by this involves a thinking that is essentially narrative. The therapist takes what he or she knows in general of a disease process, appropriate theoretical frames of reference, and relevant experience with similar patients and applies all of this generalized and abstract knowledge to a particular case, such as that of the patient whose wife thinks he should be able to do household chores and resists having his bed moved up to the first floor where he will have access to the bathroom.

Medical anthropologists have made an extremely useful distinction in looking at health care by separating disease from illness experience (Good, 1977; Good & Delvecchio-Good, 1980, 1985; Kleinman, 1988; Kleinman, Eisenberg, & Good, 1978). Although traditionally medicine has focused on the diagnosis and treatment of disease, anthropologists argue that much more attention needs to be given to treatment of the illness experience, which involves the way in which the disease affects the person's life. Physiologically, the same disease can result in a very different illness experience, depending on the patient's particular life history and life possibilities. The patient with Parkinson's disease whose wife learns all she can about the disease and welcomes her husband home is likely to have quite a different illness experience than the patient whose wife wants to relegate him to the basement.

What anthropologists have argued to the medical community during the last decade or two, occupational therapists have known for a long time: To effectively treat persons with long-term disabilities, one must treat the whole patient, which involves looking beyond the disease to how that disease is experienced by that particular patient. Treatment of a patient's illness experience is integral to good occupational therapy and it is where the heart of clinical reasoning lies; it is also where the thorniest reasoning puzzles present themselves. Reasoning about how to treat the illness experience is often the most difficult thing to teach the affiliating student or new therapist. How does a supervisor help a novice therapist to examine what is going on with this patient's wife and what therapeutic approach would best help this patient make the transition back home to this wife? Notably, when one addresses the illness experience, as opposed to the disease alone, it is often hard to establish who has the disease. Although a disease obviously belongs to one person—the patient—the illness experience, especially in the case of serious life-changing illnesses, is likely to be shared by the whole family.

Puzzling over how to treat a patient with Parkinson's disease, given how his wife is responding to the illness, involves narrative reasoning, because it involves consideration of the disease from the patient's and family's points of view. The therapist must try to imagine how it feels to the patient and to various family members to have this disease, how they are experiencing it, and how it enters and changes the life story of a patient and his or her family.

Narrative Reasoning and Story Making: Creating Clinical Stories

Therapists create as well as tell stories. The narrative nature of clinical reasoning manifests itself not only in the work therapists do to understand the effect of a disability in the life story of a particular patient, but also in the therapist's need to structure therapy in a narrative way, as an unfolding story. This is perhaps the most interesting and subtle use of narrative reasoning in occupational therapy practice. Therapy can be seen as a kind of short story within the patient's longer life story. The therapist enters and exits the patient's life, playing a part for only a short time. Often, this part occurs at a critical juncture in the patient's life, a turning point triggered by the onset or downturn of an illness. Sometimes it occurs at a critical juncture in an entire family's life, as is often true in pediatric therapy when a family is learning to adjust to a newborn with a disability or when a child with a disability begins school. If disability is considered in narrative terms as something that interrupts and irreversibly changes a person's life story, then work with a patient can be seen as one chapter in that life story.

Although this narrative language is not a familiar way for therapists to describe their own practice, it serves to highlight how intensely therapists want to make therapy itself an occasion for patients to remake life stories that can no longer continue as they once did when a disability was absent or less serious. The therapist enters the life story of a patient and has the task of negotiating with the patient what role therapy is going to play within the unfolding illness and rehabilitation story that the patient is living through. To be meaningful, occupational therapy must serve as a coherent short story within a larger narrative whole.

In each new clinical situation, then, the therapist must answer the question, What story am I in? To answer this question, the therapist must make some initial sense of the situation and then act on it. The process of treatment encourages, perhaps even compels, therapists to reason in a narrative mode. They must reason about how to guide their therapy with particular patients by imagining where the patient is now and where this patient might be at some future point after discharge. It is not enough for therapists to know how to do a set of tasks that have an abstract order based on a general or typical treatment plan; therapists must be able to picture a larger temporal whole, one that captures what they can see in a particular patient in the present and what they can imagine seeing sometime in the future. This picturing process gives them a basis for organizing tasks.

In her study of clinical reasoning among nurses, Benner (1984) noticed this narrative mode of reasoning in her subjects, although she did not focus on its narrative nature per se. The need for a narrative framework was suggested by a nurse quoted in Benner's study who worked in an intensive care nursery. She described what she considered to be the most essential kind of thinking she wanted her newly graduated students to evince at the end of their 3-month affiliation with her:

> To my mind, moving the child from Point A to Point B is what nursing is all about. You have to perform tasks along the way to make that happen, but performing the task isn't nursing.... I wanted to see a light going on—that OK, here's this baby, this is where this baby is at, and here's where I want this baby to be in six weeks. What can I do today to make this baby go along the road to end up being better? It's that kind of thing that's just happening now. They're [the student nurses] just starting to see the whole thing as a picture and not as a list of tasks to do. (p. 28)

This example emphasizes both the imagistic character of what the clinician needs to know, in contrast with the knowledge of tasks, and the context-specific nature of those images. Therapists in the Clinical Reasoning Study spoke similarly about picturing the patient and especially about having future images of who the patient could be. They believed that what they often held most vividly in mind when treating patients was not plans or objectives, but rather, pictures of the potential patient, that is, the future patient. For example, one of the pediatric therapists said, "You know, when I treat that 18-month-old child, I see the child at 3, then I see the child at 6, learning to hold a pencil. I have all these pictures in my head." The therapists described their difficulty when the patients or their families held different images of the future and their dilemma about the extent to which they should give patients or families their therapeutically based pictures, which were often more pessimistic. The therapists were frequently in the difficult position of trying to give hope to a patient while also having to let the patient know of his or her dark prognosis. The patients and their families could be extremely depressed about conditions that were even worse than they had imagined. The therapists spoke of these images as necessary but dangerous: necessary because the therapist and patient needed some guiding pictures, but dangerous because these pictures could blind the therapist or patient to what was realistically possible.

The therapists in the Clinical Reasoning Study were, like Benner's (1984) nurses, also conscious of the need to create specific images appropriate to a particular patient. General treatment goals devised from general knowledge of functional deficits and developmental possibilities were insufficient guides to practice, in the therapists' view. Instead, they worked with much more concrete guides, images, and stories, which were the "wholes" that allowed them to selectively choose what aspects of their knowledge base were appropriate to the situation. These images were organized temporally and teleologically, thus giving the therapists a sense of an ending for which they could strive.

Although these images of the future were often not formulated in words, unless there was some need to explicitly communicate them, they were part of what I call a prospective treatment story. In this prospective story, the therapists envisioned a possible and desirable future for the patient and imagined how they might guide treatment to bring such a future about.

The treatment approaches and treatment paths that the therapists tried to follow were often guided by such stories. These stories, derived from particular experiences and stereotypical (collectivized) scenarios, were projected onto new clinical situations in order to help therapists make sense of what story they were in and where they might go with particular patients. The therapists then attempted to enact their projected stories in the new clinical situations, working improvisationally to narratively pull in and build on whatever happened in a clinical session so as to add to the story's plot line. The therapists saw a possible story, which they recognized as clinically meaningful, and they tried to make that story come true by taking the individual episodes of their clinical encounters and treating them as parts of a larger, narratively unfolding whole. Prospective treatment stories were based on what therapists observed and inferred about the patient's larger life history, which involved both the patient's past and future. The therapeutic stories that the therapists imagined took their power and plausibility as part of a larger historical context that included a past that began before therapy started and a future that would extend after therapy had ended.

Notably, the prospective story cannot be equated with treatment goals and plans, although these will be incorporated into the story. Therapists try to create significant therapeutic experiences and not simply reach a set of objectives in the most efficient way possible. They are concerned that the whole process of therapy unfold in such a way that patients will have powerful experiences of successfully met challenges; such challenges will motivate them to believe in therapy and work hard at it. In listening to therapy success stories, I found it rare for the success of therapy to have been measured by the reaching of the final goal. Rather, most of the therapists counted success as the generation of therapeutic experiences along the way, in which patients developed increasing confidence and commitment to take on challenges. The whole treatment story mattered.

Therapists in the Clinical Reasoning Study also worked to create significant experiences for their patients, ones worth telling stories about, because if therapy was to be effective, then the therapists had to find a way to make the therapeutic process matter to the patient. Each therapist faced the problem of constructing therapeutic activities that were meaningful enough to elicit the patient's active cooperation. The patients had to see something at stake in therapy. Otherwise, why should they bother to try? If the patient did not try, therapy did not work. This was partly because the therapists required the patients to do things in therapy that the patients did not necessarily feel ready to do or believe to be worth the effort. But more important, the patients had to become committed because they had to take up the therapeutic activities. Therapists were often with patients only a short time—just a few weeks or less. They might teach a few skills or improve the patient's strength a bit, but generally their effectiveness depended on the use of therapy as a catalyst to help patients begin to see how they might do for themselves even when the therapist was no longer present.

For example, a therapist is working with a spinal cord–injured patient, teaching him to move checkers pieces with a mouth stick. It is not enough for this patient to learn to move these checkers pieces for the therapy to be successful; he must also take up a point of view that comes with being committed to the tremendous concentration needed to perform this previously trivial task. He must absorb a vision about why he should work so hard at something that was once so easy. This is just as critical as the skills he acquires. The therapeutic time together itself must provide a kind of existential picture of how he might live his life in the future with his disability. Therapy will not ultimately work, not in any catalytic way that patients will take home when they leave the hospital, if they are not strongly committed to the process. Without experiencing treatment activities from a committed stance, they will not see any future in them. They will not see the point.

If the patient is to become committed to the therapeutic process, then both the patient and the therapist must share a view about why engaging in any particular set of treatment activities makes sense. Coming to share such a view requires that both the therapist and the patient see how these treatment activities are going to move the patient toward some future that he or she can care about. Such a view is not reducible to a general prognosis or even to a shared understanding of a treatment plan. The therapist and patient must come to share a story about the therapeutic process; they must come to see themselves as in the same story. This is a kind of future story, a story of what has not yet happened, or has only partly happened—an as yet unfinished story.

How is such a story constructed? Generally it is not constructed through any explicit storytelling, but rather, through the sharing of powerful therapeutic experiences that point to a prospective story—a path that therapy will take. Clinical reasoning requires that the therapist (a) see possibilities for creating important experiences in which the patient will be staked, (b) make moves to act on those possibilities, (c) respond to the moves the patient makes in return, and (d) build on the experience by showing the patient a future in which this therapeutic experience becomes one building block. In the language of narrative, the experience becomes one episode in a much longer story. The therapist tells the story not in words but in actions that create an experience the patient can care about.

I follow the work of the philosophers Ricoeur (1984) and White (1987) in describing this therapeutic work as "emplotment." The clinician's narrative task is to take the episodes of action within the clinical encounter and structure them into a coherent plot. A plot is what gives unity to an otherwise meaningless succession of events. Quite simply, "emplotment is the operation that draws a configuration out of a simple succession" (Ricoeur, 1984, p. 65). What we call a story is precisely this rendering and ordering of a succession of events (e.g., a series of treatment activities) into parts belonging to a larger narrative whole. When a therapeutic process has been successfully emplotted, it is driven and shaped by a sense of an ending (Kermode, 1966). To have a single story is to have made a whole out of a succession of actions. These actions then take their meaning by belonging and contributing to the story as a whole. A story, Ricoeur wrote, "must be more than just an enumeration of events in serial order: it must organize them into an intelligible whole, of a sort such that we can always ask what is the 'thought' of this story" (p. 65).

Narratives give meaningful structure to life through time. The told narrative builds, to borrow from Ricoeur's (1984) argument, on action understood as an as yet untold story. Or, in Ricoeur's provocative phrase, "action is in quest of narrative" (p. 74). Therapists are in a quest to transform their actions and the actions of their patients into as yet untold stories.

This can be translated into more familiar clinical language through a narrative reading of treatment goals. When an occupational therapist makes an assessment of the patient, the outcome is a set of treatment goals. Goals, according to Ricoeur (1984), are not predictions of what will happen; rather, they express the actor's intentions and preferences. These goals express a therapeutic commitment. They capture what the therapist intends to accomplish over the course of therapy. Treatment goals are an expression of what the therapist has committed himself or herself to care about with a particular patient.

As occupational therapists have argued (Rogers, 1983 [see Chapter 43]; Rogers & Kielhofner, 1985), a primary task of clinical reasoning is the individualization of treatment goals. Narratively, individualization involves the construction of a particular story of the treatment process rather than reliance on a generic line of action that strings together standard goals and activities.

Therapeutic Emplotment: A Case Example

A wonderful illustration of this process of narratively structured treatment is given by O'Reilly (1990), who, as part of the Clinical Reasoning Study, described her work with a head injury group. O'Reilly recounted a situation in which she was asked to take over a failing head injury group that was poorly attended. The first thing that bothered her was its name—the Upper Extremity Group. She described her first visit to the group, "I enter the large OT/PT treatment area where I see several residents scattered about at tables and exercise equipment.... At one table, a resident diligently puts small pegs into a pegboard.... What is most memorable is the silence. Except for the clang of the pulley weights, a dropped peg or the therapist's quiet voice, there is not a sound in this room" (p. 2).

O'Reilly noticed that several of the group members were not present, and when she went to inquire, they told her, "That [expletive deleted] group is a waste of time." She tried several strategies to entice members back, but nothing worked. She puzzled:

I wonder, 'What's wrong with this group?'
I make mental lists:

1. The name—I'll talk to the residents about that.
2. The activities—no meaning, no purpose, no life-related goals, no goals that belong to the patients.
3. No interaction among members with the therapist.
4. Nobody is having fun—the residents are bored and the therapist is bored (and boring?).
5. Is there any progress that the residents experience?
6. What are the reasons for attending or not attending? and there is no direction—no theme.
(O'Reilly, 1990, p. 2)

Although O'Reilly did not use the language of story to describe the problems she noticed, this list could easily be restated in narrative terms. Her statement that the group has no direction and no theme could be recast to say that there is no plot to this group; there is no story for which the group members are a part. The group is not going anywhere, narratively speaking. Any particular group activity is not an episode in an unfolding story that members share. The activities of the group are focused on broken body parts, as the group name (Upper Extremity Group) implies. Although the exercises may help improve body functioning, they carry no intrinsic meaning to the group members, because group activities are in no sense a short story in the larger life story of the patients.

The therapist pondered what to do by beginning to think about individual group members. Her mode of puzzling represents a shift from a biomechanical framing of the members' disability to seeing their disability as having personal meaning in their lives. She described her reasoning in this way: "I think about the people. What do they want? What do they need? They are all so young; so far from home. They want to get out. They want to go home. HOME! They're all from New York. That's it! NEW YORK! I have a theme with which to begin" (O'Reilly, 1990, p. 2).

O'Reilly was reasoning in narrative terms. She was not telling a story, but she was beginning to envision a prospective story that all the group members could be a part of. She wrote:

I have a theme with which to begin, but I don't know a thing about New York. The Program Director is from New York ... I dash to her office. "New York," I blurt. "The Upper Extremity Group, they're all from N.Y. Tell me something about N.Y., anything, everything." She lists: "Empire State Building, Statue of Liberty, Long Island Ferry, the subway." Laughingly, "You could have a New York Subway Group." I reply, "We could be on the subway. They can take me to New York. What does it look like—is there graffiti? We can do graffiti. I need a new room, away from the big treatment room. Can we use the small meeting room?" Program Director replies "yes" and adds that she has a map of the N.Y. subway and will bring it in. "I'll be the conductor ... I have a blue blazer." She says, "I think I have a funny little hat that will pass for a conductor's hat." We laugh through all the possibilities of this activity. This is going to be FUN! (O'Reilly, 1990, p. 3)

In deciding to create a therapy group around a New York theme, O'Reilly could not only locate therapy in the relevant past of these patients, but also locate it within the future that they desire. This study dealt with young people in a chronic long-term care facility in Massachusetts, one that residents rarely ever leave. These patients wanted to go home.

O'Reilly invented the ingenious idea of turning a therapy room into a New York subway station. She also devised a way of generating some interest in the group:

I go straight to Mike's room and ask him to make sure everyone comes to group today. "I have a different type of activity planned, and I'd really like to talk to everyone so that we can make some plans together." Mike states that he hates the [expletive deleted] group. I tell him that I understand that and that perhaps he could gather everyone for me, and come for awhile. "Then, if you are really unhappy with the activity, you can leave." He agrees. I hand him a small bag containing poker chips and ask him to give one to each group member on the attached list and have them bring the chips to group. "Okay, but what the [expletive deleted] are these for?" "It's a surprise. See you at 1:30." (O'Reilly, 1990, p. 3)

Notably, in announcing the group, she introduced a key narrative element critical to any dramatic story—the element of suspense. In any good story, the reader will want to know what will happen next. To prepare for the meeting of the group, the therapist lined three walls of the therapy room with white paper. She labeled spots with street names and subway stops and hung a subway map on the fourth wall.

Just as the group was scheduled to begin, O'Reilly stood outside the door in a subway conductor's uniform (trying not to feel too foolish in front of other surprised hospital colleagues) and waited for group members to arrive. She, herself, also felt unsure about what would happen:

I put out materials, don my conductor's uniform and stand outside the door, on which a sign reads: NEW YORK THIS WAY. As I await the passengers, my stomach churns with anxiety and excitement, and I wonder where this subway ride will take us. (O'Reilly, 1990, p. 3)

She described the following scene:

As the members arrive, escorted by Mike, I take their tokens, explaining that it's commuter fare for a ride on the New York Subway. Nancy grins, Eileen looks puzzled. Bobby shrugs. Mike says, with a great laugh, "You are crazy!" As these travelers enter the room, I hear snickers and queries like, "what the [expletive deleted] is she doing?" and comments like, "It's better than the other room." Then snickers, laughter, recognition. They go from stop to stop, reading, commenting, all smiling! [As they turn to her, she explains] "You folks are all from N.Y. Right? This is a N.Y. subway station. You've all ridden on the subway, right? M. tells me that there's graffiti, words and pictures on the walls, in the subway. We're going to do graffiti. You do remember graffiti, don't you?" "Yeah," laughs Mike, "but nothing I could write HERE!" With that, I close the door, and say, "You can draw or write anything you want in this room. The only rule is that you use the tools that I give you." These tools have been chosen with particular concern for the motor

deficits of individual patients: "Large colored pencils and wrist weights for Mike who has a tremor, but brush and paint for Bobby who's working on gross motor skills, crayons for Nancy who needs to strengthen wrist and fingers, markers for Eileen who can't tolerate resistance." (O'Reilly, 1990, p. 4)

O'Reilly described the reaction of her "travelers" to this new activity:

Eileen asks, "Where are we supposed to be?" "Anywhere you'd like to be, and when you finish working at one place, you can move to another. It's up to you." Nancy starts: "This is neat ... just like when I was a kid." We're off!

From this point on, drawing, writing, conversation, and laughter are continuous. So much activity fills this room that it is difficult to remember details. Words, pictures, memories, and feelings cover the walls:

"This place sucks." "My ass is stuck in Mass." "Home sweet Home." And on and on.... I go from one participant to another, asking about their work or just watching. After 35 minutes, I ask the group to finish up their artwork so that we can talk a bit and plan for our next group session. Stickball wins unanimously. Since, I admit, I know nothing about stickball, I ask the group to write out rules and equipment we'll need and get it to me on Tuesday. They agree, and, in fact, begin to work immediately. As I leave to see my next client, I tell the group,"You guys can hang out here for awhile. Just be sure to take your words and pictures with you when you leave." Thinking ... clean up can wait. (O'Reilly, 1990. p. 4)

The end result of this therapeutic intervention was the beginning of the "New York Gang," as they came to call themselves. They met not only twice a week but also informally on the weekends, at which time they planned a series of events and activities. Their ventures included "making giant pretzels and cooking hot dogs to sell from a makeshift pushcart; taking a trip to a simulated Central Park; and filling a photo album with pictures of the group, home, drawings, postcards, and New York Times clippings" (O'Reilly, 1990, p. 4). The therapist had begun a story that spawned additional episodes. She set a therapeutic story in motion. The first group session that O'Reilly described in her case not only had a coherent plot, that is, a beginning, middle, and end (making graffiti), but also, because of her success, that session became just one episode in an unfolding therapeutic story in which patients became a cast of characters in the New York Gang. Even the name of the group came from the group members themselves. Specific biomechanical interventions were integrated in a meaningful way as activities allowed group members to act their part in this drama, and the task of writing things on the wall allowed each person to express an individual voice as well.

When O'Reilly initially devised the idea of doing something with a New York theme, the prospective story that she had begun to envision (and that she had concretely begun when she fixed up a room and donned a conductor's uniform) was much more than a set of treatment goals. Specific goals were incorporated in the narrative plot that she started. The success of this therapeutic intervention was ensured when the patients themselves took the story up and began to create new episodes that the therapist could not have imagined.

Narratively speaking, the shift of names from the Upper Extremity Group to the New York Gang represents a shift from a series of interactions in which therapeutic time is treated as a mere succession of activities, that is, as a procedural movement not grounded in context or in a picture of the patient, to narrative shaping of the therapeutic interaction in which therapeutic time has been emplotted by the clinician's picture of how to create an important therapeutic experience for the patients. The therapeutic efficacy of this intervention is about much more than meeting specific treatment goals. It is about creating an experience that gives the participants a vision of themselves as actors in the world, that is, as more than just patients.

Conclusion

Narrative thinking is central in providing therapists with a way to consider disability in the phenomenological terms of injured lives. Narrative thinking especially guides therapists when they treat the phenomenological body; that is, when they are concerned with their patients' illness experience and how the disability is affecting their lives.

In this article, I examined two kinds of narrative thinking. One is narrative as a mode of talk that therapists rely on to consider certain kinds of clinical puzzles. Because narratives are predominantly about human actions, they provide a particular vantage point from which one can view the nature of clinical practice and pose clinical problems. The stories that the therapists told portrayed disability from an actor-centered point of view. They were personal, even individualistic, built on the structure of actors acting. Disability itself shifted from a physiological event to a personally meaningful one, that is, to an illness experience. General physiological conditions were shadowed as background context. What was brought to center stage were the ways that particular actors, with their own motivations and commitments, had done things for which they could be praised or blamed.

The second form of narrative thinking, which occurs in occupational therapy in a more subtle way, is story making, which involves the creation rather than the telling of stories. The telling of stories is always retrospective—a way of considering past events—whereas story making is largely prospective, playing out images that therapists have of what they would like to happen in therapy. Story making as therapeutic emplotment concerns the way in which therapists work to structure therapy narratively, thus creating dramatic therapeutic events that connect therapy to a patient's life. Often, the search for a meaningful therapeutic story appears to be triggered by resistance or alienation of the patient to the initial therapeutic activities offered, as in the case of the members of the Upper Extremity Group. Whatever the impetus, therapists try to create clinical experiences in which there is a significant occurrence or event for the patient in therapy, one in which the therapy itself is a meaningful short story in the larger life story of the patient.

References

Benner, P. (1984). *From novice to expert. Excellence and power in clinical nursing practice.* Reading, MA: Addison-Wesley.

Bruner, J. (1986). *Actual minds, possible worlds.* Cambridge, MA: Harvard University Press.

Bruner, J. (1990). *Acts of meaning.* Cambridge, MA: Harvard University Press.

Burke, K. (1945). *A grammar of motives.* Berkeley, CA: University of California.

Coles, R. (1989). *The call of stories.* Cambridge, MA: Harvard University Press.

Dray, H. (1971). On the nature and role of narrative in historiography. *History and Theory, 10,* 153–171.

Dray, W. (1980). *Perspectives on history.* London: Routledge & Keegan Paul.

Dreyfus, H., & Dreyfus, S. (1986). *Mind over machine: The power of human intuition and expertise in the era of the computer.* New York: Free Press.

Forster, E. M. (1927). *Aspects of the novel.* Harcourt Brace Jovanovich.

Gardner, H. (1982, March). The making of a storyteller. *Psychology Today,* pp. 49–63.

Good, B. (1977). The heart of what's the matter: The semantics of illness in Iran. *Culture, Medicine, and Psychiatry, 1,* 25–28.

Good, B., & Delvecchio-Good, M.J. (1980). The meaning of symptoms: A cultural hermeneutic model for clinical practice. In I. Eisenberg and A. Kleinman (Eds.), *The relevance of social science for medicine* (pp. 165–196). Norwell, MA: D. Reidel.

Good, B., & Delvecchio-Good, M. J. (1985). *The cultural context of diagnosis and therapy.* Unpublished manuscript.

Kermode, F. (1966). *The sense of an ending: Studies in the theory of fiction.* London: Oxford University Press.

Kleinman, A. (1988). *The illness narratives. Suffering, healing, and the human condition.* New York: Basic.

Kleinman, A., Eisenberg, L., & Good, B. (1978). Culture, illness, and care: Clinical lessons from anthropologic and cross-cultural research. *Annals of Internal Medicine, 88,* 251–258.

Kuhn, T. (1962). *The structures of scientific revolutions.* Chicago: University of Chicago Press.

Mattingly, C. (1991). What is clinical reasoning? *American Journal of Occupational Therapy, 45,* 979–986.

O'Reilly, M. (1990). *The New York subway.* Unpublished data, Tufts University Clinical Reasoning Institute, Boston.

Putnam, H. (1979). *The meaning and the moral sciences.* Boston: Routledge & Keegan Paul.

Ricoeur, P. (1984). *Time and narrative* (Vol. 1). Chicago: University of Chicago Press.

Rogers, J. (1983). Clinical reasoning: The ethics, science and art. *American Journal of Occupational Therapy, 37,* 601–616. Reprinted as Chapter 43.

Rogers J. C., & Kielhofner, G. (1985). Treatment planning. In G. Kielhofner (Ed.), *A model of human occupation* (pp. 136–155). Baltimore: Williams & Wilkins.

Rorty, R. (1979). *Philosophy and the mirror of nature.* Princeton, NJ: Princeton University Press.

Schön, D. (1983). *The reflective practitioner. How professionals think in action.* New York: Basic.

Schön, D. (1987). *Educating the reflective practitioner.* San Francisco: Jossey-Bass.

White, H. (1987). *The content of the form: Narrative discourse and historical representation.* Baltimore: Johns Hopkins University Press.

Enhancing Occupational Performance Through an Understanding of Perceived Self-Efficacy

Read this one

MARIE GAGE, MSC
HELENE POLATAJKO, PHD, OT(C)

Occupational therapists enable clients to develop occupational performance skills with the expectation that these skills will be used outside the treatment setting and that the use of these skills will enhance their clients' occupational competence and their ability to cope with the life stresses associated with their deficits. Therefore, it is important for occupational therapists to understand the role of any factor that influences their clients' occupational performance, or their resultant ability to cope with their deficit in the community. Perceived self-efficacy is one such factor.

It is postulated that perceived self-efficacy explains part of the variance between a person's skill and the quality of that person's actual performance outside the protected clinical environment (Bandura, 1977, 1986; Shaffer, 1978). Furthermore, according to the Appraisal Model of Coping, the concept of perceived self-efficacy is one of 12 factors that influence a person's manner of coping with stressful person–environment interactions, such as those encountered by people with occupational performance deficits (Gage, 1992). Perceived self-efficacy has been found to be a significant behavioral determinant of actual performance and to influence psychological well-being (Allen, Becker, & Swank, 1990; Bandura, 1977, 1986; Bandura & Adams, 1977; Bandura & Wood, 1989; Ewart et al., 1986; Seydel, Taal, & Wiegman, 1990; Shunk, 1982; Toshima, Kaplan, & Ries, 1990; Wang & Richarde, 1987; Wassem, 1992). The most effective means of enhancing perceived self-efficacy is deemed to be through performance-based procedures (Bandura, 1977): the procedures upon which occupational therapy practice is traditionally based.

This article explores the construct of perceived self-efficacy, including origin, definition, relationship to self-esteem, parameters, history, relationship to behavior, outcome expectancy, psychological well-being, and the means of enhancing a client's perceived self-efficacy. The purpose of our review is to help occupational therapists recognize the goodness of fit between perceived self-efficacy and occupational therapy practice and thereby to identify the potential benefits of incorporating the attributes of perceived self-efficacy into day-to-day clinical practice.

Perceived Self-Efficacy
Origins of Perceived Self-Efficacy

Perceived self-efficacy is a concept originally developed as part of Social Cognitive Theory. Social cognitive theorists view human functioning as the result of triadic reciprocality: "behavior, cognitive and other personal factors, and environmental events all act as interacting determinants of each other" (Bandura, 1986, p. 18). The relative influence of each of these three factors varies from situation to situation, from person to person, and from environment to environment. Within the framework of Social Cognitive Theory, people are attributed with six basic capacities.

1. Symbolizing capacity—the ability to use symbols to transform experiences into models that guide future actions,

which in turn are guided by thoughts; thoughts are sometimes inaccurate due to misinterpretation of the incoming information.

2. Forethought capacity—the ability to anticipate the potential outcome of future actions, set goals, and develop action plans.
3. Vicarious capacity—the ability to learn through observation of others and thereby abbreviate the learning period; this ability is vital to survival.
4. Self-regulatory capacity—the ability to make choices based on personal beliefs, rather than on the expectations of the external environment. Internalized standards are used to guide behavioral choices.
5. Change capacity (plasticity)—the ability to develop or change. The vast potential for human development is shaped by both direct and vicarious experiences into many forms, constrained only by biological limitations.
6. Self-reflective capacity—the ability to think about personal experiences and derive generic knowledge about oneself and the world in which one lives. One of the most powerful types of self-reflective thought is perceived self-efficacy (Bandura, 1986).

Each of these six capacities influences the degree of self-efficacy expressed for each task by any given person.

Definition of Perceived Self-Efficacy

The concept of perceived self-efficacy (or efficacy expectations) evolved primarily from the observation that traditional cognitive psychology models did not adequately explain the discrepancy between attained skills and the quality of performance output (Bandura, 1977). Traditional models attempted to explain the discrepancy between skills and performance as a function of the actor's expectation of outcomes or "action-outcome expectancy." Action-outcome expectancy theorists postulate that, given equivalent skills, performance differences are due to differences in the actor's belief that the response will lead to a desired goal. If this belief is strong, the actor will engage in the requisite behavior; if this belief is weak, the actor will not engage in the behavior even though he or she possesses the skill to do so.

Bandura (1977) suggested that a difference in outcome expectancy does not explain the total variance between skill and performance. He suggested that perceived self-efficacy is also a significant factor. Bandura (1986) defined perceived self-efficacy as:

> people's judgments of their capabilities to organize and execute courses of action required to attain designated types of performances. It is concerned not with the skills one has but with the judgments of what one can do with whatever skills one possesses (p. 391).

Thus, Bandura (1977) asserted that one's belief in one's ability to use a specific skill partially explains why people of equivalent skill achieve at differing levels. This belief in one's

ability to perform (i.e., perceived self-efficacy) develops as a result of the interaction of each of the six attributes of Social Cognitive Theory described earlier.

Relationship to Self-Esteem

Perceived self-efficacy should not be confused with the construct of self-esteem. *Self-esteem* is defined as "the dimension of self-concept that includes a negative and/or positive sense of self" (Daub, 1988, p. 57). Self-esteem is created by the person's analysis of his or her overall competency at factors that he or she considers to be socially relevant (Mayberry, 1990). Thus, a person may perceive himself or herself to be competent at many things but have low self-esteem due to a belief that these competencies are not socially relevant. Conversely, a person may express a low degree of perceived self-efficacy for one or more tasks yet have high self-esteem. Self-esteem and perceived self-efficacy should be highly correlated only when measuring perceived self-efficacy for a task that is highly socially relevant to the subject. A Nobel Prize winner may have high self-esteem in part due to the recognition of the value of his or her contribution to society. The same Nobel Prize winner may have low perceived self-efficacy for playing racquetball or gourmet cooking. However, his or her perceived self-efficacy for the activity that resulted in the Nobel Prize should be high and should correlate strongly with a measure of his or her self-esteem. Thus, perceived self-efficacy may contribute to a sense of self-esteem, but it is an independent construct.

Parameters of Self-Efficacy

Bandura (1977) identified three parameters of perceived self-efficacy: magnitude, strength, and generality. *Magnitude* refers to the relative level of difficulty of the task that is being rated. For example, Ewart and colleagues (1986) used different jogging distances to reflect differences in the magnitude of perceived self-efficacy for a group of subjects with postmyocardial infarction. Subjects who were completely confident that they could jog 1 mile were considered to have a greater magnitude of perceived self-efficacy than those who were completely confident that they could jog only a quarter of a mile and somewhat confident that they could jog 1 mile.

Strength of perceived self-efficacy refers to the degree to which people believe they can succeed at a given level of an activity; this degree can vary from total certainty to total uncertainty. The stronger the sense of efficacy, the more likely people are to persevere in the face of adversity and the less likely it is that failure will extinguish their efficacy expectations (Bandura, 1977).

Generality of perceived self-efficacy refers to the degree to which the person's perceived self-efficacy for one activity transfers to other similar or different activities. Successful performance of some tasks results in a strengthening of efficacy expectations for that task alone, whereas success at other tasks generalizes to tasks that are different from the original task

(Bandura, 1977). Bandura does not identify the types of tasks that generalize or those that do not.

History of the Construct

Bandura postulated that, given the requisite skills and belief that the response will lead to a desired outcome, perceived self-efficacy would be an important determinant of successful performance. Bandura (1977; Bandura & Adams, 1977) tested the theory about perceived self-efficacy with an unspecified number of persons with snake phobias. Subjects were asked to state whether they were able to perform each of 18 tasks and to rate the strength of their expectations that they would succeed on a 100-point scale with 10-point intervals. The subjects were randomly assigned to one of three groups: vicarious experience, modeling (later called enactive experience), or no treatment. The subjects in the vicarious learning group observed an instructor handling snakes, while the enactive learning group first observed and then attempted the snake-handling techniques themselves. Of the subjects who achieved maximal performances during therapy (successfully achieved the snake-handling techniques), Bandura noted that not all expressed maximal efficacy expectations. Efficacy expectation and performance during the treatment sessions were examined as possible predictors of subsequent performance. Perceived self-efficacy was found to be the best predictor of subsequent performance. The higher the subjects' perceived self-efficacy at the completion of treatment, the better their performance when retested at a later date ($r = .75$, $p < .01$). This relationship existed regardless of whether the efficacy expectations were derived through vicarious or enactive experience. However, subjects who experienced enactive education produced higher, more generalized, and stronger efficacy expectations and increased performance attempts. Bandura (1977) stated that:

> on the one hand, the mechanisms by which human behavior is acquired and regulated are increasingly formulated in terms of cognitive processes. On the other hand, it is the performance based procedures that are proving to be most powerful for effecting psychological changes. As a consequence, successful performance is replacing symbolically based experiences as the principal vehicle of change. (p. 191)

Since his initial work, Bandura has examined the effect of perceived self-efficacy with a variety of subjects and found that perceived self-efficacy is a consistent predictor of performance (Bandura, 1982; Bandura, Cioffi, Taylor, & Brouillard, 1988; Bandura & Wood, 1989).

The construct of perceived self-efficacy has been applied in a variety of different clinical, educational, and organizational situations by many other authors. From January 1987 to December 1992, 933 articles referring to perceived self-efficacy have been printed in journals indexed by Psychlit alone. The following is a brief summary of the findings of a small sampling of these articles that were selected for their relevance to occupational therapy practice.

Clinical Examples

- Perceived self-efficacy for exercise was found to be correlated with an increase in exercise endurance in a sample of subjects ($n = 119$) with chronic obstructive lung disease (Toshima et al., 1990).
- Self-efficacy was found to explain 24 percent of the variance in adjustment to multiple sclerosis ($n = 62$) (Wassem, 1992).
- Self-efficacy for jogging proved superior to treadmill performance, depression, and type A personality in predicting adherence to exercise prescription in a sample ($n = 40$) of patients with coronary artery disease (Ewart et al., 1986).
- The results of a study of subjects ($n = 30$) diagnosed with arthritis indicated that a higher level of perceived self-efficacy for pain control after a cognitive behavioral education program was related to a lower level of perceived pain (O'Leary, Shoor, Lorig, & Holman, 1988).

Health Promotion Examples

- A scale, developed to measure perceived barriers to health-promotion activities, was found to be highly correlated (- .48) with perceived self-efficacy (Stuifbergen, Becker, & Sands, 1990).
- In a sample ($n = 600$) of subjects participating in the Stanford Heart Disease Prevention Program, self-efficacy was found to be a better predictor of nutritional choices than demographic factors, social influences, and health knowledge (Slater, 1989). This study also found that cognitive control (the capacity to exercise control over one's own thinking and motivation) predicted the level of perceived self-efficacy.
- Raising self-efficacy for health-promoting behaviors was found to be more effective than emphasizing the risk of not performing the health-promoting behavior in two separate studies (Seydel et al., 1990).

Education Examples

- Attributional feedback from the researcher (feedback about who was responsible for past successes), as opposed to feedback about future potential success or no feedback, was found to be related to faster mathematical skill development and higher perceived self-efficacy in a sample ($n = 40$) of children ranging in ages from 7 to 10 years (Shunk, 1982).
- Subjects who were successful using strategies taught in a "learning to learn" program led to enhanced perceived self-efficacy and generalized to other activities requiring similar learning skills for a group of 4th graders (Wang & Richarde, 1987).

Perceived Self-Efficacy as a Behavioral Determinant

A strong sense of perceived self-efficacy for an activity is crucial to successful performance because "it determines which activities people engage in, the amount of effort they expend before terminating the activity, and how long they will persevere in the face of adversity" (Bandura, 1981, p. 215). People are faced with frequent activity choices throughout their lives. The strength of their efficacy expectations for an activity affects whether they choose to engage in the activity or not. Strong efficacy expectations result in engagement in an activity; whereas weak efficacy expectations result in avoidance (Bandura, 1986). This process of activity selection has a profound effect on human development, in that activity choices enlarge or restrict one's opportunities to develop new skills, or to enhance existing ones (Bandura, 1986).

Errors in judgment regarding one's performance, whether too optimistic or too pessimistic, may result in significant consequences (Bandura, 1986). In activities with a small margin of error (e.g., driving a car), overly optimistic efficacy expectations may prove disastrous. However, in activities with a greater margin of error, activities that are unlikely to result in harm to oneself or others, appraisals of performance that exceed actual ability are quite functional (Bandura, 1989).

For example, when a patient is attempting to learn to maneuver a wheelchair, a high expectation that he or she is capable of learning to propel the chair will result in more frequent attempts and learning will advance more quickly. On the other hand, if the patient believes that he or she is unlikely to master propelling the wheelchair, he or she will avoid situations where this is a requirement and progress will be impeded. Bandura asserted (1989) that people must strive to exceed past performances, and that if efficacy expectations never exceeded past performance, the acquisition of new skills would not occur.

People with strong efficacy expectations will persevere in the face of adversity, due to a belief that they will ultimately succeed (Bandura, 1977). People with weaker efficacy expectations will quit when faced with obstacles, or refuse even to try. People who view themselves as efficacious are more likely to expect things to go right (Bandura, 1989). They approach difficult tasks as challenges to master rather than threats to avoid. People who experience success react by raising their personal goals and being more committed to the activity (Bandura & Wood, 1989). The stronger the sense of perceived self-efficacy, the higher the goals set and the stronger the commitment to attainment of the goals.

Although perceived self-efficacy is a crucial behavioral determinant, Bandura (1977) pointed out that perceived self-efficacy in the absence of skill, or a desire to perform, will not ensure successful performance. Attempts to enhance performance must be accompanied by an understanding of the influence of perceived self-efficacy on performance.

Outcome Expectations and Perceived Self-Efficacy

Perceived self-efficacy refers to a belief in one's ability to perform a certain task or behavior. It should not be confused with a belief that performance of a specified behavior will result in a specific outcome (Bandura, 1977). Rogers (1983) referred to a belief that performance of a specified behavior will result in a specified outcome as response efficacy. Both perceived self-efficacy and response efficacy affect whether or not the person will elect to perform a certain task; however, they are distinct behavioral determinants (Bandura, 1977). That is, one must believe both that a specific action will lead to a desired goal and that one is capable of performing the specific action, or one will not act.

Bandura (1986) argued that theories that emphasize outcome expectations are based on animal research where measurement of perceived self-efficacy was impossible. He stated that "convictions that outcomes are determined by one's own actions can be either demoralizing or heartening, depending on the level of self-judged efficacy" (Bandura, 1986, p. 413). Therefore, an expectation that a certain behavior will result in a certain outcome is not sufficient to ensure successful performance unless one believes one has the skills to succeed at the required task.

Relationship to Psychological Well-Being

According to self-efficacy ideology, people can give up trying and become hopeless in two different ways: they may believe that their continued attempts will not bring positive results (response efficacy), or they may believe that they are unable to perform the tasks necessary to bring about the desired results (perceived self-efficacy) (Bandura, 1982). Different combinations of these two factors result in different self-assessments:

- If persons have a strong sense of perceived self-efficacy and a strong belief in the efficacy of the response, they will act in an assured manner and be dynamic.
- If persons have a strong sense of perceived self-efficacy but a weak sense of response efficacy, they will energize themselves to make changes in the system so that they can successfully attain their goal.
- If people have a weak sense of perceived self-efficacy and a weak sense of response efficacy, they will become resigned and apathetic.
- If people have a weak sense of perceived self-efficacy and a strong sense of response efficacy, they will become despondent and self-deprecating.

The relationship between perceived self-efficacy and psychological well-being was explored by Holahan, Holahan, and Belk (1984). Perceived self-efficacy was measured by asking a group of retired university faculty members how well they handled or could in the future handle each of the items on a list of daily hassles (self-efficacy / hassles scale) and a list of negative life events (self-efficacy / life events scale). The results indicated that higher levels of perceived self-efficacy were associated with lower levels of depression for both sexes. Additionally high levels of perceived self-efficacy were associated with lower levels of psychological distress for women and fewer psychosomatic complaints for men. Overall, the results indicate a significant association between perceived self-efficacy and psychological adjustment.

Perceived self-efficacy has also been shown to negatively correlate with depression. Davis-Berman (1990) administered the Physical Self-Efficacy Scale and the General Self-Efficacy Scale to a sample of 200 elderly residents of a retirement center. The Physical Self-Efficacy Scale consists of 22 items and includes questions about reflexes, muscle tone, and sports ability. The General Self-Efficacy Scale consists of two subscales, the General Scale and the Social Self-Efficacy Scale. The scale contains questions about one's general belief in one's ability to do things and one's ability to handle oneself in social situations. All three Self-Efficacy Scales were found to be inversely and significantly ($p > .01$) correlated to depression. (General Self-Efficacy $r = -.40$, Social Self-Efficacy $r = -.23$, and Physical Self-Efficacy $r = .50$). That is, persons with lower self-efficacy scores were more likely to be depressed.

Influencing the Strength of Perceived Self-Efficacy

Perceived self-efficacy is influenced through an ongoing evaluation of success and failure with each task people participate in over the course of their lives (Bandura, 1986). Bandura (1982) stated that perceived self-efficacy develops through successful experiences that create high efficacy expectations and failure experiences that lower efficacy expectations. Thus, the development of perceived self-efficacy is a dynamic process.

Perceived self-efficacy is constantly affected by four sources of information: personal performance accomplishments, vicarious experience (watching others of similar skill perform a task), verbal persuasion, and the person's physiological state (Bandura, 1977).

Personal Performance Accomplishments

Personal performance accomplishments, also called enactive experiences, are the most influential source of information about one's perceived self-efficacy (Bandura, 1986). Success, as perceived by the person, enhances perceived self-efficacy, and failure decreases it. Failure early in the development of a new skill is more likely to decrease perceived self-efficacy than failure after a firmly entrenched belief in the skill has been developed. When people believe they are efficacious, they attribute failure to the circumstances, poor effort on their part, or the use of poor strategies (Bandura, 1986).

Vicarious Experience

A great deal of human learning begins with observing others perform tasks (Bandura, 1986). Vicarious learning is developed more readily when the observer considers the person being observed to have similar skills to himself or herself. Children watch and then imitate their parents. In this process of observing activities, some learning occurs before the person is required to attempt any of the requisite behaviors. For example, children observe their parents driving cars for years before they begin. They observe how the wheel is turned, how to start the car, what the highway signs mean, and so on. This learning decreases the number of new skills that must be learned when the children reach an appropriate age and actually begin to drive the car. They already understand the component skills and now need to learn to execute them independently (Bandura, 1986). Vicarious learning is not as powerful a source of information as enactive learning, but it is still very important.

Persuasion

Persuasion is a frequently used means of convincing someone that his or her self-assessment is incorrect. However, it is the weakest form of information with respect to altering perceived self-efficacy (Bandura, 1986). Persuasion will be effective in altering beliefs only if the current belief is close to the belief that is being proposed. Subsequent performance quickly affirms or denies the new belief. Thus, accurate assessment of the other person's ability is required if persuasion is to succeed.

Physiological State

People read their level of somatic arousal as an indication of competency (Bandura, 1977). Thus, if your heart rate increases and you begin to sweat, you interpret these reactions as an indication that the activity you are approaching is in some way threatening. Strategies that decrease the level of arousal (relaxation techniques) have been found to enable people to feel more efficacious. This feeling of efficacy in turn leads to a willingness to attempt the behavior that had previously resulted in a state of physiological arousal, and to success experiences (Bandura, 1986).

Cognitive Appraisal

Personal performance accomplishments, vicarious experience, persuasion, and physiological arousal are the types of experiences that affect perceived self-efficacy. However, the degree to which these experiences influence perceived self-efficacy is determined by the person's cognitive appraisal and integration of these experiences (Bandura, 1982; Gist & Mitchell, 1992).

Gist and Mitchell (1992) developed a model to explain the effect of these experiences on perceived self-efficacy. They suggested that the cognitive appraisal and integration process has three components. The first component is the analysis of the requirements of the task. The more complex the task and the less previous experience one has with a task, the harder it is to accurately assess one's perceived self-efficacy for the task. The second component is the analysis of the degree to which success or failure is attributed to oneself rather than others or to chance. If one believes that one is successful due to a skill one possesses, then perceived self-efficacy for the task will be heightened. However, if one believes that one was successful because of chance, the actions of others, or the environment, perceived self-efficacy will not be affected. The third component is the analysis of personal and situational resources and constraints that affect the task at hand. This appraisal process involves the assessment of personal factors such as skill, motivation, anxiety, and desire, as well as situational factors, such as distractions, support of influential others, and competing demands.

The three cognitive appraisal processes will result in the subjects' determination of the degree of perceived self-efficacy for a task, which in turn affects the person's willingness to participate or persevere with the task in the future, and hence will affect actual future performance.

Generalizability

The development of perceived self-efficacy is largely situation specific, with a tendency to generalize to similar activities (Ewart, Taylor, Reese, & DeBusk, 1983). Ewart and his colleagues studied the relationship between perceived self-efficacy and activity for a group of patients with postmyocardial infarction. These patients participated in treadmill testing and filled in a perceived self-efficacy questionnaire before the treadmill test, after the treadmill test, and after a counseling session that followed the treadmill test. The perceived self-efficacy questions covered walking, running, climbing stairs, engaging in sexual intercourse, lifting objects, and an overall estimate of ability to tolerate physical activity. Perceived self-efficacy ratings for the activities that used the same physical skills as the treadmill (walking, running, and climbing stairs) showed the greatest increase. With the addition of counseling (a form of verbal persuasion), the efficacy ratings for the other activities increased. Assistance with interpretation of the treadmill experience was necessary before generalization could occur.

Control

The degree of control the person perceives that he or she has alters the influence of success or failure on the development of perceived self-efficacy. Bandura and Wood (1989) studied the influence of perceived control on perceived self-efficacy in a simulated manufacturing environment. The degree of perceived control and the amount of success the subjects experienced were regulated through the design of the experiment. Subjects were randomly assigned to one of four groups. Each group received instructions designed to alter their perception of two constructs, personal control and performance expectations. The four groups were low perceived control with high performance expectations, low perceived control with low performance expectations, high perceived control with high performance expectations, and high per-

ceived control with low performance expectations. The groups that were given high performance standards experienced less success than those with low performance standards. Subjects who viewed the organization as controllable, regardless of whether they were in the high or low performance expectations group, had higher mean self-efficacy scores than those who thought that they had little control over the organization ($p < .02$). Subjects in the high control, high performance standards group showed increases in perceived self-efficacy over three trials, whereas subjects in the high control, low success groups showed decreases in perceived self-efficacy ($p < .05$). Subjects who were led to believe that the organization was difficult to control demonstrated low self-efficacy regardless of whether they were in the high or low performance expectation group; that is, their perceived self-efficacy was low regardless of whether or not they were experiencing success.

Discussion of the Literature

Adolph Meyer, a major contributor to the philosophical basis of occupational therapy practice, recognized the value of the feelings of satisfaction and achievement associated with successful completion of a project (1922) (see Chapter 2). Thus, from the early days of occupational therapy practice, the value of successful experiences, that is, performance accomplishments, was recognized. Activity programs were structured to ensure success because success was believed to lead the patient to try another, more difficult task. Occupational therapists have often described this process as the enhancement of self-esteem (Christiansen, 1991; Meyer, 1922 [see Chapter 2]), yet the activities the occupational therapy client performs are not always socially relevant. Therefore, it is postulated that success with occupational therapy activities leads to an increase in perceived self-efficacy for these activities, which leads to a willingness to engage in and persist in future similar tasks. If the success experiences relate to socially relevant activities an elevation in self-esteem would also be predicted.

The occupational performance literature addresses the need to understand the effect of psychosocial factors on occupational performance (Christiansen, 1991; Pedretti & Pasquinelli-Estrada, 1985; Trombly, 1989). An underlying assumption appears to be that psychological factors affect only the acquisition of skill and that once the skill has been learned it will be used outside the protected clinical environment. However, just as Bandura (1977) noted that people do not always perform optimally even when they have the requisite skills, clinicians have stated that occupational therapy clients do not always perform at the level one might predict on the basis of clinical observation of skill (Gage, 1992).

The Model of Human Occupation, a model that guides occupational therapy practice, addresses the discrepancy between skill and performance through, among other things, a concept similar to perceived self-efficacy: personal causation

(Oakley, Kielhofner, & Barris, 1985). *Personal causation* is defined as "the collective beliefs that an individual has efficacious skills, is personally in control, and will succeed in future endeavors" (Oakley et al., p. 148). This construct is equivalent to the construct of perceived self-efficacy.

When discussing the influence of inefficacy (a term that Kielhofner has used in the same view as perceived self-efficacy), Kielhofner stated that "occupational dysfunction is at the level of inefficacy when there is an interference with performing meaningful activity accompanied by dissatisfaction with performance" (1985, p. 69). He went on to state that "sources of inefficacy may be environmental constraints, disease processes, or imbalanced lifestyles" (p. 69).

The importance of the strength of the person's belief in his or her ability to perform the specific component parts of life roles is not articulated. One's perception of one's ability to perform is considered to be a major behavioral determinant (Allen et al., 1990; Bandura, 1977, 1986; Bandura & Adams, 1977; Bandura & Wood, 1989; Ewart et al., 1986; Seydel et al., 1990; Shunk, 1982; Toshima et al., 1990; Wang & Richarde, 1987; Wassem, 1992). Therefore, it is essential that the relationship of perceived self-efficacy to occupational performance be explored.

The terms *perceived self-efficacy* or *efficacy expectations* are beginning to appear in the occupational therapy literature. Crist and Stoffel (1992) (see Chapter 29), when discussing the Americans With Disabilities Act as it applies to persons with mental impairments, discussed the value of perceived self-efficacy with respect to successful employment of persons with mental disabilities. Christiansen (1991) acknowledged that the "single characteristic of the individual that has the greatest influence on performance is one's sense of competence" (p. 20), yet this concept is given only four paragraphs in the occupational therapy textbook written by Christiansen and Baum.

There is a growing recognition that clients' perceptions of performance (perceived self-efficacy) are important. In the March 1993 issue of the *American Journal of Occupational Therapy,* professional leaders discussed the needs of the profession with respect to assessment. Authors cited the need to measure client perception of performance (Law, 1993), the need to identify the psychological factors that contribute to performance deficits and strengths (Bonder, 1993), and the need to develop means of remediating these psychological factors once identified (Bonder, 1993). Trombly stated that the overall goal of occupational therapy is to "enable the client to gain a sense of efficacy" (1993, p. 254). The Canadian Occupational Performance Measure (Law et al., 1991) uses client perception of performance as one outcome variable. However, there is a need to incorporate this belief into occupational therapy practices.

The influence of perceived self-efficacy on the person's ability to cope with the effects of disability has also been articulated by Gage (1992). She was interested in determining why patients of equal physical impairment and rehabilitation potential do not progress at the same pace, and why, given similar goals, these patients attain different levels of independent function. After a review of the literature on coping, Gage formulated the Appraisal Model of Coping as a guide to assessment and intervention for occupational therapists. The Appraisal Model of Coping was based on the Cognitive Relational Theory of Coping and Emotion (Lazarus & Folkman, 1984) and Social Cognitive Theory (Bandura, 1977). *Coping* was defined by Lazarus and Folkman (1984) as the process through which people manage the demands and emotions generated by person–environment relationships.

The model presented by Gage identified 12 factors that influence the ability of persons to cope with their disability or any other life event that taxes personal resources. One of these 12 factors is perceived self-efficacy. In this model, perceived self-efficacy is considered by Gage to be particularly salient to the practice of occupational therapy because of its potential ability to explain the discrepancy between skill developed in therapy and occupational performance outside the protected clinical environment. However, the model is, as yet, conceptual and must be tested to determine the specific nature of the influence of perceived self-efficacy on coping with occupational performance deficits.

Enhancing Occupational Performance

A recognition that the client's level of perceived self-efficacy for a specific activity influences the likelihood of the client performing that activity outside the protected clinical environment has far-reaching implications for the practice of occupational therapy. This recognition brings with it an understanding that a client's ability to perform a specific skill in the clinical environment may not mean that the client will use the skill in his or her usual contextual environment. What good is treatment if it does not generalize to the use of the skill in the community?

Occupational therapists must learn how to evaluate their client's level of perceived self-efficacy and to develop techniques that not only improve clients' skills, but also enhance their self-efficacy for use of those skills in the community. As previously presented, empirical findings about the influence of perceived self-efficacy on clinical outcome are already available (Ewart et al., 1986; O'Leary et al., 1988; Toshima et al., 1990; Wassem, 1992). Although these studies do not specifically look at occupational performance activities or the influence of the occupational therapy process on perceived self-efficacy, they do provide information that is relevant to occupational therapy practice. Empirical studies have also investigated the relationship between perceived self-efficacy and the initiation or adherence to health-promoting behaviors (Seydel et al., 1990; Slater, 1989; Stuifbergen et al.,

1990). The results of these studies are increasingly relevant to occupational therapists as more and more therapists become involved with primary and secondary prevention activities. In addition, the process of occupational therapy is often one of teaching new skills or teaching new ways to perform familiar activities. Thus, articles that present data about the relationship between perceived self-efficacy and learning are also relevant to occupational therapists (Shunk, 1982; Wang & Richarde, 1987).

It is important to remember that the articles cited in this paper are just a small sampling of the perceived self-efficacy literature available to occupational therapists. Occupational therapists working in various fields are encouraged to search the literature for articles that have valuable information about perceived self-efficacy within their area of practice. Occupational therapy research studies to add to this knowledge base are encouraged. There are many possible applications that arise from the attributes of perceived self-efficacy as presented in the section of this paper titled "History of the Construct." These themes can be categorized into three major categories: assessment, outcome, and therapeutic process.

Assessment and Outcome

Previous research has demonstrated a link between clinical outcomes and perceived self-efficacy (Allen et al., 1990; Bandura, 1977, 1986; Bandura, & Adams, 1977; Bandura & Wood, 1989; Ewart et al., 1986; Seydel, Taal, & Wiegman, 1990; Shunk, 1982; Toshima et al., 1990; Wang & Richarde, 1987; Wassem, 1992). Thus, it is important to derive ways to measure perceived self-efficacy for occupational performance activities that will enable the exploration of its relationship to outcome. For example, perceived self-efficacy is thought to explain the variance between development of skill and performance of that skill in the community. It is, therefore, important to explore the influence of increases or decreases in perceived self-efficacy for occupational performance activities on treatment outcomes. The level of perceived self-efficacy that is required before a client will use the skill independently in the community must be determined. The belief that the development of a skill is not sufficient to ensure successful occupational performance in the absence of an adequate level of perceived self-efficacy leads to a need to monitor a client's perceived self-efficacy during the treatment process. The ability to demonstrate occupational competence in the clinical environment should no longer indicate successful treatment outcome. Therapists must find ways to determine whether their clients are using these skills in the community. Because perceived self-efficacy is believed to be a good predictor of future performance, therapists need to establish the level of perceived self-efficacy that is likely to result in use of the skill in the community. This level may then be useful in the determination of when to discharge from therapy. However, individual variation will always necessitate individual follow-up to ensure that a given client has been successful.

Therapeutic Process

The section of this paper titled "Influencing the Strength of Perceived Self-Efficacy" provides occupational therapists with specific strategies for increasing perceived self-efficacy in the clinical environment. For example, perceived self-efficacy is enhanced through personal performance accomplishments; that is, by actually doing the activity or very similar activities. In fact, it is suggested that perceived self-efficacy for an activity performed in the occupational therapy department will only generalize to very similar activities. Thus, occupational therapists must use realistic activities that simulate the contextual environment of the client. This will be easy for therapists working in the community who provide services in the client's home; it will be more difficult for therapists working in institutional environments. The relevance of reductionistic activities such as peg boards and puzzles must be questioned. How does the mastery of these component skills relate to changes in perceived self-efficacy and actual performance for personally important life activities?

The role of vicarious learning with respect to the development of occupational competence must also be explored. If, in fact, a great deal of human learning begins with observing others perform tasks, it would be important for clients to observe the successful performance attempts of their peers. Bandura (1977) suggested that vicarious experience is most powerful when the participants consider themselves to have similar skills. Thus, modeling by the therapist may be ineffective, and consumer self-help groups might be encouraged.

Gist and Mitchell (1992) suggest that self-efficacy beliefs are most accurate when clients are rating familiar activities because they understand the relationship between the skills required to perform the task and the skills they possess. For occupational therapy clients the knowledge of the skills they possess has often been affected by the onset of a disabling condition. Although the clients are aware of the skills required for occupational performance activities, they may believe that their disability has robbed them of these skills. Thus, the occupational therapist must provide them with a safe environment within which to experiment with their altered level of performance and to develop a new understanding of their efficacy.

Therapists often try to convince clients that they are able to go home and live independently, or return to work, only to be confronted with a barrage of reasons why the client is not yet ready. These patients are labeled as fearful or, worse yet, as malingerers. Perhaps it is simply their perceived self-efficacy for home management or work activities that has not yet reached the level necessary to engage in the activity independently. If one accepts that persuasion is the least influential method of raising efficacy expectations, then the therapist must devise new intervention techniques. The treatment plan must incorporate vicarious learning and relevant personal performance accomplishments if success is to occur. The use of such simulations as Easy Street,[1] a stay in an activities of daily living (ADL) apartment located in the protected clinical environment, or a home visit with the therapist may be a better solution than attempts to persuade.

Perceived self-efficacy increases more when the client is in control. Thus, it is important for therapists to enable clients to articulate their needs and have a real voice in the therapeutic process. Tools such as the Canadian Occupational Performance Measure (Law et al., 1991) may create a feeling of control and enhance outcomes.

Summary

Perceived self-efficacy has great relevance to the practice of occupational therapy. It is consistent with the fundamental philosophical beliefs of the profession, may enhance and predict outcomes, and has a strong empirical basis that suggest specific changes to current occupational therapy treatment practice. Occupational therapists are challenged to develop, test, and publish these linkages.

Many of the attributes of perceived self-efficacy are relevant to occupational performance. By monitoring and working to enhance perceived self-efficacy, occupational therapists may be better able to explain the variance between development of skill and performance of that skill in the community, ensure successful occupational performance in the community, predict future performance, and enable occupational competence.

Acknowledgment

Funds for this study were obtained through a Health Services Research Grant awarded to the first author by Victoria Hospital, London, Ontario, Canada.

References

Allen, J. K., Becker, D. M., & Swank, R. T. (1990). Factors related to functional status after coronary artery bypass surgery. *Heart and Lung, 19,* 337–343.

Bandura, A. (1977). Toward a unifying theory of behavioral change. *Psychological Review, 84,* 101–215.

Bandura, A. (1981). Self-referent thought: A developmental analysis of self-efficacy. In J. H. Flavell & L. Ross (Eds.), *Social cognitive development: Frontiers and possible futures* (pp. 200–239). New York: Cambridge University Press.

Bandura, A. (1982). Self-efficacy mechanism in human agency. *American Psychologist, 37,* 122–147.

Bandura, A. (1986). *Social foundations of thought.* Englewood Cliffs, NJ: Prentice Hall.

Bandura, A. (1989). Regulation of cognitive processes through perceived self-efficacy. *Developmental Psychology, 25,* 729–735.

Bandura, A., & Adams, N. E. (1977). Analysis of self-efficacy theory of behavioral change. *Cognitive Therapy and Research, 1,* 287–310.

Bandura, A., Cioffi, D., Taylor, C. B., & Brouillard (1988). Perceived self-efficacy in coping with cognitive stressors and opioid activation. *Journal of Personality and Social Psychology, 55,* 497–488.

Bandura, A., & Wood, R. (1989). Effect of perceived controllability and performance standards on self-regulation of complex decision-making. *Journal of Personality and Social Psychology, 56,* 805–814.

Bonder, B. R. (1993). Issues in assessment of psychosocial components of function. *American Journal of Occupational Therapy, 47,* 211–216.

Christiansen, C. (1991). Occupational Therapy: Intervention for life performance. In C. Christiansen & C. Baum (Eds.), *Occupational therapy: Overcoming human performance deficits* (pp.3–43). Beckenham, Kent, England: Slack.

Crist, P. A. H., & Stoffel, V. C. (1992). The Americans With Disabilities Act of 1990 and employees with mental impairments: Personal efficacy and the environment. *American Journal of Occupational Therapy, 46,* 434–443. Reprinted as Chapter 29.

Daub, M. (1988). Prenatal development through mid-adulthood. In H. L. Hopkins & H. D. Smith (Eds.), *Willard and Spackman's occupational therapy* (7th ed., pp. 50–75). Philadelphia: Lippincott.

Davis-Berman, J. (1990). Physical self-efficacy, perceived physical status, and depressive symptomatology in older adults. *Journal of Psychology, 124,* 207–215.

Ewart, C. K., Stewart, K. J., Gillilan, R. E., Kelemen, M. H., Valenti, S. A., Manley, J. D., & Kelemen, M. D. (1986). Usefulness of self-efficacy in predicting overexertion during programmed exercise in coronary artery disease. *American Journal of Cardiology, 57,* 557–561.

Ewart, C. K., Taylor, C. B., Reese, L. B., & DeBusk, R. F. (1983). Effects of early postmyocardial infarction exercise testing on self-perception and subsequent physical activity. *American Journal of Cardiology, 51,* 1076–1080.

Gage, M. (1992). The appraisal model of coping: An assessment and intervention model for occupational therapy. *American Journal of Occupational Therapy, 46,* 353–362.

Gist, M., & Mitchell, T. (1992). Self-efficacy: A theoretical analysis of its determinants and malleability. *Academy of Management Review, 17,* 183–211.

Holahan, C. K., Holahan, C. J., & Belk, S. S. (1984). Adjustment in aging: The roles of life stress, hassles, and self-efficacy. *Health Psychology, 3,* 315–328.

Kielhofner, G. (1985). Occupational function and dysfunction. In G. Kielhofner (Ed.), *A model of human occupation* (pp. 63–75). Baltimore: Williams & Wilkins.

Law, M. (1993). Evaluating activities of daily living: Directions for the future. *American Journal of Occupational Therapy, 47,* 233–237.

Law, M., Baptiste, S., Carswell-Opzoomer, A., McCall, M. A., Polatajko, H., & Pollock, N. (1991). *Canadian Occupational Performance Measure.* CAOT Publications ACE, Toronto, Canada.

Lazarus, R. S., & Folkman, S. (1984). *Stress appraisal and coping.* New York: Springer.

Mayberry, W. (1990). Self-esteem in children: Considerations for measurement and intervention. *American Journal of Occupational Therapy, 44,* 729–734.

Meyer, A. (1922). The philosophy of occupation therapy. *American Journal of Occupational Therapy, 31,* 639–642. Reprinted as Chapter 2.

Oakley, F., Kielhofner, G., & Barris, R. (1985). An occupational therapy approach to assessing psychiatric patients' adaptive functioning. *American Journal of Occupational Therapy, 39,* 147–154.

---

[1]Manufactured by Easy Street Environments, 6908 E. Thomas Road, Suite 201, Scottsdale, AZ 85251.

O'Leary, A., Shoor, S., Lorig, K., & Holman, H. R. (1988). A cognitive–behavioral treatment for rheumatoid arthritis. *Health Psychology, 7,* 527–544.

Pedretti, L. W., & Pasquinelli-Estrada, S. (1985). Foundations for treatment of physical dysfunction. In L. Pedretti (Ed.), *Occupational therapy: Practice skills for physical dysfunction* (2nd ed., pp. 1–10). St. Louis: Mosby.

Rogers, R. W. (1983). Cognitive and physiological processes in fear appeals and attitude change: A revised theory of protection motivation. In J. T. Cacioppo, R. E. Petty, & D. Shapiro (Eds.), *Social psychophysiology* (pp. 153–176). New York: Guilford.

Seydel, E., Taal, E., & Wiegman, O. (1990). Risk-appraisal, outcome, and self-efficacy expectancies: Cognitive factors in preventive behavior related to cancer. *Psychology and Health, 4,* 99–109.

Shaffer, H. (1978). Psychological rehabilitation, skills-building, and self-efficacy. *American Psychologist, 33,* 394–396.

Shunk, D. (1982). Effects of effort attributional feedback on children's perceived self-efficacy and achievement. *Journal of Educational Psychology, 74,* 548–556.

Slater, M. (1989). Social influences and cognitive control as predictors of self-efficacy and eating behavior. *Cognitive Therapy and Research, 13,* 231–245.

Stuifbergen, A., Becker, H., & Sands, D. (May 1990). Barriers to health promotion for individuals with disabilities. *Family and Community Health,* 11–22.

Toshima, M., Kaplan, R., & Ries, A. (1990). Experimental evaluation of rehabilitation in chronic obstructive pulmonary disease: Short-term effects on exercise endurance and health status. *Health Psychology, 9,* 237–252.

Trombly, C. A. (1989). *Occupational therapy for physical dysfunction* (3rd ed.). Baltimore: Williams & Wilkins.

Trombly, C. (1993). The Issue Is— Anticipating the future: Assessment of occupational function. *American Journal of Occupational Therapy, 47,* 253–257.

Wang, A., & Richarde, R. S. (1987). Development of memory monitoring and self-efficacy in children. *Psychological Reports, 60,* 647–658.

Wassem, R. (1992). Self-efficacy as a predictor of adjustment to multiple sclerosis. *Journal of Neuroscience Nursing, 24,* 224–229.

Understanding the Family Perspective: An Ethnographic Framework for Providing Occupational Therapy in the Home

LAURA N. GITLIN, PHD
MARY CORCORAN, PHD, OTR/L
SUSAN LEINMILLER-ECKHARDT, OTR/L

It has been firmly established that families provide the majority of long-term care in the home to elderly persons with cognitive and physical impairments (Pepper Commission, 1990; Stone, Cafferata, & Sangi, 1987). To support family caregivers in these efforts, there has been an increased interest in developing and testing the effectiveness of a wide range of interventions (Knight, Lutzky, & Macofsky-Urban, 1993) and in identifying the particular contributions of occupational therapy (Clark, Corcoran, & Gitlin, in press; Corcoran & Gitlin, 1992; Hasselkus, 1989). However, the growing body of literature on caregiver interventions has suggested that family members tend to underuse formal health and human services (Knight et al., 1993), may indicate little need for assistance (Collins, 1992; Smyth & Harris, 1993), and sometimes express conflict with the goals that are established by health and human service professionals (Chiou & Burnett, 1985; Hasselkus, 1991; Kaufman, 1988). Furthermore, research on caregiver interventions such as home environmental modifications (Gitlin & Corcoran, 1993; Pynoos & Ohta, 1991), respite, psychoeducational counseling, and support groups has indicated that caregivers are selective in their use of prescribed strategies and do not uniformly benefit or demonstrate reduced stress from participation in these services (Knight et al., 1993).

This chapter was previously published in the *American Journal of Occupational Therapy, 49*, 802–809. Copyright © 1995, American Occupational Therapy Association.

Recent research in caregiving that has used naturalistic inquiry has demonstrated that caregiving in the home is a complex process that is imbued with meaning and purpose. The meaning of caregiving, or how a person makes sense of his or her experiences, influences how daily care is provided in the home and how caregivers define their needs (Albert, 1992; Gubrium & Sankar, 1990; Hasselkus, 1988, 1989). Other research has noted that caregivers vary in the way they adapt to their experiences and that they identify a range of factors as stressful and cope differently depending upon the particular stressor (Corcoran, 1992; Henderson & Gutierrez-Mayka, 1992; Williamson & Schulz, 1993). These findings underscore the highly individual and unique nature of each caregiving situation. The findings also suggest the existence of a "neglect of perspective" or the disregard by health-care professionals of the client's perspective on his or her own needs in developing services (Fine, 1993, p. 2).

Despite the evidence that caregivers define, approach, and react to their caregiving role in distinct ways, occupational therapists lack a framework for developing occupational therapy services that are based on the unique needs of the family members we seek to support. A framework from which to evaluate the specific and individualized needs of families and their elderly members with disabilities is increasingly important as we move toward a health-care system that is community and home based.

Recently, there has been an increased interest in ethnography as an approach to research in gerontology (Gubrium & Sankar, 1994) and health services (DePoy & Gitlin, 1994), and as a basis for deriving clinical intervention strategies that overcome the potential conflict in perspectives between service provider and client (Hasselkus, 1990; Hill, Fortenberry, & Stein, 1990; Kleinman, 1988; Spencer, Krefting, & Mattingly, 1993). Ethnography is an approach to understanding culture or patterns of behavior and the meaning and interpretation by its participants. The purpose of ethnography is to understand another way of life as it is viewed and given meaning by participants. The ethnographer is interested in the values, meanings, and viewpoints of persons and how persons make sense of or perceive their own context.

It has been suggested that occupational therapists function in a fashion similar to ethnographers in that they strive to elicit the client's perspective and use this information to develop treatment protocols to fit the client's value and meaning structure. In her 1990 Eleanor Clarke Slagle lecture, Fine stated, "Occupational therapists are ethnographers of sorts. We have unique access to information about activities of everyday living and what it is like to live with an illness or disability. We need only to acknowledge and actualize it" (1991, pp. 500–501) (See Chapter 25). A few occupational therapists have begun to identify how to actualize an ethnographic perspective. Hasselkus (1990) described the value of using ethnographic interviewing techniques as a tool in occupational therapy practice with family caregivers. Spencer et al. (1993) also suggested that constructs derived from ethnography are relevant and useful to occupational therapy and offer an important approach to practice.

Building on these works, we have developed a framework for evaluating the needs of family caregivers that uses concepts from ethnographs. This framework is intended to advance the efforts of occupational therapists to evaluate the caregiver's *inner life* as a basis from which to make treatment decisions and derive an individualized service approach in the home (Fine, 1993). It incorporates four key terms from ethnography (informant, emic, reflexivity, and interpretation) and the principles they reflect. The strategy is to use these principles and the actions they represent to derive an understanding of the perspective of the family member, the personal meaning of providing care, how care is provided in the home, and specific aspects that are perceived to be problematic. Specific occupational therapy strategies are then constructed that fit the fundamental values and belief system of the family unit or social–cultural context of the home.

This ethnographic framework has evolved through a number of funded research and training programs awarded to the first two authors. These programs have developed and evaluated the use of this framework under a number of conditions. Systematic case analyses involving family members caring for persons with disability suggest that occupational therapy intervention strategies are integrated into family routines and effectively used when occupational therapists use these principles to guide treatment. The outcomes of this research (Corcoran & Gitlin, 1992; Gitlin & Corcoran, 1993) as well as a description of a training approach based on some of these principles (Gitlin & Corcoran, 1991) have been reported elsewhere.

We examine the four key principles constituting the framework, their ethnographic foundations, and their clinical applications. A case example illustrates the framework in action in a home situation with family members caring for a person with dementia.

Four Key Principles Of Ethnography

The four key principles of this framework, which are outlined in Table 1, are designed to enable an occupational therapist to modify traditional practice and evolve treatment strategies that target the values and meaning of the caregiver or family unit. These principles are not to be thought of as linear, step-by-step procedures for evaluation. Rather, they form a framework, or

way of thinking about the caregiving situation, and can be used in combination with formal evaluations that are traditionally conducted in the home.

Principle One: Identify an Informant in the Home

As shown in Table 39.1, the first term in ethnography that is relevant to service delivery is that of identifying an informant or informants. In ethnographic methodology, an informant is a person with knowledge of the cultural system who informs the ethnographer of the values, beliefs, and activities of the group that is being studied. This person is a key source from whom the ethnographer learns about daily practices and behaviors and gains insight into the meaning of an activity or routine.

The clinical application of the term *informant* involves the principle of viewing the family member or primary caregiver as a lay practitioner. Hasselkus (1988) has used the term *lay practitioner* to refer to caregivers because of their primary role in managing, coordinating, and providing hands-on care to older adults with impairment. Through the act *of doing* and trial and error, family members develop a practice style, gain knowledge, and develop expertise or wisdom in providing care. Smith and Baltes have defined wisdom as "expert knowledge" about "fundamental life matters." (1990, p. 495) Applied to the case of caregiving, wisdom or expert knowledge of the pragmatics of providing daily care evolves over time as lay practitioners develop knowledge of how to perform caregiving tasks. This knowledge is situation specific and reflects a professional's *know how* as opposed to his or her formal or theory-based knowledge (Albert, 1992; Benner, 1984).

As an informant, the lay practitioner is an important source of information about caregiving routines and priorities of both the caregiver and the family member who is impaired. By viewing family members as practitioners, an occupational therapist recognizes their pivotal role and responsibility in the caregiving situation and their ultimate control over what therapeutic strategies evolve and are adapted. This principle encourages the occupational therapist to view his or her own role as that of an *enabler* as opposed to a prescriber.

Table 39.1. Ethnographic Principles, Definitions, and Clinical Applications

Ethnographic Principle	Definition	Clinical Application
Informant	Individual with knowledge	Lay practitioner
Emic	Insider perspective	Uncovering personal meaning
Reflexivity	Self-reflection	Treatment planning Hypothesis development Hypothesis testing Self-questioning
Interpretation	Deriving an analytic framework	Treatment implementation: Putting it together

Principle Two: Use an Emic Approach

The second principle is the use of an *emic* approach, that is, obtaining an insider perspective or the point of view of an informant as to how things are and why. In an ethnographic framework for service delivery, the occupational therapist interviews and observes the lay practitioner(s) to identify their perspective of the meaning that shapes their act of caregiving. This step is done in an effort to gain the family members' perspective and identify the unique meaning they have assigned to caregiving. Although a wide range of questions may be useful to gain an insider perspective, those included in Section I of the Appendix are straightforward and simple. They enable a caregiver to begin to tell the story of his or her caregiving experience. Other techniques to learn the inside view include observation of the physical environment, observation of a caregiving task, and active listening to how the lay practitioner constructs his or her story of the caregiving situation. Observation of the home environment in traditional occupational therapy evaluation typically focuses on accessibility and safety. In an ethnographic approach, observation is expanded to include how caregivers set up objects for daily routines, the presence of photographs and other objects of meaning, and the extent to which caregivers have rearranged the home to accommodate the level of competence of the family member who is impaired.

Principle Three: Engage in Self-Reflection

The third principle is a dynamic activity in which the ethnographer engages in self-questioning in an attempt to understand the relationship of his or her own values and beliefs to those that exist in the cultural setting of the home. Through this constant comparison between the investigator's expectations and the way things are, insights are gained. Likewise, in working with a lay practitioner to identify and understand meaning, the occupational therapist remains reflexive or self-questioning and continually asks himself or herself four questions: (a) What do I see happening in this home? (b) Do I understand the perspective of the family members? (c) Is my vision of the family members' needs the same as those of the lay practitioner(s)? (d) In what ways are my values in this caregiving situation the same or different from those of the lay practitioner(s)?

Keeping notes as to one's own personal reactions to the caregiving situation, as well as one's discoveries, facilitates the reflexive discovery process. Through the act of self-reflection, the occupational therapist advances his or her own understanding of the family members' perspective and begins to formulate initial hunches or hypotheses about the meanings that underscore the actions of these lay practitioners. These initial hypotheses form the basis from which treatment planning emerges. As treatment progresses, the therapist continually tests these initial hypotheses by comparing observations of the family members' actions during treatment to his or her interpretive framework, discussed in Principle Four.

Principle Four: Develop a Framework for Interpreting Information

The fourth principle is based on the interpretive method used in ethnography. The interpretive process involves deriving an analytic framework from which to understand and explain behaviors and phenomena. Through interpretation, the ethnographer attempts to make sense of what is observed and uncover the underlying meanings and beliefs that guide behavior.

Likewise, the occupational therapist, on the basis of interview, observation, active listening, and reflexivity, derives an interpretation or analysis of the emic perspective, or how things work and what is important for the lay practitioner. Interpretation is a fluid, dynamic process by which the therapist continually refines his or her understanding of the family members' perspective on the basis of incoming information. The interpretative process is comparable to the clinical reasoning process by which a service provider attempts to fit the pieces together in the form of an effective treatment plan and its implementation (Fleming, 1991) In an ethnographic framework, the clinical reasoning involves skill in interpreting the meanings that underscore the family system and skill in adapting treatment strategies to fit the particular system meaning of the family unit. To refine an interpretive framework, the occupational therapist constantly observes the family members' behavior and returns to three fundamental questions: (a) What does the disability or impairment mean to the care receiver and the family member? (b) How do the family member and care receiver experience the caregiving activity? (c) On the basis of the underlying meaning that informs care, what is an appropriate treatment strategy to support the efforts of the family unit?

Refinement of the interpretive framework begins with the initiation of a home visit and does not end until the termination of treatment. As strategies are introduced, the occupational therapist evaluates how they are received and the extent to which they are incorporated into daily caregiving routines. Those strategies that are rejected by family members provide important information to the occupational therapist as to the beliefs and practices of the lay practitioner(s). Strategies that most closely match the beliefs and self-defined needs of family caregivers are those that will be embraced by family members and used effectively.

As displayed in Figure 39.1, this ethnographic framework for service delivery leads to the development of an individualized treatment approach. It uses a dynamic, iterative process, as in ethnography, in which treatments evolve and are continually refined in light of the observations and interpretations that are derived.

Case Example

A case example illustrates the four principles described previously as used in a five-visit occupational therapy intervention protocol with family members caring for an elderly person

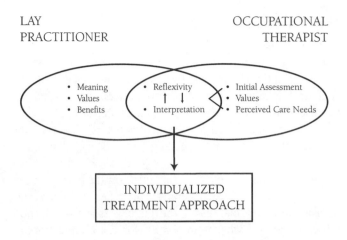

LAY   OCCUPATIONAL
PRACTITIONER   THERAPIST

- Meaning   • Reflexivity   • Initial Assessment
- Values   ↑ ↓   • Values
- Benefits   • Interpretation   • Perceived Care Needs

INDIVIDUALIZED
TREATMENT APPROACH

Figure 39.1. Ethnographic framework for service delivery.

with dementia in the home. A detailed description of the intervention protocol has been published elsewhere (Corcoran & Gitlin, 1992; Gitlin & Corcoran, 1993).

In this case, there were two informants, or lay practitioners. Mrs. P, a frail, 90-year-old spouse, and her 85- year-old sister resided together in a two-story, twin home and cared for Mrs. P's 89-year-old husband. Mr. P suffered from moderate-to-severe dementia, aphasia, and physical decline including weight loss, rigidity, and movement problems. Mr. P needed constant supervision and assistance in bathing, eating, dressing, using the toilet, grooming, and ascending and descending stairs. Mrs. P and her sister reported that Mr. P was often "uncooperative," especially when descending stairs and during meals. Mrs. P and her sister appeared fatigued, stressed, and unsure how to accomplish the daily routines that they had established for Mr. P.

In an initial home visit, the occupational therapist was struck by the enormous difficulty imposed on the two elderly women in providing personal care to a resistive man twice their size and their use of caregiving techniques and routines that impeded the family members' functions and placed them at risk of injury.

The initial evaluation of the daily challenges faced by Mrs. P and her sister indicated four major areas of concern to the occupational therapist. These concerns included: (a) the risk of falling and injury to Mrs. P, her sister, and her husband, (b) the extremely poor nutritional state of Mr. P, (c) Mrs. P and her sister's struggle to maintain good hygiene for Mr. P, and (d) the overall level of stress and physical frailty of all three family members.

On the basis of these immediate concerns and an incomplete understanding of the meaning underlying the actions of the family members, the therapist initially offered recommendations to enhance safety and decrease caregiver stress. These initial recommendations included: (a) the use of formal home care services to assist in activities of daily living, (b) the implementation of major home adaptations such as installing a stair

glide or moving Mr. P's bed downstairs to the dining room for safety, (c) medical intervention for Mr. P's poor nutritional status, (d) day care participation for Mr. P, and (e) preparation for the possibility of nursing home placement for Mr. P. These recommendations, which represent standard practice, were considered by the occupational therapist as critical for the well-being of both the care receiver and the caregivers. Each suggestion, however, was rejected by the lay practitioners (the caregivers).

Strategies to Understand the Caregivers' Perspective

The occupational therapist began to realize that Mrs. P and her sister rejected these suggestions because they presented a dramatic change to the daily routines and image of the household that they had constructed. In addition, these recommended interventions reflected only the formal provider perspective that focused on the medical and dysfunctional aspects of the situation. The occupational therapist recognized that she had an imprecise understanding of what was meaningful in this household and began to use several techniques to discover the beliefs and values that informed decision-making by the lay practitioners. She observed how objects were used in the home and the way caregiving tasks were performed, and she more closely listened to the language used by the lay practitioners to describe their daily routines. For example, the therapist noted that care objects in the home, such as a walker and commode, were kept out of sight until they were required. There were no signs or visual cues to encourage Mr. P's participation in basic self-care tasks, and the environment was not simplified to enhance his competence. As a consequence of the process of observing objects and behaviors, testing emerging hypotheses as to what was occurring in the home, and self-reflection over several home visits, the occupational therapist gained a better understanding of the emic perspective and a feasible, interpretive framework from which to develop specific, relevant solutions to fit this particular case.

Emic Perspective

The essential meaning of the caregiving activities for these two frail women was to maintain a sense of normalcy, or consistency, with the way things were before the onset of Mr. P's dementia. Their primary concern in providing care was to preserve or maintain a sense of continuity in Mr. P's role in the home. From the perspective of Mrs. P and her sister, normalcy meant getting Mr. P through his daily routines of self-care, stair use, and eating as they had always done with minimal changes so as to preserve an image of what Mr. P used to do and how he used to be. The importance of maintaining normalcy and Mr. P's previous biographical roles were reflected in their stoic determination to enforce the basic routines that had always been followed in their adult lives, the language they used to describe their difficulties in the caregiving situation, and the types of caregiving concerns that they identified. For example, they preferred to label Mr. P's behavior as "uncooperative" in daily routines and rejected medical terms that suggested that Mr. P was *unable* to behave competently because of the underlying pathology. They were concerned about his poor eating habits primarily because these habits upset their meal routines. They also identified Mr. P's uncooperative behavior and stiffness when descending the stairs as a concern because it interfered with their expectation that he sit in the living room at a specific point in time during the day, as he used to do.

Mrs. P had rejected the occupational therapist's initial recommendations based on her wish to preserve her image and understanding of who Mr. P was and what he had liked to do. As she pointed out, Mr. P was never one to participate in groups and therefore he would not like a day care situation or nursing home. Whereas the occupational therapist had been concerned with the physical well-being of the caregivers and the medical status of the care receiver, the lay practitioners chose to preserve and be concerned with the biographical status of Mr. P. and to value the preservation of this status.

Interpretation

Through observation of daily tasks, open-ended interviewing, and reflexive self-questioning that occurred over all five home visits, the occupational therapist was able to derive an emic understanding and an interpretative framework of *normalization* for this particular family (Robinson, 1993). Individualized treatment strategies emerged from an iterative process that was based on continual evaluation of things observed and said, self-reflection of the therapist's own values and concerns, and refinement of the therapist's interpretive framework.

The therapist validated and tested her emerging interpretations of the caregivers' need to preserve Mr. P's roles and a sense of normalcy by asking the caregivers validating questions, such as "Is this how you see it?" This technique invited the lay practitioners to comment on the accuracy of the therapist's hypotheses and understandings of what was meaningful and important to them. The therapist began to use the language of the lay practitioners to discuss what was happening in the caregiving situation and affirm their perspective. This communication required avoiding the use of medical or professional terminology and reframing problems with the vocabulary of the caregivers. An example was the use of the term "uncooperative" when describing Mr. P's actual inability to participate in life tasks.

On the basis of the meaning of caregiving in this home, the occupational therapist was able to offer a number of solutions to caregiving problems that were acceptable to the lay practitioners. The challenge to the occupational therapist was to uphold the biographical image of Mr. P while easing the lay practitioners' stresses and safety risks in performing caregiving tasks. In order to effectively communicate about caregiving strategies and routines, it was important for the therapist to link suggestions to the lay practitioners' goal of making Mr. P

more "cooperative." Suggestions that fit this framework involved what may appear to be small changes in technique or routine (e.g., allowing Mr. P to initiate descending the stairs with the lay practitioners walking on either side, involving other family members to provide respite for the caregivers), minor home modifications for safety, and incorporation of techniques that enhanced Mr. P's role performance (e.g., use of visual cues, finger foods, and simplified instructions during eating). These modifications were accepted by the lay practitioners and easily incorporated in the routines that they had established long ago and sought to maintain. These solutions were acceptable because the occupational therapist framed them in terms of how well they maintained Mr. P's role as a family member and status as an independent person. In addition, these solutions did not change valued routines but modified lay practice to enhance safety and minimize the chance of injury.

In addition, on the final visit, the occupational therapist shared information about dementia and its progression with the lay practitioners and put together a packet of materials about other services that they could refer to in the future. This packet included information about day care, respite services, and nursing home placement. Although these services had not been acceptable to the lay practitioners, the information packet was welcomed. This approach to education enabled Mrs. P and her sister to control the information flow and the decision as to if and when additional assistance would be required.

Implications for Occupational Therapy

From an ethnographic point of view, informal caregiving represents a cultural activity in that it has meaning to its participants and reflects the caregiver's values and beliefs about the person and his or her disability. In an ethnographic framework for service delivery, a health-care professional suspends his or her own values and beliefs as to the appropriate course of treatment in an effort to discover what actually goes on in a family that is providing care and the value and meaning that underlie these activities. The four principles provide a framework to guide the clinical reasoning that needs to occur in working with lay practitioners. Mattingly and Fleming (1994) have asserted that a primary and challenging feature of clinical reasoning in occupational therapy is distinguishing the nature of *the good* for each particular client. The good refers to an image of what is beneficial and healthy for each client and is directed partially by the meanings assigned to the disability by the client. Occupational therapists are acutely aware of the need for knowledge about their clients' meaning structures (Fleming & Mattingly, 1994) and the difficulties associated with evaluating these perspectives accurately (Fine, 1993; Spencer, 1993). The ethnographic framework for evaluating the family members' perspective presented in this article can serve as a helpful structure for integrating the client's psychosocial, physical, and emotional dimensions in treatment planning. It can be used in combination with traditional formal assessment instruments of cognition, function, or health status, and can enable occupational therapists to gain insight into distinct caregiving practices and how these practices are embedded in the social and cultural context of the family unit.

An important implication of this framework for occupational therapy practice lies in its usefulness for identifying and addressing client-therapist ethical conflicts. Differences in priorities about the focus of treatment has been identified as a major form of ethical dispute between client and therapist (Corcoran, 1993; Gitlin, 1993; Hasselkus, 1991). For instance, Hasselkus (1991) noted that the principle of *autonomy* (listed first in the *Occupational Therapy Code of Ethics* [American Occupational Therapy Association, 1991]) may conflict with a client's cultural belief that one's elder is entitled to be dependent.

The case of Mrs. P illustrates our discomfort with these ethical dilemmas. For example, Mrs. P and her sister chose to uphold their biographical image of Mr. P as an independent, functioning husband who participated in daily routines, and they rejected the use of medical terms to describe the caregiving process. That is, they chose to continue practices such as his stair climbing at the risk of great personal injury. In this case, the occupational therapist needed to respect the lay practitioners' need to uphold these biographical notions even though the frailty of the caregiving situation remained disconcerting for her. Use of an ethnographic framework will not only help the therapist identify and validate the client's beliefs about disability, but also to continually explore the nuances of his or her own belief structure through the process of reflexivity.

An ethnographic framework for interviewing and service delivery is unlike a medical model approach and will therefore feel different to an occupational therapist in several ways (Levine & Gitlin, 1990). First, the family member as a lay practitioner is viewed as a partner in determining the most appropriate way of approaching the caregiving situation. This approach has the effect of empowering and reassuring family members while helping service providers to relinquish control. Second, intervention strategies are not dictated but evolve from interactions that reflect a blend of formal and practical knowledge. Third, decisional control to adapt new caregiving strategies or coping styles resides with the lay practitioner, whereas the service provider needs to remain flexible. Fourth, service providers must develop a different measure of success that includes the family members' acceptance and modification of suggestions to fit their situation.

Conclusion

The framework presented here is in direct contrast to the medical model approach in which standard treatment protocols emerge according to the condition, its pathology, considerations of dysfunction, and the assumption of the caregiving situation as a universal stressor. The intent of the framework presented here is to enable the occupational therapist to think beyond what *ought* to be done in a home-care situation to understand and respect what family members themselves emphasize as valued practice. It provides a systematic way of thinking about occupational therapy practice with caregivers and shaping the clinical reasoning process in home-based occupational therapy.

The framework also has potential application to other practice areas in the profession of occupational therapy. For instance, therapists specializing in pediatrics may find that an ethnographic framework augments their efforts to collaborate with parents of children with disabilities. Likewise, occupational therapists practicing in the fast-paced arena of acute care may gain a useful way to establish the priorities of treatment and determine relevant discharge plans for their short-stay clients. Although this framework focuses on the caregiver, a similar process can be used to understand the perspective of the care receiver and how it may differ from that of the caregiver. In addition, the elements of this framework are appropriate for home-care situations in which the person who is impaired is the primary receiver of service.

As our health-care system undergoes dramatic revisions, the focus will be increasingly aimed at delivery of quality care in the community. Understanding individual perspectives and the unique meanings of the caregiving experience is critical to the development of services that are effective in assisting the family members in their ongoing caregiving efforts. Our experiences suggest that caregivers are receptive to the knowledge and skill of formal providers when this knowledge and skill is transmitted in a manner that is consistent with the beliefs and values of the family unit.

Appendix 39.A.
Examples of Useful Questions

I. To obtain meaning, ask lay practitioner:
   What is a typical day like for you?
   What most worries or concerns you?
   How is it now versus before?
   Tell me how you manage your day.
   What are your feelings about the future?
   What are some of your successes?

II. To verify meaning, ask lay practitioner:
   Is this how you see it?
   So you are saying that when ___ happens, you get frustrated.
   It sounds as though that really upset you.

III. To think reflexively, ask yourself:
   What do I see happening in this home?
   Do I understand the perspective of the family members?
   Is my view the same as that of the lay practitioner(s)?
   In what ways are my values in this care situation the same or different from those of the lay practitioner(s)?

IV. To derive an interpretive framework, ask yourself:
What does the disability or impairment mean to this person and the family member?
How does the family member experience the caregiving activity?
On the basis of an understanding of meaning, what is an appropriate treatment strategy to support the efforts of this family unit?

Acknowledgments

The framework presented in this article was developed on the basis of research supported by the National Institute on Aging (Grant No. AG10947). The first author's participation was also supported by a research grant awarded by the National Institute on Disability and Rehabilitation Research (Grant No. H133G00160). An earlier version of this article was presented at the Mental Health and Aging Symposium, Wills/Jefferson Hospital, Geropsychiatry, Philadelphia, Pennsylvania, October 29, 1993.

References

Albert, S. M. (1992). The autonomy of lay and professional knowledge in home health care. *Journal of Aging Studies, 6,* 227–241.

American Occupational Therapy Association. (1991). Essentials and guidelines for an accredited educational program for the occupational therapist. *American Journal of Occupational Therapy, 12,* 1077–1084.

Benner, P. (1984). *From novice to expert.* Menlo Park, CA: Addison-Wesley.

Chiou, I. L., & Burnett, C. N. (1985). A survey of stroke patients and their home therapists. *Physical Therapy, 65,* 901–906.

Clark, C., Corcoran, M. A., & Gitlin, L. N. (in press). Engaging family caregivers: How occupational therapists develop therapeutic relationships. *American Journal of Occupational Therapy.*

Collins, C. (1992). I don't need help! *Home Healthcare Nurse, 10(5),* 53–56.

Corcoran, M. A. (1992). Gender differences in dementia management plans of spousal caregivers: Implications for occupational therapy. *American Journal of Occupational Therapy, 46,* 1006–1012.

Corcoran, M. (1993). Collaboration: An ethical approach to effective therapeutic relationships. *Topics in Geriatric Rehabilitation, 9(2),* 1–29.

Corcoran, M., & Gitlin, L. N. (1992). Dementia management: An occupational therapy home-based intervention for caregivers. *American Journal of Occupational Therapy, 46,* 801–808.

DePoy, E., & Gitlin, L. (1994). *An introduction to research: Multiple strategies for health and human services.* St. Louis: Mosby.

Fine, S. B. (1991). Resilience and human adaptability: Who rises above adversity? 1990 Eleanor Clarke Slagle Lecture. *American Journal of Occupational Therapy, 45,* 493–503. Reprinted as Chapter 25.

Fine, S. B. (1993, December). Psychosocial issues and adaptive capacities. *Mental Health Special Interest Section Newsletter, 16,* 1–7.

Fleming, M. H. (1991). Clinical reasoning in medicine compared with clinical reasoning in occupational therapy. *American Journal of Occupational Therapy, 45,* 988–996.

Fleming, M. A., & Mattingly C. (1994). Giving language to practice. In C. Mattingly & M. A. Fleming (Eds.), *Clinical reasoning: Forms of inquiry in therapeutic practice.* Philadelphia: H. A. Davis.

Gitlin, L. N. (1993). Therapeutic dilemmas in the care of the elderly in rehabilitation. *Topics in Geriatric Rehabilitation, 9,* 11–20.

Gitlin, L. N., & Corcoran, M. (1991). Training occupational therapists in the care of the elderly with dementia and their caregivers: Focus on collaboration. *Educational Gerontology, 17,* 591–605.

Gitlin, L. N., & Corcoran, M. (1993). Expanding caregiver ability to use environmental solutions for problems of bathing and incontinence in the elderly with dementia. *Technology and Disability, 2,* 12–21.

Gubrium, J. F., & Sankar, A. (Eds.). (1990). *The home care experience.* Newbury Park, CA: Sage.

Gubrium, J. F., & Sankar, A. (Eds.). (1994). *Qualitative methods in aging research.* Thousand Oaks, CA: Sage.

Hasselkus, B. R. (1988). Meaning in family caregiving: Perspectives on caregiver/professional relationships. *Gerontologist, 28,* 686–691.

Hasselkus, B. R. (1989). The meaning of daily activity in family caregiving for the elderly. *American Journal of Occupational Therapy, 43,* 649–656.

Hasselkus, B. R. (1990). Ethnographic interviewing: A tool for practice with family caregivers for the elderly. *Occupational Therapy Practice, 2,* 9–16.

Hasselkus, B. R. (1991). Ethical dilemmas: The organization of family caregiving for the elderly. *Journal of Aging Studies, 5,* 99–110.

Henderson, J. N., & Gutierrez-Mayka, M. (1992). Ethnocultural themes in caregiving to Alzheimer's disease patients in Hispanic families. *Clinical Gerontologist, 11,* 59–74.

Hill, R. F., Fortenberry, J. D., & Stein, H. F. (1990). Culture in clinical medicine. *Southern Medical Journal, 83,* 1071–1080.

Kaufman, S. R. (1988). Stroke rehabilitation and the negotiation of identity. In S. Reinharz & G. D. Rowles (Eds.), *Qualitative gerontology* (pp. 82–103). New York: Springer.

Kleinman, A. (1988). *The illness narratives.* New York: Basic.

Knight, B. G., Lutzky, S. M., & Macofsky-Urban, F. (1993). A meta-analytic review of interventions for caregiver distress: Recommendations for future research. *Gerontologist, 33,* 240–248.

Levine, R. E., & Gitlin, L. N. (1990). Home adaptations for the chronically disabilities: An educational model. *American Journal of Occupational Therapy, 44,* 923–929.

Mattingly, C., & Fleming, M. A. (1994). *Clinical reasoning: Forms of inquiry in therapeutic practice.* Philadelphia: F. A. Davis.

Pepper Commission. (1990). *A call for action. U.S. Bipartisan Commission on Comprehensive Health Care.* Washington, DC: U.S. Government Printing Office.

Pynoos, J., & Ohta, R. (1991). In-home interventions for persons with Alzheimer's disease and their caregivers. *Physical and Occupational Therapy in Geriatrics, 9(3/4),* 83–92.

Robinson, C. A. (1993). Managing life with a chronic condition: The story of normalization. *Qualitative Health Research, 3,* 6–28.

Smith, J., & Baltes, P. B. (1990). Wisdom-related knowledge: Age/cohort differences in response to life-planning problems. *Developmental Psychology, 26,* 494–505.

Smyth, K. A., & Harris, P. B. (1993). Using telecomputing to provide information and support to caregivers of persons with dementia. *Gerontologist, 33,* 123–127.

Spencer, J. C. (1993). The usefulness of qualitative methods in rehabilitation: Issues of meaning, of context, and of change. *Archives of Physical Medicine and Rehabilitation, 74,* 119–126.

Spencer, J., Krefting, L., & Mattingly, C. (1993). Incorporation of ethnographic methods in occupational therapy assessment. *American Journal of Occupational Therapy, 47,* 303–309.

Stone, R., Cafferata, G. L., & Sangl, J. (1987). Caregivers of the frail elderly: A national profile. *Gerontologist, 27,* 616–626.

Williamson, G. M., & Schulz, R. (1993). Coping with specific stressors in Alzheimer's disease caregiving. *Gerontologist, 33,* 747–754.

The Patient–Therapist Relationship: Beliefs That Shape Care

CHAPTER 40

SUZANNE M. PELOQUIN, PHD, OTR

Occupational therapists can be with patients in many ways that reflect their various understandings of what it means to be competent and caring. Because the beliefs of a profession shape a therapist's sense of what it means to give care, the beliefs about competence and caring found in the occupational therapy tradition have warranted consideration (Peloquin, 1990). Three images of how occupational therapists act in practice dominate patients' stories: the images of technician, parent, and collaborator or friend. When therapists act as technicians or authoritarian parents, patients cast them negatively in stories that reflect their disappointment. When acting in either of these manners, therapists seem to value the competence articulated within the professional literature more than they value the caring aspects of *relationship* (Peloquin, 1990). Both of these enactments, however, reflect some understanding of what it means to care. The technical therapist, equating expertise with care, values the best method and the successful outcome. The parental therapist manipulates the decisions and methods that are in the patient's best interests and sees this action as caring. In each of these images of care, the therapist's competence dominates the encounter.

If choosing how to be among patients is a matter of some consideration, it follows that a number of societal beliefs and expectations also shape a therapist's choice. Those beliefs are the subject of this discussion. It seems apt for occupational therapists to consider the societal forces that surround practice. As Yerxa (1980) said, "Occupational therapy, which began in a climate of caring, has been influenced in its practice by social change" (p. 532). It is a growing truism that the current health care system is now perceived as "not oriented to the human being" (Baum, 1980, p. 514). What causes this disorientation to persons? King (1980) suggested that any sense of the meaning of caring is an intermingling of personal, professional, *and* societal beliefs. Any lack of caring that derives from a preferential valuation of competence must also reflect such an intermingling.

Nature and Scope of the Inquiry

This article constitutes part of a larger inquiry into the challenge of creating a climate of caring. Conducted between January 1990 and September 1991, the inquiry considered the following: (a) personal narratives that describe impersonal treatment; (b) the historical events and societal constructs that have shaped the patient–helper relationship; (c) empathy and the manner in which helpers learn to be empathic; (d) the nature, practice, and experience of art; and (e) the proposition that empathy might be cultivated through the use of art. Each step of the inquiry required an extensive literature review from which important themes emerged. These themes were then subjected to the reflection, analysis, and synthesis characteristic of studies in the medical humanities.

A number of phenomenological narratives about the impersonal treatment of patients served as subjects for an earlier discussion (Peloquin, 1993). That discussion produced a descriptive profile of those behaviors to which patients refer when they use the term *depersonalizing*. The central complaint found within those narratives was that when practitioners act impersonally their behaviors are discouraging. Patients say that helpers fail to see illness and disability as emotional events charged with personal meaning. They fail to attend to the experiences of patients; instead, they establish a distance that diminishes them. They withhold information, they use brusque manners, and they misuse their powers. They are insensitive, silent, and aloof. Patients conclude that their helpers may treat them, but they do not treat them well.

Alongside these descriptive narratives were a number not included in the discussion on depersonalization because they were more reflective than descriptive: (a) those written by patients who consider the beliefs that may cause their helpers to behave carelessly; (b) those written by caregivers who, after their own bout with illness and impersonal treatment, discuss societal expectations; and (c) those written by helpers who ponder the difficulties of caring. These reflections offer cues about the societal constructs that may have a hand in shaping care, and, as cues, they constitute assumptions that can direct further research.

This discussion does not address concerns in practice such as those that Bailey (1990) described as the "harmful variables" that cause therapists to leave the field (p. 23). Staff shortages, large caseloads, red tape, excessive paperwork, lack of job status, chronic conditions of the patient population, lack of respect for occupational therapy by other professionals, stress and overload, and the need to justify treatment also shape decisions about the manner in which helpers will choose to care. Many of these negative variables, although not the specific focus of this inquiry, can also be said to associate with the societal beliefs that are the subject of this discussion.

The Connections That Mean Care

A number of stories do portray helpers as caring persons who offer patients equal measures of competence and caring (Peloquin, 1989 [see Chapter 56]; Peloquin, 1990). These stories suggest that caring attitudes, gestures, and words give patients the courage to face illness and disability.

Pekkanen (1988) treated a 14-year-old boy whose electrical accident had warranted amputation of his legs; Pekkanen willed himself to feel the boy's injury from the inside out. He then understood:

> He was a tall, rangy black kid from the inner city and had been a very good junior high school basketball player. All he ever wanted to be was a basketball player, and I think that the young man took this news with more hurt, more disappointment, and more disbelief than any child I can remember.... I think it was one of the most crushing truths to come to a young man that I have ever seen. (p. 126)

A caring attitude can encourage patients. Lee (1987), a patient hospitalized with cancer, felt care in this small gesture:

> As I slept a nurse took the cloth wrapping off a sterile instrument. He smoothed out the material. He painted with a blue flow pen a moon face with wide eyes and an enormous crescent smile. He climbed over my bed. He climbed over my plants and hung this banner down from my window, using the extra-wide masking tape. It was the first thing I saw in the morning. (p. 111)

Patients also draw courage from caring words. Benziger (1969) remembered the encouragement that she took from this conversation with an occupational therapist:

> "You know, you go at your work too hard, too fast, too desperately—and too frenetically."

> "I guess I do, but that's the way I feel. Time stands still for me now, it is endless, and yet if I have something to do, I get the sense that there will not be time enough to finish it, or that someone will stop me."

> She said, "You are an intelligent person, and you will help yourself to get well quickly." "You know," I answered, "you're the first person who has mentioned intelligence versus non-intelligence, instead of sanity. You make me feel like a human being." I was grateful. I should not forget her. (p. 49)

The directness and the proffered confidence held in these words meant concern to Benziger; she would call this therapist *friend*.

Sarason's (1985) point of view is no doubt the most helpful. At the very least, he said, practitioners can *try*. Patients, he says, mostly ask helpers to try "in ways that say 'I am trying to understand because I want to be helpful.' It is those manifestations that are experienced as caring and compassionate, even though they may be more or less ineffective" (p. 188). And when "a patient, whether terminal or not, draws courage—courage to live or courage to die—from the man who stands at his bedside" (Hodgins, 1964, p. 843), surely they both feel the magic of care.

If practitioners can be both competent and caring among their patients, what societal beliefs cause them to act otherwise? Three constructs surface within the reflections of patients and practitioners as shaping forces that compromise caring expressions: (a) an emphasis on the rational fixing of problems; (b) an overreliance on methods and protocols; and (c) a health care provision system that is driven by business, efficiency, and profit.

The Emphasis on Rational Fixing

One societal belief that compromises caring actions is the emphasis on solving discrete health care problems in a logical and rational manner. When Hodgins wrote in 1964 after his stroke, he found a particular form of disregard at the heart of the problem. He described this picture of how the patient and the caregiver perceive illness:

> In stroke two basic sets of assumptions could govern treatment. One set proceeds from what the patient perceives or thinks he perceives; the other comes from what the doctor knows or thinks he knows. The two are very different sets of things. (p. 842)

Many health care narratives hold similar pictures, with helpers governing some aspects of care while neglecting others that their patients value. Sir Dominic Corrigan, a physician, argued as long as a century ago that the trouble with doctors is "not that they don't know enough, but that they don't see enough" (cited in Taylor, 1972, p. 6).

Van Eys (1988), also a physician, has regretted the hemi-sected worldview in which "diseases become problems, and patients become dissected into such problems" (p. 21). Patients resent this narrowness of focus because it feels uncaring. They complain that practitioners address their disease, the physiology and the mechanism of their bodies and dysfunctions, but not the experience of illness and unease, not its meaning, and surely not their feelings.

Disregard for parts of persons disturbs Murphy (1987), an anthropologist who wrote of his own disabling illness: "The full subjective states of the patient are of little concern in the medical model of disability, which holds that the problem arises wholly from some atomic or physiological disorder and is correctable by standard modes of therapy—drugs, surgery, radiation, or whatever" (p. 88). Sacks (1983), a neurologist who experienced impersonal care, considered this splitting insane:

the madness of the last three centuries, the madness which so many of us—as individuals—go through, and by which all of us are tempted. It is the Newtonian–Lockean–Cartesian view—variously paraphrased in medicine, biology, politics, industry, etc.—which reduces men to machines, automata, puppets, dolls, blank tablets, formulae, ciphers, systems, and reflexes. (p. 205)

Sarton (1988) remembered in her journal that after a stroke she was made to feel like "so many pounds of meat, filled with potentially interesting mechanical parts and neurochemical combinations" (p. 106).

Leder (1984) argued while in medical school that a person is never so many pounds of meat, that the human body is "not a mere extrinsic machine but our living center" (p. 34). Paradoxically, however, it seems that the body, so prized in this narrow view of illness, matters little on a day-to-day basis. Most persons, said Leder, ignore the body until it malfunctions. Then when they are ill, they beg some practitioner to fix the complex mechanism that has disrupted the flow of their personal lives. And the picture of health care practice that one then sees is "an ironic fulfillment of Cartesian dualism—a mind (namely, that of the doctor) runs a passive and extrinsic body (that of the patient)" (p. 35). The image offered by Jourard (1964), a psychologist, illuminates this Orwellian disjunction:

Each patient lies in his own cubicle, and there are attached to him all kinds of wires, connected to his brain, his muscles, his viscera. Every time these wires, which are actually electronic pick-ups, transmit signals to a computer indicating that the bladder is too full, a bowel stuffed, and patient hungry or in pain, before you could blink an eye, the computer sends signals to different kinds of apparatus which empty the bowel and bladder, fill the stomach, scratch the itch, massage the back and so on. We could even mount the bed on a slowly moving belt; the patient gets in at one end, and four or six days later his

bed reaches the exit and the patient is healed—we hope. (p. 138)

If this reduction is a prevalent view, is it fair to expect practitioners to think divergently, to routinely see and treat a self embodied instead of a body? If the general population views the body as a mechanism controlled by higher functions, as something that one has instead of who one is, why the surprise that practitioners engage only their rational functions in practice? If imagining patient experiences, sensing patient needs, and expressing personal feelings seem actions incongruent with fixing, practitioners are quite reasonable in underusing these so-called lower functions. What is the problem, then, with treating bodies when they need fixing?

Most narratives answer that "when a patient appears as a physiological mechanism, the doctor may neglect personal communication in favor of the immediate scientific task at hand" (Leder, 1984, p. 36). The preference for fixing makes it easier for a helper to neglect feelings, easier to justify being silent, curt, or aloof. The resulting problem is impersonal care. Any caregiver can focus narrowly on fixing. Gebolys (1990) remembered this incident:

A male therapist came in whistling and cheerfully setting up his equipment. He stuck the breathing tube into my mouth and told me to "breathe" which I did while he walked around the room admiring my flowers, gazing out the window and remarking at what a lovely day it was. (p. 13)

Mattingly (1991) (see Chapter 37) gave occupational therapists pause for reflection when she argued that "therapists can come to reduce their practice to a manipulation of the physical body, forgetting how much their interventions are directed to a person's life" (p. 986). Parham (1987) argued that there are such situations in occupational therapy when:

time, energy, and money are funneled into treating one small part of the total problem, a part that may be insignificant in comparison with complexities that are more difficult to understand but that have a profound impact on the life situation of the patient being served. (p. 556)

Schultz and Schkade (1992) (see Chapter 48) shared a similar concern: "The current demand for therapists to base occupational therapy on acquisition of functional skills ... may actually limit the contribution of occupational therapy and may deny patients the opportunity to make vital changes in their occupational adaptation process" (p. 918). Certainly a patient's poem, "Some Other Day" (McClay, 1977), presents an occupational therapist bent on partial fixing:

Preserve me from the occupational therapist, God
She means well, but I'm too busy to make baskets ...
"Please, open your eyes," the therapist says;
You don't want to sleep the day away."
She wants to know what I used to do,

Knit? Crochet?
Yes, I did those things, and cooked and cleaned, and
raised five children and had things happen to me.
Beautiful things, terrible things,
I need to think about them, rearrange them on the
shelves of my mind.
The therapist is showing me glittery beads.
She asks if I might like to make jewelry.
She's a dear child and she means well,
So I tell her I might.
Some other day. (pp. 107–108)

The consequence of a strong commitment to rational fixing—of the disease, the body, or the dysfunction—is a disregard that feels careless. And although practitioners mean well,
physician–educator Anthony Moore (1978) acknowledged the
problem: "Professions tend to be right in what they affirm and
wrong in what they ignore" (p. 3).

The Reliance on Method and Protocol

A second societal belief that compromises caring is an overreliance on the instruments of health care practice: the techniques, procedures, and modalities that solve the problem.
When they are ill, patients seek concern in addition to solutions. They grieve that in health care practice they find something else. Hodgins (1964) regretted the find:

For the physician, of course, it must have been wonderful,
indeed, when true specifics began to arrive on the scene to
supplant beef, iron, and wine or syrup of hypophos-
phates.... As so-called science more and more enters medicine, the heedless or routine physician will be accordingly
tempted to withdraw his humanity and wait for specifics.
(p. 843)

Hodgins considered the specifics needed for cure and the
humanity needed for care different but inseparable aspects
of care. Flagg (1923), a physician who practiced at the turn
of the century, agreed; he regretted "the unwise employment
of laboratory methods to the exclusion of personal attention" (p. 5).

When a drug or a procedure suffices, a practitioner may
think less about the need to make meaningful connections
with the patient. The problem becomes clear in Barbara
Peabody's (1986) recollection of an incident that occurred
during her son's hospitalization for acquired immunodeficiency syndrome (AIDS):

Peter woke at two A.M., just as the intern was about to give
him an injection in his left thigh.

"What do you have there?" Peter asked.

"What do you care?" the intern snapped back.

"I care very much, and I hope that's not pentamidine."

"What if it is?" the intern asked insolently.

"Because if it is, I'm not supposed to get it anymore," Peter
replied. "I think you better check my chart and you'll see
that it was discontinued on Monday."

"Oh, no, the orders are still on your chart."

"I'm sure they're not," Peter insisted. "Go back and read
them again, you'll see that I'm right."

The intern left the room and never returned. (p. 51)

Reiser (1980) told the following story about helpers whose
reliance on protocol precluded personal attention. A woman
hospitalized with a diagnosis of acute granulocytic leukemia
and severe anemia agreed to an aggressive course of
chemotherapy that made her quite ill. She was discharged
after remission, and when she was readmitted 4 months later
she refused chemotherapy. The staff decided that if she continued to refuse this treatment, she would be discharged
against medical advice. She refused and was discharged.
Reiser's perception was that she had "stepped out of the established 'system' and had to be punished for it" (p. 146).

Sacks (1983) rejected the argument that helpers must
use only treatments or protocols. When facing surgery, he
wondered:

What sort of man would Swan be? I knew he was a good
surgeon, but it was not the surgeon but the person that I
would stand in relation to, or, rather, the man in whom, I
hoped, the surgeon and the person would be wholly fused.
(p. 92)

Cassell (1985), another physician, shared a similar belief:
"Doctors who lack developed personal powers are inadequately trained.... Doctors are themselves instruments of
patient care" (p. 1).

When they are effective, however, methods and protocols
take the upper hand. Helpers side with what works, so that a
challenge to the procedure also threatens them. Martha Lear
(1980) remembered the upshot of such an identification when
her husband Hal, a urologist, requested a milder painkiller:
"The resident got angry. He said, 'There is a medication
ordered for pain for you. If you want it, you can have it. If not,
you'll get nothing.' And he walked out" (p. 41). But patients,
wrote the physician Pellegrino (1979), do not want practitioners to fuse with their skills: "Physicians have a medical education, an M.D. degree, a set of skills, knowledge, prestige,
titles. They possess many things by which they mistakenly
identify themselves" (p. 228).

Helpers wrap themselves in their procedural authority,
binding themselves so tightly in their concern for the right
method, the latest technology, that it is no wonder that their
actions then seem constricted. Helpers can never be seen as
personal if they offer knowledge or skills instead of themselves. Murphy (1987) resented the trade: "What I needed was
not a new instrument, but an old fashioned clinician with
plenty of intuition" (p. 14). Patients argue that their helpers

routinely neglect their feelings, that they have bought the argument in favor of impersonality.

But whenever anyone mentions using either selves or intuitive traits therapeutically, practitioners stir uneasily. They have a problem with being intuitive or personal. Some actually call caring *feminine*. Lear (1980) claimed that her husband felt care from women, distance from men: "They were with him constantly, those woman figures. They were gentle and good.... The male figures were with him for ten minutes a day. They were marginal figures, shadowy and cold. They touched him with instruments—stethoscopes, blood-pressure gadgets" (pp. 40–41). It seems that here too helpers try to split the inseparable; they say that men will offer cures and skills, women service and caring. But patients argue that this and all other separations are unthinkable; all helpers must care.

Hodgins (1964) argued that encounters felt as personal are often what patients need most: "[The patient] will draw courage as he perceives human understanding underlying the professional techniques of those into whose care he has been given. Human understanding, however, is not to be found in the rituals of anything called medical science" (p. 841). Unhappily, concern for more personal issues seems to matter little in this formulaic belief: Correct procedures produce the superior results that serve the patient's best interests.

Occupational therapists are among those who must admit that techniques and protocols can preempt caring. Yerxa (1980) argued that "*technique*, once employed in the service of human needs, is rapidly moving us toward a society of total technology in which our ways of thinking and being themselves become so technical that we lose sight of other ways of thinking and being" (p. 530).

King (1980) concurred, claiming that "therapists have ignored their instinct for caring" (p. 525). Heller and Vogel (1986) described Heller's experience with the tight formula in his occupational therapy treatment for Guillain-Barré syndrome:

As soon as I could sand a block of wood (with a need to rest both arms, it was written, after seven repetitions), a change was made to a coarser grade of sandpaper, increasing the amount of force required, and it was just as punishing for me to have to execute them as it had been in the beginning. (pp. 166–67)

Although Heller wanted to savor his gain and determine his next move in therapy, a protocol forbade his doing so.

Parham (1987) discussed the case of Longmore, a former faculty member at the University of Southern California Program in Disability and Society:

He was subjected to long hours of occupational therapy training for self-care skills although he had no intention of performing these time-consuming tasks independently at home. He planned to hire an attendant who would expedite the process, freeing him to use his time and energy to pursue more stimulating and productive activities. (p. 556)

Neither Heller's nor Longmore's treatments heeded Baum's (1980) reminder that interventions notwithstanding, "we are nothing more than a bystander in the life of that individual until a relationship is formed" (p. 514).

A Health-Care System Driven by Business, Efficiency, and Profit

Francis Peabody (1930), a physician, articulated the problem well when he argued that "hospitals, like other institutions, founded with the highest human ideals, are apt to deteriorate into dehumanized machines" (p. 33). Many narratives suggest that this dehumanization stems from a system of providing health care that builds on business, efficiency, and profit.

The Business of Health Care

Any business that aims to offer individual service to large numbers of people may suffer from criticisms such as Sarton's (1988):

A small incident at the hairdresser's has given me something to try to understand .... While Donna was securing my hair into curlers, an old lady who was waiting to be picked up came and stood beside us and talked cheerfully about herself and her daughters and Donna responded. It was though I did not exsist, was an animal being groomed. (p. 255)

The number of patients who seek treatment can compromise caring expressions in hospitals. As Sarason (1985) wrote, "The clinician becomes a rationer of time, and that obviously sets drastic limits on the degree to which the ever-present client need for caring and compassion can be met" (p. 170). The result of that rationing is the feeling articulated by Peter Peabody during his visits to a busy clinic: "I just feel like they don't give a damn.... I feel like I'm always being ignored, they don't care" (1986, p. 172). Additional complications associate with the business of hospitals, however, by virtue of their life-saving function. Hodgins (1964) discussed the personal estrangement that occurs with the rapid interventions warranted by life-threatening illness:

Speaking as a patient, I think this point is important: that the stroke victim is most likely to encounter, as his first medical ministrant, a physician to whom he is a total stranger. Since speedy hospitalization is usually a first goal in stroke, treatment by strangers is likely to continue. (p. 839)

Peabody (1930) explained one consequence of the lifesaving business:

When a patient enters a hospital, the first thing that commonly happens to him is that he loses his personal identity. He is generally referred to, not as Henry Jones, but as "that case of mitral stenosis in the second bed on the left".... It leads, more or less directly, to the patient being treated as a case of mitral stenosis, and not a sick man. (p. 31)

The problem is a matter of focus; the institutional eye sees the relevance of saving Henry's life and so does not capture the wider clinical picture—that although "Henry happens to have heart disease, he is not disturbed so much by dyspnea as he is by anxiety for the future" (Peabody, 1930, p. 34).

The Efficiency of the Health-Care System

Murphy (1987) has spoken to the kind of ordering that occurs in institutions, renaming the hospital an island invaded by a rationalized system of schedules and shifts: "The hospital has all the features of a bureaucracy, and, like bureaucracies everywhere, it both breeds and feeds on impersonality" (p. 21)

The impersonality is well illustrated in Saxton's (1987) account:

> The scariest part of the hospitalization for me was not the surgery but the doctor rounds. On the mornings when these rituals were scheduled, the nurses and aides awakened us much earlier than usual. Meals and wash-ups were rushed.... Then they would come, the surgeons, the residents, the interns.... They entered our ward, about fifteen adults.... Strange long words were uttered; bandages were opened and quickly closed. (p. 53)

Gebolys (1990) recalled that only on the fourth day of her hospital stay did a nurse's aide wash her hair, which was bloody and dirty from an automobile accident. The aide did so after her shift was over because the highly regulated day precluded this helping task. Sacks (1983) concluded that "the hospital, in short, is a singular mixture, where freedom and bondage, warmth and coldness, human and mechanical, life and death, are locked together in perpetual combat" (p. 24).

The battle sometimes seems insane, Murphy (1987) explained, because like most bureaucracies, the hospital has turned "capricious, arbitrary, and irresponsible as Wonderland's Red Queen" (p. 44). One feels the capriciousness in Beisser's (1989) experience with heartless caretakers:

> In one hospital, the first hour of the nurses' shift was spent in a detailed discussion of who would take coffee breaks when. Medications, patient needs, all other things paled in comparison. Sometimes people would literally leave you in midair in a lift to go on a coffee break, or leave you in some other awkward position, and just say, "It's my break time." (p. 35)

Brice (1987) recalled a nurse in the recovery room whom she asked for a blanket. The nurse, seeming much like the Red Queen, "barked 'I just brought you one; I'm not going to bring you another' and disappeared" (p. 31). People are a hospital's only possible conveyors of personal care; there can be no social life there if helpers are capricious and irresponsible. Sarton (1988) wearied of her treatment that was "bland at best, cold and inhuman at worst" (p. 103).

The Profit of Health-Care Provision

Hodgins (1964) thought that helpers produced mostly problems with the profit-driven business of health care:

> We have heard much sentimental lamentation over the disappearance of the old "family physician"—dear, lovable old Dr. Peatmoss, who delivered all the babies, saw them through diphtheria, whooping cough and scarlet fever, sat at the deathbeds of the elderly, and never sent anyone a bill. This last lovable quality is, I suppose, why he disappeared. I felt no sense of personal loss at his passing because I never knew him. I should have liked to. The physicians in my life all had very efficient accounting systems—if not actual departments. (p. 840)

Longcope (1962), a physician, had argued even earlier that a business orientation causes "the 'quantification, mechanization and standardization' which are said to characterize this country" (p. 547). Within a business orientation to health care, knowledge takes coin value, cure becomes a high-priced commodity, and ill persons are transformed into buyers. Success and solvency turn into treatment goals, productivity and efficiency into the means to achieve them. In this scheme, more accrues from procedures that cure than from manners that care. Rabin (1982), a physician with amyotrophic lateral sclerosis, remembered that his physician gave him a pamphlet outlining the course of a disease that he already knew too well. He regretted that this physician gave him no suggestions about "how to muster the emotional strength to cope with a progressive degenerative disease" (p. 307).

Practitioners face a major quandary when their patients' needs for time and compassion compete with the institution's need to prosper. When high regard falls to those who treat the most patients or accumulate the most billable units of time, moments spent noticing, listening, or communicating are harder to justify. Sarason (1985) explained: "Whose agent I was became a pressing, daily, moral problem. I know what it is to have divided loyalties, to want to give up the fight, to rationalize away the internalized conflict' (pp. 170–171). And although few helpers buy the idea that patients are mere customers, many budget their caring actions. Patients experience the cuts as hurtful. Lear (1980) wrote of her husband's regret that he had never attended to his patients' experiences. He thought: "Damn it, doctors *should* know. They should care. Say how're they treating you? How's the food? Accommodations comfortable? Staff courteous?.... He himself would never even have thought to ask. Didn't that make him negligent too? Ah. Bingo" (p. 43).

Occupational Therapists Within the System

According to Sacks (1983), occupational therapists are among those who struggle more successfully against the impersonality within the health-care provision system: "There are, of course, gaps in this totalitarian structure, when real care and affection still maintain a foothold; many of the 'lower' staff nurses, aides, orderlies, physiotherapists, speech therapists, etc. give themselves unstintingly, and with love, to their patients" (p. 24). But occupational therapists speak openly about the frustrations of clinical practice; as Howard (1991) (see Chapter 53) wrote, "occupational therapy does not exist in a vacuum" (p. 878). Growing numbers of patients are a concern. Departments must handle more patients with fewer staff members because "productivity and efficiency are becoming high-priority goals" (p. 878). Howard argued that technological approaches are thus "valued more than the holistic use of a variety of methods" (p. 880).

The climate in hospitals seems one of "cost containment" rather than caring (Howard, 1991, p. 878 [see Chapter 53]. Kari and Michels (1991) wrote of their regret that "daily life for those living within the institution can become compartmentalized and focused on receiving services to alleviate dysfunction" (p. 721). Trahey (1991) saw the combat to which Sacks (1983) referred as a "struggle to integrate quality care with a businesslike approach to fiscal soundness" (p. 397). Burke and Cassidy (1991) (see Chapter 54) called it the "disparity between reimbursement-driven practice and the humanistic values of occupational therapy" (p. 173). Boyle (1990) questioned one aspect of the dilemma:

Are occupational therapists today meeting the needs of the rehabilitation population and considering their social, political, and economic status? Or are we compartmentalizing our services on the basis of our own need for neat, tidy treatment plans that fit our expertise and the selective mission of our institution? (p. 941)

The enormity of the challenge pressed Grady (1992) to ask a more fundamental question: "Is there still enjoyment in occupational therapy, or have we become so controlled with the realities of productivity, reimbursement, and modalities that we are failing to see the process as part of the outcome?" (p. 1063) A number of therapists have spoken to the powers essential for the struggle. Knowledge is one:

All occupational therapists should have the knowledge, skills, and attitudes to position themselves to gain influence, power, and control of the systems in which they operate. To move upward in the power hierarchy, we must have knowledge (i.e., expertise), knowing (i.e., process skills), competencies, and credentials. (Nielson, 1991, p. 854)

But that competence, wrote Dickerson (1990), must be tempered by another concern: "Care must also be exercised so that therapists never sacrifice quality of care for increased profits" (p. 137).

The quality of care central to occupational therapy has traditionally included the assumption that "if therapists are to create individually designed, personally meaningful treatment programs, then they must spend considerable time and energy getting to know each patient as a person" (Burke & Cassidy, 1991, p. 173) (see Chapter 54). More and more, according to

Burke and Cassidy, occupational therapists "must use a technical, protocol-driven approach to treatment" (p. 174). "Like physicians," they wrote, "we have had to amend our traditional allegiance to the patient due to increased fiscal restraint, which requires that we now consider the economic realities of the hospitals in which we work" (p. 174).

Conclusion

Caregivers such as Vanderwoude (1988) have paused after the course of their own illness to explain: "My illness was beneficial in helping me to be more reflective, in teaching me an element of patience, and in heightening my understanding of the person facing possible terminal illness" (p. 125). Sacks (1984) was similarly convinced: "I saw that one must be a patient, and a patient among patients, that one must enter both the solitude and the community of patienthood, to have any idea of what 'being a patient' means" (p. 172). Although such an experience offers a profound form of knowing, first-person narratives can also inspire helpers to consider the manner in which they care.

Occupational therapists who choose how they will be among their patients do so within a context shaped by an intermingling of personal, professional, and societal beliefs. Occupational therapists have traditionally endorsed a practice based on competence and caring (Peloquin, 1990). Therapists who act as either technicians or authoritarian parents disappoint patients with their overvaluation of competence. Several societal beliefs can be seen to connect with such overly competent enactments: an emphasis on the rational fixing of problems, an overreliance on method and protocol, and a health-care system that thrives on business, efficiency, and profit.

A focus on fixing bodily parts and functional problems leads to a tendency to disregard a patient's understanding or feelings about illness. To a patient, the disregard feels technical rather than personal. A reliance on protocols that have success, authority, and reliability leads to a tendency to deny a patient's control, to dismiss a helper's intuition about what is right. To a patient, this preeminence of protocol feels impersonal and authoritarian. The routinization and rationalization of health-care institutions lead to discourteous behaviors. The actions feel efficient but uncaring. Therapists who act as technicians or authoritarian parents reflect society's preference for the rational fixing of problems, the implementing of successful strategies, and the management of solvent businesses. And although each of these orientations is important and worthy of affirmation in any health-care practice, overvaluation of any one of these can compromise the actions and words that mean care. Practice that values the person must build on both competence and caring.

Toward the end of his personal litany of complaints, Hodgins (1964) remembered the need that helpers also have for courage in the face of illness. He ended his address to the Academy of Physicians by suggesting that practitioners consider a picture of practice that might replenish their commitment: "Reclothe yourselves in humanity" (p. 843). It is hoped that occupational therapists will be among those who will hold fast to this image of personal caring as they practice competent care.

Acknowledgment

The research on which this article is based constitutes a portion of a dissertation that partially fulfilled requirements for a doctoral degree conferred by the Institute for the Medical Humanities, the University of Texas Medical Branch, Galveston, TX. The dissertation is entitled *Art in Practice: When Art Becomes Caring*.

References

Baum, C. M. (1980). Eleanor Clarke Slagle Lecture—Occupational therapists put care in the health system. *American Journal of Occupational Therapy, 34,* 505–516.

Bailey, D. M. (1990). Reasons for attrition from occupational therapy. *American Journal of Occupational Therapy, 44,* 23–29.

Beisser, A. (1989). *Flying without wings: Personal reflections on becoming disabled.* New York: Doubleday.

Benziger, B. F. (1969). *The prison of my mind.* New York: Walker.

Boyle, M. A. (1990). The Issue Is—The changing face of the rehabilitation population: A challenge for therapists. *American Journal of Occupational Therapy, 44,* 941–945.

Brice, J. (1987). Empathy lost. *Harvard Medical Letter, 60,* 28–32.

Burke, J. P., & Cassidy, J. C. (1991). Disparity between reimbursement-driven practice and humanistic values of occupational therapy. *American Journal of Occupational Therapy, 45,* 173–176. Reprinted as Chapter 54.

Cassell, E. J. (1985). *Talking with patients: Volume 1. The theory of doctor–patient communication.* Cambridge: MIT Press.

Dickerson, A. (1990). Evaluating productivity and profitability in occupational therapy contractual work. *American Journal of Occupational Therapy, 44,* 133–137.

Flagg, P. (1923). *The patient's viewpoint.* Milwaukee: Bruce Publishing.

Gebolys, E. (1990). Inadequacies, inequities, and inanities in modern medicine—A personal experience. *Occupational Therapy Forum, 12,* 6–7, 13–18.

Grady, A. P. (1992). Nationally Speaking—Occupation as vision. *American Journal of Occupational Therapy, 46,* 1062–1065.

Heller, J., & Vogel, S. (1986). *No laughing matter.* New York: Avon.

Hodgins, E. (1964). Whatever became of the healing art? *Annals of the New York Academy of Sciences, 164,* 838–846.

Howard, B. S. (1991). How high do we jump? The effect of reimbursement on occupational therapy. *American Journal of Occupational Therapy, 45,* 875–881. Reprinted as Chapter 53.

Jourard, S. (1964). *The transparent self: Self-disclosure and well being.* New York: Van Nostrand Reinhold.

Kari, N., & Michels, P. (1991). The Lazarus project: The politics of empowerment. *American Journal of Occupational Therapy, 44,* 719–725.

King, L. J. (1980). Creative caring. *American Journal of Occupational Therapy, 34,* 522–528.

Lear, M. (1980). *Heartsounds.* New York: Simon & Schuster.

Leder, D. (1984). Medicine and paradigms of embodiment. *Journal of Medicine and Philosophy, 9*(1), 29–43.

Lee, L. (1987). Transcendence. In M. Saxton & F. Howe (Eds.), *With wings: An anthology of literature by and about women with disabilities* (pp. 109–116). New York: Feminist Press.

Longcope, W. (1962). Methods and medicine. In W. H. Davenport (Ed.), *The good physician: A treasury of medicine* (pp. 546–559). New York: Macmillan.

Mattingly, C. (1991). The narrative nature of clinical reasoning. *American Journal of Occupational Therapy, 45,* 998–1005. Reprinted as Chapter 37.

McClay, E. (1977). *Green winter: Celebrations of old age.* New York: Reader's Digest Press.

Moore, A. R. (1978). *The missing medical text: Humane patient care.* Melbourne, Australia: Melbourne University Press.

Murphy, R. F. (1987). *The body silent.* New York: Henry Holt.

Nielson, C. (1991). The Issue Is—Positioning for power. *American Journal of Occupational Therapy, 45,* 853–854.

Parham, D. (1987). Nationally Speaking—Toward professionalism: The reflective therapist. *American Journal of Occupational Therapy, 41,* 555–561.

Peabody, B. (1986). *The screaming room: A mother's journal of her son's struggle with AIDS.* New York: Avon.

Peabody, F. W. (1930). *Doctor and patient papers on the relationship of the physician to men and institutions.* New York: Macmillan.

Pekkanen, J. (1988). M.D.: *Doctors talk about themselves.* New York: Del Publishing.

Pellegrino, E. (1979). *Humanism and the physician.* Knoxville: University of Tennessee Press.

Peloquin, S. M. (1989). Sustaining the art of practice in occupational therapy. *American Journal of Occupational Therapy, 43,* 219–226. Reprinted as Chapter 56.

Peloquin, S. M. (1990). The patient–therapist relationship in occupational therapy: Understanding visions and images. *American Journal of Occupational Therapy, 44*(1), 13–21.

Peloquin, S. M. (1993). The depersonalization of patients: A profile gleaned from narratives. *American Journal of Occupational Therapy, 47,* 830–837.

Rabin, D., Rabin, P., & Rabin, R. (1982). Compounding the ordeal of ALS. *New England Journal of Medicine, 307,* 506–509.

Reiser, D., & Schroder, A. K. (1980). *Patient interviewing: The human dimension.* Baltimore: Williams & Wilkins.

Sacks, O. (1983). *Awakenings.* New York: Dutton.

Sacks, O. (1984). *A leg to stand on.* New York: Harper & Row.

Sarason, S. B. (1985). *Caring and compassion in clinical practice.* San Francisco: Jossey-Bass.

Sarton, M. (1988). *After the stroke: A journal.* New York: Norton.

Saxton, M. (1987). In M. Saxton & F. Howe (Eds.), *With wings: An anthology of literature by and about women with disabilities* (pp. 51–57). New York: Feminist Press.

Schultz, S., & Schkade, J. K. (1992). Occupational adaptation: Toward a holistic approach for contemporary practice, Part 2. *American Journal of Occupational Therapy, 46,* 917–925. Reprinted as Chapter 48.

Taylor, R. (1972). *The practical art of medicine.* New York: Harper & Row.

Trahey, P. (1991). A comparison of the cost-effectiveness of two types of occupational therapy services. *American Journal of Occupational Therapy, 45,* 397–400.

Van Eys, J., & McGovern, J. P., Eds. (1988). *The doctor as a person.* Illinois: Charles C Thomas.

Vanderwoude, J. (1988). The caregiver as a patient. In J. Van Eys & J. P. McGovern (Eds.), *The doctor as a person* (pp. 172–184). Illinois: Charles C. Thomas.

Yerxa, E. J. (1980). Occupational therapy's role in creating a future climate of caring. *American Journal of Occupational Therapy, 34,* 529–534.

The Process of Evidence-Based Clinical Decision-Making in Occupational Therapy

EVIDENCE-BASED PRACTICE FORUM

CHRISTOPHER J. LEE, PHD
LINDA T. MILLER, PHD

There is a need for occupational therapy to conceive of evidence-based practice in a way that reflects the contextualized nature of occupational engagement. In occupational therapy, we should resist following the lead of experts in evidence-based medicine, such as Sackett and his colleagues (Rosenberg & Donald, 1995; Sackett, Rosenberg, Gray, Haynes, & Richardson, 1996; Sackett, Straus, Richardson, Rosenberg, & Haynes, 2000), who advocate that clinical decision-making must be based on systematic appraisal of the best research evidence. Instead, we argue here that evidence-based clinical decision-making in occupational therapy should encompass the diverse variety of evidence brought to the clinical context by both the client and therapist.

The following definitions of evidence-based practice are excellent examples of those espoused by medicine. Rosenberg and Donald (1995, p. 1122) define *evidence-based practice* as "the process of systematically finding, appraising, and using contemporaneous research findings for clinical decision." Similarly, Sackett et al. (1996, p. 71) describe evidence-based practice as "the conscientious, explicit, and judicious use of current best evidence in making decisions about the care of individual patients." Both of these definitions reflect a core belief that evidence-based practice entails systematic appraisal of the best research evidence. More recently, Sackett et al. (2000, p. 1) refer to evidence-based medicine as "the integration of best research evidence with clinical expertise and patient values." Although this definition acknowledges the expertise of the clinician and the values of the patient, it still clings to research as the only source of evidence. We propose that the values, beliefs, knowledge, and experiences of the clinician and client be recognized, in addition to research, as valuable sources of evidence in the clinical decision-making process.

Although the core belief about evidence-based medicine is beginning to acknowledge the expertise of the clinician and the values of the patient, it does not adequately reflect the highly contextualized and dynamic nature of occupational therapy. The practice of occupational therapy is an individualized activity shaped by a unique client–therapist relationship; it is not a static outcome that can be achieved by following a rigid procedure. Furthermore, as noted by Tickle-Degnen and Bedell (2003), the use of a single, invariant hierarchy of research evidence serves to depreciate the information provided by research methods other than randomized clinical trials. There are many kinds of research, and each variety can provide important insights into the nature of occupational performance.

Occupational therapy is highly contextualized, and evidence-based practice should reflect the different kinds of evidence that clients as well as therapists bring to the therapeutic process. When describing evidence-based practice in occupational therapy, it is important to emphasize that rehabilitation is a dynamic process. Unlike medical interventions, which can be described as standardized *procedures*, occupational therapy interventions are often more aptly described as dynamic processes. Indeed, the *Occupational Therapy Practice Framework: Domain and Process* (American Occupational Therapy Association [AOTA], 2002) (see Appendix A) clearly identifies occupational therapy as a dynamic process. To further delineate the distinction between medical practice and occupational therapy practice, consider the role of the patient or client. Medical procedures are frequently pharmacological or surgical in nature, with the patient playing a passive or receptive role. In contrast, the rehabilitation client plays a participatory role in the dynamic therapy process. Therefore, we argue that effective evidence-based practice in occupational therapy should acknowledge the diverse kinds of evidence brought to the clinical context by both the client and therapist.

Methods of Evidence

In his classic paper on the sources of evidence that serve to substantiate belief, Peirce (1877) presents four general methods of appraising belief that he identifies as the *method of tenacity,* the *method of authority,* the *a priori method,* and the *method of science.* In the clinical context, each of these methods introduces a different kind of evidence into the therapeutic process.

The method of tenacity refers to the unwavering acceptance of an idea because it is what one already believes; it is the continuing adherence to a belief on the basis of its longstanding acceptance. As Peirce (1877) comments, such "a steady and immovable faith yields great peace of mind" (p. 7). But this method of sustaining a belief requires considerable resolution and the ability to dismiss contrary opinion and evidence. As Peirce notes, "the social impulse is against it.... Unless we make ourselves hermits, we shall necessarily influence each other's opinions" (p. 8).

The method of authority refers to the uncritical acceptance of an idea because it is advocated by a respected individual, group, or institution. In large part, the method of authority perpetuates common beliefs in a culture. As Peirce (1877) notes, "It is mere accident of their having been taught as they have, and of their having been surrounded with the manners and associations they have, that has caused them to believe as they do and not far differently" (p. 10).

The *a priori* method refers to the acceptance of an idea because it is consistent with reason; that is, it is an idea that "we find ourselves inclined to believe" (Peirce, 1877, p. 10) because it seems to make sense. Although the *a priori* method "is far more intellectual and respectable from the point of view of reason than either of the others" (p. 10), it remains the case that what one person is inclined to believe as reasonable is not necessarily the same as what another person is inclined to believe. As Peirce notes, it "is always more or less a matter of fashion" (p. 11) to determine whether a conclusion is agreeable to reason.

The fourth method described by Peirce (1877) is science. Peirce viewed science as a method of overcoming the "accidental and capricious element" (p. 11) in the other methods. However, in contemporary accounts, science is no longer attributed such a degree of objectivity. For instance, in his influential historical analysis of science, Kuhn (1970) argues

that "an apparently arbitrary element, compounded of personal and historical accident, is always a formative ingredient of the beliefs espoused by a given scientific community at a given time" (p. 4). Furthermore, Kuhn notes that "few philosophers of science still seek absolute criteria for the verification of scientific theories" (p. 145) because "no theory can ever be exposed to all possible relevant tests" (p. 145). Thus, in considering science as a method of appraising belief, it is important to acknowledge the provisional nature of scientific evidence.

The methods of appraising belief described by Peirce (1877) provide a useful classification of the different kinds of evidence that may be introduced into the therapeutic process by the client and therapist. An account of the variety of client beliefs is given in the next section of the paper, followed by an account of the variety of therapist beliefs. These beliefs affect the therapeutic process; they represent the kinds of evidence warranting consideration when appraising the potential therapeutic benefit of an intervention in occupational therapy.

Client Perspective

In terms of client beliefs held on the basis of tenacity, a client with osteoarthritis, for example, may be quite emphatic in expressing her dislike for swimming pools each time a therapist suggests that she consider participating in a therapeutic aquatics program. The tenacity with which the client maintains an unwavering disdain for swimming pools is an important piece of evidence to consider in appraising the potential therapeutic benefit of an aquatics program. A second illustration of the consequence of beliefs held on grounds of tenacity stems from the fact that some beliefs are cornerstones of a client's construction of self. Consider a client for whom being independent is of utmost importance and central to his view of himself. In order to maintain his perception of personal independence, the client may underestimate the number of times he has fallen in his home when asked in an interview or in completing a questionnaire. Although evidence of a self-presentation bias, such as a misreporting of falls, can be difficult for a therapist to discover, it is important to recognize that a client's highly persistent beliefs about himself or herself pervade his or her perspective of therapeutic goals and outcomes.

In terms of beliefs held on the basis of authority, a peer with related experiences can be a compelling source of information affecting therapeutic goals and outcomes. For instance, a peer who uses a walker can represent an authoritative source of evidence about the utility of a particular type of walker, and a peer's negative evaluation of a walker can be a barrier to its use by the client despite the recommendations of the therapist.

Consider as well an example of the *a priori* method: A client is reluctant to use a walker as recommended by her therapist, preferring to use a cane. She reasons that a cane is better for her to use because it is lighter in weight and seems to offer her as much support as the walker. Although such reasoning is not rigorous, the conclusion is reasonable to the client.

Finally, scientific findings reported in the media, including the Internet, can be taken by clients as a valid basis of belief. Media reports of scientific research are intended to be compelling for the audience, and it is conceivable for a brief account of the treatment of rheumatoid arthritis in yesterday's news to affect a client's beliefs about the treatment of his or her arthritis. In sum, these examples indicate that clients bring to therapy a variety of beliefs that can be important sources of evidence to consider when appraising the eventual therapeutic benefit of an intervention.

Therapist Perspective

Therapists also demonstrate the varieties of belief described by Peirce (1877). In terms of beliefs held on the basis of tenacity, occupational therapists share a set of core beliefs about practice. Kanny (1993) identified seven core values that occupational therapists use to guide clinical decisions. These values include, for instance, an unselfish concern for the welfare of others, an affirmation of the intrinsic uniqueness of each person, and a valuing of self-direction in the pursuit of meaningful goals. Occupational therapists also hold the fundamental belief that the engagement in occupation is a vital component of health and well-being. Obviously, these professional beliefs have a substantial effect on therapeutic goals and outcomes. Insomuch as the core beliefs underlying occupational therapy are different than those of other health professions, it is reasonable for occupational therapists to hold a somewhat different conception of evidence-based practice than other health professionals.

Therapists demonstrate beliefs that are based on authority when practices are modeled in accord with the ideas of clinical specialists or individuals highly regarded for their expertise on particular issues. Institutional guidelines or mandates may also serve as a source of authority for therapists insomuch as they establish the set of common practices at a particular institution.

In clinical practice, the *a priori* source of evidence refers to the use of clinical experience to inform practice. Clinical experience is an important repository of information gained from working with other clients, and it represents an appropriate place to begin the process of accruing evidence.

Lastly, science encompasses a diverse variety of peer-reviewed research relevant to occupation. We believe that all research has the potential to contribute to a fuller understanding of occupational performance, and no one kind of research can be judged universally to be the best source of evidence.

In many discussions of research methods, randomized clinical trials, systematic reviews of randomized clinical trials, and meta-analyses of randomized clinical trials are ranked as providing the highest quality of evidence (e.g., Egan, Dubouloz, von Zweck, & Vallerand, 1998; Greenhalgh, 1997; Law & Philip, 2002; Lloyd-Smith, 1997; Porter & Matel, 1998; Sackett et al., 2000; Taylor, 1997). However, many research questions are aptly addressed by research methods other than randomized clinical trials (Tickle-Degnen & Bedell, 2003). For example, investigations of the subtle complexity of a client's personal experiences are facilitated by qualitative methods, and studies informing the appropriate use of standardized assessments are well served by descriptive and correlational methods. To state universally that experimental methods, such as randomized clinical trials, represent the highest quality of evidence disregards the multifaceted nature of clinical practice and depreciates the diverse variety of research in occupational therapy.

In sum, the conception of evidence-based practice as a systematic appraisal of the best evidence does not reflect the diverse kinds of evidence brought to the clinical context by clients and therapists. If occupational therapy is truly a contextualized activity shaped by a unique client–therapist relationship, then the full variety of client and therapist beliefs, as summarized in the evidence matrix presented in Table 41.1, should be considered in the course of goal setting and in anticipating the eventual therapeutic benefit of an intervention.

The process of evidence based clinical decision-making in occupational therapy is illustrated in Figure 41.1. The figure shows how the evidence gathered from the client, the therapist, and research inform clinical action and, subsequently, how clinical evidence informs modifications to the course of clinical action. Further, the process clearly demonstrates how the evidence cumulated with respect to each individual client becomes integrated into the therapist's repertoire of clinical experience with the potential to affect future decision-making. To this point, we have considered the elements of constructing an evidence matrix; the integration of evidence using decision strategies and the monitoring of therapeutic progress are examined below.

Table 41.1. Evidence Matrix: Varieties of Evidence Classified by Method and Perspective

Method*	Perspective	
	Client	Therapist
Tenacity	Personal Beliefs & Convictions	Professional Values
Authority	Personal Experts	Clinical Experts
A Priori	Personal Reasoning & Experience	Clinical Reasoning & Experience
Science	Publicized Science	Research Literature

*From Peirce (1877).

The Process of Evidence-Based Clinical Decision-Making in Occupational Therapy

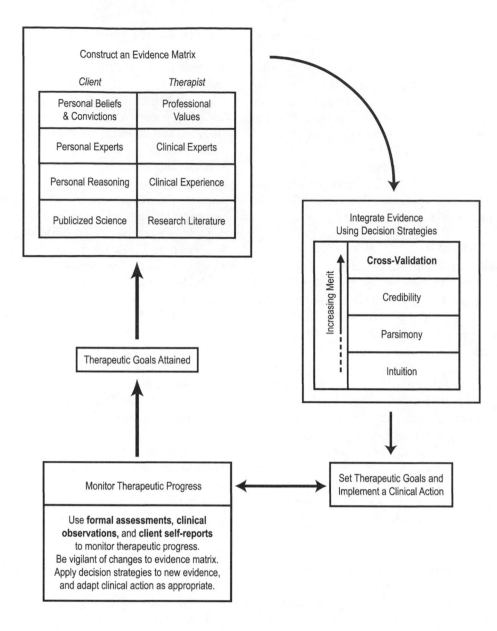

Figure 41.1. The evidence-based occupational therapy process.

Integrating Evidence Using Decision Strategies

We have suggested that in order to make appropriate decisions in clinical practice, it is necessary to integrate multiple pieces of evidence in a way that recognizes the contextualized nature of clinical practice. This necessitates a dynamic approach to integrating evidence. Each client–therapist relationship provides a unique matrix of evidence. Evidence can conflict, and it may be necessary to consider new evidence as therapy progresses. The four strategies described below, referred to as *intuition, parsimony, consensual-validation,* and *cross-validation,* have sufficient flexibility to be applied to a diverse variety of evidence.

Decisions made on intuition are those based on what feels right or seems reasonable. Such decisions are frequently diffi-

cult to justify because of their subjective nature, despite the fact that they may reflect extensive clinical experience.

Parsimony is a strategy for choosing among alternative interventions. The principle of parsimony is a general heuristic stating that if two propositions are equally tenable the simpler one is preferable. Thus, in deciding between two or more interventions of equal potential benefit, the principle of parsimony holds that the simpler intervention should be employed. In judgments of parsimony, simpler means requiring fewer assumptions. Thus, in deciding between two interventions, it is the one whose imputed benefit is based on fewer assumptions that is preferable.

For example, consider the following two hypothetical interventions aimed at improving the legibility of a child's handwriting. The first intervention involves activities for hand strengthening and activities for improving hand coordination. The second intervention emphasizes "sky writing" letters in the air in addition to hand strengthening and hand coordination activities. Both interventions assume that strength and coordination are important aspects of handwriting skill, but the second intervention makes the additional assumption that writing letters in the air facilitates the development of handwriting skill. In the situation where these two interventions appear to be equally effective, the principle of parsimony would hold that the first intervention is to be preferred. In other words, one begins with the simpler explanation of handwriting skill and switches to the more assumption-burdened explanation only when warranted by a clear demonstration that it is a more effective intervention.

A third decision strategy is consensual-validation; it reflects a belief that as more persons concur with a particular conclusion, the more likely it is to be valid. In clinical practice, consensual-validation often takes the form of informal consultation with colleagues who serve as a sounding board for clinical reasoning. In the research process, consensual-validation is provided by a formal mechanism of peer review. In general, consensual-validation is preferable to intuition or parsimony as a strategy for decision-making. Although consensual-validation should not be construed as providing objectivity, it does result in decisions that have greater acceptability to others.

Arguably, the most justifiable decisions are those based on multiple sources of evidence and multiple decision strategies. Thus, in assimilating a diverse array of evidence, it is important to look for cross-validation in different sources of evidence as well as among the conclusions afforded by intuition, parsimony, and consensual-validation. The concept of cross-validation is not novel; it has long been advocated as an approach to substantiating the validity of evidence. For example, Campbell and Fiske (1959) proposed the multitrait–multimethod matrix as an approach to validating evidence in which validity is strengthened by demonstrating convergence of findings across a variety of methodological and measurement approaches. The rationale of cross-validation rests on the premise that convergence of findings across multiple and varied sources of evidence indicates that the findings are not spurious, but rather are impervious to methodological variation. Consequently, decisions based on cross-validation are less likely to be influenced by bias or subjective interpretation.

Monitoring Therapeutic Progress

In the process of setting therapeutic goals, it is important that one or more measures be taken prior to intervention and periodically throughout the course of intervention to provide evidence of change as a function of the intervention. Such evidence can take the form of formal assessments or evaluations, informal clinical observations, and client self-reports, with a combination of these methods considered to be most valid on the premise of cross-validation. Further, one should be vigilant of changes to the evidence matrix over time, especially client and therapist beliefs and expectations pertaining to the progress and outcome of therapy. In these respects, it is important that evidence continue to be gathered throughout the clinical process to facilitate the best possible treatment.

With the eventual attainment of therapeutic goals, the process of evidence-based clinical decision-making circles back upon itself. A therapist's observations, measures, and explanations of the therapeutic progress of one client contribute to the evidence matrix of future clinical practice by becoming part of clinical experience. Furthermore, this information offers a basis for preparing more formal commentaries on clinical practice for contribution to professional journals, and especially when cumulated across clients, the process of evidence-based clinical decision-making provides a basis for integrating a program of research within clinical practice. In the longer term, such contributions to the literature of occupational therapy serve to develop clinical experience to a point of clinical expertise, providing an authoritative basis for other therapists to model therapeutic practices.

Conclusion

Occupational therapy has evolved its own professional values and beliefs. In our opinion, the approach of evidence-based medicine, as advocated by experts such as Sackett and his colleagues (Rosenberg & Donald, 1995; Sackett et al., 1996; Sackett et al., 2000), depreciates the core values and beliefs of occupational therapy. In contrast, we believe that the process of evidence-based clinical decision-making described in this paper embraces occupational therapy's professional values and beliefs. There is no doubt that research evidence is essential to the practice of occupational therapy. But in our opinion, we should resist accepting the relative infrequency of randomized clinical trials evaluating occupational therapy interventions as a weakness in the scientific grounding of occupational therapy practice. Rather, the relative infrequency of randomized clinical trials may simply reflect the limited relevance and applicability of this design to occupational therapy practices and interventions. We argue that evidence-based occupational therapy should encompass a diverse variety of evidence, and it should value all research paradigms and designs as having the potential to inform clinical practice. Evidence-based occupational therapy should integrate a client's beliefs with the therapist's experiences and draw on pertinent expertise and research. As clearly stated in the *Occupational Therapy Practice Framework: Domain and Process* (2002), "clients bring knowledge about their life experiences and their hopes and dream" (p. 615) to the clinical context (see Appendix A). The client's knowledge and experiences should be explicitly integrated into the process of evidence-based clinical decision-making in occupational therapy; otherwise, we neglect "occupational therapy's unique focus on occupation and daily life activities and the application of an intervention process that facilitates engagement in occupation to support participation in life" (p. 609).

References

American Occupational Therapy Association. (2002). Occupational therapy practice framework: Domain and process. *American Journal of Occupational Therapy, 56,* 609–639. Reprinted as Appendix A.

Campbell, D., & Fiske, D. (1959). Convergent and discriminant validation by the multitrait–multimethod matrix. *Psychological Bulletin, 54,* 81–105.

Egan, M., Dubouloz, C. J., von Zweck, C., & Vallerand, J. (1998). The client-centered evidence-based practice of occupational therapy. *Canadian Journal of Occupational Therapy, 65,* 136–143.

Greenhalgh, T. (1997). *How to read a paper: The basics of evidence-based medicine.* London: BMJ Publishing Group.

Kanny, E. (1993). Core values and attitudes of occupational therapy practice. *American Journal of Occupational Therapy, 47,* 1085–1086.

Kuhn, T. S. (1970). *The structure of scientific revolutions* (2nd ed.). Chicago: University of Chicago Press.

Law, M., & Philip, I. (2002). Evaluating the evidence. In M. Law (Ed.), *Evidence-based rehabilitation: A guide to practice.* Thorofare, NJ: Slack.

Lloyd-Smith, W. (1997). Evidence-based practice and occupational therapy. *British Journal of Occupational Therapy, 60,* 474–478.

Peirce, C. S. (1877). The fixation of belief. *Popular Science Monthly, 12,* 1–15.

Porter, C., & Matel, J. L. S. (1998). Are we making decisions based on evidence? *Journal of the American Dietetic Association, 98,* 404–407.

Rosenberg, W., & Donald, A. (1995). Evidence-based medicine: An approach to clinical problem-solving. *BMJ, 310,* 1122–1126.

Sackett, D. L., Rosenberg, W. M., Gray, J. A., Haynes, R. B., & Richardson, W. S. (1996). Evidence-based medicine: What it is and what it isn't. *BMJ, 312,* 71–72.

Sackett, D. L., Straus, S. E., Richardson, W. S., Rosenberg, W., & Haynes, R. B. (2000). *Evidence-based medicine: How to practice and teach EBM* (2nd ed.). Edinburgh, Scotland: Churchill Livingstone.

Taylor, M. C. (1997). What is evidence-based practice? *British Journal of Occupational Therapy, 60,* 470–473.

Tickle-Degnen, L., & Bedell, G. (2003). Evidence-Based Practice Forum—Heter-archy and hierarchy: A critical appraisal of the "levels of evidence" as a tool for clinical decisionmaking. *American Journal of Occupational Therapy, 57,* 234–237.

Defining Lives—Occupation as Identity: An Essay on Competence, Coherence, and the Creation of Meaning

1999 ELEANOR CLARKE SLAGLE LECTURE

CHARLES H. CHRISTIANSEN, EdD, OTR, OT(C), FAOTA

This article presents a view of occupation as the principal means through which people develop and express their personal identities. Based on a review of theory and research, it proposes that identity is instrumental to social life because it provides a context for deriving meaning from daily experiences and interpreting lives over time. The article proposes that identity also provides a framework for goal-setting and motivation. It is asserted that competence in the performance of tasks and occupations contributes to identity-shaping and that the realization of an acceptable identity contributes to coherence and well-being.

Within this framework, it is postulated that performance limitations and disfigurement that sometimes result from illness or injury have identity implications that should be recognized by occupational therapy practitioners. By virtue of their expertise in daily living skills, occupational therapy practitioners are well positioned to help address the identity challenges of those whom they serve. In so doing, they make an important contribution to meaning and well-being.

The anthropologist Bateson (1996) has written that:

> The capacity to do something useful for yourself or others is key to personhood, whether it involves the ability to earn a living, cook a meal, put on shoes in the morning, or whatever other skill needs to be mastered at the moment. (1986, p. 11)

In this article, I assert that occupations are key not just to being a person, but to being a particular person, and thus creating and maintaining an identity. Occupations come together within the contexts of our relationships with others to provide us with a sense of purpose and structure in our day-to-day activities, as well as over time. When we build our identities through occupations, we provide ourselves with the contexts necessary for creating meaningful lives, and life meaning helps us to be well.

In this article, an important distinction is made between being well and being healthy. The ultimate goal of occupational therapy services is well-being, not health. Health enables people to pursue the tasks of everyday living that provide them with the life meaning necessary for their well-being. As Englehardt said in describing the virtues of occupational therapy, *"people are healthy or diseased in terms of the activities open to them or denied them"* (1977, p. 672).

Overview

In addressing the complex topic of personal identity, I begin by reviewing key concepts from the literature, noting particularly how our use of language gives us important insights into how we think about ourselves. I then discuss how identity is thought to be formed during the crucial developmental stages of our lives, and how it seems to be of immense importance to us as we make our way through the stages of life. After this, I consider how daily occupations serve the important purpose of enabling us to experience or realize our personal identities. I then address the implications of incomplete or blemished identities on personal well-being, and conclude with observations on the implications of identity-making for the practice of occupational therapy in the new millennium.

Propositions

My presentation is based on four propositions, all centered on the assertion that one of the most compelling needs that every human being has is to be able to express his or her unique identity in a manner that gives meaning to life. This assertion was influenced greatly by an ethnographic study of adaptive strategies reported in the *American Journal of Occupational Therapy* (McCuaig & Frank, 1991). That study described a middle-aged woman [Meghan] with severe athetoid cerebral palsy who had great difficulty with voluntary movement that profoundly affected her mobility and speech. Somehow, without much professional assistance, the woman was able to devise adaptive strategies so that she could use her limited voluntary movement and assistive technology to get along in daily life. Despite rather considerable postural deformities and difficulty with hearing, she was able to live in an apartment, requiring only modest assistance of friends and neighbors to live independently.

In considering the study, I found Meghan's motivations for choosing strategies, rather than the nature of her adaptations, of greatest interest. It seemed that one very important consideration underlying her choices—especially when they were to be viewed by others—was whether or not they would show her to be an intelligent, competent woman. In short, they were issues of identity.

I remember being surprised by this observation, thinking that someone as disabled as she was would be driven by the functional necessities of life, with little reserve time or energy to be consumed by thoughts of how she might be viewed in the eyes of others. But as I thought about it more deeply, I realized that life around me was teeming with indications[1] that people (with disabilities or without) are universally concerned about their social identity and acceptance by others. The ethnographic study also pointed squarely to the reality that daily occupation was the primary means through which the woman was able to communicate her identity as a competent person.

My further thinking and study about the relationships between daily occupations and selfhood led to four premises that may be useful to the process of considering identity issues in occupational therapy. Because there is yet much work to be done in establishing the validity of theories of how identity is constructed and maintained, each proposition must be viewed as tentative.

Proposition 1: Identity is an overarching concept that shapes and is shaped by our relationships with others.

Personal identity can be defined as the person we think we are. It is the self we know. Note that this is not the same as self-concept nor is it the same as self-esteem, although these important concepts are related to identity. Baumeister (1986, 1997), an often-cited authority on the study of identity, has noted that the most obvious things in daily life are sometimes the most difficult to define. We use the word *self* in our everyday language several times a day. When we say *self*, we include

the direct feeling we have about our thoughts and feelings and sensations. This begins with the awareness of our body and is augmented by our sense of being able to make choices and initiate action. It also encompasses the abstract and complex ideas that embellish the self.

The term *self-concept* refers to the *inferences* we make about ourselves. It encompasses our understanding of personality traits and characteristics, our social roles, and our relationships. We are motivated as adults to achieve some consistency in terms of how we view ourselves, and we want this view to be favorable. In general, we strive to maintain favorable views and to dispute or avoid feedback that is discrepant from our view of self (Swann, 1987; Swann & Hill, 1982). To the extent that we perceive discrepancies between our perceived and ideal selves, we are motivated to change.

A third concept is self-esteem. This refers to the evaluative aspect of the self-concept. Self-esteem is related to identity in the sense that our esteem is related to our ability to demonstrate efficacious action, which gains social approval and thus influences our overall concept of self (Baumeister, 1982; Franks & Marolla, 1976).

Finally, *identity* refers to the definitions that are created for and superimposed on the self. Identity is a composite definition of the self, and includes an interpersonal aspect (e.g., our roles and relationships, such as mothers, wives, occupational therapists), an aspect of possibility or potential (i.e., who we *might* become), and a values aspect (that suggests importance and provides a stable basis for choices and decisions). Self-concept is entirely created in one's mind, whereas identity is often created by the larger society, even though it is often negotiated with others and refined by the individual as a result of those social negotiations (see Figure 42.1).

In summary, identity can be viewed as the superordinate view of ourselves that includes both self-esteem and the self-concept, but also importantly reflects, and is influenced by, the larger social world in which we find ourselves. This definition of identity leads logically to a second proposition.

Proposition 2: Identities are closely tied to what we do and our interpretations of those actions in the context of our relationships with others.

It is interesting to note that in North America, after an exchange of names between strangers, the next part of a conversation often turns on the expression "What do you do?" The resulting dialogue provides for shared meaning by situating each person in a context the other understands or attempts to understand through further dialogue.

This everyday exchange illustrates the close connection between doing and identity, and also points out the important role that language has in creating understanding and meaning. Were it not for our social existence, there would be no need

---

[1]Consider the prevalence (and popularity) of monograms, tattoos, vanity license plates, titles, degrees, pierced body parts, autobiographies, and unique names (changed or not).

for language and communication, and it is generally believed that thought itself is a product of language. That is, when we think, we carry on an internal dialogue with ourselves. Vygotsky (1981) maintained that language provides children with the tools to gain self-awareness and, consequently, voluntary control of their actions. Thus, our understanding of the world around us is shaped as much by language, a system of spoken and written symbols, as it is by direct experience.

For example, when we learn the word *stove* as toddlers, we are also apt to learn the words *hot* and *danger*. We may also discover that if we ignore our parents' admonitions and touch a hot stove, we may burn our fingers. At the same time, we may experience disapproval for not having behaved as our parents expected.

Piaget (1954) and others (Kagan, 1981) have shown that as infants and as toddlers, the experience of coming to know the world very much involves *doing*. As children, we learn that we can intentionally act on our environment and change it. It is this acting on the environment with observable consequence that gives us our sense of selfhood, that teaches us that we are active agents, separate from our environment.

As children explore cause-and-effect events, they learn that they can have an effect on inanimate objects, such as toys, and that they can also elicit reactions from animate objects, such as pets and other people. Mostly, a child's early experiences in this regard are positive because doting parents and grandparents tend to regard any behavior as cute and, as a consequence, are very forgiving of transgressions. Later, this tolerance becomes more selective, and parents can then also communicate disapproval when a child disobeys. Yet, already, children have become active agents in the world, exerting an effect on objects and on people. Using dolls or toy figures, they can even pretend that objects are people.

Thus, children learn that they can get the attention of others through their actions and that their actions can be approved or not. Studies have shown that *good* and *bad* are among the words most frequently spoken to young children (Kagan, 1981). Thus, very early on, a connection is made between behavior and social approval in a manner that influences our sense of self. The point to be made here is that already, at an early age, children know themselves as individuals capable of acting on the world, and they understand that their actions have a social meaning. They also begin to appreciate that their approval as individuals is often contingent on what they do (Keller, Ford, & Meacham, 1978).

This is to be the beginning of a lifetime of understanding the interdependence of self and the social groups to which we are connected. It is also the beginning of understanding ourselves as having an identity that is related to group membership. For example, as children we learn that we are members of a family, that we are male or female, and that we have other characteristics in common or in contrast with others.

Identity development continues to be influenced by social relationships as children mature. Beginning at preschool age,

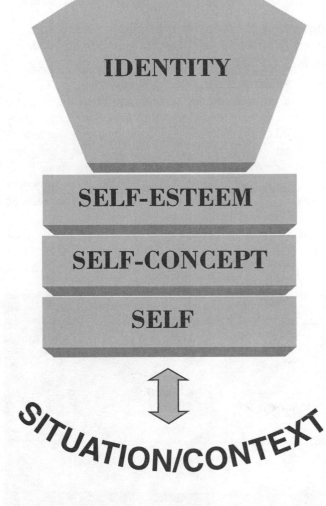

Figure 42.1. Hierarchy of identity concepts.

self-concept and identity are shaped by a person's competencies and capabilities in comparison to others and in relationship to social standards or expectations (Ruble, 1983). During adolescence, identity is shaped by more abstract concepts, such as interpersonal traits, values, and preferences (Erikson, 1968). For adults, identity is oriented toward goals, often related to becoming a certain kind of person and not becoming another kind of person (Baumeister, 1986). Adolescent and adult identity development, although based more on abstractions, is nonetheless largely influenced by social phenomena.

Because symbolic communication involves behaviors as well as language, children learn also that a raised eyebrow or an awkward silence can be among many forms of communicating disapproval. As maturity develops, the task of understanding what constitutes social approval takes on even greater importance, and becomes even more challenging, because the feedback adults receive in social settings is much more ambiguous and indirect. At this point, it should be obvious that identity has no existence outside of interpersonal relationships. Our views of our goals, our behaviors, and ourselves are inextricably tied to our relationships with others.

Proposition 3: Identities provide an important central figure in a self-narrative or life story that provides coherence and meaning for everyday events and life itself.

When we interpret events, we evaluate them for personal meaning. If they are meaningful, they have significance to us, we respond emotionally to them, and they shape our behavior and perceptions of life. When people believe that they have no identity or that their identity has been spoiled, life becomes less meaningful and can become meaningless (Debats, Drost, & Hansen, 1995; Moore, 1997; van Selm & Dittmann-Kohli, 1998).

Our interpretation of life events and situations takes place within the framework of life stories or narratives. Other people are part of our life stories, and we are part of the life stories of others. Our lives are interwoven within the lives of others and, therefore, if our identities change, this influences our life as well as the lives of others. In this sense, identities are socially interconnected and distributed, yet understood in the context of ongoing life stories.

Proposition 4: Because life meaning is derived in the context of identity, it is an essential element in promoting well-being and life satisfaction.

Each of us hopes for a satisfactory outcome for the particular goals we are pursuing at the moment as well as for the life we are leading, which we are aware will end at some point. To the extent that we can successfully weave together the various and multiple short stories that comprise our lives into a meaningful whole, we can derive a sense of coherence and meaning and purpose from our lives. I am proposing that our identities provide us with the context through which we interpret and derive meaning from the events we experience. Our identities also provide us with a view for future possibilities.

Theoretical Contexts

Having elaborated four propositions regarding identity, it is useful to create a context from which to view them and evaluate their implications for occupational therapy practice. There are three roots of selfhood that will serve as a framework for understanding. The first is the experience of reflexive consciousness, derived from the traditions of symbolic interactionism. This allows us to think about ourselves and the influence of our actions on others. The second is the interpersonal aspect of selfhood, the reality that identities are shaped within a social setting, where we receive acceptance, approval, and validation as worthwhile persons. The third is the agential aspect of identity, that aspect of demonstrating influence on the world around us that allows us to make meaning in our lives. When we create, when we control, when we exercise choice, we are expressing our selfhood and unique identities.

Reflexive Consciousness

The ability to think about ourselves and to have these thoughts modify our behavior is a distinctly human characteristic, and it depends on symbolic communication. Using symbols or language, we not only are able to categorize, think about, and act in socially influenced ways, but we also are able to reflect on ourselves from the perspective of others.

When we think about ourselves, we carry on the equivalent of an internal dialogue between two aspects of self, the experiencing self and the thought of self. These two aspects of the self can be labeled the *I* and the *me*. The *I* is the active creative agent doing the experiencing, thinking, and acting, and the *me* is the perspective or attitude toward oneself that one assumes when taking the roles of specific others or the generalized community. In this approach, the *mes,* or perspectives of the self, are the social selves—who we are in our own and

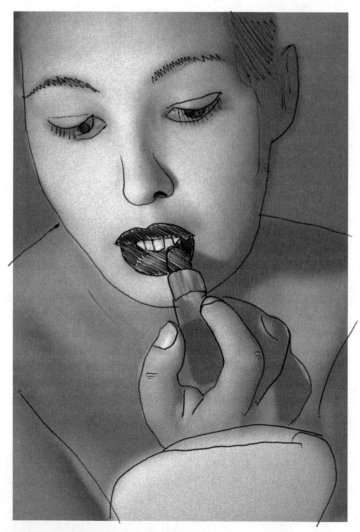

Figure 42.2. Reflexive self-consciousness—The dialogue between the *I* and the *me.* Image © 1999 PhotoDisc, Inc. Used with permission.

others' eyes. Thought of in another way, when we consider the image of ourselves reflected in a mirror, the I is looking at and thinking about the me, all the while making grooming adjustments to improve it (see Figure 42.2).

The reflexive nature of the self is exemplified by everyday language that illustrates its duality. When we speak of self-discipline, we are talking about one aspect of the self keeping the other under control. Similarly, when we observe that Sue has "let herself go," we imply that she no longer has self-control or that she no longer cares about her public identity.

The Interpersonal Nature of Selfhood

The ideas of symbolic communication and the reflexive nature of the self are derived from a tradition of social psychology known as symbolic interactionism. This tradition goes back to the turn of the century and several prominent behavioral scientists of the time, beginning with William James (1892). Later, the famous sociologist Charles Horton Cooley (1902) made the observation that our views of ourselves are very much influenced by the reactions of others to what we do. He formulated what is known as the "looking glass theory," which maintained that the reactions of others reflect their approval and disapproval and thus constitute a primary means of developing an awareness of ourselves.

The psychologist George Herbert Mead extended this thinking in the 1930s, advancing the theory even further. In *Mind, Self, and Society,* Mead (1934) held that society is created, sustained, and changed through the process of symbolic communication. In other words, social reality is constructed and negotiated through interactions with others. In these interactions, people seek to present images of the self for others to see and evaluate. The primary purposes of these social selves are to gain approval from others and to be able to gain influence, which occurs through social status and power. Mead believed that by using the reflexive processes of communication, the dialogue between I and me, we are able to imagine how we appear to others or what reactions others will have to our behaviors.[2]

Because of the dependence on others for feedback about the self, Mead (1934) believed that there is a mutual interdependence of self and society. By seeking the approval of others, a person's behavior may be moderated, but this occurs only to the extent that people are capable of exercising the self-control necessary for them to gain social approval.

Many people are reluctant to accept a view of self that suggests that every action they take is calculated to gain the approval of others because it sounds manipulative or deceptive. However, in reality, people are not able to exercise conscious control over their behaviors in a manner that permits them to plan calculated actions at every moment in every social relationship. To a certain extent, however, the rules and conventions of social interaction are such that we preserve and enhance our identity through conformity and careful reflection about the anticipated results of our behaviors on others.

As expressions of identity, people often exhibit spontaneity and creativity that test the boundaries of conformity or risk social disapproval. Unconventional behavior is often risky. This is one of the things that makes the world such an interesting place. Occasionally, acts of spontaneity and creativity are embraced and adopted by the larger group with the result that such innovations create change or progress in the culture. In this way, the reciprocal influence between self and society described by Mead (1934) is completed. That is, social expectations influence the individual, and the individual, through acts of creativity, sometimes influences the larger society. A proposal of symbolic interactionism views that the individual and society are interdependent. That is, they depend on each other for predictability and stability as well as for progress.

To summarize, the basic ideas underlying symbolic interactionism are that (a) we communicate symbolically much of the time and that the language of social life consists of both spoken and unspoken messages; (b) through our conversations with ourselves, we are able to modify our behaviors to gain social approval; and (c) the need for social approval encourages conformity, which promotes stability and predictability, but occasionally also yields individual creativity that, when adopted, serves to advance the social group.

Social Constructionism and Distributed Selves

In recent years, views of the social nature of self-identity have been extended with a school of thought called social constructionism. Theorists in this tradition propose that selves are distributed. That is, the person and their social context cannot be easily separated. Social constructionists argue that although we perceive a private and self-contained world inside our heads, it would be more accurate to describe this image as a snapshot from a constantly changing public panorama (Bruner, 1990; Gergen, 1991; Polkinghorne, 1988).

When we think of our multiple expressions of self, our children, our friendships, our marriages, our journals, and our daily interactions, we realize that our identities are indeed distributed throughout our social environments. These "pieces of self" are part of us. They define who we are, and yet they exist in other mediums, distributing identities well beyond the boundaries of a physical body. This distribution of the self only occurs through social interaction.

The social constructionist view suggests that people's identities not only are social, they also are multifaceted, yet they are perceived not so much as fragments, but as part of a comprehensive and understandable self (cf Kondo, 1990).

[2]It is worth noting that Mead's assertion that our identity is totally dependent on the feedback of others has been shown to be incomplete (Schrauger & Schoeneman, 1979), mainly because research has shown that people deceive themselves by perceiving that others evaluate them more favorably than is actually the case (Greenwald, 1980).

Ordinarily, we do not think of ourselves as fragmented, but as complex people with many dimensions of self. In short, we piece together our experiences to fashion an intelligible self, an identity that is comprehensible to both ourselves and others.

Life Stories

How is it that our identities can be complex and distributed while at the same time seem to be stable and predictable? The answer to this question lies in our understanding of our lives as evolving narratives or life stories. Through stories, we understand life events as systematically related. As Gergen and Gergen wrote: "One's present identity is thus not a sudden and mysterious event, but a sensible result of a life story" (1988, p. 255).

In a sense, our stories are unfolding and being rewritten as we live them. All narrative shares the similar characteristic of having a temporal order. That is, our life stories consist of events in progressive sequences. In order for our stories to have meaning, the events in our lives must be interpreted in ways that give them a relationship to each other. In this manner, they have coherence and unity. It helps that our everyday routines, our personality traits, and other factors, such as our genetic make-up, influence us in ways that provide a degree of consistency to our behavior. This makes it easier to interpret our life stories in an understandable way.

Making Sense of Experiences

The problem of how people make sense of their life experiences has been central to the work of McAdams (1997). He has analyzed life stories to derive insights into the processes people use to construct their identities within a coherent structure. His work suggests that one of the central purposes of the life story is to create unity and purpose in daily life. In constructing and interpreting life stories, people seek to fashion identities that make sense to themselves and others. Importantly, because people are not passive participants in their life stories, they can enact or create the events that express their identities in the manner they would like others to view them. This brings us to the third requirement of identity, that of human agency, or expressing the self through acting on the world around us.

Selfing: Shaping Identity Through Experience

It is the reflexive dialogue between the *I* and *me* that McAdams (1996, 1997) suggests ties human agency to identity. The *I*, he argues, is not a noun, but a process, which McAdams and others refer to as *selfing*. That is, by experi-

encing our actions and our lives as our own, we adopt them as part of ourselves, as belonging to the *me*. Selfing is responsible for human feelings of agency.

McAdams (1996) suggests that selfing is inherently a unifying, integrative, synthesizing process. Ego psychologists (e.g., Loevenger, 1976), building on Freud (as cited in Stachey, 1990), viewed the ego as the organizational medium of the mind that promotes healthy adaptation to life through learning, memory, perception, and synthesis (Kris, 1952). It permits the gaining of competence that White (1959) viewed as so important to successful adaptation. To quote McAdams: "The *I* puts experience together—synthesizes it, unifies it, makes it mine. The fact that it is mine—even when I see the sunset, I am seeing it; that when you hurt my feelings those were my feelings, not yours that were hurt—provides a unity to selfhood without which human life in society as we know it would simply not exist" (1997, p. 57). To *self* is to maintain the stance of the self in the world, it is the being and becoming that Fidler (Fidler & Fidler, 1978 [see Chapter 9]) has written about. In other words, selfing is the shaping of identity through daily occupations.

Occupations are more than movements strung together, more than simply doing something. They are opportunities to express the self, to create an identity.

Creating Life Meaning Through Selfing

When we create our life stories through doing, or selfing, as McAdams would say, we are living for a purpose, and deriving a sense of meaning in our lives in the process. Sommer and Baumeister (1998) have observed that people seek meaning in ordinary events along the same lines that they seek meaning in life generally. That is, they try to fulfill four basic needs. These needs are *purpose, efficacy, value,* and *self-worth*. By definition, our daily occupations, whether they pertain to work, leisure, or maintenance of self, are goal directed and, therefore, provide purpose in the moment. When we achieve success in reaching our goals, we derive a sense of efficacy and believe that we have some measure of control over our environments (Langer & Rodin, 1976).

Meaning is also derived from believing that we have done the right thing, that our actions are justifiable under the circumstances. Finally, and not least importantly, we derive meaning from our feelings of self-worth. We meet this need through the approval of others and by viewing our own traits and abilities favorably. We want to feel good about ourselves, and we want to believe that we are worthy of other people's attention and affection.[3]

---

[3]The British psychologist and philosopher Rom Harré (1983) has used the term *identity projects* to refer to self-directed development and expression of self. Identity projects may take the form of pursuit of fame or status or recognition of some kind. Or they may be concerned with the more personal aspects of ourselves and the way we think about ourselves. This may involve developing our potentials to create and to relate to others, or enriching our experience and understanding. Harré (1998) has also written extensively about the importance of discourse in shaping agency. A complete treatment of his propositions is beyond the scope of this article, but highly recommended for readers interested in a more in-depth analysis of the psychology of selfhood.

This discussion should emphasize the important relationships among identity, occupations, competence, and meaning. There is clearly an important interplay among these concepts. We cannot gain the recognition of others without competent action, nor can we meet our needs for meaning without engaging in occupation in a way that receives social validation. Moreover, the things we do, even when validated by others as competent, must be understandable to ourselves within a meaningful life context.

Identity—Goals and Occupational Performance

It may be helpful here to elaborate on the important relationship between occupations and identity. To speak of occupation is to describe goal-directed activity in the context of living. Goals work as motivators precisely because we imagine how we will be affected directly or indirectly when the goal is met. Thus, goals serve as motivators because we view them in the context of self, whether we are dressing for the day or seeking a promotion. We put on the blue blazer because we imagine what we will look like and anticipate that it will be satisfactory or appropriate for the day's activities.

Similarly, when we work late, or when we willingly take on an added responsibility in volunteer activities, we imagine ourselves as being viewed as virtuous, hardworking, and worthwhile people. We may imagine getting praised, getting a promotion, or receiving a raise or recognition as a result of those efforts. These views of our identity in the future are imagined selves, and they are powerful motivators of goal-directed action. Markus and colleagues (Markus, 1977; Markus & Nurius, 1986) have called these motivating images *possible selves*. They have suggested that a goal can have an influence on behavior to the extent that an individual can personalize it by building a bridge of self-representations between the current state and the hoped-for state.

Possible selves can consist of both positive as well as negative images. They not only may represent what we would like to become, they also may represent what we are afraid of becoming. Either type of possible self can be a motivator. Thus, we may strive to become the wealthy self, the shapely self, or the well-respected and loved self, while we dread, and thus try to avoid becoming, the lonely, depressed, or incompetent self (Ogilvie, 1987).

Possible Selves as Images of Action

Markus and her colleagues have contended that possible selves give personal meaning and structure to a person's thoughts about the future. That is, when we think about actions we might take, we project images of ourselves into those thoughts, and we view ourselves taking the actions. In other words, possible selves provide a very useful and direct mechanism for translating thoughts into actions. Goals that individuals view as important, and to which they are com-

mitted, are effective because these goals are self-relevant and self-defining.

Goals differ among people because the nature of possible selves depends on the nature of one's core self or complex identity system. Goal-directed and motivated behavior and personal identity are thus reciprocally related. Studies (Pavot, Fujita, & Diener, 1997) have shown that as we perceive ourselves becoming more like the person we want to be, our life satisfaction increases. When we do not perceive ourselves as progressing toward our desired identities, we tend to exhibit signs of unhealthy adaptation (Heatherton & Baumeister, 1991).

Social Approval and Competent Performance

Social approval and competent performance are instrumental to our thoughts of actions that will help us avoid or realize possible selves. Research shows that people will go to great lengths to alter their behavior (and indeed, even their appearance) in order to gain social approval and avoid rejection (Crowne & Marlowe, 1964).

To a large extent, our ability to gain this approval depends on our ability to portray ourselves as competent people. Through implicit expectations associated with social standing and the performance of roles, social groups help define the levels of competence necessary for acceptance, approval, and recognition.

In other words, self-appraisal is highly dependent on the extent to which we believe that we will be accepted by others. Research has also shown that it is related to efficacious action or competent performance, meaning that we must demonstrate to others that we are competent people as part of the acceptance process (Franks & Marolla, 1976).

Competent Performance

To be competent suggests that we are effective in dealing with the challenges that come our way (White, 1971). If we experience success in the challenges we undertake, we enhance our view of ourselves as competent beings (Bandura, 1977; Gage & Polatajko, 1994 [see Chapter 38]). This encourages us to explore and to engage the world in ways that give us our sense of autonomy and selfhood.

As we experience successes, our views of ourselves as efficacious or competent become strengthened. Thus, completing a task successfully adds to our sense of being competent human beings and, in a sense, prepares us for new challenges by bolstering our self-confidence. The term *self-confidence* is an interesting expression because it establishes a clear link between our identity and our belief in the things that we can do. Rogers (1982) asserted that developing a sense of the self as a competent agent in the world requires the expression of choice and control. Through choice, we express autonomy and, through control, we express efficacy. Brewster Smith summed it up nicely: "The crucial attitude toward the self is self-respect as a significant and efficacious person" (1974, p. 14).

Performance Deficits

If our identities are crafted by what we do and how we do it, then it follows that any threat to our ability to engage in occupations and present ourselves as competent people becomes a threat to our identity. On a daily basis, occupational therapists come into contact with persons whose identities are threatened by virtue of performance limitations. These identity crises may occur as the result of normal aging, which often deprives us of the sense of competence we once had, or result from congenital disorders, injuries, and diseases that leave lasting or progressive disability.

To the extent that disabilities interfere with the competent execution of tasks and roles, they threaten the establishment of an identity based on competence. In some cases, injury, disease, and disability also result in bodily disfigurement, which further assaults the person's identity and increases the challenges associated with establishing an identity that receives social approval (Goffman, 1963). Facial scars or anomalies, involuntary movements related to motor planning deficits, balance disorders, and unwanted tics are among the many observable signs of disorders that gain unwanted public attention and increase the challenge of fashioning a social identity that is acceptable to self and others.

Stigma

Goffman (1959) suggested that a socially competent performance involves more than simply getting the job done. There are certain stylistic and procedural expectations that must be fulfilled in order for the person to be considered by others to have performed competently and credibly. When we convince others that we have performed credibly, we are engaging in what Goffman called *impression management*.[4]

It is widely acknowledged within the cultures of people with activity limitations that impression management is an important strategy to undertake. It is a practiced skill to develop such social proficiency that one's impairment is hardly noticed. Indeed, there is a word for this, *passing,* which means that one has hidden one's devalued characteristics from others successfully, so that one has been able to pass as "normal" or able-bodied.

The ability to manage the impressions of others is often so compelling that actual performance may be secondary to preserving identity by leaving a good impression. Studies of prosthetic and assistive technology devices show that their acceptance and use may be as dependent on appearance and perceived social acceptability as their functional benefits (Batavia & Hammer, 1990; Pippin & Fernie, 1997; Stein & Walley, 1983).

Of course, the easiest way to avoid rejection is to increase control and the possibility of rejection by avoiding social interaction altogether. In confronting the risk of social rejection, it is not unusual to find people with observable disability to retreat to the safety and emotional security of interactions limited to close friends and associates. These people, it is reasoned, know the person beyond the disfigurement. Avoidance strategies are more understandable when one considers that social disapproval is not simply an uncomfortable situation that evokes feelings of embarrassment or shame. It is, quite directly, an assault on one's identity.

Researchers have shown that while passing is a useful strategy for avoiding stigma, it can result in an unhealthy adaptation to disability if it results in denial. Successful adaptation to one's individual differences requires the ability to acknowledge one's differences and to integrate them into an identity that permits a confident expression of self (Weinberg & Sterritt, 1986). One of the challenges of acquired disability is reintegration into social patterns that promote acceptance of self and a more comfortable relationship with able-bodied persons. This comfort leads to more positive acceptance by those persons.

Disability and Identity Adaptations

A surprising number of studies have directly or indirectly studied the identity consequences of children and adults with chronic illnesses and disabling conditions. These have often shown that preserving and developing one's identity are often at the heart of adaptational strategies (Charmaz, 1994; Estroff, 1989; Monks, 1995; Ville, Ravaud, Marchal, Paicheler, & Fardeau, 1992; Weinberg & Sterrit, 1986).

For example, a study by Charmaz (1994) of men with chronic illnesses is relevant here. She found that when men did awaken to the changes in their bodies and accept the uncertainties of their futures, they engaged in reflection and reappraisals that often improved their awareness of self and personal priorities. It is noteworthy that reappraisals of productivity, achievement, and relationships were central to this process. As a result of these reappraisals, some men changed jobs, others retired or renegotiated their work assignments, and many followed health regimens, such as exercising, more devotedly.

One recurring theme in these and other studies of adaptation to illness and disability is the role of identity in creating a sense of coherence or continuity over time. When people experience loss and change, the continuity of their lives is disrupted. Identity is the great integrator of life experience. We interpret events that happen to us in terms of their meaning for our life stories. This gives life a sense of coherence.

---

[4]It is worth mentioning that stigma affects those with whom one shares identity. Consistent with the idea of distributed selves, spouses and family members may also endure the social cost of disfigurement, poor role performance, or deviance. For example, stigma accrues to families whose members have HIV or mental illness, or who have committed suicide.

Identity, Sense of Coherence, and Well-Being

People with a sense of coherence view their lives as understandable, meaningful, and manageable. The concept emanates from Aaron Antonovsky (1979), who proposed a model that would explain how some people are able to cope with stressors without experiencing the negative consequences to health experienced by others. Antonovsky proposed that a sense of coherence was central to this ability to cope with stress, suggesting that people who interpret their experiences within a meaningful and understandable framework, and who perceive that their challenges are manageable, are better equipped to deal with life's unexpected turns.

Research on the sense of coherence during the past 20 years has shown that people with this attribute, or way of viewing the world, are healthier and better adjusted than people without a strong sense of coherence. For example, significant relationships have been found between sense of coherence and blood pressure, emotional stability, global health, subjective well-being, and coping skills (Antonovsky, 1993). Sense of coherence is different from, but related to, another factor found in coping studies called hardiness (Kobasa, 1979).

Of importance to this discussion is the finding that sense of coherence seems to measure a human dimension that intersects with identity. Because it reflects one's efficacy or sense of agency, because it reflects meaning, and because it reflects a person's sense of how the events in their lives fit together, sense of coherence is related in important ways to the issue of identity (Baumeister & Tice, 1990; Korotkov, 1998). In fact, this relationship is borne out in studies of personal projects done by Little and others (Christiansen, Backman, Little, & Nguyen, 1999; Little, 1989). This research, using personal projects analysis (cf. Christiansen, Little, & Backman, 1998), seeks to connect occupations of everyday life with personality traits. Findings have shown a relationship between identity dimensions of personal projects and sense of coherence. This provides a small but important piece of evidence supporting the hypothesis that identity and sense of coherence are related, and possibly overlapping, concepts (see Figure 42.3).

Issues of coherence, personal identity, meaning, and well-being have been nicely tied together in research reported by Wong (1998). He has used an implicit theories approach to study how people define their lives as personally meaningful. Through analysis of the responses of subjects in different age groups, he has identified nine factors that collectively provide a profile of an ideal meaningful life.[5] Four of these factors focus directly on the self. In these studies, Wong has found that when people have higher profiles on these factors, their subjective well-being increases.

We can summarize by noting that research has shown that people shape their identities through their daily occupations, which are performed in a social context that gives them

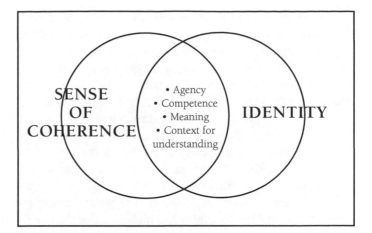

Figure 42.3. Concepts that link sense of coherence to identity.

symbolic meaning. Over time, our evolving identities and our actions are woven together to provide a coherent life story. The central place of occupations in shaping identity and creating life meaning is so powerful that one cannot help but marvel at their implications for occupational therapy practice.

Implications for Occupational Therapy Practice

Nearly 20 years ago, Bing (1981) (see Chapter 5) provided a historical review of the people and ideas that have influenced occupational therapy since its inception. In his identification of themes that have provided particular relevance for the field, he included this principle: "The patient is the product of his or her own efforts, not the article made nor the activity accomplished" (p. 501). This principle suggests that the work of therapy involves identity building.

Therapy becomes identity building when therapists provide environments that help persons explore possible selves and achieve success in tasks that are instrumental to identities they strive to achieve, and when it enables them to validate the identities that they have worked hard to achieve in the past.

Occupational Therapy as Identity Building

There is much opportunity for occupational therapy as a special and unique service that provides opportunities for people to establish, maintain, or reclaim their identities. Particularly in North America, the demographics of aging will bring the declines in function that are a threat to identity (Kunkel & Applebaum, 1992; Statistics Canada, 1993). It is no accident that late-life depression is one of the most common mental health problems in adults 60 and older. Although there are many causes of depression, late-life depression can arise from a loss of self-esteem, a loss of meaningful roles, declining social contacts, and reduced functional status (Karp, 1994; Reker, 1997). Research on

---

[5]The nine factors are achievement striving, religion, relationship, fulfillment, fairness–respect, self-confidence, self-integration, self-transcendence, and self-acceptance.

---

psychosocial theories of depression have shown that depression can be averted when people are given an opportunity to gain personal meaning from everyday activities, when their sense of optimism is renewed, and where they believe that there is choice and control in their lives (Baumeister, 1990; Brewer, 1993; Kapci, 1998; Rodin, 1986).

This was shown by investigators (Jackson, Carlson, Mandel, Zemke, & Clark, 1998) at the University of Southern California in their recent study of a program for well elderly persons. That successful program used lifestyle redesign to engage participants in occupations that provided both structure and meaning to the participants. The participants in the program showed less morbidity and higher morale than a control group, demonstrating clearly that occupations, through the mechanism of identity, provide the purpose, structure, and global meaning that is an essential need for all human beings. I suggest that the key link here is identity building.

Because issues of health and well-being are at stake, society needs services concerned with helping people establish and maintain their identities. The decline of abilities that comes with normal aging need not be interpreted or experienced as a decline in competence. The key to successful aging may very well be related to the acceptance of a changed body along with opportunities for demonstrating competence and control in mastering late-life challenges that create the beginnings so necessary for satisfactory endings. Coming to terms with the end of life may be facilitated through occupations that lead to an enduring presence of self and the sense that one can derive meaning from all that has happened during one's life.

Beyond the demographics of aging, there are other developments that call out for a profession that can help people find meaning in their lives. The recently released global burden of disease study contains some astonishing statistics. This study, completed at Harvard University but sponsored by the World Health Organization and the World Bank, is a careful epidemiological projection of the kinds of health-related problems the world will be dealing with in the year 2020 (Murray & Lopez, 1996).

The most interesting finding from the study is that unipolar major depression will become the second leading threat to life quality in the world. It is projected to increase significantly from 1990 levels in the developed countries. Besides dementia and osteoarthritis, other conditions showing major increases will be alcohol use and self-inflicted injuries. Although the projected pattern for the world in the year 2020 will show a general increase in overall health owing to the control of infectious diseases in the developing countries, many other health challenges will be of a nature that traditional medicine is currently unequipped to handle. Depression, self-inflicted injuries, and alcohol abuse have one thing in common—they are diseases of meaning; therefore, they can be linked to social conditions that permit people to lose their identity and sense of purpose and meaning in life.

Summary

In this article, I have made the claim that occupations constitute the mechanism that enables persons to develop and express their identities. I have asserted that identities are central features of understanding the world in an evolving self-narrative and that the continuity provided by identity enables life to be comprehended in a manner that helps minimize the uncertainties and stresses of daily life. I have maintained that it is the imagined self that provides the context for motivation and purpose and that competence is interpreted as the capable expression of identity within a social world. And finally, and most importantly, I have argued that that identity is the pathway by which people, through daily occupations and relationships with others, are able to derive meaning from their lives.

As a profession concerned with enabling people to engage in meaningful daily occupations, occupational therapy is positioned uniquely to meet the challenges confronting people whose identity is threatened by impairments, limitations to activity, and restrictions on their participation as social beings. We have seen that, in the years ahead, our friends and colleagues will be challenged with assaults on their identities brought by age, health problems, and social conditions.

Englehardt (1986) once described occupational therapists as technologists and *custodians of meaning*. As an outsider, he saw the same opportunity and unfulfilled promise that Adolph Meyer (1922) (see Chapter 2) described in the founding years of occupational therapy. Yet, a full and genuine appreciation of the power of occupation to enable health and well-being has not yet made its way across the landscape of the profession.

Just as individual persons create their unique identities and life meaning through occupations, so too do professions, which represent groups of people with shared purposes, values, and interests, realize their identities through collective action. Biomedicine will experience many great advances in the years ahead. But no genetic code, no chemical intervention, and no microsurgical technology will be invented to repair broken identities and the assault on meaning that accompanies them. Because of this, the new millennium will realize the health-enabling, restorative potential of occupation, and the promise of occupational therapy will be fulfilled.

Acknowledgments

This lecture is dedicated to my friend and mentor, Robert K. Bing, EdD, OTR, FAOTA; to my special colleague and friend, Carolyn Baum, PhD, OTR/L, FAOTA; to my parents; and especially to my wife, Pamela, a pediatric occupational therapist; and, not least of all, to my children, Carrie, Erik, and Kalle.

I thank Cindy Hammecker, Charles Hayden, and Natalie Sims for their invaluable assistance in the preparation of this paper. I am indebted to my colleagues Kenneth Ottenbacher, PhD, OTR, FAOTA, and Beatriz Abreu, PhD, OTR, FAOTA, for their expressions of confidence and support.

References

Antonovsky, A. (1979). *Health, stress, and coping: New perspectives on mental health and physical well-being.* San Francisco: Jossey-Bass.

Antonovsky, A. (1993). The structure and properties of the Sense of Coherence Scale. *Social Science and Medicine, 36,* 725–733.

Bandura, A. (1977). Self-efficacy: Toward a unifying theory of behavioral change. *Psychological Review, 84,* 191–215.

Batavia, A. I., & Hammer, G. S. (1990). Toward the development of consumer based criteria for the evaluation of assistive devices. *Journal of Rehabilitation Research, 27,* 425–436.

Bateson, M. C. (1996). Enfolded activity and the concept of occupation. In R. Zemke & F. Clark (Eds.), *Occupational science: The evolving discipline* (pp. 5–12). Philadelphia: F. A. Davis.

Baumeister, R. F. (1982). Self-esteem, self-presentation, and future interaction. A dilemma of reputation. *Journal of Personality, 50,* 29–45.

Baumeister, R. F. (1986). *Identity: Cultural change and the struggle for self.* New York: Oxford University Press.

Baumeister, R. F. (1990). Suicide as escape from self. *Psychological Review, 97*(1), 90–113.

Baumeister, R. F. (1997). Identity, self-concept, and self-esteem. In R. Hogan, J. Johnson, & S. Briggs (Eds.), *Handbook of personality psychology* (pp. 681–711). San Diego, CA: Academic Press.

Baumeister, R. F., & Tice, D. M. (1990). Self-esteem and responses to success and failure. Subsequent performance and intrinsic motivation. *Journal of Personality, 53,* 450–467.

Bing, R. K. (1981). Occupational therapy revisited: A paraphrastic journey. 1981 Eleanor Clarke Slagle Lectureship. *American Journal of Occupational Therapy, 35,* 499–518. Reprinted as Chapter 5.

Brewer, B. W. (1993). Self identity and specific vulnerability to depressed mood. *Journal of Personality, 61*(3), 343–34.

Bruner, J. S. (1990). *Acts of meaning.* Cambridge: Harvard University Press.

Charmaz, K. (1994). Identity dilemmas of chronically ill men. *Sociological Quarterly, 35*(2), 269–288.

Christiansen, C. H., Little, B. R., & Backman, C. (1998). Personal projects: A useful approach to the study of occupation. *American Journal of Occupational Therapy, 52,* 439–446.

Christiansen, C. H., Backman, C., Little, B. R., & Nguyen, A. (1999). Occupations and well being: A study of personal projects. *American Journal of Occupational Therapy, 53,* 91–100.

Cooley, C. H. (1902). *Human nature and the social order.* New York: Scribner.

Crowne, D. P., & Marlowe, D. (1964). *The approval motive.* New York: Wiley.

Debats, D. L., Drost, J., & Hansen, P. (1995). Experiences of meaning in life: A combined qualitative and quantitative approach. *British Journal of Psychology, 86*(3), 359–375.

Englehardt, T. (1977). Defining occupational therapy: The meaning of therapy and the virtues of occupation. *American Journal of Occupational Therapy, 31,* 666–672.

Englehardt, T. (1986). Occupational therapists as technologists and custodians of meaning. In G. Kielhofner (Ed.), *Health through occupation* (pp. 139–144). Philadelphia: F. A. Davis.

Erikson, E. H. (1968). *Identity, youth, and crisis.* New York: Norton.

Estroff, S. E. (1989). Self, identity, and subjective experiences of schizophrenia: In search of the subject. *Schizophrenia Bulletin, 15*(2), 189–196.

Fidler, G. S., & Fidler, J. W. (1978). Doing and becoming: Purposeful action and self-actualization. *American Journal of Occupational Therapy, 32,* 305–310. Reprinted as Chapter 9.

Franks, D. D., & Marolla, J. (1976). Efficacious action and social approval as interacting dimensions of self-esteem: A tentative formulation through construct validation. *Sociometry, 39*(4), 324–341.

Gage, M., & Polatajko, H. (1994). Enhancing occupational performance through an understanding of perceived self-efficacy. *American Journal of Occupational Therapy, 48,* 452–461. Reprinted as Chapter 38.

Gergen, K. J. (1991). *The saturated self: Dilemmas of identity in modern life.* New York: Basic.

Gergen, K. J., & Gergen, M. M. (1988). Narrative and the self as relationship. In L. Berkowitz (Ed.), *Advances in experimental and social psychology* (pp. 17–55). San Diego, CA: Academic Press.

Goffman, E. (1959). *The presentation of self in everyday life.* Garden City, NY: Doubleday.

Goffman, E. (1963). *Stigma: Notes on the management of a spoiled identity.* Englewood Cliffs, NJ: Prentice-Hall.

Greenwald, A. G. (1980). The totalitarian ego: Fabrication and revision of personal history. *American Psychologist, 35,* 603–613.

Harré, R. (1983). *Personal being.* Oxford, England: Blackwell.

Harré, R. (1998). *The singular self.* London: Sage.

Heatherton, T. F., & Baumeister, R. F. (1991). Binge eating as escape from self-awareness. *Psychological Bulletin, 110,* 86–108.

Jackson, J., Carlson, M., Mandel, D., Zemke, R., & Clark, F. (1998). Occupation in lifestyle redesign: The well elderly study occupational therapy program. *American Journal of Occupational Therapy, 52,* 326–336.

James, W. (1892). *Psychology: The briefer course.* New York: Henry Holt & Co.

Kagan, J. (1981). *The second year: The emergence of self-awareness.* Cambridge, MA: Harvard University Press.

Kapci, E. G. (1998). Test of the hopelessness theory of depression: Drawing negative inference from negative life events. *Psychological Reports, 82*(2), 355–363.

Karp, D. A. (1994). Living with depression: Illness and identity turning points. *Qualitative Health Research, 4*(1), 6–30.

Keller, A., Ford, L. H., & Meacham, J. A. (1978). Dimensions of self-concept in preschool children. *Developmental Psychology, 14,* 483–489.

Kobasa, S. C. (1979). Stressful life events, personality and health: An inquiry into hardiness. *Journal of Personality and Social Psychology, 37,* 1–11.

Kondo, D. (1990). *Crafting selves: Power, gender, and discourses of identity in a Japanese workplace.* Chicago: University of Chicago Press.

Korotkov, D. L. (1998). The sense of coherence. Making sense out of chaos. In P. T. Wong & P. S. Fry (Eds.), *The human quest for meaning: A handbook of psychological research and clinical applications* (pp. 51–70). Mahwah, NJ: Erlbaum.

Kris, E. (1952). *Psychoanalytic explorations in art.* New York: International Universities Press.

Kunkel, S. R., & Applebaum, R. A. (1992). Estimating the prevalence of long-term disability for an aging society. *Journal of Gerontology: Social Sciences, 475,* S253–S260.

Langer, E. J., & Rodin, J. (1976). The effects of choice and enhanced personal responsibility for the aged: A field experiment in an institutional setting. *Journal of Personality and Social Psychology, 34*(2), 192–198.

Little, B. R. (1989). Personal projects analysis: Trivial pursuits, magnificent obsessions, and the search for coherence. In D. M. Buss & N. Cantor (Eds.), *Personality psychology: Recent trends and emerging directions* (pp. 15–31). New York: Springer-Verlag.

Loevenger, J. (1976). *Ego development.* San Francisco: Jossey-Bass.

Markus, H. (1977). Self-schemata and processing information about the self. *Journal of Personality and Social Psychology, 35,* 63–78.

Markus, H., & Nurius, P. S. (1986). Possible selves. *American Psychologist, 41,* 954–969.

McAdams, D. P. (1996). Personality, modernity, and the storied self: A contemporary framework for studying persons. *Psychological Inquiry, 7,* 295–321.

McAdams, D. P. (1997). Multiplicity of self versus unity of identity. In R. D. Ashmore & L. Jussim (Eds.), *Self and identity: Fundamental issues* (pp. 46–78). New York: Oxford University Press.

McCuaig, M., & Frank, G. (1991). The able self: Adaptive patterns and choices in independent living for a person with cerebral palsy. *American Journal of Occupational Therapy, 45,* 224–234.

Mead, G. H. (1934). *Mind, self, and society.* Chicago: University of Chicago Press.

Meyer, A. (1922). The philosophy of occupation therapy. *Archives of Occupational Therapy, 1,* 1–10. Reprinted as Chapter 2.

Monks, J. (1995). Life stories and sickness experience: A performance perspective. *Culture, Medicine, and Psychiatry, 19*(4), 453–478.

Moore, S. L. (1997). A phenomenological study of meaning in life in suicidal older adults. *Archives of Psychiatric Nursing, 11*(1), 29–36.

Murray, C. J. L., & Lopez, A. D. (1996). Alternative visions of the future: Projecting mortality and disability 1990–2020. In C. J. L. Murray & A. D. Lopez (Eds.), *The global burden of disease* (pp. 325–396). Geneva, Switzerland: World Health Organization.

Ogilvie, D. M. (1987). The undesired self: A neglected variable in personality research. *Journal of Personality and Social Psychology, 52,* 379–385.

Pavot, W., Fujita, F., & Diener, E. (1997). The relation among self-aspect congruence, personality and subjective well-being. *Personality and Individual Differences, 22*(2), 183–191.

Piaget, J. (1954). *The construction of reality in the child.* New York: Basic.

Pippin, K., & Fernie, G. R. (1997). Designing devices that are acceptable to the frail elderly: A new understanding based upon how older people perceive a walker. *Technology and Disability, 7*(1/2), 93–102.

Polkinghorne, D. (1988). *Narrative knowing and the human sciences.* Albany, NY: State University of New York Press.

Reker, G. T. (1997). Personal meaning, optimism, and choice. Existential predictors of depression in community and institutional elderly. *Gerontologist, 37*(6), 709–716.

Rodin, J. C. (1986). Aging and health: Effects of the sense of control. *Science, 233*(4770), 1271–1276.

Rogers, J. (1982). Order and disorder in medicine and occupational therapy. *American Journal of Occupational Therapy, 31,* 29–35.

Ruble, D. (1983). The development of social comparison processes and their role in achievement-related self-socialization. In E. T. Higgins, D. Ruble, & W. Hartup (Eds.), *Social cognition and social behavior: Developmental perspectives* (pp. 134–157). New York: Cambridge University Press.

Schrauger, J. S., & Schoeneman, T. J. (1979). Symbolic interactionist view of self-concept: Through the looking glass darkly. *Psychological Bulletin, 86,* 549–573.

Smith, M. B. (1974). Competence and adaptation: A perspective on therapeutic ends and means. *American Journal of Occupational Therapy, 28,* 11–15.

Sommer, K. L., & Baumeister, R. F. (1998). The construction of meaning from life events: Empirical studies of personal narratives. In P. T. P. Wong & P. S. Fry (Eds.), *The human quest for meaning: A handbook of psychological research and clinical applications* (pp. 143–161). Mahwah, NJ: Erlbaum.

Stachey, J. (Ed.). (1990). *The standard edition of the complete psychological works of Sigmund Freud.* New York: W. W. Norton. Statistics Canada. (1993). *Population ageing and the elderly: Current demographic analysis.* Cat. No. 91-533E. Ottawa, Canada: Government of Canada.

Stein, R. B., & Walley, M. (1983). Functional comparison of upper extremity amputees using myoelectric and conventional prostheses. *Archives of Physical Medicine and Rehabilitation, 73,* 1169–1173.

Swann, W. B. (1987). Identity negotiation: Where two roads meet. *Journal of Personality and Social Psychology, 53,* 1038–1051.

Swann, W. B., & Hill, C. A. (1982). When our identities are mistaken: Reaffirming self-conceptions through social interaction. *Journal of Personality and Social Psychology, 43,* 59–66.

Van Selm, M., & Dittmann-Kohli, F. (1998). Meaninglessness in the second half of life: The development of a construct. *International Journal of Aging and Human Development, 47*(2), 81–104.

Ville, I., Ravaud, J. F., Marchal, F., Paicheler, H., & Fardeau, M. (1992). Social identity and the international classification of handicaps: An evaluation of the consequences of facioscapulohumeral muscular dystrophy. *Disability and Rehabilitation, 14*(4), 168–175.

Vygotsky, L. S. (1981). The instrumental method in psychology. In J. V. Wertsch (Ed.), *The concept of activity in Soviet psychology* (pp. 134–143). Armonk, NY: M. E. Sharp.

Weinberg, N., & Sterritt, M. (1986). Disability and identity: A study of identity patterns in adolescents with hearing impairments. *Rehabilitation Psychology, 31*(2), 95–103.

White, R. W. (1959). Motivation reconsidered: The concept of competence. *Psychological Review, 66,* 297–333.

White, R. W. (1971). The urge toward competence. *American Journal of Occupational Therapy, 25,* 271–274.

Wong, P. T. P. (1998). Implicit theories of meaningful life and the development of the personal meaning profile. In P. T. P. Wong & P. S. Fry (Eds.), *The human quest for meaning* (pp. 111–140). Mahwah, NJ: Erlbaum.

PART V

Guidelines for Best Practice Throughout the Occupational Therapy Process

Introduction

As supported by this text's previous part, best practice in occupational therapy is person-directed and client-centered. The entire occupational therapy process must be founded on a collaborative therapeutic relationship that is respectful of the person's unique identity, values, beliefs, and priorities. It is important to recognize that occupational therapy practitioners' own personal identity, values, and beliefs also shape care. In addition, there are special characteristics that we bring as professionals to the occupational therapy process. The *Occupational Therapy Practice Framework* describes these unique practitioner resources as including clinical reasoning skills and knowledge about engagement in occupation (American Occupational Therapy Association [AOTA], 2002). This part provides fundamental readings related to these areas of our professional expertise.

Rogers begins this presentation in Chapter 43 with a discussion on the ethics, science, and art of clinical reasoning along with a strong call for the individuation of the occupational therapy process. She poses a series of three fundamental questions, which occupational therapy practitioners should ask to ensure that interventions are congruent with the person's needs, values, goals, and lifestyle. Each question is explored in terms of the knowledge needed to answer it and the processes used to obtain this essential knowledge, providing readers with clear guidelines and concrete suggestions for improving clinical-reasoning skills. Rogers acknowledges that there is no

cookbook of clinical solutions and proposes the use of general systems theory as a framework for integrating data relevant to the uniqueness of each person and pertinent to the complexities of clinical problems. She comprehensively explores the scientific, ethical, and artistic dimensions of clinical reasoning, substantiating these issues with several practice examples that highlight the benefits of becoming an "inquisitive practitioner."

Fleming in Chapter 44 expands on Rogers' exploration of the clinical-reasoning process by reporting results of the AOTA/American Occupational Therapy Foundation's Clinical Reasoning Study. This landmark research project analyzed the reasoning processes used by therapists in solving problems in their day-to-day practice. After extensive study, four types of reasoning—procedural, interactive, conditional, and narrative—were identified. The first three are discussed extensively in this chapter, with the last being explored in depth in Chapter 37 by Mattingly. Each type of reasoning is defined, with its major characteristics, purposes, methods, values, and benefits discussed. Case examples substantiate the implementation of these principles into clinical practice and add humanness to the discussions. This chapter supports the notion that practitioners can "walk and chew gum" at the same time and that we can work with a person holistically using a "multitrack" mind. This ability to use a diversity of perspectives in a health care system that devalues holism and only values concrete reductionist procedures as a critical skill needed

throughout the occupational therapy process. Experienced occupational therapy practitioners in this study appeared to move smoothly and sometimes rapidly among the different types of reasoning or to simultaneously use multiple types of reasoning as they analyzed, interpreted, and resolved different types of clinical problems throughout the occupational therapy process.

The use of the different types of clinical reasoning also provides occupational therapy practitioners with the knowledge, skills, and attitudes needed to formulate meaningful goals with the person. However, a relevant question to ask throughout the occupational therapy process is what determines the worthiness of an occupational therapy goal. In Chapter 45, Crabtree provides a thoughtful response to this question. He recognizes that achievement of functional independence in occupational performance is often considered the ultimate desired outcome of the occupational therapy process, with our literature frequently supporting this view. However, Crabtree contends that the predominance of this goal (and the idea that this is an ideal to strive toward) reflects philosophical assumptions that are incongruent with our profession's core beliefs and founding principles. He examines the assumptions that typically underlie the functional independence construct and the concept of dependence. Crabtree questions if these traditional viewpoints about a narrow idea are truly the best expression of our profession, or should we be examining broader concepts such as the meaning and purpose of being human? Issues related to purposiveness, autonomy, wholeness, and meaningfulness are explained and contrasted with the limited possibilities of functional independence. The relevance of these concepts to the occupational therapy process and the value of helping people achieve these abilities (rather than functional independence) are strongly supported. Active reflections on Crabtree's analysis and the use of a client-centered tool such as the Canadian Occupational Performance Measure can ensure that the goals formulated for occupational therapy interventions are considerate of all that it means to be human, resulting in outcomes that are personally meaningful to the individual. Once relevant and meaningful goals are established, intervention is implemented.

The intervention tools that occupational therapy practitioners use in their daily practice are strongly influenced by sociopolitical forces and changes in the health care system. Chapter 46 by Reed critically examines the multitude of factors that determine whether a tool of practice is adopted, maintained, or discarded by the profession. Occupational therapy practitioners have used many media and methods for intervention over the years, yet the reasons for embracing or abandoning numerous media or methods are often unclear. In her Eleanor Clarke Slagle Lecture, Reed postulates that the lack of a rationale for the use of a medium or method may lead to limited understanding of its therapeutic value, for both the practitioner and the client. This lack of awareness can compromise the therapeutic potential of the selected tool of practice. She suggests that eight factors—cultural, social, economic, political, technological, theoretical, historical, and research—influence the selection or abandonment of tools of practice in occupational therapy.

Reed explores the nature of these influences, providing clear and relevant examples to highlight her points. She summarizes the effects of these eight factors by proposing 14 assumptions and providing three relevant, yet diverse, examples to illustrate how these factors and assumptions operate to affect the use of specific tools in occupational therapy practice. Reed emphasizes that the media, methods, and objectives of an activity must be consistent with each other for the activity to be purposeful and meaningful. She asserts that careful consideration of cultural, social, individual, and professional interests and values will ensure that the tools used in occupational therapy practice will have therapeutic value and be meaningful and purposeful to the individual. Reed's call for practitioners to increase their awareness of the "why" of practice to ensure their interventions are consistent with occupational therapy philosophy is a timely one.

A fundamental premise of our professional philosophy is that to achieve therapeutic goals there must be a "match" between a person who has been holistically assessed and an activity that has been thoroughly analyzed and synthesized (AOTA, 2002; McGarry, 1990; Mosey, 1996). Activity analysis and synthesis have been major tools of occupational therapy practice from the inception of the profession, and they have maintained their relevance and importance throughout the years. The need to analyze activities to determine how the demands of the activity relate to the person's skills and to successful performance is emphasized in the *Practice Framework*. While the *Practice Framework* provides a holistic view of activity analysis, in practice, this process has often focused only on the physical demands of an activity.

In Chapter 47, Creighton explores this reductionistic view of activity analysis and traces the evolution of this process to its more recent holistic conceptualization. The origin of activity analysis in the early 1900s with the initial development of structural activity analysis based on motion studies is discussed. The first systematic application of activity analysis in an occupational therapy clinic is presented. These early analyses emphasized the study of movement required by each activity and the subsequent adaptations of the activities to improve physical function or compensate for a movement deficit. Creighton describes the evolution of activity analysis between World War I and World War II and the expansion of activity analysis to include psychosocial characteristics of activities. However, she states, these analyses continued to perpetuate a physical and psychosocial split that was reflective of the dichotomy between psychiatric and physical disabilities practices. Creighton examines the refinement of activity analysis into an integrated, holistic approach in the 1970s and 1980s as frames of reference were further developed. The current view of activity analysis as a multifaceted process that also considers environmental contexts according to a frame of reference is emphasized.

The need to use holistic frames of reference to guide occupational therapy practice is further explored in Chapter 48 by Schultz and Schkade. Their discussion builds on Chapter 11's presentation of the Occupational Adaptation frame of reference by examining the practice implications of applying this model to the occupational therapy process. Schultz and Schkade's Occupational Adaptation practice model proposes that occupation adaptation is an internal phenomenon within the person. They review their model's key assumptions and explain how these are operationalized in practice. They claim that the application of the model facilitates a therapeutic climate, uses occupational activities, and incorporates all sources of motivation; therefore, practice based on this holistic model will differ from reductionistic interventions that focus solely on the acquisition of functional skills. Because this practice model directs the occupational therapy process toward the person's internal occupational environments, the person's ability to adapt to occupational challenges is developed. Schultz and Schkade provide a systematic guide for the application of Occupational Adaptation concepts and principles to a diversity of populations and practice settings. This practice guide includes relevant questions to use throughout the occupational therapy process. Using this guide will ensure that all aspects of the person including his or her occupational environment and roles; physical, social, and cultural contexts; sensorimotor, cognitive, and psychosocial factors; and relative mastery are considered in assessment, programming, and re-evaluation.

The integration of this guide with traditional occupational therapy evaluation and intervention methods is clearly explained with several clinical examples reinforcing the application of these in practice. Four practice examples illustrate how the model can be used with a diversity of individuals across the life span and along the continuum of care, supporting the efficacy, utility, and flexibility of this model. The holistic nature of this model is highly congruent with the core principles of our profession, yet it is realistically applicable to current practices. Because the desired outcome of the occupational therapy process is "engagement in occupation to support participation in life" (AOTA, 2002, p. 609), the application of this model is a helpful guide to use throughout the occupational therapy process.

A major concept identified in the Occupational Adaptation model by Schultz and Schkade was "occupational readiness." They defined this concept as "skill-based activities and other such interventions that focus on change in the person's systems in preparation for occupational activities" and explained that instruction was one method of occupational readiness. Chapter 49 by Padilla examines an instructional method that is widely used in occupational therapy practice, that is, psychoeducation. While

psychoeducation techniques have been predominantly used by occupational therapy practitioners in psychiatric rehabilitation, patient education has become an increasingly important component of any occupational therapy intervention program. As a result, a thoughtful exploration of these practices is warranted. Padilla contends that our professional literature may frequently describe psychoeducation programs, but it rarely examines the teaching approach used by practitioners when applying these techniques. He proposes that this lack of inquiry into how occupational therapy practitioners approach psychoeducation has led to educational practices that are incompatible with our profession's philosophical base and our increased understanding of and appreciation for occupation and the occupation nature of the human being.

Three approaches to teaching—the executive approach, the therapist approach, and the liberationist approach—are thoughtfully examined and critiqued. The congruence among each of these approaches and occupational therapy values is explored, with Padilla concluding that the first two approaches present fundamental incompatibilities between their assumptions and outcomes and occupational therapy philosophy. He asserts that the assumptions and outcomes of the liberationist approach are most compatible with authentic occupational therapy. The goodness-of-fit among liberationism's view of knowledge, the teacher–student relationship, the social context of learning, and the development of a critical consciousness with our profession's heritage and our renewed awareness of contextual constraints on life participation and satisfaction is analyzed. Realistic issues that challenge the application of this approach are presented, with Padilla acknowledging that the three approaches to teaching can accomplish very different objectives. As a result, the aims of a given psychoeducation program should be

evaluated to determine the appropriateness of fit with the teaching approach selected. Padilla advises that reflection on these issues can empower the therapist to adopt the liberationist approach because it is the one that places the therapist and learner as co-equals within the learning process and considers the entire context of the person's life.

While thoughtful consideration of the theoretical foundations to our teaching approaches is clearly relevant, many entry-level occupational therapy practitioners frequently struggle with the basic question of what to actually say to a person about the planned occupational therapy intervention. Chapter 50 provides clear guidelines to help address this fundamental concern. In this chapter, Peloquin presents an outstanding discussion on linking purpose to procedures during each therapeutic interaction we have with our clients. She explores the effectiveness of a collaborative approach that involves people in the intervention process and examines the increased efficacy of intervention when individuals know the purpose of each given treatment session. Peloquin presents a clear rationale for discussing the relevance and purpose of any and all procedures with clients. Her stand, that each intervention session is an opportunity to link goals through person–therapist collaboration with a structured activity that is relevant to the individual's daily life, is a strong one. Peloquin provides concrete examples and realistic suggestions for developing this collaborative approach. Providing the purpose of each activity can increase a person's knowledge about the reasons for the intervention, thereby increasing the level of active participation in the session. She contends that the need to consistently integrate goal statements with occupational therapy intervention is critically important because of three realities. These realities include current health care trends, traditional occupational therapy assumptions supportive of the collaborative process, and the often-ambiguous nature of occupational therapy's primary modality of activity. The recent health care system's emphasis on informed consent, treatment accountability, and patient rights provide strong justification for incorporating a collaborative approach into each occupational therapy session.

The influence of health care trends on the occupational therapy process is explored from a different perspective in Chapter 51 by Horowitz, who thoughtfully examines the impact that changing health care environments, emerging areas of practice, and increased demands on practitioners have on the ethical practice of occupational therapy. The reality that current practice requires occupational therapy practitioners to pay increased attention to cost-effectiveness and functional outcomes in an environment that often challenges ethical practice is well-supported by clinical examples. Horowitz reflects on the influence that personal values and ethics have on one's ability to recognize ethical issues, challenges, and dilemmas. The role of a profession's code of ethics and the societal expectation that a profession provide ethical practice in a morally responsible manner is explored. Purtilo's Six-Step Approach to ethical decision-making is reviewed. This practical process provides strategies that can effectively structure the problem-solving process needed when an occupational therapy practitioner is confronted with an ethical challenge, problem, or dilemma. Horowitz advises that using this organized approach can reduce practitioners' distress and thereby decrease the risk of burnout. A case study is provided to demonstrate the efficacy of using a structured ethical decision-making approach to solving an ethical problem. The reality that additional resources and strategies are needed to ethically respond to the complexities of everyday occupational therapy practice is well-supported by this example and Horowitz's discussion. The need for

occupational therapy practitioners to actively and continuously reflect on our profession's core values and ethics and our professional legal and social responsibilities to ensure that our actual practices remain ethically and morally congruent is strongly validated by Horowitz's analysis.

Sadly, many occupational therapy practitioners seem to forget the vital importance of this reflective process as they argue that constraints within the current care system force them to use treatment techniques and modalities in an isolated, reductionist manner (so they continue to scurry from patient set-up to patient set-up with little interaction with their clients). Fortunately, others do maintain a holistic approach grounded in our profession's core beliefs, in spite of system limitations and the use of adjunctive modalities (West & Wiemer, 1991). Ahlschwede (1992) describes an approach to treatment that is realistic in the current health care system and congruent with occupational therapy's philosophical base. She states that the time "during which a patient's hand is sandwiched between hot packs is spent discussing occupational performance or daily living components, collaborative goal setting, and patient education, or addressing psychosocial concerns or issues that the patient may have. The remainder (and majority) of each session is then spent in traditional, graded functional activities" (p. 650). It is hoped that the chapters in this section, and throughout the book, provide readers with invaluable information to facilitate the use of traditional and nontraditional occupational therapy tools of practice in a collaborative manner that adheres to our profession's ethical principles while being purposeful and meaningful to the person, for this is the art and science of occupational therapy.

Questions to Consider

1. Identify major tools of occupational therapy practice. Describe the main therapeutic purposes of these tools.

How would you explain these purposes to clients to increase their understanding of your therapeutic rationale and to enhance their participation in the occupational therapy process?

2. Think about a particularly challenging individual with whom you worked or observed in a practice setting. Analyze this person's situation using all modes of clinical reasoning and the occupational adaptation model. How could the insights that you gained from this analysis be used to guide the occupational therapy process? What psychoeducational approach would be most compatible to use with this person in this situation?

3. Review the following case entitled "Helen and the Disappearing Pegs." Identify the tools of practice and principles of intervention that were used and those that were not used in the described treatment session. Explain how the missing tools of practice could be used to increase the relevance of Helen's occupational therapy treatment. Identify a diversity of purposeful activities that could have been used in this case to facilitate Helen's crossing of the midline with her upper extremity in a functional manner. Describe how you would have explained the purposes of these activities to this client to facilitate her active participation in this treatment session.

4. Reflect on Helen's case and its relationship to ethical practice. What principles of our professional code of ethics did this occupational therapy practitioner violate? What were the likely external factors that may have contributed to this practitioner's use of a meaningless activity in a manner that ignored the individual? How could the structured approach to ethical decision-making be used to ensure that future sessions with Helen are congruent with our profession's ethical standards and core values?

Helen and the Disappearing Pegs

Helen was an elderly woman with multiple physical disabilities, including diabetes, double lower-extremity amputations, expressive aphasia, upper-extremity weakness, and decreased upper-extremity range of motion. She had a feeding tube and was dependent in all activities of daily living. She was also perceived by many to have a major cognitive deficit, for her interactions with her environment were limited to moans and attempts to remove her feeding tube and slide out of her wheelchair.

One day, while waiting with my brother in the occupational therapy clinic, we observed a therapist place numerous pegs on the right side of Helen's lapboard and a basket on the floor to the left of her wheelchair. The therapist told Helen her activity for the day was to pick up each peg and drop it into the basket. She demonstrated the desired movement and then asked Helen to begin the activity. Helen dutifully picked up a peg, crossed her midline, and dropped the peg into the basket. The therapist praised Helen and told her to continue this activity until all of the pegs were placed in the basket. She then walked away to set up another patient with a "treatment activity." Helen watched her walk away, and as the therapist began to talk to another client, Helen placed her forearm on her lapboard, and by moving her forearm across the surface, she placed all of the pegs in the basket in one fell swoop. A gasp of breath and then laughter came from both my brother and me as we witnessed her cleverness in completing her assigned task.

Helen instantly turned her gaze to us. Giving us a stern look and placing her index finger to her lips, she nonverbally commanded us to "Shh.'" We complied, and Helen serenely waited for the therapist to return. After about 20 minutes, the therapist returned to shower Helen with profuse praise for doing the activity so well. A transporter was then summoned to take Helen back to her room. As she was wheeled past us, Helen gave us a profound wink and a smile. Thereafter, each time Helen saw my brother and me, she would wink and put her finger to her lips. This supposedly cognitively disabled woman turned out to be one sharp lady with a great sense of humor. It was tragic that so few ever got to know her and that the potential of occupational therapy was never realized for her.

References

Ahlschwede, K. (1992). The Issue Is: Views on physical agent modalities and specialization within occupational therapy—A rebuttal. *American Journal of Occupational Therapy, 46*, 650–652.

American Occupational Therapy Association. (2002). Occupational therapy practice framework: Domain and process. *American Journal of Occupational Therapy, 56*, 609–639.

McGarry, J. (1990). National perspective: Our special skill—Is it lost? *Canadian Journal of Occupational Therapy, 57*, 258–259.

Mosey, A. C. (1996). *Psychosocial components of occupational therapy.* New York: Raven Press.

West, N. L., & Wiemer, R. B. (1991). The Issue Is: Should the Representative Assembly have voted as it did, when it did, on occupational therapists' use of physical agent modalities? *American Journal of Occupational Therapy, 45*, 1143–1147.

Clinical Reasoning: The Ethics, Science, and Art

CHAPTER 43

JOAN C. ROGERS, PhD, OTR/L

A therapist, employed at a regional rehabilitation center, extracts cues from the records of acute hospitals, to judge the rehabilitation potential of patients referred for admission. Another therapist, working with persons with mental retardation, selects a treatment approach based on task analysis to teach self-care skills. A third therapist, serving on a geriatric assessment team, uses scores on a mental status examination and performance ratings in daily living activities to estimate patients' ability to continue living alone in their homes. A fourth therapist reviews patients' progress in manual dexterity to formulate a recommendation for or against hand surgery. These four therapists are using their clinical reasoning skills to collect and transform data about patients into decisions that have critical implications for the quality of life of their patients.

If we questioned the therapists about their decisions, each would probably comment on their potential fallibility. Some patients, denied occupational therapy because of a perceived lack of potential for rehabilitation, would make substantial gains in functional skills if intervention were initiated. Some patients with mental retardation will not benefit from the task breakdown approach to self-care training. Some geriatric patients admitted for institutional living could have been supported adequately in the community. Some patients undergoing hand surgery will lose functional abilities. The possibility of error in our clinical judgments and the potential ensuing negative consequences urge us to develop ways of improving our assessment and treatment decisions.

Despite the obvious importance of clinical judgment in the occupational therapy process, little attention has been given to explicating the thinking that guides practice. My research, albeit with a small number of occupational therapists, suggests that our cognitive processes are regarded as intuitive and ineffable. For example, when therapists were asked how they arrived at their treatment decisions, they commonly responded by saying, "I have never really thought about it" or "I don't know how I reached that conclusion. I just know." Cognitive activity constitutes the heart of the clinical enterprise. Our failure to study the process of knowing and understanding that underlies practice precludes an adequate description of clinical reasoning. This in turn prevents the development of a methodology for systematically improving it and for teaching it.

I intend to explore here the reasoning process through which we learn about patients so that we may help them through engagement in occupation. I will construct an intellectual device for viewing clinical reasoning from the perspective of the basic questions the therapist seeks to answer through clinical inquiry. The scientific, ethical, and artistic dimensions of clinical reasoning will be elucidated as these questions are explored. The device will be useful for directing and appraising our thoughts about treating patients and for developing a clinical science of occupational therapy. In developing my thoughts, I have relied on the basic scheme of clinical judgment presented by Pellegrino (1) for medicine and have adapted it to the occupational therapy process.

The Goal of Clinical Reasoning

The goal of the clinical reasoning process has an impact on each of the steps taken to achieve the goal. Hence, an appreciation of this goal provides insight on the whole process.

Patients come to occupational therapy when they, their physicians, family members, or caregivers perceive that they are not adequately performing their daily activities. Performance in self-care, work, and leisure occupations has been compromised because of the consequences of disease, trauma, abnormal development, age-related changes, or environmental restrictions. The disruptions in occupational functions are characteristically severe and enduring as opposed to transitory. To regain a former level of performance, maintain the current level, or achieve a more optimal one, the patient enlists the aid of the therapist. The therapist's task, therefore, is to select a right therapeutic action for the patient (1). In other words, the goal of clinical reasoning is a treatment recommendation issued in the interests of a particular patient. Decision-making is highly individualized.

The occupational therapy treatment plan details what a particular patient should do to enhance occupational role performance. The therapeutic action must be the right action for this individual. This implies that it must be as congruent as possible with the patient's concept of the "good life." Treatment should be in concert with the patient's needs, goals, lifestyle, and personal and cultural values. A therapeutic program that is right for one patient is not necessarily right for another. The ultimate question we, as clinicians, are challenged to answer is: What, among the many things that could be done for this patient, ought to be done? This is an ethical question. It involves a judgment to which facts contribute but that must be decided by weighing values. A salient criterion of an ethical action is its agreement with the patient's valued goals. The clinical reasoning process terminates in an ethical decision, rather than in a scientific one, and the ethical nature of the goal of clinical reasoning projects itself over the entire sequence.

Ethical decisions regarding treatment are not made in isolation from scientific knowledge. The patient comes to the therapist for expert advice regarding adaptation to chronic dysfunction. The factual basis for decision-making is provided by the therapist. When therapists set out to solve clinical problems, they are confronted with an unknown—the patient. Scientific methodologies are used to learn about the patient. Once the patient's condition is adequately understood, scientific and empirical knowledge is applied in the efforts to enhance occupational status. Although ethical considerations can override scientific ones, they do not displace the need to secure a scientific opinion.

Clinical Questions

To ascertain the right action for each patient, clinical inquiry focuses on three questions: What is the patient's current status in occupational role performance? What could be done to enhance the patient's performance? And what ought to be done to enhance occupational competence? These are the fundamental questions that I previously alluded to as guiding the

clinical process. Each question will be considered first in terms of the knowledge needed to answer it, and, subsequently, in terms of the cognitive processes used to obtain the knowledge.

What Is the Patient's Status?

Assessment

The first question to be considered is the assessment question: What is the patient's occupational status? The occupational therapy assessment is a concise and accurate summary of a patient's occupational role performance that arises from an investigation of the patient. The occupational therapy assessment tells us what we need to know about the patient to plan a sound intervention or prevention program. To serve this function, the assessment includes several features: it indicates what is wrong with the patient, it indicates the patient's strengths, and it indicates the patient's motivation for occupation.

The word assessment is preferable to the terms diagnosis or problem definition for the evaluation of occupational status because it has a much broader meaning. Diagnosis and problem definition connote the identification of pathological, abnormal, dysfunctional, or problematic processes or states. To assess means to rate the value of property for the purpose of taxation. The word assessment, then, with its emphasis on the evaluation of the worth of something, is an appropriate term to apply to the process of collecting information to resolve clinical problems and to the statement that summarizes the results of that process. Occupational therapy is concerned with helping disabled persons to adapt to chronic disability more effectively. This may be accomplished by enhancing abilities as well as by remediating or reducing dysfunction. The occupational therapy assessment serves as the end point of evaluation and the starting point for treatment planning. To serve this pivotal function, the assessment must specify both assets and liabilities. Thus, diagnosis, or the determination of what is wrong with the patient, is only a part of the assessment.

Knowledge

The assessment process usually begins with diagnosis, because knowledge of dysfunction tells us what is wrong and requires correction or amelioration. The therapist seeks to ascertain the specific problems the patient is having in performing self-care, work, and leisure occupations. Disruptions in occupational role are commonly of two major types: an inability to perform socially defined age-appropriate tasks and an inability to coordinate these tasks effectively in daily life. To the extent that a person has disruptions in occupational role, or impairments that we can predict will result in such disruptions, that person is an appropriate candidate for occupational therapy. The occupational therapy diagnosis clearly articulates the disruption in occupational role that is of concern for treatment. For example, we might state that Tom Smith is totally dependent in hygiene and dressing and requires physical assistance with feeding. This diagnosis indicates that these are the major problems at this time.

The occupational therapy diagnosis has a temporal quality. Participation in daily living tasks may change over the course of an illness or other disorder. For example, as Tom Smith gains competence in self-care, the diagnosis may switch to dysfunctions in home management. Similarly, as an individual matures and needs and interests change, the occupational therapy diagnosis changes, and intervention is refocused. Thus, the range of problems that comprise the occupational therapy diagnosis is broad and variable, and the diagnosis may change over time.

Often, the occupational therapy diagnosis indicates not only the disruption in occupational role, but also the suspected cause or causes for this disruption. This is the etiological component of the diagnostic statement and it offers an explanation of why the individual behaves or fails to behave in some way.

The most prevalent perspective for defining the etiology of occupational role dysfunctions is based on the biopsychosocial model. This enables us to pinpoint the causes of performance dysfunctions in terms of biological, psychological, and social variables. For example, we might state that Ida Cox cannot dress herself because she has contractures in her upper extremities, thus attributing the cause to a biological variable. Or we might suggest that she cannot dress herself because of a memory problem, thus attributing the cause to a psychological variable. Or. we might conclude that the reason she is unable to dress herself is because she cannot reach her clothes from a wheelchair. In this case, the dressing dysfunction is attributed to the interaction of a biological variable, motor impairment, and a social variable, the man-made environment. Such attributions allow us to plan appropriate treatment. We can plan to remediate the contracture or memory deficit or to circumvent their effects on performance. We can remove the architectural barriers.

An occupational therapy diagnosis stemming from the biopsychosocial model is so specific that it is applicable to only one patient. For instance, an occupational therapy diagnosis might state: Homemaking disability secondary to a lack of endurance for shopping to procure groceries, and postural instability in negotiating the stairs to the laundry facilities in the basement; ability is complicated by blurred vision in both eyes as a consequence of cataracts. Such a diagnosis is unlikely to be appropriate for more than one patient. Although the diagnostic statement is highly descriptive, it is also highly prescriptive. For example, the above diagnosis suggests such interventions as: employing homemaker services, scheduling and performing activities in such a way as to control fatigue, using good light with no glare, and using mobility aids or environmental supports.

In addition to a description of what the patient cannot do and why, the occupational therapy assessment includes a description of what the patient can do and how well it can be done. Although the problem is diagnosed, it is the person who is assessed. The need to acknowledge positive factors was well expressed by the little boy who reacted to the scolding he received about his report card by saying, "Daddy, I think your eyes need fixing. You only saw the D and not the four As." Knowing a person's problems or deficits tells us little about his or her strengths. The image of the patient drawn from problem behaviors is distorted. It needs to be supplemented with snapshots of the patient's occupational competencies and strengths to enable the therapist to construct a fair and valid impression of the patient.

The assessment of occupational competence requires a wide-angled lens. Occupational performance emerges from a complex network of transactions between the internal characteristics of the individual and the external properties of the surrounding environment. Just as features of a particular situation may account for a limitation of ability, so they may also allow the expression of ability. The qualities of the environment are important enablers of human performance. You cannot swim without water or play tennis without a partner. Both the physical and the social environments influence the patient's ability to occupy time productively. To assess occupational competence, the therapist evaluates the people, places, and objects associated with the patient's occupational endeavors to determine the extent to which they support occupation.

The final requirement of the occupational therapy assessment is to summarize the patient's motivation to engage in occupation. Who among us has never pondered over the patients with excellent potential who fail to achieve and those with intractable conditions who surpass all expectations? We cannot understand the patient without an appreciation of the way in which the urge toward competence has been habitually satisfied. The ontogenetic aspects of occupation have critical implications for recovery and growth. The patient's history of occupation informs us whether the present dysfunction is extenuated by a pattern of adaptive behavior or augmented by a career of maladaptive behavior. The patient's mastery of the environment is documented in occupational achievement, while exploration of the environment is recorded in the use of time. Because time is occupied by doing things of value, the patient's use of time provides insight into the varieties of occupations that are meaningful to him or her. The patient's past is reviewed to shed light on how occupational behavior is organized and to lend perspective to activities that are important and incidental to the life plan.

Historical assessment is directed toward a deeper understanding of the patient's occupational nature. The normative sequence of occupational endeavors begins in childhood play and self-care. Participation in arts and crafts, games, academics, chores, and part-time work are added to the repertoire through young adulthood. Productive occupation in the form of employment predominates in adulthood. This often changes to leisure pursuits during later maturity. The therapist thus captures the development and balance of self-care, work, and leisure occupations in studying the sequence of preschool, school age, worker, and retiree roles.

The yield of the occupational therapy assessment is a model of the patient that describes and explains his or her unique functioning in occupation. The model superimposes current functional abilities on disabilities, and relates these to environmental demands and to past performance. It is from this comprehensive model of the patient that future capacity is predicted and treatment goals are recommended.

Process

Having described the requirements of the occupational therapy assessment, I will now turn to the cognitive processes used to formulate it. What is involved in clinical inquiry? How do we go about the task of constructing a model of the patient? The approach used here for looking at the cognitive processes that undergird practice reflects an information-processing view of cognition. The human mind is thus conceptualized as a computer that has certain information-processing capabilities. It can do some things better than others and uses certain labor-saving strategies to overcome its limitations. A primary limitation of the human mind is its small capacity for short-term or working memory. Because of this limitation, data must be selected judiciously, processed serially, and managed through simplifying strategies (2). In assessment, the clinician has as intake to the information-processing system cues gathered from the patient or about the patient. The output is the conclusions summarized in the occupational therapy assessment. The conversion of intake data to output conclusions is a critical feature of clinical reasoning.

The therapist begins the assessment by choosing a plan for studying the patient. We say to ourselves, "Of all things that I could consider about this patient, what am I going to think about?" We typically respond to this question by constructing an image of the patient from the preassessment data and use this image to direct our plan. Our preassessment image tells us what to include and what to exclude as we observe the patient. Thus, the first labor-saving device the therapist uses is to limit the parameters within which the patient will be studied.

The preassessment image of the patient is derived from the conceptual frame of reference or postulate system of the therapist. A conceptual frame of reference represents a therapist's unique view of occupational therapy. It consists of facts derived from research studies, empirical generalizations drawn from experience, theories and models accepted by the therapist, and principles of practice obtained from instructors and colleagues. My frame of reference represents what I believe about occupational therapy practice. A frame of reference operates largely as an unconscious ideology in forming the preassessment image. The therapist links his or her frame of reference with the preassessment data to construct an image of the patient that furnishes the outline for the clinical investigation.

Two salient preassessment factors are the medical diagnosis and age. By knowing even these elementary facts. we can predict certain things about a patient. For example, if we know that a patient's dominant arm has been amputated, we can anticipate problems in manual dexterity and bilateral coordination. If, in addition, we know that the patient is 6 years old, rather than 76, we can expect to direct treatment toward habilitation of hand skills as opposed to rehabilitation.

The preassessment image of the patient is used to generate a series of testable working hypotheses. The therapist reasons that, if a particular hypothesis is valid, then it should follow that such and such will be found in further study of the case. For example, a therapist learns from the occupational therapy referral that the patient is a 40-year-old woman with depression. The therapist reasons that, if this patient is depressed, she is likely to be disheveled, to have a low level of involvement in activities, and to concentrate on events associated with negative affect. In other words, by knowing that the patient is depressed, the therapist is able to view the patient as a representative of the class of depressed patients, and, thus, hypothesizes that she will exhibit characteristics of depression. The therapist then sets out to perform the procedures needed to substantiate the hypothesis.

Up to this point, the reasoning process is essentially deductive in nature. The therapist recalls some general postulates from memory and applies them to a specific patient. The open-ended question of what is wrong with the patient has now been refined to a set of better-defined problems for exploration and resolution.

The working hypotheses provide a plan for acquiring cues from the patient to test the hypotheses. A cue is any bit of information that guides or directs the assessment (3). Cues arise from the observational process that employs three general types of data-gathering methodologies: testing or measurement; questioning, including history taking and interviewing; and observation. Accurate clinical decisions are dependent on the collection of good cues. Two tests of the goodness of cues are reliability and validity.

Cues can be used to test the working hypotheses developed from deductive reasoning. By comparing each cue to the working hypotheses, sense may be made of the data. The therapist reasons, "This is what I expect to find, now what do I find?" A cue may be interpreted as confirming a hypothesis, disconfirming a hypothesis, or noncontributary to a hypothesis. Thus, as information is collected about the patient, the therapist decides repeatedly whether or not a finding is related to the patient's problems. Confidence in each hypothesis increases or decreases, based on the interpretation of additional data. Extensive case data are reduced by eliminating, or holding in reserve, data that do not appear significant. Hypothesis testing is thus another of the mind's strategies for simplifying data management. Hypotheses direct the collection of data and determine how they are organized and filed in memory. This organization prevents the mind from becoming overloaded with irrelevant facts and assists the therapist in retrieving information from memory.

Cues may also be combined to formulate new hypotheses. As cues are collected to test the validity of the deduced hypotheses, some cues may not fit well. Some of the performance problems we had expected to find will not be found, and others that we had not anticipated will become manifest. Our thinking begins to move from the classical, textbook picture of the disorder, to the disorder as it is uniquely manifested in this patient. The reasoning process now becomes inductive, with problem definition induced from empirical study of the patient, rather than deduced from the therapist's frame of reference. Additional cues may then be collected to test the inductively derived hypotheses. Clinical reasoning proceeds by developing hypotheses that pull together several inferences into a broader pattern or model of the patient.

After gleaning a clear perception of the patient's problems, the therapist then begins to search for cues indicative of the health of the patient as avidly as the search was conducted to identify dysfunction. Inductive reasoning and hypothesis testing are the basic processes through which the clinician assesses the patient's competencies, motivation for occupational achievement, and the environments in which the patient operates or will operate. These kinds of data are highly personal and hence are less likely to be deduced from knowledge of disease or disorder.

Data collection cannot continue indefinitely, and at some point the therapist decides that adequate information has been collected. How much data constitutes adequate data is dependent on the ethical consequences of an error in judgment (2,4). A recommendation to institutionalize a patient because he or she is unable to look after his or her self-care needs would require more evidence than that required for the prescription of a rocker knife. Regardless of how many data are collected, however, the database remains incomplete. The database represents only a sampling of the patient's behavior. The therapist's task is to use this incomplete information to make a judicious decision. Decision-making takes place under conditions of uncertainty.

Throughout the process of data collection, the therapist's preassessment image of the patient has been revised and elaborated, based on the accumulated cues. Once cue collection is stopped and no new information is being generated, hypothesis testing also ceases. The clinical reasoning of the therapist now resembles the dialectical process in which the therapist argues or defends the interpretation of the data in much the same way as a lawyer pleads a case in court. Does the patient have a dressing problem that is of concern? Is the cause of the patient's performance difficulties visual–perceptual problems? Is the mental status of the patient adequate for self-care? The evidence supporting or opposing each alternative is weighed with the objective of rendering one explanation more cogent than another. Inferences that are compatible are retained and others are rejected or modified as contradictions appear. Through the dialectical process the model of the individual patient is polished and repolished. In this way, the therapist arrives at a cohesive conception of the patient, and, having grasped the whole, reinterprets the parts in light of this understanding. Once a holistic picture of the patient has been devised, the function of the assessment moves from model building to decision-making.

What Are the Available Options?

The second of the three general questions guiding clinical inquiry is the therapeutic question: What can be done for this patient? Having proposed a model of the patient's occupational status, we then begin to explore the actions that could be taken to enhance occupational role performance. The intent is to generate a list of the treatment options available for the problems and assets presented by this patient. For example, suppose a patient's problems in self-care were attributed to hemiplegia subsequent to a cerebral vascular accident. To treat this problem, we might consider a neurological approach aimed at regaining controlled action in the involved arm, or a rehabilitative approach aimed at training the uninvolved arm to perform skilled activities, or a combination of these approaches. The aim, at this stage of clinical reasoning, is to foster an awareness of the range and kind of treatment possibilities. In effect, the therapist uses the model of the patient to construct a theory of practice for the patient.

Knowledge

The therapist's consideration of what could be done includes a review of the relative effectiveness of each treatment approach. If a particular treatment option is initiated, what results can be expected, and how long will it take to achieve them? Any hazards associated with the various treatments, or with no treatment, are evaluated in light of the potential benefits.

Decision-making concerning the appropriate action can approach certitude if the deleterious effects of a disorder without treatment are known, and if there is substantial evidence of how these effects can be altered by a particular treatment. We know, for instance, that if joints are not moved, contractures develop and the joints become immobile. Thus, movement becomes the scientifically acceptable treatment for preventing contractures.

For most occupational therapy approaches or procedures, however, the scientific evidence is not definitive. Rarely are the outcomes of research so specific that they allow us to know with 100 percent accuracy what will happen. Scientific findings generally emerge as probabilities rather than as certainties. They may, for example, tell us that 95 percent of the patients with right hemiplegia receiving self-care training will become independent in self-care. But when we apply this finding to Edith Jones, we do so with the recognition that her chances of becoming independent remain 50–50. The response of a patient to treatment cannot be predicted with certitude. Scientific knowledge can improve our chances of making accurate technical decisions but it cannot assure this. When the scientific evidence is inconclusive, the therapist has considerable leeway in devising treatment recommendations.

In the absence of scientific knowledge about the effectiveness of treatment options, clinicians rely on knowledge gleaned from their own clinical experience or from the experiences of others. Knowledge derived from practice rather than research indicates what works but may not indicate what works best.

Process

To draw up a list of the patient's treatment options, the therapist searches memory for relevant scientific and practice knowledge. Clinical experiences are stored and classified in memory and retrieved as needed for application to new patients. Each time a therapist treats a patient, a clinical experiment is performed in which the objective is to replicate a successful outcome of a past experiment (5). As a first step in reproducing the experiment, the therapist mentally reviews previous patients whose occupational status resembled the patient at hand. Although no two patients are exactly alike, the therapist assembles a subgroup of patients who are most similar to the patient under study (6). Treatment is selected for the new patient by analyzing and comparing the therapeutic actions and outcomes of the patients in the reference group. If there is a high degree of similarity between the patient being treated and previous patients, the therapist will select a treatment that is highly replicative. If the similarity is low, or if previous treatment was not very effective, the therapist will propose a treatment that is more inventive.

The cognitive process involved in the selection of treatment is again that of dialectical reasoning. The therapist argues one treatment option against another without recourse to new clinical data. The process of enumerating the patient's treatment alternatives relies heavily on the content of long-term memory. The more clinical experience therapists have, the more empirical data are available to guide decision-making. It is impossible for therapists to consider a treatment with which they have no familiarity. Similarly, clinicians cannot debate the scientific merits of one procedure over another, unless the procedure has been scientifically investigated and the research has been assimilated.

What Ought to Be Done?

The third and final question to be considered is the ethical question: What ought to be done to enhance occupational competence? Simply because a goal appears technically feasible for the patient does not mean that it should be set as a goal. And, simply because a treatment approach can be initiated does not imply that it should be instituted. We must avoid confusing action that can be taken with action that ought to be taken. From an ethical standpoint, decisive action must take the patient's valued goals into account. It must conform to the patient's definition of health, accomplishment, and the "good life."

Knowledge

Ethical principles arise from reflection on the nature of humanity and human dignity. Respect for individuals requires that each individual be regarded as autonomous. Each individual has a definite pattern and characteristic style for mastering the environment in the pursuit of occupational competence. The life plan is guided by personal and cultural values. Values give meaning and direction to one's life by inciting future goals and sustaining involvement in activity.

The concept of respect for the individual implies that the occupational therapy treatment plan should not interfere with the patient's intentions for recovery. To develop an appropriate plan, the patient's values are distilled from the thematic continuity of the assessment of occupational status and taken into account in the review of technically feasible treatment options. When there is a range of possibilities for treatment goals and substantial lack of certitude concerning the technical merits of treatment alternatives, the therapist has considerable latitude in shaping recommendations. Expert advice is based more on opinion than fact. Ethical decision-making requires the therapist to search for an understanding of the patient's life rather than to make an evaluation of it. This understanding facilitates the selection of options to be discussed with the patient.

The goal of the clinical encounter is to devise a therapeutic plan that preserves the patient's values and represents a mutual understanding between the therapist and patient. Occupational therapy involves habit training and often requires major restructuring of the way in which personal values are to be satisfied. If habits are to be developed, patients must choose the objects and processes that they want to master in occupational therapy. Worthwhile achievement is the end product of personally deliberated decision-making. Occupational achievement begins with the choice to develop one's capabilities. It is the patient who restores, maintains, and enhances occupational performance. The patient, not the therapist, is the agent of change. The patient's active participation is required not only in determining and prioritizing the goals of treatment, but also in deciding on the methods to be used to achieve the goals. As a result of assuming personal responsibility for treatment decisions, the patient emerges from the assessment with an increased sense of self-determination and control, and a sense of commitment to accomplishing planned goals. In the capacity of expert advisor, the therapist guides patients through the decision-making process, and helps them fuse the intellectual and emotional aspects of decision-making into choices that are right for them.

It cannot be assumed that the goals selected by a patient for himself or herself will match those the therapist would select. Each may have a different view of the "good life." Because most persons with quadriplegia secondary to a spinal cord lesion at the level of the 6th and 7th cervical vertebrae can relearn dressing skills, the therapist may reason that Tim Robbins should work toward this goal. However, Tim may conclude that he would prefer to spend his limited energy relearning how to manage his home computer.

When the therapist and patient have different goals, the potential for conflict is high, and the resolution of conflict can easily be tipped in favor of the therapist's view. Two factors contribute significantly, to the therapist holding the balance of power (1). First, the therapist has the knowledge and skills to alleviate the problems facing the patient. The patient is thus dependent on the therapist for help. Second, the patient's position of dependency is compounded by the patient's vulnerability. As a result of disease or other disorders, patients sustain insults to functions regarded as integral to human life and living. The very fact that they need help may diminish their sense of autonomy. Adaptive functioning in basic life tasks, such as eating and dressing, may be impeded. Patients may even be unable to express their own values or make rational choices. Such impairments place a patient's moral agency at risk, and often make it easy to take advantage of the patient's right to control his or her life.

Process

The methods used to answer ethical questions differ from those used in science. While scientific questions are answered by accumulating data and testing hypotheses, ethical questions are resolved by coming to grips with values and making value judgments (7). To empower the patient to act as his or her own moral agent, the therapist provides the patient with the knowledge needed to participate effectively in decision-making. The patient's choice must not only be autonomous, it must also be informed. Patients are not adequately informed to make choices, unless they can anticipate the results of their choices. The ethical and scientific dimensions of clinical reasoning are closely intermingled. The therapist presents the possible options for treatment, projects the outcomes of each option, explains how the outcomes are achieved, and outlines a time sequence for goal attainment. Together the therapist and patient consider each recommendation and evaluate the consequences of each alternative in terms of the patient's occupational potential and goals. If necessary, the therapist tempers unrealistic expectations, corrects inaccurate information, and points out any inconsistencies in rationalization. In effect, the therapist assists the patient in imagining what might occur, if treatment is to be undertaken or rejected. The strength of arguments for one action over another is assessed by dialectic. Greater weight is assigned a position according to the importance it holds for the patient. The selection of treatment becomes more difficult as the merits of one action over other actions become more ambiguous. The therapist makes known his or her preferences for the patient's treatment as well as the rationale for this decision. The patient ends the deliberation by making a choice.

Once the patient has determined the course of action, the therapist supports or confirms the decision. The therapist captures the persuasive elements of the dialectical argument, and uses them to instill in the patient a belief that treatment X is the best course of action and should be undertaken. At the same time, the therapist strives to bolster the patient's belief that he or she can carry out the treatment and achieve the goals. The reasoning process ends, therefore, in persuasive rhetoric, which we call "motivating the patient." In situations where therapists judge that they cannot lend support to the patient's choice, responsibility for providing occupational therapy services is terminated.

The therapist is privileged to help the patient select from the available opportunities those that are to be brought to fruition. As the patient executes and fulfills his or her choice, the therapist learns about the healing power of occupation. Occupational choice rekindles the will to live, and mobilizes the mind to discipline the body, in enacting the creative processes associated with reversing disability. The subtle wisdom of participation in self-initiated and self-directed occupation becomes apparent as confidence is rebuilt and hope is restored. Choices are not confined to the outset of treatment. Assessment and planning are ongoing processes and there are repeated occasions to consider if treatment should be continued, terminated, modified, or supplemented.

This discussion of the ethical dimension of clinical reasoning has been based on three cogent assumptions: 1. that patients can serve as their own moral agents; 2. that the patient's choice is the ultimate one; and 3. that the therapist acts independently. None of these conditions may be met in a particular situation, which introduces further complications into the already complex process of ethical decision-making. Surrogates may substitute for patients in the planning process because patients are too young, too impaired mentally, or too emotionally disturbed to participate in decision-making. The rights of family members and the values and resources of society may limit the choices patients can make. The conjoint decision of therapist and patient may be modified or set aside by the health-care team. These are vital issues that cannot be avoided in clinical decisions.

In summary, the data collected in clinical inquiry play three roles in clinical reasoning. First, clinical data are used to describe the patient's occupational status. This description includes an indication of the patient's adaptive skills, performance dysfunctions and their presumed causes, and competency motivation. Second, clinical data are used to conjure up a group of patients who have an occupational status and history comparable to the patient under consideration. These patients serve as a reference group for the identification of treatment options and prediction of treatment outcomes. Third, clinical data are used to identify therapeutic options appropriate to the specific needs of the patient, and to recommend a course of action consistent with the patient's values. As the clinical reasoning process moves from an assessment of occupational status, to a review of treatment options, to a selection of the right action, the scientific mode of reasoning gives way to non-scientific intellectual processes. Choosing a course of action involves many value considerations. The closer we come to making a clinical judgment, the less use is made of facts and hypothesis testing, and the more reliance is placed on the dialectical process, opinion, and persuasion.

Perfecting Clinical Inquiry

Now that what is involved in clinical study has been considered, it seem appropriate to ponder how our habits of inquiry can be improved. My suggestions are intended to be directional rather than comprehensive.

Model of the Patient

The therapist's understanding of the patient is highly dependent on the development of a model of the patient. It is pertinent to point out that studies conducted with counseling professionals have consistently supported the value of inductive theory building for practice, as opposed to the application of deductive theory. McArthur (8), for example, found that psychologists who applied existing theories in a doctrinary fashion turned out to be the poorest appraisers of personality. The critical element in devising a model of the patient is meticulous attention to the cues obtained from the patient. The ability to use assessment-related data to develop hypotheses is a vital professional skill.

Although hypotheses have adaptive value for organizing and managing data, they represent strong conceptual biases. In collecting and interpreting data, we have a tendency to overlook evidence that does not support our hypotheses. This is accompanied by an inclination to overemphasize positive evidence. In other words, we are psychologically prone to affirm our ideas, and feel less compelled to refute them (4, 9). Agnew and Pyke (10) drew a salient comparison between the blindness imposed by hypotheses and that generated by love. They commented: "The rejection of a theory once accepted is like the rejection of a girlfriend or boyfriend once loved— it takes more than a bit of negative evidence. In fact, the rest of the community can shake their collective heads in amazement at your blindness, your utter failure to recognize the glaring array of differences between your picture of the girl or boy, and the data." (p. 128) The rigid application of a conceptual bias emerged as a major concern in my study of occupational ther-

apists' thinking (11). The medical diagnosis was used to formulate the preassessment image of the patient and that image remained stable, even in the face of cues portending a revision.

Once cognizant of the pitfalls involved in hypothesis use, the therapist can initiate steps to avoid them. Obtaining a second opinion through consultation is one method commonly used to check the validity of one's interpretation. Consultants should perform their own assessments without reference to the patient's database. Objectivity will be destroyed if consultants read reports or participate in discussions about the patient before conducting their own evaluations. The consultant's final opinion, however, should be based on the total available data (5).

A fixed data collection schedule is another mechanism used to prevent premature closure of hypothesis generation. The Occupational Therapy Uniform Evaluation Checklist (12) is an example of a fixed data collection schedule. It specifies the boundaries of occupational therapy practice and lists the variables to be reviewed for assessment. The Checklist forces the therapist to examine occupational performance from a panoramic view rather than microscopically. In so doing, it fosters the search for information that might suggest hypotheses the therapist might not otherwise have entertained. Adherence to a fixed routine assures the therapist that observations will be conducted that afford a fair and adequate opportunity to disprove as well as to confirm favorite hypotheses (13).

Research on the assessment process suggests that practitioners' "favorite" hypotheses concentrate on the dysfunctional aspects of patient performance (14, 15). We seem to be more interested in exploring why Alice Thompson falls so often than in ascertaining why she maintains her balance for so long. This preoccupation with problematic behaviors probably stems from the fact that they are the reason for the patient's referral to occupational therapy and constitute the focus of interventive efforts. Our first response to the question concerning the patient's occupational status is that it is dysfunctional. Our image of the patient changes as we collect additional cues and make adjustments in the initial picture. However, once our thoughts are anchored in dysfunction, it becomes difficult to switch our focus and too few modifications may be made in the image (16). Wright and Fletcher (14) point out that the perception of strengths and weaknesses as a unit, that is, as belonging to one person, requires the therapist to integrate two dissimilar qualities and that such synthesis is difficult. The same rationale may also be used to explain why practitioners are prone to see more pathology in their patients than the patients themselves perceive. Patients live with disability and adapt to it. Professionals regard disability as something to be eliminated. From this vantage point it is hard for professionals to see how disability can have any positive implications. Unfortunately, an emphasis on negative perceptions results in a skewed image of the patient. Dysfunctions are overestimated and abilities are underestimated (14).

Research also indicates that practitioners are more likely to hypothesize that a patient's problems are caused by factors within the patient as opposed to factors in the patient's physical and social milieu (14, 15). For instance, we are more apt to attribute a patient's distress to an inability to deal with authority figures than to an unreasonable supervisor. One reason for this tendency is that we generally have a clearer picture of patients than we do of the situations in which they live, work, and play. We generally see patients in health-care settings and rarely sample their behaviors in natural settings. Thus, the patient's environment has a quality of vagueness about it compared to the patient, who appears more real. Another explanation for our neglect of the environment is that it is often impossible or very difficult to change the environment. Even if the patient's supervisor is irrational, the patient still has to learn to manage the situation or to find another job. Nevertheless, it should be recognized that our "clinic-bound" view of the patient may lead us to ignore or underestimate impediments to occupational performance residing in the environment. Furthermore, because patients often attribute their difficulties to situations rather than to themselves, there is a potential conflict between the therapist's and patient's perceptions of causation. The validity of the patient's causal attribution should not be dismissed lightly by the therapist because patients are attuned to situational exigencies by their struggle for occupational competence.

Recognizing the distortion that may occur because of the exploration of hypotheses oriented toward dysfunction rather than function, and emphasis on the person as opposed to the environment, the therapist can take steps to countermand these biases. The data collection schedule can be arranged to include both assets and liabilities for every aspect of occupational performance evaluated. Because a patient's self-perceptions of competence are as important for participation in activity as is competence itself, the checklist should also highlight the patient's subjective impressions of occupational status. The schedule can also be extended to include the physical and social environments. These additions will serve to remind us of the significance of these variables for occupation and to foster the habit of routinely evaluating them.

Integration of Data

The challenge presented to the mind by the occupational therapy assessment is intensified by the need to integrate the wide variety of information gathered about the patient. Although we may isolate aspects of human functioning for the purposes of data management, humans function as unities or wholes. Competence requires the individual to function as an integrated organism, with the physical, mental, emotional, and social dimensions of occupational behavior interacting with the surrounding human and nonhuman environment. The selection of treatment proceeds from a holistic conception of the patient. If the therapist is to manage the array of complex clinical data required to understand occupational behavior, a simplifying strategy is needed to ward off chaos in the information-processing capabilities of the human mind. Clinical judgments are not made on the basis of one or two test scores. And, although the statistical integration of clinical data may be possible in some situations, it is impractical in most. We need a labor-saving device to assist the mind in integrating data. General systems theory provides such assistance.

According to the systems metaphor, data are framed in terms of relationships among systems and systems are ordered hierarchically based on increasing levels of complexity. In the assessment of a patient with a traumatic spinal cord injury, for example, we would look at the effects of disorder on other biological systems, such as the musculoskeletal and integumentary. At the same time, the rules of systems hierarchy would direct our attention to factors in the psychological system, such as competency motivation, which will strongly influence the recovery of the biological system as well as the social reintegration of the patient. Although the assessment checklist is useful for reminding us of the spectrum of occupational performance, general systems theory provides rules for organizing the list so that the assessment data can be meaningfully related and stored in memory.

Occupational Therapy Assessment

Once an occupational therapy assessment has been made, viable therapeutic approaches are selected. The selection of treatment rests on a comparison between the patient under consideration and similar patients previously treated. Thus, the effective application of treatment requires that patients be accurately identified and grouped together according to characteristics that are salient for occupation. If the results of a clinical experiment are to be replicated, we must begin with a patient who closely resembles those used in the original experiment.

At the present time, occupational therapy has no meaningful way of systematically describing occupational role performance and of differentiating homogeneous subgroups based on occupational characteristics. The medical diagnosis is inadequate for delineating the diverse levels of occupational performance that occur in patients with the same diagnosis. It also lacks utility for identifying the similar levels of occupational performance that occur in patients with different medical diagnoses. Occupational therapy lacks a standardized way of classifying the functional disabilities that result from disease and other disorders. In the absence of an agreed-upon system for thinking about, remembering, and expressing our clinical observations, each therapist develops his or her own idiosyncratic system for describing occupational performance. To the extent that these informal descriptions facilitate a comparison of patients, based on salient occupational characteristics, the inferences resulting from the comparison will be valid. However, until a systematic scheme for describing and organizing clinical data is developed, we will not be able to communicate meaningfully with each

Selection of Treatment

We have seen that a treatment recommendation is largely based on the therapist's recall of similar cases. Some memories are more easily recalled than others (6). We are more likely to think of patients treated recently than those treated in the past. It is easier to remember patients who are seen frequently than those treated less often. Exceptional cases, either of success or failure, make strong impressions. Inferences gleaned from patients who happen to come to mind are likely to be less accurate than those derived from systematic analysis. Although we can all recount our brilliant successes, how many of us know what our batting average is? How good are we as judges of occupational potential? By keeping a score of the accuracy of our clinical predictions, our judgmental abilities can be improved. Checking our initial predictions against discharge data is something that can be readily incorporated into the clinic routine. Did the patient accomplish what I predicted he or she would? If not, why not? Because the ultimate test of treatment is what happens after discharge, mechanisms should also be sought for testing the accuracy of our discharge predictions with follow-up data.

A common error made by therapists in arriving at a clinical judgment is to assume that the patient is like oneself (17). This assumption enables us to know the patient through ourselves. In using the self as a referent, one rationalizes, "I will treat the patient as I would wish to be treated if I were in this situation." This kind of reasoning risks denying the validity of the patient's values. The therapist ascribes meaning to the patient's situation according to his or her own criteria. The patient is presented with a decision, rather than a list of options, and the choice of occupation is denied. Respect for the individual implies giving the patient the same opportunity to express and achieve what the patient sees as worthwhile as one would desire for oneself. We must be sensitive to the human spirit and curb the offering of pseudo choices of activity that have little meaning for the patient.

Instrumentation

The validity of clinical reasoning is grounded in the collection of good cues. This is a critical point to consider as we concentrate our energies on developing assessment instruments for practice. The nature of the phenomena we are interested in evaluating dictates the appropriate kind of instrumentation. As clinicians, our primary interest lies in evaluating performance in self-care, work, and leisure occupations. Our concern is with the ability to do and that doing is observable. You do not need to infer that I can dress from my grip strength, or mental acuity. You can observe my ability. Performance is not an abstract construct as is intelligence, anxiety, or sensory integration. We can see performance. Furthermore, we know that performance in occupation

depends on the environment or situation as much as it does on the patient. Recognizing the interplay between the patient and the environment leaves us with two fundamental ways of evaluating occupational performance. First, we can go into the environments where our patients live, work, and play and observe their performance. Second, we can simulate the occupational environments of our patients by providing test stimuli, such as beds, chairs, games, arts and crafts, and work and collect a series of behavior samples in our clinics. In this case, the validity of our evaluation depends on how well we approximate the places where function is to occur.

There is inherently little uniformity in the occupational environments of our patients and, if we try to establish that uniformity, we will obscure the validity of our evaluation. The strength of occupational therapy assessment lies not in placing patients in contrived and standardized situations and recording their responses, but rather, in observing them in real-life settings and evaluating their adaptive competence. Thus, development of occupational therapy instrumentation depends on a conceptualization of the task environment, because this constitutes the test stimulus that evokes behavior. Our description of occupational behavior will be incomplete until we can mesh it with a description of the task environment.

The Art

Our exploration of the intellectual technology of clinical reasoning has focused on the scientific and ethical aspects. We have not considered the art except by implication and innuendo. In the peroration, I return to the therapist who says, "I don't know how I know, I just know that I know." While the scientific dimension of clinical reasoning is directed toward specifying the correct treatment from a technical standpoint, and the ethical dimension is geared toward selecting the treatment that meets the patient's criteria of right occupational role performance, the artistic dimension pursues excellence in achieving a right action—and it does this in the face of individuality, indeterminacy, and complexity (6). Artistry involves the orchestration of broad strategies for grappling effectively with the uncertainties inherent in clinical practice.

Skill in Thinking

Artistry is knowing as it is revealed in our actions (6). It is exhibited in knowing what to do and how to do it, rather than in knowing about something. In the early stages of acquiring a skill, such as dressing or piano playing, our actions are slow and clumsy. We have to think a lot about what we are doing and we make a lot of errors. But as skill develops, our actions become smooth, flexible, and spontaneous, and our thinking becomes automatic. We get a feel for the skill and that feeling allows us to repeat our performance. You know how to touch the piano keys to play a Mozart piano concerto, and your artistry is apparent in your music. If you were to describe your "knowing how to" play the piano, you would find this difficult, if not impossible, just as someone else would find it difficult to acquire the skill of piano playing by following your instructions.

Clinical reasoning may be viewed as a skill akin to piano playing. The skill consists of reducing the ambiguities inherent in clinical practice to manageable risks, and by so doing, enabling the formulation of prudent decisions (6). In each clinical transaction, the therapist is challenged to apply the theories and techniques of occupational therapy to a particular patient. Our textbooks inform us of the implications of blindness, hemiplegia, and age-related changes, but the hiatus between theory and practice becomes readily apparent when 90-year-old John Green, accompanied by his loving wife and devoted daughter, stands before us with hemiplegia, blindness, and the beginning signs of brain failure. Who among us has not experienced the gap between what we learned in school and what we need to know in the clinic?

Clinical problems are not neat. They are messy and complex. Everything that could be known about the patient is not known and much of the data collected are flawed and imperfect. Clinical problems deal with the uniqueness of patients rather than with their similarities. And, as Gordon Allport (18) reminds us, uniqueness is not equivalent to the sum of the ways in which a person deviates from the hypothetical average human. Unlike the simple cause-and-effect problems associated with basic science, clinical problems involve a complex interplay of multiple variables, the effects of which are largely unpredictable. The outcomes of occupational therapy treatment cannot be guaranteed. Clinical problems change as patient's progress and regress and as the occupational opportunities provided by the environment fluctuate.

No one can provide "cookbook" recipes for dealing with situations in which uniqueness, uncertainty, complexity, and instability are the chief characteristics. There are no formulas or algorithms that tell us how to use the interneuronal processes associated with perception, memory, reasoning, and argument. In the clinical situation, the therapist is under pressure to act and to act now. One cannot interrupt an assessment to go to the library and read up on a critical point. In handling the uncertainties contained in clinical practice, therapists rely on their accumulated experience, conceptual and judgmental heuristics, intuition, and insight to "apply their knowledge" and make clinical judgments. In spite of defective data and incomplete information, artistic inquiry enables the therapist to make prudent decisions and to know why a treatment will work for a particular patient.

The artistry of clinical reasoning is exhibited in the craftsmanship with which the therapist executes the series of steps that culminates in a clinical decision. It is expressed in the interpersonal skills through which the therapist invites involvement in decision-making, builds trust, explains treatment alternatives, and offers encouragement. Artistry manifests itself in the adeptness with which the therapist gathers cues: by selecting questions, probing for information not volunteered, clarifying discrepancies, administering tests, and observing performance. The degree of perfection with which the data to be processed are obtained influences the reliability and validity of the data, and hence sets limits on the quality of the final judgment. The art extends to grouping cues effectively, recognizing patterns, and depositing in memory organized reference images. The knowing derived from perceptual acuity, such as that needed to discern spasticity and achievement motivation, is also contained in the art of clinical reasoning. Linking the model of the patient with the appropriate memory structures to build a theory of practice for the patient requires considerable acumen. Artistic insight reaches its peak in combining evidence and opinion to support arguments convincingly, thus bringing closure to the decision-making process. Although each of these processes is difficult to master in and of itself, getting them coordinated and "on line" so that one can think "on one's feet" is an even vaster task.

Experts and Novices

The automation of clinical reasoning is not merely a matter of thinking faster. Experts think differently from novices. Because of the limited capacity of short-term memory, the human mind can only consider five to nine units of information at a time (16). This is why we find it difficult to remember telephone numbers. If I asked you to remember 9 1 9 9 6 6 2 4 5 1, chances are you would have forgotten the number long before you arrived at a telephone to dial it. However, if you knew that the area code for Chapel Hill is 919, and that all university numbers begin with the prefix 966, it is likely that you would have remembered the number 919-966-2451 correctly. Memory is aided by organizing and chunking information into larger units. By chunking telephone digits into familiar patterns, the number of units to be remembered is reduced and falls within the capacity of working memory.

Evidence is accumulating that expert and novice problem solvers differ in their use of problem-solving strategies, such as chunking (19). The expert sees and stores cues in patterns and configurations, whereas the novice records individual cues. Experts chunk data into larger information units than novices do. The expert creates memory structures by classifying data according to how they are to be applied in practice. The novice's memory structures, on the other hand, arise from features more peripheral to functional usage. The novice relies on conceptual principles to get things out of memory. The expert retrieves knowledge on the basis of situational cues as well as on conceptual stimuli. As the reasoning process unfolds, experts monitor their own thinking and understanding, which enables them to curtail errors and omissions. The ability to think faster is thus a result of thinking more efficiently, more functionally, and more critically.

Simply because our knowledge is in our action does not mean that we cannot think about it. When skill breaks down, and we strike a discordant note, drop a stitch, or fall off a bicycle, we step back, slow down our pace, and reflect on our actions. In clinical reasoning, skill breakdown occurs when clinical data are incongruous with our expectations and experience. Artistic inquiry is spurred by perplexity. As long as we are assessing patients whom we perceive as highly similar to those we have treated in the past, the clinical encounter presents no challenges, our intuitive understanding of the situation remains tacit. However, when we are no longer able to see things as we previously saw them, or do things as we previously did them, our curiosity is engaged, our anxiety is aroused, and we become inquisitive practitioners.

Expert clinicians are those who are competent in action and, simultaneously, reflect on this action to learn from it (6). They create opportunities for introspection by critically examining their reasoning to disclose bias and inconsistency. Artistic inquiry is also initiated through reframing, that is, by looking at the clinical situation from a new perspective. For example, a therapist might reason, "What would happen if this patient with low back pain were treated by diverting attention from back pain to pleasurable activity, instead of with exercises to improve body mechanics?"

As thinking becomes less automatic and more conscious, through self-criticism and reframing, it also becomes more accessible to explanation. Although our explanations and descriptions of clinical reasoning may never be complete, they can become progressively more adequate through reflection, and the artistic dimension can be better understood. The conversion of our practice into theory revolves around a cycle of concrete experience, reflective thinking, conceptual integration, and active experimentation.

In conclusion, the clinician functions as a scientist, ethicist, and artist. The scientific, ethical, and artistic dimensions of clinical reasoning are inextricably intertwined, and each strand is needed to strengthen the line of thought leading to understanding. Without science, clinical inquiry is not systematic; without ethics, it is not responsible; without art, it is not convincing. The intentions and potentials of chronically disabled patients are difficult to discern, but a therapist of understanding will elicit them, and use them to help patients discover health within themselves.

Acknowledgments

Sincere appreciation is expressed to the following individuals for their critical review of the ideas presented in this paper: Anne Blakeney, David Hollingsworth, Teena Snow, and Joyce Sparling.

References

1. Pellegrino ED, Thomasma DC: *A Philosophical Basis of Medical Practice,* New York: Oxford University Press, 1981.
2. Scriven M: Clinical judgment. In *Clinical Judgment: A Critical Appraisal,* HT Engelhardt, SF Spicker, B Towers, Editors. Dordrecht, Holland: D. Reidel Publishing Co., 1979, pp. 3–16.
3. Cutler P: *Problem Solving in Clinical Medicine: From Data to Diagnosis,* New York: Basic Books, Inc., 1979.
4. Sober E: The art of science of clinical judgment: An informational approach. In *Clinical Judgment: A Critical Appraisal,* HT Engelhardt, SF Spicker, B Towers, Editors. Dordrecht, Holland: D. Reidel Publishing Co., 1979, pp. 29–44.
5. Feinstein AR: Scientific methodology in clinical medicine, III. The evaluation of therapeutic response. *Am Intern Med 61:* 944–966, 1964.
6. Schön DA: *The Reflective Practitioner: How Professionals Think in Action,* New York: Basic Books, Inc., 1983.
7. Brody H: *Ethical Decisions in Medicine,* Boston: Little, Brown, and Co., 1981.
8. McArthur C: Analyzing the clinical process. *J Counseling Psychol 1:* 203–208, 1954.
9. Koester GA: A study of diagnostic reasoning. *Educ Psychol Measurement 14:* 473–486, 1954.
10. Agnew NM, Pyke SW: *The Science Game,* Englewood Cliffs, NJ: Prentice Hall, 1969.
11. Rogers JC, Masagatani G: Clinical reasoning of occupational therapists during the initial assessment of physically disabled patients. *Occup Ther Res 2:* 195–219, 1982.
12. Shriver D, Mitcham M, Schwartzberg S, Ranucci M: Uniform occupational therapy evaluation checklist. In *Reference Manual of the Official Documents of The American Occupational Therapy Association,* 1983.
13. Elstein AS, Shulman LS, Sprafka SA: *Problem Solving: An Analysis of Clinical Reasoning,* Cambridge, MA: Harvard University Press, 1978.
14. Wright BA, Fletcher BL: Uncovering hidden resources; A challenge in assessment. *Prof Psychol 13:* 229–235, 1982.
15. Bateson CD, O'Quin K, Pych V: An attribution theory analysis of trained helpers' inferences about clients' needs. In *Basic Processes in Helping Relationships,* TA Wills, Editor. New York: Academic Press, 1982, pp. 59–80.
16. Matlin M: *Cognition,* New York: Holt, Rinehart, and Winston, 1983.
17. Sarbin TR, Taft R, Bailey DE: *Clinical Inference and Cognitive Theory,* New York: Holt, Rinehart, and Winston, 1960.
18. Allport GW: *Pattern and Growth in Personality,* New York: Holt, Rinehart, and Winston, 1961.
19. Feltovich PJ: Expertise: reorganizing and refining knowledge for use. *Professional Education Researcher Notes,* December 1982/January 1983, pp. 5–9.

The Therapist With the Three-Track Mind

CHAPTER 44

MAUREEN HAYES FLEMING,
EdD, OTR, FAOTA

The primary purpose of the American Occupational Therapy Association/American Occupational Therapy Foundation Clinical Reasoning Study was to identify the reasoning strategy that occupational therapists used to guide their practice. The designers of this study assumed that there was one reasoning style that is typical of clinical reasoning in occupational therapy. They decided that ethnography was the research method (Gillette & Mattingly, 1987) most likely to enable them to identify this typical or best reasoning style. However, as investigators, Mattingly and I soon realized that the occupational therapists in the study employed a variety of reasoning strategies.

During the early stages of the research project, when we were still searching for a single reasoning style, the apparent use of several forms of reasoning led us to believe that the therapists' thinking was inconsistent or scattered. Further analysis of the videotapes of treatment sessions, interviews, and group discussions with the therapist–subjects gave us deeper insight into their reasoning processes. They employed different modes of thinking for different purposes or in response to particular features of the clinical problem. The occupational therapists in the study seemed to use at least four different types of reasoning: narrative reasoning (Mattingly, 1989, 1991), procedural reasoning, interactive reasoning, and conditional reasoning (Fleming, 1989). These last three types of reasoning are discussed in the present chapter.

Another insight was that each type of reasoning seemed to be employed to address different aspects of the whole problem. Eventually, we realized that the therapist–subjects attended to the patient at three levels: (a) the physical ailment, (b) the patient as a person, and (c) the person as a social being in the context of family, environment, and culture. We then saw that each type of reasoning was employed to address a particular level of concern. The procedural reasoning strategy was used when the therapist thought about the person's physical ailments and what procedures were appropriate to alleviate them. Interactive reasoning was used to help the therapist interact with and understand the person better. Conditional reasoning, a complex form of social reasoning, was used to help the patient in the difficult process of reconstructing a life now permanently changed by injury or disease.

These three reasoning strategies appeared to be distinctly different, yet the therapist–subjects seemed to shift rapidly from one form of reasoning to another. They changed reasoning styles as their attention was drawn from the original concern to treat the physical ailment to other features of the problem, such as the particular person's response to the present activity. Using procedural reasoning, the therapist–subjects readily moved back to the physical problem that they had been pursuing earlier. They analyzed different aspects of the problem simultaneously. They used different thinking styles without losing track of some aspects of the problem while they temporarily shifted attention to another feature of the problem. We began to think about these styles of reasoning as different operations that interacted with each other in the therapist's mind. We referred to these operations as different *tracks* for guiding thinking.

Thus, we developed the notion of the occupational therapist as a therapist with a three-track mind. The track analogy helped us envision how a therapist thought about the multiple and diverse issues that pertained to the patient's problems and the therapist's ability to influence them.

Procedural Reasoning

The therapist–subjects used what we called *procedural reasoning* when they were thinking about the disease or disability and deciding on which treatment activities (procedures) they might employ to remediate the person's functional performance problems. In this mode, the therapists' dual search was for problem definition and treatment selection. In situations where problem identification and treatment selection were seen as the central task, the therapists' thinking strategies demonstrated many parallels to the patterns identified by other researchers interested in problem solving in general and clinical problem solving in particular (Coughlin & Patel, 1987; Elstein, Shulman, & Sprafka, 1978; Newell & Simon, 1972; Rogers & Masagatani, 1982). The problem-solving sequence of diagnosis, prognosis, and prescription, which is typical of physicians' reasoning, was commonly used. However, the words the therapists used to describe this sequence were *problem identification, goal setting,* and *treatment planning.*

Experienced therapists in the study used forms of reasoning similar to the problem-solving strategies identified by many investigators who study physicians. For example, therapists used all three problem-solving methods described by Newell and Simon (1972)—recognition, generation and testing, and heuristic search. They also displayed characteristics identified by Elstein et al. (1978), such as cue identification, hypothesis generation, cue interpretation, and hypothesis evaluation. They interpreted patterns of cues, much like the ones that Coughlin and Patel (1987) identified among physicians and medical students. The structural features of the hypotheses generated by the therapists were similar to those of medical students in a study by Allal (as cited by Elstein et al., 1978), that is, hierarchical organization, competing formulations, multiple subspaces, and functional relationships.

One characteristic of reasoning common to all of the physicians and medical students in the studies by Elstein et al. (1978) was generation and evaluation of competing hypotheses. Physicians always looked for more than one potential cause of the problem presented. They devoted a considerable portion of their reasoning efforts to seeking additional cues and rearranging hypotheses in their minds in order to either support or negate more than one possible cause of the presenting ailment. Competing hypothesis generation was also a strategy commonly used by the occupational therapists. The experienced therapists in this study typically generated two to four possible hypotheses regarding the cause and nature of aspects of the person's problem. They generated several hypotheses about potential treatment activities as well. However, there was a tendency among the newer therapists to seek the right answer rather than to generate hypotheses about possibilities. When they generated hypotheses, they tended to consider only one or two of them.

Elstein et al. (1978) noticed a phenomenon that they referred to as *early hypothesis generation,* which they interpreted as being an attempt on the part of the physician to define, or mentally enter, the appropriate problem space, as theorized by Newell and Simon (1972). Newell and Simon hypothesized that abstract thinkers categorized problems or phenomena in different spaces or areas of the possible source of the problem or avenue of inquiry. A similar notion was advanced by Feinstein (1973), who suggested that physicians' thinking would be improved if they systematically searched for sources of the problem using a reverse hierarchical method. Using this method, physicians would think of what area of the body was involved, then what system, then what organ, then what process, until the problem space was sufficiently defined and specific problems could be identified. Experienced therapists seemed to quickly identify and search within the appropriate problem spaces. Novice therapists had more difficulty with this task.

It makes sense that occupational therapists who work in a medical center, as did the subjects in the Clinical Reasoning Study, and for whom part of their education contained long hours of medical lectures, would use a thinking style similar to that used in medical decision-making. That therapists frequently used these logical reasoning styles was expected. However, it was surprising that therapists often did not use these styles. This phenomenon led us to search for other modes of thought that the therapist–subjects might be using.

In discussions with the therapists, a few persistent themes emerged. At first, these themes did not seem to be explicitly linked to clinical reasoning. Some seemed to be distractions from discussing reasoning. Later, we found that these seeming distractions were important to the therapists' thinking about clinical problems. Our misunderstanding of these possible distractions was a result of our initial failure to recognize that therapists viewed clinical problems from more than one perspective. After examining these perspectives, we achieved a greater understanding of how therapists think in general and how they think differently about different aspects of the patient's situation.

We were able to identify these perspectives by analyzing several of the persistent themes that flowed through the therapists' conversations. One such theme was that the therapist–subjects often questioned what aspects of the person and the disability were appropriate for them to treat. In one group discussion, we were analyzing a videotape in which a therapist was attempting to encourage an outpatient to solve a problem. The personal care attendants he hired all quit after only a few weeks of working with him. The therapist was unable to convince the patient that this was a problem. He engaged in a wide range of what therapists referred to as avoidance tactics. Clearly the therapist and the patient had differing points of view on this issue. As the problem was discussed, many therapists in the group interpreted it as a value conflict between the patient and the therapist. There were at least two value conflicts here. One was the that the therapist thought it was unsafe for the patient to live alone without someone to assist him in accessing the bed, the tub, the toilet, or his wheelchair. The patient had fallen many times while attempting these moves by himself, and his solution was to call the fire department in his small town and have someone come to his house and pick him up. The patient viewed this as a simple solution, whereas the therapist viewed it as poor judgment and irresponsibility. Another conflict was that the therapist believed that the patient should keep himself and his home cleaner. The patient did not agree with this. The group of therapists focused on whether the therapist should have pursued the discussion. The concern was whether or not the therapist, who specialized in treating physical disabilities, should have been discussing personal issues with the patient. Some group members believed that discussions of personal issues were under the aegis of psychiatric therapists only. A therapist who worked in a psychiatric setting then said that in her hospital, occupational therapists were not supposed to discuss personal issues; only psychiatrists were to discuss personal issues. In her setting, therapists could only discuss observable behaviors and relate them back to possible implications for such concerns as how one behaves at work. The discussion became more intense regarding the role of the different types of occupational therapists and what they could and could not do or discuss with their patients. It was clear that the group members had different opinions regarding the appropriate depth and range of their interaction with patients. This difference was not divided along specialty lines. One therapist said, "Well, I work in physical disabilities and I talk about all sorts of things with my patients." Others confirmed her position. The therapists were not in agreement regarding their role in discussing the more personal issues and what they considered to be intimate or embarrassing aspects of the person's thoughts, feelings, bodily functions, or history. Some believed that therapists should treat the whole person. However, others believed that their role was to treat only the physical aspects of the person's disability or functional limitation. Still other therapists were undecided about their stance on these issues.

A related issue came up weeks later in a discussion group with experienced therapists. Their concern was to identify exactly what constitutes treatment. They wanted to define which of the therapist's actions were part of the therapeutic process and which were not. These therapists were generally comfortable with the notion of treating the whole patient, but they were not sure whether their conversations with patients were part of the treatment. Because the therapists in this particular hospital tended to see patients on a fairly long-term basis, they knew the patients as individuals quite well. There seemed to be confusion regarding whether the therapist's understanding of the individual person and his or her con-

cerns was part of therapy or simply an artifact of the therapist's personality. Some therapists felt strongly that the relationship with the patient was an essential element of the therapy. Others saw it as an adjunct to therapy. Still others saw it as not a part of therapy. Some believed that personal discussions were inappropriate.

It seemed that these two related issues of what aspects of the person an occupational therapist treats and what actions of the occupational therapist constitute the therapeutic process were sources of conflict for the therapists. There were two types of conflict. The opinion held by some therapists that occupational therapists should treat the whole person conflicted with the opinion that therapists should treat only the physical problems. Another conflict was that some therapists were uncertain about which of these two points of view or perspectives was the right one. This conflict seemed to be created, at least in part, by a perceived conflict between the medical model perspective and the humanistic perspective.

Therapists who had strong beliefs that their relationship with patients was an effective part of therapy thought that those beliefs were in conflict with the perspective of the medical setting. Issues such as what constitutes therapy, the role of the therapist, turf boundaries, and the necessity for scientific evidence as a validation of practice all served to deny or devalue the importance of therapists' concerns for the patient as a person. This feeling was so pervasive that some therapists had difficulty appreciating the depth and complexity of their practice. They seemed confused and wondered whether they should accept their own interpretations of their practice or the interpretations of individuals and groups around them. The discussions were full of comments like the following:

> Well, I know I was supposed to be teaching the lady bathing techniques. After all, that's my job—that's what I get paid for. But she really wanted to talk to me about her grandchild. So I did and she felt better and we understood each other better. Besides, what was I going to say? "Don't talk to me while you take a bath"? She has been much better at learning the bathing since that session, by the way. Of course, I put on the chart, "bathing training," but I sort of felt guilty even though I know I did the right thing. I know I wasn't wasting time chatting, but it could have looked that way.

The therapists believed that the physicians, administrators, and especially the insurance companies did not value their interactions with patients. They further believed that these various authorities would criticize them for interacting with patients and taking time away from what the authorities considered the real treatment. It soon became clear that those therapists who valued their relationship with the patient persisted in interacting with them as people regardless of the requirements of the hospital and reimbursement agencies. Therapists talked to, listened to, understood, and were respected by their patients. Therapists and patients valued these interactions. Most therapists valued interacting with patients but did not report talking with patients.

This process of conducting essentially two types of practice, one focused on the procedural treatment of the person's physical body and the other focused on the phenomenological person as an individual, is discussed by Mattingly (1991). The point here is that while two practices were conducted, only one was reported—the procedural practice. The interactive practice, which was the unreported practice, we called the underground practice. Later, we saw that although often underground, this sort of practice was important both to patients and therapists. It also had a logic or reasoning strategy of its own and a particular way of guiding therapists' thoughts and actions. We called this *interactive reasoning*.

Interactive Reasoning

Interactive reasoning took place during face-to-face encounters between the therapist and the patient. It was the form of reasoning that therapists employed when they wanted to understand the patient as an individual. There were many reasons why a therapist might want to know the person better. The therapist might want to know how the person felt about the treatment at the moment or what the patient was like as a person, either out of sheer interest or in order to more finely tailor the treatment to his or her specific needs or preferences. Further, the therapist might be interested in this patient in order to better understand the experience of the disability from the person's own point of view. This is what Kleinman (1980) called the *illness perspective,* as contrasted with the *disease perspective*. The therapists wanted to know what the illness experience was like for a person. They wanted to understand the patients from their own point of view. Interactive reasoning occurred when therapists took the phenomenological perspective (Kestenbaum, 1982), although the therapists did not typically use that term to explain a shift to the humanistic point of view.

Several people have been interested in the clinical reasoning study and have analyzed various videotapes made during the data-gathering stage. Some have examined different aspects of interactive reasoning. The depth of these analyses is impressive, as is the complexity of the interactive reasoning strategies discovered. A compilation of those analyses shows us that therapists appeared to employ interactive reasoning for at least eight reasons or purposes, as follows:

1. To engage the person in the treatment session (Mattingly, 1989, identified six such strategies).
2. To know the person as a person (Cohn, 1989).
3. To understand a disability from the patient's point of view (Mattingly, 1989).
4. To finely match the treatment goals and strategies to this patient with this disability and this experience. Therapists call this process *individualizing treatment* (Fleming, 1989).

5. To communicate a sense of acceptance, trust, or hope to the patient (Langthaler, 1990).
6. To use humor to relieve tension (Siegler, 1987).
7. To construct a shared language of actions and meanings (Crepeau, 1991).
8. To determine if the treatment session is going well (Fleming, 1990).

It seems that although the therapists did not initially recognize interaction and interactive reasoning as central to their practice, they used it at least as an adjunct to practice on many occasions for various reasons. Perhaps particular interactive strategies were used for particular therapeutic reasons. Some of the reasoning styles or strategies identified and the hypothesized reasons for their use are similar to new concepts about reasoning that have been proposed by various psychologists and philosophers. Gardner (1985), for example, proposed that there are many useful ways to think and that hypothetical deductive reasoning is not necessarily the only, or even the best, way to think. Many forms of reasoning have been suggested by investigators who study how persons think about themselves and their experience within the cultural context (Berger & Luckman, 1967; Bruner, 1986, 1990). Many are concerned with how such elusive processes as values, norms (Perry, 1979), and symbolic meanings (Koestler, 1948) are used to guide, gauge, frame, and formulate thought and action (Bernstein, 1971; Dreyfus & Dreyfus, 1986; Geertz, 1983; Schön, 1983). Others examine properties of problems and relate them to particular problem-solving strategies. Some propose that features of the problem will influence individuals and, in effect, direct them to select a particular problem-solving method. Such features may include salient characteristics of a task or problem (Hammond, 1988), the context (Greeno, 1989), individual interests and talents (Gardner, 1985), or experience (Dewey, 1915).

The notion that characteristics of the presumed problem will prompt a particular thinking process seemed to be borne out in our observations of the therapists in the clinical reasoning study. The therapists shifted from one form of thinking to another. They often noted subtle cues and responded to them rapidly, then returned to another task and thinking mode without "skipping a beat," as one observer commented.

If such numerous reasoning strategies exist, and if the therapists had different purposes in mind for using interaction as a therapeutic medium, then it also seems likely that the purpose of the interaction would prompt the use of a particular reasoning strategy. For example, in trying to understand the person as a person, therapists' reasoning resembled what Belenky, Clinchy, Goldberger, and Tarule (1986) described as connected knowing, which they linked to empathy. In trying to understand the disability from the patient's point of view, therapists used a phenomenological approach similar to that advocated by Paget (1988). Therapists' interactions with patients created an understanding of the person as an individual within a culturally constructed point of view, or what Schutz (1975) called a reciprocity of motives.

When individualizing treatment, therapists appeared to be functioning intuitively rather than analytically. Hammond (1988) proposed, however, that intuitive reasoning is as effective and complex as analytical reasoning. Intuitive reasoning is employed in response to problems that are not well defined. Tasks in which there are many cues from several sources and that require perceptual rather than instrumental measurement, Hammond argued, induce the person to use intuitive methods of problem solving. He further asserted that in these situations, analytical reasoning would be less effective than intuitive reasoning.

The interactive reasoning strategies that Mattingly (1989) identified indicate that therapists use several ways to engage the patient in treatment. To be effective, some of these strategies require complex interpretations of subtle interactive cues. The 23 interactive strategies that one therapist used in treatment, which were identified by Langthaler (1990), seem to suggest that the therapist was partially influenced by psychoanalytic theorists such as Rogers (1961) and occupational therapy theorists such as Fidler and Fidler (1963) and Mosey (1970). This finding is not surprising, because occupational therapy students are required to read the works of these theorists. The complexity, subtlety, and facility with which some therapists used numerous interaction forms, however, suggest processes far more complex than could be accounted for by professional education alone.

We also had a strong sense that the therapists' reasoning about and interaction with patients was directly related to their values. Their sense of the importance of patients as individuals leads one to draw parallels to beliefs about ethical and moral decision-making, such as those expressed by Gilligan (1982), Kegan (1982), and Perry (1979). The task of monitoring the patient's feelings about the treatment and yet managing that treatment, which is often difficult and sometimes painful or distasteful, seems to require a considerable amount of what Gardner (1985) referred to as *interpersonal intelligence*. Gardner postulated two kinds of interpersonal intelligence: "The capacity to access one's own feeling life" and the "ability to notice and make distinctions among other individuals in particular among their moods, temperaments, motivations and intentions" (p. 239). Interactive reasoning requires active judgment (Buchler, 1955) on several levels simultaneously. This requires that the therapist analyze cues from the patient, transmit his or her interpretation of the patient, and interpret the patient's interpretations of the therapist's interpretations quickly and accurately. This reciprocal process is one that Erikson (1968) considered essential to identity formation and future social interaction capabilities. Possibly, the therapist's ability to interact successfully and therapeutically is strongly linked to his or her personal and professional identify. Gardner hypothesized that interpersonal

intelligence is based on a well-developed sense of self. Certainly it is linked to professional self-confidence. Novice therapists reported that in their first year of practice they did not have the confidence, nor did they believe they had the right, to interact with patients as individuals. They reported that they "stuck to the procedural" until they were confident in their use of those skills. We observed therapists even in the second year of practice going back and forth between the procedural and interactive modes of treating their patients. In the experienced senior therapists, procedural and interactive forms seemed to flow together, each enhancing the other.

We therefore found that interaction, which at first seemed like a distraction from treatment or, at best, an adjunct to it, was a necessary and legitimate form of therapy. Interactive reasoning was used effectively by most therapists to guide this aspect of their treatment. It appears that procedural reasoning guides treatment and interactive reasoning guides therapy. Although interactive reasoning is far more difficult to map than procedural reasoning, we will continue to make observations and develop theory in this area.

Conditional Reasoning

The concept of conditional reasoning is perhaps the most elusive notion in our proposed theory of a three-track mind. Yet we are firmly, if intuitively, convinced that there is a third form of reasoning that many therapists used. This reasoning style moves beyond specific concerns about the person and the physical problems placed on them to broader social and temporal contexts. The term *conditional* was used in three different ways. First, the therapist thought about the whole condition, which involved the person, the illness, and the meanings the illness had for the person, the family, and the social and physical contexts in which the person lived. Second, the therapist needed to imagine how the condition could change. The imagined new state was a conditional (i.e., temporary) state that might or might not be achieved. Third, the success or failure of treatment was contingent on the patient's participation. The patient must participate not only in the therapeutic activities themselves, but also in the construction of the image of the possible outcome, that is, the revised condition.

Conditional reasoning seems to be a multidimensional process involving complicated, but not strictly logical, forms of thinking. In using conditional reasoning, the therapist appears to reflect on the success or failure of the clinical encounter from both the procedural and interactive standpoints and attempts to integrate the two. Thinking then moves beyond those immediate concerns to a deeper level of interpretation of the whole problem. The therapist interprets the meaning of therapy in the context of a possible future for the person. The therapist imagines what that future would be like. This imagined future is a guide to bringing about a revised condition through therapy. This thinking process is essentially imagination tempered by clinical experience and expertise.

The therapists tried to imagine what the person was like before the injury. Similarly, they tried to estimate or imagine what the possibilities were for the person's future life. By imagining, therapists mentally placed the person in contexts of current, past, and future social worlds. The therapists used imagination in order to best match the treatment selections to the specific interests, capacities, and goals of the person. Thus, the therapists were able to make their current treatment relevant to the individual patient. The present treatment, therefore, was not simply a link to future performance, but also was imagined within the context of a life in process.

Perhaps this form of reasoning is best described by example. Cathy, a pediatric therapist, was the most articulate about using this form of reasoning. Cathy usually treated very young children who lived in the community and had come to an outpatient early intervention program. The child's mother or guardian was usually present, and Cathy invariably included the mother in the session. The mother might be enlisted to hold the baby in an advantageous position or to help sustain the child's interest. Cathy would often talk to the mother while simultaneously working with the child. She often asked questions like, "Does he do this at home?" "Does he usually cry in this sort of situation?" "What does he like to do?" "Does he usually have difficulty calming himself down?" These were not diagnostic history-taking questions in the medical procedural sense. Cathy said she asked these questions to construct an image of what the child was really like on a day-to-day basis. She told us that she used this image to structure her treatment and imagine possible goals for the child. As she said:

> I see this little child and his movement patterns and his difficulties, and then I imagine what he will be like in 2 years and then when he is 5 (years old) and maybe going to school. I think of what I can do to help him develop the skills that he will need to function in school and in the community and what he will be like and how his family will be with him.

Here Cathy describes a process of imagining and integrating images of the past, present, and future for this child given the variables of the child himself, his developmental delays and disabilities, his family situation, the social and educational opportunities available to him, what he might be able to do in the future, and how she might enable that future condition to come about.

Clearly, it takes professional experience to be able to project the possible developmental pattern and potential rate of success in attaining a future developmental level. It also requires a mind that is imaginative, curious, and interested in future possibilities. Conditional reasoning involves a way of thinking that may include a systems perspective and that extends to the future (Mattingly, 1989), yet it moves beyond this perspective to an analysis of present interactions (Kielhofner, 1978;

Mattingly, 1989), so that one can envision how these interactions might help create a better life for the child.

Having constructed these images, which changed slightly over time and throughout the course of treatment, the therapists used images as a way of interpreting the importance of the patient's treatment. Therapists would mentally compare the patient's abilities today and the relative success of today's treatment session against images of what the person was like before. They also compared where the patient was today to where they wanted the patient to be in the future. Each therapist would envision the patient today and estimate how close that was to where he or she thought the patient should be at this point in the course of treatment. They would mentally check to see how far the patient had come toward attaining the future the therapist had in mind. The evaluation of today's treatment was made in the context of past and future possibilities. Therefore, the particular state of things today would serve as a mental mile marker for indicating progress toward a distant, and perhaps only dimly perceived, future.

One reason that we called this conditional reasoning was because a change in the present condition was conditional on the therapist's and the patient's participation in effective therapy. This condition was dependent not only on the therapist's ability to engage the patient in treatment in the sense discussed in the interactive section, but also on building a shared image of the person's future self. This image building was often accomplished through stories or narrative, as described by Mattingly (1991). However, in many aspects of therapeutic interaction, the images that the therapists helped to build were often based in action. Pediatric therapists often included the mother in creating a mental image of the child in the future. This image was projected into the distant future, such as when a therapist wondered what an infant she was treating would be like in school several years later. Therapists projected images into the near future as well. They also used images as a way of extending therapy into the home setting. Cathy said to the child's mother, "Would he do this at home? Could he just sit quietly and look at something and have this nice position? Could the kids maybe hold him like I am doing while they watch TV?" Here she created a visual image, based on action in the present, of the child in a near-future situation. This was done not only to enhance the therapy, but also to build an image of the child as a participant in the family, rather than just as a disabled baby.

One technique for conveying these images that therapists often used was to tell patients that they were getting better and to produce evidence of this by saying such things as, "Remember when you could not do this? Now you can." Sometimes the therapists would also use this technique for themselves. Therapists commented that when they were discouraged with a patient's progress, they found it helpful to remind themselves of how far the patient had come. This technique helped both the patient and the therapist focus on the importance of their joint participation in this enterprise of treatment. It helped them through difficult, frustrating, and boring times and allowed them to place the moment in a more positive, though abstract and distant, context. Most importantly, it seemed to remind them that the condition was changing. Such changes were often quantitative, such as increased range of motion, and would be noted in the person's chart. But qualitative changes and their meanings were equally important to therapists and patients. Although these changes were not reported in the patient's chart, they did indicate progress toward that shared future image that the therapist and patient jointly constructed and worked toward. Meaningful progress was best measured through the therapist's and patient's collective memory. Therapists were not simply saying, "This is progress. Remember how bad things were before?" Instead, they were saying, "If you have come this far, maybe we will get to where you imagined you would be, even though you are discouraged today."

Putting It All Together: Treating the Whole Person

The therapists in the Clinical Reasoning Study often used two phrases to describe their treatment—*putting it all together* and *treating the whole person.* Treating the whole person did not mean that the therapists were in charge of the patient's whole medical and psychological treatment. In fact, in the traditional medical sense of the word *treatment,* occupational therapists are peripheral to the patient's treatment. The phrase was intended to convey the belief that therapists concern themselves with the patient as a person, that is, as an individual with many facets, interests, and concerns. By saying that they treat the whole person, therapists mean that they treat the person as a whole, not as the sum of ill and healthy parts.

The phrase *putting it all together* seemed to mean that although the therapists often had to think only about the disability or only of the individual patient at a given moment, they were concerned that they eventually thought and did something about the patient as a whole person, that is, person, illness, and condition. Although they used several types of reasoning and addressed several different types of concerns, therapists always wanted their reasoning to track back to making a better life for the patient as a person. Their ultimate goal was to use as many strategies as necessary to improve the individual functional performance of the person. Because functional performance requires intentionality, physical action, and social meaning, it is not surprising that persons who concern themselves with enabling function would have to address problems of the person's sense of self and future, the physical body, and meanings and social and cultural contexts—contexts in which actions are taken and meanings are made. Because these areas of inquiry are typically guided by different types of thinking, it seems necessary that therapists become facile in thinking about different aspects of human beings using various styles of reasoning. Perhaps these multiple ways of thinking guide the therapists

in accomplishing and evaluating the mysterious process of "putting it all together" for the person. This process, which enables the whole person to function as a new self in the future, seemed to be guided by a complex yet unidentified form of reasoning that was both directed and conditional.

Conclusion

The Clinical Reasoning Study showed that therapists use several different types of reasoning to solve problems and to design and conduct therapeutic processes. Further, the particular reasoning processes are selected to guide inquiry into different aspects of the person's problem or of the therapist's intervention. As part of this research process, we developed a theory about these reasoning processes and constructed concepts to which we added terminology in order to discuss these concepts among ourselves and with the therapists. Thus, we referred to the type of reasoning that was used to guide those aspects of practice that are concerned with the treatment of the patient's physical ailment as *procedural reasoning.* *Interactive reasoning,* we propose, is a type of reasoning that therapists used to guide their interactions with the person. *Conditional reasoning* is both an imaginative and an integrative form of reasoning that the more proficient therapists used to think about the patient and his or her future, given the constraints of the physical condition within the patient's personal and social context. The therapists who were part of this study confirmed our assumptions that they use different forms of reasoning for different parts of the problem and found these concepts and terms useful in understanding and explaining their reasoning and practice.

References

Belenky, M. F., Clinchy, B. M., Goldberger, N. R., & Tarule, J. M. (1986). *Women's ways of knowing.* New York: Basic.

Berger, P., & Luckman, T. (1967). *The social construction of reality.* Garden City, NJ: Anchor.

Bernstein, R. J. (1971). *Praxis and action.* Philadelphia: University of Pennsylvania Press.

Bruner, J. (1986). *Actual minds, possible worlds.* Cambridge, MA: Harvard University Press.

Bruner, J. (1990). *Acts of meaning.* Cambridge, MA: Harvard University Press.

Buchler, J. (1955). *Nature and judgement.* New York: Columbia University Press.

Cohn, E. S. (1989). Fieldwork education: Shaping a foundation for clinical reasoning. *American Journal of Occupational Therapy, 43,* 240–244.

Coughlin, L. D., & Patel, V. L. (1987). Processing of critical information by physicians and medical students. *Journal of Medical Education 62,* 818–828.

Creapeau, E. B. (1991). Achieving intersubjective understanding: Examples from an occupational therapy treatment session. *American Journal of Occupational Therapy, 45,* 1016–1025.

Dewey, J. (1915). The logic of judgments of practice. *Journal of Philosophy, 12,* 505.

Dreyfus, H. L., & Dreyfus, S. E. (1986). *Mind over machine.* New York: Macmillan.

Elstein, A., Shulman, L., & Sprafka, A. (1978). *Medical problem solving. An analysis of clinical reasoning.* Boston: Harvard University Press.

Erikson, E. H. (1968). *Identity, youth, and crisis*. New York: Norton.

Feinstein, A. R. (1973). An analysis of diagnostic reasoning, Parts I & II. *Yale Journal of Biology and Medicine, 46*, 212–232, 264–283.

Fidler, G., & Fidler, J. (1963). *Occupational therapy: A communication process in psychiatry*. New York: Macmillan.

Fleming, M. H. (1989). The therapist with the three-track mind. In *The AOTA Practice Symposium program guide* (pp. 70–75). Bethesda, MD: American Occupational Therapy Association.

Fleming, M. (Ed.). (1990). *Proceedings of the Clinical Reasoning Institute for occupational therapy educators*. Medford, MA: Tufts University.

Gardner, H. (1985). *Frames of mind: The theory of multiple intelligences*. New York: Basic.

Geertz, C. (1983). *Local knowledge: Further essays in interpretive anthropology*. New York: Basic.

Gillette, N. P., & Mattingly, C. (1987). The Foundation—Clinical reasoning in occupational therapy. *American Journal of Occupational Therapy, 41*, 399–400.

Gilligan, C. (1982). *In a different voice: Psychological theory and women's development*. Cambridge, MA: Harvard University Press.

Greeno, J. (1989). A perspective on thinking. *American Psychologist, 44*, 134–141.

Hammond, K. H. (1988). Judgment and decision-making in dynamic tasks. *Information and Decision Technologies, 14*, 3–14.

Kegan, R. (1982). *The evolving self: Problems and process in human development*. Cambridge, MA: Harvard University Press.

Kestenbaum, V. (1982). *The humanity of the ill: Phenomenological perspectives*. Knoxville, TN: University of Tennessee Press.

Kielhofner, G. (1978). General systems theory: Implications for theory and action in occupational therapy. *American Journal of Occupational Therapy, 32*, 637–645.

Kleinman, A. (1980). *Patients and healers in the context of culture*. Los Angeles: University of California Press.

Koestler, A. (1948). *Insight and outlook: An inquiry into the common foundations of science, art, and social ethics*. Lincoln, NE: University of Nebraska Press.

Langthaler, M. (1990). *The components of therapeutic relationship in occupational therapy*. Unpublished master's thesis. Tufts University, Medford, MA.

Mattingly, C. (1989), *Thinking with stories: Story and experience in a clinical practice*. Unpublished doctoral dissertation, Massachusetts Institute of Technology, Cambridge, MA.

Mattingly, C. (1991). What is clinical reasoning? *American Journal of Occupational Therapy, 45*, 979–986.

Mosey, A. C. (1970). *Three frames of reference for mental health*. Thorofare, NJ: Slack.

Newell, A., & Simon, H. (1972). *Human problem solving*. Englewood Cliffs, NJ: Prentice Hall.

Paget, M. (1988). *The unity of mistakes*. Philadelphia: Temple University Press.

Perry, W. (1979). *Forms of intellectual and ethical development in the college years*. New York: Holt, Rinehart & Winston.

Rogers, C. (1961). *On becoming a person*. Boston: Houghton Mifflin.

Rogers, J. C., & Masagatani, G. (1982). Clinical reasoning of occupational therapists during the initial assessment of physically disabled patients. *Occupational Therapy Journal of Research, 2*, 195–219.

Schön, D. (1983). *The reflective practitioner: How professionals think in action*. New York: Basic.

Schutz, A. (1975). *On phenomenology and social relations*. Chicago: University of Chicago Press.

Siegler, C. C. (1987). *Functions of humor in occupational therapy*. Unpublished master's thesis, Tufts University, Medford, MA.

What Is a Worthy Goal of Occupational Therapy?

JEFFREY CRABTREE

Our profession, particularly in the United States, as evidenced by much of its literature, appears to believe that functional independence in performance areas amounts to our ultimate goal. To cite a few examples, the American Occupational Therapy Association (AOTA, 1994a) maintained that "function in performance areas is the ultimate concern of occupation therapy" (p. 1047). DiJoseph (1982) asserted that independence, gained through purposeful activity, is the essence of occupational therapy. Dutton (1995) echoed this view, with qualifications, when she said that "while early treatment may be aimed at remediating underlying deficits such as abnormal muscle tone, the ultimate goal of clinical reasoning in occupational therapy is to restore the patient to his or her highest level of functional independence" (p. 3). Thornton and Rennie (1988), in their article describing the uniqueness of occupational therapy, stated that "the first area of consideration for occupational therapists should be the core, occupational performance, which refers to competence in self-care, work, and play activities" (pp. 52–53). Finally, the AOTA (1993) said that occupational therapists help those in the independent living movement "achieve their goals of living as purposefully and independently as possible" (p. 1088), and in long-term care, occupational therapists help people with disabilities be as independent as possible (AOTA, 1994b).

Typically, in conversation, we do not clarify what we mean when we speak of a client's function; the term *function* has become shorthand for bathing, dressing, socialization, shopping, work, play, and all of the other performance areas (AOTA, 1994b, 1994b) (see Appendix I). We tacitly exclude the many physiological and neurological functions that support cognition, respiration, homeostasis, etc.

This tacit understanding of the meaning of function grew out of our practical need to assess ability and measure treatment progress. For example, Sheldon (1935), a teacher of orthopedic physical education, developed a physical achievement record as a means to learn "what activities were really necessary to [the] personal *independence*" [emphasis added] (p. 6) of "crippled" children in a public school in New Jersey. Later, Brown (1947, 1950a, 1950b, 1951), a physical therapist who knew of Sheldon's work, writing in the *Physical Therapy Review* and in the *American Journal of Occupational Therapy*, developed an activity inventory of daily activities she felt were predictive of future function and independence. (Brown's inventory included mostly what we think of today as performance areas.) This practical need to assess ability, establish program eligibility, measure treatment progress, and the like, continues to sustain the construct of functional independence in performance areas today (Kane, Saslow, & Brundage, 1991; Ottenbacher, Hsu, Granger, & Fiedler, 1996; Shah & Cooper, 1993; Smith, 1992). Because of its pragmatic value and frequent use, the construct of functional independence in performance areas has gained nearly universal acceptance in the profession (Allen, 1992; American Occupational Therapy Association [AOTA], 1979, 1986, 1992, 1993, 1994, 1995a, 1995b [see Appendix I]; Cynkin, 1995; Dutton, 1995; Orr & Schkade, 1997; Rogers, 1982; Unsworth, 1997, to name a few references).[1]

While the construct of functional independence in performance areas seems to have permeated our professional consciousness, we have not fully examined its meaning and the assumptions underlying it, or explored the implication of its use. For example, will a person with a C-1 spinal cord lesion value functional independence in activities of daily living (ADL) the same way a person with a radial nerve injury will? Should the "ultimate" goal or concern of occupational therapy be limited to function, independence, or some theoretical combination of the two? If not, what is the ultimate goal and concern of occupational therapy? This article explores the likely assumptions that underlie the construct of functional independence in performance areas. Further, the article explores broader concerns, such as autonomy, wholeness, meaning, and purposiveness, which best express the ultimate concerns of our profession.

Assumptions Underlying the Construct of Functional Independence in Performance Areas

According to the AOTA (1995a) "function is viewed as the interaction of neural and physiological mechanisms, behavior, and environment" (p. 1019). Further, "occupational therapists address the function of the individual at the occupational performance level where the environmental supports and barriers, the individual's skills, and the individual's occupational demands interact" (AOTA, 1995a, p. 1019). Fisher (1992) maintains that while a number of professions use the concepts of function, occupational therapy uniquely frames "function in occupation, or the ability to perform the daily life tasks related to ADLs and IADL, work, and play and leisure" (p. 183). These daily life tasks, or performance areas, with their concomitant performance components, compose the proper domain of occupational therapy (AOTA, 1994a; Mosey, 1992). Implicit in this construct is the notion that human endeavors or concerns outside these performance areas are also outside the domain of occupational therapy.

However, even if all who receive occupational therapy hope to regain function in all or some performance components and areas, their desire to overcome deficits seldom stops there. Persons with performance deficits not only strive for functional independence, they seek and often attain fulfillment in the full range of human potentialities from the spiritual and familial, to the artistic and economic.

Independence refers to a state or quality of being in relation to others and the environment, but these states are not mutually exclusive. People can simultaneously be independent and dependent. A client, for example, may independently choose what she wants to wear, but because of performance deficits due to a stroke, be dependent on others to dress. Another client may be physically able to dress, but because of performance deficits due to severe depression, may refuse to dress, and because of this refusal be dependent on others. Most therapists would concede that in these examples, both clients are in ways nonfunctional and functional, dependent and independent, and that to describe these people as functionally independent or dependent does not appropriately and fully characterize these clients.

Implications for Practice

Much of what it means to be human falls outside the construct of functional independence in performance areas. One has only to recall a modern-day example, Christopher Reeve, who fractured a cervical vertebra during a horse back riding accident. From the perspective of performance areas, he has severely limited function and is dependent, yet Reeve is a successful speaker, fund raiser, actor, and film director, among only a few of his successes. At several points along the course of his rehabilitation, therapists and physicians likely measured his functional independence in performance areas to plan and execute their interventions. However, Reeve probably never accepted his so-called level of independence or his limited functions as prescriptions for how to live the rest of his life.

To Function for What Purpose?

At best, the notion of functional independence in performance areas serves our need to measure clients' performance abilities and improvement more than it serves clients' abilities to construct and express meaning (Burke & Cassidy, 1991 [see Chapter 54]; Coppola, 1998; Radomski, 1995; Spencer, 1993; Whiteneck, 1994). At worst, exclusive pursuit of functional independence risks overlooking clients' subjective constructs of purpose and meaning. Rosenblueth, Wiener, and Bigelow (1943) explain the importance of differentiating *purpose* from function:

> The basis of the concept of purpose is the awareness of 'voluntary activity'.... When we perform a voluntary action what we select voluntarily is a specific purpose, not a specific movement. Thus, if we decide to take a glass containing water and carry it to our mouth we do not command certain muscles to contract to a certain degree and in a certain sequence; we merely trip the purpose and the reaction follows automatically. Indeed ... when an experimenter stimulates the motor regions of the cerebral cortex he does not duplicate a voluntary reaction; he trips efferent, 'output' pathways, but does not trip a purpose, as is done voluntarily. (p. 19)

Thus, when we perform, we select a purpose, not a specific function of muscle and nerve. We have many functions, human and nonhuman, available to us to meet a specific purpose (to make or express a particular meaning). For example, when our purpose is to hit a soft ball, we use our many biomechanical functions in addition to the functions of the soft ball pitcher (to throw the ball), the bat (to strike the ball), and the catcher (to catch the ball when we miss).

Often therapists and clients use a variety of functions to meet a *single purpose*. For example, a person with severe loss of physical functions who chooses to live alone in an apartment (a single purpose) must harness many alternate functions. She will use the functional capacity of assistive technology such as an environmental control unit to open and close doors, turn on lights, change TV channels, and dial the telephone. In addition, she may use the strength and experience of a physical therapy assistant to reduce contractures, and use the functional ability of a personal attendant to bathe, dress, and transfer. She employs these many functions, comparatively few her own, to serve the single purpose of living in the community.

To Be Independent of What or Whom?

We know the myth of independence well; independence and self-reliance maintain a central place in all Americans including our clients. This myth seems to have crowded out of many occupational therapists' consciousness a conception of autonomy that "acknowledges the essential social nature of human development and recognizes dependence as a nonaccidental feature of the human condition" (Agich, 1990, p. 12). If, for whatever reason, we believe independence represents the ideal state of the individual, how do we reconcile our ongoing dependence on food and water, our interdependence on members of our community, and our heightened dependence on others during the beginning and end of our life cycle? As Jonas (1966) put it, "independence as such cannot be the ultimate good of life, since life is just that mode of material existence in which being has exposed itself to dependence" (p. 103).

It makes more sense to acknowledge that we are all dependent in various ways and in varying degrees. Our dependency does not significantly increase or decrease from time to time or from person to person over a lifetime. Dependency, to the extent it can be quantified, remains essentially the same throughout life, but is dispersed in different ways and at different times (Kelly, 1955). For example, a fetus is solely dependent on one person, its mother. Once the child is born, he seeks increasingly greater numbers of people and resources to satisfy his needs. As an adult, with respect to any one individual, he is likely more independent than he was with respect to his mother. However, taking all of his relationships and needs into account, the degree to which he is dependent is the same as it has always been; his dependence is now dispersed over a broad range of people and resources.

Practice Blind Alleys

Theoretically, the logic of the functional independence in performance areas construct would lead therapists to conclude that no reasonable interventions exist outside the construct's boundary. Yet, it is likely that therapists often treat people who have little function or no independence. Practically, when we impose the construct of functional independence on clients, we risk not asking simple questions like, What do independence and function mean to you? What function and independence tradeoffs do you want to make? Recognition that dependence is a natural feature of the human condition frees some people to choose among otherwise unacceptable choices. Some clients may choose to perform *independent* of some thing (perhaps a mechanical lift) and cheerfully depend on a person for transfers. Some may choose to be *independent* of some person (perhaps his or her mother) and happily depend on several assistive devices from a sock aide to a bath bench for dressing and bathing.

In practice, both the client and the reflective therapist face a dilemma created by the narrow functional independence construct. For example, after screening a client and deciding that because of the severity of his disability he will not become functionally independent in performance areas, is it appropriate, from either a reimbursement or professional ethic perspective, to treat that person? During treatment of someone that clearly can get no more functional and can gain no more independence, would not clinical reasoning based on this construct dictate the therapist discontinue therapy? In reality, therapists often shrug off this functional independence construct and continue to treat even the most nonfunctional and dependent by any construct because they and their clients have found good reasons to continue therapy.

What Does It Mean to Be Human?

While the topic human meaning is much broader and more complex than can be addressed in this article, a brief discussion of how the construct of functional independence in performance areas falls short of what it means to be a human will help to inform occupational therapy. As Mosey (1992) says, "a profession's philosophical assumptions are the basic beliefs it holds about the nature of the individual, the environment, the relationship between the individual and the environment, and the purpose and goals of the profession relative to meeting the needs of society" (p. 54). When we base treatment on the functional independence construct, we restrict our view of the human condition. At best this construct barely foreshadows what is of great and lasting importance to those we serve: Their sense of personal autonomy and wholeness and the awareness that they have and pursue purposiveness and meaning.

Autonomy in Spite of Dependence

Dworkin (1988) conceives of *autonomy* in a way that sheds light on the differences between independence and autonomy. He says that autonomy can be conceived of as a second-order capacity of persons to reflect critically upon their first-order preferences, desires, wishes, and so forth and the capacity to accept or attempt to change these in light of higher-order preferences and values. By exercising such a capacity, persons define their nature, give meaning and coherence to their lives, and take responsibility for the kind of person they are (p. 20).

Considering this definition of autonomy, persons might have a powerful automobile and enjoy driving at high speeds (a first-order preference or desire). However, because of their concern for others and awareness that speeding in an automobile is dangerous (their second-order capacity to reflect critically on first-order preferences), they may choose to drive within the speed limits, and in certain circumstances even slower than the speed limit. They are autonomous because they reflect critically on their first-order preferences and because they choose among different actions or values.

As suggested earlier, the functional independence in performance areas construct bestows on the human condition limited possibilities; it overlooks the possibility of reflecting on one's circumstances and limitations, and of choosing to rise above dependence or poor function. That people are autonomous, or have what Dworkin (1988) considers a second-order capacity to reflect critically on their first-order preferences, wishes, and values, describes a potent resource for moral action. However, perhaps more important for occupational therapy, it describes our clients' capacity to reflect critically on abilities and disabilities and choose among different self-judgments and personal meanings.

Dependence is a natural part of human existence. Dependence is only problematic when it is inappropriately or inadequately dispersed. Problems arise when one is dependent upon an unwanted thing or person, when the composition of dependencies is new or different, or when the amount of dependency on a thing or person is too great or too small. The person with a cervical spinal cord injury who had previously been a successful athlete and had appropriately dispersed his dependencies over family, friends, and community illustrates these problems. During the acute phase of his treatment, he depends on a few new people for all of his needs. He may not like one or more of the people upon whom he depends. As rehabilitation proceeds, he may disperse his dependencies over more, but still unfamiliar, people and resources. During this process, he may depend on people to bathe and feed him—occupations he took pride in doing himself. Even years after his accident and after marriage and raising a family, he may have to disperse his dependencies in ways different from his able-bodied peers.

Throughout their lives, as the above example suggests, autonomous people with performance deficits reflect on their first-order preferences, choices, and values regarding independence, and make second-order choices that help give meaning and coherence to their lives. Occupational therapy offers persons with performance deficits and dependence on others many opportunities to explore both their first-order preferences and what it will be like for them to make second-order choices.

Wholeness

Kass (1985) characterizes the relationship of health and wholeness "as 'the well-working of the organism as a whole,' or again, 'an activity of the living body in accordance with its specific excellences'" (p. 174). To the extent that wholeness refers to the integrity of a person, it is a relative sense of well-being with no prescribed limits or standards:

> Meyer (1957) describes the human as a whole being that is: constantly changing, yet it maintains a reasonably orderly internal and external structural and functional organization [that] varies according to its own complexity and the situations to be faced. It is a plastic entity with a wide range of differentiation of capacity and function; it is a center of relative but definable spontaneity and responsiveness; it is an object which constitutes itself a subject or agent, more or less self-dependent, and autonomous. (p. 6)

A young athlete, for example, may base his sense of wholeness on attaining one physical fete after another. When faced with living the rest of his life with quadriplegia resulting from a sky diving accident, he can still have a sense of personal wholeness. To paraphrase Meyer, this young person's sense of wholeness can vary depending on his complexity and the situations he faces. Despite potentially devastating personal losses, through the therapeutic use of occupation, he can reconstruct for himself a meaningful existence and a sense of wholeness based on new challenges and different performance. As this example illustrates, neither functional independence in performance areas is a sufficient condition for, nor is it a necessary condition of, wholeness. In other words, people measure their sense of personal wholeness by constructs other than whether they have certain functions or a particular level of independence.

Purposiveness

Our profession has a long history of upholding the worth of purposeful activity (Cottrell, 1996). Most authors seem to agree that people naturally engage in purposeful activity, and that purposeful activity is goal-directed. The importance of purpose from the occupational therapy perspective seems best characterized by McNary (1947) when she wrote, "An activity entered into without a purpose is not occupational therapy. Busy work and idle recreation have their place, but they are not occupational therapy" (pp. 10–11).

While our literature firmly suggests the value of purpose applied to therapy, further exploration of the construct of purpose will help clarify its application to the human condition. Plants show purposeful activity when they convert water and carbon dioxide into carbohydrates. Guided missiles programmed to seek heat show goal directedness that serves a purpose. How is human purposeful activity different from a plant's or a machine's? Is that difference important to occupational therapists?

Wright's (1971) differentiation between the terms *purposeful* and *purposive* helps answer these questions. He uses the term *purposeful* when discussing behavior of a living body or of a machine, "in the sense of being needed for the performance of functions characteristic of certain systems" (pp. 59–60). From his perspective, the purposefulness of a plant is different from the purposefulness of a human because of the uniquely different functions characteristic of each system. In this way, the purposefulness of a thing is similar to its capabilities. Wright makes an important distinction, one that we must make if we are to more closely match our philosophical assumptions and our view of the human condition. He says "behavior and other processes which are in this sense *purposeful* must be distinguished from behavior which is *purposive* in the sense of intentionally aiming at ends" [emphasis added] (Wright, 1971, p. 50). Said in a different way, humans have no control over their purposefulness, which is dictated by the functions characteristic of the human system. For example, we grasp and manipulate objects because we have a thumb that can oppose the other digits—characteristics of human beings. We do not fly because without feathered extremities and other functions characteristic of birds, human flight is not possible.

However, humans control their *purposiveness*, or intentions and meanings. While it is critically important for occupational therapists to understand the unique functions characteristic of the human, or what Wright calls human *purposefulness*, we must also identify and understand the unique *purposiveness* (or intentions and meanings) of each of those we treat. Persons can lose many functions characteristic of being human and yet retain the meanings and purposiveness that mark the depth and breadth of the human spirit. Consequently, as many occupational therapy writers have noted, we must acknowledge and support meaning and purposiveness in therapy. As stated earlier, neither functional independence in performance areas is a sufficient condition for, nor is it a necessary condition of, purposiveness. Thus, a person's meaning, experienced through purposiveness, can transcend the person's performance deficits.

Meaningfulness

The distinction between purposefulness and purposiveness is empty without considering meaningfulness. As Dunning (1973) asserts about humans, "choice is the vehicle by which he imbues his existence with essence or meaning" (p. 22). How human agents choose is a matter of fascinating conjecture, and its exploration is outside the scope of this paper. What is important to this discussion is not *how* we make choices, but *why* we make choices. Some assert that meaning making is constitutive of humans (Crabtree, 1998; Kramer & Hinojosa, 1995; Mattingly & Fleming, 1994), and further, that we don't need to be "motivated" to make meaning, it comes naturally. We make choices based upon what meaning we attribute to the alternatives, or what the options mean to us, our family, and others. Meaning, and associated intentions, explain *why* we act and why we consider one choice over others (Crabtree, 1998).

More important, from an occupational therapy point of view, we make and express meaning through occupation. Being human means that in spite of often overwhelming loss of function or demoralizing dependence on others, we, through occupation, make meaning in our lives. We can do this in part because we can reflect on our circumstances and limitations and make second-order choices that help us transcend our limitations. Furthermore, constructing and expressing meaning is neither dependent upon all functions characteristic of humans being intact, nor on the person being totally independent. Rather, they are dependent upon a sense of wholeness regardless of how limited or deficient the action.

When we help our clients reach some practical level of performance, we at least intuitively expect them to take action:

Return to work, or continue with a craft, or rejoin family and friends, not just to be performing, but because this doing is meaningful. When clients have no skill to restore, we expect they will develop new skills, again, not for the sake of simply being skillful, but because those skills help the client make and express meaning. To help our clients reach those goals, we not only evaluate their function and level of independence, but we help them tap into their sense of autonomy, purposiveness, and wholeness. We show them that through even the most mundane and commonplace performance, they can express their meanings, and that despite their limited function and dependence on others, they are part of a family and the broader community.

Conclusion

I have explored some assumptions underlying the construct of functional independence in performance areas and proposed that, despite its evolution into what some might consider the goal of practice, its restricted range and scope fall short of both the ultimate goal of occupational therapy and of a worthy vision of what it means to be human. Being human signifies far more than being independent in some task or functioning in some particular performance area. Humans choose among possible actions and values; they make choices that give meaning and purpose to their lives despite loss of function or independence. Humans seek wholeness; they strive for personal meaning and integrity despite their deficits and inabilities. Humans yearn for the "unattainable" and pursue practical goals; they marshal all possible resources against great odds to reach the most grand, and sometimes the most simple, objectives. Our construct of practice must not hold our clients back. Rather, our construct must sometimes even rise above the level of our clients' personal expectations. When we help our clients express their meanings through occupation, and when, through occupation, we help them construct meaning out of often severely limited function and sometimes total dependence, we have attained an appropriate construct of practice.

Note

1. It is important to note one significant exception—the client-centered approach (Canadian Association of Occupational Therapists, 1996; Law, Baptiste, & Mills, 1995) developed in Canada. "Client-centred practice recognizes the autonomy of individuals, the need for client choice in making decisions about occupational needs, the strengths clients bring to a therapy encounter, the benefits of client–therapist partnership and the need to ensure that services are accessible and fit the context in which a client lives" (Law, Baptiste, & Mills, 1995, p. 253). As stated in a Canadian Association of Occupational Therapists Position Statement (1994) "Occupational therapists' broad vision is to enable people who face emotional, physical or social barriers to develop healthy patterns of occupation. The aim is to enable people to choose meaningful occupations which develop their personal and social resources for health" (p. 295). Therapist presumptions about function and independence or dependence are essentially irrelevant in the client-centered construct.

References

Agich, G. J. (1990). Reassessing autonomy in long-term care. *Hastings Center Report, November/December,* 12–17.

Allen, C. K. (1992). Independence and assistance in doing activities. In C. K. Allen, C. A. Earhart, & T. Blue (Eds.), *Occupational therapy treatment goals for the physically and cognitively disabled* (pp. 4–17). Rockville, MD: American Occupational Therapy Association.

American Occupational Therapy Association. (1979). The Association-Resolution C: The philosophical base of occupational therapy. *American Journal of Occupational Therapy, 33*(11), 785. Reprinted in Appendix E.

American Occupational Therapy Association. (1986). Roles and functions in occupational therapy in early childhood intervention. *American Journal of Occupational Therapy, 40*(12), 835–835.

American Occupational Therapy Association. (1992). Constructs of practice for occupational therapy. *American Journal of Occupational Therapy, 46*(12), 1082–1085.

American Occupational Therapy Association. (1993). Statement: The role of occupational therapy in the independent living movement. *American Journal of Occupational Therapy, 47*(12), 1079–1080.

American Occupational Therapy Association. (1994a). Uniform terminology for occupational therapy—3rd edition. *American Journal of Occupational Therapy, 48*(11), 1047–1054,

American Occupational Therapy Association. (1994b). Position paper: Broadening the construct of independence. *American Journal of Occupational Therapy, 48*(11), 1035–1036.

American Occupational Therapy Association. (1995a). Position paper: Occupational performance: Occupational therapy's definition of function. *American Journal of Occupational Therapy, 49*(10), 1019–1020.

American Occupational Therapy Association. (1995b). Position paper: Broadening the construct of independence. *American Journal of Occupational Therapy, 49*(10), 1014. Reprinted as Appendix I.

Brown, M. E. (1947). Daily activity testing and teaching. *The Physiotherapy Review, 27*(4), 249–253.

Brown, M. E. (1950a). Daily activity inventory and progress record for those with atypical movement. *American Journal of Occupational Therapy, 4*(5), 195–204.

Brown, M. E. (1950b). Daily activity inventory and progress record for those with atypical movement (Part II). *American Journal of Occupational Therapy, 4*(6), 261–272.

Brown, M. E. (1951). Daily activity inventory and progress record for those with atypical movement (Part III). *American Journal of Occupational Therapy, 4*(6), 23–38.

Burke, J. P., & Cassidy, J. C. (1991). Disparity between reimbursement-driven practice and humanistic values of occupational therapy. *American Journal of Occupational Therapy, 45*(2), 173–176.

Canadian Association of Occupational Therapists. (1994). Position statement on everyday occupations and health. *Canadian Journal of Occupational Therapy, 61*(5), 294–285.

Canadian Association of Occupational Therapists. (1996). Profile of occupational therapy practice in Canada. *Canadian Journal of Occupational Therapy, 63*(2), 79–95.

Coppola, S. (1998). Clinical interpretation of "Occupational and well-being in dementia: The experience of day-care staff." *American Journal of Occupational Therapy, 52*(6), 435–438.

Cottrell, R. P. (Ed.). (1996). *Perspectives on purposeful activity: Foundations and future of occupational therapy.* Bethesda, MD: American Occupational Therapy Association.

Crabtree, J. L. (1998). The end of occupational therapy. *American Journal of Occupational Therapy, 52*(3), 205–214.

Cynkin, S. (1995). Activities. In C. B. Royeen (Ed.), *AOTA Self-Study Series. The practice of the future: Putting occupation back into therapy* (pp. 7. 1–7.52). Rockville, MD: American Occupational Therapy Association.

DiJoseph, L. M. (1982). Independence through activity: Mind, body, and environment interaction in therapy. *American Journal of Occupational Therapy, 36*(11), 740–744.

Dunning, R. E. (1973). Philosophy and occupational therapy. *American Journal of Occupational Therapy, 27*(1), 18–23.

Dutton, R. (1995). *Clinical reasoning in physical disabilities.* Baltimore: Williams & Wilkins.

Dworkin, G. (19S8). *The theory and practice of autonomy.* Cambridge: Cambridge University Press.

Fisher, A. G. (1992). Functional measures, part I: What is function, what should we measure, and how should we measure it? *American Journal of Occupational Therapy, 46*(12), 183–185.

Jonas, H. (1966). *The phenomenon of life.* Chicago: University of Chicago Press.

Kane, R. L., Saslow, M. G., & Brundage, T. (1991). Using ADLs to establish eligibility for long-term care among the cognitively impaired. *Gerontologist, 31*(1), 60–66.

Kass, L. R. (1985). *Toward a more natural science.* New York: Free Press.

Kelly, G. A. (1955). *The psychology of personal constructs,* vol. 2. New York: W. W. Norton & Company, Inc.

Kramer, P., & Hinojosa, J. (1995). Epiphany of human occupation. In C. B. Royeen, (Ed.), *AOTA Self-Study Series. The practice of the future: Putting occupation back into therapy* (pp. 8.1–8.17). Rockville, MD: American Occupational Therapy Association.

Law, M., Baptiste, S., & Mills, J. (1995). Client-centred practice: What does it mean and does it make a difference? *Canadian Journal of Occupational Therapy, 62*(5), 250–257.

Mattingly, C., & Fleming, M. H. (1994). *Clinical reasoning: Forms of inquiry in a therapeutic practice.* Philadelphia: F. A. Davis Company.

McNary, H. (1947). The scope of occupational therapy. In H. S. Willard & C. S. Spackman (Eds.), *Principles of occupational therapy* (pp. 10–22). Philadelphia: Lippincott.

Meyer, A. (1957). *Psychobiology: A science of man.* Springfield. IL: Charles C. Thomas.

Mosey, A. C. (1996). *Applied scientific inquiry in health profession: An epistemological orientation* (2nd ed.). Bethesda, MD: American Occupational Therapy Association.

Orr, C. S., & Schkade, J. (1997). The impact of the classroom environment on defining function in school-based practice. *American Journal of Occupational Therapy, 51*(1), 64–69.

Ottenbacher, K. J., Hsu, Y., Granger. C. V., & Fiedler, R. C. (1996). The reliability of the Functional Independence Measure: A quantitative review. *Archives of Physical Medicine and Rehabilitation, 77*(12), 1226–1232.

Radomski, M. V. (1995). There is more to life than putting on your pants. *American Journal of Occupational Therapy, 49*(6), 487–490.

Rogers, J. C. (1982). The spirit of independence: The evolving of a philosophy. *American Journal of Occupational Therapy, 36*(11), 709–715.

Rosenblueth, A., Wiener, N., & Bigelow, J. (1943). Behavior, purpose, and teleology. *Philosophy of Science, 10*(1), 18–24.

Shah, S. & Cooper, B. (1993). Issues in the choice of activities of daily living assessment. *Australian Occupational Therapy Journal, 40*(2), 77–82.

Sheldon, M. P. (1935). Physical achievement record for use with crippled children. *Journal of Health and Physical Education, 6*(5), 30–31, 60.

Smith, R. O. (1992). The science of occupational therapy assessment. *Occupational Therapy Journal of Research, 12*(1), 3–15.

Spencer, J. C. (1993). The usefulness of qualitative methods in rehabilitation: Issues of meaning, of context, and of change. *Archives of Physical Medicine and Rehabilitation, 74*(2), 119–126.

Thornton, G., & Rennie, H. (1958). Activities of daily living: An area of occupational therapy expertise. *Australian Occupational Therapy Journal, 35*(2), 49–53.

Unsworth, C. A. (1993). The concept of function. *British Journal of Occupational Therapy, 56*(8), 287–292.

Whiteneck, G. G. (1994). Measuring what matters: Key rehabilitation outcomes. *Archives of Physical Medicine and Rehabilitation, 75*(10), 1073–10176.

Wright, G. H. (1971, 1993). *Explanation and understanding.* Ithaca, NY: Cornell University Press.

Tools of Practice: Heritage or Baggage?

1986 Eleanor Clarke Slagle Lecture

Kathlyn L. Reed, PhD, OTR/L, FAOTA

Over the years, occupational therapists have adopted or adapted numerous media and methods. The list is so long it staggers the imagination. Yet explanations for the changing practice scene are rare. Few therapists seem to know *why* media come and go or even *when* or *how* various media or methods became part of the occupational therapy tool kit. Why do occupational therapists drop some media or methods like so much excess baggage? Is occupational therapy losing its heritage or keeping up with the times?

The question of heritage first occurred to me during Mary Fiorentino's Slagle Lecture (Fiorentino, 1975). She said she used no arts and crafts in her clinic, implying that such media were no longer useful in the treatment tool kit of occupational therapists. Many people applauded her pronouncement as if occupational therapy finally had shed its 19th-century image and joined the 20th century. Her denunciation of arts and crafts set me thinking. Why did arts and crafts become a medium of occupational therapy in the first place? What about other media and methods, such as sanding blocks or work-related programs? Discussions with colleagues produced few answers except that arts and crafts had always been taught since the days of the founders. Therefore, I decided to investigate the literature, historical documents, and old photographs to find some answers.

The objective of this article is to suggest reasons why certain media and methods have evolved as the treatment of choice in occupational therapy in a particular period of time. Likewise, a discussion of why certain media and methods fall into disfavor is relevant.

Definition of Media and Methods

A *medium* is an intervening mechanism through which a force acts or an effect is produced (Morris, 1981). In therapy the medium is the means by which the therapeutic effect is transmitted. A sanding block, a weaving loom, a vestibular board, and a large plastic ball are all media or means by which the therapeutic effect of occupational therapy is activated. Of course, the same objects can be used for other purposes not related to the therapeutic effect of occupational therapy.

Methods are the manner of performing an act or operation: a procedure or technique (*Dorland's*, 1985). In therapy the methods constitute the steps, sequence, or approach used to activate the therapeutic effect of a medium. Examples include one-handed techniques, joint protection, work simplification, and activity configuration. Thus, media and methods are two sides of the same coin. Media provide the means, and methods provide the manner through which the therapeutic effect of occupational therapy is achieved.

Definitions describe but do not determine what will become a therapeutic medium or method. To discover how an object or approach becomes identified as having therapeutic potential, one must look outside a dictionary. Analysis of media and methods over several years has suggested to me that there are eight primary factors that account for which media and methods are selected or discarded from the occupational therapy tool kit. These factors are cultural, social, economic, political, technological, theoretical, historical, and research (Christiansen, 1981; Cynkin, 1979; Di Sante, 1978; English, 1975; Jantzen, 1964; Johnson, 1983; Kielhofner, 1985; Kielhofner & Burke, 1983).

Factors in Selecting and Discarding Media and Methods

Culture is the most pervasive but hidden factor in the selection of media and methods in occupational therapy practice (Cynkin, 1979; Kielhofner, 1985). Occupational therapy was organized around the concept of improving people's abilities to deal with their daily lives. Therefore, it is logical that activities, occupations, or daily living tasks would be selected and used as media and methods. The activities, occupations, and daily living tasks are determined by the culture in which a person lives. A simple example is eating utensils. In Western culture the knife, fork, and spoon are used, but in Eastern culture chopsticks are used to get food from the serving vessel to the mouth. Thus, an occupational therapy clinic in America likely will contain eating utensils that resemble knives, forks, and spoons, but an occupational therapy clinic in Japan likely will contain chopsticks or adaptations of chopsticks.

The social factor is more conspicuous than the cultural (Cynkin, 1979; Kielhofner, 1985). Media and methods are subject to social acceptance or nonacceptance, which often is influenced by marketing and advertising strategies and changing values. The marketing strategies and changing values in turn create fads or trends that influence purchasing decisions. An example is the ongoing issue of whether handmade or machine-made products are superior in quality and value. Is there a difference in the warmth provided by a sweater made of the same yarn when one is handmade and the other made by machine? Probably not. Why then would a person pay more for one than the other? Because social factors, such as perceived value, enter the picture.

Table 46.1. Factors in the Selection and Use of Media and Methods

1. Cultural factor
    Dominant culture
    Subdominant culture
	5. Technological factor
	    New invention
	    Modification of
	       known invention

2. Social factor
    Upper-, middle-, or
       lower-class custom
    Fad or tradition
	6. Theoretical factor
	    Organismic philosophy
	    Mechanistic philosophy

3. Political factor
    Family or extended
       family politics
    Local community politics
    State or national politics
	7. Historical factor
	    Significant
	    Incidental
	
	8. Research factor
	    Supports statements
	    Refutes statements

4. Economic factor
    Budget of department
       or hospital
    Reimbursement policies	

The economic factor affects the selection or discarding of media because some media cost more to use and may or may not be reimbursable by third-party insurance. Building a 16-foot boat could be a very therapeutic occupational activity, but the cost is a little high for many therapists' budgets and probably not reimbursable through most health insurance plans.

The impact of political factors on media and methods has been well documented. Diversional methods of occupational therapy have been ruled out of reimbursable services for many years. More recently there have been disputes over the use of occupational therapy for people with hip replacements or sensory integrative dysfunction.

Technological factors can have a dramatic impact on the media and methods of occupational therapy. Perhaps the best example is the change that has occurred in splinting with the advent of plastics. Originally splints were made from plaster reinforced with wire. The process was tedious, and the product subject to frequent breakdown. Then came plastics, but they had to be heated at high temperatures and tended to become brittle with age. The advent of low-temperature plastics allowed a splint to be made in a few minutes in a small frying pan. Splints from this material last for many months without noticeable change in molecular structure.

Some media and methods develop directly from a given theoretical model. An example is the use of vestibular boards, which is a direct application of the sensory integration model. When a medium or method is associated only with one theoretical model, it is easy to determine the origin. However, some media and methods can be used within a variety of theoretical models, and thus identification becomes more difficult. Cooking, for example, can be viewed as essential to nutrition, a pleasurable reward, a social activity, a paid vocation, a leisure skill, or an educational task. How many theoretical models encompass cooking as a medium and method?

The historical factor influences media and methods because some media and methods have been associated with occupational therapy from the earliest records and their origin is now obscure. For example, the use of the bicycle jigsaw can be traced back to occupational therapy clinics in 1918, but the trail is difficult to follow beyond that point. Who built the first bicycle jigsaw, and what was the original therapeutic objective?

Finally, research influences the selection and discarding of media and methods. For example, the research on building muscle strength led to the concept of progressive resistive exercise, which in turn led to the development or adaptation of media that can be modified to provide increased resistance. Many floor looms were modified in the 1950s and 1960s to provide increased resistance to shoulder, arm, hand, and leg muscles.

These factors can be explained further in a set of assumptions about their effect on the selection and discarding of media and methods in occupational therapy. The 14 assumptions can be stated as follows:

1. Media and methods become tools of occupational therapy through one or more of the eight factors.
2. Media and methods disappear from the tool kit of occupational therapy because of one or more of the eight factors.
3. The factors may operate to change the selection or discarding of media and methods singly or, more often, in combination.
4. Occupational therapists should understand the effects of the eight factors on the media and methods used in occupational therapy practice. (See Table 46.1 for a list of subfactors.)
5. Media and methods are selected from the dominant existing culture.
6. The sociocultural meaning of a medium and its methods may change over time and be used for a different reason or be discarded.
7. When the sociocultural rationale for a medium or method is lost or changed, the medium may be used in therapy in ways that make little sense to patients or other health professionals.
8. Economic considerations affect the selection and discarding of media and methods and thus restrict their use if the price is too high or if the cost is not reimbursable.
9. Changes in political issues may restrict or facilitate both the selection and use of various media and methods in occupational therapy based on decisions to cover them under or to exclude them from health-care programs.
10. Technology introduces new possibilities or modifies existing ones, allowing new media or methods to emerge.
11. Media and methods may be selected because they operationalize an existing theoretical model recognized by the profession.
12. A medium or method may be used in more than one model. Therefore, the therapist must know why a medium or method is being used and change the explanation when a new model is adopted.
13. Historical precedent is the least desirable justification for the existence and continued use of a medium or method but the easiest to explain.
14. Selection and use of media and methods based on research and study is the most professionally responsible approach to justifying the use of a medium or method but the most difficult to obtain.

To illustrate how the eight factors and 14 assumptions operate, I have selected three media and their methods from among the many possible choices. The three are arts and crafts, sanding blocks, and work-related programs. Arts and crafts will illustrate the cultural, social, technological, and historical factors; the sanding blocks will illustrate the theoretical and research factors; and work-related programs will illustrate the political and economic factors.

Arts and Crafts

The use of arts and crafts as media and methods in occupational therapy is directly attributable to the arts-and-crafts movement that was in full swing during the formative years of occupational therapy early in this century (Levine, in press-a, in press-b [see Chapter 3]). The movement was designed as a cure for the social ills of a society struggling to deal with the impact of the Industrial Revolution. During the 1800s, Western civilization changed from an agrarian to a manufacturing economy; from a cottage industry to a mass-production society; from a consumer-driven marketplace to a producer-driven marketplace; from a patronage system to an industrial-wealth system; from pride in workmanship to concern for profit; and from an ordered society of similar cultural backgrounds to a disordered society of many cultures and customs. These factors all played a role in the demise of moral treatment. The arts-and-crafts movement provided a means of revitalizing the ideas of moral treatment in a new rationale, which the founders and early leaders of occupational therapy were quick to understand. Thus, the arts-and-crafts movement is the missing link between moral treatment, which dominated the practice of medicine in the 1800s, and the treatment models to follow.

The arts-and-crafts movement began in England. The original philosophy was based on the "conviction that industrialization had brought with it the total destruction of 'purpose, sense and life'" (Naylor, 1971). Mechanical progress had been gained at the expense of human misery and the destruction of fundamental human values. Thus, the arts-and-crafts movement "was inspired by a crisis of conscience" (Naylor, 1971). Its motivations were social and moral, and its aesthetic values derived from the conviction that a society produces the art and architecture it deserves (Naylor, 1971). To that idea could be added the thought that society produces the lifestyle it deserves.

Many people contributed ideas and thoughts to the arts-and-crafts movement, and not all agreed as to their importance. Therefore, a summary of concepts must be general. The arts-and-crafts movement did the following:

- Advocated the simplification of life and ordering of daily activity as opposed to the overcomplicated or idle life (Borris, 1986; Kornwolf, 1972; Lears, 1981; Shi, 1985; Wagner, 1904);
- Valued the "craftsman" ideal, in which occupation was pursued at its own pace and not on a production schedule (Borris, 1986; Kornwolf, 1972; Lears, 1981);
- Valued the standard of craftsmanship that gave an honest day's work for an honest day's pay, rather than exploitation of the worker or cheating by the employee (Borris, 1986; Kornwolf, 1972; Naylor, 1971);
- Favored returning to the land and the home as a means of escaping the crowded, unhealthy, unnatural conditions of the city and factory (Lears, 1981; Shi, 1985);

- Ennobled the power of handwork as useful, important, a joy, and a pleasure, as opposed to mindless, repetitive activity on an assembly line, which was viewed as drudgery (Borris, 1986; Lears, 1981);
- Promoted an appreciation of performing the process and the inherent satisfaction or pride in doing or making a product, as opposed to concern only for sale and profit (Naylor, 1971);
- Encouraged respect for the inherent properties of materials and opposed any deception designed to make a material look like something it was not (Kornwolf, 1972);
- Considered functionalism and fitness of purpose the best guide to decoration, as opposed to ornamentation that served no purpose (Borris, 1986; Kornwolf, 1972);
- Believed that manual training of children would increase knowledge of moral aesthetics and improve work skills, as opposed to intellectual learning only (Borris, 1986; Lears, 1981);
- Valued the creative spirit in the artist and abhorred the mindless copying of designs (Borris, 1986);
- Attempted to improve the standards of taste and aesthetics, as opposed to allowing moral decay (Borris, 1986; Shi, 1985); and
- Viewed people as more than mere machines; human beings as having morals, values, and a sense of purpose (Kornwolf, 1972; Shi, 1985).

One early influence of the arts-and-crafts movement on occupational therapy came from Jane Addams. In 1900 she started the Hull House Labor Museum, because she wanted young people to see that the complicated machinery of the factory had evolved from the simple tools that their parents had used in the old country before immigrating to America. She wanted to interest young people in the older forms of industry so they would see "a dramatic representation of the inherited resources of their daily occupation" (Addams, 1945). The Labor Museum not only showed how spinning, weaving, pottery, and many other crafts were done, but also provided classes to teach people how to do the crafts. Addams admonished educators, saying that "educators have failed to adjust themselves to the fact that cities have become great centers of production and manufacture, and manual labor has been left without historic interpretation or imaginative uplift" (Addams, 1900, p. 236). Thus, when the training courses for attendants were started in 1907, in conjunction with the Chicago School of Civics and Philanthropy, there was an emphasis on the idea that occupation should be used as a means of education and that education was to substitute for custodial care of the mentally ill (20th Biennial Report, 1909).

In 1914, Eleanor Clarke Slagle started the Community Workshop under the auspices of the Illinois Society of Mental Hygiene. Its purpose was to serve as a clearinghouse for cases of doubtful insanity whom the courts considered as showing promise of a return to usefulness if given a proper environment and trade (Favill, 1917). The environment was the Hull House Labor Museum. In 1917 the Community Workshop became the Henry B. Favill School of Occupations. The following year, the first course in curative occupations and recreation was offered (Special Courses, 1917). Again the Labor Museum at Hull House served as the laboratory until the school was moved to the headquarters of the Illinois Society of Mental Hygiene in late 1919.

Another person to incorporate the ideas of the arts-and-crafts movement into treatment was Herbert J. Hall. In 1904 Hall began his studies of alternate treatments to the "rest cure" for neurasthenia. He was assisted by Jessie Luther, OTR, the first curator of the Hull House Labor Museum (Luther, 1902). Hall states that the "modern Arts and Crafts idea appealed very strongly, because of the growing interest in the movement and because of the clean, wholesome atmosphere which surrounds such work, and because of the many-sided appeal which such a work as the making of pottery, for instance, has to most educated minds" (Hall, 1905). Hall believed that faulty living was the cause of neurasthenia and that what was needed was a change in occupation and habits. Manual work based on the life of the artisan (craftsman ideal) was recommended itself because it was simple. The "simple life," he felt, was best for neurasthenics because it offered the least food for the nourishment of neurasthenia and provided a structure of normality. Today the person with neurasthenia would be classified as suffering from stress or burnout. The "simple life" would be called stress reduction, and the "craftsman ideal" would be called time management.

In 1906 Hall received a grant from the Procter Fund of Harvard University for $1,000 to "assist in the study of the treatment of neurasthenia by progressive and graded manual occupation." His study at Marblehead, Massachusetts, probably was the first grant-funded research project on the use of occupation as a means of treating patients. He reported that 59 of 100 patients improved, 27 were much improved, and 14 received no relief (Hall, 1910).

The arts-and-crafts philosophy was summarized in the "Philosophy of Occupation Therapy" by Adolf Meyer (1922) (see Chapter 2). He said, "Our industrialism has created the false idea of success in production to the point of overproduction, bringing with it a kind of nausea to the worker and a delirium of the trader..."—in other words, loss of the craftsman ideal. Meyer said, "The man of today has lost the capacity and pride of workmanship and has substituted for it a measure in terms of money." In other words, there was a loss of respect for hand work. And he said that there is "a real pleasure in the use and activity of one's hands and muscles." In other words, one can find pride and satisfaction in performing and doing. Furthermore, "Our body is not merely so many pounds of flesh and bone figuring as a machine."

A final example of the influence of the arts-and-crafts movement on occupational therapy is the regional location of the arts-and-crafts societies that developed to organize the work of the arts and crafts movement. The three major areas

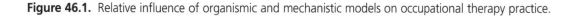

	1880	1890	1900	1910	1920	1930	1940	1950	1960	1970	1980	1990

Organismic

End of Moral Treatment (1880)

Rise of the Arts-and-Crafts Movement (1890)

Rise of the Developmental Model (1940)

Rise of Systems Model / Return of Humanism (1970)

Mechanistic

Flexner Report (1910)

Rise of the Orthopedics Model (1920)

Rise of the Biomedical Model (1940)

Dominance of the Psycho-analytic Model (1950)

Dominance of the Behaviorism Model (1970)

Medical Schools Increase Science Study (1910)

Figure 46.1. Relative influence of organismic and mechanistic models on occupational therapy practice.

of the country that responded to the arts-and-crafts movement were New England, Chicago and the Midwest, and the Pacific area (Clark, 1972). There is a strong correspondence between these three areas and the areas where there are large numbers of occupational therapists today.

The specific location of the societies also influenced occupational therapy. Thirteen states had at least one known arts-and-crafts society in 1904 (West, 1904). Of the 13, nine (69 percent) developed early programs in occupational therapy before 1920. All 13 states have occupational therapy programs today (West, 1904).

Considering its influence, what happened to the arts-and-crafts movement? It was overtaken by World War I. The rules of the game changed for many people. The war effort provided its own sense of purpose. Some industries did hire craftsmen to improve designs, and machine-made products did improve in quality. City life improved as sanitation efforts made inroads against the piles of garbage. The expanding population meant that machine manufacture was the only means of providing products for everyone. Hand production was just too slow and too expensive.

How did the changes influence occupational therapy? What factors were changing the role of arts and crafts in practice? The cultural scene had shifted: Society was no longer struggling to adapt to city life, and the factory system had been integrated in the fabric of American life. The number of people living on the land would continue to decrease over the coming years. People had become used to the technological changes the factory had produced. Machine-made goods were acceptable and could be made in quantities unknown under the handmade system. Young therapists did not remember the arts-and-crafts movement and did not

know what it represented. They only knew that arts and crafts always had been a part of occupational therapy's tool kit. Finally, a new philosophy was overtaking the profession. The humanistic ideas of the founding years were being challenged as unscientific and unmeasurable. The profession was being reformulated in such a manner that the arts-and-crafts philosophy made little sense. Not until the 1960s would the founding ideas resurface. Figure 46.1 illustrates the changing theory and philosophy of the arts-and-crafts ideology.

Sanding Blocks

Sanding blocks, or sandblocks, are a common sight in many occupational therapy clinics. Nearly all occupational therapists become acquainted with them during their education, and many have made sanding blocks. Yet, few can describe the origin and original purpose of the sanding block or trace the changes in thinking about their use over the years.

Woodworking and sanding can be traced to the beginning of occupational therapy history. The initial use of sanding blocks, however, is unclear. The first mention of them appears in 1934 in an article by Henrietta McNary. In the same article, the first description of an adapted sanding block also appears. Its purpose was to improve opposition. The last article in our literature on a sanding block, a reciprocal sanding device, appears in 1965 (Mathews, 1965). In all, 14 different types of sanding blocks are presented. These are listed in Table 46.2.

The dates of the articles on sanding blocks coincide with the rise and fall of the orthopedic and kinesthetic treatment models of occupational therapy. The orthopedic model followed the arts-and-crafts model. It was concerned with muscle strengthening and range of motion. Stretching contractures, exercise, and physical tolerance also were included.

Table 46.2. Types of Sanding Blocks

1. Proximal sanding blocks
   (Abbott, 1957; *Photographs,* 1947)

2. Proximal interphalangeal sanding block
   (Abbott, 1957; *Photographs,* 1947)

3. Metacarpal phalangeal sanding blocks
   (Abbott, 1957; *Photographs,* 1947)

4. Distal sanding block
   (Abbott, 1957)

5. Opponens sanding block
   (Abbott, 1957)

6. Shoulder abduction sanding block
   ("Adapted," 1957; Bennett & Driver, 1957)

7. Spring squeeze sanding block
   (Gurney, 1959)

8. Grip sanding block
   (Hightower et al., 1963)

9. Reciprocal sanding device
   (Mathews, 1965)

10. Weighted sander or progressive resistive exercise sander
    (Svensson & Brennan, 1954)

11. Bilateral sander, horizontal or vertical handles
    (*Photographs,* 1947)

12. Wrist exercise sander (Blodgett, 1947)

13. Hemiplegia sander (Forbes, 1951)

14. Graduated sanding blocks—graduated straight
    handles or graduated round knob handles
    (*Photographs,* 1947)

Table 46.3. Purposes or Objectives of Sanding Blocks

Sanding blocks were adapted to provide the following:
1. Different hand grip position for active or passive stretching:
   a. Handles were added and enlarged.
   b. Holes or grooves were drilled or carved for finger and thumb placement.
   c. Straps were added to hold the hand in place.
   d. Gloves were used to position the hand.
   e. Construction was altered to provide a different grip than that normally used.
2. Dynamic exercise of wrist, elbow, or shoulder—usually range of motion
3. Increased grip strength of hand and fingers
4. Bilateral activity of the upper extremities
5. Reciprocal activity of the upper extremities
6. Improved trunk stability
7. Standing and physical tolerance

These concepts form the basis of the objectives for which the sanding block was used. A summary of these purposes or objectives is found in Table 46.3.

The use of sanding blocks has not disappeared, but the theories underpinning their development and use have been superseded by the sensorimotor and sensory integration models. As a result, some unusual uses of sanding blocks have surfaced. For example, one therapist was observed giving a patient a sanding block with no sandpaper and an incline plane made of formica. Because the patient did not want to make anything, the therapist explained that the purpose of the activity was bilateral exercise. In this example, the fundamental concepts of occupational therapy, performance through doing and the use of occupation toward some purpose, were overlooked or separated from the application. The medium of sanding blocks and the methods of setting up the activity to obtain selected objectives had been separated from the original concepts so the meaning and purpose of the activity were lost. The *motion* of sanding is a necessary but not sufficient part of the *activity* of sanding. The media, the methods, and the objective of an occupation must be consistent with each other. Three out of three—

medium, method, and objective—must be the rule, not the exception.

Sanding blocks illustrate the factors of theory and research. The many adaptations of the sanding block are based on the theoretical concepts of the orthopedic and kinesthetic treatment models, which stress positioning the body part in the desired pattern of motion and then encouraging that motion to stretch, strengthen, or increase the motion of a particular body part or parts. Research supported the concept that increased amounts of resistance applied to a given muscle group would strengthen the muscle group involved. This concept became known as progressive resistive exercise.

Work-Related Programs

Work-related programs were a part of the early ideology of occupational therapy. The term *work-related programs* is used to represent all efforts to enable people to engage in productive occupations through occupational therapy, whether the effort is aimed at vocational education, vocational guidance, prevocational evaluation and training, vocational training or retraining, vocational readiness, work hardening, work adjustment, or career education.

Hall was very interested in helping patients find an alternate occupation that would be less stressful and more suitable to the person's needs. The "work cure" was based on the assumption that by substituting or bringing about "by a gradual process the conditions of a normal life, a life of pleasant and progressive occupations, as different as possible from the previous life, a person could overcome the mental and nervous problems in his life" (Hall, 1905).

George E. Barton said he was going to "try to prove that the hours of idleness in convalescence could be filled with pastimes which would be useful not only to pass the time, but to prepare the person for remunerative labor later on to get a job, a better job, or to do a job better than it was before" (Barton, 1914). Consolation House was created to serve the needs of people who were learning to put their lives back together and who needed assistance to find an occupation suitable to their abilities but not limited by their disabilities.

Slagle had experience in assessing people's fitness for a job at the Community Workshop at Hull House. At the founding conference of occupational therapy in Clifton Springs, New York, she spoke of a family of five who had been supported by charities for many years. After 1 year at the Community Workshop, the family was self-sufficient (Dunton, 1917).

Thomas B. Kidner, Vocational Secretary to the Military Hospitals Commission in Ottawa, Canada, was well acquainted with the vocational side of occupational therapy. In June 1918, he was loaned by the Canadian government to the United States as a special adviser on rehabilitation to the Federal Board for Vocational Education (FBVE). The FBVE had been created the previous year to establish a federal-state program in vocational education. In 1918 it had been given the authority and responsibility for the vocational rehabilitation of veterans ("Editorial," 1922). Elizabeth G. Upham (later Davis), who had been instrumental in starting the occupational therapy course at Milwaukee Downer College, also joined the FBVE in 1918. She wrote two documents illustrating the role of occupational therapy with the disabled veteran (Upham, 1918a, 1918b) and recommended that the FBVE be given control of military patients as soon as possible in order to prepare them for adjustment to normal life (Davis, no date). Had her recommendation been accepted, occupational therapy's role in vocational preparation would have been larger than it has been. Both Kidner and Upham left the FBVE in 1919.

The medical department of the army also had a plan for the rehabilitation of disabled soldiers. It had created a system of orthopedic reconstruction hospitals that included vocational workshops and employment bureaus (Gritzer & Arluke, 1985). The dispute over who would do what came to the floor of the U.S. Senate in July 1918. The medical department of the army was granted the exclusive right to all aspects of functional restoration and medical control over curative work. This action bound occupational therapy to medicine's domain. The FBVE, on the other hand, was given responsibility for vocational rehabilitation. The separation became more divided in 1920 when the Industrial Rehabilitation Act was passed without any coverage for medical services. Bulletin #57 of the FBVE makes it quite clear than any occupational work not related to the vocation for which the injured person is being trained is evidently given for its therapeutic value. Therapeutic use of work was viewed as part of the injured person's physical rehabilitation rather than vocational rehabilitation and therefore was not covered under the act ("Industrial rehabilitation," 1920). Thus, occupational therapy was cut off from many of its work-related programs by a political compromise over which it ultimately had little control. Work-related programs were not reestablished until 1943 when the Vocational Rehabilitation Act was changed to include coverage for medical services (Lassiter, 1972). In 1954, the Vocational Rehabilitation Act was further modified to include coverage for the training of rehabilitation personnel, including occupational therapists. In addition there were monies for research and demonstration projects (Lassiter, 1972). Among the demonstration projects were prevocational evaluation and training centers in which occupational therapists played a significant role. However, by the 1960s these projects became too expensive to continue, and the role of occupational therapy in work-related programs again went into a period of decline. Finally in the 1980s the interest returned. A position paper was written and a grant was funded to increase occupational therapists' awareness of the role of occupational therapy in work-related programs. Some of the current interests are assessment of work potential and aptitude skills, physical capacities assessment and work hardening, job evaluation, work experience, career exploration and job-seeking skills, independent living, and industrial consultation.

The level of occupational therapists' interest and opportunities in work-related programs has waxed and waned over the past 80 years. The fluctuations can be traced to politics and economics. When both were favorable or neutral, occupational therapists provided many examples of programs designed to help a person to gain or regain productive skills. However, when the politics and economics made it difficult for occupational therapists to provide such skill assessment and skill training, their activity in work-related programs decreased. The challenge will be to shape the political and economic factors in favor of occupational therapy if therapists want to maintain their role in helping people attain or regain productive skills.

Occupational Analysis

As illustrated thus far, the selection and discarding of media and methods in occupational therapy has not been accidental. Factors converge and diverge to increase or decrease the likelihood that a particular medium and its methods will be selected or discarded in the practice of occupational therapy. Culture sets the major parameters, but changes in society frequently alter the cultural set. Political and economic factors often work in combination. Political factors can be influenced by occupational therapists, but some events may occur over which therapists have little control. The results may be felt most keenly economically when reimbursement patterns result in changes in coverage of occupational therapy services. Technology may lead to dramatic changes in media or methods. Theoretical factors often introduce new media and methods into the treatment setting. Sometimes the new theory or model brings new media and methods with it; at other times just the explanation and the use of an existing medium or method changes. History often is used to explain the existence of media or methods when the origin has been lost through time. Research offers a better explanation for the use of media and methods but is more difficult to obtain.

All of these factors need to be considered when examining why certain media and methods appear in a clinic or practice setting. Can practicing occupational therapists explain why each medium or method is used in their practice setting? Is the explanation the best one, or is the explanation of history used by default? Perhaps a more systematic use of occupational or activity analysis should be promoted which includes the selection and discarding of factors as well as considerations such as range of motion, sensory stimulation, or amount of social interaction obtained.

Central to each of the factors are the concepts of interests and values. A culture, individuals, and professionals have interests and values. An interest is defined as a set that guides behavior in a certain direction or toward certain goals (Chaplin, 1975). A value is a social end or goal that is considered desirable to achieve (Chaplin, 1975).

In occupational therapy there seem to be three major areas to consider in interest and values. These are culture and society, the individual, and the profession. The eight factors that affect selection and discarding of media and methods can be organized under the cultural and social interest and values and professional interests and values. Under the *cultural and social* area are the cultural, social, economic, political, and technological factors. Under the *professional* are the theoretical, historical, and research factors. Under the *individual* are factors that must be determined by assessment of each individual. These are the roles performed by the individual and the functional abilities, skills, and capacities of the individual. When the three areas of cultural-social, individual, and professional interests and values are considered, there should be less chance of using media and methods that are out-of-date in society, not meaningful to the individual, and of questionable use to the profession.

Summary

This article presents and illustrates the major factors that influence the selection and discarding of media and methods in occupational therapy. The eight factors are the cultural, social, economic, political, technological, theoretical, historical, and research factors. The factors may operate in various combinations or alone to influence the use of a specific medium or method in practice. Therapists are encouraged to know these eight factors and in particular to be familiar with (a) what media and methods occupational therapists use, (b) why occupational therapists use those media and methods, (c) from where the media and methods come, (d) with whom the media and methods should be used in treatment, (e) how the media and methods are used, (f) when the media and methods are used, and (g) how much of the medium or method should be used. Educators, in particular, need to teach why a medium or method is used as well as how. Researchers need to provide more information as to why certain media and methods became part of our tool kit. Practitioners would be wise to follow the statement. If you know how, be sure you know why and be sure the why is consistent with the philosophy of occupational therapy.

References

Abbott, M. (1957). *A syllabus of occupational therapy procedures and techniques as applied to orthopedic and neurological conditions.* New York: American Occupational Therapy Association.

Adapted sand block. Part I. (1957). *American Journal of Occupational Therapy, 11,* 198.

Addams, J. (1900). Social education of the industrial democracy. *Commons, 5,* 17–28.

Addams, J. (1945). *Twenty years at Hull House, with autobiographical notes.* New York: Macmillan.

Barton, G. E. (1914). A view of invalid occupation. *Trained Nurse & Hospital Review, 52,* 327–330.

Bennett, R. L., & Driver, M. (1957). The aims and methods of occupational therapy in the treatment of the after-effects of poliomyelitis. *American Journal of Occupational Therapy, 11,* 145–153.

Blodgett, M. L. (1947). Sanding for exercise. *American Journal of Occupational Therapy, 1,* 6.

Borris, E. (1986). *Art and labor: Ruskin, Morris, and the craftsman ideal in America.* Philadelphia, PA: Temple University Press.

Chaplin, J. P. (1975). *Dictionary of psychology* (2nd ed.). New York: Dell.

Christiansen, C. H. (1981). Editorial: Toward resolution of crisis: Research requisites in occupational therapy. *Occupational Therapy Journal of Research, 1,* 115–124.

Clark, R. J. (1972). *The arts-and-crafts movement in America: 1876–1916.* Princeton, NJ: Princeton University Press.

Cynkin, S. (1979). *Occupational therapy: Toward health through activities.* Boston: Little, Brown.

Davis, E. U. (no date). *Just another biography.* Unpublished manuscript.

Di Sante, E. (1978). Technology transfer: From space exploration to occupational therapy. *American Journal of Occupational Therapy, 32,* 171–174.

Dorland's illustrated medical dictionary (26th ed.). Philadelphia, PA: W. B. Saunders, p. 809.

Dunton, W. R. (1917). *The growing necessity for occupational therapy.* New York: Teachers College. (In AOTA Archives, Moody Library, Galveston, TX).

Editorial: The 6th annual meeting. *Archives of Occupational Therapy, 1,* 419–427.

English, C. B. (1975). Computers and occupational therapy. *American Journal of Occupational Therapy, 29,* 43–47.

Favill, J. (1917). *Henry Baird Favill: 1960–1916.* Chicago: Rand McNally, p. 87.

Fiorentino, M. R. (1975). Occupational therapy: Realization to activation—1974 Eleanor Clarke Slagle lecture. *American Journal of Occupational Therapy, 29,* 15–21.

Forbes, E. S. (1951). Two devices for use in treating hemiplegics. *American Journal of Occupational Therapy, 5,* 49–51.

Gritzer, G., & Arluke, A. (1985). *The making of rehabilitation: A political economy of medical specialization, 1890–1980.* Berkeley, CA: University of California Press.

Gurney, G. W. (1959). Spring-squeeze sandblock. *American Journal of Occupational Therapy, 13,* 278.

Hall, H. J. (1905). The systematic use of work as a remedy in neurasthenia and allied conditions. *Boston Medical & Surgical Journal, 112,* 29–32.

Hall, H. J. (1910). Work-cure: A report of 5 years' experience at an institution devoted to the therapeutic application of manual work. *Journal of the American Medical Association, 54,* 12–14.

Hightower, M. D., et al. (1963). Grip sander. *American Journal of Occupational Therapy, 17,* 62–63.

Industrial rehabilitation—A statement of policies to be observed in the administration of the Industrial Rehabilitation Act. (1920). *FBVE Bulletin, 57.*

Jantzen, A. C. (1964). The role of research in occupational therapy. *Proceedings of the 1964 Annual Conference* (pp. 2–9). New York: American Occupational Therapy Association.

Johnson, J. A. (1983). The changing medical marketplace as a context for the practice of occupational therapy. In G. Kielhofner (Ed.), *Health through occupation: Theory and practice in occupational therapy* (pp. 163–177). Philadelphia, PA: F. A. Davis.

Kielhofner, G. (Ed.). (1985). *A model of human occupation: Theory and application.* Baltimore, MD: Williams & Wilkins.

Kielhofner, G., & Burke, J. P. (1983). The evolution of knowledge and practice in occupational therapy: Past, present and future (pp. 3–54). In G. Kielhofner (Ed.), *Health through occupation: Theory and practice in occupational therapy.* Philadelphia, PA: F. A. Davis.

Kornwolf, J. D. (1972). *M. H. Baillie Scott and the arts-and-crafts movement.* Baltimore, MD: Johns Hopkins Press.

Lassiter, R. A. (1972). History of the rehabilitation movement in America. In J. G. Cull & R. E. Hardy (Eds.), *Vocational rehabilitation: Profession and process* (pp. 5–58). Springfield, IL: Charles C Thomas.

Lears, T. J. J. (1981). *No place of grace: Antimodernism and the transformation of American culture: 1880–1920.* New York: Pantheon.

Levine, R. E. (in press-a). Guest editorial: Historical research: Ordering the past to chart our future. *Occupational Therapy Journal of Research.*

Levine, R. E. (in press-b). The influence of the arts-and-crafts movement on the professional status of occupational therapy. In W. Coleman (Ed.), *Written history monograph.* Rockville, MD: American Occupational Therapy Association. Reprinted as Chapter 3.

Luther, J. (1902). The labor museum at Hull House. *Commons, 7,* 1–13.

Mathews, T. (1965). Reciprocal sanding device. *American Journal of Occupational Therapy, 19,* 354–355.

McNary, H. (1934). Anatomical considerations and technique in using occupations as exercise for orthopedic disabilities: III. Wrist and fingers. *Occupational Therapy Rehabilitation, 13,* 24–29.

Meyer, A. (1922). Philosophy of occupational therapy. *Archives of Occupational Therapy, 1,* 1–10. Reprinted as Chapter 2.

Morris, W. (Ed.). (1981). *American heritage dictionary of the English language.* Boston: Houghton Mifflin, p. 815.

Naylor, G. (1971). *The arts-and-crafts movement: A study of its sources, ideals, and influence on design theory.* Cambridge, MA: MIT Press.

Photographs of occupational therapy adapted equipment as developed in Veterans Administration and Army hospitals. (1947). Washington, DC: Department of Medicine & Surgery, Veterans Administration.

Shi, D. E. (1985). *The simple life: Plain living and high thinking in American culture.* New York: Oxford University Press.

Special courses in curative occupations and recreation. (1917, December). Chicago: Chicago School of Civics and Philanthropy Special Bulletin.

Svensson, V. W., & Brennan, M. C. (1954). Adapted weighted resistive apparatus. *American Journal of Occupational Therapy, 8,* 13.

20th biennial report of the board of public charities of the state of Illinois, July 1, 1906–June 30, 1908. Springfield, IL: Illinois State Journal Co., p. 58.

Upham, E. G. (1918a). Training of teachers for occupational therapy for the rehabilitation of disabled soldiers and sailors. *Federal Board for Vocational Education Bulletin, 6,* 1–76.

Upham, E. G. (1918b). Ward occupations in hospitals. *Federal Board for Vocational Education Bulletin, 25,* 1–57.

Wagner, C. (1904). *The simple life.* New York: Grosset & Dunlap.

West, M. (1904). The revival of handicrafts in America. *Bureau of Labor Bulletin, 55,* 1573–1622.

CHAPTER 47

The Origin and Evolution of Activity Analysis

CYNTHIA CREIGHTON, MA, OTR

In 1911, industrialization had resulted in unprecedented economic growth for the United States. The average employee worked a 9- to 12-hour shift, 6 days per week, for a wage of approximately $2 a day. The automobile assembly line had not yet been invented.

Two books that would revolutionize industry were published that year: *The Principles of Scientific Management* (Taylor, 1911) and *Motion Study* (Gilbreth, 1911). Taylor, past president of the American Society of Mechanical Engineers, proposed in his text that management in business and industry be approached as a true science with clearly defined rules and principles. An important element of Taylor's new system of management was the study and standardization of jobs to increase productivity. Soon, efficiency experts were observing and timing workers in shops and factories nationwide. As a laborer shoveled ore or cut metal, the consultant identified the fundamental operations, the most efficient tools, and the optimum speed for the task.

---

[1] Lillian Gilbreth also applied motion study methodology to organizing the Gilbreth's home and raising 12 children while earning her doctorate at Brown University. The American public came to know the family through the books *Cheaper by the Dozen* and *Belles on Their Toes,* written by two of the children.

Gilbreth (1911), 10 years younger than Taylor and also an engineer, was the first to use the term *analysis* when discussing the systematic study of jobs. He believed that the worker's movements should be the focus of such studies. Gilbreth outlined the steps in analyzing a task as follows: "1. Reduce ... practice to writing. 2. Enumerate motions used. 3. Enumerate variables which affect each motion" (p. 5). Three categories of variables were considered in a motion study: characteristics of the worker (e.g., physical build, experience, temperament), characteristics of the surroundings (e.g., lighting, tools), and characteristics of the motion (e.g., direction, length, speed). Gilbreth documented these in chart form and in photographs. The purpose of analyzing a job was to identify and teach the "definite best" (most productive and least fatiguing) method of performance (p. 93).

Gilbreth (1911) also discussed adapting activity to make it more efficient:

> A careful study of the worker will enable one to adapt his work, surroundings, equipment and tools to him. "This will decrease the number of motions he must make, and make the necessary motions shorter and less fatiguing." (p. 10)

In his own bricklaying business, he made adaptations such as reversing the position of materials for left-handed workers and placing stock on a scaffold so the bricklayer no longer had to stoop when picking it up. In 1913, he began founding small museums of devices designed to simplify work and prevent fatigue (Gilbreth & Gilbreth, 1920).

Gilbreth and his wife, Lillian,[1] became well known both at home and abroad as consultants to the business community (Yost, 1949). In 1914 and 1915, Gilbreth visited hospitals in Europe to analyze surgeons' work. World War I had begun, and he met disabled veterans and learned about the groundbreaking research of Jules Amar.

Amar (1918) was a French physiologist appointed by his government to investigate scientific management and apply its principles to the training and re-employing of wounded soldiers. At that time, France led the world in the study of human physiology and the development of instruments to measure physiological functions; Amar began analyzing jobs in terms of their physiological requirements. He described the planes of motion in which work was performed and measured movements with simple goniometers. To document strength requirements, Amar attached spring dynamometers to tools such as a file, a plane, and a spade. He measured energy expenditure during work, using oxygen consumption, pulse rate and blood pressure, and urine and blood byproducts as indicators. The results of the analyses were applied in a three-part program to re-educate soldiers (many of them with amputations). At the beginning of the convalescent period, exercise and crafts were used to strengthen stump muscles and build endurance. The patient was then fitted with a prosthesis or splint and taught to use it in vocational tasks.

Occupational Therapy and Motion Study

When Gilbreth returned from his travels, he and his wife presented papers to several professional groups about the application of motion study to "re-education of the crippled soldier" (Gilbreth & Gilbreth, 1920). The theme of the papers was as follows:

> In considering any type of activity to which it is proposed to introduce the cripple, we first analyze this activity from the motion study standpoint, in order to find exactly what motions are required to perform the activity and in what way these motions may be adapted to the available, or remaining, capable members of the cripple's working anatomy or eliminated by altering the device or machine itself. (pp. 45–46)

One in this series of papers was presented in March 1917 at the founding conference of the National Society for the Promotion of Occupational Therapy (NSPOT) at Consolation House in Clifton Springs, New York (NSPOT, 1918). Titled "The Conservation of the World's Teeth," it recommended that disabled veterans be retrained as dental assistants (Gilbreth & Gilbreth, 1920). During the meeting, Frank Gilbreth and Jules Amar were elected honorary members of the Society (NSPOT, 1918).

The Gilbreths clearly believed that engineers were best qualified to analyze and adapt jobs for people with disabilities (Gilbreth & Gilbreth, 1920). Still, in their presentations after the Consolation House conference, they began acknowledging the contributions of George Barton and William Rush Dunton, Jr. (first and second presidents of the National Society). Barton and Dunton, in turn, began incorporating motion study into their work and their writings. A paper about Barton's practice with convalescents at Consolation House stated that he:

> considers what motions are possible or impossible, desirable or undesirable; then he finds some occupation which involves those possible and desired motions.... Failing to find such an occupation in his own knowledge, the "Director" turns to his "materia medica"—a huge fifteen-hundred

page catalog of tools and machines—from which, by a visualization of each tool, how it is used and what motions are necessary for its use, he "compounds" his "prescription." (Newton, 1919, pp. 4–5)

Dunton (1919) discussed the work of both Amar and the Gilbreths in his second occupational therapy textbook and provided a bibliography of the Gilbreths' publications on motion study.

When the United States entered World War I, activity analysis was included in the new occupational therapy programs and in training courses that were developed to serve returning American soldiers. In early 1918, Elizabeth Upham wrote a curriculum plan for a proposed government course to train teachers of occupational therapy.[2] The plan, presented to the U.S. Senate and the Federal Board for Vocational Education, stated that students should study "1. Analysis of industrial, commercial and agricultural occupations in terms of therapeutic values. 2. Modification of processes, special devices and tools for special needs and fatigue prevention" (Dunton, 1918, p. 89). Upham's required reading list included selections from Amar's research.[3] Later that year, Upham became director of the first university-based occupational therapy school, at Milwaukee Downer College, Milwaukee (Reed & Sanderson, 1980).

The first systematic application of activity analysis in an occupational therapy clinic may also have been in 1918, at Walter Reed General Hospital in Washington, DC. Bird Baldwin (1919a), director of the new occupational therapy department, described the selection of therapeutic activities for patients as follows:

> First, the work must be one which involves as an essential part the movements required by the prescription, or in which these movements recur from time to time as the work is performed by the normal individual. In order to discover the activities in which certain specific movements were thus involved, a survey was made of all the shop and ward activities, and insofar as it was possible by observation and practice, each activity was analyzed into its constituent movements. (p. 449)

Baldwin's activity analyses were detailed but addressed primarily joint position and action. For example, his analysis of engraving described the position of each body part: Fingers flexed at all joints, thumb extended at the interphalangeal and metacarpophalangeal joints to guide the tool, shoulders rigid and slightly abducted. Other important requirements, such as muscle strength and vision, were not delineated, although they were clearly considered when patients' programs were planned (Baldwin, 1919b). Activities were also adapted by changing the tools or methods used

---

[2]The term *occupational therapist* was not yet in use. Practitioners in the new discipline were called *teachers of occupation* or *reconstruction aides*.

[3]An English translation of Amar's most recent text had been published in 1918, making his ideas more accessible to American students.

when this was indicated to improve the patient's physical function or compensate for deficits.

Between the Wars

In the 1920s, after the NSPOT had become the American Occupational Therapy Association (AOTA), a standing committee of the organization began publishing a series of papers designed to help therapists establish new departments in curative workshops and state psychiatric hospitals (AOTA, 1924). Dunton and Association president Thomas Kidner were among the influential members of the committee. Their reports included guidelines for analyzing crafts[4] in terms of joint motion and muscle strength (AOTA, 1928). Crafts requiring active motion with strength were listed for each body joint, and actions of the two sides of the body were differentiated. No attempt was made to quantify the requirements (e.g., in degrees of range or grades of strength). These craft analyses remained a standard reference for occupational therapists working with physically disabled patients for many years.

In psychiatric occupational therapy, activity analysis took the form of classification of crafts according to their characteristics or applications. Louis Haas, another member of AOTA's standing committee, developed an early system of classification that was widely accepted (Haas, 1922). He analyzed and rated activities in terms of the types of tools and materials used, the noise involved, the potential for modifying methods, the appeal to various ages and sexes, and the simplicity or complexity of processes. As was typical in psychiatry, he was most interested in the characteristics of activities that would address patients' emotional and social needs (e.g., channel aggression, promote self-esteem).

World War II stimulated renewed interest in motion study, now sometimes called *work simplification*. Frank Gilbreth had died, but Lillian Gilbreth published a paper in an occupational therapy journal recommending that engineers and rehabilitation professionals work closely together to help handicapped soldiers (Gilbreth, 1943). The army's War Department (1944) printed a technical manual on occupational therapy that contained the most detailed activity analyses to date. In addition to the traditional breakdown of joint motions, this manual listed activities for strengthening individual upper-extremity and lower-extremity muscles. Charts rating the intensity of motion at each joint during the performance of various tasks were also included.

Activity Analysis Comes of Age

In 1947, Sidney Licht, a physician who had been chief of physical medicine in an army hospital during the war, wrote a paper calling for more precise analysis of activities used in occupational therapy for physical dysfunction. He suggested the name *kinetic analysis* for the study of specific motions required in an occupation. Licht stated that a kinetic analysis should be based on actual observation of an experienced worker using proper body mechanics. It should describe the starting position and cycle of motion for the activity. The type of muscle contraction and degrees of joint range should be specified, as should the size and shape of tools used. Although Licht's terminology was not generally adopted, the elements of such an analysis are addressed today.

Through the 1960s, occupational therapists continued to analyze activities either in terms of physical requirements or in terms of emotional and social properties. In the 1970s and 1980s, however, a new way of thinking about the theory base of the profession led to major changes in activity analysis. Theorists began to delineate frames of reference within which occupational therapy intervention occurred (e.g., developmental, biomechanical, behavioral). Because each frame of reference included a unique perspective on the selection and uses of activity, each required a different type of activity analysis. Llorens' (1973) analysis of activities for treatment of cognitive-perceptual-motor dysfunction focused on the sensory systems stimulated and the motor responses produced. Trombly and Scott (1977) differentiated biomechanical analysis (emphasizing range of motion and strength) from neurodevelopmental analysis (emphasizing postures and patterns of movement). Cubie (1985) discussed volitional, habituation, and performance analysis within the Model of Human Occupation. The cognitive requirements of tasks were Allen's focus (1985).

Conclusion

Today, activity analysis is viewed as a multifaceted process (Cynkin & Robinson, 1990; Hopkins & Smith, 1988; Lamport, Coffey, & Hersch, 1989; Mosey, 1986). A comprehensive analysis first places the activity within a cultural and environmental context. Then both its generic properties (e.g., steps, tools used, cost, safety considerations) and its characteristics related to a specific frame of reference are described. The activity is discussed as it is normally performed and as modified for remedial or compensatory applications with patients.

Okoye (1988) provided an example of activity analysis as it is currently applied in occupational therapy. She discussed the importance of the computer as a medium for skill development, education, and prevocational training in our computer age. She presents a form for analyzing a computer-based treatment activity in which the therapist lists the hardware and software needed and answers a series of questions about the characteristics of the activity. The form delineates the neuromotor requirements for accessing the computer (posture, alignment, coordination) and the basic cognitive and sensory integrative functions necessary (visual discrimination,

---

[4]During this period, the term *crafts* was used more broadly than it is today. Early craft analyses included work-related and recreational activities such as tennis, typing, gardening, and bookbinding.

---

attention, problem solving), because the persons most likely to have difficulty are those with severe physical or multiple handicaps. For each requirement identified, the therapist lists alternative positioning, equipment, or methods for access (e.g., breakaway keyboard, audio reinforcement, software with slower speed options).

Although the original link with industrial engineering and other fields doing time and motion studies in the pursuit of productivity has been severed, occupational therapists continue to use activity analysis essentially as the founders did: to improve the functioning and quality of the lives of persons with disabilities.

Acknowledgment

This work was supported in part by Grant #H133G00139 from the National Institute on Disability and Rehabilitation Research.

References

Allen, C. K. (1985). *Occupational therapy for psychiatric diseases*. Boston: Little, Brown.

Amar, J. (1918). *The physiology of industrial organization and the re-employment of the disabled*. London: Library Press Limited.

American Occupational Therapy Association. (1924). Report of Committee on Installations and Advice. *Archives of Occupational Therapy, 3*, 299–318.

American Occupational Therapy Association. (1928). Report of Committee on Installations and Advice. *Occupational Therapy and Rehabilitation, 7*, 29–43, 131–136, 211–216, 417–421.

Baldwin, B. T. (1919a). Occupational therapy. *American Journal of Care for Cripples, 8*, 447–451.

Baldwin, B. T. (1919b). *Occupational therapy applied to restoration of function of disabled joints*. Washington, DC: Walter Reed General Hospital.

Cubie, S. H. (1985). Occupational analysis. In G. Kielhofner (Ed.), *A Model of Human Occupation: Theory and application*. Baltimore: Williams & Wilkins.

Cynkin, S., & Robinson, A. M. (1990). *Occupational therapy and activities health: Toward health through activities*. Boston: Little, Brown.

Dunton, W. R. (1918). Rehabilitation of crippled soldiers and sailors: A review. *Maryland Psychiatric Quarterly, 7*, 85–101.

Dunton, W. R. (1919). *Reconstruction therapy*. Philadelphia: Saunders.

Gilbreth, F. B. (1911). *Motion study*. New York: Van Nostrand.

Gilbreth, F. B., & Gilbreth, L. M. (1920). *Motion study for the handicapped*. London: Routledge.

Gilbreth, L. M. (1943). The place of motion study in rehabilitation work. *Occupational Therapy and Rehabilitation, 22*, 61–64.

Haas, L. J. (1922). Crafts adaptable to occupational needs: Their relative importance. *Archives of Occupational Therapy, 1*, 443–445.

Hopkins, H. L., & Smith, H. D. (Eds.). (1988). *Willard and Spackman's occupational therapy* (7th ed.). Philadelphia, Lippincott.

Lamport, N. K., Coffey, M. S., & Hersch, G. I. (1989). *Activity analysis handbook*. Thorofare, NJ: Slack.

Licht, S. (1947). Kinetic analysis of crafts and occupations. *Occupational Therapy and Rehabilitation, 26*, 75–78.

Llorens, L. A. (1973). Activity analysis for cognitive-perceptual-motor dysfunction. *American Journal of Occupational Therapy, 27*, 453–456.

Mosey, A. C. (1986). *Psychosocial components of occupational therapy*. New York: Rover.

National Society for the Promotion of Occupational Therapy. (1918). *Proceedings of the first annual meeting of the National Society for the Promotion of Occupational Therapy*. Towson, MD: Author.

Newton, I. G. (1919). *Consolation House*. Clifton Springs, NY: Consolation House.

Okoye, R. L. (1988). Computer technology in occupational therapy. In H. L. Hopkins & H. D. Smith (Eds.), *Willard and Spackman's occupational therapy* (pp. 340–345). Philadelphia: Lippincott.

Reed, K. L., & Sanderson, S. R. (1980). *Concepts of occupational therapy*. Baltimore: Williams & Wilkins.

Taylor, F. W. (1911). *The principles of scientific management*. New York: Harper & Brothers.

Trombly, C. A., & Scott, A. D. (1977). *Occupational therapy for physical dysfunction*. Baltimore: Williams & Wilkins.

War Department. (1944). *Occupational therapy*. Washington, DC: U.S. Government Printing Office.

Yost, E. (1949). *Frank and Lillian Gilbreth*. New Brunswick, NJ: Rutgers University Press.

Occupational Adaptation: Toward a Holistic Approach for Contemporary Practice, Part 2

SALLY SCHULTZ, PHD, OTR
JANETTE K. SCHKADE, PHD, OTR

This paper introduces a practice model based on the occupational adaptation frame of reference (Schkade & Schultz, 1992). The occupational adaptation practice model emphasizes the creation of a therapeutic climate, the use of occupational activity, and the importance of relative mastery. Practice based on occupational adaptation differs from treatment that focuses on acquisition of functional skills because the practice model directs occupational therapy interventions toward the patient's internal processes and how such processes are facilitated to improve occupational functioning. The occupational adaptation model is holistic. The patient's occupational environments (as influenced by physical, social, and properties) are as important as the patient's sensorimotor, cognitive, and psychosocial functioning, and the patient's experience of personal limitations and potential is validated. The integration of these concepts drives the treatment process. Through a description of treatment with a variety of patients, this paper presents the model's diversity and illustrates the relationship between the concepts. The occupational adaptation practice model reflects the uniqueness of occupation therapy and integrates the profession's historical practice with contemporary interventions and methods.

This chapter was previously published in the *American Journal of Occupational Therapy, 46,* 917–925. Copyright © 1992, American Occupational Therapy Association.

This paper presents the implications for practice of the theoretical concepts discussed in "Occupational Adaptation: Toward a Holistic Approach for Contemporary Practice, Part 1" (Schkade & Schultz, 1992) (see Chapter 11). The present paper discusses the occupational adaptation construct presented in Part 1 and illustrates how that construct becomes operationalized in therapy. Although the occupational therapy literature contains many references that discuss the relationship between occupation and adaptation (Breines, 1986; Clark, 1979; Fidler, 1981; Fidler & Fidler, 1978 (see Chapter 9); Fine, 1990 (see Chapter 25); Gilfoyle, Grady, & Moore, 1990; Kielhofner, 1985; King, 1978 (see Chapter 10); Kleinman & Bulkley, 1982; Lindquist, Mack, & Parham, 1982; Llorens, 1984, 1990; Mosey, 1968; Nelson, 1988; Reed, 1984; Reilly, 1962 (reprinted in Chapter 8); Yerxa, 1967, 1989), this paper proposes treatment that is based, not on a relationship between occupation and adaptation, but on *occupational adaptation,* a single internal phenomenon within the patient (Schkade & Schultz, 1992 [see Chapter 11]). Parts 1 and 2 are offered to enhance the understanding of occupational therapy as a vital intervention.

The proposed practice model is based on the occupational adaptation construct. This normative construct, which is conceptualized as both a state and a process, was discussed in Part 1 (Schkade & Schultz, 1992 [see Chapter 11]). The present paper focuses on interventions based on this construct with its associated concepts and assumptions. Occupational adaptation treatment is directed at improving the patient's occupational adaptation process, a normative process that is used throughout the life span as the person faces occupational challenges. Numerous events and conditions, such as traumatic injury, chronic illness, physical abuse, congenital anomalies, chemical dependency, and mental illness, can greatly impair the patient's occupational adaptation process. Traditional approaches in occupational therapy have focused treatment on improving the patient's sensorimotor, cognitive, and psychosocial systems, which together compose the patient's person system. The occupational adaptation practice model leads the therapist into a new layer of intervention, that is, treatment directed at affecting the patient's internal ability to generate, evaluate, and integrate adaptive responses in which relative mastery is experienced. Although the importance of improvement in the person system is a given, we suggest that the most beneficial effect of occupational therapy may occur when the occupational therapist focuses on the internal workings of the patient's occupational adaptation process, because that process leads to the patient's ability to adapt and to approach each occupational challenge with greater success and satisfaction.

Many occupational therapists have shifted their orientation away from phenomenological processes to focus on functional performance that can be measured more objectively (Mattingly, 1991). The current demand for therapists to base occupational therapy on acquisition of functional skills illustrates this trend. We believe, however, that a focus on the patient's functional skills may actually limit the contribution of occupational therapy and may deny patients the opportunity to make vital changes in their occupational adaptation process until they are discharged from the treatment setting. At home, former patients often discard techniques and assistive devices that they have received and design more efficient or effective methods for meeting their needs and going about their activities with greater satisfaction. The patient's resulting occupational adaptation may bear little resemblance to the occupational therapy that was received.

The Occupational Adaptation Practice Model does not disregard the necessity of functional skills. However, in this model, the occupational adaptation process has a more direct link to future occupational functioning than does the acquisition of specific functional skills. Therefore, the model focuses primarily on the patient's internal process of occupational adaptation. Because the present paper incorporates the assumptions and terminology introduced in Part I (Schkade & Schultz, 1992), a review of that paper will be necessary for complete understanding of the perspectives presented in the present paper. Additionally, four concepts that are required to apply the concepts introduced in Part 1 must be defined: occupational activities, occupational readiness, occupations of daily living, and therapeutic climate.

Occupational activities are discrete activities that are occupational (i.e., active, meaningful, and process-oriented with a tangible or intangible product) and are incorporated into treatment because they can promote the occupational adaptation process. *Occupational readiness* includes skill-based activities and other such interventions that focus on change in the person systems in preparation for occupational activities (e.g., the use of preparatory techniques, instruction, or assistive devices necessary for the patient to engage in occupational activity). *Occupations of daily living* are the unique patterns of occupations in which the person regularly engages as a result of the interaction between his or her occupational environments and related occupational roles. *Therapeutic climate* is the product of an interdependent exchange wherein the therapist, as the primary facilitator, functions as the agent of the patient's occupational environment and the patient functions as the agent of his or her unique person systems. The climate defines the role of each party, the goal of therapy, and the expected outcome; both parties are empowered to make their optimal contribution.

Occupational Adaptation: A Practice Model

The Occupational Adaptation Practice Model is based on the same essential beliefs stated by the founders and leaders of the occupational therapy profession: (a) human beings have an occupational nature and can influence their health through occupation: (b) human development is a continuous process of adaptation; (c) biological, sociological, and psychological factors may interrupt and impair the adaptation process at any point in the life cycle; and (d) appropriate occupation can facilitate the adaptive process (American Occupational Therapy Association [AOTA], 1979; Meyer, 1922; West, 1989). Occupational adaptation practice focuses on identifying and treating impairment or interference in the patient's occupational adaptation process. The following discussion identifies the conditions and parameters of practice that is based on the occupational adaptation frame of reference discussed in Part 1 (Schkade & Schultz, 1992).

Facilitating the Therapeutic Climate

Through exchange of knowledge, experience, ability, analysis of motivation, and shared vision, the therapeutic climate is created. Practice based on this frame of reference (Schkade & Schultz, 1992) requires the therapist to establish a close therapeutic relationship with the patient (Fidler & Fidler, 1963; Peloquin, 1990). The treatment process is an ongoing collaboration with mutual identification of goals between therapist and patient. It depends on an exchange of "needs, visions, and expectations" (Peloquin, 1990, p. 13). Such an exchange is made possible through the roles of agency that are assumed by the patient and the occupational therapist. The role of the patient is to function as his or her own agent. The role of the therapist is to function as the agent of the patient's occupational environment. This approach directs the therapist to base treatment on the patient's occupational environments and the associated expectations of occupational performance. Treatment guided by mutual agency may free each party to act in a way that empowers both to make optimal contributions to the treatment process.

Aspects of the therapeutic climate will change over time. In the initial stages of therapy, the therapist's role is greater than the patient's, but as therapy progresses, the patient's role becomes greater. Although the therapist is the primary catalyst in this evolutionary process, the concept of agency empowers each party to assume a unique and vital role. As the therapist fulfills the identified role and function, therapeutic use of self may become the most important element in both the process and outcome of therapy.

The overarching goal of therapy is improvement in the patient's internal occupational adaptation process (Schkade & Schultz, 1992). To meet this goal, the therapy program must be directly related to the patient's occupations of daily living.

Assumption: *For maximal effect on occupational adaptation, the activities, tasks, methods, and techniques of intervention must* *be centered on occupational activity that promotes satisfaction for the patient and society.*

Perspective on Motivation

The therapist incorporates all sources of motivation, such as the patient's desires, potential, limitations, and societal expectations, to facilitate the therapeutic climate. The experience of mastery is accepted as a major component of motivation. In this practice model, mastery is conceptualized as a relative phenomenon rather than an absolute condition; therefore, the term *relative mastery* is used. Relative mastery is incorporated in occupational adaptation practice as a patient-centered concept because it measures performance from the patient's orientation. This perspective is based on the beliefs that each person is endowed with a desire for mastery, that the occupational environment also has a demand for mastery, and that together these internal and external motivational forces provide an interactive press for mastery (Schkade & Schultz, 1992).

Assumptions: (a) Change in the occupational adaptation process occurs as a result of both internal and external sources of motivation that interact to prompt a striving for mastery. (b) Mastery is more than the ability to perform a discrete task; it is a reflection of the patient's experience as an occupational being. (c) Relative mastery has three major properties: efficiency, effectiveness, and satisfaction to self and others. These properties are operative explanations of the interactive influence of internal and external motivation.

The occupational adaptation practice model is organized around a set of concepts and assumptions that add a unique perspective to the current body of knowledge on the efficacy of occupational therapy. The following statements summarize this perspective. First, the patient's level of relative mastery is directly related to the degree that the internal occupational adaptation process is activated and affected by therapy. Second, a change in the patient's occupational adaptation process is more predictive of future occupational functioning than is the patient's ability to perform discrete functional tasks. Third, the patient's internal occupational adaptation process is the optimal pathway for occupational therapy to affect occupational functioning. The assumptions of the Occupational Adaptation Practice Model are considered to be universal regardless of age, race, culture, gender, condition, or other classifications.

Occupational Adaptation Practice Guide

The systematic guide for applying the occupational adaptation concepts and assumptions to a variety of settings and populations (see the Appendix) is based on the normative construct of occupational adaptation presented in Part 1 (Schkade & Schultz, 1992). The flow of the practice guide matches our understanding of the occupational adaptation process and how that process may be affected by therapeutic intervention.

The format of the guide provides the therapist with a sequence of questions to be asked, rather than an identification of specific treatment methods or techniques. The intent of this format is to free the therapist to address the uniqueness of each patient and each treatment setting. Specific interventions will vary greatly. It is hoped that therapists will find the practice guide useful in the development of population-specific practice models. The occupational adaptation practice guide has three main parts: data gathering and assessment, programming, and evaluation: The following discussion provides further explanation of the practice guide and an example of each part of the guide.

Occupational Adaptation Data Gathering and Assessment

An occupational adaptation assessment is conducted in the following sequence. First, information is collected about the patient's occupational environments and the respective occupational role expectations (past, present, and future). Next, the effect of the presenting problem (e.g., illness, condition, behavior) on the patient's person systems (i.e., sensorimotor, cognitive, and psychosocial functioning) is evaluated. Traditional occupational therapy tests and instruments are used as indicated. On the basis of the accumulated information, the patient and the therapist determine the relative match between the patient's current occupational functioning and the role expectations of the occupational environments. Last, the therapist estimates the patient's present potential for occupational adaptation and how this potential can be facilitated over the course of occupational therapy intervention. Identifying the sources of dysfunction in the components of the occupational adaptation process and their effect on relative mastery is an underlying theme of occupational adaptation practice. Such identification enables the therapist to clarify the points in the patient's occupational adaptation process where intervention will be most effective. During the initial phase of therapy, the therapist's essential task is to transform the patient's assessment into an occupational adaptation treatment program that reflects the patient as an occupational being. The following example demonstrates responses for patients with similar person systems but different occupational roles:

> Two patients complain of pain, edema, and limited range of motion due to traumatic tendon and nerve damage in their dominant hands. For Patient A, the mother of four young children, the greatest concern might be performing the occupations of preparing meals, doing laundry, and bathing her children. Assessment of the person systems reveals sensorimotor deficits in range of motion, strength, sensation, and dexterity; no cognitive impairment; and psychosocial anxiety about ability to carry out her occupational role. The primary treatment focus would become her work environment and the role of mother. In contrast,

Patient B's greatest concern might be returning to her occupation as a secretary. The person system assessment is comparable to that of Patient A. Although both patients present with similarities in the status of their person systems, there are substantial differences in their occupational environments (work) and the relative role expectations.

Occupational Adaptation Programming

The occupational adaptation assessment is used to design an intervention program focused on helping the patient achieve the highest level of internal occupational adaptation. The program is designed to improve the occupational adaptation process to help the patient narrow the gap between present occupational functioning and the role performance required by both the patient and the occupational environments. As the gap narrows, it is expected that the patient's experience of relative mastery will improve. All therapy activities and methods should be consonant with these two effects. On the basis of a thorough review of the occupational adaptation assessment and patient and family collaboration, a primary occupational environment is selected and the expected role performance within that occupational environment is identified as the primary treatment focus.

The resulting treatment program for Patients A and B would vary because the primary treatment focus is different for each. The activities and associated tasks planned by the patient and therapist would give the patient the maximum opportunity to improve her internal occupational adaptation prowess relative to the primary treatment focus.

Improvement in the patient's occupational adaptation process is accomplished through a therapy program that includes both *occupational readiness* and *occupational activity*. It is expected that both aspects of treatment would be indicated for most patients. Examples of occupational readiness are progressive resistive exercise, assertiveness training, social skill development, and passive or active range of motion. Occupational activities allow the patient and the therapist to put into meaningful action the benefit derived from occupational readiness. Both the occupational readiness and the occupational activities used in treatment must be directly related to the primary treatment focus.

For Patient A, the occupational readiness should focus on addressing edema, range of motion, dexterity, and sensory loss relevant to meal preparation or other appropriate role expectations. The therapist may use a variety of occupational readiness techniques such as assistive devices, alternative methods, and a home exercise program. Occupational activities would be progressive. For example, therapy may be initiated with the patient preparing a simple lunch with the therapist and then may progress to a real-life situation in which the children are present and the demand for occupational adaptation is increased. In this more challenging occupational environment, the opportunity for experiencing relative mastery is enhanced,

and motivation is therefore increased.

For Patient B, occupational readiness would also focus on addressing edema, range of motion, dexterity, and sensory loss. However, the specific form would be relevant to the type of secretarial work performed by the patient. Occupational activities for this patient may range from putting a floppy disk into a computer to completing segments of real work brought from her office. As with Patient A, occupational activity enhances the opportunity for experiencing relative mastery and increasing motivation.

Throughout the course of therapy, the therapist must continually critique the therapy program to ensure that its design offers the patient the optimal opportunity to improve the occupational adaptation process. Changes in relative mastery indicate that the therapy program is appropriately designed.

Assumption: Although the patient may be improving in functional skills, change in occupational adaptation may not be occurring. An increase in relative mastery is the best indicator that change in the occupational adaptation process is taking place.

Evaluation of the Occupational Adaptation Process

In the Occupational Adaptation Practice Model, treatment effectiveness depends on a view of the patient as a whole person with a unique occupational nature. For example, even though the chief complaint may be physical, other aspects of the patient's occupational environments and relative roles may affect treatment outcome more than physiological deficits. Consequently, the therapist should consider the patient as a whole occupational system when documenting progress. In addition to reporting traditional measures of patient improvement, such as level of functional independence, the therapist should note the patient's change in occupational adaptation by documenting the patient's energy level, adaptive response mode, adaptive response behavior, and resulting relative mastery (Schkade & Schultz, 1992). Holistic evaluation and documentation are essential for an understanding of the effect of programming on the patient's occupational adaptation process and potential for occupational performance.

Occupational adaptation is an internal phenomenon and therefore seems to be less measurable than observable behaviors that can be counted or functional skills that can be objectively measured. However, a systematic approach based on both observable and phenomenological criteria could be generated to measure change in occupational adaptation. We believe that change in the occupational adaptation process is manifested by three predictable outcomes: improvement in self-initiation, generalization, and relative mastery. Many practitioners have observed these outcomes and have noted their positive effect on the patient's empowerment.

Assumption: As the internal occupational adaptation process changes, the following outcomes result: (a) the patient begins to initiate changes in the way occupational activities are approached; (b) *the patient begins to spontaneously generalize knowledge and competencies acquired in therapy to other occupational activities; and (c) the patient begins to experience greater relative mastery.*

Periodic measurement of these outcomes may show the changes that are occurring in the patient's occupational adaptation process. Self-initiation and generalization may be readily measured by frequency counts. However, the measurement of relative mastery requires a different approach, such as a framework that practitioners may use to measure relative mastery as an outcome of change in occupational adaptation (see Figure 48.1). Although it is a phenomenological experience, relative mastery can be translated into quantitative information, as is described below.

The three properties of relative mastery, as discussed in Part 1 (Schkade & Schultz, 1992 [see Chapter 11]), are efficiency, effectiveness, and satisfaction to self and others. A procedure to measure change in relative mastery involves three steps. First, the patient and the therapist select one or more occupational activities for outcome measurement. The activity selected is drawn from those identified as part of the primary treatment focus during the initial occupational adaptation assessment. The occupational activity selected to measure change in relative mastery must not be one in which the patient has had direct training or experience in occupational therapy. A degree of novelty in the occupational activity is necessary for the therapist to determine whether the associated outcomes of

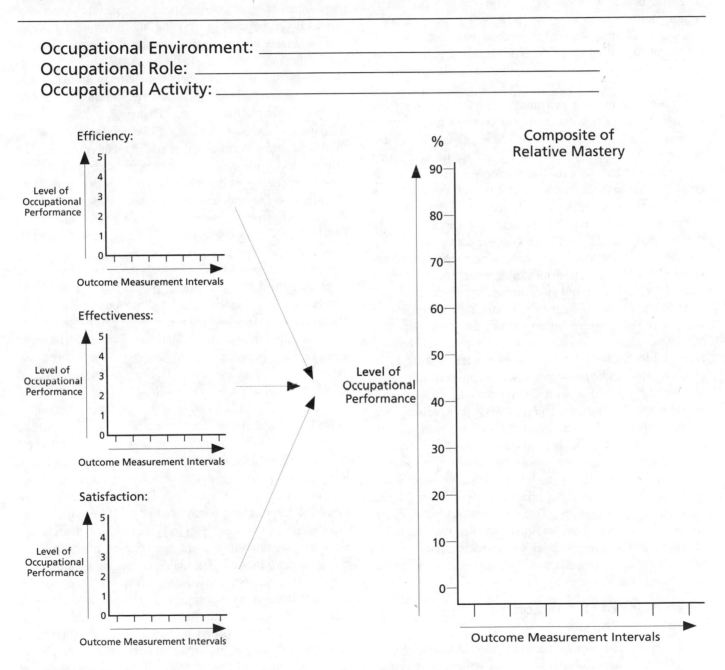

Figure 48.1. Measurement of relative mastery.

self-initiation and generalization are occurring. Second, the patient and the therapist determine the criteria that describe the levels of expected occupational performance for each property of relative mastery (i.e., what will constitute the five levels of efficiency, effectiveness, and satisfaction). Third, the patient and therapist decide how often measurement is to occur. After each measurement of relative mastery, the patient and the therapist collaborate to plot the results. The relative weight of each property is determined by the patient.

Assumption: The patient will weigh the three elements of relative mastery according to personal priorities.

For example, a patient with many competing responsibilities may weigh efficiency as the most important property, whereas a patient with few demands on time may place more importance on satisfaction. The patient determines the relative weight of each property given the selected occupational environment and relative role expectations. One can calculate the composite measure of the patient's relative mastery by adding the ordinal data points from each property and computing a composite percentage for relative mastery. For example, if on the first occurrence of outcome measurement the patient rated efficiency as 1, effectiveness as 2, and satisfaction as 4, the sum would be 7. One would compute a composite percentage of relative mastery by dividing the calculated value into the highest possible total value (7÷15 = 47%). The percentage is then plotted (see Figure 48.1). A comparison of the composite percentage on admission with the percentage at different points during therapy provides a measure of change in relative mastery over time. Such comparison may be useful in determining whether the patient is ready for discharge, requires continued inpatient treatment, or requires referral to outpatient rehabilitation services. An analysis of performance within each of the three properties of relative mastery may clarify where therapy should be concentrated for greater effect on relative mastery and the overall occupational adaptation process. A graphic representation of outcome effect may provide the patient, the therapist, family members, and concerned professionals with a visual record of therapeutic effect (see Figure 48.1).

Two caveats should be kept in mind about this method of measuring relative mastery. First, the measurement assumptions have not been fully tested. Second, a 5-point scale was used within each property of relative mastery to suggest one approach to measurement. Different treatment settings or patient conditions may call for either a smaller or greater number of levels. This decision is left to the discretion of the therapist. Examples of program evaluation can be found in the illustrations that follow.

Illustrations of Occupational Adaptation Practice

The following examples are excerpts from the course of therapy with four hypothetical patients. They are provided to illustrate various aspects of practice applications based on the occupational adaptation frame of reference. Familiarity with Part 1 (Schkade & Schultz, 1992 [see Chapter 11]) is required for a complete understanding. The treatment presented in these examples is based on three factors: the normative construct of occupational adaptation discussed in Part 1, the conditions and parameters of occupational adaptation practice discussed in the present paper, and the questions posed in the occupational adaptation practice guide (see the Appendix 48.1).

Example 1: Outpatient Rehabilitation for Carpal Tunnel Syndrome

For the patient in this example, occupational therapy was initiated after surgery. As the patient began to experience increased occupational functioning, the therapist transferred more and more of the responsibility for planning and managing the therapeutic outcome to the patient. With the therapist's facilitation, the patient designed a home program that would incorporate essential movement patterns and precautions into her occupations of daily living. This process increased the magnitude of the patient's agency and empowered the patient to make changes in her occupational adaptation process. The primary focus throughout treatment was on helping the patient experience greater relative mastery in her occupational environment of work and role of mother. The patient placed the most importance on the property of satisfaction. As the patient began to change her approach to occupational challenges, such as doing the laundry, her overall relative mastery increased. She found that the splints recommended by the therapist helped her to maintain proper wrist position and enabled her to make necessary hand motions with less pain. However, although her efficiency and effectiveness were increasing, her satisfaction was not. In response, the therapist encouraged the patient to reassess her occupational role expectations. The patient revealed that before surgery, she had always taken great pride in methodically folding and putting away the laundry. She now realized that the task took so much of her energy and ability that it gave her little satisfaction. She began to see folding laundry as an unnecessary task and a performance expectation that, if eliminated, would allow her to focus on occupational activities with greater potential for satisfaction. Her assessment had a similar effect on the occupational role expectations relative to her occupational environment. Family members began to verbalize their desire to do tasks that would help prevent exacerbation of the patient's carpal tunnel syndrome. The children changed their expectations of their mother and began to help with the laundry, although they had never done so before. Other tasks that were related to performance expectations were also modified by the patient. The patient's change in occupational role expectations relative to the occupational environment had a positive influence on the patient's satisfaction and her overall experience of relative mastery.

Example 2: Inpatient Rehabilitation for Traumatic Brain Injury

The patient in this example had deficits in upper extremity movement and sensation in his dominant arm. The initial therapy program emphasized activities designed to promote sensorimotor functioning and independence in self-care. The primary occupational environment was self-maintenance, and the relative role was that of independent adult. Although he was making satisfactory progress in self-care, discussion with the patient revealed that the treatment program was not meaningful. The patient was experiencing little relative mastery. The therapist suggested a change in the occupational environment and role. The patient and the therapist selected the patient's work and the role of architect to guide treatment. Occupational activities were incorporated to provide a fit with what the patient found meaningful. Occupational challenges were included that engaged his occupational adaptation process. For example, the patient's drafting tools were brought in and the patient and therapist observed the patient's adaptiveness, identified the sources of interference with relative mastery, and designed a plan to help the patient become more adaptive and increase relative mastery.

Example 3: Inpatient Rehabilitation for Post–Cerebral Vascular Accident

After 1 month of rehabilitation, this patient's occupational skills were little improved. Aphasia and depression continued to interfere with therapy. It seemed to the therapist and the patient's wife that the patient was not fulfilling his potential. To the extent possible, the therapist reviewed the treatment program with the patient. The patient showed little response to any of the activities being used and was not experiencing any relative mastery. The therapist determined that, although the patient needed much more occupational readiness, it was essential to begin occupational activity to increase motivation. Further discussion with family members resulted in a new treatment plan that emphasized occupational activity. Gardening became the primary modality for occupational therapy because it had been the patient's main leisure occupation. Occupational readiness training that emphasized strength and sensorimotor skills related to gardening was begun by a certified occupational therapy assistant. The occupational therapist emphasized to the patient the connection between the exercises and the new program. Occupational activity was incorporated when possible (e.g., following oral and written directions in the care of seedlings, managing the plants in the clinic, using more complex gardening tools, tending plants in the outdoor garden). Sensorimotor, cognitive, and psychosocial systems improved through occupational readiness and occupational activity. Relative mastery also began to improve; efficiency was the biggest obstacle for the patient. The therapist encouraged the use of the gardening modality by other members of the treatment team. Speech therapy began to focus on words associated with gardening.

Physical therapy engaged the patient by relating necessary exercises to his hobby. A plan was designed with the patient and the family to extend the gardening occupation into his occupational environments and related roles upon discharge.

Example 4: Public School Special Education for Behavior Disorder, Attention Deficit, and Fine Motor Problems

The 15-year-old student was referred to the occupational therapist for handwriting and attention problems. She had a severe behavior disorder, an attention deficit disorder, and fine motor problems. She came from a dysfunctional family and was failing in school. Her intelligence was within average range. She was described as explosive, physically aggressive, and at risk for dropping out of school. She had no vocational interests or goals. The therapist's occupational adaptation assessment revealed that the student was occupationally dysadaptive in all of her occupational environments and roles and experienced no relative mastery. When faced with an occupational challenge, the student used primary energy most of the time. Her fine motor deficits interfered with performance tasks. Her adaptive response behaviors were largely hyperstabilized, which usually resulted in her being fixated with no action occurring. She would finally respond, "I can't do it." At other times, she was hypermobile and approached tasks randomly with no apparent plan of action. She perseverated in the use of existing but ineffective adaptive response modes. Her ability to generate, evaluate, and integrate adaptive responses was dysadaptive. She was markedly inefficient and ineffective and experienced little satisfaction.

The therapist collaborated with the special education teacher to develop a holistic program to treat the student's occupational dysadaptation. Occupational readiness was instituted with a variety of media designed to improve the student's fine motor skills, develop interests, and increase self-control. As the therapeutic climate evolved, the student began to express how, as a child, she had always loved to style her doll's hair. As her interest in hairstyling became more apparent, the therapist expanded the occupational readiness program by giving her information about the role expectations of a hairstylist and the knowledge required to be licensed and by giving her home-therapy assignments to visit and discuss work with practicing hairstylists. As a result of the occupational readiness, the student decided she wanted to become a hairstylist. Occupational readiness was further tailored to be consistent with her goal: A home program that emphasized fine motor tasks and other coordination activities specific to her work goal, and relevant behavioral goals such as timeliness, dependability, and impulse control were instituted in the classroom.

In addition, the therapist guided the student into extracurricular activities to widen her exposure to occupational challenges (e.g., decorating for the school dance, collecting and sorting food for a community food pantry). She began to display more mature adaptive response behaviors and to modify her existing adaptive response modes. For example, as the student became more aware of her dysadaptation, she began to anticipate the ways in which her adaptive response modes were obstacles to relative mastery and to generate alternative modes and modified responses. These changes in her occupational adaptation process resulted in greater relative mastery. The most dramatic improvements occurred in satisfaction to self and others.

As therapy continued, the student integrated these changes and began to generalize her new occupational adaptation process. She was able to see the relevance of school and the need to develop her fine motor skills, self-control, and social skills as part of her future life goals. The fine motor exercises were improving her handwriting and she noted her improved efficiency in the use of hair-styling tools and equipment.

Additional occupational activity was begun in which the student began to style other students' hair. She achieved positive recognition and acceptance from her peers for her competency in this activity. Her relative mastery increased substantially. As therapy progressed, the teacher noted to the therapist that the student was modifying her way of doing things by attempting to plan her approach to tasks, displaying more organization, and showing more neatness and pride in her handwriting. Behavioral problems in the classroom declined. The student had begun to initiate changes in how she responded to other occupational challenges (e.g., occupational performance at home and at her part-time job).

The occupational therapist discontinued direct service but periodically monitored the student's progress. She made suggestions to the teacher on ways to provide the student opportunities to increase relative mastery in the occupational environment of school. To the student she suggested ways to increase her awareness of her adaptive response behaviors, to develop new adaptive response modes, and to evaluate and affect her relative mastery when faced with new occupational challenges.

Conclusion

The Occupational Adaptation Practice Model integrates the beliefs, principles, and techniques that have been addressed by many theorists and are reflected tacitly in the practice of many clinicians. The uniqueness of the Occupational Adaptation Practice Model lies in the adherence to a theoretical framework that concentrates treatment on the patient's internal occupational adaptation process. The construct of occupational adaptation discussed in Part 1 (Schkade & Schultz, 1992 [see Chapter 11]) provides an overall explanation of this process and how the patient generates, evaluates, and integrates adaptive responses. We believe that interventions that affect relative mastery are instrumental in helping the patient become more adaptive, thus enhancing the potential for a productive and satisfying life.

In treatment based on the occupational adaptation frame of reference, the occupational environment is as important as the patient's physical or mental condition and is conceptualized as a blend of the physical, social, and cultural influences that affect the patient. The style of patient-therapist interaction is process oriented rather than performance driven. The therapist's primary gauge of effectiveness is change in the patient's internal occupational adaptation as opposed to improvement in self-care or other function-oriented criteria. The concept of relative mastery is introduced as an outcome of change in occupational adaptation. The occupational adaptation practice model views mastery as a relative phenomenon that can, however, be understood in terms of three predictable outcomes. Such outcomes are identified and methods for measurement are proposed. The effect of relative mastery on treatment is described in practical illustrations that provide an overview of occupational adaptation concepts and assumptions and their effect on the nature of practice. These illustrations clarify the construct of occupational adaptation, the conditions and parameters of occupational adaptation practice, and use of the occupational adaptation practice guide.

We believe that the occupational adaptation frame of reference (Schkade & Schultz, 1992 [see Chapter 11]) and model for practice have potential benefits for the occupational therapist. First, they may formally articulate the current practice of therapists who use a similar approach but have lacked a formal structure, thus validating what has been perceived as intuitive by many therapists. Second, they may provide a fresh perspective for therapists who have practiced within the medical model but are searching for a practice model that is more holistic. Third, the model offers a generic perspective; it is not specific to any particular dysfunction or condition. Consequently, the model is applicable to many settings, such as schools, hospitals, and home health care. It is an appropriate practice model for patients with a variety of conditions such as behavioral problems, physical dysfunction, developmental disability, or psychosocial dysfunction.

The concepts and assumptions presented in this paper and in Part 1 (Schkade & Schultz, 1992 [see Chapter 11]) remain to be formally tested. We hope that these writings will lead to increased scholarly debate and research on the integrative nature of occupation and adaptation with regard to the discipline and the practice of occupational therapy.

Acknowledgments

We acknowledge the impetus, support, and challenging critical comments provided by the doctoral planning committee at Texas Woman's University: Grace Gilkeson, EdD, OTR, FAOTA; Adelaide Flower, MA, OTR; Harriett Davidson, MA, OTR; Carol Freeman, MA, OTR; Nancy Griffin, EdD, OTR; Nancy Nashiro, PhD, OTR; Jean Spencer, PhD, OTR (Chair); and Virginia White, PhD, OTR. We also appreciate the input from Lela Llorens, PhD, OTR, FAOTA; Anne Henderson, PhD, OTR, FAOTA; and Kathlyn Reed, PhD, OTR, FAOTA, who provided thoughtful reading of earlier versions.

Appendix 48.1
Occupational Adaptation Guide to Practice

Occupational Adaptation Data Gathering/Assessment

- What are the patient's *occupational environments* and *roles*?
- Which role is of primary concern to patient and family?
- What occupational performance is expected in the primary *occupational environment* and *role*?
- What are the *physical, social, and cultural* features of the primary *occupational environment* and *role*?
- What is the patient's *sensorimotor, cognitive,* and *psychosocial* status?
- What is the patient's level of *relative mastery* in the primary *occupational environment* and *role*?
- What is facilitating or limiting *relative mastery* in the primary *occupational environment* and *role*?

Occupational Adaptation Programming

- What combination of occupational readiness and occupational activity is needed to promote the patient's *occupational adaptation process*?
- What will help the patient assess *occupational responses* and use the results to affect the *occupational adaptation process*?
- What is the best method to engage the patient in the occupational adaptation program?

Evaluation of the Occupational Adaptation Process

How is the program affecting the patient's *occupational adaptation process*?

- Which *energy level* is used most often (*primary* or *secondary*)?
- What *adaptive response* mode is used most often (*preexisting, modified,* or *new*)?
- What is the most common *adaptive response behavior* (*primitive, transitional,* or *mature*)?
- What outcomes does the patient show that reflect change in the *occupational adaptation process*?
  - Self-initiated adaptations?
  - Enhanced *relative mastery*?
  - Generalization to novel activities?
- What program changes are needed to provide maximum opportunity for occupational adaptation to occur?

Note: The italicized terms are constructs in the Occupational Adaptation Frame of Reference (Schkade & Schultz, 1992 [see Chapter 11]).

References

American Occupational Therapy Association. (1979). The philosophical base of occupational therapy. *American Journal of Occupational Therapy, 33,* 785.

Breines, E. (1986). *Origins and adaptations: A philosophy of practice.* Lebanon, NJ: Geri-Rehab.

Clark, P. N. (1979). Human development through occupation: A philosophy and conceptual model for practice, part 2. *American Journal of Occupational Therapy, 33,* 577—585.

Fidler, G. S. (1981). From crafts to competence. *American Journal of Occupational Therapy, 35,* 567–573.

Fidler, G. S., & Fidler, J. W. (1963). *Occupational therapy: A communication process in psychiatry.* New York: MacMillan.

Fidler, G. S., & Fidler, J. W. (1978). Doing and becoming: Purposeful action and self-actualization. *American Journal of Occupational Therapy, 32,* 305–310. Reprinted as Chapter 9.

Fine, S. (1990). Resilience and human adaptability: Who rises above adversity?—1990 Eleanor Clark Slagle Lecture. *American Journal of Occupational Therapy, 45,* 493–503. Reprinted as Chapter 25.

Gilfoyle, E., Grady, A., & Moore, J. (1990). *Children adapt* (2nd ed.). Thorofare, NJ: Slack.

Kielhofner, G. (Ed.). (1985). *A Model of Human Occupation: Theory and application.* Baltimore: Williams & Wilkins.

King, L. (1978). Toward a science of adaptive responses—1978 Eleanor Clarke Slagle Lecture. *American Journal of Occupational Therapy, 32,* 429–437. Reprinted as Chapter 10.

Kleinman, B. L., & Bulkley, B. L. (1982). Some implications of a science of adaptive responses. *American Journal of Occupational Therapy, 36,* 15–19.

Lindquist, J. E., Mack, W., & Parham, L. D. (1982). A synthesis of occupational behavior and sensory integration concepts in theory and practice, part 1. Theoretical foundations. *American Journal of Occupational Therapy, 36,* 365–374.

Llorens, L. (1984). Theoretical conceptualizations of occupational therapy: 1960–1982. *Occupational Therapy in Mental Health, 4*(2), 1–14.

Llorens, L. (1990). Foreword. In E. Gilfoyle, A. Grady, & J. Moore, *Children adapt* (2nd ed., pp. xi–xii). Thorofare, NJ: Slack.

Mattingly, C. (1991). What is clinical reasoning? *American Journal of Occupational Therapy, 45,* 979–986.

Meyer, A. (1922). The philosophy of occupational therapy. *Archives of Occupational Therapy, 1,* 1–3. Reprinted as Chapter 2.

Mosey, A. (1968). Recapitulation of ontogenesis: A theory for practice of occupational therapy. *American Journal of Occupational Therapy, 22,* 426–432.

Nelson, D. (1988). Occupation: Form and performance. *American Journal of Occupational Therapy, 42,* 633–641.

Peloquin, S. M. (1990). The patient–therapist relationship in occupational therapy: Understanding visions and images. *American Journal of Occupational Therapy, 44,* 13–21.

Reed, K. (1984). *Models of practice in occupational therapy.* Baltimore: Williams & Wilkins.

Reilly, M. (1962). Occupational therapy can be one of the great ideas of 20th-century medicine. *American Journal of Occupational Therapy, 16,* 1. Reprinted as Chapter 8.

Schkade, J. K., & Schultz, S. (1992). Occupational adaptation: Toward a holistic approach for contemporary practice, part 1. *American Journal of Occupational Therapy 46,* 829–837. Reprinted as Chapter 11.

West, W. (1989). Perspectives on the past and future, part 1. *American Journal of Occupational Therapy, 43,* 787–790.

Yerxa, E. (1967). Authentic occupational therapy–1996 Eleanor Clarke Slagle Lecture. *American Journal of Occupational Therapy, 21,* 1–9.

Yerxa, E. (1989, October 30). What is this thing called occupation? *Advance for Occupational Therapists,* p. 5.

Teaching Approaches and Occupational Therapy Psychoeducation

CHAPTER 49

RENÉ PADILLA, MS, OTR/L

Patient education has become an important feature of any treatment program. In the last two decades the mental health literature has increasingly used the term "psychoeducation" in reference to techniques found useful in the treatment and rehabilitation of patients with severe and persistent mental illness and their families (Spencer et al., 1988; McFarlane, Lukens, & Link, 1995; Pollio, North, & Douglas, 1998; Lubin, Loris, Burt, & Johnson, 1998). One of the earliest definitions of the term stated that psychoeducation is "the use of educational techniques, methods, and approaches to aid in the recovery from the disabling effects of mental illness or as an adjunct to the treatment of the mentally ill, usually within the framework of another ongoing treatment approach or as part of a research program" (Barter, 1984, p. 23). This definition was further refined by Goldman (1988), who stated that psychoeducation is "education or training of a person with a psychiatric disorder in subject areas that serve the goals of treatment and rehabilitation, for example, enhancing the person's acceptance of his illness, promoting active cooperation with treatment and rehabilitation, and strengthening the coping skills that compensate for deficiencies caused by the disorder" (p. 667).

A basic assumption of psychoeducation is that information can enhance understanding of the illness, needed treatment resources, and supportive services available (Greenberg et al., 1988). Outcomes reported often include increase in daily living skills and adaptive capacities and the creation of more productive alliances among patients, families, and mental health professionals, making treatment more efficient and cost-effective (Dixon, Adams, & Lucksted, 2000). Although the specific elements and construction of the various programs vary, all programs have a common characteristic in that they are professionally created and led, often by a multidisciplinary team (Solomon, 1996; Pollio, North, & Foster, 1998; Dixon, 1999). These teams frequently include an occupational therapy practitioner (Dixon, 1999).

Psychoeducational procedures dominate the treatment used by occupational therapists in psychiatric rehabilitation (Hayes & Halford, 1993). Emphasis in occupational therapy intervention in mental health is often placed on life skills training through behavioral approaches (Fine, 1980; Barris, 1985; Bartlow & Hartwig, 1989; Klasson, 1989). Occupational therapy literature frequently describes the content of psychoeducational programs but rarely examines the teaching approach therapists use in them. Presumably, the behavioral emphasis on life-skills training is viewed as consistent with basic occupational therapy philosophy, and therefore the teaching methods used are not carefully scrutinized. However, several studies have recently brought into question the generalizability to community life of skills learned in occupational therapy treatment (Wallace et al., 1992; Hayes & Halford, 1993). Of ever more concern is the possibility that occupational therapy treatment has no greater relative effectiveness than training provided in psychoeducation by paraprofessionals (Liberman et al., 1998). It is necessary, therefore, to begin carefully questioning how we are approaching psychoeducation and justifying it as a method compatible with our basic philosophical principles and our growing understanding of occupation.

Basic Principle: The Occupational Nature of the Human Being

In order to evaluate the compatibility of various teaching approaches with occupational therapy, it is necessary to first briefly review some foundational philosophical beliefs of the profession. This review is not intended to be exhaustive, but to highlight general principles that should be present in any and all services we provide in order for them to be recognized as unique to occupational therapy.

A fundamental belief of occupational therapy is that "Man is an active being whose development is influenced by the use of purposeful activity" (American Occupational Therapy Association [AOTA], 1995-a, p. 10). (See Appendix E.) Central to this concept is the human capacity for intrinsic motivation, self-initiation, and choice (Dickerson, 1996). Yerxa (1967) emphasized that occupational therapy recognizes this notion by supporting the patient's choice of activity, stating that "it is impossible to force any human being to initiate without his choosing to do so; choice is one of the keys to our unique therapeutic process. It is also a necessity if we are to achieve the ultimate goal of occupational therapy, that is, the ability of the person to function in his environment with self-actualization. For no matter how well-conceived the therapeutic program, the resulting achievement of the client's function depends both upon his capacities and his choice to use them" (1967, p. 23). According to Yerxa (1967), the therapeutic process is one in which clients are able to gradually "experience their possibilities" and become increasingly informed about reality in order to make choices for which they can anticipate the results. In this process, clients are able to self-actualize.

From its inception, occupational therapy chose occupation as its unique method to help clients function with self-actualization (AOTA, 1995-b). The term "occupation" has been the subject of debate throughout the history of the profession because of the complexity it represents. Derived from the Latin root "occupaio," meaning "to seize or take possession," occupation conveys action and anticipation (Englehardt, 1977) and the taking of control over one's life (Reilly, 1966). For some, the term refers to the active participation in self-maintenance, work, leisure, and play (AOTA, 1993). For others, occupation is synonymous with "purposeful activity" (Henderson et al., 1991). Occupations are also considered to be "the ordinary and familiar things that people do every day" (AOTA, 1995b, p. 1015). Occupation has been described as the behavior which results from the volitional and adaptive interaction of the human being with the environment (Kielhofner, 1995), and as "a complex dynamic involving individuals and their purposive behavior within environmental contexts that have meaning and which change over time" (Nelson, 1996, p. 775). Occupation has also been explained as self-initiated, goal-directed, and socially sanctioned daily pursuits which are often personally satisfying and which shape, in part, one's perception of quality of life (Yerxa et al., 1990). Finally, occupation has been recognized as a principal way through which human beings learn to live in a community and contribute meaningfully to society (Grady, 1995). (See Chapter 30.)

Although a singular definition is elusive, we can summarize here by saying that the term occupation represents the adaptive process through which human beings take charge of their own lives and actively realize their own particular meaning both as individuals and as contributors to their communities. Ultimately, any occupational therapy intervention should contribute to this end (Yerxa, 1966). This, then, is the philosophical filter through which we must examine all therapeutic approaches used in treatment, including educational ones.

Approaches to Teaching and Occupational Therapy Philosophy

As with occupation, "teaching" is also a multidimensional concept that defies definition. Although there are numerous schools of thought, each with its own set of philosophical values and educational techniques, they can be classified into three very basic and broad approaches to teaching, including the "executive," the "therapist," and the "liberationist" approaches (Fenstermacher & Soltis, 1998). Each of these approaches must be examined in light of psychoeducation and of occupation, the treatment of choice in occupational therapy.

At first glance, each of the teaching approaches is representative of a conception of education that seems compatible with occupational therapy philosophy. Translating them to our work with clients, we might say that the executive conception is that we must shape clients to the current norms and conventions of society. The therapist conception is that we must encourage the development of each client's individual potential. Finally, the liberationist conception is that we must teach clients the knowledge that will focus their thinking on what is real and true about the world so they may contribute to it in a meaningful way. Upon closer examination, however, to some extent these three conceptions are mutually incompatible, and not all are consistent with the core values of occupational therapy. These inconsistencies become even more striking when we consider the occupational therapy practitioner as the teacher and the clients of occupational therapy the students in the psychoeducation process.

Executive Approach

In this approach, the teacher is the "executor" of education and therefore is responsible for determining what is to be taught and then planning and delivering lesson content. In addition, the teacher acts as a manager of the students in the classroom or educational setting so that they proceed through prescribed learning activities in the way the teacher believes is most appropriate. In a similar way as executives in business firms do, the teacher in this model makes decisions about what people will do, when they will do it, how long it is likely to take, and what standard of performance determines whether to move to the next task or repeat the old one. Essentially, the executive teacher manages people and resources (Berliner, 1983).

The executive teacher, then, is far more than a content expert, though the content of learning is an important consideration. Emphasis in this approach is placed on the teacher's skill, such as being able to act friendly with the students in order to enlist their participation and maintain a cooperative relationship (Sedlak, Wheeler, Pullin, & Cusik, 1986). Further emphasis is placed on the teacher's ability to maintain students engaged in the learning task through cues, corrective feedback, and reinforcement (Waxman & Walberg, 1991). In other words, this conception of teaching emphasizes direct connection between what the teacher does and what the student learns—student learning is the product of the teacher's effectiveness in communicating or transmitting knowledge. In summary, the teacher assumes the responsibility for moving specific knowledge and skills from some outside source into the mind of the learner.

When comparing assumptions of the executive approach to occupational therapy values, certain conflicts arise. The teacher/therapist functions more like a manager of a production line, where students/clients are molded and shaped in order to reach a predetermined standard. This standard is set by the teacher/therapist. In this approach, it is the students/clients who are involved in the process of education, while the teacher/therapist stays outside the process, directing it.

Psychoeducation programs designed and carried out within the framework of the executive approach emphasize a step-by-step curriculum. This curriculum is established by professional experts who, based on their expertise, have identified the knowledge clients need in order to be successful. Therefore, these programs often offer a lock-step progression of learning. For example, a program of this type might first introduce lectures by experts about various mental health disorders, followed by lectures about the usual treatment of such disorders. Some "practical" topics such as how to manage one's medication routine while at work, or even how to manage stress might be included in these programs. Worksheets to be completed by the client may be included as a method to maintain the client's attention. Two main characteristics are, however, that the teacher/expert takes responsibility for deciding which topics should be presented, and student/client adapts to the pre-established program which stresses attention to tasks and sequenced performance.

The executive approach is attractive to institutions and professionals because it provides a very efficient, clear, and straightforward means to move some specified knowledge into the mind of the client. The approach also makes it possible to make someone ultimately responsible for progress: the teacher/therapist. The teacher/therapist's effectiveness is measured by his/her ability to bring about learning by knowing precisely when and how to reinforce clients for behaviors that increasingly approximate the goals set for them.

The executive approach seems to disregard some fundamental elements of occupational therapy philosophy, such as the nature and interests of students/clients and their ability to influence their own health through occupation. Although psychoeducational experiences offered within this approach may include numerous purposeful activities or tasks, the evaluation of purposefulness lies within the teacher/therapist, not the student/client. Therefore, other core values of occupational therapy are ignored, including the student/client's choice to use his/her own capacities, to be self-directed, and to become self-actualized. Further, little consideration is given to each student/client's unique life context because the emphasis of the executive approach is on generic skills that all members of the class or group should master. This behaviorist, cause-and-effect conception of teaching and learning converts the client's therapeutic progress into a series of concrete and isolated events. The student/client must depend on the wisdom and knowledge of the teacher/therapist to not only sequence the events correctly, but to structure how these events are presented so that the client can produce the desired result. In this process, students/clients are not permitted to fully take charge of their own lives and actively realize their own particular meanings individually and as contributors to life in community. In fact, this approach relies on the maintenance of a relationship of dependence.

Therapist Approach

In contrast to the executive approach which emphasizes the content to be learned and the skills of the teacher, the therapist approach to teaching emphasizes the individual differences among students or learners. These differences are seen as impediments or facilitators of learning, and a core assumption is that who the learner is cannot be separated from what is learned and how it is learned (Fenstermacher & Soltis, 1998).

In the therapist approach, teaching is the process of guiding and assisting the learner to select the content and pursue the learning. Unlike the executive approach where teaching had mostly to do with preparing the content, the therapist teacher is more involved in preparing the learner for the tasks of choosing, working on, and evaluating what is learned. The purpose of teaching in the therapist approach is to enable the learner to become an authentic human being. This authenticity is cultivated by acquiring knowledge that is related to the quest for personal meaning and identity. Therefore, the learner's characteristics become the central focus of the teaching. The therapist teacher accepts responsibility for helping students make the choice to acquire specific knowledge, and then supports students as they advance their sense of self. In summary, in the therapist approach to teaching, the teacher is not one who imparts knowledge and skill to another, but one who helps another gain his own knowledge and skill. The teacher's task is to direct the learner inward so that the learner is then able to take responsibility for choices of actions that result from mastery of the content of learning (Rogers, 1964; Noddings & Shore, 1984).

Because the central concern in the therapist approach to teaching is the student/client's choice, this approach seems more akin to occupational therapy values. Rooted in humanist psychology from which occupational therapy has also derived much inspiration, the therapist approach to teaching stresses the uniqueness of individuals. Freedom, choice, personal growth, and the development of emotional and mental health are goals shared between the therapist approach to teaching and occupational therapy. The concern for the learner becoming an authentic human being finds particular echo in occupational therapy philosophy. Both perspectives view a self-actualized human being as one who possesses a balanced and integrated personality, and such traits as autonomy, creativeness, independence, altruism, and a healthy goal directedness (Maslow, 1962; Rogers, 1969; Fine, 1991; Kielhofner, 1997). (See Chapter 25.)

Given that the central concern of the therapist approach to teaching is the learner's individual growth, emphasis is placed on the learner's unique experience, or "experiential learning" (Rogers, 1969). The teacher or therapist does not impart knowledge. Instead, the teacher or therapist can only guide, suggest, and encourage while the learner self-initiates and becomes fully and actively involved in the learning that has personal meaning to him or her. Thus, what is important is not what is taught, but rather, what is learned.

Psychoeducation provided from the therapist approach to teaching directs learners inward toward the self so that they can thereby reach outward and choose the content to be acquired and the actions to pursue. The most efficient way to provide this form of psychoeducation is likely to be individual, as each client uniquely seeks to find meaning through his or her actions. Any group instruction with specific objectives to learn a predetermined content would necessarily negate the search for individuality and displace the client from the center of the therapeutic/learning process. Group instruction would not only homogenize the learners, it would emphasize the therapist teacher's control over the direction of learning.

The therapist approach to teaching is quite attractive to occupational therapy practitioners because it seems filled with dignity and hope for each human being. A concern which arises with this approach, however, is that its language of purpose, freedom, emotions, feelings, and subjective experience seem to center students/clients on themselves, incorporating caring for others only to the degree students/clients find it meaningful (Nodding, 1995). In this process, the common good, life in community, and responsibility toward contributing to a democratic society seem secondary.

Liberationist Approach

While the executive approach emphasizes teacher skill in transmitting specific knowledge and the therapist approach emphasizes the learner's ability to choose and acquire knowledge, a third approach can be identified that brings the knowledge, or content of learning itself, to the forefront. The aim of the liberationist approach to teaching is to free the student's mind from the limits of everyday experience, convention, and stereotype (Fenstermacher & Soltis, 1998). In contrast with the executive approach where knowledge is to be obtained and "had," or the therapist approach where knowledge is to be used for personal growth, in the liberationist approach, knowledge is to be experienced critically (Peters, 1973; Bruner, 1987; Nodding, 1995, 1999). A foundational belief of the liberationist approach is that knowledge inherently calls for particular actions and therefore, the teacher must teach by modeling such actions. In other words, in order to understand science, teachers and students must *do* science rather than simply learn *about* science; in order to understand literature, teachers and students must actively engage in creating literature; and so on. It is not the teacher as expert nor the student as personal meaning-seeker who determine what and how to learn. In the liberationist approach, it is the content or subject itself that calls for specific ways of learning and acting.

The liberationist approach places great emphasis on the general manner in which teachers and learners face learning. Honesty, integrity, fair-mindedness, along with curiosity and judicious skepticism, are to be developed at the same time as knowledge because learning comes about *by the way you learn* as well as from what you learn. The liberationist teacher must, therefore, teach these traits indirectly by modeling them as he or she learns alongside the students.

One thrust of liberationist thinking is related to the nature of knowledge itself, as explained above. Another thrust, however, is consideration of the social context in which learning occurs. This consideration is much broader than the group of students and teacher that surround each learner—it extends to the whole social world. Liberationism sees the whole world as a place of constant struggle and oppression in which people who have power assert themselves, and those who see themselves as inferior accept a fate of powerlessness. Liberationist thinkers argue that education is too often an instrument of an oppressive social system in which teachers have power and students do not, thus reproducing the broader context of society (Freire, 2000). The purpose of liberationist teaching is, then, to free the minds of students from the unconscious grip of oppressive ideas about their socioeconomic class, gender, race, or ethnicity because these ideas debilitate them and cut them off from a better life.

The two thrusts of liberationist teaching—that knowledge should be experienced, and that education should help one challenge oppression—come together in the notion of "critical consciousness" (Freire, 1974). To develop a critical consciousness, students and teachers must dialogue and collaborate, and together develop their images of a better, new reality. A critical consciousness arises when together teacher and students can step away from the unconscious acceptance of things the way they are and perceive the world critically in the midst of oppression. From this perspective, the ultimate aim of education is for students to liberate themselves to fully participate as equals in the classroom and in society (McLaren, 1989; Popkewitz, 1991; Noddings, 1999).

Liberationist thinking poses some interesting challenges to both the notion of psychoeducation and to occupational therapy practice. The development of a critical consciousness calls for not only the learning of various bodies of knowledge, but of the conceptual systems that underlie such knowledge (Freire, 2000). These conceptual systems are made of assumptions and values which should be questioned and examined critically. Therefore, from this perspective, psychoeducation (and the occupational therapy process itself) should begin with a questioning of the values which assume there even is a need for such education or treatment. Learning should not only involve the learner with the content and process of learning, but with the premises behind the need to learn (Mezirow, 2000). This can be an uncomfortable process, as it often will call into question the reasons that justify occupational therapy intervention.

Learning from the liberationist perspective does not end with an understanding of the values and assumptions that underlie knowledge. This approach calls for all participants (teacher and students alike) to critically examine their own values and assumptions because these play a significant role in the way in which each person perceives knowledge and the surrounding world. Only by understanding how these personal values and assumptions limit humans can the learner's mind be truly liberated. Of particular focus in the liberationist approach is the critical questioning of the values and assumptions learners hold that perpetuate a social system of oppression. In this approach, the development of self is only a step toward the development of the common good. The common good arises only when "...the person searches to be fully human by humanizing his fellow men and standing in solidarity together—a critical consciousness that knows one cannot be human as long as others are less than that" (Freire, 2000, p. 34). This solidarity can only be achieved through community.

From a liberationist perspective, psychoeducation would take on the form of dialogue in which both clients and occupational therapy practitioner openly discuss how their beliefs and actions contribute to their life in community, and to an oppressive or liberated society. The encounters between the occupational therapy practitioner and clients would be on an even plane, where the focus is not on the client's individual needs nor the practitioner's assessment of the client's need for development, but as "co-conspirators to humanize their life in community" (Mezirow, 2000, p. 26). The practitioner cannot be external to this process, but must be fully engaged with the client in the construction of meaning and of the future of society.

In this context, psychoeducation on stress management, for example, would include an examination of not only the physiology of stress and techniques to manage it, but also an examination of how each of us contributes to our own stress, each other's stress, and that of others. An essential discussion would include why we permit that cycle to continue. Further, an examination of how stress comes from and impacts our shared community in particular and society as a whole would be accompanied by an exploration of actions that we each can take, both as individuals and as a group, to effect a change not only in our own lives, but in society as a whole. Finally, that action should be undertaken together. This might lead us, for example, to make calls or write letters to government representatives, to participate in public protests, or to become involved in a community service program.

Conclusions

The three different ways of thinking about teaching presented here accomplish very different objectives. The executive approach emphasizes the transmission of information, the therapist approach emphasizes the search for personal meaning, and the liberationist approach emphasizes contribution to the common good. Psychoeducation undertaken from each of these approaches, then, also accomplishes different objectives. Given that occupational therapy practitioners often are involved in psychoeducational programs, the objectives of such programs must be evaluated in light of both the teaching approach and the philosophical values that should undergird all occupational therapy intervention.

Psychoeducation provided by occupational therapy practitioners from an executive approach appears to create the most obvious conflict of values. The practitioner stands in the center of this relationship, holding the power to decide what knowledge the client needs and how he/she will learn it. The emphasis on the therapeutic context rather than on the client's real life fragments the meaning such education may have, and stresses development of components of function rather than the integration of such components. Some may argue that many clients with mental conditions do not have the cognitive capacity to make sophisticated choices for themselves or others, and need first to develop abilities upon which to build choice. The result of this reasoning is occupational therapy intervention focused on developing components of function (for example, increasing attention or endurance). We know, however, that component-driven therapy is not effective (Trombly, 1995; Lin, Wu, Dengen, & Coster, 1997). (See Chapter 16.) At any rate, the choice of psychoeducation would be inappropriate for clients with severe cognitive impairments because they would not be able to process cognitive information anyway. Because the executive approach de-emphasizes client agency, this form of psychoeducation cannot be considered authentic occupational therapy (Yerxa, 1966).

The therapist approach to teaching seems more compatible with occupational therapy values because, in contrast to the executive approach, it does emphasize client agency. However, because this approach is maintained through client unique-ness in making individual choices, the approach does not fully realize the occupational therapy value of contributing to the growth of social beings. Psychoeducation from this perspective would only address life in community if the client were to express such concern. Further, psychoeducation from this perspective would occur at the individual level because any group approach would homogenize people and de-emphasize their uniqueness. Therefore, the fullness of occupational therapy values may not be realized.

Finally, the liberationist approach to teaching offers a unique perspective to occupational therapy which challenges practitioner and client together to explore their relationship and critically examine the assumptions behind the notions of illness and need for therapy. The liberationist approach calls for the occupational therapy experience to be fully recognized as a real life experience in community, rather than preparation or training for life away from that relationship. Unlike the executive or therapist approaches explained above, the liberationist approach places the occupational therapy practitioner and the client as co-equals within the therapeutic learning process, so that as both learn together they form a learning community. In this sense, the occupational therapy process is one in which the client is brought into community, not only trained or prepared for it. The client's life or context cannot be seen as separate from the therapeutic one. Instead, we must understand how the therapeutic context fits into the wider life context of the client. Most importantly, we must critically consider whether the therapeutic experience is serving to actually liberate the client toward the fullness of life in society, or whether it is contributing to perpetuate in the client and in society the sense of being different and less than worthy to be included and seen as inherently equal.

Although the differences among these three approaches may at times seem subtle, they point to dramatically different outcomes of the therapeutic process. Ultimately, they bring into question the way in which we build a relationship with our clients and should guide how and why we use psychoeducation in the quest for providing authentic occupational therapy.

References

American Occupational Therapy Association. (1995-a). The philosophical base of occupational therapy. *American Journal of Occupational Therapy, 49,* 1026. Reprinted as Appendix E.

American Occupational Therapy Association. (1995-b). Position paper: Occupation. *American Journal of Occupational Therapy, 49,* 1015–1018.

American Occupational Therapy Association. (1993). Position paper: Purposeful activity. *American Journal of Occupational Therapy, 47,* 1981–1082.

Barris, R. (1985). Psychosocial occupational therapy education. *Mental Health Special Interest Section Newsletter, 7,* 4: 1–2.

Barter, J. (1984). Psychoeducation. In J. Talbott (Ed.), *The chronic mental patient: Five years later.* New York, NY: Grune & Stratton.

Bartlow, P., & Hartwig, C. (1989). Status of practice in mental health: Assessment and frames of reference. *Australian Occupational Therapy Journal, 36,* 180–192.

Berliner, D. (1983). The executive functions of teaching. *Instructor.* September: 29–39.

Bruner, J. (1987). *Actual minds, possible worlds.* Cambridge, MA: Harvard University Press.

Dickerson, A. (1996). Should choice be a component in occupational therapy assessment? *Occupational Therapy in Health Care, 10,* 3: 23–32.

Dixon, L. (1999). Providing services to families of persons with schizophrenia: Present and future. *Journal of Mental Health Policy and Economics, 2,* 3–8.

Dixon, L., Adams, C., & Lucksted, A. (2000). Update on family psychoeducaticm for schizophrenia. *Schizophrenia Bulletin, 26,* I: 5–20.

Englehardt, H. (1977). Defining occupational therapy: The meaning of therapy and the virtues of occupation. *American Journal of Occupational Therapy, 31,* 666–672.

Fenstermacher, G., & Soltis, J. (1998). *Approaches to teaching, 2nd ed.* New York, NY: Teacher's College Press.

Fine, S. (1991). Resilience and human adaptability: Who rises above adversity? The 1991 Eleanor Clarke Slagle Lecture. *American Journal of Occupational Therapy, 45,* 493–403. Reprinted as Chapter 25.

Freire, P. (2000). *Pedagogy of the oppressed (30th Anniversary Edition).* New York: Continuum Publications.

Freire, P. (1974). *Educating for critical consciousness.* New York: Continuum Publications.

Goldman, C. (1988). Toward a definition of psychoeducation. *Hospital and Community Psychiatry, 39,* 666–668.

Grady, A. P. (1995). Building inclusive community: A challenge for occupational therapy. The 1995 Eleanor Clarke Slagle Lecture. *American Journal of Occupational Therapy, 49,* 300–310. Reprinted as Chapter 30.

Greenberg, L., Fine, S., Cohen, C., Larson, K., Michaelson-Baily, A., Rubinton, P., & Glick, I. (1988). An interdisciplinary psychoeducation program for schizophrenic patients and their families in an acute-care setting. *Hospital and Community Psychiatry, 39,* 277–282.

Hayes, R., & Halford, W. (1993). Generalization of occupational therapy effects in psychiatric rehabilitation. *American Journal of Occupational Therapy, 47,* 161–167.

Henderson, A., Cermak, S., Coster, W., Murray, E., Trombly, C., & Tickle-Degnen, L. (1991). The issue is: Occupational science is multidimensional. *American Journal of Occupational Therapy, 45,* 370–372.

Kielhofner, G. (1995). *A model of human occupation: Theory and application, 2nd ed.* Baltimore, MD: Williams & Wilkins.

Kielhofner, G. (1997). *Conceptual foundations of occupational therapy, 2nd ed.* Philadelphia, PA: F.A. Davis.

Klasson, E. (1989). A model of the occupational therapist as case manager: Two case studies of chronic schizophrenic patients living in the community. *Occupational Therapy in Mental Health, 9,* 63–89.

Liberman, R., Wallace, C., Blackwell, G., Kopelowicz, A., Vaccaro, J., & Mints, J. (1998). Skills training versus psychosocial occupational therapy for persons with persistent schizophrenia. *American Journal of Psychiatry, 111,* 1087–1091.

Lin, K., Wu. C., Dengen, L., & Coster, W. (1997). Enhancing occupational performance through occupationally embedded exercise: A metaanalytic review. *Occupational Therapy Journal of Research, 17,* 25–47.

Lubin, H., Loris, M., Burt, J., & Johnson, D. (1998). Efficacy of psychoeducational group therapy in reducing symptoms of posttraumatic stress disorder among multiply traumatized women. *American Journal of Psychiatry, 155,* 1172–1177.

Maslow, A. (1962). *Toward a psychology of being.* New York: Van Nostrand.

McFarlane, W., Lukens, E., & Link, B. (1995). Multifamily groups and psychoeducation in the treatment of schizophrenia. *Archives of General Psychiatry, 52,* 679–687.

McLaren, P. (1989). *Life in schools: An introduction to critical pedagogy in the foundations of education.* New York: Longman.

Mezirow, J. (2000). *Learning as transformation: Critical perspectives on a theory in progress.* San Francisco, CA: Jossey-Bass.

Nelson, D. (1996). Therapeutic occupation: A definition. *American Journal of Occupational Therapy, 50,* 775–782.

Noddings, N. (1995). *Philosophy of education.* New York: Westview Press.

Noddings, N. (1999). *Justice and caring: The search for common ground in education.* New York: Teachers College Press.

Noddings, N. & Shore, P. (1984). *Awakening the inner eye: Intuition in education.* New York: Teachers College Press.

Peters, R. (1973). *The philosophy of education.* London: Oxford University Press.

Pollio, D., North, C., & Foster, D. A. (1998). Content and curriculum in psychoeducation groups for families of persons with severe mental illness. *Psychiatric Services, 49,* 816–822.

Popkewitz, T. (1991). *A political sociology of educational reform: Power/knowledge in teaching, teacher education, and research.* New York: Teachers College Press.

Reilly, M. (1966). A psychiatric occupational therapy program as a teaching model. *American Journal of Occupational Therapy, 20,* 60–67.

Rogers, C. (1969). *Freedom to learn.* Columbus, OH: Charles E. Merrill.

Sedlak, M., Wheeler, D., Pullin, C., & Cusik, A. (1986). *Selling students short: Classroom bargains and academic reform in the American high school.* New York: Teacher's College Press.

Solomon, P. (1996). Moving from psychoeducation to education of families of adults with serious mental illness. *Psychiatric Services, 47,* 1364–1370.

Spencer, J., Glick, L., Haas, G., Claekin, J., Lewis, A., Peyser, J., DeMane, N., Good-Ellis, M., Harris, E., & Lestelle, V. (1988). A randomized clinical trial of inpatient family intervention: Effects at 6-month and 18-month follow-ups. *American Journal of Psychiatry, 145,* 1115–1121.

Trombly, C. (1995). Occupation: Purposefulness and meaningfulness as therapeutic mechanisms: The 1995 Eleanor Clarke Slagle Lecture. *American Journal of Occupational Therapy, 49,* 960–972. Reprinted as Chapter 16.

Wallace, C., Liberman, R., MacKain, S., Blackwell, G., & Eckman, T. (1992). Effectiveness and replicability of modules for teaching social and instrumental skills to the severely mentally ill. *American Journal of Psychiatry, 149,* 654–658.

Waxman, H., & Walberg, H. (1991). *Effective teaching: Current research.* Berkeley, CA: McCutchan.

Yerxa, E. (1967). Authentic occupational therapy: The 1966 Eleanor Clarke Slagle Lecture. *American Journal of Occupational Therapy, 21,* 1–9.

Yerxa, E., Clark, F., Frank, G., Jackson, J., Parham, D., Pierce, D., Stein, C., & Zemke, R. (1990). An introduction to occupational science: A foundation for occupational therapy in the 21st century, *Occupational Therapy in Health Care, 4,* 2: 1–17.

CHAPTER 50

Linking Purpose to Procedure During Interactions With Patients

Suzanne M. Peloquin, PhD, OTR

This chapter describes a rationale and some methods for incorporating statements of purpose, or goal statements, into the daily practice of occupational therapy. Given the clinical pressures generated by brief lengths of stays in care facilities, occupational therapists need to recommit themselves to meaningful relationships with their patients. The need for this renewed commitment sharpens when one considers three realities basic to practice: current trends in health care, traditional occupational therapy assumptions, and the often ambiguous nature of activity, occupational therapy's primary modality. Each of these realities provides a context within which the process of discussing goal statements with patients will be explored.

Rosen (1974, p. 292) used the term *therapy set* to refer to statements or directives that inform patients about a therapeutic procedure, motivate them to cooperate, and heighten their expectations of the benefits to be derived from treatment. When this treatment approach is used, patients (a) understand what they are doing and why they are doing it and (b) feel encouraged to engage in the process.

As applied to occupational therapy, a communication in psychiatric practice that encourages informed patient involvement might be the following:

> We'd like to have you join us in the 9 am craft group today. You will probably experience this as a pleasant hour since you enjoy working with your hands. Our main interest in having you attend this group, however, is that your participation will give you an opportunity to use several skills, such as your ability to concentrate, to solve problems, and to organize your thoughts.

Effectiveness of the Collaborative Approach

Although the purpose of this article is not to investigate the effectiveness of enlightening patients about and involving them in their therapy, but to explore a rationale for the use of such a collaborative approach in occupational therapy practice, some brief discussion of the effectiveness of the approach seems indicated. Rosen (1974) cited several studies involving subjects receiving desensitization therapy procedures accompanied by different forms of "therapy set." He indicated that two primary approaches dominated the research on the effectiveness of informing and involving the patient. The first group of studies investigated the extent to which varied instructions might alter subjects' expectations for a therapeutic outcome. The second group of studies explored the effects of changing subjects' knowledge of the procedure through instructions. In the first approach, control groups were given a general therapeutic orientation, whereas experimental groups were given instructions that might influence their expectations of the treatment outcome positively. Small between-group differences that failed to achieve statistical significance were reported in these studies (Lomont & Brock, 1971; McGlynn, 1971; McGlynn & Mapp, 1970; McGlynn, Mealiea, & Nawas, 1969; McGlynn, Reynolds, & Linder, 1971; McGlynn & Williams, 1970; Woy & Efran, 1972). In the second approach, groups given therapeutic orientation were compared with groups who believed they were being studied for physiological reactions only. In this approach, subjects' knowledge of the purpose of the procedure was being manipulated. Most studies of this type demonstrated significant effects attributable to the type of instruction given (Borkovec, 1972; Leitenberg, Agras, Barlow, & Oliveau, 1969; Miller, 1972; Oliveau, Agras, Leitenberg, Moore, & Wright, 1969; Rappaport, 1972). Subjects who knew that the purpose of the treatment was therapeutic had better therapeutic outcomes.

In his own study, Rosen (1974) concluded that subjects aware of the purpose of procedures designed to make them less afraid of snakes demonstrated significantly higher mean behavioral changes, that is, became more desensitized to the offending stimulus, than subjects unaware of the purpose. Those informed that test procedures were therapeutic demonstrated more confident behavior in approaching snakes than those told that the procedures were simply experimental.

The collaborative approach's focus on patients' expectations resembles a construct called "expectancy of therapeutic gain." Historically, this construct emerged from research on the placebo effect described in the medical literature (Wilkins, 1973). Cartwright and Cartwright (1958) explained that in the 1950s the concepts of anticipation, belief, confidence, and conviction emerged in psychotherapy, giving rise to the concept of the placebo effect. Frank (1959) said that a patient's expectancy of benefit from treatment may in itself have enduring and profound effects on his or her physical and mental health. Krause, in 1967, wrote that the client's beliefs about treatment determine his or her valuation of the process, and that this valuation determines his or her motivation to participate. Kielhofner (1985) echoed this conviction in his conceptualization of volition as the human subsystem that provides the energy and desire for choosing an action, that energy being generated by what a person believes to be interesting and valuable.

Wilkins (1973) proposed that an individual's expectancy of therapeutic gain may be treated as either (a) an attitude that the individual brings to a situation concerning how much benefit he or she will receive or (b) a state that can be induced by instructions delivered about the effectiveness of procedures to which he or she will be exposed. The idea of the collaborative approach is predicated on the assumptions that instructions can induce an expectancy of therapeutic gain and that creating a state of expectancy potentiates the therapeutic procedure.

There is justification for the use of the collaborative approach in occupational therapy when one considers its efficacy; there is additional justification for its use when one reflects on current demands in health-care practice.

Current Demands in Health Care

In light of the current emphasis on bioethical issues such as informed consent and patients' rights, there is sound reasoning for incorporating a collaborative approach into each occupational therapy procedure. Engelhardt (1986) described the patient's status as that of a stranger in a strange land:

Patients, when they come to see a health care professional, are in unfamiliar territory. They enter a terrain of issues that has been carefully defined through the long history of the health care professions. A patient is unlikely to present for care with as well-analyzed and considered judgments as those possessed by health care professionals.... The patient in this context is a stranger, an individual in unfamiliar territory who does not fully know what to expect or how to control the environment.... Things no longer happen as usual; they no longer take place in their taken for granted ways. As an outsider in a strange culture, the patient always runs the risk of being a marginal person. (pp. 256–257)

The caregiver must explain this new and strange land to the patient, thereby reducing the patient's sense of being a marginal person. The caregiver must augment the patient's sense of belonging by providing him or her with access to information and by giving him or her control in the form of consent over the treatment process (Engelhardt, 1986).

Current emphasis on patients' rights reminds those in positions of power that the ultimate power is changing hands. Patients have the right to know the precise relevance and nature of their treatment and to choose it or reject it on the basis of their understanding of its value to them (Bloomer, 1978). This patient/consumer right gives the practitioner a powerful incentive for explaining procedures and for collaborating with patients throughout treatment.

Clinicians face a demand from agencies, both accrediting and reimbursing, to be accountable for the treatment they provide. They face requests from patients and their families to prove the utility of their service and to clarify the expected outcome of their treatments. Current trends to exact statements of purpose from therapists can be perceived as the public's validation of a professional and ethical response that is their due.

Traditional Occupational Therapy Thinking

Even before the emergence of current trends, traditional occupational therapy assumptions supportive of the collaborative approach were well represented in the literature. The assumptions can be summarized as follows: The patient is rational. The patient is a collaborator with the therapist. The patient is free to choose or reject therapeutic services. The therapist, in turn, is a teacher and a motivator in the therapy process.

Excerpts from *Willard and Spackman's Occupational Therapy* highlight these assumptions. McNary (1947) wrote: "An activity entered into without a purpose is not occupational therapy" (p. 10). If the patient is the one entering into the activity, it is he or she who must understand the purpose. It then becomes the therapist's responsibility to share that information. Edgerton (1947) said that "the ability to relate an activity to the need of the individual is one of the characteristics that distinguishes the occupational therapist from the . . . crafts instructor" (p. 42). Here is a clear endorsement of any procedure that communicates the relevance of a therapeutic activity. If occupational therapists resent having their role minimized by others, they must take measures to ensure that they are not sabotaging themselves by failing to define their work so that others will recognize it unmistakably as therapy.

Wade (1947) said that "if the patient is unable to participate actively in the plan, its existence should be kept in his consciousness as a justification for the task" (p. 90). When meaningful collaboration with the patient is not possible, the therapist still retains responsibility for explaining the plan on some level. When the patient is elderly, psychotic, young, or cognitively impaired, it may seem easier to abandon explanations in favor of expediting the procedure. Therapists are encouraged to do otherwise. At whatever level of comprehension is possible, caregivers need to inform. The information may be brief, simple, and even reductionistic. The information is nonetheless "placed in the patient's consciousness." When in doubt about the potential for awareness, one communicates.

An anecdotal contribution to *Reader's Digest* ("Speedy Recovery," 1987) illustrates a response that even patients assumed to be minimally aware can furnish. A nurse's aide described her patient as a 96-year-old woman immobilized after a stroke. The aide's task was to get the patient out of bed. She communicated her plan to her assistant as follows: "I'll take an arm and a leg on this side, you take an arm and a leg on that side and then...." The explanation was interrupted by the patient's saying in a weary voice. "Oh, God, she's not even going to make a wish!" (p. 53).

This anecdote clearly reminds therapists that the presence of a significant disability does not justify excluding the patient from an active understanding of any procedure. Exclusion constitutes treatment of the patient as a marginal person. The publication of this anecdote as a humorous short in a popular magazine reflects perhaps the universality of the situation. The treatment is all too familiar. The poignancy of the story lies in the fact that the patient's best defense was that of taking the offensive by being more humane and personable than the caregiver.

Current literature supports these examples taken from the past. Reed and Sanderson (1983) described several attitudes and assumptions about the occupational therapy process consistent with those underlying the idea of the collaborative approach. They emphasized salient points made more subtly 40 years ago by encouraging therapists to regard the client as a "*valuable, worthwhile person,* even if the client does not respond readily to the program" (p. 153). Here stands a declaration of the patient's right to challenge services offered on the basis of his or her understanding of them. A consequent responsibility for the therapist is to maintain the patient in high regard and to respond to the challenge with information. "The client has a right to be informed, but also the information should be in a manner that is comprehensive and at a rate that can be absorbed by the client" (p. 154).

Reed and Sanderson (1983) drew up a list of patient's rights that included the following:

1. A person has the right to decide whether to seek and accept health care services within legal limitations.

2. A person has the right to determine the state of health and level of wellness that person will seek to attain and maintain, as long as the decision does not threaten or endanger the health and wellness of other persons.

3. A person has the right to be consulted regarding the objectives, goals, and methods to be used in individual health care plans. (p. 71)

These three rights merit observance during daily sessions when specific treatments are being proposed. The patient's right to be consulted and to decide needs to be reinforced daily. Providing the patient with the necessary information at each session can operationally reaffirm his or her rights.

Motivating the patient becomes an inevitable therapist responsibility if one endorses the patient's right to choose. Reed and Sanderson (1983) identified the last step of the occupational therapy process as being "to facilitate and influence client participation and investment" (p. 81). This step constitutes a directive to communicate the rationale, the importance, and the relevance of the therapy process in such a manner as to facilitate the patient's investment in a successful outcome.

Traditional occupational therapy has been a process of teaching, motivating, and collaborating with the patient during therapeutic activity. More recently, proponents of a psychoeducational approach to occupational therapy have contrasted it with traditional occupational therapy. Fine and Schwimmer (1987) described the psychoeducational approach to occupational therapy as a derivation from social learning theory:

The life skills curriculum (LSC) is further differentiated from its traditional counterpart by structuring the educational format and techniques, emphasizing the patient's active participation in setting and evaluating treatment goals, identifying learning needs and influencing the teaching-learning process, planning the integration and continuity of problem-solving and communication skills among all groups, providing multiple opportunities to practice skills through graded repetition and homework assignments, and matching treatment tasks to patient's problems and priorities. (p. 3)

Excerpts from traditional and more current literature, cited earlier, support the premise that traditional occupational therapy (a) has incorporated the tenets of social learning theory to a considerable extent and (b) has promoted active involvement in goal formulation all along.

The Public's Knowledge of Occupational Therapy

The rationale for using the collaborative approach sharpens considerably when we reflect on the profession's unclear image. "Occupational therapy is not understood well by the average client because it is not a common profession, such as medicine, nursing, engineering, law, teaching or the ministry" (Reed & Sanderson, 1983, p. 161). Practitioners often find themselves explaining the word *occupational,* differentiating occupational therapy functions from those of other therapies, and otherwise clarifying their professional roles. If the public expects physicians, nurses, and engineers, whose professions are better understood, to clarify their procedures, the expectation increases for those representing less well understood professions.

Occupational therapy is often not understood; it can, in fact, often be misunderstood. A particularly noteworthy example of that misunderstanding appears in Joyce Rebeta-Burditt's novel *The Cracker Factory* (1977). In the story a young female patient, a self-described alcoholic, writes from the psychiatric hospital to a friend:

I should write to you every day. I could not only unravel the Gordian knot in my psyche, but appear to be busy and involved when Brunhilde, the misplaced Viking lady, comes tapping on my door every afternoon in an effort to intimidate me into going to Occupational Therapy. She marches around the seventh floor telling all the patients that their doctor has "ordered" Occupational Therapy and they must come IMMEDIATELY. She herds them out in the hall where they mill around until she lines them up in two columns and goose steps them out the door....

Patients are forever trying to hide by taking a shower or even [having] a fit, but she doesn't care. Wet or screaming, it makes no difference. She drags them along anyway....

I go sometimes and hate myself for it. I sit and dab grout on a metal shell and try to decide what color ashtray I'm going to mess up that day. I listen to the conversations around me, and the tape recorder in my head jots down snatches and fragments and I smile and pretend that I am not listening in. (pp. 114–115)

Fiction will often exaggerate or satirize those aspects of our functioning that create interesting reading material, such as the domineering qualities of Brunhilde and the perceived irrelevance of occupational therapy. Fiction also mirrors reality. In this case the reality is that occupational therapy is sometimes misunderstood.

The consequence of this misunderstanding can be significant. Patients uninformed of the purpose of occupational therapy are free to infer its meaning based on their observations. The result may well be compliance with the procedure. It might as easily be noncompliance accompanied by hostility. One probability is that patients who are uninformed or misinformed will be less able to generalize to their life situations those concepts the therapist had hoped might be learned in therapy.

The Ambiguous Nature of Activity

Because occupational therapists use activity as a primary modality, they increase the risk of being misunderstood. Any single activity can have many therapeutic possibilities. Proficiency in activity analysis enables clinicians to recognize the multiple goals that can be attached to any one activity. Therapists need to apply that theoretical concept clinically and consider its practical consequences. Therapeutic methods can easily confuse patients. A patient can be given leather stamping as a task to achieve a wide range of goals, including (a) the enhancement of grip strength, (b) the redirection of nervous energy through gross-motor release, or (c) the use of organizational and problem-solving skills in the planning of a balanced design. If the only focus patients have is the one they can infer while doing the task, the relationship between the leather-stamping activity and the treatment plan may elude them. Because they do not clearly understand the therapeutic concepts supporting the activity, they may be less apt to apply them to their personal life situations.

A pleasant staff development exercise that illustrates the multifaceted aspect of any activity is the following: Divide the total group into five working subgroups. Provide each small group with a bowl of sliced oranges. The primary activity will be to eat the oranges. From the list given in the appendix to this paper, provide each group with a different set of written directions. Allow each group to complete the activity as directed. Following the group activity, ask a representative from each group to share both the directions given and the results of their activity. Reports from the representatives will reflect the different end points that one task with different directions can have. The exercise can stimulate reflection on the importance of clarifying the specific focus of a planned activity.

Methods of Providing a Collaborative Approach

A collaborative approach can be used creatively. Therapists can provide feedback formally or informally, use the printed or the spoken word, and communicate the purpose of occupational therapy procedures at various phases in the treatment process. Any method used that communicates the purpose of or the expectations for the treatment can qualify.

In an earlier article (Peloquin, 1983), I endorsed integrating information about the expectations and relevance of the occupational therapy program into the structure of an initial interview format in an acute-care psychiatric setting. The three-part interview stresses the continuous provision of feedback to the patient. My conviction remains that, if nothing else, we give patients methods of self-help when we provide them with informative goal statements that they can readily apply to their personal environments after discharge.

One way to enlighten patients is to give them printed materials. A general description of the occupational therapy program might be a suitable accompaniment to the initial contact between a patient and a therapist. The descriptive introduction might include a statement of the various purposes of the occupational therapy program. Next, a brief, goal-oriented paragraph at the top of an occupational therapy schedule might serve as a motivational reinforcement. Posters listing typical occupational therapy goals for various groups can be displayed in both residential and treatment areas. In more financially comfortable settings, pamphlets or video messages discussing the programmatic goals of occupational therapy might be used as part of a general hospital orientation.

Feedback can be provided in formal groups and individual orientations. On a daily basis, a brief discussion can either precede or follow each activity group. More articulate patients can be asked to help clarify the purposes and expectations of various groups for new patients. Less organized patients can be reminded informally on the way to and from groups about the specific purpose of each group. Brief personal contacts reminding patients about individualized goals can occur during large parallel groups.

It might be helpful to include here a few illustrations of how the collaborative approach can be incorporated into occupational therapy. Each illustration includes vocabulary that can be adjusted upward or downward to match the intellectual level of the patient population being addressed. Any verbal delivery of the feedback needs to reflect, in its tone, rate, and inflection, the therapist's perception of the patient as intelligent. A singsong or overly didactic delivery, suggesting condescension, could vitiate or at least compromise the purpose of the feedback. A respectful intent requires respectful delivery.

An introductory explanation of a psychiatric occupational therapy program might read, in part, as follows:

Occupational therapy adds to your total treatment by encouraging you to use activities and occupy your time in a therapeutic way. Purposeful activity has an organizing and beneficial effect on an individual. Because it involves the total person, activity meets several mental health needs.

Occupational therapy offerings here include crafts, exercise, greenhouse, relaxation, communication, and life skills groups. By participating in these activities you help ready yourself to return to your community. During group and individual sessions, you can set goals and practice skills essential to your coping more effectively outside of the hospital.

You will have daily opportunities to plan and organize tasks, to solve problems, to improve your physical condition, to interact effectively with others, to make decisions, to boost your self-confidence, to learn new ways of relaxing and coping with different life situations. Activity becomes therapy because of the adaptive skills you practice when you are active.

A poster mounted in the clinical area to provide information about a typical occupational therapy craft group might list some of the following goal statements:

Why Crafts?

To improve your concentration
To organize your thoughts
To have you solve problems
To help you make decisions
To exercise your work skills
To boost your self-confidence
To increase your independence
To help you interact with others
To increase your sense of control
To keep you alert and involved.

A poster describing the purposes of a communication group might read as follows:

Why Communication Group?

To improve your listening skills
To help you share and interact
To increase your self-awareness
To help you identify your feelings
To help you express yourself
To help you better deal with anger
To increase your assertiveness
To help you clarify your thoughts
To help you make or keep friends.

A discussion at the end of a particular group might follow a basic outline such as the following, addressing a different goal from day to day. The following format has been used with groups of adults having cognitive problems:

1. *Explain the purpose of the group:* "One of the goals for this particular group is to have you use your cognitive or thinking skills. During the course of this hour each of you has had some opportunity to use a number of thinking skills, such as concentrating, problem solving, decision making, comprehending instructions, or organizing your activity."
2. *Set the stage for a discussion:* "Take a minute to think about the thinking skills you used while working on your project. I'll be asking a few of you to share with the rest of us how you used your skills during the past hour."
3. *Facilitate a brief discussion of skills used, making sure to clearly link for patients the various task steps they completed with the cognitive skills they used:* Examples of therapist responses might be
    a. "That's right, Jim. You had to follow several complex verbal instructions today. I also noticed that you were doing a lot of planning and organizing for the design you want to put on your belt tomorrow."
    b. "Lorene, you're feeling that you didn't use your thinking skills today, but I noticed that you had to make

several color choices when you were painting. That's decision making. You also had to pay attention to the shapes you were painting. That required you to concentrate on what you were doing. You really were using thinking skills for the better part of the hour."

4. *Summarize what was accomplished and encourage patients to return to the next session.*

Formulating and providing a set of goals in collaboration with the patient can be a creative process evolving from the basic premise that patients have rights, capabilities, and a vested interest in knowing the relevance of therapy. Using the collaborative approach can potentiate our therapeutic activities by communicating their value to patients in the real world outside the treatment setting. An old proverb says, "Give a man a fish and you have fed him for a day; teach a man to fish and you have fed him for a lifetime." Sharing goal statements with patients can give them an understanding of a process that can provide a link to improved functioning.

Summary

There is a rationale for a collaborative approach with patients in the daily practice of occupational therapy. Effective collaborative procedure (a) provides patients with knowledge about what they are doing and why they are doing it and (b) encourages patients to engage in the process.

The effectiveness of this approach has not been established conclusively, but studies suggest that subjects exposed to the therapeutic purpose of desensitization procedures tend to have better therapeutic outcomes than those unaware of the purpose. Current emphasis on the patient's right to be informed and on the therapist's responsibility to inform reflects the public's growing insistence that practitioners explain the utility of the treatments they provide to the patient.

Excerpts from past and present literature indicate that assumptions underlying the practice of traditional occupational therapy reflect similar assumptions underpinning the use of a collaborative approach. These assumptions describe the patient as rational, as having rights, and as a collaborator in therapy. The therapist is assumed to be a teacher and a motivator in the therapeutic process, the person who articulates the relevance of therapy and encourages the patient's participation.

The general public often lacks understanding of the occupational therapy process. Additionally, the versatility and multiple possibilities associated with any activity can confuse the patient about its purpose. The uninformed patient might be less inclined to participate in therapy and less able to generalize helpful concepts from the experience.

Feedback to patients can be provided in a number of creative ways throughout treatment. Providing such feedback need not require a major time investment, but can represent the therapist's renewed commitment to the therapeutic alliance and to the goal directedness of occupational therapy practice.

Acknowledgments

I thank Lillian Hoyle Parent, MA, OTR, FAOTA, for her support and encouragement in the preparation of this paper.

The topic of this paper featured in a workshop entitled "Goal Formulation: Clinical Leverage in Challenging Times," which I co-presented with Debora Davidson, MS, OTR. The workshop was sponsored by the Department of Occupational Therapy at the University of Texas Medical Branch Hospitals, L. Randy Strickland, EdD, OTR, FAOTA, Director.

Appendix 50.A

1. You have been given orange sections as a help in your discussion. The tangible and sensual experience of the orange will enable you to complete your task. As you are eating the sections, discuss as a group the various memories you have that are associated with eating oranges. Appoint a spokesperson who will later present a 30–60 second summary of your discussion.

2. You have been given orange sections as a help in your discussion. The actual taste of the orange will help you to better focus on your task. As you are eating the sections, discuss as a group as many dishes or recipes as you can think of that use oranges. Appoint a spokesperson who will later present a 30–60 second summary of your discussion.

3. You have been given orange sections as a help in your discussion. The visual and tactile experience of the orange will help you in your task. As you are eating the sections, discuss as a group as many functions as you can think of that an orange might have aside from its function as a food item. Appoint a spokesperson who will later present a 30–60 second summary of your discussion.

4. You have been given orange sections as a help in your discussion. The sight of the orange will help you in your task. As you are eating the sections, discuss as a group as many other natural items as you can think of that share a similar color. Appoint a spokesperson who will later present a 30–60 second summary of your discussion.

5. You have been given orange sections as a help in your discussion. The smell of the orange will help you in your task. As you are eating the sections, discuss as a group as many other items as you can think of that share a similar odor, or that have the orange scent. Appoint a spokesperson who will later present a 30–60 second summary of your discussion.

References

Bloomer, J. S. (1978). The consumer of therapy in mental health. *American Journal of Occupational Therapy, 32,* 621–627.

Borkovec, T. D. (1972). Effects of expectancy on the outcome of systematic desensitization and implosive treatments for analogue anxiety. *Behavior Therapy, 3,* 29–40.

Cartwright, D. S., & Cartwright, R. D. (1958). Faith and improvement in psychotherapy. *Journal of Counseling Psychology, 5,* 174–177.

Edgerton, W. B. (1947). Activities in occupational therapy. In H. Willard & C. Spackman (Eds.), *Occupational therapy* (pp. 40–59). Philadelphia: Lippincott.

Engelhardt, H. T., Jr. (1986). *The foundations of bioethics.* New York: Oxford University Press.

Fine, S. B., & Schwimmer, P. (1986, December). The effects of occupational therapy on independent living skills. *Mental Health Special Interest Section Newsletter,* pp. 2–3.

Frank, J. D. (1959). The dynamics of the psychotherapeutic relationship. *Psychiatry, 22,* 17–39.

Kielhofner, G. (1985). The human being as an open system. In G. Kielhofner (Ed.), *A model of human occupation: Theory and application* (pp. 2–11). Baltimore: Williams & Wilkins.

Krause, M. S. (1967). Clients' expectations of the value of treatment. *Mental Hygiene, 51,* 359–365.

Leitenbheerg, H., Agras, W. S., Barlow, D. H., & Oliveau, D.C. (1969). Contributions of selective positive reinforcement and therapeutic instructions to systematic desensitization therapy. *Journal of Abnormal Psychology, 74,* 113–118.

Lomont, J. F., & Brock, L. (1971). Cognitive factors in systematic desensitization. *Behavior Research and Therapy, 9,* 187–195.

McGlynn, F. D. (1971). Experimental desensitization following three types of instructions. *Behavior Research and Therapy, 9,* 367–369.

McGlynn, F. D., & Mapp, R. H. (1970). Systematic desensitization of snake-avoidance following three types of suggestion. *Behavior Research and Therapy, 8,* 197–201.

McGlynn, F. D., Mealiea, E. L., & Nawas, M. M. (1969). Systematic desensitization of snake avoidance under two conditions of suggestion. *Psychological Reports, 25,* 220–222.

McGlynn, F. D., Reynolds, E. J., & Linder, L. H. (1971). Systematic desensitization with pre-treatment and intra-treatment therapeutic instructions. *Behavior Research and Therapy, 9,* 57–63.

McGlynn, F. D., & Williams, C. W. (1970). Systematic desensitization of snake-avoidance under three conditions of suggestion. *Journal of Behavior Therapy and Experimental Psychiatry, 1,* 97–101.

McNary, H. (1947). The scope of occupational therapy. In H. Willard & C. Spackman (Eds.), *Occupational therapy* (pp. 10–22). Philadelphia: Lippincott.

Miller, S. B. (1972). The contribution of therapeutic instructions to systematic desensitization. *Behavior Research and Therapy,* 159–169.

Oliveau, D. C. (1969). Systematic desensitization in an experimental setting: A follow–up study. *Behavior Research and Therapy, 7,* 377–380.

Oliveau, D. C., Agras, W. S., Leitenberg, H., Moore, R. C., & Wright, D. E. (1969). Systematic desensitization, therapeutically oriented instructions and selective positive reinforcement. *Behavior Research and Therapy, 7,* 27–33.

Peloquin, S. M. (1983). The development of an occupational therapy interview/therapy set procedure. *American Journal of Occupational Therapy, 37,* 457–461.

Rappaport, H. (1972). Modification of avoidance behavior: Expectancy, autonomic reactivity, and verbal report. *Journal of Consulting and Clinical Psychology, 39,* 404–414.

Rebeta-Burditt, J. (1977). *The cracker factory.* New York: Macmillan.

Reed, K. L., & Sanderson, S. R. (1983). *Concepts of occupational therapy.* Baltimore: Williams & Wilkins.

Rosen, G. M. (1974). Therapy set: its effects on subjects' involvement in systematic desensitization and treatment outcome. *Journal of Abnormal Psychology, 83,* 291–300.

Speedy recovery. (1987, July). *Reader's Digest,* p. 53.

Wade, B. D. (1947). Occupational therapy for patients with mental disease. In H. Willard & C. Spackman (Eds.), *Occupational therapy* (pp. 81–117). Philadelphia: Lippincott.

Woy, J. R., & Efran, J. S. (1972). Systematic desensitization and expectancy in the treatment of speaking anxiety. *Behavior Research and Therapy, 10,* 33–49.

Wilkins, W. (1973). Expectancy of therapeutic gain: An empirical and conceptual critique. *Journal of Consulting and Clinical Psychology, 40,* 69–77.

CHAPTER 51

Ethical Decision-Making Challenges in Clinical Practice

BEVERLY P. HOROWITZ,
PHD, CSW, OTR/L, BCG

Changing health care environments, organizational charts, and occupational therapy department structure require practitioners to be effective problem solvers in fast-paced environments (Horowitz, 2001a, 2001b). Increased practice opportunities in school-based programs, home health care, and private practice also support increased professional autonomy and modified supervisory patterns and teamwork strategies. Simultaneously, demographic changes and increasing appreciation of the need to improve access to health care services challenges health care providers, including occupational therapists, to increase their understanding of diverse populations and to provide culturally competent care (Wells & Black, 2000). Professional education and clinical experience enables practitioners to amass resources, including clinical assessments and instruments to promote clinical reasoning for "best practice."

In today's health care environment practitioners face complex ethical problems and/or dilemmas, including the "business–administrative and community dimensions" often involved in ethical issues involving patient care (Purtilo, 1999, p. 28). Supportive peer relationships are optimal for effective problem solving to resolve ethical dilemmas, particularly when practitioners face problems that challenge their personal and/or professional values and professional integrity. However, organizational cultures in many of today's busy health care settings, with combinations of per-diem, part-time, and full-time staff, is not always conducive to cohesive departments or close collegial relationships, both of which are beneficial when practitioners face ethical problems. Ethical decision-making in these environments requires practical problem-solving strategies to guide practitioners to evaluate all relevant information, define the presenting problem, determine tentative courses of action, and finally select and implement an ethical resolution (Darr, 1997; Purtilo, 1999; Scott, 1998).

One common ethical dilemma arises when providing health care services to uninsured individuals, Practitioners face conflicts between professional and ethical responsibilities to equitably support the health and well-being of our patients and the realities of health care business practices that typically require administrative review to ensure payment for services as a prerequisite for treatment. Often uninsured patients receive limited services, are transferred to alternative settings, or are denied non-emergency services. We face a different type of dilemma when we observe an experienced colleague whose personal problems are intruding upon their professional competence. What is our obligation to our colleagues, institutions, and patients? How do we respond? While these are dissimilar situations, each situation asks us to consider our individual and professional values and ethics, and presents a professional challenge.

Values and Ethics and Ethical Decision-Making

In our increasingly heterogeneous society, individuals have diverse personal beliefs and values and are influenced by internalized principles that guide their relationships with people (Wells & Black, 2000). These personal values, often coupled with cultural and religious perspectives, support concepts of morality, the guidelines and standards that protect our human values and accompany our social interactions (Horowitz, 1996; Purtilo, 1999).

Personal biases and prejudice, whether conscious or unconscious, similarly influence moral perspectives, our view of the world, and our ability to both understand and work with diverse populations. Prejudice and biases extend beyond the usual "isms" (e.g., racism, ageism, sexism) to attitudes related to parenting, sexual orientation, leisure, work ethics, and retirement. Reflection on our own values, perspectives, and biases enables us to understand personal values that are the basis of our morality (Diller, 1999; Horowitz, 1996, 2001a, 2001b).

Ethics is the systematic study of what may be called the "nature of morality" (Bailey & Schwartzberg, 1995, p. 2; Horowitz, 1996; Purtilo, 1999). It provides an organized framework to understand and discuss personal and social values, individual and social behavior, and methods for resolving conflicts between values and ethical principles in our daily lives. Religion, culture, family, and community influence individual values and moral principles; however, we are also influenced by our forbearers and history, including perspectives on morality, ethical principles, and ethical behavior. Deontologic and teleologic ethical theories are two theoretical approaches with particular relevance for health care practitioners (Horowitz, 2001a, 2001b, 1996; Purtilo, 1999). Deontology can be summarized as an absolutist duty-driven theory, associated with philosopher Immanuel Kant (1724–1804). It holds that behavior needs to be based upon moral obligation or "duty," and that one's conduct can be perceived as following correct or incorrect moral precepts, regardless of the consequences. In contrast, teleological theory, often identified with "utilitarianism," associated with John Stuart Mill and Jeremy Bentham, is less concerned with determining correct or incorrect conduct, and more concerned with the consequences of conduct and behavior (Purtilo, 1999; Rhodes, 1989).

These perspectives continue to reflect dialog on ethical behavior today, in both our personal and professional lives and provide a foundation for understanding ethical principles of fidelity, justice, beneficence, nonmaleficence, veracity, autonomy, and self-determination (Horowitz, 1996; Purtilo, 1999). Teleologic, or utilitarian theories, influence our thinking, when we focus our attention on the consequences of either individual or social behavior or policies, and seek actions that bring about the "best balance of benefits over burdens" for our patients and their families. In contrast, when we choose between two courses of action, and select one because we feel it to be morally correct, we are responding to deontologic ethical theory (Horowitz, 1996, 2001a, 2001b; Purtilo, 1999, p. 48).

However, how do we recognize ethical issues, challenges, and dilemmas? Ethical issues commonly face us. These issues present moral principles that may pose challenges to individual values, but do not necessarily pose a problem. This may include a concern regarding advance directives for one particular client (e.g., Do Not Resuscitate Orders), or a hospital admission policy that requires insurance documentation for entry into a rehabilitation program. They may also involve situations where we perceive threats to moral values, requiring systematic analysis and decision-making to determine a course of action. Ethical dilemmas are more complex ethical problems that cause ethical distress. Here, there is no one best course of action, rather a problem that involves conflicting values, where each possible action results in conflicting values, for example, a conflict between the principles of autonomy versus nonmaleficence, or fidelity versus beneficence (Horowitz, 2001a, 2001b; Purtilo, 1999).

Codes of Ethics, Legal Issues, and Social Responsibility

Society expects health care professionals to be of high moral standing with similar expectations of fiduciary provider–patient/client relationships, built upon trust, privacy, and confidence (Kutchins, 1991; Levy, 1976; Lo, 1995). Licensed health care professionals commonly are required to be of "good moral character" and maintain high professional standards, with legal sanctions for misconduct, establishing policy to codify this expectation (New York State Department of Education, 1993, p. 11). Health professionals are expected to: (1) Avoid misrepresentation, including implications for documentation; (2) Be faithful and honest in relationships with patients and colleagues; (3) Provide competent professional services to promote health and well-being; (4) Be cognizant of precautions to prevent harm; and (5) Provide patients with accurate information about treatment, including treatment options (American Occupational Therapy Association, 2000a; Hansen, 2001; Horowitz, 2001a; Lo, 1995).

Health care professional codes of conduct typically emulate the ancient physicians' Hippocratic Oath and codes of the professions of law, medicine, and clergy. They publicly enunciate shared values, historically represent a means of self-regulation, and acknowledge the importance of public trust in the health professions. In this tradition, the Occupational Therapy Code of Ethics (AOTA, 2000a) sets forth the following principles of occupational therapy:

1. Concern for the well-being of clients;
2. Avoid harm;
3. Respect for the rights of clients;
4. High standards of competence;
5. Compliance with policies of the profession and laws regulating practice;
6. Provide accurate information about occupational therapy services; and
7. High professional conduct.

These principles reflect shared professional values, including altruism; equality and impartiality; freedom, including professional independence and the commitment to freedom of choice for all people; justice; dignity; valuing each person's uniqueness; truthfulness; prudence; discipline; discretion; and vigilance (American Occupational Therapy Association

Commission on Standards and Ethics, 1996; Horowitz, 1996). However, while these professional principles provide an ethical framework for practice, practitioners need to distinguish ethical problems and dilemmas from clinical, administrative, or legal issues, and determine appropriate approaches for differing problems and needs.

Practitioners generally have experience identifying and resolving clinical and administrative problems. Health care organizations have written operating procedures and supervisory personnel who provide administrative direction. Practitioners often have access to texts, journals, and monographs that address clinical reasoning and practice issues for persons with a range of diagnoses across the life span. Additionally, technological advances and the information explosion enable increasing numbers of practitioners to hve ready access to varied computer databases, professional listserves and journals to obtain current information on best practice (Horowitz, 2001b).

There is a wealth of information available on ethical decision-making. However, occupational therapy practice focuses on clinical interventions to address client goals, often with a focus on promoting functional capability and occupational performance. Additionally, our health care environment requires practitioners to balance clinical–ethical considerations, organizational policies and expectations, third-party payer requirements, clinical demands, financial pressures, and personal and professional values (Crabtree, 1991; Darr, 1997, Hofland, 1994; Horowitz, 2001a, 2001b; Kyler-Hutchison, 1996; Scott, 1997). These pressures may ultimately affect clinical decision-making and interfere with collaborative treatment planning with clients and families (Haas, 1995). Like many disciplines, accredited occupational therapy programs are required to include course material that enables students to appreciate and understand ethical principles and relationships between ethics and practice (Accreditation Council for Occupational Therapy Education, 1998). Professional organizations, including the American Occupational Therapy Association, provide resources for practitioners to increase their knowledge of methods of resolving ethical dilemmas in practice (Accreditation Council for Occupational Therapy Education, 1998; American Speech-Language Hearing Association, 2001a, 2001b; Hansen, 2001; Scott, 1997). Occupational therapy practitioners are skilled analysts of human behavior and problem solvers, but have less experience and professional support to increase ethical decision-making capabilities in most practice settings.

Ethical problems arise when we find ourselves facing moral challenges. They commonly occur when we find ourselves in situations that force us to reflect upon our personal and professional beliefs, values, and responsibilities. Ethical dilemmas result when we perceive ourselves caught between conflicting values and ethical principles that require choices between competing "morally correct" solutions and courses of action (Purtilo, 1999, p. 72). One such dilemma

may develop in the context of strong professional relationships with patients. For example, in the course of regular treatment a severely ill patient may choose to ask her therapist questions about her medical condition and prognosis instead of seeking this information from her physician. How should the therapist respond? What is her responsibility? Ethical principles instruct us to be honest and truthful and not provide false hope, or inaccurate information. However, the principle of beneficence simultaneously asks us to be concerned with "doing good," and the principle of nonmaleficence instructs us to prevent harm, including potential negative consequences of interventions. Crafting an appropriate ethical solution requires reflection on personal values and perceived conflicting ethical principles, and determination of alternative choices and available courses of action. Here, the challenge is to utilize broad-based clinical skills and clinical judgment to answer questions we can honestly answer, empower the patient to speak with her physician, and address those health care needs within our domain to maximize quality of life and well-being.

In other situations, ethical problems may have corresponding legal implications (Horowitz, 1996; Scott, 1997; Wenston, 1987). For example, ethical concepts regarding confidentiality need to be understood in the context of both professional ethics as well as the law. For example, therapists who inappropriately disclose confidential patient information regarding HIV may find themselves reported for violations of both the AOTA Code of Ethics as well as violations of state statutes (Kyler-Hutchison, 1995; Liang, 2000). Inappropriate disclosure of medical information regarding HIV status in some states can result in civil and criminal penalties (Liang, 2000). Additionally, conduct considered professionally unethical increasingly also violates criminal or licensure law. Specific examples are noted in The Occupational Therapy Code of Ethics in Principle 1, which prohibits exploitation of recipients of services "sexually, physically ... or in any manner," and in Principle 5, which requires accurate representation of "qualifications, education, experience, training, and competence" (American Occupational Therapy Association, 2000a; Scott, 1997). Relationships and similarities between ethical standards and legal requirements are clear when state law delineates specific unprofessional conduct, as in New York State. Two examples of unprofessional conduct listed by New York State's Board of Regents include: "willful or grossly negligent failure to comply with substantial provisions of Federal, State, or local law ..."; and "willfully making or filing a false report ..."; or "practicing beyond the scope permitted by law ..." corresponding to Principles 5 and 6 in AOTA's Code of Ethics, which commit occupational therapists to comply with all laws regulating practice, and to accurately document information about occupational therapy services (American Occupational Therapy Association, 2000a; New York State Department of Education, 1993, p. 30).

In addition to being knowledgeable about ethical practice, occupational therapy practitioners need to fully understand licensure requirements and their scope of practice, professional standards of practice, and requirements of varied accrediting agencies. We are expected to comply with the full range of laws, from Constitutional law to criminal law and administrative law (including regulations of federal agencies such as the Equal Opportunity Commission (EEOC), Centers for Disease Control (CDC), and Occupational Safety and Health Administration (OSHA). Additionally, we need to be knowledgeable about health care law, regulations, and policy, particularly those with direct impact upon practice (American Occupational Therapy Association, 2000b; Bailey & Schwartzberg, 1995; Horowitz, 2000; Liang, 2000; Scott, 1997). Major federal legislation with significant impact upon occupational therapy practice include: Public Law 94–142, PL 99–457, and PL 105–17 (special educational needs of disabled children and toddlers), the Omnibus Reconciliation Act of 1987 and 1990 (nursing home reform and services), Medicare and Medicaid regulations (rehabilitation services, including occupational therapy), and the Americans with Disabilities Act (ADA) (PL 101–336) (civil rights legislation for disabled persons in the areas of education), employment, public accommodations, transportation, and telecommunications (Bailey & Schwartzberg, 1995; Dunn, 2000). State insurance law and state Medicaid policy directly affect coverage of occupational therapy services for clients across the life span. Therapists involved in nontraditional practice need to be particularly cognizant of legal issues, including licensure regulations, malpractice law, laws and regulations regarding consultation, and contract law (Bailey & Schwartzberg, 1995; Horowitz, 1996; Kornblau, 1992; Scott, 1997).

Strategies for Ethical Decision-Making

Ethical problems and dilemmas can occur in everyday practice, in clinical or administrative settings, educational environments, or within professional relationships. Professional Codes of Ethics, such as AOTA's Code of Ethics, socialize and commit practitioners to shared values and responsibilities to guide professional conduct. They are optimally utilized in combination with a systematic approach to ethical decision-making. This process guides data gathering for problem identification, data analysis, determining an optimal course of action, and individual reflection on action outcomes. Ethical decision-making frameworks optimally include opportunities for self-reflection and feedback to guide the overall process, modify problem analysis, and conceptualize potential courses of action (Horowitz, 1996, 2001a, 2001b; Scott, 1998).

Purtilo's Six-Step Approach (Purtilo, 1999) provides one practical ethical decision-making strategy that addresses the needs of health care practitioners in varied contexts. It includes:

1. Data gathering and getting the story straight;
2. Problem identification;
3. Problem analysis utilizing ethical theory and principles;
4. Exploration of practical options;
5. Selecting and executing a course of action; and
6. Evaluation of the process and the outcome.

This six-step process organizes and structures the problem-solving process to prevent practitioners from allowing emotional reactions and time pressures to direct their behavior. Step 1 asks practitioners to gather all relevant information, determine the accuracy of the information they obtain, and the context in which information was gathered. In Step 2 the problem analysis process promotes self-questioning. It asks, What is the morally correct course of action? How does one maintain professional integrity within this situation? Who has primary responsibility for resolving this situation? Step 3 requires practitioners to utilize their knowledge of ethical principles, including teleologic (utilitarian) and deontologic approaches, to determine the kind of ethical problem or dilemma they face, including competing values and principles. Formulations of all possible, practical solutions, including anticipated consequences, follow in Step 4. At this point in the process, with data and analysis in hand, one needs to consider available options, selecting among those deemed most appropriate. Practitioners then need to act (Step 5) and initiate a response to the ethical problem or dilemma. While individuals may or may not successfully execute actions to resolve their dilemma, this structured ethical decision-making approach constructively increases information about the problem or dilemma, thereby reducing distress and potential "burnout." The last step (Step 6) is evaluative. It poses the questions: What went well? What could be done differently? How did this action affect you? Affect other people's perceptions of you? Are you empowered for future ethical decision-making (Purtilo, 1999)?

Ethical Decision-Making in Practice

In practice, ethical problems and/or dilemmas may occur in response to conflicts between values and ethical principles; ethical principles set forth within the AOTA Code of Ethics; and responsibilities to employers, patients/clients, our profession, and ourselves (American Occupational Therapy Association, 2000; Bailey & Schwartzberg, 1995; Kyler-Hutchison, 1996; Purtilo, 1999). We may observe an impaired friend and colleague unable to provide competent treatment, resulting in an ethical dilemma and personal conflict between being faithful (fidelity) and the principle "do no harm" (nonmaleficence). Or, we find ourselves employed in a medical center with budget constraints; increasing demand for services; knowledgeable, inquiring consumers; and a waiting list of patients, from patients with acute head injuries to medically ill developmentally delayed children. The reality of scarce resources poses challenges to health care professionals, often with resulting conflicts between principles of justice and equity for needy patients, principles of fidelity (faithfulness) to colleagues and employers, and the principles of veracity (honesty) and beneficence (bringing about good) in relationships with patients and families.

Case Study

The following case study demonstrates the utility of a structured ethical decision-making approach. Occupational therapist Evelyn McNeil has recently become employed as a school-based practitioner in a suburban primary school in New York State. Ms. McNeil has a reputation as an expert clinician, and has experience in a wide range of pediatric rehabilitation settings, with children with chronic illness. She attends continuing education programs, including local workshops to increase clinical skills utilizing sensory integration evaluation procedures and treatment approaches. However, her knowledge about school-based practice is limited.

The Kennedy Elementary School, where she provides occupational therapy services, is a suburban primary school serving preschool children and students from grades 1 through 3. This neighborhood school is recognized as a model school and encourages interdisciplinary approaches between educators and therapists. Children served have varied diagnoses and problems; many are developmentally delayed. Parents are encouraged to volunteer within the classroom, and there are positive partnerships among the parent–teacher associations, faculty, and school administration.

Ms. McNeil works closely with teachers and parents and believes in the efficacy of sensory integrative treatment to promote educational and therapeutic goals for her young students. She promotes the benefits of occupational therapy, use of standardized sensory integration evaluation, and use of a sensory integration (SI) practice model to enable children with sensory modulation disorders to more appropriately respond to "environmental demands and be more successful learners" (Dunn, 2000, p. 35). Ms. McNeil also conducts in-service programs and writes guidelines for suggested classroom activities for children with a range of disorders and needs. In order to promote her strengths, she distributes business cards and in-service materials. These materials highlight her expertise as an occupational therapy specialist in pediatrics with advanced training and expertise in SI practice. Her success promoting occupational therapy has resulted in strong administrative support, a series of public relations stories on the occupational therapy program, and decisions to apply for grant funding to increase building space and equipment for optimal implementation of SI treatment. This competitive grant application requires Ms. McNeil to provide an updated curriculum vitae, including verification of licensure and her credentials as a pediatrics specialist with expertise in use of SI evaluation and treatment methodologies.

Are there ethical problems and potentially legal issues in this scenario? While occupational therapists can utilize a range of practice models, including the sensory integrative practice model, without advanced certification, occupational therapists can obtain certification by Sensory Integration International to document competence to administer and interpret the Sensory Integration Praxis Test (SIPT) (Sensory Integration International, 2001). Ms. McNeil does not have this certification, nor does she hold board certification in pediatrics from the American Occupational Therapy Association. Clearly, she appears to be indicating a level of expertise that she does not possess.

Misrepresenting credentials to colleagues and her employer is a breach of faith. The AOTA Code of Ethics (Principle 6) commits practitioners to the principle of veracity and states, "Occupational therapy personnel shall accurately represent their credentials, qualifications, education, experience, training, and competence." In addition to violating the spirit of Principle 6, Ms. McNeil disregarded Principle 7, which states, "Occupational therapy personnel shall treat colleagues and other professionals with fairness, discretion, and integrity," and the ethical principle of fidelity. This misrepresentation can potentially cause the Kennedy School administration significant embarrassment and professional harm given their support of her work and efforts to obtain funding for an enlarged treatment area to support her use of a sensory integration practice model. In addition in New York State, unsubstantiated claims of "professional superiority" are also considered unprofessional conduct (New York State Department of Education, 1993, p. 31).

The ethical problems presented in this case study were avoidable. Ms. McNeil worked diligently to promote occupational therapy and her program. However, she neglected ethical implications implicit in the words "specialist" and "expertise," and ramifications of her marketing strategy. Colleagues, employers, and consumers recognize and value practitioners who have achieved advanced clinical competencies (Scott, 1998). Advanced competencies and specialization typically denote additional training, certification through advanced professional examination, or completion of recognized continuing education programs. Thus, misuse of these words is confusing, particularly given recent efforts to enable occupational therapists to develop and receive acknowledgement of advanced competencies through the American Occupational Therapy Association's Board Specialty Certification Program in Pediatrics and the availability of certification from Sensory Integration International to document competence in administering the Sensory Integration and Praxis Text (American Occupational Therapy Association, 2000c; Sensory Integration International, 2002).

Today's demanding outcome-oriented health care programs focus on efficient, effective treatment approaches. Treatment programs are often short; client caseloads high. Evidence of continuing education is increasingly required to maintain licensure, to meet administrative employer requirements, or to demonstrate professional competency. School systems and school-based practitioners face different challenges, but also have limited resources; growing numbers of children with identified needs for occupational therapy services; and administrative, taxpayer, and consumer questions regarding outcomes.

Busy practitioners thus commonly focus their attention on clinical issues, often with less attention to the full meaning and consequences of other professional decisions. Small occupational therapy departments often promote practitioner autonomy and reduced routine on-site collegial communication and interactions. Pragmatic strategies to enable individual practitioners to integrate and apply their personal and professional values, and knowledge of ethical principles, including the AOTA Code of Ethics, for ethical decision-making are increasingly valuable. These strategies provide practical guidelines to analyze ethical problems and dilemmas in our changing world, empower decision-making and action, and encourage reflection on the relationships among practice, our core values and ethics, and professional social responsibilities and legal obligations.

References

Accreditation Council for Occupational Therapy Education. (1998). *Standards for an accredited education program for the occupational therapist.* Bethesda, MD: American Occupational Therapy Association.

American Occupational Therapy Association. (2000a). Occupational therapy code of ethics (2000). *American Journal of Occupational Therapy, 54,* 614–616.

American Occupational Therapy Association. (2000c). *The specialty certification programs in geriatrics, pediatrics, or neurorehabilitation.* Bethesda, MD: Author.

American Occupational Therapy Association. (2000b). Standards of practice for occupational therapy. Retrieved September 5, 2000, from (www.aota.org/otsp.asp).

American Occupational Therapy Association, Commission on Standards and Ethics. (1996). *1966 occupational therapy code of ethics reference guide.* Bethesda, MD: Author.

American Speech-Language Hearing Association. (2000a). Code of Ethics. Retrieved September 3, 2001, from (www.professional.asha.org/library/code_of_ethics.htm).

American Speech-Language Hearing Association. (2000b). Standards and implementation for professional service programs in audiology and speech-language pathology (Effective Jan. 1. 2002). Retrieved September 8, 2001, from (www.professional.asha.org/contents.htm.#professionals)

Bailey, D., & Schwartzberg, S. (Eds.). (1995). *Ethical and legal dilemmas in occupational therapy.* Philadelphia: FA Davis.

Crabtree, J. (1991). The effect of referral for profit on therapists and client's autonomy and fair competition. *American Journal of Occupational Therapy, 45,* 464–466.

Darr, K. (1997). *Ethics in health services management* (3rd ed.). Baltimore: Health Professions Press.

Diller, J. (1999). *Cultural diversity: A primer for the human services.* Albany: Wadsworth Publishing.

Dunn, W. (2000). *Best practice occupational therapy in community service with children and families.* Thorofare NJ: Slack.

Hansen, R. (2001). Guidelines to the occupational therapy code of ethics. Retrieved 2001 from (www.aota.org/memhers/area2/links/lasp?).

Haas, J. (1995, January/February). Ethical considerations of goal setting for patient care in rehabilitation medicine. *American Journal of Physical Medicine and Rehabilitation,* S16–S20.

Hofland, B. (1994). When capacity fades and autonomy is constricted: A client-centered approach to residential care. *Generations, 18,* 31–37.

Horowitz, B. (2001a, April). *Strategies for ethical decision-making.* Paper presented at the annual American Occupational Therapy Association Conference, Philadelphia, PA.

Horowitz, B. (2001b, October). *Professional ethics: It's academic.* Paper presented at the annual conference of the National Council of State Boards of Examiners for Speech-Language Pathology and Audiology, Pittsburgh. PA.

Horowitz, B. (1996). Ethical issues and gerontic occupational therapy practice. In O. Larson, R. Stevens-Ratchford, L. Pedretti, & J. Crabtree (Eds.), *The role of occupational therapy with the elderly* (pp. 144–165). Rockville, MD: AOTA.

Kornblau, B. (1992). Legal issues in occupational therapy consultation. In E. Jaffe & C. Epstein (Eds.), *Occupational therapy consultation* (pp. 594–621). St. Louis: Mosby Yearbook.

Kutchins, H. (1991). The fiduciary relationship: The legal basis for social workers' responsibilities to clients. *Social Work, 36,* 106–113.

Kyler-Hutchison. P. (1996). Issues in ethics. In AOTA Commission on Standards and Ethics, *1996 occupational therapy code of ethics reference guide* (pp. 43–44). Bethesda: AOTA.

Levy, C. (1976). *Social work ethics.* New York: Human Sciences Press.

Liang, B. (2000). *Health law and policy.* Boston: Butterworth Heinemann.

Lo, B. (1995) *Resolving ethical dilemmas: A guide for clinicians.* Baltimore: Williams & Wilkins.

New York State Education Department, Office of Professional Credentialing. (1993). *Occupational therapy and occupational therapy assistant handbook.* Albany: Author.

Purtilo, R. (1999). *Ethical dimensions in the health professions* (3rd ed.). Philadelphia: Saunders.

Rhodes, M. (1989). *Ethical dilemmas in social work practice.* Milwaukee, Wisconsin: Family Service America.

Sensory Integration International. (2002). *Certification programs.* Retrieved January 9, 2002 from (www.sensoryint.com/certification.html).

Scott. R. (1997). *Promoting legal awareness in physical occupational therapy.* St. Louis: Mosby.

Scott, R. (1998). *Professional ethics: A guide for rehabilitation professionals.* St. Louis: Mosby.

Wells, S., & Black, R. (2000). *Cultural competency for health professionals.* Bethesda, MD: AOTA.

Wenston, S. (1987). Applying philosophy to ethical dilemmas. In G. Anderson & V. Glesnes-Anderson (Eds.), *Health care ethics* (pp. 22–33). Rockville, MD: Aspen Publishers.

PART VI

Current Realities and Future Directions for Best Practice in Occupational Therapy

Introduction

The influence of historical movements, sociopolitical forces, and health care system trends on occupational therapy has been comprehensively discussed in many of the chapters in this text. From the profession's early struggle to define practice to the debate on physical agent modalities, occupational therapy has faced several challenges and changes throughout its first century of growth (Schemm, 1994; Shannon, 1977; West, 1984). Our profession has a strong history of divergent viewpoints as occupational therapy practitioners have always strove to balance the art and science of care (Law, 2002; Schemm, 1994; Wood, 1995). However, over the years, the growing concern that the challenges faced by occupational therapy would result in the loss of the heart and soul of our profession if we did not actively work to sustain this balance between the art and science of practice was actualized in the spread of reductionistic practices (Shannon, 1977; Whiteford, Townsend, & Hocking, 2000).

Twenty years ago, West (1984) expressed concern that the term *activity*, while clearly a core principle of our philosophical base, has become "narrow and impoverished, bearing little resemblance to its rich, original connotations" (p. 22). This concern was clearly valid, as many occupational therapy practices became apparent clones of their physical therapy or social work counterparts, emphasizing physical modalities or verbal therapies (Haase, 1995; Whiteford et al., 2000). The infrequent use of meaningful occupation and purposeful activity in

treatment resulted in the loss of the uniqueness and distinctive benefits of occupational therapy. The critical need for occupational therapy practitioners to integrate our fundamental theoretical principles with client information to collaborate and design natural, real-life occupations to ensure that individuals, caregivers, reimbursing agencies, policymakers, and the public view occupational therapy as a viable and distinct profession, separate from physical therapy and social work, has been widely discussed in our literature (Haase, 1995; Wood, 1998). Grady (1992) has asked "have occupational therapists become so controlled by the realities of productivity, reimbursement, and modalities that we are failing to see the process as part of the outcome and therefore also measurable, reimbursable, and valuable?" (p. 1013).

The chapters in this part explore this question, examining the current realities influencing our profession while sustaining a commitment to our founding beliefs, which emphasize the value of the therapeutic relationship and the use of occupation throughout the occupational therapy process. It is hoped that some of the issues discussed in this part (e.g., reimbursement-driven practice, professional competition) will quickly become dated and irrelevant. However, given the slowness of societal change and the resistance of entrenched systems, it is likely that many of the issues raised by these authors will remain pertinent as we continue practicing in the first quarter of our profession's next century. Therefore, this part's emphasis on the need for occupational therapy

practitioners to become politically astute and market savvy to ensure that our profession remains viable, now and in the future, is very realistic. On a positive note, it also is hoped that all occupational therapy practitioners will embrace the principles of the *Occupational Therapy Practice Framework* (American Occupational Therapy Association [AOTA], 2002), thereby enabling us to fulfill the visions of a world of occupational justice and participation in life for all, as put forth by several of this part's authors.

This part begins with an exploration of the value of our professional history to current and future occupational therapy practice that was first presented in 1981. In this classic Presidential Address, Johnson examines in Chapter 52 the "old" values of humanism, caring, and the therapeutic relationship and the "new" directions of science, logic, and depersonalization. She examines the conflict between being humanistic and caring while striving to meet demands to be scientific and objective, expressing concern that the profession is moving toward reductionism and away from holism. A historical review of the characteristics of the founders of occupational therapy and the evolution of the profession up to 1981 is provided. As Johnson notes, during this time period, there had been growth in the profession with respect to the types of clients served, settings in which occupational therapy practitioners provide service, and our professional repertoire of tools of practice. She cautions that this growth may have sacrificed depth for breadth. Johnson challenges occupational therapy practitioners to question their work so that they can maintain holistic values while developing knowledge and skills in a scientific sense. She calls for increased professional support for entry-level therapists, administrators, researchers, and educators to ensure they are able to meet the challenges of their roles. Increased research also is needed to substantiate the value of occupational therapy by developing a solid unifying theoretical foundation. Personal poignant examples highlight Johnson's presentation, emphasizing the depth of meaning inherent in these professional values, considering the complexities of occupational therapy practice. She concludes that the combination of old values of humanism and holism with new values of science, research, and knowledge will enable occupational therapy practitioners to acquire new competence and attain professional unity.

A critical review of this address more than 20 years later will help readers realize how astute Johnson was regarding the danger that reductionism presented to our profession. Regrettably, many practitioners did not heed her call to maintain our core values while expanding our competencies, and reductionistic practices grew throughout the 1980s and 1990s (Whiteford et al., 2000). Fueling this trend toward reductionism during this period were major changes within the health care delivery system, which resulted in increased demands on occupational therapy practitioners from reimbursers. The next two chapters explore the effect of reimbursement on occupational therapy service delivery. Howard in Chapter 53 begins by examining the extent to which third-party reimbursement dictates day-to-day practice. The history and meaning of reimbursement with respect to occupational therapy practice is explored through a thoughtful and comprehensive analysis of the literature. According to this review, occupational therapy's definition, scope of practice, professional roles,

management of occupational therapy departments, and professional ethics have been modified over the years in response to changes in reimbursement.

Howard thoroughly explores each of these affects on occupational therapy, analyzing the profession's response to changes in reimbursement including licensure, public relations, and political actions. Societal forces that influence reimbursement policies and subsequently affect occupational therapy practice are examined. Howard contends that third-party payers currently control the definitions of occupational therapy, rewarding the use of the medical model, which leads to changes in our professional language and how we define ourselves to accommodate these pressures. Implications of reimbursement-driven practice and the resulting values conflict experienced by many occupational therapy practitioners working in the current health system are explored. Howard concludes that practitioners must understand the precipitants to the imposition of reimbursement standards on occupational therapy practice. This knowledge will enable occupational therapy practitioners to be proactive with respect to issues of health care policy so that they can maintain viable marketable professional roles, which remain grounded in occupational therapy's humanistic base.

The conflict between the values of reimbursement-driven practice and the humanistic values of occupational therapy are further explored in Chapter 54 by Burke and Cassidy. They consider the opposing forces faced by practitioners today, whose practices are fundamentally based on occupational therapy's humanistic philosophy, yet these practices are located in a health care environment that is determined by economics. The philosophical foundations of our profession are reviewed, and the question as to how these individually oriented, humanistic values can survive within the current health care system with numerous economic,

political, and social factors affecting this philosophy of care is analyzed. The impact of economically driven practice on occupational therapy treatment approaches and service delivery models and the conflicts between evaluation and intervention based on individual needs versus evaluation and intervention based on reimbursement are explored. The need for occupational therapy practitioners to shift their allegiance from being solely focused on the patient to also include concern for employers' economic viability and the fiscal constraints of reimbursement is emphasized by the authors as being a reality in current practice. Burke and Cassidy analyze the expansion of the "consumer" of occupational therapy services to include the government, HMOs, third-party payers, health corporations, and school administrations, resulting in increased pressures for accountability and leading to the development of several vested interests that can lead to ethical conflicts and practice dilemmas. A number of relevant practice dilemmas that result from these ethical conflicts and a series of thought-provoking questions for occupational therapy practitioners to consider as they attempt to manage these dilemmas are presented. A series of directives that will lead to occupational therapy's inclusion in the health care marketplace are provided. The challenge to practitioners is to effectively implement these directives while maintaining a humanistic and holistic philosophy of practice.

Chapter 55 by Schwartz offers a way to deal effectively with the challenges, demands, and frustrations of reimbursement-driven practice. She presents the excellence perspective as a way to ensure quality of care, as well as efficient care. The excellence perspective is contrasted with the efficiency perspective, which emphasizes productivity. The history of the efficiency perspective is presented, and its introduction to health care management is examined. The adoption of the efficiency perspective in health care resulted in a change from a humanistic emphasis to a business administration focus. The incongruence between a business mode and the provision of humanistic health care presents a dilemma as to how to achieve quality as well as efficiency. Schwartz proposes the excellence perspective as an alternative to the efficiency perspective, stating that if one stresses excellence as his or her primary goal, productivity will also be enhanced. Because leadership is a critical factor in successful implementation of the excellence perspective, she identifies ways that leaders can shape organizations in which members strive for excellence. A case study of a hospital program that exemplifies many of the characteristics of the excellence perspective with leaders that epitomize the leadership qualities fundamental for success is provided. The excellence perspective can be used as a guide for program innovation, as it is congruent with occupational therapy's concern for quality patient care and with the health care system's concern for productivity. Occupational therapy practitioners must develop leadership skills and knowledge of management to be able to articulate consumer needs and design and implement programs based on excellence.

Peloquin further explores in Chapter 56 methods for maintaining excellence in practice, which focuses on sustaining the art of practice in occupational therapy. She thoughtfully reviews the literature on the art and science of occupational therapy, examining fundamental principles and assumptions of our profession. While mastering the art of practice has always been challenging, current demands from a changing health care system limit the ability of occupational therapy practitioners to develop and engage in meaningful relationships with their patients. Decreased lengths of stay, increased documentation requirements, and heightened emphasis on productivity take time and

energy away from caring, thereby constraining therapeutic relationships. According to Peloquin, the health care system focuses on the science of practice and does not value, nurture, or reward the art of practice. Therefore, occupational therapy practitioners must obtain sustenance and nurturance of their art from other sources. She suggests that practitioners use literature to affirm the value of the art of practice as it can provide sustaining images to support their commitment to the therapeutic relationship and in using occupation as therapy.

Providing several poignant examples from fiction, Peloquin accentuates the power of images and the written word to occupational therapy practitioners reflecting on the art of practice. Insightful reading of literature containing both positive and negative images of the profession and its practitioners can increase readers' awareness of the type of therapist they would like to emulate. Self-reflection on character strengths and weaknesses is vital to maintaining the art and soul of occupational therapy. Peloquin's unique suggestion to use literature to increase self-awareness is an effective tool because it can be used individually at one's own convenience. Given the multiple demands on practitioners' time, this can be an efficient method of sustaining the art of practice in a challenging health care system. Sustaining the art of practice in occupational therapy will be critical if our profession is to successfully meet the demands of its next century.

The next two chapters eloquently present the authors' thought-provoking viewpoints on occupational therapy practice in the 21st century. Yerxa presents an American perspective, and in Chapter 58, Polatajko presents a Canadian perspective on dreams, dilemmas, and decisions for occupational therapy practice in this century. Yerxa puts forth the assumption that the 21st century will have several unique characteristics that will be important to occupational therapy practitioners and the

consumers of our services. These characteristics—increase in chronicity; knowledge of human purpose; complexity of daily living; awareness of demands from the environments in which people live and work; emphasis on personal power, autonomy, self-direction, and self-responsibility; and a new conceptualization of health as people's capacities to achieve goals through a repertoire of skills—are briefly described. A clear link between each characteristic and the philosophy and unique body of knowledge of the profession of occupational therapy is provided. Based on the congruence between these characteristics and occupational therapy, Yerxa asserts that this century will begin a millennium of occupation, for occupational therapy practitioners can effectively meet the needs reflected in each of the identified characteristics.

Yerxa strongly emphasizes the value of authentic occupational therapy and reflects on the potential of occupational science to enrich and broaden occupational therapy practice. Implications for the future of occupational therapy are discussed, and the need for occupational therapy practitioners to establish their priorities in the "millennium of occupation" is examined. She calls for occupational therapy practice to emphasize the potential of people with disabilities, with practitioners serving as advocates and allies for individuals and their families. Yerxa concludes that the knowledge, skills, and values of occupational therapy practitioners, as founded in our early philosophical base, will enable us to ensure that people with chronic illnesses and disabilities will develop the skills they need to achieve their goals of competency. Social barriers to this self-definition will be removed, enabling them to thrive in their environments throughout the next century.

Polatajko continues this theme of viewing people with disabilities in a "new light" in the 21st century, thereby requiring occupational therapy to shift its emphasis in this millennium. She proposes that, in the future, the world will eliminate the concept of *handicap* by creating an environment where individuals with different abilities and disabilities can live meaningful lives with dignity. In this new world, the focus of occupational therapy will change from reducing impairments to preventing handicaps through empowerment. The definitions of handicap, impairment, and disability are provided and contrasted. The relationship of occupation to these concepts is examined, and a review of the basic assumptions and core values of occupational therapy are reviewed. Polatajko realistically discusses the limits of current occupational therapy practice, which is heavily influenced by the medical model, and puts forth her vision that an occupational therapy profession, which emphasizes the full potential of occupation, can assume a leadership position in the 21st century. Adopting occupation as the core concept of our profession and entrenching occupation into our professional value system are essential to achieve the ultimate goal of practice, which is the empowerment of occupational competence. Clear figures illustrate what occupational therapy is in a medical model and what it can become in an occupational competence model. Polatajko concludes that occupational therapy practitioners are uniquely positioned to eliminate handicaps and enable all to achieve occupational competence during the next millennium.

The criticality of the need for occupational therapy practitioners to adopt occupation as the core of our profession and to become known as occupational experts is strongly validated by Gutman in Chapter 59. In this challenging (and at times alarming) work, Gutman asks the provocative questions, Who possesses the domain of function? Who is competing for this domain? She begins her discourse by providing a historical perspective as to how occupational therapy initially developed and mastered our domain of functional activities of daily living

(ADL). How the exclusivity of our profession's mastery of this domain is now being challenged in response to external forces is clearly articulated. The reality that several other professions are now competing vigorously to claim the domain of functional ADL as within their profession's area of expertise is bluntly discussed. Readers unfamiliar with the 1997 practice guidelines of the American Physical Therapy Association will likely be taken aback by the striking similarities between these guidelines and AOTA's *Uniform Terminology* and *Practice Framework*.

Gutman does not exaggerate the enormity of the implications of the fact that these guidelines are written to define physical therapy's domain of concern to legislators, policymakers, and reimbursers. She does not minimize the reality that these guidelines pose a serious threat to the survival of the occupational therapy profession. Recent attempts by state physical therapy associations and the District of Columbia Physical Therapy Association to have these guidelines adopted as the official Practice Act language by their respective legislatures underscores the urgency of Gutman's concern. As she notes, the validity of physical therapy's claim to the domain of function is increasingly being supported by research studies demonstrating the efficacy of physical therapy services in improving ADL and IADL.

The recent development of occupation-based nursing practices and the increase in occupation-focused nursing research literature is also examined by Gutman. The reality that these practices and this literature reflect a fundamental lack of basic awareness about the existence of occupational therapy as a rehabilitation profession capable of providing these needed services is a grave concern. The final encroachment on occupational therapy's domain of concern presented by Gutman is neuropsychology. She reviews how the traditional neuropsychologist's role has changed in response to external forces, resulting in a focus on functional ADL.

Gutman provides numerous examples that clearly demonstrate the overlap among the rehabilitation practices of nurses, neuropsychologists, and occupational therapy practitioners. Most worrisome is the research that has been generated and disseminated by all three of these professions—physical therapy, nursing, and neuropsychology—as they strive to prove that their practices are most effective. This established efficacy can legitimize their claim to the domain of function and justify exclusive reimbursement for their profession's service delivery. Gutman's frank discussion of this outright competition for the domain of function ends with several critical suggestions to support, develop, generate, and disseminate research that can be used to preserve occupational therapy's ownership of our profession's core area of expertise.

The role of research in demonstrating the efficacy of a profession's practices and its concomitant validation of a profession's worth to society was clearly articulated by Gutman. This call for research is echoed loudly and clearly in Holm's 2000 Eleanor Clarke Slagle Lecture in Chapter 60. In this presentation, Holm critically examines our profession's lack of evidence demonstrating that our practices are valid or effective. This inability to provide data supportive of our interventions presents several ethical dilemmas as occupational therapy practitioners provide services based on limited evidence. Holm begins her discussion by examining the changes that have occurred in the health care environment over the past quarter-century that affected how occupational therapy services are provided. Most significant has been the increased emphasis on the need to justify service through the provision of evidence that supports what occupational therapy practitioners do in daily practice. This societal press for evidence-based practice is one that practitioners must respond to if we are to remain a viable profession.

Holm defines evidence-based practice and provides an excellent overview of the standards used to measure the strength of evidence. She contends that the confidence level that a practitioner has in his or her clinical decisions should be congruent with the strength of the evidence available on the given intervention. The strength of evidence for occupational therapy intervention is examined along a five-level hierarchy. Concrete examples and realistic clinical scenarios highlight the implications of her key points for everyday practice, emphasizing the relevance and need for "in-the-trenches" occupational therapy practitioners to use evidence-based practice.

The critical difference between preferred practice and evidence-based practice is emphasized. Holm's stance that the acquisition of evidence to support best practice must be conducted in actual practice settings (not in university ivory towers) is particularly noteworthy when one reflects on Gutman's prior discussion about the evidence-based, function-oriented practices of other health care professionals. The necessity for all occupational therapy practitioners to increase their research competencies to ensure our profession's survival is well supported throughout Holm's treatise. To help practitioners develop these abilities and integrate them with active clinical reasoning, five questions are posed. Holm suggests that affirmative answers to these questions indicate positive steps toward evidence-based practice. She honestly addresses systemic and personal barriers to evidence-based practice, reframing them as sources of motivation. Holm concludes by challenging all occupational therapy practitioners to take the ethical step of advancing our profession's base of evidence to ensure that occupational therapy practice is based on solid research.

Holm's call for research seems timely and reflective of recent societal trends and our profession's developing sophistication. Yet this need for research to support "what we do and how we do it" is not a new phenomenon. In 1967, West presented her visionary Eleanor Clarke Slagle Lecture that has remained startlingly current (see Chapter 61). In this lecture, West puts forth a call for research, community-based practice, and social activism to be sure that occupational therapy practitioners respond proactively to change. It is interesting to note that West gave this address at the 1967 AOTA National Convention in Minneapolis, site of the 2004 AOTA Annual Conference. If one deleted West's references to the 50th anniversary of our profession and the initiation of Medicare, Head Start, and community mental health programs and substituted the term "age of terrorism" for "nuclear age," one could reasonably conclude that this speech was given at this most recent conference.

West's call to move beyond our traditional limited identification with the medical model to a broad conceptualization of health, which includes prevention of illness and disability, maintenance and promotion of well-being, and the facilitation of normal growth and development, is striking in its timeliness. Her identification of the role of the occupational therapy practitioner as a health agent in community-based settings and her argument that practitioners must aggressively adapt and redesign their roles to be viable in a changing society and an evolving health care system remains amazingly contemporary almost 40 years later. West's stance that occupational therapy practitioners must advocate for equal access to health care and equal opportunities for comprehensive, holistic health services for all continues to be relevant today. Her discussion of the development of pediatric health care services, the initiation of the Head Start program, and the rise of the community mental health movement provides an interesting historical perspective for readers. Most significant is West's identification of the practice possibilities afforded by these trends and at these sites. She realistically explores the rich opportunities for occupational therapy practitioners in providing prevention, early intervention, and health promotion services. However, West expresses fear that few practitioners will appreciate these trends, and our profession will remain wedded to a traditional medical model, which severely limits our contributions to society. She calls for occupational therapy practitioners to develop a professional consciousness and collective responsibility to think about the social and cultural causes of disease and disability and to become active in health care planning and community-oriented services. The sad reality that the majority of occupational therapy practitioners did not heed this call and that West's fear was realized cannot be denied. Although many occupational therapy practitioners do work in early intervention programs, few have a primary prevention focus, and the role of occupational therapy in community mental health has diminished to an impenetrable level (Brown, 2002).

West concluded her Eleanor Clarke Slagle Lecture with the hope that a future generation of occupational therapy practitioners would look back and see a profession that was dynamically sharing a professional consciousness and collective responsibility. Current practitioners now have the opportunity to fulfill this dream. As West noted, societal trends are unmistakable and irreversible, and it is up to all practitioners to be collectively responsible to respond to these changes by assuming new roles and adopting new practices. Our profession's recommitment to its core values, as evidenced in the *Practice Framework*, now provides the shared vision that West had aspired toward to help current and future occupational therapy practitioners seize the opportunities put forth by her almost four decades ago.

In her Eleanor Clarke Slagle Lecture, West also expressed hope that one day a "better definition" of our profession would be developed. The *Practice Framework* (see Appendix A) and the recently adopted *Scope of Practice* (see Appendix B) and *Definition of Occupational Therapy* (see Appendix C) provide a holistic view of our profession that I think would please West. In addition, our profession's growing recognition of the need to critically examine the foundations of our profession and expand our knowledge base would also likely be welcomed by West. Chapter 62 by Blanche and Henny-Kohler provides a thought-provoking analysis about the development of this knowledge through occupational science. The authors discuss the interaction between the philosophy of occupational therapy and the science of occupation. The reality that occupational science has received a mixed reception globally is honestly presented. The relationship between occupational therapy and occupational science is explored, with the authors contending that the development of our own science is pivotal to our profession's ownership of its knowledge and professional identity throughout the world. They propose that the regional ideologies of different geographic areas affect occupational therapy philosophy, occupational science, and daily occupational therapy practice. A review of key concepts and definitions related to philosophy, ideology, and science provide a foundation for the presentation of two models that depict the relationship between regional ideology and occupational therapy. The first model focuses on the interaction between the international influence of occupational science and the daily activities of occupational therapy practitioners in different geographic regions. The international relevance of occupational science research on occupational therapy service delivery is thoughtfully explored. The second model put forth by Blanche and Henny-Kohler centers on the relationship among occupational therapy philosophy, occupational science, and regional ideology. In this model, the

authors propose that all of these factors influence and nourish each other. This interrelationship and its inherent value are clearly presented. The authors conclude by emphasizing the importance for our profession of developing a global identity by importing knowledge from occupational science and developing basic and applied knowledge in occupational therapy practice. This shared identity is based on recognition that occupational therapy and occupational science share a core global belief in empowering people to be autonomous.

The uniqueness of our profession's identity and the value of occupational science research to our profession's development are examined in depth in Chapter 63. In this seminal work, Pierce declares that a time of congruence has arrived that can result in the emergence of a powerful profession offering occupation-based practice. This congruence is the result of two major forces converging. The first is the exponential growth in our profession's knowledge base about occupation. The second force is society's increased valuation of functional outcomes. The reality that other professions have noticed the potential of this second force cannot be ignored. The danger of other professions imitating occupational therapy practice and claiming our profession's area of expertise was thoroughly examined by Gutman in Chapter 59. Pierce echoes Gutman's concerns and challenges occupational therapy practitioners to face this competition by simply being the best at what we do. We must expeditiously translate our substantial knowledge about occupation into the realization of superior occupation-based practice.

Pierce proposes that, to effectively achieve this outcome, our profession must build three bridges to bring the full potential of occupation to fruition. She describes these bridges—a generative discourse on the use of occupation in practice, practice demonstration sites, and effective education—in a

straightforward, realistic manner. To enable occupational therapy practitioners to forge these bridges, Pierce puts forth three conceptual tools. These tools, including the dimensions of power, sources of therapeutic power, and the occupational design process, are explored in depth. Their congruence with the core values of our profession is highly evident. The efficacy of using this occupation design approach to provide occupation-based practice, which considers the complexities of the person's occupational experience and the uniqueness of the therapeutic process, is clearly supported by the literature and practice examples. Pierce's discussion about how the subjective and contextual dimensions of the occupational experience interact with the elements of the occupational design process to produce the therapeutic power of occupation highlights the unique knowledge base of our profession. The reality that all occupational therapy practitioners must actively call on and use this uniqueness in daily practice if we are to be recognized as providers of occupation-based practice cannot be ignored. It is my hope that Pierce's thoughtful discourse (along with other chapters in this text) motivate readers to seize the opportunities afforded by the period of "congruence" described by Pierce.

The tremendous current and future potential of occupational therapy, as envisioned by Pierce, Johnson, West, Yerxa, Polatajko, and other leading occupational therapy scholars, is exciting. Because our profession has renewed its commitment to fundamental beliefs about the therapeutic power of occupation, we now have a fortified foundation for the fulfillment of these visions. While several authors in this part realistically recognized present constraints on occupational therapy practice and potential threats to our profession's viability, it is important to note that they also emphasized the need to reaffirm the core values of occupational therapy to successfully counter these limitations and perils. This reaffirmation of our profession's fundamental beliefs and core values brings this last part on current realities and future directions full circle back to the text's first part on historical and philosophical foundations. It is hoped that the chapters selected for this text sustain the readers' commitment to our profession's founding principles as they face the inevitable challenges of practice today and throughout the 21st century. Occupational therapy practitioners upholding this professional heritage by holistically using occupation in a manner meaningful to a person and relevant to his or her contexts will contribute greatly to society, enabling people with disabilities and chronic illnesses to be self-directed, engage in occupational roles, and fully participate in life. This was the vision of the founders of occupational therapy in the early 20th century, and it is the ongoing promise of our profession as we proceed through the 21st century.

Questions to Consider

1. Reflect on your personality, your assets, and your limitations. What character strengths will assist you in maintaining the art of practice in a changing health care system? What character weaknesses may make it difficult to maintain this art of practice? What resources are available to help you work on your limitations and strengthen your assets to meet the demands of current and future practice, while sustaining a commitment to the fundamental, holistic beliefs of occupational therapy?

2. What is your vision of occupational therapy? How can occupational therapy practitioners work to sustain the art and science of practice in the 21st century? How will recent and impending federal and state legislation affect current and future occupational therapy practice? How can current societal movements and sociopolitical trends serve as a foundation for the enhancement of holis-

tic care to enable people with disabilities and chronic illnesses to fully participate in life?

3. Compare and contrast the guidelines for physical therapy practice with AOTA's *Practice Framework* (see Appendix A), *Scope of Practice* (see Appendix B), and *Definition of Occupational Therapy Practice* (see Appendix C). Why are leaders in our field expressing concern about the similarity between our professions' language and defined practice? How can occupational therapy practitioners ensure that consumers, caregivers, reimbursers, policymakers, and the public recognize occupational therapy's professional expertise about the domain of function as unique? How can our existing knowledge in occupational science and evidence-based practice be used to support our claim to this domain of concern? What additional knowledge is needed to strengthen our stance that we are functional experts providing specialized occupation-based services?

4. Review the following case entitled "The Student Who Dared to Care." What are the major value conflicts experienced by Carina? What are the potential ethical dilemmas exhibited in this case? How can an occupational therapy practitioner balance the psychosocial and physical needs of a client in a health care system that does not recognize the need for holism? What are practice models and alternative delivery systems supportive of holistic occupational therapy service delivery?

The Student Who Dared to Care

Carina was an occupational therapy student who had just finished her first Level II Fieldwork experience at a physical disabilities setting and was now completing her final 6 weeks of academic coursework. Carina spoke to me of her experience during this fieldwork placement and of her struggle to

maintain the art of practice in today's health care system. She has generously agreed to share her story in this text.

Carina had been assigned to evaluate and formulate a treatment plan for a 40-year-old woman, Charlotte, diagnosed with late-stage cancer. Charlotte was cooperative with the evaluation but felt she did not need therapy, as she was very sick, weak, and in a lot of pain. Carina consulted with her supervisor, who suggested she work on endurance and ADL with this client, two times per week for 30-minute sessions. The first time Carina met with Charlotte, she asked her about her interests and learned that Charlotte liked to read and listen to music. Carina then attempted to get Charlotte to sit up to do basic grooming activities. Charlotte was unable to sit up to brush her hair due to low endurance. Carina encouraged her to try to sit up for just a short period of time without performing an activity. She agreed to try, and during the next few sessions, Carina read several paragraphs from a collection of short stories while Charlotte maintained a sitting position. Carina also loaned her portable CD player to Charlotte so she would be able to listen to music between treatment sessions. During each session, Carina encouraged Charlotte to try to sit longer and do basic grooming tasks, such as combing her hair and brushing her teeth. At this point, Carina experienced mixed feelings about her role in helping this individual.

The physical disabilities setting emphasized increased endurance and ADL performance as the only appropriate goals for this client, yet Carina saw Charlotte had other needs to be met. Charlotte needed someone to listen to her as she spoke of her pain, her concern for her daughters, about giving up hope, and the reality of dying. Carina sought to help this client by listening and validating her feelings. However, this was not supported in this setting because psychosocial issues were not considered an appropriate focus of occupational therapy treatment for people with physical disabilities or illnesses (even terminal ones). Throughout her affiliation, Carina struggled to treat this person holistically, addressing Charlotte's feelings, as well as her physical symptoms. She met with Charlotte two or three times per week for a few minutes at a time, just to talk. This was not scheduled treatment time, but it provided Charlotte with an opportunity to reflect on her battle with cancer and her impending death. These actions also enabled Carina to develop her ability to meet clients' psychosocial needs, as well as their physical ones. Carina's fieldwork supervisor continued to emphasize the need to only work on ADL and endurance, while Carina recognized that Charlotte was dying, and her immediate need was for someone to listen to her concerns and not give her false hope. Charlotte died during this hospitalization. This polar difference in viewpoints resulted in significant tension during this fieldwork experience, but Carina did not waver.

Carina's ability to treat Charlotte in a holistic manner in a health care system, which did not encourage, reward, or nurture holism, is a tribute to her humanism and her developing skill as an occupational therapist. Her commitment to the fundamental beliefs of occupational therapy, and her willingness to focus on the art of practice, in addition to the science of practice, certainly enabled Charlotte to receive greater benefits from her occupational therapy interventions and, as Carina hoped, helped make her last days of life easier and more meaningful.

References

American Occupational Therapy Association. (2002). Occupational therapy practice framework: Domain and process. *American Journal of Occupational Therapy, 56,* 609–639. Reprinted in Appendix A.

Brown, E. J. (2002, September 9). The psychosocial drought: Is OT education "failing" psychology? *Advance for Occupational Therapy Practitioners, 50,* 13–15.

Grady, A. P. (1992). Nationally Speaking—Occupation as a vision. *American Journal of Occupational Therapy, 46,* 1062–1065.

Haase, B. (1995). Clinical interpretation of "Occupationally embedded exercise versus rote exercise: A choice between occupational forms by elderly nursing home residents."

American Journal of Occupational Therapy, 49, 403–404.

Law, M. (2002). Distinguished Scholar Lecture: Participation in the occupation of everyday life. *American Journal of Occupational Therapy, 56,* 640–649.

Schemm, R. L. (1994). Looking back: Bridging conflicting ideologies: The origins of American and British Occupational Therapy. *American Journal of Occupational Therapy, 48,* 1082–1088.

Shannon, P. (1977). The derailment of occupational therapy. *American Journal of Occupational Therapy, 31,* 229–234.

West, W. L. (1984). A reaffirmed philosophy and practice of occupational therapy for the 1980s. *American Journal of Occupational Therapy, 38,* 15–23.

Whiteford, G., Townsend, E., & Hocking, C. (2000). Reflections on a renaissance of occupation. *Canadian Journal of Occupational Therapy, 67,* 61–70.

Wood, W. (1995). Weaving the warp and weft of occupational therapy: An art and science for all times. *American Journal of Occupational Therapy, 49,* 44–52.

Wood, W. (1998). Nationally speaking: Is it jump time for occupational therapy? *American Journal of Occupational Therapy, 52,* 403–411.

Old Values–New Directions: Competence, Adaptation, Integration

CHAPTER 52

JERRY A. JOHNSON,
EdD, OTR/L, FAOTA

One of the truly exciting and stimulating benefits that derives from being president of an organization like the American Occupational Therapy Association is the opportunity to be exposed to the problems and concerns of 20,000–25,000 people and to be involved in the resolution of some of those issues. It is an incredible experience, and one can never be quite so provincial or so quick to render judgment after having held such a position.

One of the privileges of no longer serving as president is the opportunity to reflect upon the experience and its meaning for my life. For me, that has meant devoting a considerable amount of time exploring the values of our profession, the directions in which the profession seems to be headed, my values, and the way that I want to spend the remainder of my life.

So, when invited to make this presentation, I accepted immediately. The topic seemed so natural in relation to my thoughts about our profession and about me, and it offered an opportunity to address issues of personal concern and professional interest. When it was time to write, however, the process was slow and arduous. Concepts that seemed clear were, upon examination, ambiguous. Connections between and among competence, adaptation, and integration were more tenuous than I had assumed. Concepts were supported by beliefs and anecdotal experience, rather than by hard scientific evidence.

In the final analysis, it was my own internal conflict that made writing difficult. The title of this presentation, "Old Values–New Directions," epitomized a conflict between the old, enduring values of humanism, caring, belief in the individual, and concern for the client, and the new values and new directions pointing toward science, rigor, objectification, logic, analysis, dehumanization, and depersonalization. This conflict seems to represent a decision: a choice between being humanistic and caring, or being scientific and objective.

Thus my challenge today is to discuss this conflict, not because I have answers, but in the hope that clarification of the issues surrounding the conflict may help us find a satisfactory means of resolving it. I believe that the conflict is serious, that it has the potential to divide our profession, with one group opting for the old values and the comfortable, traditional approaches to practice, and the other seeking to move in the direction of scientific advancement. Intuitively, I feel that the creativity and sensitivity that are generally characteristic of occupational therapists offer hope for resolution of the conflict. However, we must be consciously aware of our fears as well as of our aspirations if we are to succeed in our endeavors.

To address this complex matter of conflict, I will first give you my interpretations of the concepts to be addressed. Then I will discuss values and their meaning for us as professionals. Next, I will review the "discovery" and evolution of occupational therapy as it occurred factually and conceptually. Finally, I will describe the nature of the conflicts, as I understand them, and offer some general thoughts about their resolution.

Definition of Terms

I will explain my interpretations of each of the words contained in the title of my presentation so that there will be a common understanding of the context within which I use each concept.

For the terms *old* and *values,* I have opted for the interpretation that suggests our values have been in existence for a long time and are familiar or known from the past. As such they have intrinsic worth, exist as social principles, and are held in high esteem.

New directions, when contrasted with *old values,* suggests that we are dealing with a phenomenon that has not existed before or has only recently been observed, experienced, and made manifest. *Direction* is defined as the way a person or thing faces or points, or a line or point toward which a moving person or thing goes. Thus the term *new directions* suggests that we are facing a particular way, a way that is new and unfamiliar and that may change our course by replacing the more comfortable and enduring values that we esteem.

Definitions of *competence, adaptation,* and *integration* offer interesting possibilities for interpretation within the context of a potential shift in our direction. *Competence* is defined as being fit or able, or as having capacities equal to expectations or requirements. When expectations or requirements shift, *adaptation,* or change, is necessary if we are to conform to new or revised circumstances, and if we are to achieve a better adjustment to a different environment. *Integration* suggests that the parts can be brought together and made whole, or renewed.

In summary, we confront the possibility of a change in our directions, a change that is currently perceived in our literature as moving toward science and reductionism and away from humanism and holism. However, competence, adaptation, and integration suggest that there may be hope for satisfactory resolution of the conflict between old values and new directions. This is the context from which I will speak today.

The Meaning of Values

The literature about professions and professionalization suggests that professionals conceptualize certain problems, or perplexing questions, that are of primary concern to members of their profession. Resolution of these problems becomes the focus of the profession's attention and energy and determines actions to be taken by its members in every sphere of practice, education, research, political activity, decision-making, and other endeavors. These problems, or questions, significantly affect the standards for content of educational programs, as well as the organization, location, and structure of the profession's services. They are influential in attracting and recruiting prospective students and may influence the degree to which

there is high attrition or "burn-out" at certain levels of professional achievement or practices. These problems, or perplexing questions, frequently reflect the values of the profession's members and may heavily influence the directions of the profession.

The directions that our profession has taken seem to be predicated on values, rather than on the basis of problems or perplexing questions. Our literature consistently reflects some of our values:

1. The value of the individual as a total person (1);
2. The value of purposeful activity (2), the value of occupation (3) in producing change and recovery;
3. The value of goal-oriented activity designed for a given individual's skills and abilities (3);
4. The value of permitting patients to choose meaningful activities (1)—activities that might, as Susan Tracy suggested, run parallel to the activity or occupation in which they would have been normally engaged (4);
5. The value of seeing the individual interacting within the framework of the environment (5); and
6. The value we place upon ourselves, our feelings, and our interactions with the patient/client as vital, integral, and caring components of the therapeutic process.

Rarely do occupational therapists do things *to* clients; rather, we engage in a collaborative process *with* them. Each party assumes responsibility and understands that the ultimate goal is for clients to achieve the fullest degree of responsibility for their lives of which they are capable.

These values appear throughout our literature. Although the language has changed, their meaning to us as occupational therapists has not. These are our espoused values (6), and the assumptions upon which they rest are that life is more than mere existence and that health is more than the absence of disease. For us, as therapists, health is a dynamic state of being that is reflected in the behaviors of people who have optimized their resources and who are living their lives fully, creatively, and expressively.

In my experience it seems that people are attracted to a profession because that profession, in its practice, demonstrates actions and behaviors that reflect its values, values that probably are common to and shared by both individuals in the profession and the profession itself.

As I considered this, I reflected on the experiences that brought me into occupational therapy as well as the experiences that reinforced my values and belief in the inherent and potential powers of our profession.

I was the older of two children; my father was a lawyer; my mother, a school teacher. About the time I was 4 or 5, my father became an active alcoholic. His addiction rapidly worsened, and within a very short time span, our lives seemed to shift dramatically while many of our resources went into alcohol. It finally became necessary for my mother to seek employment. Divorce was out of the question both because of the prejudices of the time and because alimony was not permitted under state laws.

As his drinking patterns increased in severity, so did violence. Many nights I ran to town—barefooted, in my pajamas—to get the police to come stop the threats or the fighting—hoping that no one would be killed or seriously injured before I could return home with help. The police would attempt to reason with my father and to calm him; if that failed, he was sometimes whipped soundly. If that approach, too, failed, he would be taken to jail to sober up. It then became my responsibility to go to his cell to bargain with him: If we would let him come home, would he stay sober?

During one of these visits I saw a woman in a cell who was very psychotic. She had been jailed because there was no place to restrain her, no drugs to sedate her, and she had to be declared insane by the court before she could be transferred to a distant state hospital for treatment.

Later, during my college years, I spent two summers with the American Friends Service Committee in institutional service units. The purpose of these units was twofold:

1. To promote understanding among people by having representatives of varied races and religions work for a common goal, which was
2. To improve treatment of the mentally ill in state hospitals.

I spent one summer in a Texas hospital and another summer in a hospital in Ohio. In both hospitals I was assigned to wards with the most disturbed, paranoid, suicidal, or homicidal patients. Most of them had been hospitalized for a long time; few had any contacts with family or friends.

Treatment consisted of insulin or electric shock, isolation in empty cells, restraints—which usually meant being chained to a bench—or occasional beatings. There were no occupational therapists to come to the wards, and generally, the patients could not leave the wards.

We used games, discussion, and behavior modeling to bring about change, and I realized our effectiveness only after returning to visit later. During that visit one of the patients described to me, in exquisite detail, what it meant to her when I took a crayon and paper in for her to use while I talked with her when she was disturbed and shackled to a bench.

As I thought about these and other experiences, I realized how strongly developed my sense of value was about humane treatment and concern for the individual patient. So, as I reviewed the literature in preparing this presentation, it was not surprising to find these and similar values occurring repeatedly. This led me to believe that others had had similar experiences. In retrospect, many of the values we have that relate to caring may well come from experiences in state hospitals and other long-term care facilities where there was only the staff to care about patients and in which sometimes caring was the only treatment medium available.

I suspect that many of you selected occupational therapy as your career choice because you, too, found that your values could be reinforced and channeled in satisfying ways through the therapist/client relationship. We care—and we believe in what we do. This I know from personal experience as well as from visits with so many of you during my terms as president.

To summarize this discussion of values and their meaning for us, I believe that competent, thoughtful, caring people are drawn to a profession like occupational therapy for several reasons:

1. Commitment to the conceptual, perplexing questions that the profession addresses (which in my earlier experience related primarily to humane care of the ill and disabled);
2. Shared concern for the values espoused by and seen in a profession's practice, particularly as that practice reflects attempts to resolve specific questions; and
3. Opportunity to commit one's creativity, energies, and life to resolution of problems that matter—that make a difference in the quality of life and the quality of the environment.

The commitment to our values is deep and strong, but there may be pitfalls for us as professionals if values are not expressed within a context of scientific thought. So let us move to a discussion of the "discovery" and evolution of occupational therapy and see how our values fit into a larger scheme.

The "Discovery" and Evolution of Occupational Therapy

The concepts and observations upon which our profession was founded were formulated when medicine and related sciences lacked knowledge and tools to understand or eliminate the causes of many illnesses, diseases, and social problems. Many illnesses, such as tuberculosis or mental illness, required prolonged hospitalization or institutionalization. Problems such as abject poverty resulted in placements in poor farms. These conditions resulted in decreased or impaired activity and often necessitated removal of the "sick" or impoverished individual from home and family.

Physicians, having limited knowledge and without the technology available today, had to develop and systematically use their powers of observation and judgment. In the absence of diagnostic tests, they relied upon intuition to connect scientific or systematic observations and empirical evidence with limited knowledge to make a diagnosis. (The term *empirical evidence* as used herein refers to reliance on practical experience without reference to scientific principles; empiricism is the dependence of a person on his or her own experience and observation, disregarding theory, reasoning, and science. At times it may be necessary to rely upon one's experience and observations because there are no scientific principles to explain the phenomenon.) It was necessary to diagnose and treat within a broad context and to look for external (to the body) or environmental causes and cures. It was acknowledged that microbes or germs produced illness or disease, but many physicians believed that external stress, produced perhaps by work or other environmental conditions, created the conditions in which germs or microbes were triggered into action.

Consequently, focus on a broad spectrum of interrelationships led to the following conclusions:

1. A relation existed between the environment and a person's state of health;
2. Recovery from illness or depression was influenced by activity; and
3. More specifically, when certain conditions were present, improvement occurred following engagement in activity or occupation.

It was thus hypothesized that activity, or occupation, and improvement in one's medical condition were related. Most members of society, lacking disciplined skill in observation and trust in their intuitive powers, would likely describe the same phenomenon as "busy work."

Our founders were physicians, architects, social workers, secretaries, teachers of arts and crafts, nurses, and of course, the first occupational therapists. Each brought a different perspective and came from a unique background and orientation, yet each observed the effects of occupation in their individual environments and believed in its curative powers. In some ways, this gathering of "specialists" represented the context in which systems theory has been most effective—that is, in situations when a group of specialists representing different perspectives and backgrounds meet to consider the resolution of complex problems.

The individuals who gave life to our profession were visionaries, persons with strong convictions and the courage to uphold and support their convictions. The men who participated in our "discovery" were humanists as well as scientists, exerting leadership to change the course of illness and medical care. Female founders were also unique: educated and dedicated professionals, exerting leadership to change social conditions and to promote healing—people who opted for a life that did not conform to the expectations of women as held by society at that time. These pioneers had competence, discipline, and the determination to succeed.

They seemed to share similar characteristics: the ability to define problems broadly and to organize an effective response to such problems; the ability to act and to reflect upon what they learned from their actions, thereby modifying their behaviors as necessary; the ability to transmit their goals and the rationale underlying these goals to others. They also had power—power granted not by the sanction of society but power that comes from within: intuitive power; power created by belief and conviction, as they are honed by knowledge and observation; the power of disciplined

minds and compassionate spirits. These qualities are demonstrated in their writing, their decisions, their interactions with others, and, most importantly, in their legacy to us. Their lives were devoted to bringing about change in the human condition. Their experience convinced them that occupation was the vehicle by which such change could be made possible.

Rene Dubos, whose life has been devoted to study of the interrelationships between living organisms and their environment, suggests that great discoveries are often intuitive and occur when surprising outcomes result from an observed phenomenon (7).

Robert Merton, the noted sociologist of science from Columbia University, "has shown in his writings that almost all major ideas arise more than once, independently, and often virtually at the same time." (8) Our professional literature reflects the concepts expressed by Dubos and Merton.

In this sense, our founders made not only a surprising discovery when they observed that occupation influenced recovery from illness, but they also translated that discovery into action by forming the National Society for the Promotion of Occupational Therapy.

At this point an interesting turn occurred. Once occupational therapy was identified, the demand for services quickly followed. The literature that I reviewed became silent about the scientific aspects of this great "discovery."

World War I was followed by legislation mandating occupational therapy services in rehabilitation. The depression brought with it demands for retraining the unemployed. World War II, followed by the Korean War, the Vietnam War, and the "wars" on poverty, stroke, heart disease, cancer, and other disabling conditions, created a great demand for occupational therapists (9). We responded.

Our tools, techniques, and values were quickly adapted to new categories of clients. We moved into many new environments to provide services: hospitals, rehabilitation centers, community mental health centers, private practice, community treatment centers, physicians' offices, nursing homes, home health, well-baby clinics, and school systems. We managed by training aides and volunteers or by becoming consultants and by supervising others.

Not only did we move into new environments, but we also adapted our repertoire of tools. We used arts and crafts, splinting and orthotics, therapeutic use of self, prevocational exploration, neurodevelopmental and kinesiological theories and techniques, activities of daily living, and more recently, exercise routines previously used in physical therapy.

Sensory-integrative therapy emerged, but it came primarily from a research base. Its adherents used a test (the Southern California Sensory Integrative Test) designed to diagnose and treat certain deficits. Treatment programs oriented to specific problems were planned and an attempt was made to formulate and organize both diagnosis and treatment into a theoretical framework.

Change, "meeting needs," and adaptation have been a way of life for us. We have been responsive to society's demands and to the needs of our clients. Indeed, those needs and demands have had priority over the needs of the profession and of its members.

We met the ever-changing challenges for delivery of services and created many jobs. This ensured the survival of our profession, the importance of which cannot be minimized. We adapted well and our efforts have without question produced a significant result: a greater demand for occupational therapists than we have ever been able to supply.

This growth was not accomplished without a price, however, and today we are beginning to pay that price.

The conditions under which our profession rapidly developed were such that demand for services quickly increased and has continued unabated. There was little time for our founders' visions to be nurtured, expanded, or understood intellectually or conceptually—rather, there was demand that the ideas, the convictions, the values be put into action immediately.

Part of the price we now pay is that our directions frequently seem to be predicated not upon the observations and concepts of our founders but upon external sources and influences: the influence of medicine, the perceived power of the federal government, sources of reimbursement for treatment, and limited vision and lack of confidence in our potential, as reflected in a narrow concept of practice and cluttered professional education programs specifying breadth rather than depth. Argyris and Schon, in *Theory and Practice: Increasing Professional Effectiveness,* state that factors such as these reflect the demands or expectations of special interest groups but that they are external to the nature of professional practice and education (6).

With each new direction we have taken, the shortage of qualified personnel has increased. To respond to the problem of personnel shortages, we have experimented and continue to experiment with a variety of ways to recruit, certify, and retread personnel for entry into our profession. Some plans have been creative and innovative; others were taken in anticipation of government action (if we fail to act, the government will). Attempts to "fill the gap" have been an obsession with us.

Abraham Maslow is reported to have once said that "If the only tool you have is a hammer you tend to see every problem as a nail" (10). We seem to have taken this approach, believing that if we can just recruit enough students, provide amnesty for enough persons who have "dropped out," or promote enough COTAs to OTRs, our problems will be solved.

Dubos proposes an interesting perspective that seems applicable to our situation. As a proponent of adaptation, he warns that, if adaptation is carried too far, without awareness of the consequences, the desired change may be harmful rather than helpful. He illustrates this point by describing how the body adapts to air pollution on a short-term basis, but

develops chronic bronchitis or emphysema if the stress of short-term adaptive processes must continue indefinitely. In crowded social environments, individuals put on blinders and no longer perceive the crowd; in so doing, however, they sacrifice a certain quality of interpersonal life (7).

Dubos provided this additional description. He related that Pasteur once taught the physiology of architecture at the Ecole des Beaux Arts in Paris. To demonstrate the importance of good ventilation, he conducted the following experiment. He placed a bird in a bell jar in which the oxygen was not renewed so that it gradually diminished. The bird adapted by decreasing its activity and remaining almost immobile. Pasteur then removed the bird and replaced it with a new one, abruptly introducing it to an atmosphere low in oxygen. The new bird began to move about and promptly died. Not only did this demonstration illustrate the importance of good ventilation, but it also demonstrated that we unconsciously adapt to unfavorable circumstances, but only if they occur slowly (7).

The principles of human adaptation presented by Dubos can be applied to professions as well as to people. We have adapted over time to medical and social need and demand but without recognizing the consequences of our adaptive behavior. Some of these consequences as they now confront us are listed below.

First, we have not considered the impact of introducing new therapists, who are still maturing and are educated only at the baccalaureate level, into the stress-producing environments that exist today. We have had time to acclimate ourselves and have acquired some of the requisite knowledge, skills, and tools through experience, but new therapists are often introduced to the environment abruptly.

Second, our sole focus on meeting needs of the disabled and of society has led to the neglect of the importance of fostering, nurturing, and supporting people who move into more demanding, challenging, and often lonely positions as administrators, clinical specialists, researchers, and curriculum directors. One has only to see the number of vacancies for curriculum directors or researchers to understand the nature of the problem. When therapists move into these positions, almost every segment of our profession wants and needs something from them: participation in a task force, continuing education opportunities, membership on or chairing a committee. Yet, as a profession, we offer little support to people in these positions.

Clinical or entry-level therapists sell a commodity that is primarily patient oriented: skill in diagnosing certain kinds of problems relating to performance; a treatment procedure, methodology, or technique; a splint or an adaptive device. The commodity that a researcher, a faculty member, or an administrator sells is an idea, a concept. Regardless of the commodity that we offer, however, we need documentation of its worth, its value, its potential dangers, and the conditions under which it is most effective. We have been so busy selling the commodity that we have neglected the work that must be done to substantiate the value of that commodity. The more we move up and extend our contacts, the more documentation for support is required.

My personal experience and explorations lead me to suggest that people in general, people as professionals, and professions composed of people, all need to be nurtured. Many forms of sustenance are required to strengthen and prepare or to renew and revitalize us, especially in times of rapidly changing conditions and high stress, both of which are found in abundance today.

Finally, the third consequence of our overadaptation to society's needs and demands is reflected in the fact that we have defined our problem as one of insufficient human resources at the entry level—or lack of nails—rather than defining conceptual problems and perplexing questions. A theoretical framework cannot emerge from the problem of insufficient personnel. Nor does the availability of jobs attract thoughtful persons who want to commit themselves, their energies, and their resources to a career.

The absence of well-defined theories limits our scope, our focus, and our research. It puts us in the position of relying on such things as role-delineation studies—studies of past performance and activity to support our endeavors. These studies do not provide a base of knowledge to support us. The absence of a solid theoretical foundation also causes us to overemphasize old values and their "rightness." It leads, I believe, to our condemnation of medicine for its lack of humanitarianism, its dehumanizing approach, its reductionism—because this further justifies our position.

So, as our evolution has brought us face-to-face with society's expectations for research and of the need for scientific support (or at least examination) of our therapeutic rationale and procedures, *we* fall back on old values and seek to defend our positions.

We face a painful conflict, and we are ill prepared for the new directions with their implications for change in our lives. The tragedy is that we are also ill prepared to defend our services and our education.

How, then, has our conceptual development progressed, and what hope is there for us?

A review of our literature suggests that conceptual development was initiated by our founders. It then was generally dormant until Dr. Reilly, in 1961 (see Chapter 8), translated the vision and "discovery" of our founders into a hypothesis:

That man, through the use of his hands as they are energized by mind and will, can influence the state of his own health.

She attributed this hypothesis to our founders and said of it:

"The splendor of its vision goes far beyond rating it as an idea conceived once in a lifetime or even once in a century. Rather, it falls in the class of one of those great beliefs which has advanced civilization. Its magnificence lies in the optimistic vote of confidence it gives to human nature. It

implies that there is a reservoir of sensitivity and skill in the hands of man which can be tapped for his health. It implies the rich adaptability and durability of the central nervous system which can be influenced by experiences. And more than all this, it implies that man, through the use of his hands, can creatively deploy his thinking, feelings and purposes to make himself at home in the world and to make the world his home."

Dr. Reilly continues: "For a profession organized around this hypothesis it sets few limits to its growth. It merely endows a group with the obligation to acquire reliable knowledge leading to a competency to serve the belief. Because this is a hypothesis about health, it requires that this knowledge be made available for the guidance of physicians and that it be made applicable to a wide range of medical problems."

Reilly concluded her lecture with a suggestion that the hypothesis would begin its proof when we identified the drive in Man for occupation and would continue as we shaped our services to fill that need. We "belong," she said, "to a profession that requires the mind to look at the history of man's achievements throughout civilization. It requires the spirit to respond to the wonders of what man has accomplished with his hands." (11)

Consider for a moment the beauty and power of Reilly's statement—and the potential that it offers to each of us as we join with our clients to assist them in fulfilling this potential in their lives. This is our heritage, our legacy, our challenge. It gives us a direction that can be sought regardless of the environment in which we work. It offers tremendous potential for channeling our values into productive outcomes. It requires no distinction of age or category of disease. It is universal.

This hypothesis, too, lay dormant for a period of time, although work in related areas was progressing.

Most recently, in the fall of 1980, Kielhofner et al. published a series of four articles in which a model of human occupation emanating from Reilly's hypothesis was proposed (12). It is suggested in this model that occupation, or function, is central to human life and that the occupational therapist is uniquely qualified to address deficits or problems causing dysfunction. The purpose of occupational therapy is to facilitate the transition of persons with illnesses or disabilities from a state of dependency and dysfunction to or toward a state of full participation and meaningful function in the environments in which they live. Consequently, we address the problems or deficits unique to each individual as well as the social system in which he or she functions and lives.

We have targeted for ourselves a level of performance that is high indeed: an approach to holistic treatment that requires consideration of many complex factors, frequently crossing interdisciplinary lines to understand and grasp the principles of:

1. Normal development in all spheres throughout the life span;
2. Pathology and its relation to function and dysfunction;
3. Adaptation and change;
4. Learning and acquisition of competence;
5. Integrative processes; and
6. Human interaction within the context of the environment.

We now add to this list of requirements an understanding of the principles of occupational behavior and general systems theory. And, as if this is not enough, we must also understand research—because it is by and through research that we determine whether or not our theoretical constructs have substance and produce the results that we claim. The knowledge acquired from research and its findings may enable us to explain, with some degree of assurance, how, under what conditions, and when therapeutic intervention is effective. It makes possible prediction, with some degree of certainty, to say when and with whom our methods of intervention will be beneficial. It may even lead to some degree of control over factors that produce or aggravate disability and dysfunction.

Research can be viewed as a form or system of communication, for it is the language of scientists and of critical thinkers. When persons from other disciplines examine and understand the methods by which we have critically evaluated and analyzed what we do, they can have confidence in what we say we produce or accomplish.

I believe that the works of Reilly and Kielhofner et al. (as well as that of Ayres, although in a slightly different context) are significant contributions to the conceptual development needed by our profession. This work is very rudimentary, but it begins to formulate the conceptual questions to be addressed, uniquely, by our profession. It also offers potential for drawing the separate and disparate parts of our profession together under one conceptual umbrella and for connecting these parts not only to each other but to the whole.

We have identified for ourselves a goal that is extremely complex and of enormous magnitude for we must have knowledge to understand the cause of dysfunction, to diagnose dysfunction as it affects performance and occupation, to identify and establish the appropriate program and process for specific individuals that will result in adaptation and ultimately integration, to bring about change in society and in technology so that both share responsibility for adapting to the needs of humans—and all living things on this earth.

Without question, this goal, this sense of direction, offers a service needed by society now and one that will be needed in ever increasing ways as technology expands. As Dubos said, the most tragic problem confronting industrialized nations is that society is increasingly unable to provide people with a function that has a profound meaning for their lives.

How, then, can we pursue this goal—and make it a reality rather than a vision or a set of values for people who want to do good things?

Thoughts for the Future

I have no certain answers for us, but I can share with you some of my thoughts, my tentative suggestions. I, like you, have intuitive feelings, beliefs, and some empirical evidence from my observations and practice that suggest we have the potential to offer "A sufficiently vital and unique service for medicine to support and society to reward." (11) Ideally, this will be a stimulus for our most creative thinking so that, together, we can find appropriate answers for us and for our profession.

First, it is important to recognize the conflict that confronts us: our desire to retain values that have been an integral part of our profession and, on the other hand, our recognition of the importance of science and research—accompanied by our fears about the directions in which science and research may take us. The potential changes have frightening implications for us—professionally and personally. None of us can help but wonder, "What will happen to me in this process of change?" Will there be a place for me to continue working, and how will I fit? What will happen to my program, my patients, my students, my job?" These questions must be addressed.

Second, I believe that we must redefine the problems that our profession is to address. We must have a sense of direction, a series of perplexing questions to which we, as a profession, commit ourselves. The problem is not one of a shortage of people; it is a shortage of ideas, of concepts, of critically defined questions and problems that attract people, that captivate their imaginations and tap their creativity, that use their intellectual capacity, that say to them, "Here is a problem, a perplexing question of great social value and individual meaning. Join us. Become an occupational therapist and help us find answers." Saving lives is important—but what is the redeeming value of saving lives if they cannot be lived with dignity and meaning?

This has been brought home to me through two recent experiences. In the first instance, I was driving home one day and, as I turned a corner near my house, I saw an older woman sitting on the ground, near the corner. She waved, and I waved back. A moment later it occurred to me to stop and walk back to see about her. She greeted me with obvious relief and said, "I thought no one would ever stop." She had stumbled and fallen and could not get up by herself. After asking about injuries, I helped her get to her feet, and we talked a bit. As I started to leave, she asked if I knew how old she was. "Oh, perhaps 60," I replied. "No," she laughed, "I'm 96." Then she stood tall and straight, looked down at me, and said, "I take a walk every day—but today I stumbled on something I didn't see and fell." Being a bit shaken at her age, my fear of potential injury to her, and not knowing quite what to do, I asked if she would like me to walk home with her.

"Oh, no," she replied, with tears welling in her eyes and a look of terror crossing her face, "I live with my daughter, and if I can't walk by myself, she'll put me in a nursing home—I don't want to be put away." How tragic that people must devote their energies and spend their last years struggling to avoid being put away.

In the second experience, I have, with my family, watched helplessly as a rapidly progressive nervous system degeneration has deprived my mother of her ability to use her body, to communicate, to function.

Medical science and humanistic, caring physicians have literally saved her life but neither the art nor the science of medicine has freed her of the indignity of her illness: incontinence; total loss of speech and ability to form words with her lips; contractures, rigidity, and spasticity in her hands, arms, trunk, and body that prohibit other forms of communication except through limited signs and signals; difficulties with eating, chewing, swallowing, and even keeping the food in her mouth. She is totally dependent on the sensitivity, awareness, and understanding of others to comprehend and respond to every need that she has; her sharp, alert, functioning mind is locked inside a useless body. She knows all that goes on; she hears, sees, cries, laughs, thinks, and feels—but our ability to comprehend is so limited.

I have watched as caring family and friends come to visit. Interaction is so limited and so uncomfortable that sometimes we come in twos or threes and end up talking to each other as though mother is not there. Or we are afraid, perhaps of tiring her or perhaps of our own discomfort and helplessness—and so we move into another room to sit and talk.

I, too, share this sense of helplessness and know how difficult it is to "treat" the members of one's family. I recognize the limitations of my own knowledge of the art and science of our practice. Still, this experience has given me a new appreciation for the potential of our profession as well as a greater realization of the complexity of the issues that we seek to address.

In addition to identifying the problems, the perplexing questions, to which we address ourselves, we must develop plans and strategies, or "road maps," to guide us as we commit ourselves and our resources to the process of seeking answers. It is necessary to recognize that each set of questions may produce some answers, but answers will also create new questions. Our search may be unending.

Third, we should set aside our condemnations of medicine and science, our contempt for basic research and reductionism. Instead, we should focus our energies and resources on those things *we* need to do. As I have learned to recognize and read the messages my own body sends to my unaware mind, I increasingly recognize that my anger is not usually about something "out there," but is a result of my frustration, pain, or anxiety about my own feelings of inadequacy, or impotence, my inability to accomplish or fulfill personal needs or certain expectations. We can learn, wisely, from the experiences of others, and avoid their pitfalls, but let us use our energies creatively and constructively to fulfill our purposes.

Fourth, I believe that we need to recognize and acknowledge the power of knowledge. We work in environments where one is measured against standards of knowledge and where power, emanating from knowledge, resides with those who have knowledge. Our own professional goals, as they are implicitly reflected in our values, require a high level of achievement, knowledge, and experience. We need to recognize the value that knowledge, of itself, has, how it can support *all* of us, and how it can nurture and open doors for us.

It is easy to be frightened by knowledge—by those who are perceived as being knowledgeable. My graduate students are frightened of my knowledge and of the control over their lives that it may give me. I, in turn, am frightened at their knowledge of clinical practice—and fearful of exposing my ignorance. It is only when we both acknowledge our fears and know that we can each make a unique contribution to strengthen the totality of our mutual experience that we move forward together.

Fifth, we need to acknowledge the validity of our professional value system. These values are expressed in the total context of our lives: How we care for ourselves and each other, how we treat our environment, and how we behave toward our colleagues, our friends, our families, and all the other creatures and living things that inhabit this earth we call home. We value freedom to make choices; independence to exercise those decisions; physical ability to come and go as we please; health; the warmth and meaning of home, friends, and privacy; the opportunity to engage intellect and creativity in meaningful activity; and the inherent spirituality and dignity that enables us to appreciate love and beauty—in all its forms.

Each of us, as professionals and as individual members of society, must retain and support our values. We value people, and their right to dignity. We value their desire to integrate themselves into life to the extent possible for them—and we seek to help them enter the mainstream of life: to shop in markets, to attend movies, to listen to the music of great symphonies, to see and feel the beauty of ballet, to work, to play, to watch, to feel. Government should not have to be responsible for bringing about such attitudes; we should accept that responsibility because it is just and right for us to do so, because we believe that every human being has the right and the responsibility to participate in life to the extent he or she is capable and desires to do so.

Still, we must also recognize some of the limitations inherent in acting on values alone or without the requisite knowledge base. A healthy respect for knowledge enables us to translate values into action effectively, thereby increasing our chances of producing lasting results.

Finally, we need to put our fears of specialization to rest. Dubos says that most of the great discoveries have been intuitive and have come from phenomenologists: people who see a problem as a whole without looking at its inner mechanisms or detailed parts (7). The discovery itself usually comes in the form of a surprise, an unexpected outcome of an event, observation, or experiment. As I said earlier, occupational therapy was just such a discovery—the observation that patients and clients who engaged in activity or occupation seemed to recover.

However, Dubos states that the great discovery alone may not be sufficient. There must also be people who are logicians and analysts, people who are committed to understanding and explaining how, when, and under what conditions the unexpected outcome, the surprise occurs. This process has two parts at work in occupational therapy. One is that of looking at the whole organism in relation to its environment. This is a complicated relationship, according to Dubos, that requires a complex response by the organism. The complexity of this problem (which Dubos calls adaptation, and we call occupational therapy) "may well require development of a new scientific approach because existing scientific methodologies may not be applicable to its resolution.... This new science would have to learn to predict the total organism's response to very complex situations." (7)

The second part of this process is an examination of the individual and of his or her deficits and assets, followed by a plan that promotes improved function through reduction of deficits and strengthening of assets. In this and other instances, Dubos stresses the importance of the reductionist approach to provide explanations. Further, both Dubos and general systems theorists emphasize the relevance, and indeed critical importance, of bringing specialists from many areas together to solve problems. The science of adaptation, says Dubos, "must be viewed from the perspectives of medicine, technology, architecture, and social life because not only must humans adapt to new conditions, but technology and environments must also be adapted to human needs."(7)

The discovery of our founders and the work of Reilly, Kielhofner et al.; and of Ayres and others provide the sketchy outlines of a model that may ultimately provide a unifying theoretical or conceptual force in our profession, integrating under one umbrella our concepts and treatment approaches in areas as diverse as pediatrics and gerontology as disparate as physical dysfunction, sensory integration, and psychiatry; and even providing a coherent, logical place for hand specialists, feeding specialists, and activity specialists. We need generalists *and* specialists, for each has a contribution to make. The potential contribution of each increases the value of the whole if appropriate connections and linkages can be established through research and theory development.

Our traditional values, when supplemented and supported by knowledge, offer us the potential to become a powerful presence in our society—powerful in that we provide a resource that enables individuals to live their lives as they want, to become what they want to be.

I believe that we do not have to sacrifice our old values for new ones but that we can merge the old and the new, thereby strengthening each. Our old values, when combined with the new, emphasizing science and knowledge, can forge powerful new directions for our profession. In so doing, we will acquire new competence. The process of adaptation will bring about change, but integration can provide us with a unity and wholeness that we have not yet achieved.

Perhaps, as we think of old values and new directions, of the concepts and meaning of competence, adaptation, and integration, we should heed the advice of Pericles when he spoke to the Athenians:

> Fix your eyes on the greatness of your profession as you have it before you day by day; fall in love with her, and when you feel her greatness, remember that her greatness was won by people with courage, with knowledge of their duty, and with a vision that all things are possible. (13)

Acknowledgments

The author gratefully acknowledges the guidance and direction given by Fanny B. Vanderkooi and Florence M. Stattel as she entered the occupational therapy profession, as well as the contributions of Ann P. Grady, Gail Fidler, Donna King, Elizabeth J. Yerxa, the faculty and students at Washington University, and other friends and colleagues for their intellectual stimulation and challenge, friendship, and support of her personal, conceptual, and professional development.

References

1. Yerxa EJ: Authentic occupational therapy. *Am J Occup Ther 21:* 6, 1967.
2. Ayres AJ: Occupational therapy for motor disorders resulting from impairment of the central nervous system. *Rehab Lit* October 1960.
3. Wiest A: *Activity Book for the Ill, Convalescent, and Disabled of All Kinds as Well as the Hand of the Physician,* Stuttgart: Ferdnand Emke, Anje Ruil, *Am J Occup Ther 21:* 280–324, 1967.
4. Tracy S: *Studies in Invalid Occupations,* Boston: Whitcomb and Burrows, 1910.
5. Yerxa EJ: *The Present and Future Audacity of Occupational Therapy,* unpublished paper presented at Washington University, St. Louis, MO, October 1980.
6. Argyris C, Schon D: *Theory in Practice: Increasing Professional Effectiveness,* San Francisco: Jossey Books, Pub., 1980.
7. Dubos R, Escandi JP: *Quest: Reflections on Medicine, Science, and Humanity,* New York: Harcourt, Brace, Jovanovich, 1979.
8. Merton RK: On the shoulders of giants, quoted in Gould SJ: *The Panda's Thumb,* New York: W.N. Norton & Co., 1980.
9. Johnson JA: Commitment to action. *Am J Occup Ther 30:* 135–148, 1976.
10. Maslow A: *Quest,* May–June, 1977.
11. Reilly M: Occupational therapy can be one of the great ideas of 20th century medicine. *Am J Occup Ther 16:* 1–9, 1962 Reprinted as Chapter 8.
12. Kielhofner G, et al.: A model of human occupation, Parts 1–4, *Am J Occup Ther 34:* 572–581; 34: 657–670; 34: 731–737; 34: 777–788, 1980.
13. Quotation from Hislop H: The not-so-impossible dream, *Phys Ther 55:* 1069–1080, 1975.

How High Do We Jump?
The Effect of Reimbursement
on Occupational Therapy

CHAPTER 53

BRENDA S. HOWARD, OTR

To what extent does reimbursement influence the practice of occupational therapy? Many occupational therapists agree that reimbursement affects clinical practice. Documentation, length and frequency of treatment, use of treatment modalities, and the need for regulation are all cited in the everyday conversation of clinicians as being related to reimbursement, at least in part. Less visible, and sometimes less comfortable, influences of reimbursement may be clinicians' ability to treat some diagnoses and not others, the development of specialty areas of treatment as new avenues of reimbursement open up, and the lack of development of some specialties because of limited reimbursement. However, the influences behind the initiation and continuance of third-party dictation of clinical practice and the question of how far dictation of practice really goes are rarely explored.

An understanding of the history and directions of reimbursement in the United States and of the depth of influence these reimbursement trends have on the development of occupational therapy will help occupational therapists put the influence of reimbursement into perspective.

History of Occupational Therapy in Relation to Reimbursement

"Historically, the reimbursement method for occupational therapy has driven its delivery system" (Foto, 1988a, p. 564). The history of occupational therapy reimbursement may be divided into three eras of change: the institution of modern health insurance, beginning in the 1920s and ending in the 1950s; the events leading up to and following the initiation of Medicare and Medicaid in the 1960s; and the control of costs that has begun in the current era of prospective payment (Baum, 1985).

The occupational therapy profession was born out of the Moral Treatment movement in the second half of the 19th century. Moral Treatment signified a change from custodial care of mentally ill people to care based on the "law of love" (Bockoven, 1971, p. 223). Adolph Meyer, whose work preceded the profession, linked occupational therapy to Moral Treatment by describing diseases as problems of adaptation, appropriate use of time as the remedy for habit deterioration, and occupational therapy as the means of teaching the structuring of time (Meyer, 1922/1977 [see Chapter 2]). In fact, the first definition of the profession, written in 1918, was "a means of instruction and employment in productive occupation" (Hopkins & Smith, 1978, p. 10). Meyer's philosophy of occupation in mental health strongly influenced the philosophy and history of occupational therapy as a whole (Hopkins & Smith, 1978).

In the decades following the Civil War, although occupational therapy was still in its infancy, the philosophy of Moral Treatment, as used in mental health, was already declining. This decline was largely due to a shift in popular thought from a moral–emotional model to a technological–pathological approach in which the scientific method was embraced (Bockoven, 1971). This happened in spite of the established efficacy of Moral Treatment (Bockoven, 1971; Peloquin, 1989 [see Chapter 4]). Mental health also shifted to an organic, pathology-based frame of reference in the early 1900s (Bockoven, 1971).

This chapter was previously published in the *American Journal of Occupational Therapy, 45,* 875–881. Copyright © 1991, American Occupational Therapy Association.

519

The shift in popular philosophy affected not only mental health practice but the entire medical community (Bockoven, 1971). The Flexner Report, published in 1906 (see Feldstein, 1987), marked a change in the philosophy underlying medical treatment. Generated by the American Medical Association in an effort to upgrade the quality of medical schools (Feldstein, 1987), the Flexner Report emphasized a unifactorial, biomedical, scientific model of disease. As a result of the report, medicine shifted to more scientific, laboratory-based concepts (Waitzkin, 1978).

During the formative years of the profession, occupational therapy persisted in its view that adaptation to and engagement in the environment were strong components of health, in spite of differing popular philosophy (Bockoven, 1971). However, the financial constraints of the depression years precipitated a significant turning point in the profession's development. In the middle of the 1930s, the American Occupational Therapy Association (AOTA) asked the American Medical Association to establish standards for training institutions and take over accreditation of occupational therapy schools. It was this decisive step that formally placed occupational therapy in the position of a medical ancillary (Rerek, 1971). This action, although it achieved its purpose of survival, limited nonmedical practice opportunities for the future in that occupational therapy was now tied to the health-care industry by educational standards and financial concerns. Thus, the profession's struggle between its roots in Moral Treatment and the medical model/scientific method began.

From the 1940s to the 1960s, occupational therapy was involved in the rehabilitation movement, which began with the return of World War II disabled veterans. New antibiotic medications and advanced methods in surgery helped injured soldiers survive their wounds, and rehabilitation helped them to be independent with the resulting disabilities. Rehabilitation was also economically advantageous. During this time, association with the rehabilitation movement (and possibly with the medical community) made occupational therapists "uncomfortable with their simple operating principle that it was good for disabled people to keep active" (Mosey, 1971, p. 235). New treatment methods (e.g., orthotics, vocational evaluation, neuromuscular facilitation), borrowed from other professions, were added to the occupational therapists' repertoire at a pace so rapid that it was impossible to assimilate these changes into the profession's theoretical base (Mosey, 1971).

The rehabilitation movement was accompanied by changes in payment for health-care services. Before this, health insurance had been based in local, private systems. Increases in the cost of medical care exceeded the limitations of this system. National health insurance was debated, but instead payment for health care was installed as an employee benefit controlled by private industry. The American Medical Association successfully campaigned against national health insurance, in conjunction with organized labor, which wanted to retain health insurance as a bargaining tool (Somers & Somers, 1961). The medical profession fought national health care coverage because it viewed "involvement of the federal government as a fatal intrusion in the hallowed doctor–patient relationship and believed that it would lead to the increasing bureaucratization of medicine" (Luft, 1978, p. 3). By the middle of the 1960s, physicians no longer had enough political power to stop government-supported health insurance (Luft, 1978), in part due to the increased political power of consumer groups (Freidson, 1975). With more support for government involvement in health care, Medicare and Medicaid were born in 1966. With their advent, the established traditions of payment and organization in health care were permanently altered (Freidson, 1975).

Few changes in the provision of services were anticipated with the start of Medicare. Diasio (1971) recognized that Medicare and Medicaid would allow the development of occupational therapy in community health care for the elderly and the poor. Reilly (1966) feared that an increased use of paramedical staff, including therapists, would cause funds for their wages to be spread thin, causing salary stagnation and the dreaded threat of symbiosis with physical therapy. As occupational therapists clarified their role, however, and as the use of more paramedical staff (therapists included) resulted in a shortage of therapists, Reilly's fears did not come true (Baum, 1985).

From the 1960s to the early 1980s, occupational therapy continued to enjoy a political climate favorable to health care, and its services grew (Davy, 1984a). However, costs began to escalate as health-care facilities took advantage of available capital. Consequently, Congress set limits on Medicare reimbursement as part of the Tax Equity and Fiscal Responsibility Act of 1982 (Public Law 97–248). In the following year the Social Security Amendments of 1983 (Public Law 98–21) were enacted, which set the stage for the phasing in of the prospective payment and diagnosis-related group (DRG) forms of reimbursement (Russell, 1989).

With the cost constraints of the late 1970s and 1980s and the inception of prospective payment, occupational therapists found that accurate documentation was crucial to reimbursement (AOTA, 1989). In addition, demand for inpatient occupational therapy services decreased, and demand for outpatient services increased (Foto, 1988a). Shorter hospital stays have resulted in higher volumes of patients for occupational therapy services; further, the new payment system encourages provision of "the fewest number of services possible" (Baum, 1985, p. 779) to meet goals. All of this has led to concern over how to maintain service quality (Baum, 1985). For example, occupational therapists have found that their poorer clients receive limited support from government programs for therapy services. Thus, clinicians must struggle to provide helpful services during limited contact with these patients (Foto, 1988a).

In 1986, Congress passed the Occupational Therapy Medicare Amendments (Section 9337 of Public Law 99–509) in response to the need for more community-based treatment. These amendments extended full coverage to occupational therapy services under Medicare Part B. Payment was authorized for patients in skilled nursing facilities, rehabilitation agencies, home health care, and private practice (AOTA, 1989). Medicare Part B coverage has provided financial support for the expansion of private practice and contractual occupational therapy services in the past few years.

The Effect of Changes in Reimbursement on the Profession

The current environment of cost containment leaves occupational therapists "caught between the pressures of patients' demands for quality care and the drive to contain costs," which "creates professional and emotional conflict" (Foto, 1988a, p. 564). The effect of reimbursement on the definition of occupational therapy and on practice, management, professional ethics, and the profession's response will be discussed in the following paragraphs.

The Definition of Occupational Therapy

The definition of occupational therapy has been shaped by changing reimbursement patterns. In a special issue of the *American Journal of Occupational Therapy* (Davy, 1984c), detailed articles supplied information on coverage available for various practice areas of occupational therapy. This implied that what occupational therapists can do, and therefore what they are, is defined at least in part by what is reimbursed. In addition, what is not covered is outlined so that therapists do not perform noncovered services, or at least do not define what they do in a noncovered manner. In the same issue, Davy (1984b) described the great lengths to which the profession has gone to get itself defined by insurance companies in order to ensure coverage.

Further substantiation of this point is found in *Medicare Outpatient Physical Therapy and Comprehensive Outpatient Rehabilitation Facility Manual* (Department of Health and Human Services, 1989). Section 503 of this document, entitled "Guidelines for Submitting Claims for Outpatient Occupational Therapy Services," defines the services that are covered under Medicare Part B. One important feature of this document is its definition of what is not occupational therapy. If it is not in the guidelines, it is not paid for. Therefore, clinicians cannot perform or document services that are not in the guidelines if they wish to obtain reimbursement under Medicare Part B. Because this document is becoming a standard used by most insurance companies, its significance in defining occupational therapy is substantial. Fortunately for the profession, occupational therapists assisted in its development at the government's request (AOTA, 1989).

Practice

Because the descriptions of the coverage available in various practice areas are used by occupational therapists in documenting their services, occupational therapists must now treat within the boundaries of these descriptions. Clinicians may therefore find themselves changing or limiting their modes of treatment to comply with reimbursement restrictions. For example, the occupational therapy guidelines for Medicare Part B specifically state that daily feeding programs are not considered skilled occupational therapy once the adapted procedures have been implemented (AOTA, 1989). Therefore, an occupational therapist may design a feeding program for a patient in a skilled nursing facility with Medicare Part B coverage but may have limited financial support for continued intervention. Patients with Medicare coverage are not the only ones affected. Outpatient care is another clinical area in which limitations in various forms of reimbursement dictate occupational therapy service provision: "Many times, because of a patient's lack of health insurance, we must turn even the most appropriate treatment candidates away from our [outpatient] departments" (Burke & Cassidy, 1991, p. 174 [see Chapter 54]). Not only the frequency but also the nature of treatment has changed. Clinicians are now asked to provide diagnosis-based treatment protocols that will guarantee coverage for services. These protocols may or may not fit in with individual patient needs (Burke & Cassidy, 1991 [see Chapter 54]).

At a deeper and more disturbing level, changing reimbursement patterns have caused shifts in the definition of occupational therapy that have led, in turn, to changes in professional roles (e.g., occupational therapists' role with the chronically ill). Reilly (1971) explained the disparity that led to this change:

> There is an enormous obstruction outside the control of the profession that seriously impairs the delivery of service. It is the absence of economic support to chronic medicine. The commitment and hence the capitalization in medicine is directed toward the reduction and prevention of pathology and the treatment of acute phases of illness. Occupational therapy makes its investments in the health residual which follows pathology and hence focuses on the chronic aspect of the illness and is concerned with health rather than pathology. (p. 245)

Indeed, program design and treatment of acute phases of chronic illness are currently among the few occupational therapy services for persons with chronic illness that are supported by Medicare (AOTA, 1989).

New directions in reimbursement provide the capital for the development of new and existing clinical areas. Foto (1988a) gave examples of occupational therapy's ability to provide what insurance companies now want (e.g., wellness programs, reduced hospital stays, treatment at a lower level of care [therapist rather than physician] where appropriate, the return of patients to the highest possible functional level). She wrote, "Since occupational therapists offer these services, we should be in demand. But we must educate the industry . . ." (Foto, 1988a, p. 564). Her statements suggest that shifts in reimbursement will shape occupational therapy by the profession's need or desire to be where the reimbursement is. For example, records of facilities developed recently indicate that they include skilled nursing homes, outpatient services, and home health care (Russell, 1989). Could it be that, with the 1986 change in Medicare Part B reimbursement, these areas are once again profitable for occupational therapy? One could argue that the recent surge in the number of contracting agencies providing therapies for these clinical areas is another direct result of improved reimbursement. The type and quality of therapy services also appears to have changed with this resurgence: Agencies are reimbursed on a treatment unit basis, so therapists must account for their time by units of productivity. This means that little time is left to develop programs for services to chronically ill people or nonreimbursable nursing home residents.

The current climate of cost containment may have an effect on available treatment technology. This trend is hard to predict due to the varied nature of regulation and the effects of national values and lobbying groups on federal legislation. Aaron and Schwartz (1984) speculated that in the case of high-technology equipment, "the demand will be fully met in some cases; in others, constraints on expenditures will reduce either quality or quantity" (p. 115). What will this mean for occupational therapy? It may mean that patients will have to be prioritized for available equipment and that treatments that rely on high-technology equipment will go up in cost because of lower supply and higher demand. This could lead to greater access to technology for those who can pay and less access for the poor.

Management

Changes in reimbursement have also meant changes in management style for occupational therapy departments. Productivity and efficiency are becoming high-priority goals, because departments must handle more patients with fewer staff. Changes to increase productivity may include attempting to meet treatment goals in fewer treatment sessions; performing evaluations and treatments that focus on decreasing lengths of stay by addressing primarily the problems that are keeping patients in hospitals; and use of occupational therapy assistants, aides, volunteers, and part-time staff to meet treatment goals at the lowest cost possible. An emphasis on efficiency could require computer documentation for faster charting and evening and weekend treatment to speed recovery (Scott, 1984). Such programs for increased productivity need to be studied to determine their efficacy and to determine whether they allow patients sufficient time for the rest needed to recover.

In addition to changes in program design, productivity concerns cause managers to justify staff positions based on reimbursement data. Foto (1988b) suggested the use of the Medicare cost report to justify hiring more staff. This report covers not the number of treatments given, but the number of treatments reimbursed. Foto's suggestion highlights the fiscal constraints under which managers are operating and the extent to which reimbursement issues are linked to clinical issues.

Ethics

Reimbursement constraints can influence changes in professional ethics. The Occupational Therapy Code of Ethics, Principle 1, Item H, states: "The individual shall establish fees, based on cost analysis, that are commensurate with services rendered" (AOTA, 1988, p. 795). In light of cost constraints and the need to justify staff, there is a risk that this principle may be interpreted loosely, resulting in ethical abuses. Possible abuses include overbilling for services (e.g., rounding up times), providing services that are not necessary for functional goals, overpricing of services, overworking employees to maintain revenues, and focusing efforts on those programs that bring in revenue but are not clinically effective (Mullins, 1989).

Reimbursement concerns raise new ethical questions: Is it ethical to make changes in the provision of services based on the patient's method of payment, or on the basis of reimbursability rather than diagnosis? Discrimination in providing health services may work both ways: The nonreimbursable patient may receive subminimal care, which compromises quality, and the patient with ample reimbursement may be treated beyond the limit of goals for cost containment. The free market medical system provides few checks and balances:

> The market is the provider's best friend. It gives providers license to supply inaccurate information, to limit service only to those patients with an ability to pay, to charge whatever they wish, and to reduce quality of care to achieve greater profitability. (Sloan, Blumstein, & Perrin, 1988, p. 237)

The Profession's Response

The responses of occupational therapy as a profession to changes in reimbursement fall into three categories: regulation, public relations, and political action. Although the justification for regulation (licensure) of health care professionals has been consumer protection (Sloan et al., 1988), an equally important consequence for occupational therapy is improved reimbursement (see Moyers, 1988). Licensure of occupational therapists exists in 46 states (Javernick, 1991).

Increased dialogue and public relations efforts with third-party payers will distribute control of the health-care industry more equally between providers and payers (Hertenstein, 1989). Occupational therapists who enter into dialogue with insurance companies must be prepared to address the insurance industry's needs (Foto, 1988a) and use the industry's language of functional independence and patient dignity to discuss occupational therapy services (Foto, 1988b). By addressing insurance industry concerns, occupational therapists may find it necessary to compromise on clinical issues. Other responses to reimbursement concerns include mobilizing to accommodate managed care, breaking through coverage barriers of health maintenance organizations (Foto, 1988b), and recruiting new occupational therapists so that services will continue to be available at a lower cost level (Baum, 1985).

Political action within the profession consists of lobbying for a better understanding of occupational therapy issues among legislators (Baum, 1985; Foto, 1988b). Being politically active is crucial to taking a proactive stance in managing change in health care (Foto, 1988b).

Discussion

Occupational therapy does not exist in a vacuum; societal influences are a dominant factor in precipitating change. Neither research nor pure theory appears to have the impact on occupational therapy practice that society does. The societal influence of reimbursement for health care has substantially affected occupational therapy in definition, practice, management, ethics, and the profession's response. Reimbursement has altered occupational therapy by at least four means: control, understanding (e.g., of disease), language, and values.

Control

It is a Marxist premise that increased concentration of capital in the hands of the few leaves others unempowered (Waitzkin, 1978). With capital for health care centralized in insurance companies and government programs, it is to be expected that these third-party payers exert great control over the health-care system. Control in occupational therapy has been altered by placing the definition of the profession, in part, in the hands of those who hold the capital. In other words, occupational therapy is being controlled to some extent by payers who participate in defining it. Examples, mentioned earlier, include the proliferation or demise of specialty areas according to reimbursability (as with the increase in hand therapy and work hardening and the decrease in inpatient care and contact with pediatric clients); changes in service provision according to coverage (e.g., limited provision of services to patients with limited reimbursement); and the need to justify the number of staff members in occupational therapy departments by the number of treatments reimbursed.

Understanding

Virchow, who studied social epidemiology and social medicine, focused on two major themes regarding the understanding of disease. He believed that the origin of disease is multifactorial (not just physical) and that successful improvements in health care must be the result of concurrent improvements in economic, political, and social reforms (as cited by Waitzkin, 1978). One can extrapolate from Virchow that it is necessary to maintain a consistent understanding of the whole health-care system, the ways it seeks to remediate disease, and the economic and political changes that affect the system.

Shifts in popular ideology have caused occupational therapy to change its understanding of itself. For example, the modern urgency for research attempts to establish occupational therapy within the biomedical/scientific model, indicating how far occupational therapy understanding has shifted from its connection to Moral Treatment philosophy. Research, therefore, becomes not just a measure of efficacy, but a method to justify occupational therapy according to the dominant model in health-care practice. Because reimbursement rewards the unifactorial medical model, it becomes difficult to survive economically while clinging to a philosophy based on multifactorial causes of disease. Compromise—by assimilating aspects of the medical model—allows for survival, but limits options for social effectiveness.

Language

Sapir and Whorf (Sapir, 1929) developed a hypothesis of linguistic relativity that held that the way things are talked about affects understanding of them. When this hypothesis is applied to occupational therapy, the way the profession is discussed changes how it is perceived. Subtle changes in occupational therapy philosophy have occurred simply through changes in the language with which thoughts are framed. By using the language of insurance companies (e.g., *skilled occupational therapy*) in documentation and definition, occupational therapy shifts into new clinical dimensions (e.g., use of objective tests and measurements) and discards old practices (e.g., use of activity for its intrinsic qualities). Framing occupational therapy in the appropriate language makes it acceptable and reimbursable to third-party payers. Language has affected management in particular; the words *cost containment*, *productivity*, and *efficacy* now occupy and shape the department manager's thoughts (Gray, 1983; Mullins, 1989).

Values

In our society, individualism and private enterprise are valued. With cost containment, the prevailing values in health care become clearer: Technology and the scientific method are valued more than the holistic use of a variety of treatment methods; the young and productive are valued more than the old and frail; and acute treatment is valued more than chronic care (Waitzkin, 1987). Reimbursement within a system that embraces these values shapes the practice of occupational therapy. What our profession valued at its inception contrasts with the values of the current health-care system; the tension between societal values and the values of the profession continues to be a source of conflict for many clinicians.

Implications

How high do we jump? Should reimbursement dictate clinical practice? No one sector of society should control the health-care field or any aspect of it. Accountability is a necessary part of participation in health care to ensure a broader distribution of power so that all interested parties may be assured of representation. The fact remains, however, that third-party payers have exerted substantial control over the profession, with an unclear understanding of how occupational therapy has influenced trends in reimbursement. It is also unclear how much say patients have in occupational therapy practice.

Occupational therapists occasionally need to step outside of the health-care arena and view the interplay among the various sources of control in health care, so that reasons for actions and reactions will become clearer. For example, when clinicians understand the financial pressures that their health care institutions face, it is easier to view frustrations with service provision to individual patients as symptoms of a larger problem. It is also imperative to view the profession from the point of view of the other players—the patient, the insurance carrier, and other disciplines—so that cooperation and dialogue are welcomed when occupational therapy's role in the health-care system is negotiated.

Occupational therapists also need to understand who they are as occupational therapists. Proactive, systematic vocational planning is then possible (Howard, 1990). Vocational planning includes defining ethical practice, framing the definition in language that is not easily bent, and lobbying for it through public relations activities and political action. It also includes examining the conflicting goals of quality service and cost containment and setting guidelines by which to practice within the boundaries of both.

The occupational therapist may use other means to maintain a fair distribution of power. Baum (1985) recommended looking to payment sources other than third-party payment to free occupational therapists to be self-directive. She mentioned workers' compensation, liability insurance, corporate funds, public health funds, and Social Security as a few examples. Another option is to practice in nontraditional (i.e., nonmedical) settings that allow greater impact on patient populations without reimbursement constraints. Occupational therapists working as employee health directors in industry are an example of nontraditional practitioners with an impact on prevention. A third means of vocational planning is volunteerism. If higher salaries and staff shortages are contributing to escalating costs and limited access for poor and rural patients, then volunteering is one option. Although most occupational therapists do not have the opportunity for full-time volunteer work, some are able to donate an hour a week to a free clinic. Others are able to offer a week or two a year of consultation services to programs for needy people. Still others participate in local and national advocacy groups for persons with disabilities.

We as occupational therapists must be aware that social factors influence the direction of the profession. Reimbursement issues not only frustrate clinical practice but participate in shaping occupational therapy. We must be aware of the causes of constraints on practice in order to be proactive in issues of health-care policy.

References

Aaron, J., & Schwartz, W. B. (1984). *The painful prescription: Rationing hospital care.* Washington, DC: Brookings Institution.

American Occupational Therapy Association. (1988). Occupational therapy code of ethics. *American Journal of Occupational Therapy, 42,* 795–796.

American Occupational Therapy Association. (1989, September 16). *Insuring payment through documentation: A common sense approach* [American Occupational Therapy Association workshop presented in Indianapolis].

Baum, C. M. (1985). Growth, renewal, and challenge: An important era for occupational therapy. *American Journal of Occupational Therapy, 39,* 778–784.

Bockoven, J. S. (1971). Legacy of Moral Treatment—1800s to 1910. *American Journal of Occupational Therapy, 25,* 223–225.

Burke, J. P., & Cassidy, J. C. (1991). The Issue Is—Disparity between reimbursement-driven practice and humanistic values of occupational therapy. *American Journal of Occupational Therapy, 45,* 173–176. Reprinted as Chapter 54.

Davy, J. D. (1984a). Nationally Speaking—Status report on reimbursement for occupational therapy services. *American Journal of Occupational Therapy, 38,* 295–298.

Davy, J. D. (1984b). Preferred provider organizations. *American Journal of Occupational Therapy, 38,* 327–329.

Davy, J. D. (Guest Ed.). (1984c). Reimbursement [Special issue]. *American Journal of Occupational Therapy, 38*(5).

Department of Health and Human Services. (1989, May). *Medicare outpatient physical therapy and comprehensive outpatient rehabilitation facility manual* (DHHS Publication No. 9, Transmittal No. 87). Washington, DC: Health Care Financing Administration.

Diasio, K. (1971). The modern era—1960 to 1970. *American Journal of Occupational Therapy, 25,* 237–242.

Feldstein, P. J. (1987). Policies of the American Medical Association: Self-interest or public interest? In H. D. Schwartz (Ed.), *Dominant issues in medical sociology* (pp. 549–558). New York: Newbery Award Records.

Foto, M. (1988a). Nationally Speaking—Managing changes in reimbursement patterns, Part 1. *American Journal of Occupational Therapy, 42,* 563–565.

Foto, M. (1988b). Nationally Speaking—Managing changes in reimbursement patterns, Part 2. *American Journal of Occupational Therapy, 42,* 629–631.

Freidson, E. (1975). *Doctoring together: A study of professional social control.* Chicago: University of Chicago Press.

Gray, B. (1983). *The new health care for profit: Doctors and hospitals in a competitive environment.* Washington, DC: Brookings Institution.

Hertenstein, R. D. (1989). Third-party concerns. *Cancer, 64* (July Suppl.), 319.

Hopkins, H. L., & Smith, H. D. (Eds.). (1978). *Willard and Spackman's occupational therapy* (5th ed.). Philadelphia: Lippincott.

Howard, B. S. (1990, December 3). Systematic vocation for OTs. *OT Forum,* pp. 8–12.

Javernick, J. A. (1991, March 28). Wyoming therapists gain licensure. *OT Week,* pp. 2, 16.

Luft, H. S. (1978). *Poverty and health.* Cambridge, MA: Ballinger Publishing.

Meyer, A. (1977). The philosophy of occupation therapy. *American Journal of Occupational Therapy, 31,* 639–642. Original work published 1922. Reprinted as Chapter 2.

Mosey, A. C. (1971). Involvement in the rehabilitation movement—1942–1960. *American Journal of Occupational Therapy, 25,* 234–236.

Moyers, P. (1988, June) *Licensure fund raising campaign.* Open form letter distributed at the June 1988 Indiana Occupational Therapy Conference, Mitchell, IN.

Mullins, L. L. (1989). Hate revisited: Power, envy, and greed in the rehabilitation setting. *Archives of Physical Medicine and Rehabilitation, 70,* 740–744.

Occupational Therapy Medicare Amendments (Public Law 99–507), § 9337.

Peloquin, S. M. (1989). Looking Back—Moral Treatment: Contexts considered. *American Journal of Occupational Therapy, 43,* 537–544. Reprinted as Chapter 4.

Reilly, M. (1966). The challenge of the future to an occupational therapist. *American Journal of Occupational Therapy, 20,* 221–225.

Reilly, M. (1971). The modernization of occupational therapy. *American Journal of Occupational Therapy, 25,* 243–246.

Rerek, M. D. (1971). The depression years—1929 to 1941. *American Journal of Occupational Therapy, 25,* 231–233.

Russell, L. B. (1989). *Medicare's new hospital payment system: Is it working?* Washington, DC: Brookings Institution.

Sapir, E. (1929). The status of linguistics as a science. *Language, 5,* 207–214.

Scott, S. J. (1984). The Medicare prospective payment system. *American Journal of Occupational Therapy, 38,* 330–334.

Sloan, F. A., Blumstein, J. F., & Perrin, J. M. (Eds.). (1988). *Cost, quality, and access in health care.* San Francisco: Jossey-Bass.

Social Security Amendments of 1983 (Public Law 98–21).

Somers, H. M., & Somers, A. R. (1961). *Doctors, patients, and health insurance.* Washington, DC: Brookings Institution.

Tax Equity and Fiscal Responsibility Act of 1982 (Public Law 97–248).

Waitzkin, H. (1978). A Marxist view of medical care. *Annals of Internal Medicine, 89,* 264–278.

Waitzkin, H. (1987). A Marxian interpretation of the growth and development of coronary care technology. In H. D. Schwartz (Ed.), *Dominant issues in medical sociology* (2nd ed., pp. 613–624). New York: Newbery Award Records.

Disparity Between Reimbursement-Driven Practice and Humanistic Values of Occupational Therapy

CHAPTER 54

JANICE POSATERY BURKE,
MA, OTR/L, FAOTA
JOANNE C. CASSIDY, MED, OTR/L

In January 1990, clinicians, educators, and researchers met at the Directions for the Future Symposium in San Diego to delineate, discuss, and debate a wide range of economic, political, and social issues that are influencing the evolution of occupational therapy practice and education. By examining these factors in an open and thorough way, therapists believe they will be able to develop proactive positions that will ensure the continued well-being of the field.

In this paper, we will consider two distinctly opposing forces that dramatically affect and present considerable obstacles to occupational therapists. On the one hand, occupational therapists are taught to embrace a fundamental, humanistically based philosophy of practice that emphasizes the importance of the individual. On the other hand, they are expected to practice in an economically defined health-care environment, where issues of reimbursement for service are highly valued and are among the key factors to be considered when making evaluation and treatment decisions.

Humanistic-Valued Practice

Adolf Meyer is among the early leaders of the field credited with advocating treatment that centers on a "profound respect for the patient and his efforts to get through this life with a maximum of gratification and a minimum of discomfort" (Muncie, 1959, p. 1322). During the early years of the profession's development, this notion formed the keystone of professional practice. This approach directed therapists to emphasize work, play, and social activities and placed with therapists a moral obligation and responsibility as agents of society to any person whose future as a member of that society was jeopardized (Bockoven, 1971). With this perspective, occupational therapists placed the utmost respect on "human individuality and on a fundamental perception of the individual's need to engage in creative activity in relation to his fellow man" (Bockoven, 1971, p. 223). This initial orientation is still very much a part of current practice, as evidenced by the preamble to the *Occupational Therapy Code of Ethics* (American Occupational Therapy Association [AOTA], 1988), which states that therapists "are committed to furthering people's ability to function fully within their total environment" (p. 795).

Additional concepts and concerns such as habit training were added to our repertoire of characteristically humanistic-based practice and directed us toward an involved role with our patients. As a primary aspect of treatment, habit training was used to enlist patients' interests as they established a sense of personal usefulness. To do so, therapists were taught to consider the person as well as the environment and the effect each had on the other (Ryon, 1925; Slagle, 1934).

Throughout its professional development, occupational therapy has continued to remain strongly oriented to the individual. Information was accumulated that would allow therapists to administer evaluation and treatment that would be highly sensitive to and inclusive of an individual's culture, values, and beliefs. Therapists found that involvement of the patient in his or her own treatment was the most natural way to ensure behavioral change. The patient's goals were used to form the basis of the treatment session, and the patient's active involvement was enlisted to ensure a successful outcome. It followed that if therapists were to create individually designed, personally meaningful treatment programs then they must spend considerable time and energy getting to know each patient as a person. In this way, the therapist could determine what was needed.

Our conflict in the 1990s lies in how these individually oriented, humanistic values can survive within the current climate of health care. What economic, political, and social factors are impinging on our deeply ingrained humanistic philosophy of care, and how shall we act in relation to those forces?

Shifting Our Allegiance

In the current practice of occupational therapy, we have been forced to shift our allegiance from focusing solely on the patient to a more expanded concern that incorporates the needs of our employers to remain financially solvent. This shift has increased our attention to efficient discharges, shortened lengths of stay, maintenance of high census, development of referral networks, and provision of care in the least costly way. Like physicians, we have had to amend our traditional allegiance to the patient due to increased fiscal restraint, which requires that we now consider the economic realities of the hospitals in which we work. We must interweave the moral commitment we have to the individual with the economic responsibilities we have to our employer (Cassidy, 1988). This dilemma surfaces daily in outpatient care, where patterns for reimbursement for services are typically narrowly defined and limited in scope. This has resulted in an environment in which conflicting forces are at work: People have a need for the service, and therapists are trained to provide the needed service, but there is no viable mechanism available to pay for the service. Many times, because of a patient's lack of health insurance, we must turn even the most appropriate treatment candidates away from our departments. In present-day practice, "the economics of the system rather than the need or condition of the patient dictates the amount and level of occupational therapy service" (Perinchief, 1988, p. 166).

Another effect of this economically driven situation is that we are faced with the pressure of providing a certain treatment protocol that is based on diagnosis. The frequency of treatment is dictated not by the patients' needs but rather by administrative directive. To follow this directive guarantees a charge for the cost of rehabilitation while that patient is eligible for such charges based on third-party reimbursement criteria (Neuhaus, 1988).

In reimbursement-driven practice, many decisions are predicated on factors outside of the therapist. Indeed, changing reimbursement patterns have demanded new service provision models. We must therefore ask ourselves whether we as occupational therapists will be able to create new treatment models that meet reimbursement guidelines and still maintain our strong commitment to individuals, holistic care, and occupational role performance.

More and more it appears that we must use a technical, protocol-driven approach to treatment. This mechanistic approach clashes with our preferred approach to the person as an individual, because, according to Neuhaus (1988), we must practice "in a climate where technology and cost containment may overshadow the needs of the individual patient" (p. 288). The conflict is further complicated, because "it is difficult to set realistic priorities that have some meaning for the patient when the patient's length of hospital stay has been determined on the basis of a diagnostic category that denies the individuality of the patient in general as well as the specific needs of that particular person" (Neuhaus, 1988, p. 291).

These obvious practice dilemmas raise key questions, such as (a) Does providing cost-effective care mean giving up quality of care and a commitment to quality-of-life issues? (b) Do we have enough time to get to know the person, develop individually valued goals, elicit motivation and participation, and provide opportunities for individually meaningful successes? and (c) Are we uncomfortable with providing what we may consider to be less than quality care and compensating in other ways, such as prescribing additional or special adaptive devices and equipment?

Identifying the Consumer

The term *consumer* is no longer reserved for the patient alone; it now extends to the government (policy makers, legislators, health-care systems), health maintenance organizations, third-party payers, for-profit hospital corporations, and school administrators. With this expanded roster of agents to whom the therapist is held accountable comes the pressure of a complex of concerns and vested interests that increase the likelihood of ethical conflicts (Hansen, 1990).

Demonstrating our effectiveness to third-party reimbursers requires that we be able to explain and justify treatment to a variety of administrators and health and education officials. Again, the nature of our practice conflicts with how outsiders view efficacy. Occupational therapy goals are oriented to the individual, and the outcomes of treatment are individually significant; by their nature, these outcomes are not statistically significant. Conversely, in economics, belief systems are built when proof is generated in large numbers that can be generalized to the population.

Where reimbursement issues are concerned, other persons, including families who may be paying a significant portion of the bill, will also need to understand and have trust in the rationale behind our treatment methods if they are going to invest their money in such treatment. In addition to paying for our services, families will have to invest their interest and time by actively participating in treatment with their family member. This unusual demand on our part contrasts with the more traditional and authoritarian position taken by other health-care practitioners. Rather than being asked to stand aside and relinquish control, families are required to actively participate in the problem solving, decision-making, and implementation of treatment. Surprised by this demand for involvement, families may grapple with the perceived value of such therapy. Their confusion is typified by their repeated inquiries for an explanation of our service, especially in terms of the outcomes they can expect for their family member. Many therapists find these inquiries difficult to handle. Their reluctance to promise outcomes stems from their respect for the individual and their knowledge of the complex factors that influence behavior and skill development.

The need to influence public policy makers, legislators, and insurance regulatory bodies to ensure our inclusion in standards and regulations for health care and associated policy decisions (e.g., education, home care, employment) requires us to move in many other unfamiliar ways. Will we be able to convince them that occupational therapy is a primary and essential service (Cassidy, 1988)? Our ability to do this may be influenced by how different and almost simplistic our practice looks, with its focus on daily living skills, as compared with the high-tech professions and environments in which we practice (Burke, 1984).

The subtle complexity of everyday activities (Fleming, 1990) may appear to be less important or to require less professional skill when compared with the operating suite, a physical therapy hydrotherapy unit, or a dialysis unit. Our practice, which uses common sense objects in everyday ways, may cause others to diminish our importance and our skill as part of a modern health-care team (Fleming, 1990).

Our role in home care exemplifies this dilemma. In home care reimbursement regulations, occupational therapy is considered a secondary service. This means that an occupational therapist is unable to open a case and provide intervention to the increasing number of homebound patients who are leaving acute care settings before they have been able to fully benefit from occupational therapy. Because therapists are working under the restricted timetables of acute care, they will frequently sketch out a brief plan to justify further occupational therapy for a given patient who is homebound. When the patient is discharged and assigned to a home health agency the occupational therapy plan is reviewed by a primary service provider, typically a nurse or a physical therapist. Upon reading the plan to provide training for daily living skills, a nurse or physical therapist will often ignore the unstated expertise that is required to teach daily living skills and instead assume by the very commonness of the goals and activities that his or her own treatment plan will suffice toward the accomplishment of these goals.

Summary

The humanistic-driven versus reimbursement-driven issues that we have outlined present complex ethical dilemmas to occupational therapists concerned with "assuring the best quality of life possible for their patients" (Hansen, 1990, p. 4). As we approach the 21st century, we find ourselves increasingly involved in a careful examination of the "ethical parameters of our practice" (Hansen, 1990, p. 7). As called for by AOTA's Directions for the Future plan (Fleming, Johnson, Marina, Spergel, & Townsend, 1987), we must make some decisions and act in ways that will lead to our appropriate inclusion in the health-care marketplace. Some of those ways are outlined in the directives below.

Establish mechanisms to ensure that patients receive occupational therapy. Ideally, the acute care role for which we are best suited is triage. In triage, we would assess the person's level of need and his or her readiness to engage in rehabilitation. On the basis of assessment findings, a patient would be assigned to a rehabilitation setting, nursing home, outpatient care setting, or home health-care agency. This would depend on our ability to secure our role as essential service providers.

Resolve personnel issues, especially in the areas of retention and recruitment. Therapists may not be attracted to or be able to stick with positions in acute and rehabilitation care centers because of their frustration with the medical model; the associated lack of support for the kind of service we want to give; and the burnout we experience from the high-paced, mechanically and technically centered care. Implementation of strategies such as the triage system outlined above may help us to mitigate our personnel shortages.

Increase the social commitment to the value of health. Current societal values associated with health care provision are reflected in an unequal provision of service based on economic and social class, including racial and ethnic distinctions. Why are some people turned away from health and rehabilitation programs while others are allowed to receive care for varying periods of time and in a variety of settings? Once we affirm that all people have an equal right to equal health care, we will be able to provide occupational therapy in a way that is consistent with our humanistic philosophy.

Develop an acute awareness of and knowledge about health-care reimbursement. Information on "the limitation of that coverage and of the alternatives for coverage" (Perinchief, 1988, p. 166) is critical in planning and implementing optimum treatment programs. Such information can help therapists succeed in their "unspoken contract with the patient to provide optimum care, which includes ensuring that the service provided is reimbursable" (Moyers, 1990, p. 15). Additionally, a thorough investigation of alternative and less costly service provision models, such as consultation, and the effect of these models on patient care status must be acted on.

Educate consumers. As consumers assume the responsibilities of their role, they will harness their power and position with reimbursement sources. Educated consumers will be able to turn their anger and frustration at being denied rehabilitation or occupational therapy for home health care into efforts to call, write, lobby, and otherwise influence their lawmakers and their insurance agencies. By doing so, consumers ensure that the health policies and procedures reflecting their true preferences for care are appropriately developed and included in laws and regulations governing health care.

References

American Occupational Therapy Association. (1988). Occupational therapy code of ethics. *American Journal of Occupational Therapy, 12,* 795–796.

Bockoven, J. S. (1971). Occupational therapy—A historical perspective. Legacy of Moral Treatment—1800's to 1910. *American Journal of Occupational Therapy, 25,* 223–225.

Burke, J. P. (1984). Occupational therapy: A focus for roles in practice. *American Journal of Occupational Therapy, 38,* 24–28.

Cassidy, J. C. (1988). Access to health care: A clinician's opinion about an ethical issue. *American Journal of Occupational Therapy, 42,* 295–299.

Fleming, M. (1990). *A common sense practice in an uncommon world.* Paper presented at the institute on Clinical Reasoning, Tufts University–Boston School of Occupational Therapy, Medford, MA.

Fleming, M. H., Johnson, J. A., Marina, M., Spergel, E. L., & Townsend, B. (Eds.). (1987). *Occupational therapy: Directions for the future.* Rockville, MD: American Occupational Therapy Association.

Hansen, R. (1990). Ethical considerations. In C. B. Royeen (Ed.), *AOTA self study series: Assessing function* (No. 10). Rockville, MD: American Occupational Therapy Association.

Moyers, P. (1990). Reimbursement for functions assessment. In C. B. Royeen (Ed.), *AOTA self study series: Assessing function* (No. 8). Rockville, MD: American Occupational Therapy Association.

Muncie, W. (1959). The psychobiological approach. In S. Arieti (Ed.), *American handbook of psychiatry* (Vol. 11, pp. 1317–1335). New York: Basic.

Neuhaus, B. E. (1988). Ethical considerations in clinical reasoning: The impact of technology and cost containment. *American Journal Of Occupational Therapy, 42,* 288–294.

Perinchief, J. (1988). Influences of the health-care system on occupational therapy practice. In H. Hopkins & H. Smith (Eds.), *Willard and Spackman's occupational therapy* (7th ed.) (pp. 165–167). Philadelphia: Lippincott.

Ryon, W. G. (1925). Habit training for mental patients. *Occupational Therapy and Rehabilitation, 4,* 235–239.

Slagle, E. (1934). Occupational therapy: Recent methods and advances in the United States. *Occupational Therapy and Rehabilitation, 13,* 289–298.

Creating Excellence in Patient Care

CHAPTER 55

KATHLEEN BARKER SCHWARTZ,
EdD, OTR, FAOTA

Occupational therapists today are working in health-care organizations that operate from an efficiency perspective. That is, administration's goals are concerned with increasing efficiency in order to succeed financially. Experts argue that this approach can put quality at risk (Snoke, 1987; Starr, 1988). This paper proposes an alternative approach—the excellence perspective—as a way to address quality and at the same time sustain productivity.

The chapter traces the evolution of the efficiency perspective and provides a critique of this approach as applied to health-care organizations. It examines the historical origins of the excellence perspective and describes its use in business and its potential for health care. To illustrate how the excellence perspective can be successfully applied to health, a case study of an inpatient unit in a large teaching hospital in northern California is presented.

The Efficiency Perspective and Health-Care Management

The efficiency perspective originated in industry with principles introduced by Frederick Winslow Taylor in the early 1900s (Copley, 1923). Taylor declared that "scientific management" would enhance productivity by increasing worker performance and increase profitability by reducing labor costs (Taylor, 1919). A critical feature of scientific management was the creation of a class of managers who were guided primarily by concerns for efficiency and profit (Hoxie, 1916). In response to Taylor's ideas, labor unions argued that if scientific management took hold, the craftsman would lose his autonomy and become little more than an animated tool of management (Montgomery, 1984).

Taylor's ideas did take hold. Indeed, scientific management ideology provides the foundation for the efficiency perspective in management today (Drucker, 1954). A basic assumption of this perspective is that resources are finite and must be carefully controlled in order to achieve productivity. Control of scarce resources such as time, money, and staff is accomplished through a hierarchical organizational structure in which formal authority is delegated to managers who are responsible for monitoring efficiency and profitability (Perrow, 1970).

Although the efficiency perspective has exerted considerable influence in industry and business since 1920, the perspective has taken much longer to permeate health-care management. Although there is evidence to show that the doctrine of scientific management was preached to doctors as well as to businessmen (Haber, 1964), there is little data to show that the efficiency perspective was influential in the formative years of American hospitals.

Health-care institutions were not identified with the business concern of profitability in the early years of the 20th century. The health-care system at that time consisted of either charity or voluntary hospitals whose goals were humanitarian in nature (Starr, 1982). In many instances, doctors had authority over both the administrative and the clinical aspects of hospital care and thus fulfilled the roles of technical expert and manager. This was in contrast to industry where the skilled worker, or "doer," became separated from the manager, or "thinker" (Reich, 1983). One prominent Chicago physician evidently was mindful of events in industry when he warned his colleagues, "If we wish to escape the thralldom of commercialism, if we wish to avoid the fate of the tool-less workers, we must control the hospital" (Holmes, 1906, p. 320).

Indeed it was a shift in control and purpose that brought the efficiency perspective to health-care organizations. By 1970, the humanitarian emphasis had shifted to a concern for the best way to run hospitals as businesses (Drucker, 1973). The health-care industry expanded from hospitals into rehabilitation centers, outpatient services, nursing homes, and community programs. Accompanying this expansion was growth in the private insurance industry and in federal insurance programs through Medicare and Medicaid. The physician–manager role eroded and governance became separated from clinical management. Hospital administrators with master's degrees in business administration took over the business functions of hospitals, guided by the efficiency perspective.

The efficiency perspective has been justified on the grounds that health care in the United States is big business, and therefore health-care organizations should be run according to a business model, which emphasizes efficiency. Given modern concerns about rising costs in health care, the need for the efficiency perspective was deemed obvious: This approach enables management to focus on the goals of productivity and cost control.

Differences between business and health care, however, raise questions as to the goodness of fit with the efficiency perspective. One important difference lies in the mission of the organization. In business, profits are the top priority. In health care, quality patient care is the predominant goal. Some for-profit health-care facilities do exist, but a large proportion of health-care institutions remain nonprofit. Even the nonprofit facilities, however, have begun to shift their emphasis away from quality and toward cost reduction as a result of the cost-containment movement.

This shift in focus has highlighted a growing conflict between practitioner and administrator. Differing professional orientations place the administrator trained from a business perspective on the side of efficiency and the practitioner trained from a humanistic perspective on the side of quality. Whereas the administrator focuses on the efficient use of funds and increased productivity, the health-care practitioner desires freedom to act in the full interests of the patient and resources to provide the most advanced treatment ("Balancing Health Care Costs," 1988).

One way to address this dilemma of efficiency versus quality is to reframe the question: Can all organizations achieve quality as well as efficiency? Some management theorists argue that this is possible, if organizations use the excellence perspective.

The Excellence Perspective and Health-Care Management

The origins of the excellence perspective can be traced to the work of Mary Parker Follett (Follett, 1924; Fox & Urwick, 1973). Follett articulated her management philosophy in the first part of the 20th century, at the same time that scientific management was gaining popularity. She proposed that businesses would be effective only when they created an environment that stimulated each member to make his or her fullest contribution. Indeed, she argued that the strength of an organization depended on its ability to create a "working unit," in which shared values and common interests could evolve (Follett, 1987). Follett proposed that the best way to create organizational environments that fostered such working units was through shared decision-making and participative governance, a position in direct opposition to the authoritarian approach advocated by Taylor.

Follett's interest in creating an environment in which people could contribute fully was probably due in part to her own experience as a woman. She was also influenced by the idealistic leanings of several of her instructors at Harvard and by her professional experience as the founder of a group of community centers called the Roxbury League (Cabot, 1934; Crawford, 1971). The prescience of Follett's vision has recently been acknowledged (Mullins, 1979; Parker, 1984). March (1965) claimed Follett was ahead of her time: Her ideas did not fit in with the management wisdom of her age, an age dominated by the efficiency perspective.

Contemporary management theorists challenge the efficiency perspective. They argue that it has not helped American business, which is suffering from declines in product quality and in productivity (Reich, 1983). They urge that we move away from the concern of efficiency and toward a focus on excellence (Peters & Austin, 1985; Peters & Waterman, 1982). They claim that if one emphasizes excellence as the primary goal, then productivity is not sacrificed but, rather, is enhanced (Walton, 1985).

Studies of successful businesses that exemplify the excellence perspective show several common elements (Deal & Kennedy, 1982; Waterman, 1987). A key element is the definition of a vision that can guide the direction and activities of an organization. This vision should be shared, that is, the organization's members must value its mission. Leadership is a critical factor (Kouzes & Posner, 1989). It is the leader with a vision who helps shape the organization. Leaders create an environment that fosters collaboration, one that encourages and recognizes the contributions of all members. Case studies show that organizations committed to a shared goal, with leaders who direct the organization's resources toward that goal, create an environment that achieves quality and productivity (Posner, Kouzes, & Schmidt, 1985).

Since the first writings on this management perspective were published, much interest has been expressed, as has some criticism. Questions arise as to how an organization creates a vision, which is a vague concept at best. How does an organization convince its members to work toward a shared goal? How does one become the kind of leader who can shape an environment that enables members to achieve excellence and productivity? Recent writings by organizational theorists who support this perspective have attempted to answer these questions (Bradford & Cohen, 1984).

For example, Kouzes and Posner (1989) used data from their research based on 1,372 questionnaires and interviews to describe how leaders bring forth the best in themselves and others. The authors discussed the concept of vision, which they said is not mysterious and which can be defined as mission, goal, purpose, or simply the desire to make something happen that will contribute to quality. Kouzes and Posner described the ways that effective leaders create an environment in which members want to achieve excellence: (a) they enable others to see the possibilities a vision holds; (b) they are willing to take risks and experiment with new ideas; (c) they enable others to act and therefore to feel strong, capable, and committed; (d) they lead by example, through actions that support their words; and (e) they encourage others through genuine acts of caring. The authors' book is replete with descriptions of acts of leadership that contributed to excellence in performance. Examples are cited from both the public sector and private industry.

Deal, Kennedy, and Spiegel (1983) addressed the specific application of the excellence perspective to health-care institutions. They asserted that although this perspective is not abundant in health care, some organizations do exemplify excellence. As examples, they described a prestigious urban teaching hospital and a community rehabilitation facility. Although these organizations differ in size (large versus small), mission (acute care versus long-term care), and financial status (nonprofit versus for profit), they share certain elements. Deal et al. found each organization was committed to being the best. For one, this meant the best teaching hospital; for the other, the best rehabilitation facility. This vision was shared by all members and shaped by leaders who committed the necessary resources to achieve this goal. Individual contributions were encouraged and recognized. Within the rehabilitation facility, the occupational therapy department was well respected for its contribution to excellence. Its members were encouraged to contribute and, in fact, developed several patient-care programs. The director of occupational therapy had recently been promoted to vice president; at that level she anticipated having a greater opportunity to further her vision of excellence in patient care (D. Robinson, personal communication, October 30, 1982).

Case Study

The Asian and Pacific American Psychiatric Inpatient Program at San Francisco General Hospital in San Francisco, California, opened in 1980. It later served as the model for the development of four other inpatient programs to serve Latinos, Blacks, women, and patients with AIDS-related psychiatric illnesses. These five programs, designed to provide culturally sensitive psychiatric care to minority and ethnic patients, were recently awarded a certificate of significant achievement by the American Psychiatric Association (American Psychiatric Association, 1987).

It all began when Francis Lu, MD, participated in a 1979 National Institute for Mental Health conference on ethnic and minority curriculum development. Out of that conference grew his idea about how to provide the best culturally sensitive care to ethnic and minority patients. Lu envisioned an Asian-focus unit in which patients of that ethnic background would come together with professionals of the same background. He believed that acutely disturbed patients could benefit from services provided by professionals who spoke the same language and understood cultural values and beliefs. This view is supported by experts who argue that successful treatment can only occur when the professional comes to understand the patient's story, that is, the way a person views himself or herself in the world (Coles, 1989; Taylor, 1989).

Dr. Lu laid the groundwork for this idea through discussions with the hospital's administration. The department of psychiatry at San Francisco General Hospital is a joint undertaking of the city and county of San Francisco and the University of California, San Francisco. Lu persuaded the administration that his idea would assist the hospital to better address the needs of San Francisco's diverse population. He proposed that a core group of mental health professionals who shared a similar vision could provide more effective diagnosis and treatment. He argued that for the same cost as traditional treatment, higher quality care would be achieved. No special grants or funding were requested; however, Lu did gain administrative support for the concept of a focus unit as well as a commitment to provide funds for recruitment. Leaders in the Asian community were approached, and they expressed their support for the idea. According to the 1980 census, 21.3 percent of San Francisco's residents are Asian American.

The unit began with two professionals of Asian origin, Lu and one nurse. The staff grew to consist of a program director, a senior attending physician, nurses, social workers, and an occupational therapist—all of Asian descent. Those who came to work on the unit did so because they shared the vision of an Asian-focus patient care unit. The unit offered professionals the opportunity to contribute their knowledge of Asian languages and culture. Once the vision was established, the professionals shaped the unit's direction and goals. The goals were (a) to provide culturally sensitive psychiatric care, (b) to provide multi-disciplinary training opportunities, and (c) to develop a body of research to improve both patient care and education.

The way patient treatment was conducted was determined by the developing unit's vision and goals. The staff employed treatment approaches most likely to provide excellent patient care that was culturally sensitive. An ethnomedical approach to diagnosis and treatment was viewed as more consistent with the unit's goal than the traditional biomedical model. This ethnomedical approach not only focuses on diagnosis and precipitating incident but explores information regarding previous life and stresses in the home country; the escape experience and refugee events; and language, cultural, financial, and racial problems encountered in the United States. The staff also explores beliefs the patient might hold about illness, for example, the belief that disease is caused by an excess or deficiency of yin and yang. This approach provides treatment based on an understanding of the patient's perceived symptoms and difficulties (Lee, 1985).

The milieu is designed to make patients comfortable. Rice and tea are routinely served with meals. Ethnic newspapers, books, and music tapes are available. Family members are allowed to bring home cooked food during their visits. Great importance is placed on family involvement and linkages with the community once the person is discharged. Evelyn Lee, EdD, became program director in 1982. Lu described Dr. Lee as a charismatic and caring leader who has energetically directed the unit toward its mission to provide psychotic and severely depressed Asian American patients with an environment that understands their pain and their cultural background (F. Lu, personal communication, November 30, 1989).

Lisa Lai, OTR, was hired in 1982 as the unit's occupational therapist. Lai has relied on general principles of occupational therapy coupled with creativity and her knowledge of Asian language and culture. Occupational therapy treatment uses occupation that is both meaningful and purposeful; Lai uses an approach to treatment that takes into account both patients' functional needs and their values and beliefs. For example, the cooking group features recipes from various Asian and Pacific countries. Support for treatment that addresses both the meaning and the purpose of occupation has been a growing theme in the professional literature (Yoder, Nelson, & Smith, 1989). Lai asserts that treatment that combines professional expertise with a sensitivity to the language and values of patients can result in major changes in patients' status and responsiveness to treatment (L. Lai, personal communication, November 30, 1989).

In summary, the Asian-focus unit exemplifies many of the characteristics of the excellence perspective. It began with an idea, a vision, that would join others in the pursuit of excellence in patient care. This vision represents the shared values and beliefs of the professionals within the unit. Its leaders epitomize the leadership qualities of the excellence perspective: They have enabled others to see the possibilities of their vision, they have experimented with new ideas, and they have encouraged professionals within the unit to make individual contributions. They lead through example and encourage through caring. Development of the Asian-focus unit was hard work; it took several years to achieve the cohesion it has now. Its evolution required patience, a commitment of resources from the administration, and energy and understanding from the professionals within the unit. Recruitment has been and remains an issue. The unit must attract and retain competent professionals with an Asian background and language capability who share the same sense of mission. Although the program has gained national recognition for its innovative approach, there is a feeling expressed by some within the facility that the program promotes a segregated approach to treatment, one that separates patients as well as staff. This belief assumes that the focus units maintain a separate mission from the rest of the organization. Another viewpoint, however, is that the focus units simply offer one way to achieve the overall mission of the hospital, which is to provide quality patient care for the residents of San Francisco. Further research is planned to document the effectiveness of the focus unit in patient treatment (Lee & Lu, 1989).

Discussion

One might ask, if the excellence approach leads to higher-quality patient care, why is it not used by more health-care organizations? The answer, in part, is that people act in ways that are most comfortable. As this paper has shown, the efficiency perspective is predominant in health care. Efficiency has become the primary goal; quality patient care is a secondary goal. Common wisdom dictates that if one focuses on efficiency, one gets productivity and reasonable patient care. Excellence in patient care has been presumed to be something that could only be achieved at a financial risk. Research has contributed to disproving this assumption, but common wisdom dies hard. We must also examine the nature of leadership in health-care organizations. Administrators tend to be conservative, particularly in a climate that is so heavily focused on cost containment and short-term financial performance. The majority of leaders using the excellence perspective are from organizational cultures noted for being more innovative, such as high technology. Finally, there can be little energy for innovation in an environment where the vision is survival. Only when one replaces that vision with one of excellence can energy be freed for making changes that can contribute to quality patient care as well as to productivity.

Implications for Occupational Therapy

As this case study has shown, health-care professionals were the leaders in developing a program to achieve quality patient care. Because many administrators are preoccupied with finances, it will probably fall to health professionals to continue to lead the focus on excellence. Occupational therapists can contribute to this effort by developing ideas to increase the quality of services within our domain.

As the profession of occupational therapy plans for its future, one vision that emerges is that of the multifaceted occupational therapist, a person who is a competent clinician, a supporter of and contributor to research, and a strong manager–leader (Directions for the Future, 1990). This vision says we can no longer afford to have occupational therapists who are knowledgeable only about patient evaluation and treatment. Instead, we need people who are able to articulate the profession's contribution and introduce new ideas that can lead practice. This requires leadership ability and management knowledge. Occupational therapists can use the excellence perspective as a guide to program innovation. It is a perspective that fits with the occupational therapist's concern for quality patient care and the administration's concern for productivity.

Acknowledgments

I express my appreciation to the staff and patients of the Asian and Pacific American Psychiatric Inpatient Program at San Francisco General Hospital, San Francisco, California. In particular I would like to cite the assistance of Francis Lu, MD, Assistant Clinical Professor of Psychiatry, University of California, San Francisco; Evelyn Lee, EdD, Assistant Clinical Professor of Psychiatry, University of California, San Francisco; Lisa Lai, OTR, Staff Occupational Therapist, San Francisco General Hospital; and Judy Levin, OTR Senior Occupational Therapist, San Francisco General Hospital.

References

American Psychiatric Association. (1987, Oct 16). *Six exceptional programs for the mentally ill share hospital and community awards.* News release.

Balancing health-care costs and quality. (1988, June). *Occupational Therapy News,* p. 3.

Bradford, D. L., & Cohen, A. R. (1984). *Managing for excellence.* New York: Wiley.

Cabot, R. (1934). Mary Parker Follett: An appreciation. *Radcliffe Quarterly, 18,* 81.

Coles, R. (1989). *The call of stories.* Boston: Houghton Mifflin.

Copley, F. B. (1923). *Frederick W Taylor: Father of scientific management.* New York: Harper & Brothers.

Crawford, D. (1971). Mary Parker Follett. In D. Crawford (Ed.), *Notable American women 1607–1950* (pp. 639–641). Cambridge, MA: Belknap Press.

Deal, T. E., & Kennedy, A. A. (1982). *Corporate cultures.* Reading, MA: Addison–Wesley.

Deal, T. E., Kennedy, A. A., & Spiegel, A. H. (1983). How to create an outstanding hospital culture. *Forum, 26,* 21–34.

Directions for the Future. (1990, January). Meeting of the American Occupational Therapy Association, San Diego, CA.

Drucker, P. F. (1954). *The practice of management.* New York: Harper & Row.

Drucker, P. F. (1973). *Management: Tasks, responsibilities, practices.* New York: Harper & Row.

Follett, M. P. (1924). *Creative experience.* New York: Longmans, Green.

Follett, M. P. (1987). Freedom and coordination. Lectures in business organization. In A. Brief (Ed.), *Ancestral books in the management of organizations.* New York: Garland.

Fox, M., & Urwick, L. (Eds.). (1973). *Dynamic administration: The collected papers of Mary Parker Follett.* London: Pitman.

Haber, S. (1964). *Efficiency and uplift.* Chicago: University of Chicago Press.

Holmes, B. (1906). The hospital problem. *Journal of the American Medical Association, 38,* 320.

Hoxie, R. F. (1916). *Scientific management and labor.* New York: D. Appleton.

Kouzes, J., & Posner, B. (1989). *The leadership challenge.* San Francisco: Jossey–Bass.

Lee, E. (1985). Inpatient psychiatric services for Southeast Asian refugees. *Southeast Asian Mental Health.* Washington, DC: National Institute for Mental health.

Lee, F., & Lu, F. (1989). Assessment and treatment of Asian American survivors of mass violence. *Journal of Traumatic Stress, 2,* 93–120.

March, J. (Ed.). (1965). *Handbook of organizations.* Chicago: Rand McNally.

Montgomery, D. (1984). *Worker's control in America.* London: Cambridge University Press.

Mullins, L. (1979). Approaches to management. *Management Accounting, 57,* 15–18.

Parker, L. D. (1984). Control in organizational life: The contribution of Mary Parker Follett. *Academy of Management Review, 9,* 736–745.

Perrow, C. (1970). *Organizational analysis.* Monterey, CA: Brooks/Cole.

Peters, T., & Austin, N. (1985). *A passion for excellence: The leadership difference.* New York: Random House.

Peters, T., & Waterman, R. (1982). *In search of excellence: Lessons from America's best-run companies.* New York: Harper & Row.

Posner, B. Z., Kouzes, J. M., & Schmidt, W. H. (1985). Shared values make a difference. *Human Resource Management, 24,* 293–309.

Reich, R. B. (1983). *The next American frontier.* New York: Times Books.

Snoke, A. W. (1987). The hospital administrator. *Hospital Topics, 65,* 23–29.

Starr, P. (1982). *The social transformation of American medicine.* New York: Basic.

Starr, P. (1988, March 20). Increasingly, life and death issues become money matters. *New York Times,* p. E1.

Taylor, F. W. (1919). *The principles of scientific management.* New York: Harper & Brothers.

Taylor, S. E. (1989). *Positive illusions.* New York: Basic.

Walton, R. E. (1985). From control to commitment in the workplace. *Harvard Business Review, 63,* 77–84.

Waterman, R. H. (1987). *The renewal factor.* New York: Bantam.

Yoder, R. M., Nelson, D. L., & Smith, D. A. (1989). Added-purpose versus rote exercise in female nursing home residents. *American Journal of Occupational Therapy, 43,* 581–586.

Sustaining the Art of Practice in Occupational Therapy

CHAPTER 56

SUZANNE M. PELOQUIN, PHD, OTR

Occupational therapists have seen an effort within their profession to unearth historical roots, to articulate a philosophical base, to elucidate models for practice, and to validate theoretical concepts through research. The search for a professional identity and for professional credibility is essential; it has also been intense. The purpose of this article is to explore a concept that has been underrepresented in occupational therapy literature over the last decade: the art of the practice of occupational therapy.

The art of occupational therapy is the soul of its practice. Therapy as an art is an old theme; literature as a nurturer of the soul is an older theme still. The occupational therapy literature with its many references to paradigms, constructs, and variables reflects a considerable effort to articulate the profession's scientific basis. A profession committed to balance can perhaps sustain its art by reflecting on the images of caring and helpful occupation seen in fictional literature.

The Art of Occupational Therapy

In 1972, the American Occupational Therapy Association (AOTA) Council on Standards defined *occupational therapy* as "the art and science of directing man's participation in selected tasks to restore, reinforce and enhance performance, facilitate learning of those skills and functions essential for adaptation and productivity, diminish or correct pathology, and to promote and maintain health" (p. 204). Years later, AOTA's Representative Assembly accepted a more comprehensive definition that begins as follows:

> Occupational therapy is the use of purposeful activity with individuals who are limited by physical injury or illness, psychosocial dysfunction, developmental or learning disabilities, poverty and cultural differences or aging process in order to maximize independence, prevent disability and maintain health. (1981, p. 798)

Definitions evolve over time to reflect changes in priorities and orientations. It is not surprising that the descriptive phrase "art and science," which validates a blend of practice components, was deleted between 1972 and 1981 as the profession's emphasis turned toward scientific research and accountability.

In spite of this deletion from the profession's official definition, the practice of occupational therapy remains a blend of art and science. There is an art to the practice of any therapeutic endeavor. Mosey (1981) discussed art relative to the practice of occupational therapy. She first defined the art of practice negatively, stating that the art of practice is not (a) a desire to help others, (b) the skilled application of scientific knowledge, or (c) simply being a systematic or sympathetic practitioner. Mosey wrote, "The capacity to establish rapport, to empathize, and to guide others to know and make use of their potential as participants in a community of others illustrates the art of occupational therapy" (p. 4). Without art, she claimed, occupational therapy would become the application of scientific knowledge in a sterile vacuum.

Mosey (1981) elaborated those characteristics commonly held by practitioners she called "masters in the art of practice" (p. 23). The artful practitioner perceives the individual as indivisible into various parts or subsystems. Although practitioners reduce the human organism into subsystems in order to understand the patient more clearly, the art of practice reintegrates those subsystems to see a whole person. Meeting the patient as an individual enables the practitioner to empathize with the patient and to accept his or her feelings, ideas, and values. The meaning that the patient places on his or her life, relationships, and environment guides the therapist–patient collaboration toward growth, independence, and the use of potential.

The science of practice, Mosey (1981) said, is a phenomenon fundamental to all professions. In occupational therapy practice, science is the gathering of data through systematic clinical observations or through more formalized research projects to help develop new theories or to verify, refine, or refute existing theories relevant to the practice. The art and the science of occupational therapy together constitute its practice.

Devereaux (1984) (see Chapter 35) identified the caring relationship as the art rather than the science of health care. She wrote, "Occupational therapists are specialists in making care happen. We know how to enrich all the transactions in the relationship with the patient. These become caring gestures" (p. 794) (in Chapter 35). Devereaux characterized the particular caring of occupational therapists as singular among professionals: helping the patient reconnect to those occupations that are meaningful to him or her. She said, "Occupational therapists care by helping people disengage from despair and dysfunction and by helping them look forward, to see their loss as being able to be ameliorated through adaptation and occupation" (p. 794) (in Chapter 35).

Within the context of her definition of caring, Devereaux (1984) (see Chapter 35) highlighted a major assumption that informs the theory and the practice of occupational therapy: that adaptation occurs through the use of occupation. According to Reed and Sanderson (1983), occupational therapy theory and practice build on several assumptions. Although it is difficult to summarize these assumptions, Reed and Sanderson demonstrated that it is possible. They categorized a long list that included assumptions about: (a) human beings; (b) occupational performance; (c) health, wellness, and illness; (d) the receipt of health-care services; (e) the provision of health care; (f) occupational therapy; and (g) the therapeutic use of occupations. In the art of practice, as occupational therapists engage meaningfully with patients, they discuss assumptions. They formulate treatment plans based on mutual assumptions chosen from among several possible categories. A cluster of assumptions gleaned from Reed and Sanderson's comprehensive list

seems central to the caring connection described by Devereaux. These assumptions relate to occupation and figure prominently in any dialogue with patients about their connection with meaningfulness:

> Each individual must perform some occupation or have the occupations performed for the person to survive.
>
> A person adapts or adjusts (grows and develops) through the use of and participation in various occupations.
>
> Occupations may be divided into three major areas: self-maintenance, productivity, and leisure.
>
> A balance of occupations is facilitatory to the maintenance of a satisfying life.
>
> Occupations permit a person to fulfill individual and group needs.
>
> Occupations must be relevant and useful to the individual in relating to the environment. (p. 70)

The art of practice supports the entire structure of occupational therapy. Caring, informed by assumptions about occupation, constitutes the base for those elements Devereaux (1984) (see Chapter 35) considered essential to an effective relationship in occupational therapy: (a) competence, (b) belief in the dignity and worth of the person, (c) belief that each person has the potential for change and growth, (d) communication, (e) values, (f) touch, and (g) sense of humor. Caring transforms a science of occupation into a therapeutic practice.

Mastery of the art of practice in the fullness described by Mosey (1981) and Devereaux (1984) (see Chapter 35) is a challenge. One need only reflect on the current demands faced by practitioners to acknowledge the difficulty. The brief length of patients' stays, the demands for productivity, the documentation criteria for third-party reimbursers and accrediting agencies, and the requirements for research and quality assurance all demand the time and energy required for caring. Occupational therapy practitioners need affirmation that the art of practice is valued and that those assumptions about occupation that are communicated through caring are relevant to patients. Today's health-care system does not tend to nurture the art; it does not encourage consistent patient–therapist dialogue about assumptions.

Associates of occupational therapy in medicine have been vocal in their articulation of the struggle to retain the humane side of practice. Engel (1977) wrote of physicians' disenchantment with an approach to disease that neglects the patient, with a dominance of procedures over patient sensitivities, and with a biomedical emphasis that disregards human meaning. Pellegrino (1979) claimed that the concepts of discreteness of disease processes and specificity of therapeutic agents have transformed the ethos of medicine. Therapeutics as we know it today, a little more than a century old, has been beneficial for humankind on the whole. But the impact of scientific advances and technological successes has profoundly compromised the relationship between patient and physician.

Patients resent the fragmentation of their care. Public distress has resulted in a series of measures to acknowledge the patient, the person, and his or her rights: quality assurance, the patient's bill of rights, legal concern with informed consent, and the regulation of experimentation on human beings. These measures systematize a defense against a powerful medical system that tends to forget or ignore the individual patient. The health-care system demands scientific competence; the legal system demands acknowledgment of individual rights. There is no escaping the reality: Practitioners must engage in the science of practice in order to function in the health-care system. And yet, patients and professionals alike recognize the sterility of a human-service practice devoid of its art, its caring. Rights can be legislated, but caring cannot. The art of practice, not so valued or nurtured by the health-care system, requires sustenance from other sources.

Literature: Toward an Affirmation of the Art of Practice

A new field, literature and medicine, suggests a source of sustenance for the art of occupational therapy practice. Jones (1987) characterized literature and medicine as a recent phase in the medical humanities experiment in medical education. She identified two approaches to literature that justify its incorporation into medical education: the aesthetic and the moral. Trautmann (1978) described the aesthetic approach: "to teach a student to read, in the fullest sense" (p. 36). The fictional world, she said, reveals "relationships between people and within a single personality" (p. 33). In reading fiction, one "must look at words in their personal and social contexts" (p. 36). Trautmann said that through literature one can make the leap to empathy, to compassion. Through literature, one can achieve affirmation of personal dignity—affirmation of a personhood threatened by the health-care system.

Coles (1979), a physician, described the second approach to literature, the moral approach. He wrote that "the point of a medical humanities course devoted to literature is ethical reflection" (p. 445). Coles believed that novelists and clinicians alike focus on the everyday life and on the unique nature of the human being. He said that there is a continuing tension between one's idealism and life's demands. Novelists, he said, can move one to scrutinize assumptions, expectations, and values, to reflect on a life either as it is being lived or as one hopes to live it.

Images from fictional literature viewed within the context of either the aesthetic or the moral approach can nurture the art of occupational therapy practice. The art of practice, is, after all, intrinsically centered on images—images of relationships, of qualities that make relationships meaningful, of occupation's meaning in a life.

The aesthetic approach to literature can help, in its scrutiny of relationships, to validate the meaningfulness of "the capacity to establish rapport, to empathize, and to guide others to know and make use of their potential as participants in a community of others" (Mosey, 1981, p. 4). The moral approach can prompt reflection about practice elements and about assumptions that inform practice. Both approaches can validate the practitioner's commitment to the art, to caring, and to caring connections.

Yerxa and Sharrott (1986), in their endorsement of a liberal arts education for occupational therapists, wrote:

> Occupational therapy's knowledge base requires an understanding of medical conditions, but it is not the medical condition per se that is of the greatest significance; rather, it is the occupational nature of the human being. Thus, although our knowledge, in practice, is primarily applied to people who are ill and disabled, the science of occupation and its concern with the play–work continuum, adaptation, and competence development applies to all people, disabled or not. (p. 158)

Literature, read in its fullest sense and reflected upon, can contribute to an understanding of the human condition.

Mosey (1981) described the process of learning the art of practice: "The individual who strives to bring art to practice must be able to engage in the often uncomfortable process of learning more about one's self, changing one's self, and gaining knowledge about how one's values and expectations may differ from those of others" (p. 25). In the world of fiction one can find a mirror reflecting back, for recognition and appraisal, one's self, one's values, and one's expectations. One can also find in the world of fiction a window opening onto a world of others, their values, and their expectations. Literature can facilitate learning the art of practice.

Fiction: A Reflection of the Art of Practice

The concept of reading fiction to enhance the art of practice will no doubt elicit varied responses from widely diverse occupational therapy practitioners. Avid, discriminating readers use the process already, but nonreaders may not be intrinsically motivated to turn to fiction without a clear indication that the process can enhance their skill in the art of practice. Although the process seems particularly suited to the educational system, it is equally adaptable to any continued learning endeavor.

The fictional world is populated by occupational therapists and patients. Some images from that world reflect practitioners inept in the art of practice and patients vocal about that ineptitude. Fiction also contains images that seriously challenge assumptions about occupation. If one expects sustenance from the literature, one needs to know how to handle the negative images.

Reading in a fuller sense can be affirming, even if the fictionalized occupational therapist happens to be a rogue or a villain. If one can agree that the character's interpersonal style lacks care, that agreement affirms one's endorsement of a different style: "I'll be (or I am) a different kind of occupational therapist." This can be affirming. Reading in the fuller sense, one can find other characters whose interactional styles are favorably represented. To reflect on characteristics worth emulating is to once again affirm one's belief in caring and in the art of practice.

An encounter in the fictional world with a blatant repudiation of an assumption about occupational therapy may be disturbing. By reading in the moral sense, that is, reading to examine human values, one can step out of one's own world of assumptions to consider those of others. This experience can enrich later dialogues with patients. The exploration of another world through fiction can enable one to better understand real patients whose values differ from one's own. The reflection and the broadening of view made possible through fiction can facilitate the meeting of each patient as an individual.

In *The Cracker Factory* (Rebeta-Burditt, 1977), an occupational therapist working in a private psychiatric hospital is characterized in a most unflattering manner. The protagonist in this story is Cassie, a young woman admitted to the hospital because she is depressed and abusing alcohol. Cassie does not single the occupational therapist out for criticism; the therapist is one of several characters seen as oppressive. Cassie describes her hospital experiences satirically. She depicts the occupational therapist in an interactionally challenging scene: attempting to motivate patients to come to a therapy group. Cassie names the therapist "Brunhilde, the misplaced Viking Lady" and "the Dictator of OT" (p. 114). Both names suggest an abuse of power. One expects ferocious and bloody battle with a Viking and arbitrary orders from a dictator. The names, unfortunately, seem apt. The therapist "marches around the seventh floor telling all the patients that their doctor has 'ordered' Occupational Therapy" (p. 114). Rather than discussing with individual patients the merits of therapy or its relevance to them personally, she invokes the power of the doctor's order. She "herds them out in the hall" and "goosesteps them out the door" (p. 114). There is no evidence of rapport here, no humor, no recognition of patients as individuals. Harshness dominates the scene.

The occupational therapist insists that the patients "must come IMMEDIATELY" (p. 114). When patients try to hide from her by taking a shower, "She doesn't care. Wet or screaming, it makes no difference. She drags them along anyway" (pp. 114–115). A caring touch is replaced by dragging and goose-stepping. Notably absent are a respect for patients' dignity and an acknowledgment of patients' rights. There is clearly no empathy. Instead, there are threats: "If you don't go to OT, it will be written down on your chart and you won't get out of here" (p. 114). Cassie's perception of the motivational attempt is one of intimidation. The reader is forced to agree.

Practitioners may recognize in this portrayal the familiar struggle inherent in the motivational process. Ultimately, the patient has the right to refuse all treatment, for whatever reason. Furthermore, the patient has every right to dispute or to reject any and all assumptions about the therapeutic process. Meanwhile, the concerned practitioner, invested in the patient as a person, tries to communicate possible benefits, to convey a deep personal interest, to attempt to collaborate, and to walk away from the motivational effort only when convinced that the patient has sufficient information to have made a real choice.

Powerful images from *The Cracker Factory* stimulate reflection about the motivational attempt. Does even the best attempt feel, to the patient, like a battle? If so, what interpersonal elements might signal a truce? Cassie's view clearly reminds therapists that a patient who has little control over an environment perceives those in control as dictators. What therapist characteristics might impress a patient differently? *The Cracker Factory* provides a clue to anyone reading in the fuller sense.

One favorite nurse escapes Cassie's sharp criticism: the nurse she calls Tinkerbell. Tink does not invoke rules or orders. She makes exceptions to the rules when possible. Cassie comes in from the cold, after a late-night Alcoholics Anonymous meeting, and Tink tosses her a set of keys saying, "The kitchen is officially closed but you may go in if you like" (p. 221). Cassie is "delighted, feeling like a friend" (p. 221). Tink takes time to establish rapport, to be with Cassie, to talk with her. She asks personal questions, and she encourages Cassie to share. When Cassie says of herself, "I doubt I'll ever have the ability to be that open," Tink says, "Give it time.... When you're more comfortable, you'll loosen up" (p. 222). When Cassie asks Tink a personal question, Tink agrees to answer, saying, "Okay, Cassie, I'll play fair" (p. 223). She shares a personally painful situation. Unlike Brunhilde, whom Cassie describes as not caring, Cassie tells Tink, "You care," to which Tink nods and replies, "I care" (p. 227). But Tink admits personal shortcomings. She says, "I have limitations like everyone else" (p. 227). She tells Cassie, "I prefer involvement on a limited basis, caring on my terms, the way I handle it best, the way I'm most effective" (p. 227). Tink's disclosure of personal weaknesses has therapeutic value. She can say, "Cassie ... from where I'm standing, I have a clear view of *your* strengths" (p. 227). Tink's display of humanity reinforces Cassie's humanity. In Cassie's worldview, Tink is a caring person; the occupational therapist is not. The art in Tink's practice of nursing contrasts harshly with the absence of art in the occupational therapist's practice.

Interactional characteristics make a difference to patients in fiction and in reality. The exaggeration and striking contrast between one occupational therapist and one nurse used in *The Cracker Factory* can generate powerful responses and productive thinking. The kind of reflection that is prompted by an encounter with forceful fictional characters can nurture the art of practice.

Images of Occupation and Caring Connections

In addition to specific images of occupational therapists in literature, there are images of occupation and of caring people associated with occupation. Two literary pieces, Kesey's *One Flew Over the Cuckoo's Nest* (1962) and Shem's *The House of God* (1978), have achieved a measure of notoriety for their portrayals of health-care environments in which professional caring is painfully compromised.

Kesey's novel depicts a state mental institution. The story is told from the point of view of the Chief, an electively mute, chronically ill American Indian patient. The Chief's delusional system and active visual and auditory hallucinations contribute to the image that patients are caught in a gigantic unyielding machine designed to socialize them into conformity. The typical hospital day is monotonous: Acutes and Chronics alike submit to the order imposed by the Big Nurse. The Chief describes the atmosphere: "There's something strange about a place where the men won't let themselves loose and laugh, something strange about the way they all knuckle under to that smiling flour-faced old mother [Big Nurse]" (p. 48). He describes group discussion among the patients as "telling things that wouldn't ever let them look one another in the eye again" (p. 49). He characterizes the therapies offered as being all the same and unable to engage the patient: "Ten, -forty, -forty five, -fifty, patients shuttle in and out to appointments in ET or OT or PT" (p. 38). The environment is devoid of meaningful occupation and meaningful interpersonal exchange; the result is dehumanizing.

Shem describes an equally maladaptive environment in *The House of God*. Roy Basch is an intern at the House of God, a hospital where the "emphasis was on doing everything always for everyone forever to keep the patient alive" (pp. 25–26). The House of God is filled with gomers, "human beings who have lost what goes into being human beings" (p. 38). Within this environment, interns and residents lack support from their supervisors, struggle against exhaustion, and grapple with life, death, and ethical issues. Tired interns focus on getting sleep: "I wish she would die so I could just go to sleep" (p. 135). They try to learn "enough medicine to worry less about saving patients and more about saving themselves" (p. 150). They always seem on the edge of sanity and control. Roy says, "I'm scared that one of these nights, with nobody else around, when someone starts to abuse me, I'm going to lose control and beat the shit out of some poor bastard" (pp. 232–233). There is no balance of occupations, no rest, and no leisure. Roy describes his inner state at his worst point: "I had been as far from the world of humans as I could get.... I had been sarcastic. I'd avoided feeling everything, as if feelings were little grenades" (p. 361). Roy Basch, denied a balance of occupations and cut off from meaningful human exchange by the demands and stresses of work, lives in an environment as dehumanized as that portrayed by the Chief.

Kesey and Shem provide hope for both the Chief and Roy Basch: there is a way out of these maladaptive environments and these dehumanizing worlds. Other people lead the way out, people who can laugh, who can relate, who can touch. People help the Chief and Roy to make connections with helpful occupations.

In *One Flew Over the Cuckoo's Nest,* McMurphy enters the Chief's world: "He sounds big. I hear him coming down the hall, and he sounds big in the way he walks.... He talks a little the way Papa used to, voice loud and full of hell" (p. 16). McMurphy laughs. The Chief says, "I realize all of a sudden it's the first laugh I've heard in years" (p. 16). McMurphy's activity level is contagious. He plays cards and Monopoly, he pitches pennies, he commandeers a tub room for a game room, he socializes and gambles incessantly, he struggles with Big Nurse over the use of the TV. The longer McMurphy stays, the more in touch with reality the Chief becomes. McMurphy organizes two activities (or occupations) in particular that seem to make meaningful connections for others: a basketball game on the ward and a fishing trip.

McMurphy "talk[s] the doctor into letting him bring a ball back from the gym" (p. 174). In response to the nurse's objections, the doctor observes: "A number of the players, Miss Ratched, have shown marked progress since that basketball team was organized; I think it has proven its therapeutic value" (p. 175). The team increases a feeling of solidarity among the patients. The Chief, though not on the team, says, "We got to go to the gym and watch our basketball team" (p. 176). The game "let most of (them] come away feeling there'd been a kind of victory" (p. 176) despite their 20-point loss. The image of this patients' team is familiar to most occupational therapists: "Our team was too short and too slow, and Martini kept throwing passes to men that nobody but him could see" (p. 176). The adaptive effects represented in this image of the game validate a major occupational therapy assumption about the human condition.

When basketball season is over, McMurphy plans a fishing trip. He deceives authorities into thinking that two maiden aunts will sponsor the expedition. Instead, he engages the help of a prostitute. The Chief focuses his attention increasingly on McMurphy's energy and strength. When he speaks for the first time in years, he speaks to McMurphy. After having been withdrawn for years, the Chief yearns to reach out. He thinks, "I just want to touch him because he's who he is" (p. 188). McMurphy signs the Chief up for the fishing trip. The Chief reflects: "I was actually going out of the hospital with two whores on a fishing boat; I had to keep saying it over and over to myself to believe it" (p. 191).

Images of the fishing trip powerfully present the competence, mastery, and connectedness with others possible through occupation. The activity meets both group and individual needs. The trip is an occupation enjoyable to these men both in the doing and in the end product: the successful catch. Fiction here validates on a dramatic level what a formal analysis might predict about this particular activity for a group of institutionalized patients. Each person on the expedition benefits in some way from the activity. The Chief's experience is representative of that of the others. On the ride he says, "I could feel a great calmness creep over me, a calmness that increased the farther we left land behind us" (p. 208). He recalls that he "was as excited as the rest" (p. 209). He fishes independently: "I was too busy cranking at my fish to ask him [McMurphy] for help" (p. 210). The clearest representation of the healing effect of the experience is the spread of McMurphy's laughter. The Chief says, "I notice Harding is collapsed beside McMurphy and is laughing too. And Scanlon from the bottom of the boat.... It started slow and pumped itself full, swelling the men bigger and bigger. I watched, part of them, laughing with them" (p. 212). The Chief explains that McMurphy knows about laughter: "He knows you have to laugh at the things that hurt you just to keep yourself in balance, just to keep the world from running you plumb crazy" (p. 212). From within the context of a dehumanizing state institution, a real person, capable of relating and capable of touching lives, makes connections for these men using occupations that help them heal. This image can nurture the art of occupational therapy practice.

In *The House of God,* Roy Basch's experience cuts him off from a number of caring peers. Two people manage to help Roy reconnect through occupations. Roy's girlfriend, Berry, quietly reflects back to him the changes she sees. Toward the end of the novel she says, "Roy, I'm worried.... You're isolated.... You're hypomanic.... For me, tonight, you're a dead man. There's no spark of life" (p. 349). She organizes a trip to see a performance of the mime Marcel Marceau. Roy tries to get out of going at the last minute, so Berry has four of Roy's friends literally carry him out of the hospital to the performance. Seeing the mime perform, Roy reflects, "All of a sudden I felt as if a hearing aid for all my senses had been turned on. I was flooded with feeling" (p. 359). Later he says, "Berry welcomed me back to her, and I felt her caring arms around me for the first time. Awakening, I began to thaw" (p. 360). The performance, in its dramatic portrayal of the human struggle, touches Roy and reconnects him with his innermost self. He says, "I realized that what had been missing [from the House of God experience] was all that I loved. I would be transformed. I'd not leave that country of love again" (p. 363). Soon after the performance, Roy describes his internship: "I hated this. The whole year sucked" (p. 374). Berry asks him, "Why not become a psychiatrist?... Being with people was all that kept you going this year, Roy. And 'being with' is the essence of psychiatry" (p. 374). Berry, having connected Roy to a powerful experience that enabled him to feel again, suggests an occupation in which his need to feel and care might be allowed to grow.

This healing image is also one that validates the art of occupational therapy practice.

The Fat Man is a caring resident in *The House of God.* In some ways a renegade like Kesey's McMurphy, the Fat Man shares survival skills in an insane world. He teaches interns to "buff" charts and to "turf" hopeless cases elsewhere (p. 61). He models caring behaviors among patients who can comprehend the care. He invokes 13 laws of the House of God, all raucous and outrageous, but aimed to counterbalance the senseless thrust of an institution to apply technological procedures regardless of human cost. One law reads: "The only good admission is a dead admission" (p. 420). Patients love Fats, and Roy asks, "As crass and as cynical as you are?" (p. 213). Fats answers, "That's why: I'm straight with 'em and I make 'em laugh at themselves.... I make them feel like they're still part of life, part of some grand nutty scheme instead of alone with their diseases" (pp. 213–214). Roy reflects on this: "I was touched. Here was what medicine could be: human to human. Like all our battered dreams" (pp. 215–216).

The Fat Man sees his residency as only a part of the nutty scheme of things. He attends to other satisfying occupations. He dabbles with inventions such as his "anal mirror" (p. 107). Fats expounds on his invention: "The anus is a great curiosity to almost all mankind" (p. 107). Roy is never quite sure how tongue-in-cheek this invention idea really is. But the idea reflects a comic relief, a reprieve from the daily grind. Fats models a life outside the House of God. He manages a private practice out of his home, saying, "What's the sense of being a licensed doc if you don't use it 'to relieve pain and suffering'? This GP work is terrific—these are my neighbors, my people" (p. 372). His life connects beyond his occupation at the dehumanizing House of God. Fats touches others; he can also be touched. When an intern commits suicide, Roy recalls that "the Fat Man was crying. Quiet tears filled his eyes, fat wet tears of desperation and loss" (p. 313). Fats can touch Roy: When he comes to apologize for the recent distance between them, he links pinkies with Roy. Roy remembers, "It was perfect, a magical moment.... He'd sensed my emptiness, and he'd responded. His touch meant I wasn't alone. He and I were connected" (p. 373).

Fats also helps the interns consider meaningful occupational connections. Toward the end of their rotation, he works with the interns to select specialty areas. Using chalk and a blackboard, he lists the advantages and disadvantages that the interns see in each specialty. The exercise, one largely of values clarification, helps Roy. He says, "By the end of the Fat Man's colloquium, the remarkable had happened: on paper, Psychiatry was the clear winner" (p. 381). Fats is able to touch the lives of the interns. Through caring gestures he helps connect them with meaningful occupations.

Conclusion

Reflection about the art of occupational therapy is less widespread in the professional literature than is reflection about the science of occupational therapy. This is a matter of concern in that occupational therapy is a blend of art and science. The art of practice includes the ability to establish rapport, to empathize, and to facilitate choices about occupational and human potential within a community of others. Engaging in the art of practice commits the therapist to an encounter with an individual who is a collaborator in his or her plan for treatment. Collaboration includes a discussion of each patient's personal goals and of professional and personal assumptions about both the human condition and the meaning of occupation in a life. Without the caring elements that ground the therapist–patient relationship and the dialogue that grounds collaborative treatment planning, occupational therapy would be reduced to a sterile science of occupation.

The current health-care system does not encourage the art of practice. Medical practitioners, propelled by the scientific model, have recently returned to a consideration of their lost art. Systematized patient defenses against the depersonalization and fragmentation of their care have affirmed the popular need for care in addition to cure. Practitioners looking to sustain their art have had to turn to sources other than the health-care system. The new discipline of literature and medicine attempts to support a humane medical practice through the insightful reading of fiction, and it has the potential to sustain the art of occupational therapy practice as well. By reading fictional literature in its fullest, aesthetic sense, one can reflect on and affirm the importance of relationships and caring in practice by comparing and contrasting those various personal characteristics most conducive to helping. Reading fictional literature in its moral sense can enable practitioners to explore values and assumptions about the human condition and, more specifically, about the importance and meaning of occupation in a life. This reading process is adaptable to the educational system as well as to any other continued education format.

Examples from three fictional works illustrate that both positive and negative images of occupational therapy and occupation can affirm commitment to artful practice. Reading fiction can validate the competence, mastery, and human connectedness with others possible through occupation. Reading fictionalized stories of occupational therapists and other caregivers can affirm those personal qualities of warmth, genuineness, humor, and empathy that are essential in the establishment of a helpful bond.

The art of occupational therapy practice requires validation, though perhaps not in the same manner as does its science. The reading of fictional literature can provide occupational therapists with sustaining images: images of relationships, images of qualities that make relationships meaningful, and images of the meaning of occupation in a life. Reflection on these images can reaffirm one's commitment to the art of providing occupation as therapy.

Acknowledgments

I extend special thanks to Dr. Anne Hudson Jones, Institute for the Medical Humanities, The University of Texas Medical Branch, whose flexibility and encouragement made it possible to integrate course material with occupational therapy issues. I also thank Doreen S. McCarty for typing the manuscript.

References

American Occupational Therapy Association Council on Standards. (1972). Occupational therapy: Its definition and functions. *American Journal of Occupational Therapy, 26*, 204–205.

American Occupational Therapy Association Representative Assembly minutes—1981. (1981). *American Journal of Occupational Therapy 35*, 792–802.

Coles, R. (1979). Medical ethics and living a life. *New England Journal of Medicine, 301*, 444–446.

Devereaux, E. B. (1984). Occupational therapy's challenge: The caring relationship. *American Journal of Occupational Therapy, 38*, 791–798. Reprinted as Chapter 35.

Engel, G. L. (1977). The need for a new medical model: A challenge for biomedicine. *Science, 196*, 129–135.

Jones, A. H. (1987). Reflections, projections, and the future of literature and medicine. In D. Wear, M. Kohn, & S. Stocker (Eds.), *Literature and medicine: A claim for a discipline* (pp. 29–40). McLean, VA: Society for Health and Human Values.

Kesey, K. (1962). *One flew over the cuckoo's nest*. New York: New American Library, Signet Books.

Mosey, A. C. (1981). *Occupational therapy: Configuration of a profession*. New York: Raven Press.

Pellegrino, E. D. (1979). In M. J. Vogel, & C. E. Rosenberg (Eds.), *The therapeutic revolution: Essays in the social history of American medicine* (pp. 245–266). Philadelphia: University of Pennsylvania Press.

Rebeta-Burditt, J. (1977). *The cracker factory*. New York: Bantam Books.

Reed, K. L., & Sanderson, S. R. (1983). *Concepts of occupational therapy*. Baltimore: Williams & Wilkins.

Shem, S. (1978). *The House of God*. New York: Dell Publishing.

Trautmann, J. (1978). The wonders of literature in medical education. In D. Self (Ed.), *The role of the humanities in medical education* (pp. 32–44). Norfolk, VA: Teagle & Little.

Yerxa, E., & Sharrott, G. (1986). Liberal arts: The foundation for occupational therapy education. *American Journal of Occupational Therapy, 40*, 153–159.

Dreams, Dilemmas, and Decisions for Occupational Therapy Practice in a New Millennium: An American Perspective

ELIZABETH J. YERXA, EDD, OTR, FAOTA

Humankind is poised to take a giant step into the 21st century. Will the year 2000 bring a great leap forward into a more humane, healthy, enlightened global community, or will it begin a downward spiral, toward an irretrievable loss of the dream for a good life? Scientists, philosophers, public policy makers, optimists, and pessimists are debating their visions of the future, looking into crystal balls filled with light or darkness.

This chapter was previously published in the *American Journal of Occupational Therapy, 48,* 586–589. Copyright © 1994, American Occupational Therapy Association.

Assumptions

As I enter this debate I bring a set of assumptions. The 21st century will possess characteristics that are of great importance to occupational therapists and the persons we serve.

First, the next century will begin an *era of chronicity* beyond that which the world has ever known. The population of persons with impairments will increase markedly, as will the number of persons at risk. This era of chronicity will result from the successes of medical technology, the aging of the populace, and the preservation of biological life on an unprecedented scale (Robinson, 1988).

Second, *new knowledge* emanating from the sciences, philosophy, literature, and the arts will affirm the significance of the uniqueness, individuality, and wholeness of each person (Edelman, 1992; Thelen, 1990). This new knowledge will enlighten scientists about life-span development and the evolution of our species. Research, at last, will emphasize human purpose, action, goal-directedness, interests, curiosity, and consciousness, as well as the joy, despair, or boredom that persons experience when they engage in their daily rounds of activity (Csikszentmihalyi, 1975).

Third, daily life will increase in *complexity* (Toffler, 1981). Successful accomplishment of the activities of daily living will be much more challenging because of increased urbanization, the diversity of cultures interacting, the multiplicity of social role expectations, high technology, and the difficulty of educating children for competency in an instantaneously changing environment.

Fourth, the future will bring an *increased emphasis on personal power, autonomy, self-direction, and self-responsibility,* with a decrease in the influence of traditional paternalistic political and social systems. Persons will demand to control their own destinies and to participate in the decisions that affect them.

Fifth, the 21st century will see a *new conceptualization of health,* a shift away from the old idea that health means the absence of disease, pathology, or impairments. The new idea of health is reflected, for example, in Pörn's (in press) philosophy. He defined health as persons' capacities to achieve their goals and purposes through possession of a repertoire of skills.

Sixth, the new era will bring an *increased awareness of attending to the demands of the environments in which persons actually live and work.* Persons will learn such skills as mathematical computation, not by classroom drills and tests divorced from the pulsating rhythms of life, but in the real world of the supermarket, office, and shopping mall.

Research has demonstrated not only that transferring skills from the academic environment to the real world is difficult but that the skills learned are different (Lave, 1988). Thus learning a skill in a classroom might develop competency for schoolwork but not for the challenges of daily life.

Dreams

Within this context of the future, being an optimist and an occupational therapist (and the two characteristics usually do go together), I have a dream. My most audacious dream is that the 21st century will begin the millennium of occupation. Occupation, as engagement in self-initiated, self-directed, adaptive, purposeful, culturally relevant, organized activity, speaks to my assumptions about the future in compelling ways. The era of chronicity requires that some profession, recognize and reclaim the potential of persons with chronic conditions or at risk of developing them, so that these persons can achieve their purposes and so that social barriers to their self-definition will be removed. I nominate occupational therapy as that profession.

The new understanding emanating from the sciences about individuality and wholeness needs to be synthesized with the 70 years of knowledge about human activity, development, learning, and evolution that are embedded in the rich history of occupational therapy. We knew it all the time! For example, we knew that infants are driven by their unique curiosity to explore the world, learn from their experiences, and thus shape their nervous systems (Reilly, 1974). Engagement in occupation cannot be divorced from the meaning it possesses for the person.

The increased complexity of daily life for all persons demands a profession that knows a great deal about daily routines and how persons manage and thrive in their environments. My global travels have shown that occupational therapists everywhere focus on engagement in daily life, regardless of other differences in practice. Alvin Toffler (1981), the futurologist, proposed that all persons, not just those with impairments, will need "life organizers" (p. 377) to help them deal with the complexity of daily life in the 21st century. I nominate occupational therapists to be tomorrow's life organizers, using our knowledge of activities of daily living to help persons get their lives together in a complex world.

As for the increased emphasis on autonomy and personal responsibility, occupational therapists have always involved patients or other participants in formulating and carrying out their programs. In fact, authentic occupational therapy cannot take place unless the patient becomes his or her own agent of competency via occupation. Many other health-care professionals do not know how to help the patient do this because they are trained in an old paternalistic model of acute care. In his book, *Medicine at the Crossroads,* Konner recommended that physicians adopt a "new model" of the physician–patient bond called the "patient as colleague" (1993, p. 14) model, in which the physician and patient exchange views and plan treatment or prevention together. Occupational therapists who have used a similar approach for decades can catalyze change in the entire health-care system through their skill and example. In this way more persons will take responsibility for their own health.

A vision of health as the possession of a repertoire of skills to achieve one's own purposes fits with occupational therapy's traditional emphasis on skill, mastery, and competence that can be attained regardless of pathology or impairment. It also suggests that occupation that develops skills can prevent illness and influence health by developing competency and making life worth living. This view of health is compatible with Reilly's (1962) (see Chapter 8) great hypothesis that human beings, through the use of their hands as energized by mind and will, can influence the state of their own health. Such a perspective on health implies that every human being has resources that can be reclaimed through occupational therapy (Montgomery, 1984).

Research demonstrating that persons need to learn skills in the environments in which their skills will be used supports occupational therapists who create a "just right challenge" (p. 251) from the environment so that the person can make an adaptive response (Robinson, 1977). It also supports the importance of providing occupational therapy in the home, community, supermarket, shopping mall, workplace, or school, not in artificial environments such as clinics or hospitals. I opened my eyes to the importance of the real-life environment when I provided occupational therapy to children with cerebral palsy in a home program after 2 years of similar work in a hospital. Not only was it easier for children to learn skills when the skills did not have to be transferred to a different environment (as was necessary in the hospital), but as an occupational therapist, I could experience the challenges of their daily lives and employ them in increments that assured both a just-right challenge and a high probability of success (Burke, 1977).

Biological evolution, in all creatures, advances in relation to real environmental challenges, not *before* such challenges occur (Jordan, 1991). Nature does not plan ahead; only when an organism is faced with a real environmental challenge can it adapt. Occupational therapists who provide service in real-life environments are not only practical but are employing the most sophisticated form of intervention supported by neurobiology, evolutionary biology, and anthropology.

Decisions and Dilemmas

What implications do these perspectives of the future hold for occupational therapy practice? Arnold Beisser (1988), a physician who became almost totally paralyzed as a result of poliomyelitis, described his experience as follows:

> More important [than the physical helplessness] was being *separated from so many of the elemental routines that occupied*

people.... I no longer felt connected with the familiar roles I had known in family, work, sports. *My place in the culture was gone.* (pp. 166–167) [Italics added]

Occupational therapists will need to establish their priorities for practice in the millennium of occupation. I recommend a decision in favor of the vital, fundamental issues that are most important to the person and society: survival, work, contribution, participation, delight in one's own actions. Focus on these will influence health through development of a repertoire of skills that reconnects persons to the elemental routines of their culture, restoring their place in the world. The dilemma is that the organization of the U.S. health-care system provides most of its resources for acute care, modalities, and techniques in an artificial environment that values short-term, measurable, physical changes and is not prepared to address these fundamental issues. As a result, the experiences recorded by articulate persons with disabilities—Lewis Puller (1991), Robert Murphy (1990), Arnold Beisser (1988), and Andre Dubus (1991)—as well as our research on persons with disabilities living in the community (Burnett & Yerxa, 1980)—show major unmet needs for help in dealing with such elemental issues as skills for living in the community, being part of one's culture, and having something satisfying to do. These authors and our research subjects did not mention occupational therapy in connection with their difficulties in daily living or their need to develop a new repertoire of skills at home or at work. If occupational therapy was mentioned at all it was as a minor aspect of acute care in the hospital.

The era of chronicity cries out for practice founded on an optimistic view of persons, their resources, and potential; one that emphasizes what is right, such as intrinsic motivation, rather than what is wrong, such as organ impairment. In spite of the Americans With Disabilities Act of 1990 (Public Law 101–336), persons with disabilities are too often stigmatized as second-class citizens or disposable persons. Unfortunately, this social attitude is so pervasive that persons with disabilities may be denied many social opportunities or internalize the stigma themselves, leading to depression and denial. This is a major dilemma. In the future world of genetic engineering and probable euthanasia, persons with disabilities are at risk of being eliminated as they were in Nazi Germany. Through new knowledge of occupation practiced by occupational therapists, these persons will be able to achieve their own purposes and to contribute to the variety and richness of society. Occupational therapists who are allies and advocates for persons with disabilities will help change society's attitudes from "those people are inferior" to "these people are fundamentally human, just like the rest of us." Through occupation this profession will reaffirm its commitment to persons with chronic conditions, a commitment initially made by Adolph Meyer (1922) (see Chapter 2) and Eleanor Clarke Slagle (1922) (see Appendix D).

A final implication is that occupational therapy practice will be enriched and broadened by new interdisciplinary knowledge of occupation, which some of us have named *occupational science.* Tomorrow's world needs a profession that views persons as both unique and whole, who create themselves through engagement in activity as driven by their interests and curiosity. Thus occupation, rather than being trivial, will be seen as the essential connector between the developing human organism and its environment, a creator of unique neural networks, motor patterns, and life-affirming mastery.

Science and philosophy's new interest in the wholeness of human beings belies the specialism that has permeated society and medicine. Persons have been divided into minds and bodies to fit into specialists' categories of mental health and physical disabilities. One of the greatest strengths of occupational therapy education has been its insistence on preparing students to look at persons as having not only muscles and joints but feelings, perceptions, families, communities, and unique patterns of daily activity. Ours is one of the few health professions that is educated to think this way, whose practitioners can serve anyone who needs to develop skills in the presence of a challenge labeled physical, psychiatric, developmental, or environmental. Our science and clinical experiences will help reconnect the human mind and body. Strengthening our generalist outlook with new knowledge will make our profession much more adaptable to the changing conditions of tomorrow's world environment. Evolutionary biology has taught us that specialists such as dinosaurs perish when their environment changes, whereas generalists such as cockroaches and human beings survive and prosper (Jordan, 1991).

A dilemma is created by the U.S. health-care system's low priority on providing resources for those labeled mentally ill and the resulting attrition in the numbers of occupational therapists adopting such practice. New knowledge of occupation that relates to skill, adaptation to changing circumstances, temporality, management and organization of the environment, and obtaining satisfaction through one's own action has a great deal to offer persons who are given psychiatric diagnostic labels. The millennium of occupation will reaffirm the commitment to improving the life opportunities of all persons regardless of diagnostic labels, because it is the right thing to do in a compassionate society and because occupational therapists have the knowledge and skill to make it happen. In the millennium of occupation, occupational therapists will enable human beings as whole persons to be reconnected with their culture through skills. Persons with disabilities will no longer be endangered or be isolated on islands of abnormality, but will perceive themselves as skilled, competent, and capable of mastery. The era of chronicity will be answered by the millennium of occupation. Health will ultimately be perceived not as the absence of impairment but as possession of a repertoire of skills to achieve one's own purposes. Robert Murphy (1990), an anthropologist paralyzed by a spinal cord tumor, at the end of his "journey into the world of the disabled," said that

the essence of the well-lived life is the defiance of negativity, inertia and death. Life has a liturgy that must be continually celebrated and renewed; it is a feast whose sacrament is consummated in the paralytic's breaking out from his prison of flesh and bone, and in his quest for autonomy. (p. 230)

Occupational therapists, in the new millennium of occupation, can provide a key to the prison and tools for the quest for autonomy.

References

Americans With Disabilities Act of 1990 (Public Law 101–336). 42 U. S. C., § 12101.

Beisser, A. (1988). *Flying without wings: Personal reflections on being disabled.* New York: Doubleday.

Burke, J. P. (1977). A clinical perspective on motivation: Pawn versus origin. *American Journal of Occupational Therapy, 31,* 254–258.

Burnett, S., & Yerxa, E. J. (1980). Community-based and college-based needs assessment of physically disabled persons. *American Journal of Occupational Therapy, 34,* 201–207.

Csikszentmihalyi, M. (1975). *Beyond boredom and anxiety: The experience of play in work and games.* San Francisco: Jossey-Bass.

Dubus, A. (1991). Broken vessels. *Essays by Andre Dubus.* Boston: David R. Godine.

Edelman, G. (1992). *Bright air, brilliant fire. On the matter of mind.* New York: Basic.

Jordan, W. (1991). *Divorce among the gulls: An uncommon look at human nature.* San Francisco: North Point.

Konner, M. (1993). *Medicine at the crossroads.* New York: Pantheon.

Lave, J. (1988). *Cognition in practice.* New York: Cambridge University Press.

Meyer, A. (1922). The philosophy of occupational therapy. *Archives of Occupational Therapy, 1,* 1–10. Reprinted as Chapter 2.

Montgomery, M. A. (1984). Resources of adaptation for daily living: A classification with therapeutic implications for occupational therapy. *Occupational Therapy in Health Care. 1,* 9–33.

Murphy, R. F. (1990). *The body silent.* New York: Norton.

Pörn, I. (In press). Health and adaptedness. *Theoretical Medicine.*

Puller, L. B. (1991). *Fortunate son. The autobiography of Lewis B. Puller, Jr.* New York: Grove Weidenfeld.

Reilly, M. (1962). Occupational therapy can be one of the great ideas of 20th-century medicine. *American Journal of Occupational Therapy, 16,* 1–9. Reprinted as Chapter 8.

Reilly M. (1974). *Play as exploratory learning.* Beverly Hills, CA: Sage.

Robinson, A. (1977). Play: The arena for acquisition of rules for competent behavior. *American Journal of Occupational Therapy, 31,* 248–253.

Robinson, I. (1988). The rehabilitation of patients with long-term physical impairments: The social context of professional roles. *Clinical Rehabilitation, 2,* 339–347.

Slagle, E. C. (1922). Training aids for mental patients. *Occupational Therapy and Rehabilitation, 1,* 11–14.

Thelen, E. (1990). Dynamical systems and the generation of individual differences. In J. Colombo & J. W. Fagan (Eds.), *Individual differences in infancy: Rehability, stability, and prediction.* Hillsdale, NJ: Erlbaum.

Toffler, A. (1981). *The third wave.* New York: Bantam.

Dreams, Dilemmas, and Decisions for Occupational Therapy Practice in a New Millennium: A Canadian Perspective

CHAPTER 58

HELENE J. POLATAJKO, PHD, OT(C)

My dreams for occupational therapy in the new millennium are predicated on what I imagine the world will be like in that millennium. Although I would like to believe that the world will be free of war, disease, illness, indeed all sources of human misery, I do not believe that to be the destiny of humanity. Rather, I believe that there will always be some phenomena that will result in less-than-ideal situations for humankind. Whether these phenomena will result in disability or handicap, however, is another issue.

I Dream of a World Free of Handicap

In my dream, the world will be free of handicap in the new millennium. Free not because we have learned to rehabilitate those with disabilities but because we have learned to create an environment that allows those with different abilities to live with dignity. Free not because we have allowed those with disabilities to end their lives but because we have enabled those with different abilities to have meaningful lives. Free not because we have learned to prevent disability but because we have learned to eliminate handicap. In other words, I dream of a world that honors, respects, and values differences, a world that enables living with different abilities.

Before I go on describing my dream and its implications for occupational therapy, let me clarify how I am using the terms *disability* and *handicap* and how they relate to each other. In attempting to establish an international classification for the long-term functional and social consequences of disease, the World Health Organization (WHO) identified three distinct and independent classifications: impairment, disability, and handicap. *Impairment* is defined as "any loss of psychological, physiological, or anatomical structure or function resulting from any cause" (1980, p. 27). *Disability* is defined as "any restriction or lack (resulting from an impairment) of ability to perform an activity in the manner or within the range considered normal for a human being" (p. 28). *Handicap* is "a disadvantage for a given individual, resulting from an impairment or disability, that limits or prevents the fulfillment of a role that is normal (depending on age, sex, and social and cultural factors) for that individual" (p. 29). In the vernacular of occupational therapy, handicap is a disadvantage that limits or prevents occupational role performance. Although WHO considers these classifications to be independent, there is, as apparent from the WHO definitions, a causal relationship among them (see Figure 58.1). It should be noted, however, that not all impairment leads to disability, nor does all disability lead to handicap. Indeed, because handicap is viewed as a disadvantage, and disadvantage is a social construct, disability must be seen as neither a necessary nor a sufficient condition for the creation of a handicap. In my dream the world will be free of handicaps because of occupational therapy—not the occupational therapy we know now, but the occupational therapy that surely must evolve because *occupation* is a powerful idea. To quote Thomas Jefferson, "It is neither wealth nor splendour, but tranquility and occupation, which give happiness" (cited in Foley, 1967, p. 399).

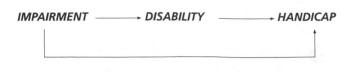
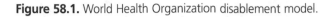

Figure 58.1. World Health Organization disablement model.

The great psychologist Hebb (1966) noted long ago that "living things must be active" (p. 248); that the need for activity and the avoidance of boredom, the result of inactivity, are important determinants of human behavior. Recently, two courageous young persons, one Canadian and one American, provided dramatic personal testimony of the vital importance that activity or the lack of it, has in determining human behavior.

In Canada, a 25-year-old woman caught national media attention when she fought the legal system for the right to refuse life-sustaining treatment. Having spent 2½ years in a hospital bed because of a disease that resulted in the permanent loss of all her independent function, including respiration, Nancy B. pleaded for the right to die. She told the judge that a life without the ability to do is not worth living ("Woman makes plea," 1991). She won her case. On February 13, 1992, Nancy B. died.

In the United States, 29-year-old Larry McAfee had a motorcycle accident that left him unable to walk, eat, or even breathe independently. After a year of intensive rehabilitation, out of finances, Larry was also doomed to a life in a hospital bed where, he said, "I used to just lie there on my back, being just so bored" (Schindehette & Wescott, 1993, p. 85). Two years later, "broken in spirit after being warehoused in a series of institutions, McAfee fought for the legal right to shut off his life-sustaining respirator" (Schindehette & Wescott, 1993, p. 85). Larry McAfee won his case. However, he is alive and well and living in the first independent-care home in the state of Georgia. While engaged in his fight to die, he discovered that he had options other than boredom, that in an environment that enabled occupation he could have an active, meaningful life. But Larry McAfee warned, "if ever I have to return to an institution, then I prefer death" (Schindeherte & Wescott, p. 86).

I Dream of a World Where Occupation Is a Powerful Idea

My dream for occupational therapy in the 21st century is that we will not only know unequivocally that occupation is a powerful idea but also choose to act on that idea, for "any powerful idea is absolutely fascinating and absolutely useless until we choose to use it" (Bach, 1988, p. 119).

Occupational therapy is in an exciting, transitional phase—a paradigm shift, as Kielhofner has described it (1992). If we make the right decisions now, if we frame the emerging paradigm well, I believe that the occupational therapy of the future will be quite different from the one we know today.

The occupational therapy we know now fails to realize the full potential of occupation. As Kielhofner (1992) and numerous others have pointed out, practice today is heavily influenced by the medical model. Practice is focused, primarily, on reducing impairment through the therapeutic use of purposeful activity. To quote Henderson et al. (1991), "the use of purposeful activity is the core of occupational therapy" (p. 370). In Canada, a similar emphasis on the therapeutic use of activity prevails. The definition of occupational therapy adopted by our national association begins with "Occupational therapy is the art and science which utilizes the analysis and application of activities" (Canadian Association of Occupational Therapists [CAOT], 1991, p. 140).

I Dream of a Discipline Focused on Occupation

In my dream, the occupational therapy of the future will realize the full potential of occupation. Practice will be grounded firmly in an occupational model. The focus of practice will shift from reducing impairment through purposeful activity to preventing handicap through occupational enablement.

My dream is predicated on two developments in our discipline, both called for by Ann Grady in her presidential address at the 72nd Annual Conference of the American Occupational Therapy Association. Grady asked occupational therapists to revisit and reaffirm the concepts and visions held by the founders of the discipline, to "reaffirm the idea that being meaningfully occupied provides direction for individuals and that successful engagement in the activity leads to individual satisfaction and promotes health and well-being" (1992, p. 1062), and to "provide the leadership needed to continue developing knowledge based on our founders' vision and to find myriad ways to apply that knowledge to the challenges of practice in the 21st century" (p. 1065).

For my dream to come true, we, as occupational therapists must:

* Affirm that occupation is a powerful idea
* Adopt occupation as the core concept
* Entrench occupation in our value system
* Become experts in enabling occupation.

My dream is that our continued study of occupation will make it possible, in the new millennium, for us to move beyond the rhetoric of the day and translate our values into action.

In my 1992 Muriel Driver Lecture, I articulated what I and a group of colleagues believe to be the core values of occupational therapy (see Appendix F). I elaborate on these briefly below and describe what I think it means to translate these into action as we embrace occupation as the core concept of our discipline. (For a more extensive discussion, see Polatajko, 1992.)

The values statement concerns itself with the core elements of this discipline. The first two, the individual and human life, are shared with all health-care disciplines. The third, occupation, distinguishes occupational therapy from the rest. Occupational therapists view humans as occupational beings with a basic need to do.

Translating the Rhetoric Into Action

Translating these values into action means, first of all, acknowledging some basic assumptions about occupation.

Occupation is a basic survival need. Occupation is essential to the well-being of every person much in the same way that sleep and food are; occupational deprivation, like sleep deprivation or food deprivation, results in serious mental and physical deterioration of the person and may even result in death—often at the individual's own hand.

Occupation is an extremely complex, multilevel, *multifaceted construct*. Occupation has cognitive, affective, physical, and environmental attributes and is individually determined; therefore, the study of occupation requires the investigation of the occupation, the person performing that occupation, the environmental context, and their interaction.

Occupational competence is the result of a goodness of fit among the person, the occupation, *and the environment*. Competence is defined as adequacy or sufficiency, answering all the requirements of an environment (Pridham & Schutz, 1985). That is, the occupational competence of any given person is determined by the interaction among the skills necessary to perform the occupation, the abilities of the person, and the demands of the environment in which the occupation is to be performed (see Figure 58.2).

Translating these values into action also means that:

Practice is client driven. The client's right to autonomy is taken seriously, and the client is understood to be a prosumer (defined by Toffler [1981, p. 11] as a fusion of producer and consumer) of occupational therapy services, keenly interested in exercising choice over the services that he or she accepts and accepting only those services that can be tailored to meet his or her needs.

Practice is founded on an ideology of empowerment (as defined by Rappaport, 1981). The role of occupational therapist is understood to be one of enhancing possibilities for persons to control their own lives at both a personal and a social level.

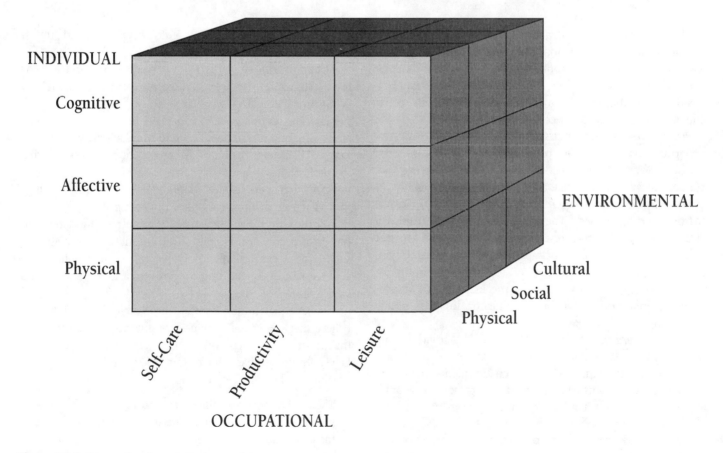

Figure 58.2. Occupational competence model.

Note. Reprinted with permission from Polatajko, H. J. (1992). Naming and framing occupational therapy: A lecture dedicated to the life of Nancy B. *Canadian Journal of Occupational Therapy, 59,* 189–200. Reprinted with permission of CAOT Publications.

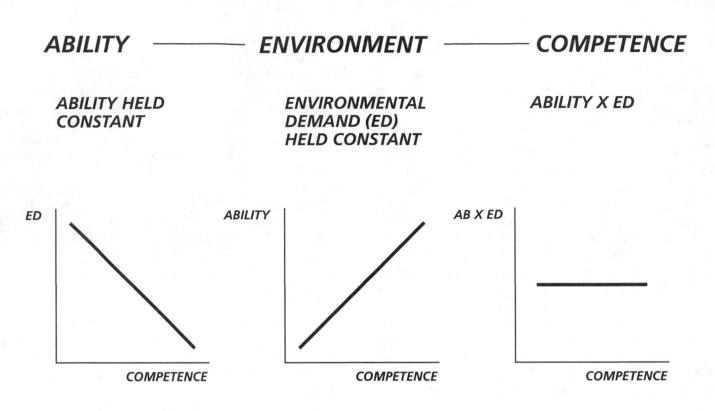

ABILITY ——— **ENVIRONMENT** ——— **COMPETENCE**

ABILITY HELD CONSTANT

ENVIRONMENTAL DEMAND (ED) HELD CONSTANT

ABILITY X ED

ED

ABILITY

AB X ED

COMPETENCE

COMPETENCE

COMPETENCE

Figure 58.3. Ability and environment interaction.

The ultimate goal of practice is wholly and solely the enablement of occupational competence. The purpose of practice is to alter the person's ability, the occupation, or the environment so that the person can achieve the necessary balance between ability and the environmental demands to enable occupational competence (see Figure 58.3).

Practice is context focused. Given the ideology of empowerment and the nature of occupation, services must be oriented toward, if not provided in, the person's context, that is, his or her physical, social, and cultural environment.

Practitioners take on many roles in enabling occupational competence. The traditional roles of hands-on clinician, administrator, researcher, and educator are not always adequate to enable occupational competence. Often, particularly when competence requires environment changes, new forms of practice are necessary, such as program designer, consultant, public educator, lobbyist, policy maker, and social critic.

Practitioners use many and any tools. Activity is only one of many tools used to enhance occupational competence. Practitioners use a variety of tools to enable clients; these may include technology, assistive devices, environmental adaptation, attitudinal shift, family education, social education, and policy change.

The domain of concern of the discipline is occupation. The body of knowledge of the discipline is centered on occupation. Scholarly inquiry is focused on understanding the phenomenon of occupation and the determinants of occupational competence. Given the complex nature of occupation,

the study of occupation is multidisciplinary and multimethodological.

Occupational therapists are experts in occupation. As my dream comes true there will be a great deal of change for occupational therapy (see Figure 58.4). These changes will present all occupational therapists—present practitioners, administrators, researchers and educators alike—with dilemmas that each of us will have to resolve for ourselves and that the profession will have to resolve as a whole.

As my dream comes true there will be a great deal of change that will create dilemmas, not only for occupational therapists, but for the world in general. Once the central importance and power of occupation is realized, it will necessitate a shift in such basic notions as quality of life and human rights. This shift has already begun, as shown by the cases of Nancy B. and Larry McAfee.

I believe that mine is not an impossible dream. Rather, I believe that we, as a discipline, are uniquely poised to make this dream come true—to lead the way in health care. Steven Lewis, former Ambassador of Canada to the United Nations, speaking at the CAOT conference in June 1991, said:

> There is no other discipline that is so eclectic, so far ranging and whose core principles are at the very heart of where the health care system is going.... You are the only health profession that has fully embraced the concepts of health promotion, prevention, community-based care and the individual as centre to the process. ("Perspectives '91," 1991, p. 11)

OT...	Will no longer be...	But...
Ideology	Treatment	Empowerment
Model	Medical	Enabling
Goal	Impairment Reduction	Occupational Competence
Function	To Cure	To Enable
Role	Clinician	Multifaceted
Setting	Institution	Occupational Context
Hallmark	Activity	Occupational Perspective
Activity	**THE Means**	**THE End**

Figure 58.4. Changes for occupational therapy in the coming millennium.

As with all change, this change will be experienced with some hesitation, discomfort and, I hope, excitement. But when my dream comes true, I believe that occupational therapists will be instrumental in helping the world to enable all to achieve occupational competence and therefore eliminate handicap.

Appendix 58.A

Occupational Therapy Values Statement

Occupational Therapy Values
As Occupational Therapists,
We value

- The individual
- Human life
- Occupation.

About the individual,
We believe that humans are occupational beings, that

- Every individual has intrinsic dignity and worth.
- Every individual has the right to autonomy.
- Each individual is a unique whole.
- Each individual has abilities and competencies.
- Each individual has the capacity for change.
- Individuals are social beings.
- Individuals shape and are shaped by their environment.

About human life,
We believe that all human life has value, that
- The value of human life is based on meaning, not perfection.
- Quality of life is as valued as quantity.

About occupation,
We believe that occupation is a basic human need, that

- Occupation is an essential component of life.
- Occupation gives meaning to life.
- Occupation organizes behavior.

- Occupation has developmental and contextual dimensions.
- Occupation is socioculturally determined.

(Conceptual Framework Think Tank, 1992)

University of Western Ontario–Occupational Therapy

Adapted from H. J. Polatajko (1992). Naming and framing occupational therapy: A lecture dedicated to the life of Nancy B. *Canadian Journal of Occupational Therapy, 59,* 193. Adapted with permission of CAOT Publications.

References

Bach, R. (1988). One. New York: Dell.

Canadian Association of Occupational Therapists. (1991) *Canadian occupational therapy guidelines for client-centered practice.* Toronto: Author.

Foley, J.P. (1967). *The Jeffersonian cyclopedic comprehensive collection of the views of Thomas Jefferson.* New York: Russel & Russel.

Grady, A.P. (1992). Nationally Speaking—Occupation as vision. *American Journal of Occupational Therapy, 46,* 1062–1065.

Hebb, D.O. (1966). *A textbook of psychology.* Philadelphia: Saunders.

Henderson, A., Cermak, S., Coster, W., Murray, E., Trombly, C., & Tickle-Degnen, L. (1991). Occupational science is multidimensional. *American Journal of Occupational Therapy, 45,* 370–372.

Kielhofner, G. (1992). *Conceptual foundations of occupational therapy.* Philadelphia: Davis.

Perspectives '91—Taking the initiative. (1991). *National, 8*(5), 11.

Polatajko, H.J. (1992). Naming and framing occupational therapy: A lecture dedicated to the life of Nancy B. *Canadian Journal of Occupational Therapy, 59,* 189–200.

Pridham, K.R., & Schutz, M.E. (1985). Rationale for a language for naming problems from a nursing perspective. *Image: The Journal of Nursing Scholarship, XVII*(4), 122–127.

Rappaport, J. (1981). In praise of paradox: A social policy of empowerment over prevention. *American Journal of Community Psychology, 9*(1), 1–25.

Schindehette, S., & Wescott, G. (1993, January 18). *Deciding not to die. People,* pp. 85–86.

Toffler, A. (1981). *The third wave.* Toronto: Bantam.

Woman makes plea to end life. (1991, November 29). *The Globe and Mail,* Section A, p. 4.

World Health Organization. (1980). *International classification of impairments, disabilities and handicaps (ICIDH).* Geneva, Switzerland: Author.

The Domain of Function: Who's Got It? Who's Competing for It?

CHAPTER 59

SHARON A. GUTMAN, PhD, OTR/L

Historically, professions develop and expand by creating areas of expertise or domains of concern. If a profession is to survive and grow, its area of expertise must be both needed and valued by the society. Professions attempt to protect their domain from competitors through various strategies: (a) demonstrating effectiveness of the profession's practices—through scientific methods—to both the scientific community and the public, (b) creating educational standards and certification examinations that ensure the competence of its professional membership, and (c) using media exposure to inform the public that the profession holds greater mastery over a specific domain than do its competitors (MacDonald, 1995).

However, historical and socioeconomic conditions often cause competing professions to assume a specific domain that had been developed and mastered by another profession (Abbott, 1988). Such is the case with the domain of functional activities of daily living (ADL). Historically, the profession of occupational therapy had developed and mastered the domain of functional ADL since the profession's inception in the early 1900s (Dunton, 1915; Hall, 1917). Occupational therapy emerged in response to the overmedicalization of patients without thought given to function in the community upon discharge (Barton, 1914, 1915). With its mission to help persons with disabilities to function optimally in self-care, home management, and work or school activities in their homes and community environments, occupational therapists had identified an unmet need in the health-care system and sought to build a profession around it (Hall & Buck, 1915).

In recent years, several other professions have begun to compete rigorously for the domain of functional ADL in response to three historical, socioeconomic events: (a) the Pew Health Professions Commission's (1993) call for a multiskilled therapist, (b) the World Health Organization's (1980) charge for rehabilitation services to become more functionally oriented, and (c) the emergence of managed care organizations that began to withhold reimbursement for services that did not enhance the health-care consumer's functional independence (Wolf & Gorman, 1996). As a result, rehabilitation professionals other than occupational therapists (e.g., physical therapists, nurses, speech-language pathologists, neuropsychologists) began to develop and use globally ADL scales, such as the Functional Independence Measure (Hamilton, Granger, Sherwin, Zielezny, & Tashman, 1987), to measure patients' functional outcomes (Ellenberg, 1996).

Physical Therapy

In the past 4 years, the attempt to assume functional ADL into practice guidelines has been increasingly observed within the profession of physical therapy. Traditionally, physical therapy has not defined function synonymously with ADL. In the physical therapy literature between 1980 and the present, function has been described as muscle function and strength (Brandsma, Schreuders, Birke, Piefer, & Oostendorp, 1995), spinal mobility (Schenk, 1996), gait function (Sanz et al., 1996), postural stability (Gill-Body, Popat, Parker, & Krebs, 1997), nerve function (Exelby, 1996), and musculoskeletal alignment and joint function

This chapter was previously published in the *American Journal of Occupational Therapy, 52,* 684–689. Copyright © 1998, American Occupational Therapy Association.

(Shamus & Shamus, 1997). Historically, areas of overlap with occupational therapy in which physical therapists defined function more similarly to ADL have included work activities needed on the job, as defined in work hardening settings (Delitto, Erhard, & Bowling, 1995); sports activities needed to return to athletics or leisure pursuit (McConnell, 1996); and functional transfers and ambulation aids (Johnson, Sayer, Hirn, & Durham, 1994). However, suggestions to consider the "limitations in role functioning such as duties in the home or at work" (Mossberg & McFarland, 1995, p. 1043) have increasingly appeared in physical therapy literature in the past several years.

In the American Physical Therapy Association's (APTA's, 1997) practice guidelines, the call to assume ADL and instrumental activities of daily living (IADL) is unambiguous. The APTA guidelines instruct physical therapists to assess and provide intervention regarding "assistive and adaptive devices" (p. 2-5); "community and work (job/school/play) integration or reintegration (including IADLs)" (p. 2-7); "environmental, home, and work (job/school/play) barriers" (p. 2-8); and "self-care and home management (including ADLs and IADLs)" (p. 2-22). The guidelines also state that when assessing any physical problem, the physical therapist should evaluate "the impairment or functional limitation during attempts to perform self-care, home management, community and work (job/school/play) integration or reintegration, and leisure tasks, movements, or activities" (p. 2-5). For example,

> Environmental, home, and work (job/school, play) barriers are the physical impediments that keep patients/clients from functioning optimally in their surroundings. The physical therapist uses the barriers tests and measures to identify any of a variety of possible impediments, including safety hazards (e.g., throw rugs, slippery surfaces), access problems (e.g., narrow doors, thresholds, high steps, absence of power doors or elevators), and home or office design (e.g., excessive distances to negotiate, multistory environments, sinks, bathrooms, counters, placement of controls or switches). The physical therapist uses these tests ... to suggest modifications to the environment (e.g., grab bars in the shower, ramps, raised toilet seats, increased lighting) that will allow the patient/client to improve in the home, workplace, and other settings. (p. 2-8)

> Self-care includes ADLs, such as bed mobility, transfers, gait, locomotion, developmental activity, dressing, grooming, bathing, eating, and toileting. Home management includes more complex IADLs such as maintaining a home, shopping, cooking, performing heavy household chores, managing money, driving a car or using public transportation, structured play (for infants and children), and negotiating school environments. (p. 2-22)

The APTA (1997) guidelines were written to articulate the profession's practices to its members and to health-care policymakers and reimbursement agencies. "The guide provides administrators and policy makers with the information they need to make decisions about the cost-effectiveness of physical therapy intervention" (p. 3-1) in comparison to professions sharing the same functional domain. Moreover, the guide states to reimbursement agents that the described physical therapy practices—"unless performed by a physical therapist—is not physical therapy; nor should it be represented or reimbursed as such" (p. 3-1). This limitation of the domain of functional ADL to physical therapists has enormous implications to the survival of the occupational therapy profession. Why would a managed care agent—who likely does not understand the difference between physical therapy and occupational therapy—reimburse occupational therapy services if they appear to duplicate physical therapy services? The APTA guidelines further provide ammunition for the Pew Health Professions Commission's (1993) call for multiskilled therapists.

Even more disconcerting is that physical therapists have begun to provide the research evidence demonstrating that physical therapy services enhance patients' functional ADL performance. Taub and Wolf (1997) found that physical therapy services helped nine patients 1 year after stoke to regain use of their affected arm to brush their teeth, comb their hair, retrieve and drink a glass of water, eat with a fork or spoon, and handwrite. These functional gains were fully maintained 2 years after the completion of the 2-week physical therapy treatment. Similarly, in a study of 801 long-term nursing home patients with stroke who received physical therapy (but not occupational therapy) services, Moseley (1996) found that physical therapy was significantly related to improved eating independence, transferring, and dressing. Carmick (1997) demonstrated how the use of neuro-muscular electrical stimulation and a dorsal wrist splint were effectively used to help a child with spastic hemiparesis to learn to independently tie his shoelaces without the need for any assistive device, including the splint. Martlew (1996) found that physical therapy service was significantly correlated with the ability to face loss of lifestyle, role, and social support in 10 hospice patients. Additionally, hospice patients reported that physical therapy services enabled them to become more functional (i.e., independently use a commode, spend small amounts of time shopping for personal needs, engage in limited gardening work). Yoshioka (1994) reported that hospice patients who received physical therapy services were more able to get in and out of bed or a chair, could toilet independently, could bathe with minimal assistance, and could independently self-feed.

Research demonstrating the efficacy of physical therapy services in the improvement of ADL and IADL places the onus on the occupational therapy profession to produce research demonstrating that its services are both more effective and cost-efficient than are physical therapy services that address ADL. Without such research support for occupational therapy practice, managed care agents may consider occupational therapy to be a duplication of physical therapy and exclude occupational therapy from their list of reimbursable services.

Nursing

Historically, nursing has shared an overlap with occupational therapy regarding self-care. Traditionally, nursing practice has been based on a model of care in which the role of the nurse was to attend to medical needs in a way that provided comfort, support, and education to patients and family members (Alsaro, 1994). ADL that fell within nursing's domain have included bathing, grooming, toileting, and dressing (Atkinson & Murray, 1990). The nurse's approach to patient self-care skills, however, has philosophically differed from that of the occupational therapist. Although the nursing model of care called for allowing the patient to become dependent on the nurse for the completion of self-care activities, occupational therapists have attempted to teach the patient to accomplish self-care activities as independently as possible using environmental adaptations (Brown, 1992; Kielhofner, 1995).

In the past several years, the relationship of the patient as a passive recipient and the nurse as an active health-care authority has changed with regard to the nurse's role in the teaching of self-care skills (Brooker & Butterwork, 1991). Members of the nursing profession have written extensively regarding a change in role from an active provider to a motivator or coach who uses environmental cues and adaptations to elicit the patient's independent self-care performance (Hoeffer, Rader, McKenzie, Lavelle, & Stewart, 1997; Thomas, 1994).

The nurses' use of environmental cues and adaptations marks a further change in the way that they perceive the patient's function as a factor of the environment. Monsen, Floyd, and Brookman (1992) suggested that the interaction of the person with the environment is essential to move the patient toward adaptation or greater integrity of function. Similarly, Hummelvoll and Barbosa da Silva (1994) proposed that:

> within this [new] model of care, understanding clients in relation to their life [and environmental] context becomes the focus [of nursing care], as well as trying to comprehend what effect suffering has on their [the clients'] ability to function. The relationship between nurse and client [should] consider such precepts as ... self-esteem, choice, meaning, values, and insight. (p. 7)

Moreover, nurses are beginning to perceive their role (particularly in nursing homes and long-term-care residences) as providers of occupation. Nolan, Grant, and Nolan (1995) suggested that "if the quality of care elderly patients receive is to improve, nursing staff must see the provision of activity as an integral part of their role and function" (p. 528). Sherry (1994) stated:

> When planning therapeutic interventions, we [nurses] need to consider how what we do will help our patients reconnect with family, friends, and, at least, some portion of their predisabiity lifestyle. We [nurses] have a responsibility to become familiar with each patient's work, interests, and hobbies, to better direct therapies to those motor skills and activities of relevance to individual quality of life. To the 76-year-old with a cerebrovascular accident, or stroke, who has never cooked a day in his life, learning kitchen skills will be meaningless, but if you teach him how to throw a softball to his 5-year-old grandson, you've helped him reconnect to his world. (p. 61)

The question must be asked: If nurses have identified occupation as an unmet need in elderly patients—a need that nurses believe that they should fulfill—why has occupational therapy not been provided first, and why are nurses not familiar enough with occupational therapy practice to make a referral to an occupational therapist?

Similarly, Antonson and Robertson (1993) completed a study of consumer-defined need in an elderly population living in the community and identified ADL (i.e., self-care, home management, maintaining a social network) as another unmet need that nurses could fulfill. Again, no mention of referrals to occupational therapists was made. Nurses have even developed an assessment for home safety (Ross & Bower, 1995)—as though home safety was another unmet need that has never been considered by another rehabilitation profession.

More disconcerting is that as health-care services have moved further into the community and nurses have transitioned into case management positions, nurses have fortuitously placed themselves as the gatekeeper of other rehabilitation services (Newell, 1996). If nurses are not aware of the role of occupational therapists, they will likely continue to identify occupation (e.g., home safety, self-care, home management, community mobility, social interaction) as unmet needs that nurses could adequately fulfill.

Neuropsychology

One further threat to occupational therapy's domain of functional ADL has recently emerged from the profession of neuropsychology. Historically, neuropsychologists have been involved in the determination of diagnostic validity and reliability of standardized tests (Diller, 1987; Vanderploeg, 1994). In the 1980s, advances in neurodiagnostic tests (e.g., computerized tomography, nuclear magnetic resonance imaging, positron emission tomography) have decreased the need for the neuropsychological examination as an aid to neurologic diagnosis (Trexler, 1987). Because neuropsychologists could not justify their existence in health care on the basis of diagnosis alone, they began to shift toward the development of rehabilitation strategies and behavior therapies (Vanderploeg, 1994).

As economic shifts in health care have continued to promote functionally oriented client outcomes, the neuropsychology literature has become increasingly populated with discussions about ways to participate in rehabilitation by addressing many of the same therapeutic concerns that have traditionally been part of occupational therapy's domain—functional ADL. Areas of rehabilitation that neuropsychologists have identified as inadequately addressed include IADL training, environmental–architectural management, functional cognitive difficulties, and visuoperceptual deficit training (Bradley, Welch, & Skilbeck, 1993; Wood, 1992).

One area that neuropsychologists have developed within their domain of concern is cognitive protheses in which computers are adapted to help persons with neurologic impairments to complete routine ADL in their home and work environments (Gianutsos, 1992). Bergman (1991a, 1991b) and Bergman and Kemmerer (1991) demonstrated how persons with traumatic brain injury (TBI) have benefitted from a customized computer system that wakes them up via a computer sound board; auditorily guides morning grooming and dressing routines; assists in the preparation of meals through written step-by-step recipe directions customized for specific memory deficit; prompts the completion of household chores, such as restocking the refrigerator every week; signals the time and day of appointments; documents telephone calls through a message center software program; and assists in money-management activities (e.g., writing checks, balancing a monthly budget).

Similarly, Cole and Dehdashti (l990a, 1990b, 1992) described how several patients with TBI have become independent in home management (i.e., paying bills, preparing meals, creating shopping lists, completing household chores) using a customized computer prosthetic system. Cole, Dehdashti, Petti, and Angert (1992) further articulated how a customized computer prosthetic system can be designed to consider the reorganization of a patient's workspace to accommodate physical and visuoperceptual impairment:

> The keyboard layout was modified to compensate for visual field restrictions in which the patient had difficulty accessing the function keys located on the top left of the keyboard. Through software reconfiguration the functions of these keys were reassigned to the numeric keypad to the right of the main keyboard area.... Visually neglected keys were also highlighted with colored tape to enhance the patient's visual attendance. Screen information was programmed to appear to the right of center to accommodate the patient's left neglect.... The menu structure was remodified to decrease the patient's confusion regarding multiple options by maintaining only those functions deemed necessary by the therapist and patient and deleting all others.... Menu bar font size was also permanently increased and color-coded to further enhance recall. (pp. 31-32)

Some occupational therapists have begun to create customized computer prosthetic systems designed to assist persons with neurologic impairment to be independent in their homes and work sites (O'Leary 1991; Stanciff, 1997). In fact, it would seem more logical for an occupational therapist trained in activity analysis, environmental adaptation, and ADL role resumption to create computer prosthetic systems than a neuropsychologist having no background in these. Yet, neuropsychologists are largely engaged in this clinical work and research. Neuropsychologists have aptly created a way to shift their professional role from diagnostician to clinician involved in the rehabilitation of functional ADL in the home and community (Gianutsos, 1992). And like physical therapists, neuropsychologists are quickly generating the research that demonstrates effectiveness for their clinical practices and providing justification for reimbursement from managed care organizations (Gauggel & Niemann, 1996).

Suggestions to Preserve Occupational Therapy's Domain of Function

Professions use varying strategies to defend their domain from competitors. One common strategy is to demonstrate expertise in a specific domain to the public and scientific community through the creation of educational standards and credentialing or licensure of its membership (MacDonald, 1995). A second common strategy is to provide efficacy studies that demonstrate the effectiveness, cost-efficiency, safety, and consumer satisfaction of the profession's clinical practices (Mosey, 1996). Although occupational therapists have skillfully maintained high entry-level educational standards and secured licensure for members in most states, members of the profession have not generated a body of research that supports the efficacy of occupational therapy practices.

Two dominant reasons likely account for occupational therapy's lack of clinically based efficacy studies: (a) The profession has not produced enough researchers at the doctoral and advanced master's degree level who have both the training to produce outcome studies and the skills to compete for highly sought-after research grant monies, and (b) entry-level education does not socialize occupational therapy students into the role of research participant. In this era of competition for managed health-care dollars, the profession can no longer afford to produce entry-level therapists whose sole role is to treat patients. Entry-level occupational therapy schools must socialize students to perceive themselves as research participants who can contribute to a research project through the generation of clinical questions and data collection. The gap between the academy and the clinic could be bridged by teams of clinicians, students, and academicians working together to implement efficacy studies. Level II fieldwork affiliations could be broadened to encompass student research experiences with skilled occupational therapy researchers who are in the stages of an efficacy study.

More importantly, members of the profession must unite to defend occupational therapy's domain against interlopers competing for limited health-care dollars. Although American Occupational Therapy Foundation (AOTF) university-affiliated research centers have produced some of the finest research to date, limiting funding to a small cadre of researchers fosters competition among the profession's resources at a time when the profession must capitalize on all of its available assets and underutilized reserves. AOTF funding of a large number of university-affiliated research centers is needed to generate a sufficient body of efficacy studies required to maintain occupational therapy's role in a tightening health-care system. This may be particularly important for less experienced researchers and academic research centers that require the initial financial support necessary to produce a body of pilot studies needed to access larger funding streams (outside of AOTF).

Alternatively, projects that foster collaboration—rather than competition—among the profession's most highly skilled researchers could be organized for the profession's benefit. For example, an AOTF think tank composed of the most talented occupational therapy researchers could be established to begin the generation of a large body of research that supports the profession's clinical practices. Several think tanks could be established in various regions of the country; such think tanks could use a rotating membership to pool a variety of talents in specialty areas within the profession. AOTF think tanks could also provide a unique training ground for novice researchers and newly minted doctoral-level members of the profession by providing the opportunity for novice researchers to work alongside experienced researchers. Positions within a think tank for new doctoral-level occupational therapists could be established as AOTF postdoctoral training, which is severely needed if occupational therapists are to learn the steps necessary to compete for research dollars with more experienced researchers from other professions whose grant funding histories have already been well established.

Additionally, research that supports the efficacy of occupational therapy practice must be disseminated to the very professionals and organizations that have the potential to limit occupational therapy service, particularly managed care organizations, nursing case managers, and hospital administrators. Dissemination of occupational therapy outcomes studies could be achieved by publishing articles in nonoccupational therapy journals and presenting papers at nonoccupational therapy conferences. The present challenge that occupational therapists face is to produce and disseminate a large body of outcomes research that demonstrates to managed care agents, nursing case managers, and hospital administrators that occupational therapy practices are more effective than those of other professions at returning persons to the home and community, with decreased hospital readmissions and decreased need for costly attendant care. The time has never been greater for the profession to demonstrate through scientific methods what occupational therapists have always known intuitively: that occupational therapists hold unique expertise in the domain of function, that occupational therapy practices are more effective and cost-efficient than that of other professions in assisting people to obtain optimal functioning in their environments, and that occupational therapy services produce high consumer satisfaction.

References

Abbott, A. (1988). *The system of professions: An essay on the division of expert labor.* Chicago: University of Chicago Press.

Alsaro, R. (1994). *Application of nursing process: A step-by-step guide* (3rd ed). Philadelphia: Lippincott.

American Physical Therapy Association. (1997). Guide to physical therapy practice [Special issue]. *Physical Therapy, 77*(11).

Antonson, M. G., & Robertson, C. M. (1993). A study of consumer-defined need amenable to community nursing intervention. *Journal of Advanced Nursing, 8,* 1617–1625.

Atkinson, J., & Murray, M. E. (1990). *Understanding the nursing process* (4th ed). New York: Macmillan.

Barton, G. E. (1914). A view of invalid occupation. *Trained Nurse and Hospital Review, 52,* 327–330.

Barton, G. E. (1915). Occupational therapy. *Trained Nurse and Hospital Review, 54,* 138–140.

Bergman, M. M. (1991a). Computer-enhanced self-sufficiency: Part 1. Creation and implementation of a text writer for an individual with traumatic brain injury. *Neuropsychology 5,* 17–23.

Bergman, M. M. (1991b). The necessity of a clinical perspective in the design of computer protheses. *Journal of Head Trauma Rehabilitation, 6,* 100–104.

Bergman, M. M., & Kemmerer, A. G. (1991). Computer-enhanced self-sufficiency: Part 2. Uses and subjective benefits of a text writer for an individual with traumatic brain injury. *Neuropsychology 5,* 25–28.

Bradley, V. A., Welch, J. L., & Skilbeck, C. E. (1993). *Cognitive retraining using microcomputers.* Hillsdale, NJ: Erlbaum.

Brandsma, J. W., Schreuders, T. A. R, Birke, J. A., Piefer, A., & Oostendorp, R. (1995). Manual muscle strength testing: Intraobserver and interobserver reliabilities for the intrinsic muscles of the hand. *Journal of Hand Therapy 8,* 185–190.

Brooker, C., & Butterwork, C. (1991). Working with families caring for a relative with schizophrenia: The evolving role of the community psychiatric nurse. *International Journal of Nursing Studies, 28,* 189–200.

Brown, J. (1992). Nurses or technicians? The impact of technology on oncology nursing. *Canadian Oncology Nursing Journal, 2,* 12–17.

Carmick, J. (1997). Case Report: Use of neuromuscular electrical stimulation and a dorsal wrist splint to improve the hand function of a child with spastic hemiparesis. *Physical Therapy, 77,* 661–671.

Cole, E., & Dehdashti, P. (1990a). Interface design as a prosthesis for an individual with brain injury. *Special Interest Group on Computers and Human Interaction Bulletin, 22*(1), 28–32.

Cole, E., & Dehdashti, P. (1990b, June). A multifunctional computer-based cognitive orthosis for a traumatic brain injured individual with cognitive deficits. *Proceedings of the Rehabilitation Engineering Society of North America, 29*–30.

Cole, E., & Dehdashti, P. (1992, June). Prosthetic software for individuals with mild traumatic brain injury: A case study of client and therapist. *Proceedings of the Rehabilitation Engineering Society of North America,* 170–172.

Cole, E., Dehdashti, P., Petti, L. A., & Angert, M. (1992, October). Computer software as an orthosis for brain injury. *Proceedings of the National Institutes of Health Neural Prosthesis Workshop,* 31–32.

Delitto, A., Erhard, R. E., & Bowling, R. W. (1995). A treatment-based classification approach to low-back syndrome: Identifying and staging patients for conservative treatment. *Physical Therapy 75,* 470-489.

Diller, W. R. (1987). Neuropsychological rehabilitation. In M. J. Meier, A. L. Benton, & L. Diller (Eds.), *Neurological rehabilitation* (pp. 3–17). New York: Guilford.

Dunton, W. R., Jr. (1915). *Occupational therapy: A manual for nurses.* Philadelphia: Saunders.

Ellenberg, D. B. (1996). Outcomes research: The history, debate, and implications for the field of occupational therapy. *American Journal of Occupational Therapy, 50,* 435–441.

Exelby, L. (1996). Peripheral mobilizations with movement. *Manual Therapy 1*(3), 118–126.

Gauggel, S., & Niemann, T. (1996). Evaluation of a short-term computer-assisted training programme for the remediation of attentional deficits after brain injury: A preliminary study. *International Journal of Rehabilitation Research, 19,* 229–239.

Gianutsos, R. (1992). The computer in cognitive rehabilitation: It's not just a tool anymore. *Journal of Head Trauma Rehabilitation, 7*(3), 26–35.

Gill-Body, K. M., Popat, R. A., Parker, S. W., & Krebs, D. E. (1997). Rehabilitation of balance in two patients with cerebellar dysfunction. *Physical Therapy 77,* 534–552.

Hall, H. J. (1917). Remunerative occupations for the handicapped. *Modern Hospital, 8,* 383–386.

Hall, H. J., & Buck, M. C. (1915). *The work of our hands: A study of occupations for invalids.* New York: Moffat & Yard.

Hamilton, B. B. Granger, C. V., Sherwin, F. S., Zielezny, M., & Tashman, J. S. (1987). A uniform national data system for medical rehabilitation. In M. J. Fuhrer (Ed.), *Rehabilitation outcomes: Analysis and measurement* (pp. 137–147). Baltimore: Brookes.

Hoeffer, B., Rader, J., McKenzie, D., Lavelle, M., & Stewart, B. (1997). Reducing aggressive behavior during bathing cognitively impaired nursing home residents. *Journal of Gerontological Nursing, 23*(5), 16–23, 53–59.

Hummelvoll, J. K., & Barbosa da Silva, A. (1994). A holistic-existential model for psychiatric nursing. *Perspectives in Psychiatric Care, 30*(2), 7–14.

Johnson, J. H., Sayer, M. A., Hirn, G., & Durham, N. C. (1994). Referral patterns to physical therapy in elderly hospitalized for acute medical illness. *Physical and Occupational Therapy in Geriatrics, 12*(2), 1–12.

Kielhofner, G. (Ed.). (1995). *A model of human occupation: Theory and application* (2nd ed.). Baltimore: Williams & Wilkins.

MacDonald, K. M. (1995). *The sociology of the professions.* London: Sage.

Martlew, B. (1996). What do you let the patient tell you? *Physiotherapy, 82,* 558–565.

McConnell, J. (1996). Management of patellofemoral problems: *Manual Therapy 1*(2), 60–66.

Monsen, R. B., Floyd, R. L., & Brookman, J. C. (1992). Stress-coping-adaptation: Concepts for nursing. *Nursing Forum, 27*(4), 27–32.

Moseley, C. B. (1996). Rehabilitation effectiveness among long-term nursing home stroke residents. *Physical and Occupational Therapy in Geriatrics, 14*(4), 27–41.

Mosey, A. C. (1996). *Applied scientific inquiry in the health professions: An epistemological orientation* (2nd ed.). Bethesda, MD: American Occupational Therapy Association.

Mossberg, K. A., & McFarland, C. (1995). Initial health status of patients at outpatient physical therapy clinics. *Physical Therapy 75,* 1043–1053.

Newell, M. (1996). *Using nursing case management to improve health outcomes.* Gaithersburg, MD: Aspen.

Nolan, M., Grant, G., & Nolan, J. (1995). Busy doing nothing: Activity and interaction levels amongst differing populations of elderly patients. *Journal of Advanced Nursing, 22,* 528–538.

O'Leary, S. (1991). Computer access considerations for patients with traumatic brain injury. *Journal of Head Trauma Rehabilitation, 6*(3), 89–91.

Pew Health Professions Commission. (1993). *Health professions for the future: Schools in service to the nation.* San Francisco: Author.

Ross, F. M., & Bower, P. (1995). Standardized assessment for elderly people (SAFE)—A feasibility study in district nursing. *Journal of Clinical Nursing, 4,* 303–310.

Sanz, M. C. M., Aparicio, A. V., Ballabriga, S. N., Moreno, E. C., Garcia, T. M., & Tolon, J. G. (1996). Electromyographic activity in the upper limb using the Brunnstrom method. *Rehabilitation, 30,* 327–338.

Schenk, R. (1996). Manual therapy rounds. A combined approach to lumbar examination. *Journal of Manual and Manipulative Therapy, 4*(2), 77–80.

Shamus, J. L., & Shamus, E. C. (1997). A taping technique for the treatment of acromioclavicular joint sprains: A case study. *Journal of Orthopaedic and Sports Physical Therapy, 25,* 390–394.

Sherry, D. (1994). Activities of daily living: Rehabilitation's three Rs. *Home Healthcare Nurse, 12*(6), 61.

Stancliff, B. L. (1997). OT uses computers to reach mental health clients. *OT Practice, 2*(11), 15–18.

Taub, F., & Wolf, S. L. (1997). Constraint induced movement techniques to facilitate upper extremity use in stroke patients. *Topics in Stroke Rehabilitation, 3*(4), 38–61.

Thomas, L. H. (1994). A comparison of the verbal interactions of qualified nurses and nursing auxiliaries in primary, team, and functional nursing wards. *International Journal of Nursing Studies, 31,* 231–244.

Trexler, L. E. (1987). Neuropsychological rehabilitation in the United States. In M. J. Meier, A. L. Benton, & L. Diller (Eds.) *Neurological rehabilitation* (pp. 437–460). New York: Guilford.

Vanderploeg, R. D. (1994). Interview and testing: The data-collection phase of neuropsychological evaluations. In R. D. Vanderploeg (Ed.), *Clinician's guide to neuropsychological assessment* (pp. 2–42). Hillsdale, NJ: Erlbaum.

Wolf, L. F, & Gorman, J. K. (1996). New directions and developments in managed care financing. *Health Care Financing Journal, 17*(3), 1–5.

Wood, R. L. (1992). A neurobehavioral approach to brain injury rehabilitation. In N. von Steinbuchel, D. Y. von Cramon, & E. Poppel (Eds.), *Neuropsychological rehabilitation* (pp. 55–65). New York: Springer-Verlag.

World Health Organization. (1980). *International classification of impairments, disabilities and handicaps: A manual of classification related to consequences of disease.* Geneva, Switzerland: Author.

Yoshioka, H. (1994). Rehabilitation for the terminal cancer patient. *American Journal of Physical Medicine and Rehabilitation, 73,* 199–206.

Our Mandate for the New Millennium: Evidence-Based Practice

2000 ELEANOR CLARKE SLAGLE LECTURE

CHAPTER 60

MARGO B. HOLM,
PHD, OTR/L, FAOTA, ABDA

The health-care environment of the past quarter-century went through numerous evolutionary processes that affected how occupational therapy services were provided. The last iterations of these processes included requests for the evidence that supported what we were doing. This year's Eleanor Clarke Slagle Lecture (a) examines the strength of the evidence associated with occupational therapy interventions—what we do and how we do it—(b) raises dilemmas we face with our ethical principles when some of our practices are based on limited evidence, and (c) proposes a framework of continued competency to advance the evidence base of occupational therapy practice in the new millennium.

This chapter was previously published in the *American Journal of Occupational Therapy, 54,* 575–585. Copyright © 2000, American Occupational Therapy Association.

If the next several patients you were to see asked you, "How do you know that what you do and how you do it really works?" would you be able to provide them with research evidence similar to that found in the pamphlets that come with your prescription medications? The evidence would include a summary of research on each occupational therapy intervention option you are considering. It would delineate the percentage of patients who benefited from each option and the percentage of those who did not. It would also clearly describe *what* each intervention consists of and *how* each is to be implemented for yielding the best outcomes for particular patient populations. Additionally, the data that support the recommended frequency and duration for each intervention would be included. It is unlikely that you could provide such evidence today. Will you be able to provide the evidence by 2010? As professionals, we have gone on record committing ourselves to evidence-based practice in Principle 2.B of our *Occupational Therapy Code of Ethics*, which states, "Occupational therapy personnel shall fully inform the service recipients of the nature, risks, and potential outcomes of any interventions" (American Occupational Therapy Association [AOTA], 1994, p. 1037). *Can we meet this commitment?*

In this year's Slagle Lecture, I will use a common definition of evidence-based practice and discuss why it has meaning for the context in which our profession finds itself today. First, I will use a five-level measuring stick (see Table 60.1) to examine the strength of the evidence or the lack of evidence associated with occupational therapy interventions—*what* we do and *how* we do it—the same measuring stick that is also being used by referring physicians, educational services administrators, and health maintenance organization purchasers of services as they appraise our evidence. Second, I will raise throughout the lecture dilemmas that face us when we try to reconcile some of the principles in our Code of Ethics with the practice of occupational therapy based on limited evidence. Third, I will use the framework of continued competency to discuss what is needed to practice occupational therapy, based on research evidence, in the new millennium.

Evidence-Based Practice

As we are all aware, the health-care environment of the past quarter-century underwent numerous evolutionary processes that greatly affected *how* occupational therapy services were provided! For example, in many practice settings, we were

Table 60.1. Hierarchy of Levels of Evidence for Evidence-Based Practice

Level	Description
I	Strong evidence from at least one systematic review of multiple well-designed randomized controlled trials
II	Strong evidence from at least one properly designed randomized controlled trial of appropriate size
III	Evidence from well-designed trials without randomization, single group pre–post, cohort, time series, or matched case-controlled studies
IV	Evidence from well-designed nonexperimental studies from more than one center or research group
V	Opinions of respected authorities, based on clinical evidence, descriptive studies, or reports of expert committees

Note. From "Evidence-Based Everything," by A. Moore, H. McQuay, & J.A.M. Gray (Eds.), 1995, *Bandolier, 1*(12), p. 1. Copyright 1995 by Bandolier. Reprinted with permission.

confronted with prospective payment reimbursement, capitation models, reduced staffing ratios, and job losses. Additionally, we are now being judged by the functional outcomes our patients achieve. The fact that patient outcomes are improved with occupational therapy services is no longer sufficient to justify our services, unless we can also explain *what* we do and *how* we do it so that others can replicate our interventions and achieve similar outcomes with comparable patients with like needs, wants, and expectations. The emphasis on justifying our practice patterns has been reflected in the increasing numbers of requests for the research-based evidence that supports what we are doing.

So, what is evidence-based practice? It has been defined as "integrating individual clinical expertise" with the "conscientious, explicit and judicious use of current best evidence in making decisions about the care of individual patients" (Sackett, Rosenberg, Gray, Haynes, & Richardson, 1996, p. 71). Thus, in our Code of Ethics we have also affirmed our commitment to evidence-based practice in Principle 3.D, "Occupational therapy personnel shall perform their duties on the basis of accurate and current information" (AOTA, 1994, p. 1037). *Can we meet this commitment?*

Gray (1997) described the evolution of evidence-based practice as progressing from providing services as efficiently and cheaply as possible, to "doing things better," then to "*doing things right*," and finally to "doing the right things" (p. 17). He has also proposed that evidence-based practice for the new millennium must focus on "doing the right things right" (p. 17). In other words, the necessary shift to the evidence-based practice of occupational therapy will require us to justify *why* we do *what* we do in addition to *how* we do it. Of course, Gray's proposal implies that for any given patient population, we *know* what is "right" and, furthermore, that we *know* the "right" way to do what we do. Silverman (1998) put it another way: "How do we go about drawing a line between 'knowing' and 'doing' … and when do we know

enough about the … consequences of our interventions to proceed with confidence" (p. 5)?

As occupational therapy practitioners, we have always used multiple sources of evidence, or "ways of knowing," to guide our "doing," including evidence derived from the oral tradition, our own beliefs and values, patient preferences, assessment data, the opinions of experts, and research evidence (Brown, 1999; Bury & Mead, 1998). Historically, our evidence resided within individual practitioners and was handed down from practitioner to practitioner; thus, it was not accessible to all. With the advent of occupational therapy textbooks and journals, opinions of experts and research evidence have been published and are now accessible to all. Although each source of evidence has inherent value for some aspect of our practice, no single source of evidence, or even all of them together, enables us to know enough to proceed to our "doing" with absolute confidence.

Information Overload and Hierarchies of Evidence

Our level of confidence in our clinical decisions should be based, in part, on the strength of the evidence we use. Fortunately, the evidence that is available has been expanding at an exponential rate; however, this expansion has created two problems: (a) There is too much evidence to sift through, and (b) the quantity of evidence does not equal quality of evidence. Shenk (1997) addressed the problem of expansion when he noted, "Just as fat has replaced starvation as [the] number one dietary concern, information overload has replaced information scarcity" (p. 29). An editorial in the *Journal of the American Medical Association* (*JAMA*) expressed concerns about the second problem: the quality of the evidence in which we may place our confidence. Rennie (1986) lamented that publication alone does not mean quality. The author noted wryly that there is

> no study too fragmented, no hypothesis too trivial, no literature citation too biased or too egotistical, no design too warped, no methodology too bungled, no presentation of results too inaccurate and too contradictory, no analysis too self-serving, no argument too circular, no conclusion too trifling or too unjustified, and no grammar and syntax too offensive for a paper to end up in print. (p. 2391)

It is because of the glut of evidence and concerns about quality control that ranking systems, or hierarchies, were developed to rate the strength of the research designs being used to generate the evidence (Moore, McQuay, & Gray, 1995; Sackett, Haynes, & Tugwell, 1985; Sackett, Richardson, Rosenberg, & Haynes, 1997). These *hierarchies of evidence* were designed to help practitioners sort through the options and select the "current best evidence" available to guide decisions about *what* to do and *how* to do it for a particular patient or patient population.

Examples of Occupational Therapy Evidence

Although evidence hierarchies vary somewhat in their rigor, the rank order of the levels of evidence is similar, with the best evidence ranked at Level I and less convincing evidence ranked at lower levels (see Table 60.1). Each level represents the research strategies that were used to structure the investigations. At the top of the hierarchy are those designs deemed (a) least vulnerable to bias, (b) more generalizable, and (c) more likely to yield patient outcomes that can confidently be attributed to the intervention being studied (see Table 60.1). Therefore, if it is current, and available, you want the "best" evidence, which is a Level I research design. The evidence hierarchy, or measuring stick, that I will use has five levels (Moore et al., 1995). At the top of the hierarchy, or Level I, are studies in which we, and those we must convince about the efficacy and effectiveness of occupational therapy, should have the most confidence. They are also the studies that we must strive to plan, implement, and publish.

Level I Evidence

Level I studies are defined as "strong evidence from at least one systematic review of multiple well-designed randomized controlled trials" (Moore et al., 1995, p. 1). Level I systematic reviews usually take one of two forms: (a) meta-analytic studies or (b) systematic reviews. Both methods (a) require adherence to rigorous procedures, with well-defined study criteria for inclusion, and (b) are usually restricted to studies that use randomized controlled clinical trials. Additionally, both methods use statistical analyses to evaluate the data from each study and the studies in total.

So, what does this mean for everyday practice? Picture yourself in this scenario: You work on a neurorehabilitation unit and a new medical resident asks you, "Why does my patient need both a physical therapy exercise program and occupational therapy? What evidence do you have that cooking tasks, adapted checkers games, and those other things you do make any difference in upper-extremity motor performance?" An appropriate response would be the provision of *current best evidence* in the form of a Level I study. Occupational therapy researchers Lin, Wu, Tickle-Degnen, and Coster (1997) carried out a meta-analytic study of 17 articles, including four articles on studies of patients with neurological impairments. They found that in studies designed to improve the motor performance of patients with neurological impairments, the outcomes were significantly better when the patients' exercises were embedded into everyday tasks than when the patients only performed rote exercises. This study is just one example of evidence that you can use to support *what* we do and *how* we can do it to yield improvements in patients with neurological impairments and upper-extremity motor deficits.

What about Level I current best evidence for other areas of practice? A meta-analytic study of the efficacy of sensory integration treatment was recently conducted by an occupational therapy researcher (Vargas & Camilli, 1998). This rigorous meta-analysis of 22 studies considered every possible influence on the outcomes of sensory integration treatment, including (a) adherence to sensory integration treatment criteria, (b) total treatment hours, (c) diagnosis and age, (d) design and sampling, (e) number of outcomes and measurement categories, (f) professional affiliation of the researchers, (g) geographic location of the studies, and (h) publication years. The results of the study, however, provide us with a stark reminder of the difference between preferred practice and evidence-based practice.

Many therapists prefer to use a sensory integration approach to intervention with both children and adults. But *current* best evidence, namely those studies published since 1983, indicated "an absence of sensory integration effects in recent studies and the equivalence of sensory integration and alternative treatments," neither of which yielded improvement in the sensory–perceptual area (Vargas & Camilli, 1998, p. 197). In other words, the experimental groups' outcomes following sensory integration interventions were no better than those of the control groups that received no treatment, regardless of the outcome being measured. When compared with alternative types of treatment, outcomes of the sensory integration groups were equivalent but not very effective. Although we may *prefer* to ignore the findings of this study, our actions would be in conflict with Principle 2.B of our Code of Ethics in which we commit to "fully inform the service recipients of the nature, risks, and potential outcomes of any interventions" (AOTA, 1994, p. 1037), especially if their effectiveness is in question. Tickle-Degnen (1998) developed excellent sample dialogues for communicating mixed or nonsupportive evidence about proposed interventions to patients.

The failure of these studies to demonstrate the superiority of sensory integration techniques over no treatment does not negate the possibility that (a) the outcome measures were insensitive to the changes produced, (b) the wrong outcomes were measured, or (c) the effects were obscured by the application of sensory integration techniques to inappropriate populations. Another possibility is that the statistical power, or sample size, may have been inadequate. Ottenbacher and Maas (1999) pointed out that often the effect sizes in our studies, or the magnitude of the difference between the experimental and control groups, indicate that our interventions do yield clinically worthwhile differences. However, we often do not have large enough samples to reject the null hypotheses, and therefore we conclude wrongly that our interventions are not effective (Mulligan, 1998; Ottenbacher & Maas, 1999; Vargas & Camilli, 1998).

Just as our practices change over time, so too should the evidence base of our practice. It will be important to revisit the evidence to see whether new sensory integration interventions being used in clinics and promoted in workshops, new measures such as those related to the family's perspective suggested by Cohn and Cermak (1998), or larger sample sizes can provide better support for *what* we do and *how* we do it when using sensory integration interventions.

Now, put yourself into this second scenario: The budget administrator in your hospital is questioning the use of life skills groups with a chronic mental health population. You do a computer search, and using the Cochrane Database of Systematic Reviews (www.update-software.com/cochrane/cochrane-frame.html), you find a review entitled, "Life Skills Programmes for People With Chronic Mental Illness" (Nicol, Robertson, & Connaughton, 1999). The review examined life skills programs that focused on interpersonal skills, self-care, time management, financial management, nutrition, and household skills as well as use of community resources. Unfortunately, only two randomized clinical trials were found that met the criteria, and both were conducted more than 15 years ago. Even though evidence was sparse and not what one would call current, it was the best evidence available, and the reviewers proceeded to conclude that:

> there is next to no evidence that life skills training programmes are of value to those with serious mental illnesses … [and] until such time as any evidence of benefit is available it is questionable whether recipients of care should be put under pressure to attend such programmes. (Nicol et al., p. 10/21)

The reviewers went on to state, "If life skills training is to continue as a part of rehabilitation programmes a large, well designed, conducted and reported pragmatic randomized trial is an urgent necessity" (p. 2/21), but then they added, "There may even be an argument for stating that maintenance of current practice, outside of a randomize d trial, is unethical" (p. 2/21).

Providing this current best evidence for life skills training with a chronic mental health population to any budget administrator could pose a threat or an opportunity. The threat comes if only the reviewers' *conclusions* are noted, namely that occupational therapy life skills groups are ineffective for chronic mental health populations at best and unethical at worst. If we provide no new evidence that counteracts the findings of the Cochrane reviewers, then it could be implied that we are in tacit agreement with the recommendation. If we take this stance, however, the threat could be generalized to other settings or populations in which life skills programs are used. We then would have to ask ourselves the next logical question: "If there is no evidence that life skills programs make any difference with chronic mental health populations (with whom they have been used since time immemorial), what evidence is there that life skills programs are effective with developmental disability or traumatic brain injury populations?" Our opportunity lies in responding to the reviewers' *recommendation* to design, carry out, and report the findings from a

large, randomized controlled trial, a design that is also known as a Level II study in our evidence hierarchy. This is the next level of evidence.

Level II Evidence

The evidence needed to confirm or reject the Cochrane database findings about life skills programs is not found in the ivory towers of universities but, rather, in occupational therapy clinics and community-based practices. The study suggested by the Cochrane reviewers was a Level II research design, which consists of "strong evidence from at least one properly designed randomized controlled trial of appropriate size" (Moore et al., 1995, p. 1). For example, to conduct a randomized controlled trial in a clinic, this would mean that after a practitioner has collected baseline performance data on a patient, any patient who meets the criteria already established for participation in a life skills program would be randomly assigned to one of three groups: (a) a control group or attention group (no occupational therapy), (b) an alternative therapy group (e.g., a social work group that talks about life skills), or (c) an occupational therapy life skills group. Typical y, randomized clinical trials include large numbers of participants. These participants can be accrued either slowly over time at one site or more quickly through collaboration among multiple clinical sites. The latter, multisite studies can dampen the spirits of even the most enthusiastic of researchers because of scheduling problems, budgeting issues, and philosophical differences. The problems with randomized control trials at single or multiple sites can be ove rcome by planning carefully, educating therapists in systematic data collection methods, ensuring that research intervention protocols are delivered in a standardized manner, and monitoring adherence to research procedures.

The common argument against doing randomized trials is the belief that patients who are randomized to the control or placebo conditions will not benefit or progress if they do not participate in occupational therapy treatment, for example, the sensory integration interventions or life skills groups. However, Portney and Watkins (1993) noted that:

> in situations where the efficacy of a treatment is being questioned because current knowledge is inadequate, it may actually be more ethical to take the time to make appropriate controlled comparisons than to continue clinical practice using potentially ineffective techniques. (p. 29)

Three examples of Level II randomized controlled occupational therapy clinical trials, which accurately followed intent-to-treat principles—in other words, carried out their statistical analyses on the basis of the number of participants that entered the study, not only those who completed it—were published in *JAMA* (Ray et al., 1997), *Lancet* (Close et al., 1999), and the *Journal of the American Geriatrics Society (JAGS)* (Cummings et al., 1999). These studies examined the impact of occupational therapy interventions on falls reduction among nursing home residents and community-based frail older adults. In the large multicenter nursing home study published in *JAMA*, the proportion of recurrent fallers in the experimental facilities was significantly less (p = .03) than in the control facilities (Ray et al., 1997). In addition to the physician and nursing components, the occupational therapy interventions consisted of wheelchair positioning and maintenance and resident and staff instruction on safe transfers.

In the study of community-based older adults with a history of falls published in *Lancet*, the experimental group had significantly fewer falls (p = .05) at the 12-month follow-up than the control group. The experimental group had received a home visit and a follow-up phone call by an occupational therapist that focused on home safety and modification of the home environment (Close et al., 1999).

In the study published in the *JAGS*, community-based older adults who presented to hospital emergency rooms after falls were randomly assigned to either a post–acute event occupational therapy intervention group or a control group. The occupational therapy intervention consisted of home safety recommendations, education, and minor home modifications. At the 12-month follow-up, the risk of falling, the risk of recurrent falls, and the odds of being admitted to a hospital were significantly lower in the occupational therapy group than in the control group (Cummings et al., 1999).

These three studies provide strong Level II evidence of the efficacy of occupational therapy for falls reduction among nursing home residents and community-based frail older adults. These are but three examples of Level II studies that you can provide to nursing home administrators, outpatient rehabilitation coordinators, or emergency room physicians as supporting evidence that *what* we do and *how* we do it can make a significant positive difference to older adults at risk for falling.

Level III Evidence

However, what happens when Level I and Level II studies are not available? According to Gray (1997), "The absence of excellent evidence does not make evidence-based decision making impossible; in this situation, what is required is the best *evidence available*, not the best evidence possible" (p. 61). For example, picture yourself in this third scenario: The new physiatrist at your rehabilitation facility came from a setting where the occupational therapists used Bobath axial rolls for patients with stroke who had hemiplegia and shoulder subluxation, and she writes specific orders for their use. You are not convinced that the axial rolls work very well, and you prefer the type of sling that you have been using for the past 10 years—the same one that your physical disabilities professor preferred. In addition, the axial rolls seem to increase your patients' shoulder pain. Even though you found no Level I or Level II studies in your literature search, you located four studies that meet Level III criteria (Brooke, Lateur, Diana-Rigby, & Questad, 1991; Hurd, Farrell, & Waylonis, 1974; Williams, Taffs, & Minuk, 1988; Zorowitz, Idank, Ikai, Hughes, & Johnston, 1995).

Level III studies derive their "evidence from well-designed trials without randomization, single group pre–post, cohort, time series or matched case-controlled studies" (Moore et al., 1995, p. 1). Although you are pleased to find that the best evidence available indicated that the Bobath axial roll made no difference, or even increased shoulder displacement (Zorowitz et al., 1995), you also find that the sling that you prefer fared no better. In fact, you find that the evidence for use of an axial roll, a sling, or a wheelchair trough for reducing shoulder displacement is mixed at best, and some of the most recent evidence indicates that the sling you prefer actually increases vertical asymmetry (Brooke et al., 1991). At that moment, Principle 1.C of our Code of Ethics comes to mind—"occupational therapy personnel shall take all reasonable precautions to avoid harm to the recipient of services" (AOTA, 1994, p. 1037)—only now its relevance has new meaning. You have learned two lessons from your search: (a) You are appalled to learn that your preferred intervention may have done harm, and (b) you have learned that although you are not from a state that requires continuing education for licensure, the relevance of one aspect of our Code of Ethics (Principle 3.C) is now clearer: "Occupational therapy personnel shall take responsibility for maintaining competence by participating in professional development and educational activities" (AOTA, 1994, p. 1037).

Next, imagine that you are an occupational therapy practitioner employed by a skilled nursing facility. You frequently encounter new residents who qualify for rehabilitation services because of a 3-day hospital stay. However, because they have a primary diagnosis of dementia of the Alzheimer type and severe memory impairments, their ability to benefit from any rehabilitation is frequently challenged. A Level III study combining occupational therapy compensatory strategies and behavioral techniques featured in *JAGS* (Rogers et al., 1999) may have the type of evidence you are looking for. The study found that during a 1-week occupational therapy skill intervention condition using compensatory strategies and a structured environment, the residents with dementia significantly increased the proportion of time they engaged in self-dressing and significantly decreased their disruptive behaviors compared with the usual care. During the 3-week occupational therapy habit training condition that followed, residents were able to maintain their gains. Additionally, during both occupational therapy intervention conditions, the use of labor-intensive physical assists decreased significantly. A Level III study such as this can be used to provide fiscal intermediaries with supporting evidence that *what* we do and *how* we do it can benefit even nursing home residents who are severely disabled and cognitively impaired.

The next Level III study could be helpful if you find yourself in the following scenario: You work for a private therapy company that provides services to several group homes for adults with developmental disabilities. The owner of the homes tells you that he had been "surfing the Net" and had found the Cochrane Database Systematic Review on the ineffectiveness of life skills groups. Given the conclusions of the reviewers, he wants to know what evidence you have that indicates that the life skills groups yo u a re implementing are effective. You tell him that you also read the review and point out that applying the findings from the Cochrane review to his clients might not be in their best interest because the participants in the studies described in the review had chronic mental illness and were in hospital-based programs—a population very different from his community-based clients with developmental disabilities. You explain that since reading the review, you have been using the methods and outcomes described in a Level III study by Neistadt and Marques (1984), whose participants also had developmental disabilities. You then show him the data you have collected over the past 3 months, documenting the specific life skills groups each client in his facilities has participated in as well as their outcomes. You note that all clients have made gains.

A fourth example of a Level III study pertains to school-based practice and pediatrics wherein occupational therapy practitioners are frequently associated with *fine motor* skills training. This association with fine motor skills is not surprising, though, because when you use the key words fine motor to search through the 10 million journal articles indexed in MEDLINE, 1 of the 10 subject headings you are presented with, and the only profession, is *occupational therapy*. A Level III intervention study by Case-Smith et al. (1998) found that preschoolers with fine motor delays who received direct occupational therapy services improved their fine motor skills and related functional performance significantly, and the rate of gain was greater than that of their peers who had no fine motor delays (p. 788). The next time you need to convince your educational services administrator about the benefits that occupational therapy can offer to preschool populations with fine motor delays, bring this supporting evidence, along with a Level IV study by Mc Hale and Cermak (1992).

Level IV Evidence

According to Moore et al. (1995), Level IV studies consist of "evidence from well-designed non-experimental studies from more than one center or research group" (p. 1). Sometimes our inquiry into the need for, or effectiveness of, an intervention begins with a multisite descriptive study. The Level IV study by McHale and Cermak (1992) described the time allocated to fine motor activities and tasks in six elementary school classrooms. Minute-by-minute data collection indicated that 30 percent to 60 percent of the day was dedicated to fine motor tasks, with writing tasks predominating. This study provides the context and relevance of occupational therapy interventions for preschoolers with fine motor delays—preschoolers who will soon become elementary school students.

Level V Evidence

The lowest level of the hierarchy of evidence is Level V, which is defined as "opinions of respected authorities, based on clinical evidence, descriptive studies or reports of expert committees" (Moore et al., 1995, p. 1). Unlike Level IV descriptive studies, Level V studies do not need to be from multiple centers or research groups. Studies that use qualitative designs are also identified as Level V studies. One such study published recently in the *Occupational Therapy Journal of Research (OTJR)* (Bye, 1998) involved in-depth interviews of therapists who worked with terminally ill patients. For a profession that is used to facilitating functional gains in patients rather than in preparing them for death, this Level V study provides a framework for guiding the practice of occupational therapy in end-of-life care. The study had as its core aim "Affirming Life: Preparing for Death" (Bye, 1998, p. 8). Interventions focused on "building against loss," achieving "normality within a changed reality," regaining "client control" over daily routines and activities, providing "supported and safe" environments, and finding "closure in some aspects of their lives" (p. 8). It is Level V studies like this one that enable researchers to describe and probe aspects of our practice that cannot be accomplished with Level I and Level II studies and simultaneously pave the way for future research. Level V evidence also can help us define new programs that have the potential to benefit populations not typically associated with rehabilitation or occupational therapy and point the way to new areas of inquiry and program development.

Also included in Level V evidence are the opinions of respected authorities. Although all the other examples of evidence I have cited were based on research, or from external sources, Level V evidence allows for the evidence *residing within the practitioner.* When we use opinion-based evidence, we are grounding our clinical reasoning and therapeutic decisions and actions in the advice of experts, established practices, continuing education information, or reference texts by known leaders in the field (Brown, 1999; Bury & Mead, 1998). It is not unusual for fieldwork students, entry-level practitioners, and practitioners changing practice areas to rely primarily on the opinions of master practitioners, supervisors, or therapists with specialty certification. It is also not unusual for us to continue to provide interventions that are based on the wisdom of the "form in the file drawer," which represents established practices that have "always been done that way."

When we use Level V evidence based on clinical experience and expertise to guide decision-making with our patients, we must be aware of how our own values, beliefs, and biases influence our decisions. In a study of physicians' perceptions of their patients' preferences, patients were asked to rate four preferred courses of action for a life-threatening illness, and their physicians were asked to predict their patients' preferences as well as to state their preferences for themselves. Unfortunately the physicians' predictions of their patients' preferences more closely matched their own preferences than those of their patients (Schneiderman, Kaplan, Pearlman, & Teetzel, 1993). It is because of the potential power associated with clinical expertise that ethicists Lidz and Meisel (1983) remind us that we must not view the decision-making process with patients as one of merely persuading the patient to accept what we believe to be the proper course.

However, it is precisely our clinical experience, clinical expertise, and clinical reasoning that Sackett et al. (1996) referred to in their definition of evidence-based practice when they speak of "*integrating individual clinical expertise* [italics added]" with the "use of current best evidence in making decisions about the care of individual patients" (p. 71). I would like to emphasize that if we are to practice evidence-based occupational therapy, evidence can only be used to inform clinical expertise, not replace it, and clinical expertise must be used in conjunction with the best available evidence, not substituted for it (Bury & Mead, 1998; Sackett et al., 1996).

We have made a commitment in our Code of Ethics to "collaborate with service recipients or their surrogate(s) in determining goals and priorities throughout the intervention process" (AOTA, 1994, p. 1037). It is in the fulfillment of this commitment that patient and practitioner together must consider the evidence before them and make informed decisions about the occupational therapy interventions that will best meet the patient's needs, wants, and expectations. *Can we meet this commitment?*

Collective Evidence

I have applied a five-level measuring stick to some of our evidence and cited examples of evidence associated with each level. But what about the strength of our collective evidence as a scholarly profession? To get a snapshot of the bigger picture, I applied the same hierarchy to all articles published in *OTJR* for the past 5 years (1995–1999). I chose the *OTJR* because it is "devoted to the advancement of knowledge through scientific methods" (Abreu, Peloquin, & Ottenbacher, 1998, p. 757). As you can see in Table 60.2, over the past 5 years, the preponderance of the evidence in our research journal was at Level V, which is defined as "opinions of respected authorities, based on clinical evidence, descriptive studies or reports of expert committees" (Moore et al., 1995, p. 1). Obviously, a journal must receive manuscripts before they can be published. As our collective research competence improves, so will the levels of evidence that we are able to generate and submit for publication.

Evidence-Based Practice and Continued Competency

At graduation, more than one class has heard the speaker say something similar to, "Half of what we taught you will not be true in 5 years. Unfortunately, we do not know which half" (Sackett et al., 1997, p. 38). Therefore, a commitment we have made to ourselves and to our service recipients in our Code of

Table 60.2. Hierarchy of Evidence Applied to Articles Published in the *Occupational Therapy Journal of Research,* 1995–1999

Level	Design	Number of Articles
I	Systematic reviews, meta-analytic studies	1
II	Randomized controlled trials	6
III	Trials without randomization	21
IV	Nonexperimental studies from more than one center	11
V	Opinions of respected authorities, descriptive studies	41

Note. Based on hierarchy by Moore, McQuay, and Gray (1995).

Ethics is to "take responsibility for maintaining competence by participating in professional development and educational activities" (AOTA, 1994, p. 1037). The importance of continued competency to occupational therapy practitioners was confirmed in a recent report entitled "Continued Competency in Occupational Therapy: Recommendations to the Profession and Key Stakeholders" by the National Commission on Continued Competency in Occupational Therapy (NCCCOT) (Mayhan, Holm, & Fawcett, 1999). From a survey of a stratified random sample of 550 of the 88,885 occupational therapists and 550 of the 33,512 occupational therapy assistants in the database of the National Board for Certification in Occupational Therapy (response rate = 33 percent), the NCC-COT found that more than 85 percent of the respondents endorsed the importance of continued competency for occupational therapy practitioners. Members of the NCCCOT also conducted in-depth interviews with representatives of other stakeholders in the future of our profession. These stakeholders included employers, payers, institutional and individual private accreditation program representatives, consumer advocates, and health policy analysts. These stakeholders shared the common perception that our continued competency is important to consumer protection and that individual occupational therapy practitioners have "the primary and ultimate responsibility for assuring their own continued competency" (Mayhan et al., 1999, p. 54).

Although we must be able to demonstrate competency in the core functions delineated in our *Standards of Practice* (AOTA, 1998) and the functions associated with the professional roles we fulfill (AOTA, 1993), we must also develop competence in research skills. Because of the changes in clinical practice as well as the changes in the evolving evidence base of occupational therapy, if we do not develop the research skills necessary to make use of the current best evidence for our patients, the result will be a progressive decline in our clinical competency.

In a special issue of *the American Journal of Occupational Therapy (AJOT)* devoted to professional competence, Abreu et al. (1998) led off their article with a prediction that in a practice environment that is continually changing, the survival of the profession depends, in part, on the "capacity of therapists to achieve competence in scientific inquiry and research" (p. 751). Then, using the levels of research competence identified by the American Occupational Therapy Foundation (1983) and Mitcham (1985), they explicated descriptors of the associated knowledge, skills, and attitudinal research competencies for practitioners at the beginning, intermediate, and advanced levels of occupational therapy research. What is necessary for continued competence in research and for our professional survival is for all of us to increase the number and level of our research competencies—not just to "maintain competence" as is the wording in our Code of Ethics but, rather, to improve our competence. *Can we meet this challenge?*

How Do I Become an Evidence-Based Practitioner?

At the *individual* level, each of us could fulfill all the research competencies identified by Abreu et al. (1998) and still not be an evidence-based practitioner, unless we also use the evidence and use it appropriately. This means that even if the evidence is clear and we decide that we can easily fit it into our preferred practice patterns, if it is not appropriate or acceptable to the patient, it is not evidence-based practice for that patient. As individuals, we must examine our practices to determine whether we are "integrating individual clinical expertise" with the "conscientious, explicit and judicious use of current best evidence" (Sackett et al., 1996, p. 71) by asking ourselves five questions. If we can answer affirmatively to any of the questions, we are making the right moves toward evidence-based practice.

Question 1: Do I Examine What I Do by Asking Clinical Questions?

The process of evidence-based practice begins by identifying the interventions that we use frequently in our practices with particular populations of patients, or for particular problems in performance, and then posing questions. Richardson, Wilson, Nishikawa, and Hayward (1995) identified the anatomy of a clinical question as having four parts: (a) the patient, population, or problem; (b) the intervention, which may include frequency and duration; (c) the outcome of interest; and (d) the comparison intervention. An example of a clinical question using this format might be: (a) In patients who have sustained a cerebrovascular accident, (b) does the use of a resting splint on the affected hand for 3 hours each day (c) reduce tone and increase function (d) compared with no splinting?

Question 2: Do I Take Time to Track Down the Best Evidence to Guide What I Do?

To answer your clinical question, you must track down the evidence. This involves computer searches with key words and syntax that will efficiently locate the best evidence as well as hand searches (Booth & Madge, 1998). Typical databases you might search are MEDLINE, CINAHL, the Cochrane Database of Systematic Reviews, the ACP Journal Club,

Evidence-Based Medicine, DARE, ERIC, PsycLit, and OT SEARCH. In addition to published articles, OT SEARCH includes manuscripts that have not been published but provide evidence that should be considered. You will also need to conduct hand searches of appropriate journals because not all articles on a specific topic will automatically show up in a database search and because not all journals are indexed. In addition to electronic and journal resources, there are human resources who can help you, and reference librarians should be at the top of the list. Additionally, researchers in related disciplines can be helpful because they may have access to important unpublished data, or they may be able to put you in touch with their colleagues who have been conducting studies relevant to the evidence you are trying to track down.

Question 3: Do I Appraise the Evidence or Take It at Face Value?

To appraise the evidence, of course, includes everything you hated about any research course you took, or why you may have avoided taking any. Appraising the evidence requires that you analyze each section of an article and apply the evidence hierarchy to determine at which level the study meets the established criteria. Article analysis is central to evidence-based practice, but it can also be very difficult. One of the structured article review instruments, such as those found on the Web sites of The Cochrane Collaboration, the University of Alberta, Mc Master University, and York University, can help you get started, or you can develop a review tool based on the 1993–1994 *JAMA* article series entitled, "User's Guide to the Medical Literature." When you get to the section of the article that includes the statistics, get out the snacks and bring up Trochim's data analysis Web site at Cornell University to reduce your anxiety and start you on your way to understanding the numbers before you (Trochim, February 20, 2000).

Question 4: Do I Use the Evidence to Do the "Right Things Right?"

One way to use the evidence before you is to develop a clinical guideline for your practice and format it according to the six "rights" identified by Graham (1996): Is "the right person, doing the right thing, the right way, in the right place, at the right time, with the right result" (p. 11)? The clinical guideline for "doing the right things right" is developed by using the evidence you locate to delineate the six "rights":

1. Who is the *right* person to implement the intervention? What level of competence is required? Is special certification required? Can an occupational therapy assistant implement the intervention?
2. What is the *right* thing to do? What does the evidence tell you? Does the patient agree?
3. What is the *right* way to implement the intervention? Does the evidence suggest a protocol or specifications that must be met? Can the patient's dignity and privacy be

maintained equally in all contexts in which the intervention could be implemented? Does the frequency or duration of the intervention make a difference?

4. What is the *right* place in which to implement the intervention? Is the home better than the clinic? Is the clinic better than the classroom? Is equipment required that dictates where the intervention must take place?

5. What is the *right* time to provide the intervention? Does time since onset of disability or admission to rehabilitation services make a difference? Does delaying the intervention make a difference? Does the time of day make a difference? Does time until, or since, discharge make a difference?

6. What is the *right* result? Did the intervention do what it was intended to do? Is the patient satisfied with the result? Are you satisfied with the result? After you have implemented the evidence-based guideline, ask yourself Question 5.

Question 5: Do I Evaluate the Impact of Evidence-Based Practice?

To assess the impact of the evidence-based clinical guideline you developed in response to Question 4, you would begin with a chart audit to determine whether the guideline was actually used and, then, whether it was used as intended. Finally, patient outcomes, cost-effectiveness, patient satisfaction, and therapist satisfaction must also be considered. The impact of the latter, therapist satisfaction with evidence-based practice, is pivotal, especially given the barriers to evidence-based practice.

Barriers and Motivation for Evidence-Based Practice

As Law and Baum (1998) noted in an issue of the *Canadian Journal of Occupational Therapy* dedicated to evidence-based practice, there are many barriers to its practice at both the system level and the individual level. The barriers cited include lack of administrative support, lack of access to research evidence, lack of skill in finding the evidence, lack of skill in interpreting the evidence, and lack of time. These barriers were reiterated in a Level V study of Canadian therapists' perceptions of evidence-based practice (Dubouloz, Egan, Vallerand, & von Zweck, 1999). The authors found that although therapists perceived evidence-based practice as a way of looking for understanding of the interventions they used, it also generated feelings of inadequacy related to research skills. Additionally, there were attitudinal barriers in that the therapists perceived that the evidence they would find might threaten the ways they preferred to practice.

Gray (1997) suggested a formula that we might find helpful as we seek to identify factors that will influence our performance of evidence-based practice (see Figure 60.1). He perceived that the performance of evidence-based practice is directly influenced by motivation multiplied by competence

$$\text{Performance} = \frac{\text{Motivation X Competence}}{\text{Barriers}}$$

Figure 60.1. Factors affecting the performance of evidence-based practice (Gray, 1997, p. 7).

divided by the barriers we need to overcome. Many factors in the context in which we practice today can be barriers to us; however, I am choosing to reframe them under motivation. Therefore, legislation, regulation, prospective payment system for skilled nursing facilities, capitations on reimbursement, new patient populations, new practice environments, new collaborations, and a new episodic reimbursement system for rehabilitation hospitals and exempt rehabilitation units can all be entered into the formula as motivation. I perceive them as motivators because they provide for us the impetus to describe, examine, and publish the evidence derived from what we do and how we do it. Also under motivation add the principles in our Code of Ethics that require us, for ethical practice, to "collaborate with service recipients," "fully inform...[them] of the nature, risks, and potential outcomes of any intervention," and "avoid harm" to them as well as to "perform... duties on the basis of accurate and current information" and "take responsibility for maintaining competence" (AOTA, 1994, p. 1037).

At a minimum, competence in this formula refers to competence in searching for, appraising, and applying existing evidence in everyday practice. For professional survival, however, we must be able to generate, publish, and make accessible to all the evidence that we now have to search for. This requires that we learn to gather evidence systematically in our practices as well as learn the knowledge, skills, and attitudes associated with occupational therapy research at the beginning, intermediate, or advanced levels of competence (Abreu et al., 1998).

Although one could dwell on barriers in the work environment and in the laws, regulations, and reimbursement systems, the barrier over which we have most influence is our own attitudes. On the basis of the findings of the Canadian study (Dubouloz et al., 1999), we have been alerted ahead of time that it may not be the external barriers but, rather, our own attitudinal barriers that may hinder the practice of evidence-based occupational therapy in the United States in the new millennium.

However, there are four encouraging examples of our movement toward evidence-based practice in the United States. Perhaps in response to the evidence-based practice initiatives of our Canadian and British colleagues, the new *Standards for an Accredited Educational Program for the Occupational Therapist* developed by the Accreditation Council for Occupational Therapy Education (ACOTE) require that occupational therapist graduates be able to "provide evidence-based effective therapeutic intervention related to performance areas" (ACOTE, 1999, p. 579). Furthermore, the AOTA Executive Board passed a motion that an evidence-based panel be formed to review and evaluate research that relates to *The Guide to Occupational Therapy Practice* (Moyers, 1999, 2000) in order to make the document evidence based. Additionally, the *AJOT* Associate Editor for Evidence-Based Practice, Linda Tickle-Degnen, instituted the Evidence-Based Practice Forum in which she guides practitioners through some aspect of evidence-based practice.

The best practice example, however, is from the notice in the *Coverage Policy Bulletin* of Aetna US Healthcare in which coverage of cognitive rehabilitation was recently announced. Although the studies were not Level I or Level II studies, the evidence was convincing. It states in the bulletin:

> The efficacy of cognitive therapy so far has been measured by its objective influence on function and the subjective value of these changes to the individual. Although current evidence supports cognitive therapy as a promising approach, definitive conclusions regarding its efficacy must await large-scale, well-conducted, controlled trials. (Aetna US Healthcare, 2000)

We can provide that evidence!

Conclusion

Eleanor Clarke Slagle was a proponent of habit development. Therefore, I will suggest two new habit patterns that we need to develop if we are to address proactively the realities of our professional exigencies. Each suggested habit pattern is followed by a question.

Habit 1: Evidence-Based Practice Now

Although the evidence for *what* we do and *how* we do it may be difficult to find, we have an obligation to become competent in, and make a habit of, searching for the evidence, appraising its value, and presenting it to those we serve in an understandable manner.

Question 1. After reading this lecture, could you provide your next several patients with a summary of the research evidence on the occupational therapy intervention options you are considering for them so that together you could make the best decisions?

Habit 2: The Evidence Base of Occupational Therapy in the New Millennium

We also have an obligation to improve our research competencies, to develop the habit of using those competencies in everyday practice, and to advance the evidence base of occupational therapy in the new millennium. Only then can we be sure that as we seek to do the "right things right," we are fulfilling our ethical responsibility to perform our "duties on the basis of accurate and current information" (AOTA, 1994, p. 1037). I will close by asking you to think ahead one decade.

Question 2. If in the year 2010 you stand accused of practicing occupational therapy based on research, will there be enough evidence to convict you?

Acknowledgments

I thank the following colleagues for their hearty critiques of my thinking and of the Slagle manuscript: Lynette S. Chandler, PhD, PT; Denise Chisholm, MS, OTR/L; Louise Fawcett, PhD, OTR/L, FAOTA; Sharon Gwinn, MS, OTR/L; Tamara Mills, OTR/L; Sharon Novalis, MSOT, OTR/L; Varick Olson, PhD, PT; Beth Skidmore, OTR/L; Ronald G. Stone, MS, OTR/L; George Tomlin, PhD, OTR/L; and especially to my mentor, Joan C. Rogers, PhD, OTR/L, FAOTA, ABDA.

References

Abreu, B., Peloquin, S. M., & Ottenbacher, K. (1998). Competence in scientific inquiry and research. *American Journal of Occupational Therapy, 52,* 751–759.

Accreditation Council for Occupational Therapy Education. (1999). Standards for an accredited educational program for the occupational therapist. *American Journal of Occupational Therapy, 53,* 575–582.

Aetna US Healthcare. Cognitive rehabilitation. *Coverage Policy Bulletin.* Retrieved March 6, 2000 from the World Wide Web: http://www.aetnaushc.com/cpb/data/CPBA0214.htm

American Occupational Therapy Association. (1993). Occupational therapy roles. *American Journal of Occupational Therapy, 47,* 1087–1099.

American Occupational Therapy Association. (1994). Occupational therapy code of ethics. *American Journal of Occupational Therapy, 48,* 1037–1038.

American Occupational Therapy Association. (1998). Standards of practice for occupational therapy. *American Journal of Occupational Therapy, 52,* 866–869.

American Occupational Therapy Foundation. (1983). The Foundation—Research competencies for clinicians and educators. *American Journal of Occupational Therapy, 37,* 44–46.

Booth, A., & Madge, B. (1998). Finding the evidence. In T. Bury & J. Mead (Eds.), *Evidence-based health care: A practical guide for therapists* (pp. 107–135). Woburn, MA: Butterworth-Heinemann.

Brooke, M., Lateur, B., Diana-Rigby, G., & Questad, K. (1991). Shoulder subluxation in hemiplegia: Effects of three different supports. *Archives of Physical Medicine and Rehabilitation, 72,* 582–586.

Brown, S. J. (1999). *Knowledge for health-care practice: A guide for using research evidence.* Philadelphia: Saunders.

Bury, T., & Mead, J. (1998). *Evidence-based health care: A practical guide for therapists.* Woburn, MA: Butterworth-Heinemann.

Bye, R. A. (1998). When clients are dying: Occupational therapists' perspectives. *Occupational Therapy Journal of Research, 18,* 3–24.

Case-Smith, J., Heaphy, T., Marr, D., Galvin, B., Koch, V., Ellis, M. G., & Perez, I. (1998). Fine motor and functional performance outcomes in preschool children. *American Journal of Occupational Therapy, 52,* 788–800.

Close, J., Ellis, M., Hooper, R., Glucksman, E., Jackson, S., & Swift, C. (1999). Prevention of falls in the elderly trial (PROFET): A randomised controlled trial. *Lancet, 353,* 93–97.

Cohn, E. S., & Cermak, S. A. (1998). Including the family perspective in sensory integration outcomes research. *American Journal of Occupational Therapy, 52,* 540–546.

Cummings, R. G., Thomas, M., Szonyi, G., Salkeld, G., O'Neill, E., Westbury, C., & Frampton, G. (1999). Home visits by an occupational therapist for assessment and modification of environmental hazards: A randomized trial of falls prevention. *Journal of the American Geriatrics Society, 47,* 1397–1402.

Dubouloz, C.-J., Egan, M., Vallerand, J., & von Zweck, C. (1999). Occupational therapists' perceptions of evidence-based practice. *American Journal of Occupational Therapy, 53,* 4 45–458.

Graham, G. (1996, June). Clinically effective medicine in a rational health service. *Health Director,* 11–12.

Gray, J.A.M. (1997). *Evidence-based health care: How to make health policy and management decisions.* New York: Churchill Livingstone.

Hurd, M. M., Farrell, K. H., & Waylonis, G. W. (1974). Shouldersling for hemiplegia: Friend or foe? *Archives of Physical Medicine and Rehabilitation, 55,* 519–522.

Law, M., & Baum, C. (1998). Evidence-based occupational therapy. *Canadian Journal of Occupational Therapy, 65,* 131–135.

Lidz, C. W., & Meisel, A. (1983). *Informed consent and the structure of medical care. In Making health-care decisions: The ethical and legal implications of informed consent in the patient–practitioner relationship* (Vol. 2). Washington, DC: U.S. Government Printing Office.

Lin, K., Wu, C., Tickle-Degnen, L., & Coster, W. (1997). Enhancing occupational performance through occupationally embedded exercise: A meta-analytic review. *Occupational Therapy Journal of Research, 17,* 25–47.

Mayhan, Y. D., Holm, M. B., Fawcett, L. C. (Eds.) & National Commission on Continued Competency in Occupational Therapy. (1999). *Continued competency in occupational therapy: Recommendations to the profession and key stakeholders.* Gaithersburg, MD: National Board for Certification in Occupational Therapy.

McHale, K., & Cermak, S. A. (1992). Fine motor activities in elementary school: Preliminary findings and provisional implications for children with fine motor problems. *American Journal of Occupational Therapy, 46,* 898–903.

Mitcham, M. D. (1985). *Integrating research competencies into occupational therapy: A teaching guide for academic and clinical educators.* Rockville, MD: American Occupational Therapy Foundation.

Moore, A., McQuay, H., & Gray, J. A. M. (Eds.). (1995). Evidence-based everything. *Bandolier,* 1(12), 1.

Moyers, P. A. (1999). The guide to occupational therapy practice. *American Journal of Occupational Therapy, 53,* 247–322.

Moyers, P. A. (2000). Letters to the editor—Author's response. *American Journal of Occupational Therapy, 54,* 113–114.

Mulligan, S. (1998). Patterns of sensory integration dysfunction: A confirmatory factor analysis. *American Journal of Occupational Therapy, 52,* 819–828.

Neistadt, M. E., & Marques, K. (1984). An independent living skills training program. *American Journal of Occupational Therapy, 38,* 671–676.

Nicol, M. M., Robertson, L., & Connaughton, J. A. (1999). Life skills programs for people with chronic mental illness. *Cochrane Database of Systematic Reviews, 3: The Schizophrenia Group.* Retrieved January 26, 2000 from the World Wide Web: http://www.update-software.com/cochrane.htm

Ottenbacher, K. J., & Maas, F. (1999). Quantitative Research Series—How to detect effects: Statistical power and evidence-based practice in occupational therapy research. *American Journal of Occupational Therapy, 53,* 181–188.

Portney, L. G., & Watkins, M. P. (1993). *Foundations of clinical research: Applications to practice.* Norwalk, CT: Appleton & Lange.

Ray, W. A., Taylor, J. A., Meador, K. G., Thapa, P. B., Brown, A. K., Kajihara, H. K., Davis, C., Gideon, P., & Griffin, M. R. (1997). A randomized trial of a consultation service to reduce falls in nursing homes. *Journal of the American Medical Association, 278,* 557–562.

Rennie, D. (1986). Guarding the guardians: A conference on editorial peer review. *Journal of the American Medical Association, 256,* 2391–2392.

Richardson, W. S., Wilson, M. C., Nishikawa, J., & Hayward, R. S. (1995). The well-built clinical question: A key to evidence-based decisions. *ACP Journal Club, 123,* A-12.

Rogers, J. C., Holm, M. B., Burgio, L. D., Granieri, E., Hsu, C., Hardin, J. M., & McDowell, B. J. (1999). Improving morning care routines of nursing home residents with dementia. *Journal of the American Geriatrics Society, 47,* 1049–1057.

Sackett, D. L., Haynes, R. B., & Tugwell, P. (1985). How to read a clinical journal. In D. L. Sackett, R. B. Haynes, & P. Tugwell (Eds.), *Clinical epidemiology: A basic science for clinical medicine* (pp. 285–322). Boston: Little, Brown.

Sackett, D. L., Richardson, W. S., Rosenberg, W., & Haynes, R. B. (1997). Critically praising the evidence. In D. L. Sackett, W. S. Richardson, W. Rosenberg, & R. B. Haynes (Eds.), *Evidence-based medicine: How to practice and teach EBM* (pp. 38–156). New York: Churchill Livingstone.

Sackett, D. L., Rosenberg, W. M., Gray, J. A. M., Haynes, R. B., & Richardson, W. S. (1996). Evidence-based medicine: What it is and what it isn't. *British Medical Journal, 312,* 71–72.

Schneiderman, L. J., Kaplan, R. M., Pearlman, R. A., & Teetzel, H. (1993). Do physicians' own preferences for life-sustaining treatment influence their perceptions of patients' preferences? *Journal of Clinical Ethics, 4,* 28–32.

Shenk, D. (1997). *Data smog.* San Francisco: Harper Edge.

Silverman, W. A. (1998). *Where's the evidence?: Debates in modern medicine.* New York: Oxford University Press.

Tickle-Degnen, L. (1998). Quantitative Research Series—Communicating with clients about treatment outcomes: The use of meta-analytic evidence in collaborative treatment planning. *American Journal of Occupational Therapy, 52,* 526–530.

Trochim, W. (February 20, 2000). *What is the research methods knowledge base.* Retrieved from the World Wide Web: http://trochim.human.cornell.edu/kb/index.htm

Vargas, S., & Camilli, G. (1999). A meta-analysis of research on sensory integration treatment. *American Journal of Occupational Therapy, 53,* 18 9–198.

Williams, R., Taffs, L., & Minuk, T. (1988). Evaluation of two support methods for the subluxated shoulder in hemiplegic patients. *Physical Therapy, 68,* 1209–1213.

Zorowitz, R. D., Idank, D., Ikai, T., Hughes, M. B., & Johnston, M. V. (1995). Shoulder subluxation after a stroke: A comparison of four supports. *Archives of Physical Medicine and Rehabilitation, 76,* 763–771.

CHAPTER 61

Professional Responsibility in Times of Change

1967 ELEANOR CLARKE SLAGLE LECTURE

WILMA L. WEST, MA, OTR

We are now convened for the final day of a conference in celebration of the 50th anniversary of our professional life. Behind us lie five decades of individual and group endeavor—endeavor to develop a profession, to define and refine a service, to improve an image and extend its acceptance, to recruit others to our ranks and train them for perpetuation of our ideals, to research new and better ways of accomplishing our goals.

At this milestone in our history, one could be tempted to look back through the years and analyze the functional relationship between endeavors and accomplishments. Such stock-taking would surely yield an inventory of assets in many areas of effort in which we might feel mutual pride. It would also, however, show liabilities for which we remain collectively responsible. Still other accounts might appear as outstanding or receivable, thus implying the necessity for continued effort in the commitment to further progress. Depending on the perspective and purpose of the individual doing the analysis, this measure of our first 50 years might be impressive, discouraging, or inconclusive with respect to net accomplishment.

Santayana has warned that "He who neglects history will be condemned to repeat it." However, awareness and understanding of effort input with reference to success or failure of outcome are most functional when new approaches are being brought to the solution of old problems. If, on the other hand, changing or new conditions prevail and hence a different set of problems is presented, there is diminishing value in more than brief review of the methods of other people and times. The example of the inadequacy of conventional defenses in a nuclear age is the obvious one, but professional personnel in medical and educational fields today face a dilemma equal to that of the military in recognizing that old ways of solving problems are no longer adequate.

Let us turn, then, from any comfortable reflection on our past to the infinitely more exciting exercise of projecting our future. Wisely approached, this can be as scientific as a retrospective analysis and surely it is a more dynamic course if we wish to have a part in determining our future rather than merely accepting one on assignment or default of others.

One cannot be in the practice of any of the health professions today without being keenly aware of the many forces shaping his future roles and responsibilities. Nor can he neglect his duty to examine the implications of these forces in three dimensions: for himself as a professional person, for the profession of which he is a member, and for the professional organization which represents and promotes his individual and group interests. In brief, the questions currently confronting us are: What is happening in both our immediate and larger worlds? and, What does this mean to us?

The general stage for this discussion may be set by an analogy from another field that is strikingly similar to that of medicine. Francis Keppel, former commissioner of the Office of Education, Department of Health, Education, and Welfare, says that America is entering a third revolution in education. In the first revolution, education of the masses was achieved by the establishment of the public school system. Later, equality of education for all people became the rallying cry for school reform. Now the astounding advances in technology demand specialized and high-quality education for all regardless of race, creed, or social class.[1]

Today this country is well into a similar multistaged reorganization of health and medical care in which equal availability and high quality of health services are sought for all people. The bipartisan endorsement of providing services to meet two of man's most fundamental needs—for education and health care—has removed the question from the arena of welfare and politics and placed it in the larger domain of basic human development.

Whether one agrees with these trends wholly, partially, reluctantly, or not at all, one fact is virtually undeniable today: comprehensive health care, among others of man's needs, is beyond individual attainment for far too many people. If we accept this fact, we can accept the organization of increasingly costly and complex programs designed to reduce disease and disability among victims of economic disparity and to raise the health standards of our country as a whole.

"Governmental involvement (then) in the financing and organization of health services is here to stay and there is every indication that it will increase."[2] I submit, however, that governmental participation and individual responsibility are neither incompatible nor mutually exclusive. In fact, we must go even further in pursuit of a rationale that is in tune with both our changing times and a high standard of personal and professional integrity. I therefore tend to agree with another commentator on this subject who has said that "placing health in the category of the rights of man involves the transformation of a social desire into a moral imperative."[3] This imperative has been stated as follows by the New York Academy of Medicine: "That *all people* should have...*equal opportunity* to obtain a *high quality* of *comprehensive health care.*"

It is difficult to see how anyone could mount an argument against the humanitarian elements of this high goal. In the sense that the primary orientation of the professions is to the community interest, there *must* be concern for all people on the basis of equal opportunity and with a standard of the highest possible quality that it is within our ability to provide. Implications of most of the key phrases in this all-encompassing objective are clear. However, the last dimension—comprehensive health care—bears elaboration because it is with reference to this focus that we will examine how our profession can best adapt its philosophy and practice to future requirements.

At our annual conference in Minneapolis last year, the theme was "Dimensions of Change." Many of us, I am sure, recall the message of several thoughtful speakers who helped us read signs among today's maze of medical plans and programs that are as complex and confusing as the newest multi-story interchange of highways around our large cities. I hope we also recall the repeated emphasis on *health,* as well as illness, on *prevention* of disease and disability, in addition to seeking the cures not yet discovered, on *maintenance and promotion of well-being,* not just being satisfied that there is an "absence of infirmity,"[4] on *continuity of care,* in lieu of only episodic attention to emergency conditions, and on *comprehensive health services* that must replace the diagnostic or categorical approach of conventional medicine.

The trends in these directions are unmistakable. They are also irreversible. To recognize them, however, is only the first step. We must also interpret their meaning for each of our specialty areas and aggressively adapt or redesign our roles to provide a more viable future service.

No one person can or should do this for all facets of his profession. Each must, however, do it for his own focus of interest and with all the professional outlook and insight he can muster. I can best relate these changing trends and their implications to the field of pediatrics, with which I have been most closely involved in recent years. I shall attempt to do so in the general framework of comprehensive health care for children and, more specifically, with reference to selected groups which present us with some very challenging opportunities to develop a preventive role for our profession. I shall conclude with some thoughts on the implications of these and other changes for the profession as a whole.

Comprehensive Health Care for Children

What is meant by comprehensive health care for children? This is a term that is variously defined, but on the conceptual level, I prefer the following statement to all others that I have read: "By comprehensive, we mean a constellation of health services that focuses on the patient as an individual human being rather than as a collection of assorted organ systems, some of which are diseased."[5] On the practical level, we believe this ideal must be translated into programs which include health supervision in the various parameters of growth and development and the regular use of specific devices for screening deficits and dysfunctions. Comprehensive health care for children, we feel, is committed to enhancing normal development as insurance against disease or, failing that objective, to the earliest possible casefinding of those conditions which have their origin in prenatal causes or in the disabling illnesses of infancy and the preschool years.

Both the number and scope of programs designed to provide health care for children are greater today than ever before. The idea behind them, however, is hardly a new one. For it was in 1890 in France that the first nursing conferences and milk stations were established to provide preventive health services for lower socioeconomic segments of the child population. At that time the motive was to reduce the enormously high infant and preschool child mortality, but from these early beginnings, clinic services of similar types have developed throughout the world. In the United States, the milk stations of the World War I era subsequently became known as well-baby clinics and today, in many areas, are called child health conferences.

It is interesting to trace the broadening philosophy of these forerunners of modern comprehensive health care for children. Because such enterprises were designed to provide health supervision of well children, one of their primary functions was to screen children for evidence of abnormality or illness that might warrant referral for care.

A classic text on preventive medicine and public health[6] tells us that the child health conference was originally necessary because a large segment of the population was unable to pay for health supervision. However, it also goes on to point out that even today such services cannot be transferred to the private practitioner. The reason, the authors state, is that education and training of medical students is still largely oriented to the patient with cellular pathology, with the result that many practitioners today have limited interest in and knowledge of the principles and techniques of health supervision of growing children. Furthermore, child health personnel even in recent years have been largely preoccupied with the development of treatment and training programs for handicapped children.

And so, it seems, have occupational therapists in pediatrics. Thus we, too, have been slow to develop a role in prevention that might greatly enhance our total professional contribution to health care. Although our traditional commitment to medicine and our orientation to illness and treatment are understandable, our greater development of a preventive role, which is "an integral part of all medical practice, wherever it may be and under whatever auspices"[7] is long overdue.

There is even a sense of urgency to the situation that cannot be escaped. Consider for example the number and diversity of settings in which new health-care programs for children are constantly being developed. The well-child clinics or child health conferences that have already been mentioned are standard services of state and local health departments, but they are only one of several locales where continuing health supervision of children is assuming ever greater importance.

Probably the best known among others that I will discuss here are the Head Start programs that have received extensive publicity in the brief 2 years since their inception. Although the initial focus of these efforts was on enrichment of experience in preparation for school, a spin-off benefit of major importance has been identification and treatment of health deficits. It is of significance to us that the range of these deficits goes far beyond the dental and nutritional problems inevitable in the target populations and includes a high incidence of retarded or deviant physical and psychosocial development. As we well know, the chances for remediation of many such problems are infinitely better at age 3 or 4 than at beginning school age which, until now, has provided our earliest large-scale screening opportunity.

Another very new program of the Office of Economic Opportunity which was launched late this past summer could provide an even richer locus for occupational therapy in a preventive role. This is the development of Parent and Child Centers that is currently taking place in 36 American communities to provide services for disadvantaged families who have preschool children. A prime objective of these centers will be the use of techniques and processes both to prevent deviations and deficits and to stimulate development to the maximum potential. Among the skills and experience sought for staff are the ability to recognize and understand the developmental stages of young children and prescribe a plan for progress to meet each child's individual needs.[8]

To pediatric occupational therapists who have been concerned with the larger objective of optimal child growth and development as well as with restoration of impaired function, the possibilities inherent in these new centers must indeed be exciting. Think, for example, of the broad range of activities that could be used to provide multisensory input directed to the development of intellectual, emotional, social, and physical skills. The graded and guided use of activities for such purposes is so integral a part of occupational therapy that this would seem to be a most fitting application of our skills to plan, elicit, interpret, and modify both performance and behavior.

There are other groups of children for whom health surveillance could provide either prevention or earlier treatment. Sparked by the increasing prevalence of daytime employment of both parents or the absence of one parent and employment of the other, day care facilities have become a way of life for thousands of young American children. The larger of these, the day care centers, are units with seven to 75 or more children, a staff of one or more persons, and an organized program. In these settings today, ages of children usually range upwards from 2 1/2 years, this being the minimum age for most children to participate in group play or other organized activities. What an opportunity there is here to prevent, restrict, or retard development of problems we now see only when they are entrenched and disabling, often to a severe degree.

A final example is a group of children which has received special attention during the past year and is already providing the occupational therapist with a role in screening, evaluation, and programming as well as in treatment. This is the group served by the Children and Youth projects sponsored by the Children's Bureau.

Organized in areas of economic and social disruption, these projects are designed to provide comprehensive health care for large numbers of children who, under existing circumstances, have only marginal opportunity to develop a healthy mind and body. Now, however, a broad range of health professionals is being assembled to provide services which should greatly improve their future outlook.

Included in the authorized core staff for children and youth projects is an occupational therapist whose job description reads quite differently from the specifications for other pediatric roles. If a few of these promising new positions can be filled by therapists with vision as well as skill, there are few limits on the extent to which they will be permitted to develop a broader role. For example: in New York City, two pediatric neurologists on a children and youth project added an occupational therapist to assist them in screening for neurological deficits; in Dallas and in Denver, pediatricians directing diagnostic clinics use their therapists to evaluate motor performance and behavior adjustment and to participate in programming based on team findings and recommendations; and in several other areas of the country, therapists are involving children in activities which permit assessment in numerous areas of function and providing selected experiences to promote development of neuromuscular, emotional, and intellectual competencies of children.

These, then, are some of the programs made possible by the federal-state alliance to extend and improve health services for increasing numbers of people. They require of all professions a careful appraisal of changes that may be necessary as we jointly seek creative and workable solutions to both old and new problems. Although we have centered attention on one specialty of our profession, it is intriguing to think about how the number and kinds of changes in pediatrics today will inevitably, in time, affect every other age group and specialty field of occupational therapy.

Furthermore, there are equally radical changes occurring simultaneously in patterns of delivering health and medical services to all people. Witness, for example, the burgeoning community mental health programs and consider the implications of trends in that specialty of our profession. Are there not elements here, paralleling the new kinds of community-based services in pediatrics, which are dictating programs concerned with the maintenance and promotion of health as well as the treatment of illness? And hence, are there not here, too, strong indications for increased emphasis on the preventive role of occupational therapy?

Of course there are, and many progressive occupational therapists in both these and other specialties of our profession have already taken steps to keep pace with trends that require new or expanded roles. Furthermore, they have done so with such effectiveness that they have created roles and functions that greatly improve the image of our profession. In a sense, therefore, my commentary only reflects what I consider to be the best abroad in practice today, with a few thoughts on where, how, and why it seems particularly urgent that we intensify our efforts in these directions and at this time. I fear, however, that there are yet too many among us who do not sufficiently appreciate current trends and who therefore are not lending their efforts to hasten and make credible more functional roles throughout the profession. The platform at a general session of our annual conference and assured publication in our professional journal lend temptation to speak frankly to one's colleagues. And, the occasion of a golden anniversary provides a good point at which to cross the treacherous terrain of prophecy and hazard a glimpse of where our best future directions may lie. He who does so will always run the chance of suggesting some wrong turns, but he who does not has missed both an opportunity and a responsibility to share with others his views on areas of mutual concern.

We Are Committed to Our Profession as a Whole

I would like, now, to discuss some ramifications of these thoughts in terms of the profession as a whole rather than in the framework of any one or more specialty areas of practice. For, regardless of our individual concerns with separate fields, it is to the whole profession that we are jointly committed to and for which we must cooperatively work. My remaining remarks will explore some of the reasons why it seems important that this be so.

What is the relevance to us as a professional group of the changes I have discussed, of other changes that are taking place in patterns of providing health services, and of the implications these have for traditional and transitional roles in our profession? Is it enough that there is a growing number of clinicians in each of our specialty fields who are continually sharpening conventional skills and also developing new ones? Can we rely on the work of a small but increasing number of researchers among us to confirm the scientific basis of our practice? Does the greater sophistication of today's authors sufficiently raise the level of our professional literature? Will the growing number of our members who are obtaining graduate degrees insure a higher quality of performance in the future? Are changes that are being effected by the more progressive among our educators adequate to the preparation of tomorrow's therapists? In short, will the leadership of these and other significantly contributing individuals suffice? Indeed, should it have to?

Decidedly not. What is absent from this kind of thinking is the concept of group responsibility—responsibility for awareness and interpretation of those changes which affect any part of our profession, and responsibility for whatever group action is appropriate to facilitate or hasten adjustment to change. Thus, although we clearly recognize that "All occupations are dependent on the individual contributions" of those who practice them, we must also realize that "the effectiveness of an occupation is not gauged by individual efforts alone; the total efforts of occupational members working together with some degree of cooperation must also be considered. The public image of an occupation, then, is in part individual and in part collective. ... Moreover, the goals of an occupation are only in a limited sense individual, for the individual responsibility of practitioners and a consciousness of the aims of the occupation are very much a function of collective action."[9]

There are, of course, many terms for the kind of collective action here referred to. Among them is what I shall call professional consciousness and responsibility. This is an attribute that we in occupational therapy have to a quite considerable degree. It has served us well in the 50 years of our professional development to date, primarily, I believe, because we have used it more in the sense of professional responsiveness to public interest and need than for purposes of protecting or promoting our constituent individuals and groups. These two major purposes of a profession—meeting external obligations to society on the one hand, and internal loyalties to members on the other—may often be in conflict. That they have not created serious problems or dichotomies for us up to this time may be viewed as a mixed blessing, for readings in the sociology of development of the professions make it clear that it is.only a matter of time until they do. Factors which may have delayed this apparently inevitable process include our extremely small size and the relative homogeneity of a profession with only incompletely developed specialties.

Trend Toward Decreased Professional Unity

With the passage of time, however, we are experiencing both an increase in size and a proliferation of special skills among our members. As these two dimensions grow, we become increasingly subject to the influence of factors which will tend to decrease professional unity and promote segmentation in accordance with divergent interests and strengths as they develop among us. Although it will undoubtedly create some problems, this trend is by no means undesirable. On the contrary, it usually brings with it both an improved service, which results from increased knowledge and skill of specialists, and a growing professional influence which can be used to improve the status of those who provide that service.

There are signs that the era of segmentation is already upon us; witness for example, the increasing number of special interest meetings and concurrent sessions scheduled at this year's annual conference. While neither deploring the problems nor lauding the advantages an increase in this trend will bring, I hope that we will retain an attitude of general professional consciousness and concern for as long as we exist. Conviction of the need for this lies in the belief that "the chief factor. ... in the accomplishments of any profession is the unified, aggressive efforts of its members."[10]

Numerous theories have been put forth to explain why persons pursuing an occupation come together and associate in a formal manner. These include everything from the likely initial motivation for exchange with those doing the same work, to such presently accepted objectives as raising standards of competence, formulating codes of ethics, improving education, undertaking protective and promotional activities, and many others. The activities of associations as major interest groups which participate in planning and policy decisions on matters of concern to them are generally thought of as a devel-

opment of recent years undertaken to counter the influence of governmental regulations on professional activities; in fact, however, these date back at least three centuries when, as one writer says, "it was characteristic of the times that powers and duties of so extensive a nature were granted to vocational associations that they may be regarded as organs of the state." Thus they are illustrative of the influence a well-organized profession can have on public decisions and policies.

I make no case for our professional association to aspire to this degree of power. I do, however, believe that both as individuals and as a professional group we should be assuming a far more frequent and contributing part in the planning of health services. It will, in fact, be mandatory that we do so if, as I said earlier, we are to have a part in shaping our own development.

Izutsu believes that "it is not too late to achieve positions of leadership that will determine the future" of our profession.[12] However, he also lists several steps that we must take if we are to remain equal to changing patterns in the organization and delivery of health services. Among these are the development of leaders not only to plan for therapy but to think in the broad spectrum of social planning; training of therapists in public health principles and procedures; and exposure, in our training, to community-oriented settings and other health team members in lieu of training primarily in hospital settings.

Professionally, We Often Resist Change

I do not suppose any of us knows, with any degree of certainty, the ideal future course for our profession. We do, however, see many signs that it must keep changing if it is to stay abreast of the larger world of which it is a part. Change is seldom easy or comfortable. Yet there is little about the world in which we live today that is more characteristic of it than the continual and fast-moving changes which transcend every aspect of our lives.

Although each of us makes the necessary adaptation to these changes as they affect our personal concerns and activities, we are slower as a group to adjust our professional directions and developments to that which is new. We are often, in fact, resistant to the suggested need for change and all that it implies in the necessity for new learning and the establishment of new roles and functions. We are also reluctant to explore new potentials, to experiment, to take an occasional risk.

From Therapist to Health Agent

Increasingly, today, I believe we should identify with the field of health services, thus broadening our traditional, more limited identification with medicine. We should enlarge our concept from that of being a therapist to one of functioning as a health agent with responsibility to help ensure normal growth and development. We should think more about roles in prevention as well as in treatment and rehabilitation, about socioeconomic and cultural as well as biological causes of disease and dysfunction, and about serving health needs of people in many other settings than the hospital.

One occasion on which this was expressed in a very effective way by a number of our colleagues was the conference on research in occupational and physical therapy held last February in Puerto Rico. In one of the discussion groups, there was studied avoidance of the term "patient," which many felt limited their concern to illness, and a plea for consideration of health as only one aspect of the developmental process of man which should not be isolated from other factors impinging on life. This kind of thinking and discussion culminated in the group's consideration of its topic in the framework of what they called "the continuum of health services which reflect the needs of man in his environment."[13]

A broad frame of reference? Admittedly, but it is also entirely in keeping with our traditional philosophy of concern for the person rather than just his disability. For us, therefore, the idea possesses what might be called "instant validity." It now needs rapid if not instant implementation.

We are living today in a world that is vastly different from that when occupational therapy began. It matters not so much that it has taken 50 years to reach this day, as that the next 50 see more, and more rapid, progress than the last. It matters less that we are still struggling to define our profession than that we build a broader base for the better definition that will one day be written. It matters most of all that we recognize the responsibility of the profession to change with changing demands for its services, to adapt via new approaches, to assume different roles, to develop the preparation for them, and to recruit in a new mold rather than by recasting the prototype of an earlier time.

On the eve of her retirement from active work in our national organization, Eleanor Clarke Slagle was paid the following tribute:

> Those of us who have been privileged to follow the winding trail of those years know of struggles, of courage in facing criticism, of disappointments and rewards, of patient waiting, persistent faith, and devoted work. The questing youth of our profession accepts both with commendation and condemnation what has been so painstakingly accomplished through this quarter century. But when they too can look back over an equal span of service in this field, they, and occupational therapy, will still be moving to the measure of the thought of Eleanor Clarke Slagle.[14]

That "equal span of service" has now passed so we, too, are looking back over the second quarter of a century which immediately precedes the present day. It seemed fitting that we do so in the context of both our practice to which she gave so much, and our professional association which she helped to organize, served as an officer in four capacities, and directed as its executive for many years. I, for one, hold to much that she obviously held high among her goals for the profession. Among those goals, I feel sure, was one related to the need for professional responsibility at all times. In times of change such as these, that need and our response to it will be of great importance in determining the next 50 years of our professional life. At the turn of the 21st century, when yet another generation looks back on these times, they may they see that ours was a dynamic posture of professional consciousness and responsibility.

References

1. Keppel, Francis, *The Necessary Revolution in American Education.* New York: Harper and Row (1966).
2. Burns, Evalina, "Policy Decisions Facing the United States in Financing and Organizing Health Care," *Public Health Reports,* 81, No. 8 (August 1966).
3. Dearing, W. P., "Prepaid Group Practice Medical Care Plans," *Public Health Reports,* 77, No. 10 (October 1962).
4. Preamble to the Constitution of the World Health Organization.
5. Kissick, William L., "Trends in the Utilization of Rehabilitation Manpower," *Manpower Utilization in Rehabilitation in New York City,* New York: New York City Regional Interdepartmental Rehabilitation Committee (September 1966).
6. Sartwell, P.E., Ed., *Maxcy-Rosenau Preventive Medicine and Public Health,* 9th ed. New York: Meredith Publishing Co. *(1965).*
7. Freeman, Ruth B., "Impact of Public Health on Society," *Public Health Reports,* 76, No. 4 (April 1961).
8. *Criteria for Parent and Child Centers,* Washington, D.C.: Office of Economic Opportunity (July 19, 1967).
9. Vollmer, Howard M. and Mills, Donald L., *Professionalization,* Englewood Cliffs, New Jersey: Prentice-Hall, Inc. (1966).
10. Stinnett, T. M., "Accomplishments of the Organized Teaching Profession," *The Teacher and Professional Organizations,* Washington, D.C.: The National Education Association (1956).
11. Carr-Saunders, A. M. and Wilson, P. A., "The Rise and Aims of Professional Associations," *The Professions,* Oxford: The Clarendon Press (1933).
12. Izutsu, Satoru, "The Changing Patterns of Patient Care" (A Position Paper) *Research Conference in Occupational Therapy and Physical Therapy,* New York: American Physical Therapy Association (1967).
13. Group Report, "Research in Patient Care," *Proceedings of the Research Conference in Occupational Therapy and Physical Therapy,* New York: American Physical Therapy Association (To be published).
14. "In the Past, Pride—In the Future, Faith," A Documentary of the Heritage, Growth, and Outlook of the American Occupational Therapy Association. Produced by the Association for its 41st Annual Conference, New York, New York (October 21, 1958).

Philosophy, Science, and Ideology: A Proposed Relationship for Occupational Science and Occupational Therapy

CHAPTER 62

Erna Imperatore Blanche, PhD, OTR
Enrique Henny-Kohler

Occupational science, the first science founded by occupational therapists, was born out of a need for a body of knowledge that focused on the multifaceted nature of engagement in occupations and its use in therapy. Occupational science has received a varied reception by occupational therapists around the globe. Whereas in some countries it has been enthusiastically embraced by the OT community, in other countries its value has been ignored, misunderstood, or questioned. In these countries, some comments have included "It sounds like something we have already heard," "What is new in this science?" and "How can we apply information developed in a foreign reality to the reality of our own regional or national problems?"

Trying to answer these questions leads into explaining why occupational science is neither something completely novel nor something completely foreign to occupational therapists practicing around the globe. Questions such as these show the confusion between our understanding of the traditional philosophical beliefs that have supported occupational therapy since its inception, the basic postulates of occupational science, the systematic character of scientific inquiry, and the external components that contribute to the development of a science in a specific context. In occupational therapy, as in any profession, a key external component is the ideology of a specific country or region.

"Lack of understanding of the relationship among the philosophy of occupational therapy; the science of occupation; and the ideology of a country, region, or community can affect the development of occupational therapy and occupational science outside the USA. Effects of decreased understanding include less development of occupational science research outside the countries of its origin, underutilization of the knowledge base of occupational science to assist in the daily practice of occupational therapy, missed opportunities in developing occupational science in a richer multicultural context, and continued importation of techniques and knowledge from sources outside the field of occupational therapy and outside the culture or geographic region.

This paper focuses on the interaction among philosophy, science, and ideology, and their mutual influence on the development of professional ideas and practice. First, the relationship of occupational therapy and occupational science will be illustrated. Next, the nature of philosophy, science, and ideology will be defined. Last, two models will be proposed for developing a comprehensive system of knowledge across countries, cultures, and regions. Furthermore, the models will illustrate the relationship between occupational science and occupational therapy and the importance of developing a global identity through the development of basic and applied knowledge by occupational therapists everywhere.

The Relationship Between Occupational Therapy and Occupational Science

Professional ideas are generated as a result of the interaction among philosophy, science, and ideology in each particular culture or region. In occupational therapy, the scientific information contributing to daily practice has traditionally originated from other disciplines such as sociology, psychology, or medicine. This information was adapted by occupational therapists to fit their professional philosophical belief system and their culture. Occupational therapists often have embraced techniques developed outside the profession without questioning how these techniques and ideas alter occupational therapy's unique professional identity. Importing scientific information from outside without questioning its fit with our profession may result in conflicts with our philosophical beliefs and further questioning of occupational therapists' unique practice role. Therefore, developing occupational science as our own science becomes pivotal for taking control of our own knowledge development and professional identity around the globe.

Can a science evolving initially in North America, Europe, and Australia be applied around the globe? Can occupational therapists, by embracing this science, continue to hold a global professional identity? The daily practice of occupational therapy in specific regions in the globe may influence the development of occupational science in the same way as occupational science may influence the daily practice of occupational therapy in each region. We will use two models to describe the relationship between the international aspects of occupational science and the daily practice of occupational therapists. The first model focuses on the identity of occupational therapists as formed by international and regional factors. The second model focuses on the interaction of scientific development, ideology, and daily regional practice. Before describing the models, we will define some basic terms.

Defining Philosophy, Science, and Ideology

Philosophy

Philosophy is often defined by reference to its relationship to sciences. Philosophy is considered to be "the mother of the sciences" (*Encyclopedia Americana*, p. 925). The following is appropriate to describe the relationship between the philosophy of occupational therapy and occupational science: "As mankind has gradually acquired more extended knowledge of phenomena, and systematic relations among these have been sufficiently made out, special branches of learning have become consolidated and have separated themselves from the general body of thought called philosophy" (*Encyclopedia Americana*, p. 925). The origins of occupational science are rooted in occupational therapy's basic philosophical assumptions about occupation. The early philosophy of occupational therapy pioneers continues to influence the identity of occupational science and occupational therapy by shaping our research questions and our daily clinical practice.

Bunge (1999), an Argentinian-born philosopher of science, distinguishes between philosophy and philosophy-of. For him, philosophy is defined as "the discipline that studies the most general concepts (such as those of being, becoming, mind, knowledge, and norm) and the most general hypotheses (such as those of the autonomous existence and knowa-

bility of the external world)" (Bunge, 1999: 210). Philosophy-of is defined as philosophizing or drawing moral philosophy from nearly any subject. The philosophy-of a given subject may be undertaken from the vantage point of art, science, religion, or technology. A philosopher can be anyone who has the capacity to reason (Bunge, 1999).

The philosophy of occupational therapy is a philosophy-of that focuses on a group of ideas about the importance of purposeful activity in humans' daily interactions in the social and physical environment. Occupational therapists around the globe share the basic philosophical belief that mundane daily occupations powerfully influence health and provide meaning to people's lives (Christiansen and Baum, 1997; Bontje, 1998; Golledge, 1998; Yerxa, 1998 [see Chapter 34]), but have lacked the scientific knowledge to support this assertion. Occupational science offers a system (which may include methodologies) to study the essence and veracity of this philosophy. Occupational science has gone beyond this shared philosophical belief, both clarifying and extending, to explore new questions whose answers can support occupation-based practice and foster innovative occupational therapy practice.

Science

Science is "the critical search for or utilization of patterns in ideas, nature, or society" (Bunge, 1999: 256). Occupational science originated as a basic social science. It has more recently been described as a human science that is both basic and applied, and that is concerned with the study of form, function, and meaning of occupations inside as well as outside the therapeutic context (Zemke and Clark, 1996).

Basic sciences are defined as the "disinterested search for new scientific knowledge" (Bunge, 1999: 258). The questions explored in basic sciences focus on the interests of the researcher which generate new information. For example, Newton's curiosity about gravity was pursued because of his own interest, not because it would be useful to explain the dynamics of movement or the effects of gravity on a planet. Applied science, on the other hand, is defined as the searching for practical applications (Bunge, 1984). However, as in the example of Newton, basic sciences influence applied sciences and the techniques developed by applied sciences (Bunge, 1984). Both basic and applied science, in turn, influence the way national and regional problems are viewed and the solutions that are provided to solve problems. Many societies turn to science to seek solutions to issues that trouble them. Bunge (1984) argues that the importance of developing basic science in a region lies in its influence on the solutions provided to national and regional problems. For example, research in occupational science could provide a different view of underemployment (Toulmin, 1995) or substance misuse, and hence different ideas about how these problems could be solved. Understanding the specific patterns of time use in daily life that produce a sense of boredom versus a sense of freedom may provide important insights into the motivation for engaging in occupations not acceptable to society as a whole, such as illegal ones.

Ideology

Ideology is the third concept that influences and is influenced by the development of science. Although the philosophical beliefs shared by occupational therapists around the globe are similar, ideologies of therapists in each region are different. An ideology is a group of somewhat coherent ideas held by societal members that might not necessarily be true (Bunge, 1984). It is defined as "a system of factual statements and value judgements that inspires some social movement or some social policy" (Bunge, 1999: 128). An ideology can be religious, secular, comprehensive, and/or sociopolitical. According to Bunge (1999), social actions must be examined in relation to the motivating ideology. Ideologically sanctioned actions affect the public well-being through the choices and beliefs they inspire. Ideologies are centrally placed in the intersection of the culture, economics, and politics of a given society (Bunge, 1984).

Social sciences cannot be ideologically neutral, in that it is important to be aware of the region's ideology when studying phenomena that have a social value. A specific ideology can either stimulate or stagnate the study of social phenomena (Bunge, 1984). Ideology goes beyond the definition of culture as an organization of social relationships, activities, and thought processes, and includes the economical and political system of the specific region. Bunge (1984) classifies ideologies as religious, sociopolitical, and those concerned with humanity and nature.

An ideology influences the goals and values utilized in the design of treatment techniques and in the service delivery models developed (Bunge, 1984). Service delivery is defined as the practical application of techniques to individuals in need of intervention (Bunge, 1984). Hence, the practice of occupational therapy in very different ideological environments will also be very different. For example, Chilean occupational therapists tended to develop practice arenas in public hospitals and marginal community settings when the dominant political ideology endorsed Christian and socialist values, whereas clinical practice in Chile under capitalism tended to develop practice delivery systems in the private sector. This tendency for the practice of occupational therapy to reflect regional ideologies can also be seen in other geographical regions of the globe.

An ideology can also influence the philosophical beliefs in a specific region. For example, some of the philosophical beliefs shared by occupational therapy include the view of the individual as autonomous and independent in daily life and the need to maintain a healthy balance among work, rest, and play. Although occupational therapists have valued the ability to be independent in activities of daily living, in certain cultures accepting the care of others is accepting their love, and interdependence is valued more than independence, suggesting a philosophical prioritization which may differ regionally.

With regard to the maintenance of a healthy balance among daily occupations, this concept is based on a society's view of work. The view of work depends on the society's ideology and the historical period. For example, in the USA, the view of a balance among work, rest, and play is strongly influenced by the Protestant work ethic. This view of work as good and primary and of play as frivolous is not necessarily shared around the globe. Also, this view of work, rest, and play has shifted over time. Americans, after spending increasingly more time at work, have become concerned about the lack of free time (Gibbs, 1989). Gibbs (1989) in *Time* magazine claimed that Americans may be running out of time to enjoy life. The article stated that work had become "trendy" and that most people felt there was not enough time to do all necessary chores and, hence, felt increasingly deprived (Gibbs, 1989). Occupational scientists in the USA are influenced by this ideology. Thus, their research reflects issues that are relevant to US culture—for example, the importance of play in adults' daily lives (Blanche, 1999). In a response to Gibbs (1989) and the ideological value placed on work in the USA, Blanche (1999) studied patterns of process-oriented (focused on the doing, not the outcome), enjoyable occupations chosen by adults in the USA. The study's results showed specific patterns of process-oriented occupations that become pivotal during transitional periods in a person's life (Blanche, 1999). Occupational therapists can use this information to develop innovative practice arenas or interventions addressing the need for balance in Americans' daily occupations described by Gibbs (1989). However, although the patterns identified by Blanche (1999) are probably universal, there are some variables that need to be considered before importing the results. First, the need to find process-oriented occupations may not be as imperative in less technological societies, and second, the expression of process-oriented, enjoyable occupations will depend on the regional, cultural, and ideological values in which they exist. Therefore occupational therapists outside the USA would need to evaluate these scientific findings in light of their own regional ideologies before importing them into their daily occupational therapy practice.

A Proposed Model of the Relationship Between International and Regional Daily Activities

The interaction among daily activities as viewed by occupational therapists in specific regions and the international aspects of a view from occupational science help form our global occupational therapy identity. Goldstein (1997) describes three aspects of the interaction between daily occupations and international events that can be used to explain the interaction between daily occupational therapy practice and the international influence of occupational science. First, international relations furnish scripts for daily lives in different regions in the globe. For example, in a nation such as the USA, the activities of recycling take on the meaning of preserving a global environment to a generation raised in this context, in contrast to those raised to see waste as a symbol of wealth. Second, everyday choices influence the nature of international relations. Our individual choices to add recycling occupations to our daily routine can affect the way our country is perceived by others on the globe. Third, individual identities are shaped by the interaction of daily lives and the international context. We can begin to see ourselves as members of a global ecosystem, perhaps a global community, through the interactions of our local daily occupations and international relations.

Using this model one can illustrate the relationship between occupational science as part of the international context and occupational therapy as the practice of daily occupations occurring in a specific region (Figure 62.1). The international relations of occupational science and therapy would include the formal and informal communications that occur among occupational therapists in different countries, including the work of the World Federation of Occupational Therapists (WFOT). International relations would also include the philosophy of occupational therapy. The international context includes those international relations and the

influence of occupational science on the profession. The everyday choices that influence the nature of international relations refer to the occupational therapy practitioner's choices and practices.

The identities that are shaped by the interaction of daily lives and the international context refer to the individual professional identity of each occupational therapist, shaped by daily choices of practice in a local/regional community and the information received from international sources such as the WFOT and international publications describing the latest developments in occupational therapy and occupational science. Figure 62.1 illustrates these proposed relationships. Some examples of how these interactions may occur are provided in what follows.

Research in occupational science can provide scripts for the daily practice of occupational therapy around the world. For example, research focusing on the effect of sensory integrative dysfunction on occupational choice of children in Los Angeles can provide a guideline that may shape practice in other parts of the world. Conversely, the everyday practice of occupational therapy can influence the global nature of occupational science and occupational therapy. This influence occurs when therapists in different countries simultaneously apply and question information imported from

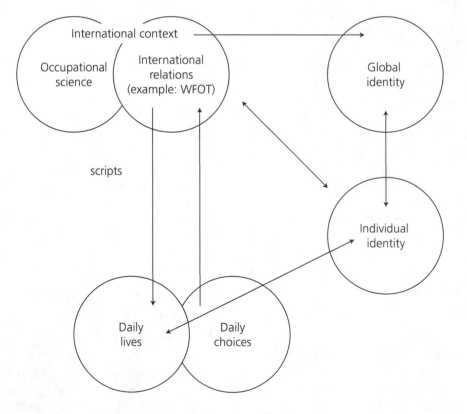

Daily occupational therapy practice

Figure 62.1. The interaction between daily occupations and international events (used to explain the interaction between daily occupational therapy practice and the international influence of occupational science).

other parts of the world into their daily practice. Research that describes to what degree the results can be generalized helps therapists determine which imported practices can be applied to culturally/regionally relevant occupational therapy situations and which can be disregarded where there is no fit with regional practices. Using the example of occupational science research about children in Los Angeles and its application to the global community, one can say that such research would provide answers that initially should be re-evaluated in each region. The original research would serve as a guideline by providing a question about the interaction between sensory integration dysfunction and occupational choices, and a possible methodology for exploring this question regionally. Another example illustrating the influence of occupational therapy practice in different regions on occupational science and global identity is the forensic practice of occupational therapists. The *WFOT Bulletin* dedicated most of the articles in one issue (November 1997) to occupational therapy services in forensics. In that issue Taylor et al. (1997) outline the role of occupational therapists in the forensic system in Alberta, Canada; Leroux (1997) outlines their role in France; Idzinga (1997) outlines their role in The Netherlands; Colpaert et al. (1997) outline their role in Belgium; and Busuttil (1997) outlines their role in Malta. Each of these articles illustrates the daily activities of occupational therapists in forensic systems in each region. By raising questions of social concern, these articles could influence future research in occupational science. For example, some questions that could be raised from these practices and that could be answered with occupational science research include, What are the patterns of activities performed by inmates? and What is the relationship between patterns of activities and satisfaction? Hence, the global identity of occupational therapy and occupational science may develop from the interaction between the daily lives of occupational therapists around the world and imported knowledge generated in the international occupational science community. Replicating research in different parts of the globe can support or reject the global character of some of our philosophical assumptions and would shape our global identity. As occupational therapists embrace the value of occupational science to their practice and continue to grow and shape their professional identities as a result of it, we must, in addition, consider the interplay of the profession's development and the influence of the region, culture, and history where it is practiced. The roots of regional or cultural beliefs can often be found in their ideology and philosophy.

A Proposed Model for Developing a Comprehensive Knowledge System

In answer to the initial question of the relevance of occupational science to occupational therapy practice in global communities, we have argued that philosophy, science, and ideology are key considerations. The generation of knowledge in

specific regions is illustrated in the following model. The relationship among philosophy, science, ideology, and other components describes the systematic character of scientific development in relation to occupational therapy practice in a global community. This model is presented in Figure 62.2.

In this model, philosophy, science, ideology, and service delivery systems are influenced by one another. Philosophy has an impact on scientific development by providing a "cosmovision" (Bunge, 1984). Cosmovision is the global view of reality and the way it can be understood. The cosmovision of occupational therapy philosophy is that occupation is important to the health and well-being of the individual. Conversely, scientific development influences philosophy through the production of new theories. For example, the occupational science assumption made by Clark (1997), referring to the "recursive relationship between occupation and narrative" as shaping personal identity (Clark, 1997: 102), was not previously part of the philosophy of occupational therapy. However, one can say that the patient's history has always been important to the practicing occupational therapist. Hence, this philosophical assumption has been redefined in occupational science and is presently influencing the philosophy and practice of occupational therapy.

Basic science is nourished with the problems studied in applied science. At the same time, basic science develops knowledge that informs applied science. Scientific development in applied sciences informs practice through the development of specific techniques, which in turn influence service delivery strategies. In this model, ideology influences the scientific development through the questions that are presumed to be important to study. Ideology also influences the development of specific techniques and the way the services are delivered by providing the values and goals of those services within a society (Bunge, 1984).

In this model, it is important to recognize our core philosophical values and ideology. In the global community, establishing a relationship with the evolving basic sciences has the potential to inform practice in occupational therapy, while being situated in the region's ideology (which includes culture, economics, and politics).

We suggest that occupational therapists in many countries who wish to import knowledge from evolving sciences in other countries work to develop their own scientific community at the same time. How can this be accomplished? There are three potential cultural styles that direct the development of scientific and cultural knowledge of a specific region that can be applied to our views of professional knowledge (Bunge, 1984). These are dependent (or colonialism), independent (or nationalism), and interdependent styles (or universalism). In the dependent style cultural goods and services are imported freely. For occupational therapy this is mainly the importing of techniques. This style tends to inhibit the development of the regional culture's knowledge and scientific inquiry. The second, independent

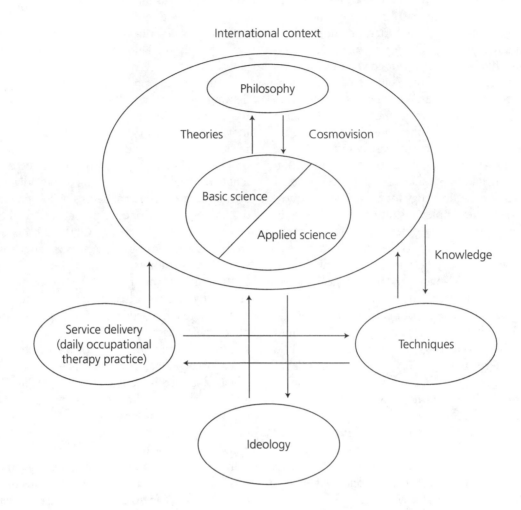

International context

Philosophy

Theories · Cosmovision

Basic science

Applied science

Knowledge

Service delivery
(daily occupational
therapy practice)

Techniques

Ideology

Figure 62.2. The relationship among philosophy, science, and ideology.

Note: This model is based on M. Bunge (1984) *Ciencia y desarrollo.* Buenos Aires: Siglo Veinte, p. 32.

style protects traditional cultures and discourages importing goods, practices, knowledge, and services. In this case, local occupational therapists lack the interaction which has been the basis for our global identity formation. The interdependent style favors the formation and development of national/regional research programs and educational systems; specifies that this formation of national scholars might be attained with the temporary help of foreign experts; and establishes an international exchange of cultural goods for knowledge production (such as books and assessment instruments). This last style is the one that is most often used in occupational therapy.

However, it still has weaknesses. One of those weaknesses is the required translation of publications and the ability to finance opportunities for international exchanges. Even with these limitations, this last model is the one offering the optimal system for global exchange and for developing a global identity among its participants.

Summary

Philosophy, science, and ideology interact in many ways. In this sense, the philosophy of occupational therapy influences and is influenced by the development of occupational science and ultimately influences the global identity of occupational therapists.

We believe that occupational science and occupational therapy share many philosophical beliefs, one of which is empowering people to become autonomous. Hence, occupational science empowers occupational therapists to become autonomous by inviting them to join in the development of their own science. Accepting this invitation requires an analysis of the relationship between international occupational science and occupational therapy, and their regional ideology. This analysis will ideally enable occupational therapists throughout the world to participate in developing further the global philosophy, science, and ideology of occupational science and occupational therapy.

References

Blanche E (1999). *Play and Process: The Experience of Play in the Life of the Adult*. Ann Arbor, MI: UMI.

Bontje P (1998). Trends in occupational therapy—a worldwide perspective. *World Federation of Occupational Therapists Bulletin 37:* 43–50,

Bunge M (1984). *Ciencia y desarrollo*. Buenos Aires: Ediciones Siglo Veinte.

Bunge M (1999). *Dictionary of Philosophy*. New York: Prometheus Books, pp. 210, 256, 258.

Busuttil J (1997). Forensic occupational therapy in *Malta: A historical. overview.* World Federation of Occupational Therapists Bulletin 36: 25–6.

Colpaert A, Cattier Y, Valentine C (1997). Experiences of creative workshops in Belgian prisons. *World Federation of Occupational Therapists Bulletin 36:* 20–4.

Christiansen C, Baum C (1997). Understanding occupation: Definitions and concepts. In C Christiansen, C Baum (eds) *Enabling Function and Wellbeing* (2nd edition). Thorofare, NJ: Slack, pp. 2–25.

Clark F (1997) Appendix III: Occupational science. In P Crist, CB Royeen (eds) *Infusing Occupation into Practice, Comparison of Three Clinical Approaches in Occupational Therapy*. Bethesda, MD: American Occupational Therapy Association.

Encyclopedia Americana—International Edition (1985). Danbury, CT: Grollier.

Gibbs N (1989). How America has run out of time. *Time* (24 April): 58–61, 64, 67.

Goldstein I (1997). International relations and everyday life. In R Zemke, F Clark (eds) *Occupational Science, The Evolving Discipline*. Philadelphia, PA: FA Davis, pp. 13–21.

Golledge J (1998). Distinguishing between occupation and activity. Part I: Review and explanation. *British Journal of Occupational Therapy 61*(3): 100–5.

Idzinga R (1997). Occupational therapy, forensics, and the care and treatment of addicts. *World Federation of Occupational Therapists Bulletin 36:* 1619.

Leroux V (1997). Lérgothérapie fonctoinnelle en milieu carcéral: une creation de poste. *World Federation of Occupational Therapists Bulletin 36:* 1 I–15.

Taylor E, Brintnell S, Shim M, Wilson S (1997). Forensic practice for occupational therapists—the Alberta experience. *World Federation of Occupational Therapists Bulletin 36:* 6–10.

Toulmin S (1995). Occupation, employment, and human welfare. *Journal of Occupational Science: Australia 2*(2): 48–58.

Yerxa E (1998). Health and the human spirit for occupation. *American Journal of Occupational Therapy 52:* 412–18. Reprinted as Chapter 34.

Zemke R, Clark F (eds). *Occupational Science, The Evolving Discipline*. Philadelphia, PA: FA Davis.

CHAPTER 63

Occupation by Design: Dimensions, Therapeutic Power, and Creative Process

DORIS PIERCE, PHD, OTR/L, FAOTA

Two forces are converging, creating conditions both challenging and potentially fruitful for occupational therapy. The profession's knowledge base describing occupation is growing exponentially. At the same time, functional outcomes of intervention are being increasingly valued within the health-care environment. Other professions imitate and claim our areas of expertise in the most flattering and dangerous ways. To benefit from the convergence of these forces, occupational therapy must expeditiously translate understanding of occupation into powerful occupation-based practice. Three bridges must be built: a generative discourse, demonstration sites, and effective education.

The occupational design approach offers important conceptual tools with which to rapidly build these bridges to powerful practice. Described here are subjective and contextual dimensions of occupational experience; elements of the occupational design process; and how these factors produce therapeutic power through the appeal, intactness, and accuracy of interventions.

Within occupational therapy, there is explosive growth in our understanding of occupation, the field's primary modality (American Occupational Therapy Association [AOTA], 1995; Clark et al., 1991; Kielhofner, 1992; Nelson, 1997; Primeau, 1996; Schkade & Schultz, 1992 [see Chapter 11]; Yerxa et al., 1989; Zemke & Clark, 1996). Simultaneously, the health-care system is increasingly valuing functional, or occupational, outcomes. A potential time of congruence is approaching if occupational therapy can expeditiously translate an expanding knowledge of occupation into powerful occupation-based practice.

Occupational therapy is already responding to the stronger emphasis on functional outcomes in health care by moving away from medical model, component-based practice and toward more whole, top–down, occupation-based practice (Coster, 1998; Law, 1998). Other professions are also responding. They honor the validity of occupation in the most flattering and dangerous ways by imitating our focus and claiming it as their own area of expertise (Wood, 1998). In the face of aggressive competition for our traditional areas of practice, the key to our success is simple: just be the best at what we do. We must use occupation in the most powerful therapeutic ways possible. We must consistently target functional occupational patterns as outcomes. And, we must be eloquent about our unique clinical perspective.

When occupational science first made its promise to occupational therapy that basic research into typical occupations would enhance therapeutic efficacy (Clark et al., 1991; Yerxa et al., 1989), some doubted (Mosey, 1992). How would a scattershot of various studies into occupation effectively move the field forward? In critical need of research on clinical issues, could we afford investment of time and energy in basic research? These are good, tough questions. The usefulness to occupational therapy of basic research into occupation could be relatively limited if it is not complemented by specific strategies to bring this knowledge into practice.

To bring the full potential of occupation to bear in the lives of clients requires three critical bridges: a generative discourse regarding occupation-based practice, demonstration sites, and effective education. Building such bridges requires new conceptual tools. The occupational design approach described here offers the following concepts to support the translation of basic knowledge of occupation into practice applications: the subjective and contextual dimensions of occupational experience, occupational design process, and three sources of therapeutic power in occupation-based interventions. Before exploring these new concepts, let us look more closely at the three bridges, or the three creative loci in the life of the profession where knowledge of occupation can be most forcefully and rapidly applied to enhance the power of practice (see Figure 63.1).

Three Bridges to Build: Translating Knowledge of Occupation Into Powerful Occupation-Based Practice

Bridge: A Generative Discourse on the Use of Occupation in Practice

The first bridge needed is an active discourse regarding the relation between theories and research describing typical occupations and their application in practice. This discussion must go on in public and private ways, from scholarly publications to the mind of the therapist during intervention. The discourse must be highly productive of useful new concepts. That is, we must be able to talk the talk of how occupation is used in practice frequently, fluently, and in a way that spurs a rapid evolution of innovative practice thinking.

We require language for articulating how the translation from knowledge to practice occurs. The most obvious explanation of how we use knowledge of occupation in practice is that by understanding occupation more fully, therapists are better prepared to use and interpret it in working with clients. The meaning of this statement, however, is not particularly transparent. Similarly, reasoning from a depth of background in how humans experience occupation is not a simple form of clinical thinking. Basing day-to-day practice on the study of occupation as it occurs in typical and atypical conditions is a demanding, theoretical, action-oriented, and fluid style of intervention. It is difficult to describe.

Generative discourse has already begun to produce an occupation-based practice language. For example, one clarifying concept that has emerged is the distinction between the use of occupation as the means of intervention versus the end of intervention (Cynkin, 1995; Gray, 1998 [Reprinted as Chapter 15]; Trombly, 1995 [see Chapter 16]). Current research on functional outcomes and the development of

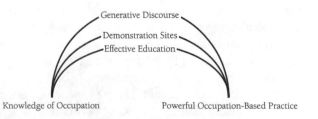

Figure 63.1. Three bridges required to rapidly translate knowledge of occupation into powerful occupation-based practice.

Note. From *Occupation by Design* by D. Pierce, 2003. Philadelphia: F. A. Davis. Reprinted with permission from publisher.

top–down assessments will also provide new language to practice (Coster, 1998). Drawing heavily from anthropology is a fruitful strategy for importing humanistic theories to describe human experience, as is demonstrated by clinical reasoning and narrative research (Clark, 1993; Clark, Carlson, & Polkinghorne, 1997; Mattingly & Fleming, 1994). As this generative discourse about the use of knowledge of occupation in practice grows, occupational therapy will find the more technical, static structures of frames of reference a poor fit. The language of occupation-based practice will be more dynamic and reflective. A flourishing, generative discourse on the use of occupation in practice is an essential bridge for putting our knowledge of occupation to work, ultimately to enhance the efficacy of intervention.

Bridge: Practice Demonstration Sites

The field requires a thousand bridges in the form of practice demonstration sites that explore, create, model, and disseminate how it is that knowledge of occupation can be effectively brought to bear in different types of practice. This is where occupational therapy must walk the walk of occupation in practice.

Demonstration sites that are productive of new concepts regarding occupation-based practice will be marked by four indicators. They will depend on insightful clinical reasoning based in the study of occupation. Powerful intervention will be provided through custom-designed, naturalistic occupational experiences. Collaborative identification of desired, functional occupational patterns will provide the goals of intervention. And, lastly, these sites will be successful in communicating within the system of health care and establishing a sufficient referral and reimbursement base.

These programs already exist (Clark et al., 1997; Jackson, Carlson, Mandel, Zemke, & Clark, 1998). It is critically important that the field benefit from the accumulating expertise at such exemplary sites through publication of their successes. Descriptions of these programs are important to our shared sense of the potential variety and number of powerful, occupation-based, life-enhancing programs possible. In these changing and competitive times in health care, the bridge of successful practice demonstration sites is critical to the profession's survival.

Bridge: Educating Sophisticated Practitioners to Use Knowledge of Occupation in Practice

The field requires educational programs that have been specifically constructed with a focus on teaching effective occupation-based practice (Yerxa, 1998). Presently, students enter the field with cultural values that give higher status to technical, medical knowledge than to the highly theoretical yet commonsense knowledge of how what we do shapes who we are. If uninfluenced, these values produce graduates who respect the knowledge base of other professions more than they do their own. Students require much more rigorous education regarding occupation. The profession can no longer afford to give lip service to occupation in the curriculum while handing over the largest portion of the student's study time to component-focused and physiological knowledge.

Reprioritizing and shifting the balance of curriculum content so that students will emerge with the necessary skills for effectively applying an understanding of occupation in practice will deeply challenge occupational therapy education. Hard decisions will be required: Less anatomy and more ethnography of disability? less infant reflexes and more family theory? For some educators, these are shocking ideas. But the curriculum is not infinitely expandable. Too often, students enter the field feeling overwhelmed by their fragmented understanding of many different knowledge bases. It is the responsibility of educators, not students, to resolve the tough issues in our knowledge base in order to offer centrally integrating concepts.

To accomplish such a rapid refocusing of mission in our educational programs will require several efforts from educators: clear recognition that teaching specific intervention techniques will not provide a lasting education in today's fast-changing health-care environment; faculty development around knowledge of occupation in practice; commitment to preparing students with insight into occupational experience and its use in intervention; and reconfiguration of curricular structures. In this process, education will draw on the conceptual language springing from the generative discourse on occupation-based practice as well as from conceptual discoveries at demonstration sites. Students prepared in this way will be innovative, entrepreneurial, and drawn to sites at which exemplary practice is taking place.

The graduate who brings a deep preparation in occupation's use in practice will be able to not only walk the walk of occupation-based intervention, but also talk the walk. That is, graduates will be able to explain why their occupation-based interventions are effectively designed for a specific person with a specific goal. Such a sophisticated graduate will be ready to adapt interventions to a variety of persons, disabilities, and settings. She or he will use the language of occupation's therapeutic power in a way that is compelling, understandable to others, and anchored in everyday experience. Not only will graduates prepared in an occupation-focused curriculum use more powerful interventions, but they also will be more eloquent about why such an approach is effective.

Bridge-Building Tools: Dimensions of Occupation, Sources of Therapeutic Power, and Occupational Design Process

As stated, in order to thrive the profession requires three bridges to move knowledge of occupation into powerful applications in practice: a generative discourse, demonstration practice sites, and education that focuses on occupation-based intervention to produce sophisticated practitioners. In this effort, the following conceptual tools should prove useful: an

understanding of the dimensions of occupational experience, language articulating the sources of therapeutic power in occupation-based interventions, and a process for design of therapeutic occupations.

Dimensions of Occupation: Sources of Therapeutic Power

To use occupation most effectively in practice, the therapist must understand its dimensions sufficiently to be able to conceptualize their occurring effects as they unfold during therapy. Here, I offer six primary dimensions of occupation (three subjective, three contextual) and the occupational design process. I will describe how these concepts translate into three primary sources of therapeutic power in occupation-based interventions (Pierce, 1997a, 1998, in press; Zemke & Pierce, 1994) (see Figure 63.2).

The important point here is not that these are the definitive dimensions of occupation or the final statement regarding the sources of its therapeutic power in practice. Other categories could have been constructed to describe occupation and its application, although many of the same concepts would surely have been included. The value of the occupational design approach presented here is that it broadly describes both the complex whole of a person's occupational experience and the elements of the therapeutic process in order to provide the therapist with conceptual sources of therapeutic power upon which she or he can easily reflect before, during, and after intervention.

Appeal: Designing with productivity, pleasure, and restoration. Appeal is the degree to which the client finds the therapeutic occupation desirable in terms of the levels of productivity, pleasure, and restoration he or she experiences (Pierce, 1997a, 1998). Designing intervention that has high appeal requires a knowledge base in how humans typically experience occupations along these subjective dimensions. This depth of knowledge must be matched by the therapist's skills for creating an informed perspective on the uniqueness of each client, especially through observation and interview. Interventions that blend pleasure, productivity, and restoration in a careful mix that is most likely to be appealing to that person at that time can then be created collaboratively.

Beyond work, play, and self-care. Since the beginning of the profession, occupational therapists have thought of occupation within familiar categories provided by our western cultural history, such as work, play, leisure, and self-care. These commonsense categories (Geertz, 1983) carry great wisdom, tapping essential differences in human activity. As occupational scientists have begun to examine these categories more closely, however, they appear to be simplistic, value laden, decontextualized, and insufficiently descriptive of subjective experience (Pierce, 1997b; Primeau, 1996). There is an important place for these historical terms, certainly. Yet, they are not fully adequate to support masterful design of interventions based in knowledge of occupation.

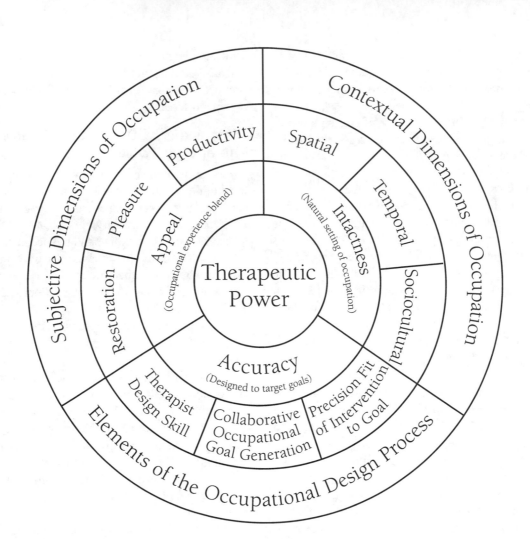

Appeal + Intactness + Accuracy = Therapeutic Power

Figure 63.2. The occupational design approach: Conceptual tools for building occupation-based practice.
Note. From *Occupation by Design* by D. Pierce, 2003. Philadelphia: F. A. Davis. Reprinted with permission from publisher.

By moving beyond the old categories, we can begin to examine how the subjective experience of occupation is made up of a unique mix of pleasure, productivity, and restoration. These three characteristics echo the familiar activity classes of play, work, and rest found in the occupational therapy literature. However, the radical difference is in the inclusive nature of the word *and*. In this approach, pleasure, productivity, and restoration are not categories among which one must choose to describe an occupation. Rather, they are three characteristics that exist simultaneously, to some degree, in all occupational experience. Every occupational experience is a blend of the three. This blending is central to the art of therapy to produce the most appealing therapeutic occupation for a client.

Productivity's contribution to the appeal of an occupation. Humans love to be productive. Give us a game, a goal, a project, or an inspiring product to build and we are off and running. Productivity seems to be central to our nature, perhaps built in by its support of our evolutionary success.

Productivity extends beyond work to include the goal-focused dimension of all occupations. It often yields great personal satisfaction. To tap productivity in powerful intervention design, therapists must acquire a knowledge base that addresses productivity in theoretical and descriptive depth. Topics that might be included in such study are the history of industrialization and the Protestant work ethic (Gellner, 1988); the tie of work and identity (Christiansen, 1999); pride of craftsmanship (Cross, 1990; Dickie, 1998); the nature of unpaid work, such as housework and caregiving (Hasselkus, 1991; Primeau, 1992); typical career progressions and retirement (Healy, 1982); the dynamics of stress (Keller, Shiflet, & Bartlett, 1994); games and sports (Harris & Park, 1983); learning; and self-actualization (Maslow, 1954). If a client appears to be motivated by a therapeutic occupation high in the experience of productivity, the therapist can then draw on this knowledge of productivity's elements to design an intervention with a satisfying outcome and clear goal achievement.

Pleasure's contribution to the appeal of an occupation. Occupational therapists have always operated from an intuitive understanding of what is pleasurable in intervention. Making intervention pleasurable is a key to engagement. Perhaps this is why we still retain our use of play, crafts, cooking, and other usually pleasurable activities in our intervention repertoires, despite our difficulties in fitting such activities into medical settings. Because they are pleasurable, they are effective (Pierce, 1997b).

Pleasure is nearly the opposite of goal-focused productivity. Pleasure is process-focused. Pleasure is the degree of enjoyment a person experiences in an occupation. Influenced by our productivity-oriented society, occupational therapy has neglected research into pleasure in intervention, focusing instead on the seriousness and respectability of the study of purposefulness and intervention outcomes. It is natural when entering into a contract with clients to assist them in reaching certain goals that we should be primarily concerned with the productivity of that effort. Yet, the efficacy of our intervention also depends on its pleasure. Pediatric occupational therapists are especially aware of this and, so, depend heavily on play (Parham & Fazio, 1996). Even for those clients who can complete interventions through a determined commitment to outcomes, the addition of pleasure to the intervention has beneficial effects on mood, health, and recovery. Areas of understanding that would support a therapist's creative use of the pleasurable dimension of occupation to enhance the appeal of intervention include sensory and limbic system processing (Guyton, 1991; Martin, 1996), arousal (Fisher, Murray, & Bundy, 1991), thrill-seeking activities, play across the life span (Cohen, 1987; Cross, 1990; Rubin, 1980), crafts and hobbies (Fidler & Velde, 1999), comedy and humor (Huizinga, 1950), the link between highly physical activity and endorphins (Davis, 1984), and aesthetics (Goodman, 1951). Applying a developed understanding of pleasure to intervention design is bound to enhance the appeal, and thus the efficacy, of interventions.

Restoration's contribution to the appeal of occupation. Restoration is the subjective aspect of occupational experience that restores our energy levels and ability to continue to engage in our daily lives. Restoration is the most neglected and poorly understood of the three subjective dimensions of occupation. Though therapists may speak often about restoring persons, this is unlikely to slow the pace and demand of intervention. Despite Meyer's (1922) (see Chapter 2) seminal description of rest as a primary occupation to be considered by the emerging field of occupational therapy, little has evolved from this idea in subsequent occupational therapy literature.

An understanding of the restorative dimension of occupation must be based in an appreciation of the basic, life-giving occupation of sleep (Coren, 1996; Hobson, 1989; Pierce, 1997b). Indeed, sleep is one occupation without which we would soon die. Because culture has long construed sleep as a ceasing of consciousness, occupational therapy has followed suit by being concerned solely with waking occupations. However, research from the relatively new specialty of sleep medicine is changing the conceptualization of sleep from unconsciousness to a different form of consciousness (Carskadon & Dement, 1994; Moorcroft, 1989). To grasp the patterns that exist in the round of daily activity, that round must be viewed in its full 24-hour circadian rhythm (Moore-Ede, Sulzman, & Fuller, 1982). Sleep quality affects neural plasticity, healing, immune function, cognitive capacities, physical abilities, and mood (Coren, 1996; Pierce, 1997b). As an occupation, sleep is fascinating. It shows clear neurophysiological fluctuations, developmental changes, and susceptibility to environmental influence and disruption (Bliwise, 1994; Schnelle, Alessi, Ouslander, & Simmons, 1993; Sheldon, Spire, & Levy, 1982). Disturbances in this occupation are specifically named as medical diagnoses, such as sleep apnea (Carskadon & Dement, 1994). Many of our clients have undiagnosed sleep problems due to respiratory disorders, neurophysiologic disorganization, medications, disruptive sleep environments, shift work, poorly managed schedules, or extended stays in intensive care units. Until occupational therapists understand enough about sleep to assure that it is providing an adequate base for other occupations, efficacy in treating waking occupational patterns will not reach its full potential.

Waking occupations that are highly restorative are also important to intervention. For a client who is very disorganized, depleted, or discouraged, intervention may need to be not highly productive, but highly restorative. Clinical judgment is required to discern what occupations a specific person may experience as restorative. People find waking restoration in different ways: quiet-focus occupations, such as needlework or woodworking; being in nature; viewing art; listening to music; quiet and solitude; socializing; a physical workout; self-care activities; or prayer and meditation. Of course, eating and drinking are also essential to restoration, though they can be done in ways that range from highly restorative to barely maintaining physiologic function. Occupational therapy is only at the beginning of exploring this important dimension in designing powerful, appealing intervention.

Masterful design of appealing intervention. Designing appealing intervention, and thus enhancing intervention power, requires a sophisticated understanding of the productive, pleasurable, and restorative dimensions of the subjective experience of occupation. Taken one at a time, the importance of each of the three dimensions' contribution to the appeal of an occupation in intervention is easily argued. The true potency of using an occupational design approach lies, however, in the carefully blended combination of the three. High appeal is one source of therapeutic power. As such, appeal is a tool for the rapid building of the three bridges to strong occupation-based practice: a generative discourse, demonstration sites, and effective education.

Intactness: Designing With Spatial, Temporal, and Sociocultural Context

Intactness is the degree to which a therapeutic occupation occurs in the usual spatial, temporal, and sociocultural conditions in which it would usually occur for that client if it were not being used as intervention (Pierce, 1997a, 1998). Intactness can also be thought of as the naturalization of therapeutic occupation through the use of typical context. In the client's own settings, the challenges, barriers, adaptations, and potential problem solutions are more clearly evident than they can be in virtual and unfamiliar environments, such as the clinic. In the customary context, the objects, cues, and complete sequences involved in an occupation of concern are physically real to both the therapist and the client. The client is not required to reason from a simulated experience to the real challenge encountered later in full context. The custom-fit nature of a client's usual settings increases the generalizability and validity of the intervention.

In keeping with the individualistic western culture from which it springs, occupational therapy has traditionally focused more on the intraindividual characteristics of occupation than on the contextual dimensions. For this reason, it is likely that enhancing appeal through design with pleasure, productivity, and restoration will come more easily to therapists than will designing for intactness through the use of the client's typical context. Strengthening the intactness of intervention is likely to shift intervention toward enhanced understandability for clients, greater holism, more community-based interventions, and increased efficacy.

Spatial context as an element of intactness. In occupational therapy, the spatial dimension of occupation that is beyond immediate physiology has been little explored, with some exceptions in the areas of tools, adaptive devices, and architectural adaptations (Trombly, 1989; Wilcock, 1998; Zemke & Horger, 1995). To effectively use the spatial context of occupation in intervention, occupational therapists require a more sophisticated appreciation of how spaces and objects support, shape, and inhibit individual experience (Holohan, 1986; Pierce, 2000; Rowles, 1991 [see Chapter 26]).

The most primary spatial aspect of human occupation is our embodiedness (Frank, 1986). Evolution has shaped the human with unique capacities to interact with the physical world: the upright pelvis, the senses, the hand, and the fertile and ceaseless conceptualizations of the neocortex. We experience our lives from within a framework of human neurophysiology: sensation, perception, ideation, and movement (Ayres, 1985). Occupational therapists are masters at understanding how occupational experience is shaped by human embodiedness, especially as it is affected by disability.

Human cultural adaptation is marked by the innumerable physical objects involved in our behavior (Hodder, 1989). A rich material culture is central to our nature as occupational beings. We survive and express ourselves through our objects: clothing, crops, vehicles, shelters, tools, toys, foods, medicines, communication devices, written materials, and aesthetic and ritual objects (Dickie & Frank, 1996). Ethnic traditions are marked by unique material culture and the action routines that support it, passed down through generations. Spaces, tools, and products can express identity: People often become deeply attached to them (Csikszentmihalyi & Rochberg-Halton, 1981). The qualities of the spaces in which people work and live, including the light, sound, size, smell, and perceptions of safety or threat there, are not abstractions to them (Holohan, 1986). They are places full of personal meaning and cultural symbols (Altman & Low, 1992; Rowles, 1991 [see Chapter 26]). Mapping and interpreting novel spaces begins the moment people encounter them (Evans, 1980; Kaplan & Kaplan, 1981; Neisser, 1991). Routines are overlaid on familiar spaces, enabling us to reach for toothbrush and then toothpaste in their usual spots without pausing as we think about other things. It is not within an abstract space, but within a familiar and experientially patterned place that humans engage in most of their occupations.

Using the spatial dimension to enhance the intactness of occupation-based intervention requires the therapist to comprehend spatial experience from the client's perspective. How is embodiedness affecting experience? What are the usual spaces in which occupations of interest in the intervention occur, and how are the routines mapped over those environments? What objects are of importance in the occupational pattern of the client in terms of function, identity, and personal meaning? What do the spaces and objects tell the therapist about the client? Are there barriers in cherished places that may be disrupting desired occupational patterns? How are the client's typical occupational patterns laid out within home, workplace, or neighborhood? By developing such insights into the spatial dimension of a client's daily experience, the therapist can design powerfully intact therapeutic occupations.

Temporal context as an element of intactness. Occupational therapists deal constantly with the temporal structures of human occupation in intervention, yet the occupational therapy literature on the temporality of human experience is extremely limited. The most basic temporal pattern of our occupations is the circadian rhythm (Moore-Ede et al., 1982; Swaab, Fliers, & Partiman, 1985). Entrained to the light, we move in a general synchrony of fluctuations in energy level and the relatively predictable round of activities required to meet our physiological needs, such as sleeping and eating meals. With the advent of electric lighting, the predominant pattern of rising with the sun and going to bed with the dark loosened somewhat, but most people continue in the same light–dark-driven pattern that has presumably regulated human occupation since the beginning of time (Coren, 1996; Pierce, 1997b).

The temporality of the life span is also basic to our experience of occupation. In western cultures we see birth as a beginning and death as an ending to our mortal existence. This linear and finite view of time poses existential challenges for the individual's construction of an optimal occupational pattern over a lifetime. Some cultures see time in a more cyclic way, emphasizing the repeating patterns of similar events (Hall, 1983). The temporality of physiological and personal maturation also impose a general developmental shape on the occupational patterns of persons at different ages (Pierce, 2000; Royeen, 1994). Occupational therapists are commonly trained in developmental theories descriptive of life patterns across the life span. Such theories, however, are extradisciplinary and do not focus on changes in occupational experience with age.

Within these broad circadian and developmental templates, people construct a unique occupational pattern each day, orchestrating and completing a series of occupations (Clark, 1993; Segal & Frank, 1998). Within situational constraints, we manage the pace, duration, sequence, and timing of each occupation (Zerubavel, 1981). Habits and routines emerge from repeated patterns, simplifying management of the sequences (Zemke, 1994). Depending on the quality of engagement, time can feel like it is moving quickly or slowly. Memory allows reflection on the temporal patterns of our occupations and planning ahead in anticipation of their sequences and orchestration. Narratives are constructed and reconstructed to package experience in valued, storied configurations (Clark, 1993; Larson & Fanchiang, 1996). The cumulation of these daily patterns of experience over days or years can yield skill, adaptation, identity, and insight.

Using temporality to provide more powerfully intact intervention will require the therapist to reflect on the client's usual temporal experience of the occupation being used in intervention or being targeted as an outcome. By matching the pace, sequence, timing, circadian rhythm, and developmental structures of a therapeutic occupation to those most natural to the client, the power of the intervention is enhanced. Therapists tend to be intuitive about doing this, scheduling, for example, activities of daily living training for mornings and feeding sessions at mealtimes. However, by bringing this dimension of occupation in intervention more cogently to mind, it can be used, improved, researched, and taught more effectively than it can be while remaining on a more intuitive level of clinical action.

Sociocultural context as an element of intactness.
The sociocultural dimension of occupational context is fairly well-understood in occupational therapy compared with the temporal and spatial dimensions of occupational context.

Occupational therapy has drawn strongly from the social sciences, especially anthropology, since the time of Reilly (1974), appropriating such informative key concepts as relationship, family, kinship, community, class, race, ethnicity, gender, stigma, values, ritual, symbol, adaptation, narrative, history, economics, and politics. Skillful use of these conceptual aspects of the sociocultural context is critical to the impact of occupation-based intervention.

A fairly concrete aspect of the sociocultural dimension of occupation is the degree to which it is interactive. A unique class of occupations, called co-occupations, can occur only in interaction with a partner (Pierce, 1997a). Teaching, caregiving, and playing tennis are examples of co-occupations. Some occupations occur as shared or parallel experiences, such as watching television with others. Occupations can also occur in complete solitude.

A critical aspect of the sociocultural dimension of occupation in intervention is power relations (Foucault, 1980). Recognizing status and power dynamics between the client and others, such as the therapist, family members, other service providers, insurers, and institutions, is important to negotiating systems of care and advocating effectively for a client. Feminist theory can also make important contributions here, explicating the power relations that lie in the social construction of gender (Smith, 1987). Intact intervention requires that the client feel, at minimum, the degree of power over the therapeutic occupation that he or she would if the therapist were not involved. Significant intervention gains targeting the most important goals of a client can only be accomplished by letting go of the directive expert viewpoint and adopting a learning–collaborative view of intervention (Law, 1998; Rosa & Hasselkus, 1996).

Shared social and cultural expectations also shape our use of space and time. There is public space and private space, public time and private time (Hall, 1976, Zerubavel, 1981). Spaces can be crowded or empty of other people. Time can be social or solitary. Interpersonal space and timing of interactions are highly expressive of our identities in relation to others through eye contact, distance, touch, action synchrony, and turn taking (Hall, 1976). The complex symbolic meanings of places is passed down in the history of culture. Holidays, the 7-day week, and the workweek–weekend cycle strongly shape our occupational patterns through the established calendar (Zerubavel, 1981). Each culture has its own unique customs for constructing, valuing, and using the space and time within which its members experience occupations.

In terms of the sociocultural dimension, therapists are generally both insightful and intuitive in constructing intervention that is natural and well designed for and with individual clients. The founders of the field were attuned to such sociocultural concepts as habit training and return to a productive worker role after disability (Slagle, 1922; Quiroga, 1995). The framework of occupational behavior (Reilly, 1974) imported many informative social science concepts into the profession's literature that enhanced understanding of the sociocultural dimension. More and more, awareness of diversity is being drawn on to enhance intervention. In regard to the spatial, temporal, and sociocultural contexts of occupation, it is in designing within the sociocultural dimension that occupational therapy interventions are most powerfully intact.

Designing contextually intact therapeutic occupations. By understanding the contextual dimensions of occupational experience, the therapist can design occupation-based intervention that is more effective through its intactness. Of course, because of institutional and pragmatic constraints, it is not possible to consistently enact intervention in perfectly intact context. Intervention must approximate intactness to the degree feasible. And, being attuned to intactness, the therapist will be ready to move toward intactness in both small and large ways when opportunities arise. Questioning and seeking out the most intact temporal, spatial, and sociocultural conditions for each therapeutic occupation is a direct avenue to more powerful intervention. Thus, the idea of spatially, temporally, and socioculturally intact intervention contributes another useful tool for rapidly building bridges to strong occupation-based practice.

Accuracy: Designing to Target Client Goals Effectively

Accuracy is the degree to which the therapeutic occupation precisely targets collaboratively developed occupational goals. A good illustration of the variable degrees of accuracy that can occur is to consider the way in which group interventions can sometimes fit the goals of some clients in the group better than it does others. The accuracy of occupation-based interventions depends on therapist design skill, collaborative generation of occupational goals, and precision fit of the intervention to the goal.

Therapist design skill. Occupational therapists require highly sophisticated design skills. The average workday of an occupational therapist is a series of high challenges to design skill (Pierce, in press). An essential process of successful occupational therapy is consistently producing creative solutions to fit the life problems and goals of individual clients, doing this thinking much of the time during complex action.

As other professions have discovered, to produce graduates who can consistently design effective and creative outcomes that fit client needs, it is necessary to be explicit and deliberate in teaching these skills. Architects in training learn the process of design through the studio method (Boyer & Mitgang, 1996; Koberg & Bagnall, 1991; Schön, 1987). In addition to other classes, architecture students share a studio in which assigned design problems are worked on under the supervision of an experienced architect. Discussions, frequent group critiques, and formal design juries are used to develop the students' abilities to explicitly discuss the phases and strategies of the creative process in which they are engaged (Jones, 1981; Straub, 1978; Wade, 1977). Consumers are expected to give input throughout the development of architectural designs.

Engineering's educational approach focuses on successful problem solving, although the creative process itself has received little explicit attention in engineering curricula until recently (Fogler & LeBlanc, 1995). While immersed in content, such as physics or electrical theory, engineering students are simply presented with challenging problems to solve outside of class. The World Solar Car Race, for instance, is a now-famous engineering school problem. Engineers are especially skilled at planning and implementing large, multitask projects.

In medical education, problem-based learning is being used to enhance students' abilities to address the puzzles of daily practice through learning situations that emphasize self-directed and small group work on cases (Boud & Feletti, 1991; Royeen, 1995). The common features of the three professions' educational approaches are the students' engagement in constructed challenges, the requirement of creative thinking, and learning contexts that approximate practice settings.

Informed by the educational strategies of architecture, engineering, and medicine, occupational therapy can become better at educating practitioners in skillful occupational design. Of these three examples of professional education, architecture's studio approach provides the strongest match to occupational therapy because both professions emphasize process, an arts aesthetic, consumer involvement, and the ability to reflect on and discuss the creative thinking required for effective practice (Koberg & Bagnall, 1991; Mattingly & Fleming, 1994; Pierce, in press). Drawing on the curricular strategies of other professions, occupational therapists can be equipped with highly developed design skills of self-motivation, problem analysis, idea generation and selection, complex implementation, and process evaluation. Such sophisticated design skills can equip graduates to consistently create accurate, and thus therapeutically powerful, occupation-based interventions.

Collaborative occupational goal generation. Highly accurate interventions must target occupational patterns as the end, or goal, of intervention and create those goals in collaboration with the client. An occupational pattern is an observable shape or regularity in the recurrences of similar occupations in a person's life (Pierce, 1997a, 1997b; Zemke & Pierce, 1994). Therapists, clients, and caregivers frequently identify occupational patterns as goals; for example, a school-based intervention goal could be for a student to independently use the lunchroom. To target broad, functional occupational patterns as an end of intervention, a substantial knowledge of typical occupational patterns across the life span is essential. The therapist must understand how the targeted occupational patterns are a part of identity, social acceptance, function, and health.

Trombly (1995) (see Chapter 16), Gray (1998) (see Chapter 15), and Cynkin (1995) described the use of occupation and activity as the means and ends of intervention. Setting occupational pattern goals with clients is using occupation as the end of intervention. Top–down, or occupation-focused, assessments contribute significantly to occupational therapists' ability to target occupational patterns as ends of intervention (Coster, 1998). If the intervention accurately targets an occupational outcome desired by the client, even the most mechanistic approach to intervention can be considered occupation-based. To set occupational goals that are well fit to the client requires strong collaborative goal-setting skills (Law, 1998; Rosa & Hasselkus, 1996). For this, a willingness of the therapist to release the powerful position of expert decision-maker is essential. Highly developed abilities to interview, observe, and assist in prioritizing the client's and caregivers' needs are also required.

Precision fit of intervention to goal. Precision fit is simply a measure of how well the therapeutic occupation directly addressed the goals. The fit of the intervention to the goals can be weakened by many conditions common to intervention settings: limitations to intervention flexibility, such as standard protocols; inadequate time for intervention planning; attempting intervention in unsuitable environments or without adequate materials; or serving clients with diverse goals through group interventions. Even under such conditions the therapist can more effectively create therapeutic occupations that provide a powerful match to the client's needs by reflecting on the precision of the fit. This is hardly a new concept for occupational therapy, although it bears repeating.

Fitting a therapeutic occupation to client need is as old as the field. What is new here is the idea of reflecting on the *degree* of fit. Questioning whether an occupation-based intervention is being used is an ongoing theme of discussion in the profession (Wood, 1998). Less common is the questioning of *how well* the occupation used met a particular client's goals, what interfered in that effort, and what activity or setting might have fit the targeted goals better. Reflecting on the preciseness of fit after an intervention is a valuable form of productive dreaming about ideal intervention. Used consistently, such reflection will yield growth for the therapist and enhanced efficacy for clients.

Accuracy: Therapist design skill, collaborative goals, and precision fit. Accuracy will boost the therapeutic power of any intervention. Powerful effects are produced by combining highly developed design skills, collaborative goals as the ends of intervention, and a therapeutic occupation that is precisely fit to those goals. Occupational therapists are the consummate professionals in this holistic approach to intervention. Thus, to the previous conceptual tools of appeal and intactness is now added a third important tool for making the bridge from knowledge of occupation to strong occupation-based practice—accuracy.

A Field's Translation: From Knowledge of Occupation to Designing for Therapeutic Power

The present is, paradoxically, both a fruitful and a dangerous time of congruence between our expanding knowledge base regarding occupation and the increased valuing of functional outcomes in health care. Occupational therapy must critically examine and recreate its traditions in theory and practice if it is to live up to its potential for providing clients with powerful interventions based on a deep understanding of occupational experience. To match the pace of change in health care, the profession must deliberately and rapidly build bridges between theoretical research on occupation and the powerful use of occupation in practice. A generative discourse around occupation-based practice, demonstration sites, and effective education are the bridges that are needed. Offered here are new conceptual tools for these bridge-building efforts: the subjective and contextual dimensions of occupation and the design process through which they can be translated into therapeutic occupations high in occupational appeal, intactness, and accuracy.

Acknowledgment

The ideas I present here are an outgrowth of years of discussion with Ruth Zemke, PhD, OTR, FAOTA, of the University of Southern California. Few are so fortunate in their colleagues.

References

Altman, I., & Low, S. M. (1992). *Place attachment.* New York: Plenum.

American Occupational Therapy Association. (1995). Position paper: Occupation. *American Journal of Occupational Therapy, 49,* 1015–1018.

Ayres, A. J. (1985). *Developmental dyspraxia and adult onset apraxia.* Torrance, CA: Sensory Integration International.

Bliwise, D. L. (1994). Normal aging. In M. H. Kryger, T. Roth, & W. C. Dement (Eds.), *Principles and practices of sleep medicine* (pp. 26–39). Philadelphia: Saunders.

Boud, D., & Feletti, G. (1991). *The challenge of problem-based learning.* New York: St. Martin's.

Boyer, E., & Mitgang, L. (1996). *Building community: A new future for architecture education and practice.* Princeton, NJ: Carnegie Foundation for the Advancement of Teaching.

Carskadon, M. A., & Dement, W. C. (1994). Normal human sleep: An overview. In M. H. Kryger, T. Roth, & W. C. Dement (Eds.), *Principles and practices of sleep medicine* (pp. 16–25). Philadelphia: Saunders.

Clark, F. (1993). Occupation embedded in a real life: Interweaving occupational science and occupational therapy, 1993 Eleanor Clarke Slagle Lecture. *American Journal of Occupational Therapy, 47,* 1067–1078.

Clark, F., Azen, S., Zemke, R., Jackson, J., Carlson, M., Mandel, D., Hay, J., Josephson, K., Cherry, B., Hessle, C., Palmer, J., & Lipson, L. (1997). Occupational therapy for independent-living older adults: A randomized controlled trial. *Journal of the American Medical Association, 278,* 1321–1326.

Clark, F., Carlson, M., & Polkinghorne, D. (1997). The Issue Is—The legitimacy of life history and narrative approaches in the study of occupation. *American Journal of Occupational Therapy, 51,* 313–317.

Clark, F. A., Parham, D., Carlson, M. E., Frank, G., Jackson, J., Pierce, D., Wolfe, R. J., & Zemke, R. (1991). Occupational science: Academic innovation in the service of occupational therapy's future. *American Journal of Occupational Therapy, 45,* 300–310.

Cohen, D. (1987). *The development of play.* New York: New York University Press.

Coren, S. (1996). Sleep thieves. New York: Free Press.

Coster, W. (1998). Occupation-centered assessment of children. *American Journal of Occupational Therapy, 52,* 337–344.

Cross, G. (1990). *A social history of leisure since 1600.* State College, PA: Venture.

Csikszentmihalyi, M., & Rochberg-Halton, E. (1981). *The meaning of things: Domestic symbols and the self.* New York: Cambridge University Press.

Cynkin, S. (1995). Activities. In C. Royeen (Ed.), *The practice of the future: Putting occupation back into therapy* (pp. 7-1–7-52). Bethesda, MD: American Occupational Therapy Association.

Davis, J. (1984). *Endorphins.* Garden City, NJ: Dial Press.

Dickie, V. (1998). Households, multiple livelihoods, and the informal economy. *Scandinavian Journal of Occupational Therapy, 5,* 109–118.

Dickie, V., & Frank, G. (1996). Artisan occupations in the global economy: A conceptual framework. *Journal of Occupational Science: Australia, 3,* 45–55.

Evans, G. (1980). Environmental cognition. *Psychological Bulletin, 88,* 259–287.

Fidler, G. S., & Velde, B. P. (1999). *Activities: Reality and symbol.* Thorofare, NJ: Slack.

Fisher, A. G., Murray, E. A., & Bundy, A. C. (1991). *Sensory integration: Theory and practice.* Philadelphia: F. A. Davis.

Fogler, H. S., & LeBlanc, S. E. (1995). *Strategies for creative problem solving.* Englewood Cliffs, NJ: Prentice Hall.

Foucault, M. (1980). *Power/knowledge: Selected interviews and other writings 1972–1977.* New York: Pantheon.

Frank, G. (1986). On embodiment: A case study of congenital limb deficiency in American culture. *Culture, Medicine, and Psychiatry, 10,* 189–219.

Geertz, C. (1983). *The interpretation of cultures.* New York: Basic.

Gellner, E. (1988). *Plough, sword, and book: The structure of human history.* Chicago: University of Chicago Press.

Goodman, N. (1951). *The structure of appearance.* Cambridge, MA: Harvard University Press.

Gray, J. M. (1998). Putting occupation into practice: Occupation as ends, occupation as means. *American Journal of Occupational Therapy, 52,* 354–364. Reprinted as Chapter 15.

Guyton, A. C. (1991). *Basic neuroscience.* Philadelphia: Saunders.

Hall, E. T. (1976). *The hidden dimension.* New York: Anchor Books, Doubleday.

Hall, E. T. (1983). *The dance of life: The other dimension of time.* New York: Anchor Books, Doubleday.

Harris, J., & Park, R. (1983). *Play, games, and sports in cultural contexts.* Champaign, IL: Human Kinetics.

Hasselkus, B. R. (1991). Ethical dilemmas in family caregiving for the elderly: Implications for occupational therapy. *American Journal of Occupational Therapy, 45,* 206–212.

Healy, C. (1982). *Career development.* Newton, MA: Allyn & Bacon.

Hobson, J. A. (1989). *Sleep.* New York: Scientific American Library.

Hodder, I. (1989). *The meaning of things: Material culture and symbolic expression.* Boston: Unwin-Hyman.

Holohan, C. J. (1986). Environmental psychology. *Annual Review of Psychology, 37,* 381–407.

Huizinga, J. (1950). Homo ludens: A study of the play element in culture. Boston: Beacon.

Jackson, J., Carlson, M., Mandel, D., Zemke, R., & Clark, F. (1998). Occupation in lifestyle redesign: The well elderly study occupational therapy program. *American Journal of Occupational Therapy, 52,* 326–336.

Jones, J. C. (1981). *Design methods: Seeds of human futures.* New York: Wiley.

Kaplan, S., & Kaplan, R. (1981). *Cognition and environment: Functioning in an uncertain world.* New York: Praeger.

Keller, S., Shiflet, S., & Bartlett, J. (1994). Stress, immunity, and health. In R. Glaser & J. Kielcolt-Glaser (Eds.), *Handbook of human stress and immunity* (pp. 217–244). New York: Academic.

Kielhofner, G. (1992). *Conceptual foundations for occupational therapy.* Philadelphia: F. A. Davis.

Koberg, D., & Bagnall, J. (1991). *The all new universal traveler: A soft-systems guide to creativity, problem-solving, and the process of reaching goals.* Los Altos, CA: William Kaufmann.

Larson, E. A., & Fanchiang, S. P. C. (1996). Nationally Speaking—Life history and narrative research: Generating a humanistic knowledge base for occupational therapy. *American Journal of Occupational Therapy, 50,* 247–250.

Law, M. (Ed.). (1998). *Client-centered occupational therapy.* Thorofare, NJ: Slack.

Martin, J. H. (1996). *Neuroanatomy: Text and atlas.* Norwalk, CT: Appleton & Lange.

Maslow, A. (1954). *Motivation and personality.* New York: Harper and Row.

Mattingly, C., & Fleming, M. (1994). *Clinical reasoning: Forms of inquiry in a therapeutic practice.* Philadelphia: F. A. Davis.

Meyer, A. (1922). The philosophy of occupation therapy. *Archives of Occupational Therapy, 1,* 1–10. Reprinted as Chapter 2.

Moorcroft, W. H. (1989). *Sleep, dreaming, and sleep disorders.* New York: University Press of America.

Moore-Ede, M. C., Sulzman, F. M., & Fuller, C. A. (1982). *The clocks that time us.* Cambridge, MA: Harvard University Press.

Mosey, A. C. (1992). The Issue Is—Partition of occupational science and occupational therapy. *American Journal of Occupational Therapy, 46,* 851–853.

Neisser, U. (1991). Two perceptually given aspects of the self and their development. *Developmental Review, 11,* 197–209.

Nelson, D. L. (1997). Why the profession of occupational therapy will flourish in the 21st century, 1996 Eleanor Clarke Slagle Lecture. *American Journal of Occupational Therapy, 51,* 11–24.

Parham, L. D., & Fazio, L. (Eds.). (1996). *Play in occupational therapy for children.* St. Louis, MO: Mosby.

Pierce, D. (1997a). Sources of power in therapeutic applications of object play with young children at risk for developmental delays. In L. D. Parham & L. Fazio (Eds.), *Play in occupational therapy practice.* St. Louis, MO: Mosby.

Pierce, D. (1997b). The neurologic base of primary occupational patterns: Productivity, pleasure, and rest. In C. B. Royeen (Ed.), *AOTA Self-Paced Clinical Course: Neuroscience foundations of occupation* (pp. 1–28). Bethesda, MD: American Occupational Therapy Association.

Pierce, D. (1998). The Issue Is—What is the source of occupation's treatment power? *American Journal of Occupational Therapy, 52,* 490–491.

Pierce, D. (2000). Maternal management of the home as a developmental play space for infants and toddlers. *American Journal of Occupational Therapy, 54,* 290–299.

Pierce, D. (2003). *Occupation by design.* Philadelphia: F. A. Davis.

Primeau, L. A. (1992). A woman's place: Unpaid work in the home. *American Journal of Occupational Therapy, 46,* 981–988.

Primeau, L. A. (1996). Work and leisure: Transcending the dichotomy. *American Journal of Occupational Therapy, 50,* 569–577.

Quiroga, V. A. M. (1995). *Occupational therapy: The first 30 years 1900 to 1930.* Bethesda, MD: American Occupational Therapy Association.

Reilly, M. (1974). *Play as exploratory learning.* Beverly Hills, CA: Sage.

Rosa, S., & Hasselkus, B. (1996). Connecting with patients: The personal experience of professional helping. *Occupational Therapy Journal of Research, 16,* 245–260.

Rowles, G. D. (1991). Beyond performance: Being in place as a component of occupational therapy. *American Journal of Occupational Therapy, 45,* 265–271. Reprinted as Chapter 26.

Royeen, C. B. (1994). The human life cycle: Paradigmatic shifts in occupation. In C. Royeen (Ed.) *The practice of the future: Putting occupation back into therapy* (pp. 1–24). Bethesda, MD: American Occupational Therapy Association.

Royeen, C. B. (1995). A problem-based learning curriculum for occupational therapy education. *American Journal of Occupational Therapy, 49,* 338–346.

Rubin, K. H. (1980). *New directions for child development: Children's play.* San Francisco: Jossey-Bass.

Schkade, J. K., & Schultz, S. (1992). Occupational adaptation: Toward a holistic approach for contemporary practice, part 1. *American Journal of Occupational Therapy, 46,* 829–837. Reprinted as Chapter 11.

Schnelle, J. F., Alessi, C. A., Ouslander, J. G., & Simmons, S. F. (1993). Noise and predictors of sleep in a nursing home environment. In J. L. Albarede, J. E. Morley, T. Roth, & B. J. Vellas (Eds.), *Facts and research in gerontology, Vol. 7: Sleep disorders in the elderly* (pp. 89–99). New York: Springer.

Schön, D. (1987). *Educating the reflective practitioner.* San Francisco: Jossey-Bass.

Segal, R., & Frank, G. (1998). The extraordinary construction of ordinary experience: Scheduling daily life in families with children with attention deficit disorder. *Scandinavian Journal of Occupational Therapy, 5,* 141–147.

Sheldon, S., Spire, J., & Levy, H. (1982). *Pediatric sleep medicine.* Philadelphia: Saunders.

Slagle, E. C. (1922). Training aids for mental patients. *Archives of Occupational Therapy, 1,* 11–19.

Smith, D. E. (1987). *The everyday world as problematic.* Boston: Northeastern Press.

Straub, C. C. (1978). *Design process and communications: A case study.* Dubuque, IA: Kendall/Hunt.

Swaab, D. F., Fliers, E., & Partiman, T. S. (1985). The suprachiasmatic nucleus of the human brain in relation to sex, age, and senile dementia. *Brain Research, 342,* 37–44.

Trombly, C. (1989). *Occupational therapy for physical dysfunction* (3rd ed.). Baltimore: Williams & Wilkins.

Trombly, C. A. (1995). Occupation: Purposefulness and meaningfulness as therapeutic mechanisms, 1995 Eleanor Clarke Slagle lecture. *American Journal of Occupational Therapy, 49,* 960–972. Reprinted as Chapter 16.

Wade, J. W. (1977). *Architecture, problems, and purposes.* New York: Wiley.

Wilcock, A. (1998). *An occupational perspective of health.* Thorofare, NJ: Slack.

Wood, W. (1998). Nationally Speaking—It is jump time for occupational therapy. *American Journal of Occupational Therapy, 52,* 403–411.

Yerxa, E. J. (1998). Occupation: The keystone of a curriculum for a self-defined profession. *American Journal of Occupational Therapy, 52,* 365–372.

Yerxa, E. J., Clark, F., Frank, G., Jackson, J., Parham, D., Pierce, D., Stein, C., & Zemke, R. (1989). An introduction to occupational science: A foundation for occupational therapy in the 21st century. *Occupational Therapy in Health Care, 6*(4), 1–18.

Zemke, R. (1994). Habits. In C. Royeen (Ed.), *The practice of the future: Putting occupation back into therapy* (pp. 1–24). Bethesda, MD: American Occupational Therapy Association.

Zemke, R., & Clark, F. (1996). Preface. In R. Zemke & F. Clark (Eds.), *Occupational science: The evolving discipline* (pp. vii–xviii). Philadelphia: F. A. Davis.

Zemke, R., & Horger, M. (1995). Hands: Tools for crafting human adaptation. In C. Royeen (Ed.), *Hands on: Practical interventions for the hand* (pp. 1–36). Bethesda, MD: American Occupational Therapy Association.

Zemke, R., & Pierce, D. (1994). [Data set on occupational event log: Student sample]. Unpublished raw data.

Zerubavel, E. (1981). *Hidden rhythms: Schedules and calendars in social life.* Los Angeles: University of California Press.

Introduction

This text concludes with nine appendices that supplement several of the text's chapters and areas of focus to serve as additional resources for readers. The first appendix contains the complete *Occupational Therapy Practice Framework: Domain and Process*. This seminal American Occupational Therapy Association (AOTA) document clearly articulates the professional domain of occupational therapy and the process that practitioners use to deliver therapeutic services.

The occupation-based, person-directed focus of the *Framework* is continued in the next two appendices which contain the AOTA's *Scope of Practice* document and the *Definition of Occupational Therapy* for the AOTA Model Practice Act. Both provide clear, succinct overviews of the field of occupational therapy, emphasizing the use of therapeutic occupation to external audiences.

The inherent worth and vital importance of occupation-based practice is reinforced in the next appendix which presents the *Address in Honor of Eleanor Clarke Slagle*. Appendix E offers *The Philosophical Base of Occupational Therapy*, while Appendix F pre-sents AOTA's official statement defining the *Core Values and Attitudes of Occupational Therapy Practice*, providing a strong affirmation of our profession's philosophical base. Appendix D also affirms occupational therapy's philosophical base and core values, but in addition it provides readers with a rare look at our profession's historical roots. This appendix contains an *Address in Honor of Eleanor Clarke Slagle* that was delivered by Adolf Meyer at a testimonial banquet on September 14, 1937, in Atlantic City, New Jersey. This event, on the eve of Slagle's retirement from professional life, featured a speech by the First Lady of the time, Eleanor Roosevelt. Regrettably, Mrs. Roosevelt's complete testimony to Slagle is not available, but fortunately Meyer's remains accessible. Meyer's intimate knowledge of Mrs. Slagle's significant contributions to our profession, and to the clients she worked with, led to this stirring tribute to the woman who "personified" occupational therapy.

The next three appendices provide readers with information that will facilitate the practical application of key occupational therapy's concepts and principles. Appendix G includes the *Lifestyle Performance Profile*, which outlines key areas for assessment according to the practice model presented in Chapter 13 by Gail Fidler. Evaluation and intervention guidelines relevant to "Part III: Contextual Considerations for Engagement in Occupation and Participation" are presented in the next appendix, which includes AOTA's *Position Paper on Occupational Therapy and the Americans With Disabilities Act (ADA)*. Knowledge of ADA is critical to ensure that occupational therapy practitioners work collaboratively and effectively with consumers to empower them in their work environments (as described in Chapter 29 by Crist and Stoffel) and in their communities of choice (as presented by Grady in Chapter 30). The final appendix, *Broadening the Construct of Independence*, provides a relevant expanded definition of independence that emphasizes a self-directed state of being that enables participation in a life of one's choice. Most important, this definition recognizes society's responsibility to ensure that all citizens have the rights and access to full societal participation.

Occupational Therapy Practice Framework: Domain and Process

Occupational therapy is an evolving profession. Over the years, the study of human occupation and its components has enlightened the profession about the core concepts and constructs that guide occupational therapy practice. In addition, occupational therapy's role and contributions to society have continued to evolve. The *Occupational Therapy Practice Framework: Domain and Process* (also referred to in this document as the Framework) is the next evolution in a series of documents that have been developed over the past several decades to outline language and constructs that describe the profession's focus.

The Framework was developed in response to current practice needs—the need to more clearly affirm and articulate occupational therapy's unique focus on occupation and daily life activities and the application of an intervention process that facilitates engagement in occupation to support participation in life. The impetus for the development of the Framework was the review process to update and revise the *Uniform Terminology for Occupational Therapy—Third Edition* (UT-III) (American Occupational Therapy Association [AOTA], 1994). The background for the development of the Framework is provided in a section at the end of this document. As practice continues to evolve, the field should consider the continued need for the *Occupational Therapy Practice Framework: Domain and Process* and should evaluate and modify its format as appropriate.

The intended purpose of the Framework is twofold: (a) to describe the domain that centers and grounds the profession's focus and actions and (b) to outline the process of occupational therapy evaluation and intervention that is dynamic and linked to the profession's focus on and use of occupation. The domain and process are necessarily interdependent, with the domain defining the area of human activity to which the process is applied.

This document is directed to both internal and external audiences. The internal professional audience—occupational therapists and occupational therapy assistants—can use the Framework to examine their current practice and to consider new applications in emerging practice areas. Occupational therapy educators may find the Framework helpful in teaching students about a process delivery model that is client centered and facilitates engagement in occupation to support participation in life. As occupational therapists and occupational therapy assistants move into new and expanded service arenas, the descriptions and terminology provided in the Framework can assist them in communicating the profession's unique focus on occupation and daily life activities to external audiences. External audiences can use the Framework to understand occupational therapy's emphasis on supporting function and performance in daily life activities and the many factors that influence performance (e.g., performance skills, performance patterns, context, activity demands, client factors) that are addressed during the intervention process. The description of the process will assist external audiences in understanding how occupational therapists and occupational therapy assistants apply their knowledge and skills in helping people attain and resume daily life activities that support function and health.

The *Occupational Therapy Practice Framework: Domain and Process* begins with an explanation of the profession's domain. Each aspect of the domain is fully described. An introduction to the occupational therapy process follows with key statements that highlight important points. Each section of the process is then specifically described. Numerous resource materials, including an appendix, a glossary, references, a bibliography, and the background of the development of the Framework are supplied at the end of the document.

Domain

The Domain of Occupational Therapy

"A profession's domain of concern consists of those areas of human experience in which practitioners of the profession offer assistance to others" (Mosey, 1981, p. 51). Occupational therapists and occupational therapy assistants focus on assisting people to engage in daily life activities that they find meaningful and purposeful. Occupational therapy's domain stems from the profession's interest in human beings' ability to engage in everyday life activities. The broad term that occupational therapists and assistants use to capture the breadth and meaning of "everyday life activity" is *occupation*. Occupation, as used in this document, is defined in the following way:

> [A]ctivities…of everyday life, named, organized, and given value and meaning by individuals and a culture. Occupation is everything people do to occupy themselves, including looking after themselves…enjoying life…and contributing to the social and economic fabric of their communities…. (Law, Polatajko, Baptiste, & Townsend, 1997, p. 32)

Occupational therapists' and occupational therapy assistants' expertise lies in their knowledge of occupation and how engaging in occupations can be used to affect human performance and the effects of disease and disability. When working with clients, occupational therapists and occupational therapy assistants direct their effort toward helping clients perform. Performance changes are directed to support engagement in meaningful occupations that subsequently affect health, well-being, and life satisfaction.

The profession views occupation as both means and end. The process of providing occupational therapy intervention may involve the therapeutic use of occupation as a "means" or method of changing performance. The "end" of the occupational therapy intervention process occurs with the client's improved engagement in meaningful occupation.

Both terms, *occupation* and *activity*, are used by occupational therapists and occupational therapy assistants to describe participation in daily life pursuits. Occupations are generally viewed as activities having unique meaning and purpose in a person's life. Occupations are central to a person's identity and competence, and they influence how one spends time and makes decisions. The term *activity* describes a general class of human actions that is goal directed (Pierce, 2001). A person may participate in activities to achieve a goal, but these activities do not assume a place of central importance or meaning for the person. For example, many people participate in the activity of gardening, but not all of those individuals would describe gardening as an "occupation" that has central importance and meaning for them. Those who see gardening as an activity may report that gardening is a chore or task that must be done as part of home and yard maintenance but not one that they particularly enjoy doing or from which they derive significant personal satisfaction or fulfillment. Those who experience gardening as an occupation would see themselves as "gardeners," gaining part of their identity from their participation. They would achieve a sense of competence by their accomplishments in gardening and would report a sense of satisfaction and fulfillment as a result of engaging in this occupation. Occupational therapists and occupational therapy assistants value both occupation and activity and recognize their importance and influence on health and well-being. They believe that the two terms are closely related yet recognize that each term has a distinct meaning and that individuals experience each differently. In this document the two terms are often used together to acknowledge their relatedness yet recognize their different meanings.

The domain of occupational therapy frames the arena in which occupational therapy evaluations and interventions occur. To make the domain more understandable to readers and easier to visualize, the content of the domain has been illustrated in Figure 1. At the top of the page is the overarching statement—Engagement in Occupation to Support Participation in Context or Contexts. This statement describes the domain in its broadest sense. The other terms outlined in the figure identify the various aspects of the domain that occupational therapists and occupational therapy assistants attend to during the process of providing services. The three terms at the bottom of the figure (*context, activity demands,* and *client factors*) identify areas that influence performance skills and patterns. The two terms in the middle of the figure (*performance skills* and *performance patterns*) are used to describe the observed performance that the individual carries out when engaging in a range of occupations. No one aspect outlined in the domain figure is considered more important than another. Occupational therapists are trained to assess all aspects and to apply that knowledge to an intervention process that leads to engagement in occupations to support participation in context or contexts. Occupational therapy assistants participate in this process under the supervision of an occupational therapist. The discussion that follows provides a brief explanation of each term in the figure. Tables included in the appendix provide full lists and definitions of terms.

ENGAGEMENT IN OCCUPATION TO SUPPORT PARTICIPATION IN CONTEXT OR CONTEXTS

Performance in Areas of Occupation
Activities of Daily Living (ADL)*
Instrumental Activities of Daily Living (IADL)
Education
Work
Play
Leisure
Social Participation
(For definitions, refer to Appendix, Table 1)

Performance Skills	Performance Patterns
Motor Skills	Habits
Process Skills	Routines
Communication/Interaction Skills	Roles
(For definitions, refer to Appendix, Table 2)	*(For definitions, refer to Appendix, Table 3)*

Context	Activity Demands	Client Factors
Cultural	Objects Used and Their Properties	Body Functions
Physical	Space Demands	Body Structures
Social	Social Demands	*(For definitions, refer to Appendix, Table 6)*
Personal	Sequencing and Timing	
Spiritual	Required Actions	
Temporal	Required Body Functions	
Virtual	Required Body Structures	
(For definitions, refer to Appendix, Table 4)	*(For definitions, refer to Appendix, Table 5)*	

*Also referred to as basic activities of daily living (BADL) or personal activities of daily living (PADL).

Figure 1. Domain of Occupational Therapy. This figure represents the domain of occupational therapy and is included to allow readers to visualize the entire domain with all of its various aspects. No aspect is intended to be perceived as more important than another.

Engagement in Occupation to Support Participation in Context

Engagement in occupation to support participation in context is the focus and targeted end objective of occupational therapy intervention. Engagement in occupation is seen as naturally supporting and leading to participation in context.

When individuals engage in occupations, they are committed to performance as a result of self-choice, motivation, and meaning. The term expresses the profession's belief in the importance of valuing and considering the individual's desires, choices, and needs during the evaluation and intervention process. Engagement in occupation includes both the subjective (emotional or psychological) aspects of performance and the objective (physically observable) aspects of performance. Occupational therapists and occupational therapy assistants understand engagement from this dual and holistic perspective and address all the aspects of performance (physical, cognitive, psychosocial, and contextual) when providing interventions designed to support engagement in occupations and in daily life activities.

Occupational therapists and occupational therapy assistants recognize that health is supported and maintained when individuals are able to engage in occupations and in activities that allow desired or needed participation in home, school, workplace, and community life situations. Occupational therapists and occupational therapy assistants assist individuals to link their ability to perform daily life activities with meaningful patterns of engagement in occupations that allow participation in desired roles and life situations in home, school, workplace, and community. The World Health Organization (WHO), in its effort to broaden the understanding of the effects of disease and disability on health, has recognized that health can be affected by the inability to carry out activities and participate in life situations as well as by problems that exist with body structures and functions (WHO, 2001). Occupational therapy's focus on engagement in occupations to support participation complements WHO's perspective.

Occupational therapists and occupational therapy assistants recognize that engagement in occupation occurs in a variety of contexts (cultural, physical, social, personal, temporal, spiritual, virtual). They also recognize that the individual's experience and performance cannot be understood or addressed without understanding the many contexts in which occupations and daily life activities occur.

Performance in Areas of Occupation

Occupational therapists and occupational therapy assistants direct their expertise to the broad range of human occupations and activities that make up peoples' lives. When occupational therapists and assistants work with an individual, a group, or a population to promote engagement in occupations and in daily life activities, they take into account all of the many types of occupations in which any individual, group, or population might engage. These human activities are sorted into categories called "areas of occupation"—activities of daily living, instrumental activities of daily living, education, work, play, leisure, and social participation (see Appendix, Table 1). Occupational therapists and occupational therapy assistants under the supervision of an occupational therapist use their expertise to address performance issues in any or all areas that are affecting the person's ability to engage in occupations and in activities. Addressing performance issues in areas of occupation requires knowledge of what performance skills are needed and what performance patterns are used.

Performance Skills

Skills are small units of performance. They are features of what one does (e.g., bends, chooses, gazes), versus underlying capacities or body functions (e.g., joint mobility, motivation, visual acuity). "Skills are observable elements of action that have implicit functional purposes" (Fisher & Kielhofner, 1995, p. 113). For example, when observing a person writing out a check, you would notice skills of gripping and manipulating objects and initiating and sequencing the steps of the activity to complete the writing of the check.

Execution of a performance skill occurs when the performer, the context, and the demands of the activity come together in the performance of the activity. Each of these factors influences the execution of a skill and may support or hinder actual skill execution.

When occupational therapists and occupational therapy assistants, who have established competency under the supervision of occupational therapists, analyze performance, they specifically identify the skills that are effective or ineffective during performance. They use skilled observations and selected assessments to evaluate the following skills:

- Motor skills—observed as the client moves and interacts with task objects and environments. Aspects of motor skill include posture, mobility, coordination, strength and effort, and energy. Examples of specific motor performance skills include stabilizing the body, bending, and manipulating objects.

- Process skills—observed as the client manages and modifies actions while completing a task. Aspects of process skill include energy, knowledge, temporal organization, organizing space and objects, and adaptation. Examples of specific process performance skills include maintaining attention to a task, choosing appropriate tools and materials for the task, logically organizing workspace, or accommodating the method of task completion in response to a problem.

- Communication/Interaction skills—observed as the client conveys his or her intentions and needs and coordinates social behavior to act together with people. Aspects of communication/interaction skills include physicality, information exchange, and relations. Examples of specific communication/interaction performance skills include gesturing to indicate intention, asking for information, expressing affect, or relating in a manner to establish rapport with others.

Skilled performance (i.e., effective execution of performance skills) depends on client factors (body functions, body structures), activity demands, and the context. However, the presence of underlying client factors (body functions and structures) does not inherently ensure the effective execution of performance skills. (See Appendix, Table 2, for complete list of performance skills.)

Performance Patterns

Performance patterns refer to habits, routines, and roles that are adopted by an individual as he or she carries out occupations or daily life activities. Habits refer to specific, automatic behaviors, whereas routines are established sequences of occupations or activities that provide a structure for daily life. Roles are "a set of behaviors that have some socially agreed upon function and for which there is an accepted code of norms" (Christiansen & Baum, 1997, p. 603).

Performance patterns develop over time and are influenced by context (See Appendix, Table 3).

Context

Context refers to a variety of interrelated conditions within and surrounding the client that influence performance. These contexts can be cultural, physical, social, personal, spiritual, temporal, and virtual. Some contexts are external to the client (e.g., physical context, social context, virtual context); some are internal to the client (e.g., personal, spiritual); and some may have external features, with beliefs and values that have been internalized (e.g., cultural). Contexts may include time dimensions (e.g., within a temporal context, the time of day; within a personal context, one's age) and space dimensions (e.g., within a physical context, the size of room in which activity occurs). When the occupational therapist and occupational therapy assistant are attempting to understand performance skills and patterns, they consider the specific contexts that surround the performance of a particular occupation or activity. In this process, the therapist and assistant consider all the relevant contexts, keeping in mind that some of them may not be influencing the particular skills and patterns being addressed. (See Appendix, Table 4, for a description of the different kinds of contexts that occupational therapists and occupational therapy assistants consider.)

Activity Demands

The demands of the activity in which a person engages will affect skill and eventual success of performance. Occupational therapists and occupational therapy assistants apply their analysis skills to determine the demands that an activity will place on any performer and how those demands will influence skill execution. (See Appendix, Table 5, for complete list of activity demands.)

Client Factors

Performance can be influenced by factors that reside within the client. Occupational therapists and occupational therapy assistants are knowledgeable about the variety of physical, cognitive, and psychosocial client factors that influence development and performance and how illness, disease, and disability affect these factors. The occupational therapist and occupational therapy assistant recognize that client factors influence the ability to engage in occupations and that engagement in occupations can also influence client factors. They apply their understanding of this interaction and use it throughout the intervention process.

Client factors include the following:

- Body functions—"physiological function of body systems (including psychological functions)" (WHO, 2001, p. 10). (See Appendix, Table 6, for complete list.) The occupational therapist and occupational therapy assistant under the supervision of an occupational therapist use knowledge about body functions to evaluate selected client body functions that may be affecting his or her ability to engage in desired occupations or activities.
- Body structures—"anatomical parts of the body such as organs, limbs, and their components" (WHO, 2001, p. 10). (See Appendix, Table 6.) Occupational therapists and occupational therapy assistants under the supervision of an occupational therapist apply their knowledge about body structures to determine which body structures are needed to carry out an occupation or activity.

The categorization of client factors outlined in Table 6 is based on the *International Classification of Functioning, Disability and Health* proposed by the WHO (2001). The classification was selected because it has received wide exposure and presents a common language that is understood by external audiences. The categories include all those areas that occupational therapists and assistants address and consider during evaluation and intervention.

Process

The Process of Occupational Therapy: Evaluation, Intervention, and Outcome

Many professions use the process of evaluating, intervening, and targeting intervention outcomes that is outlined in the Framework. However, occupational therapy's focus on occupation throughout the process makes the profession's application and use of the process unique. The process of occupational therapy service delivery begins by evaluating the client's occupational needs, problems, and concerns. Understanding the client as an occupational human being for whom access and participation in meaningful and productive activities is central to health and well-being is a perspective that is unique to occupational therapy. Problems and concerns that are addressed in evaluation and intervention are also framed uniquely from an occupational perspective, are based on occupational therapy theories, and are defined as problems or risks in occupational performance. During intervention, the focus remains on occupation, and efforts are directed toward fostering improved engagement in occupations. A variety of therapeutic activities, including engagement in actual occupations and in daily life activities, are used in intervention.

Framework Process Organization

The *Occupational Therapy Practice Framework* process is organized into three broad sections that describe the process of service delivery. A brief overview of the process as it is applied within the profession's domain is outlined in Figure 2.

Figure 3 schematically illustrates how these sections are related to one another and how they revolve around the collaborative therapeutic relationship among the client and the occupational therapist and occupational therapy assistant.

To help the reader understand the process, key statements highlight important points about the process outlined below.

The process outlined is dynamic and interactive in nature. Although the parts of the Framework are described in a linear manner, in reality, the process does not occur in a sequenced, step-by-step fashion. The arrows in Figure 3 that connect the boxes indicate the interactive and nonlinear nature of the process. The process, however, does always start with the occupational profile. An understanding of the client's concerns, problems, and risks is the cornerstone of the process. The factors that influence occupational performance (performance skills, performance patterns, context or contexts, activity demands, client factors) continually interact with one another. Because of their dynamic interaction, these factors are frequently evaluated simultaneously throughout the process as their influence on performance is observed.

Context is an overarching, underlying, embedded influence on the process of service delivery. Contexts exist around and within the person. They influence both the client's performance and the process of delivering services.

Evaluation		
Occupational profile—The initial step in the evaluation process that provides an understanding of the client's occupational history and experiences, patterns of daily living, interests, values, and needs. The client's problems and concerns about performing occupations and daily life activities are identified, and the client's priorities are determined.		
Analysis of occupational performance—The step in the evaluation process during which the client's assets, problems, or potential problems are more specifically identified. Actual performance is often observed in context to identify what supports performance and what hinders performance. Performance skills, performance patterns, context or contexts, activity demands, and client factors are all considered, but only selected aspects may be specifically assessed. Targeted outcomes are identified.		
Intervention		
Intervention plan—A plan that will guide actions taken and that is developed in collaboration with the client. It is based on selected theories, frames of reference, and evidence. Outcomes to be targeted are confirmed.		
Intervention implementation—Ongoing actions taken to influence and support improved client performance. Interventions are directed at identified outcomes. Client's response is monitored and documented.		
Intervention review—A review of the implementation plan and process as well as its progress toward targeted outcomes.		
Outcomes (Engagement in Occupation To Support Participation)		
Outcomes—Determination of success in reaching desired targeted outcomes. Outcome assessment information is used to plan future actions with the client and to evaluate the service program (i.e., program evaluation).		

Figure 2. Framework Process of Service Delivery as Applied Within the Profession's Domain.

The external context (e.g., the physical setting, social and virtual contexts) provide resources that support or inhibit the client's performance (e.g., presence of a willing caregiver) as well as the delivery of services (e.g., limits placed on length of intervention in an inpatient hospital setting). Different settings (i.e., community, institution, home) provide different supports and resources for service delivery. The client's internal context (personal and spiritual contexts) affects service delivery by influencing personal beliefs, perceptions, and expectations. The cultural context, which exists outside of the person but is internalized by the person, also sets expectations, beliefs, and customs that can affect how and when services may be delivered. Note that in Figure 3, context is depicted as surrounding and underlying the process.

The term client is used to name the entity that receives occupational therapy services. Clients may be categorized as (a) individuals, including individuals who may be involved in supporting or caring for the client (i.e., caregiver, teacher, parent, employer, spouse); (b) individuals within the context of a group (i.e., a family, a class); or (c) individuals within the context of a population (i.e., an organization, a community). The definition of client is consistent with *The Guide to Occupational Therapy Practice* (Moyers, 1999) and is indicative of the profession's growing understanding that people may be served not only as individuals, but also as members of a group or a population. The actual term used for individuals who are served will vary by practice setting. For example, in a hospital, the person might be referred to as a "patient," whereas in a school, he or she might be called a "student." Clients may be served as individuals, groups, or populations. Although the most common form of service delivery

within the profession now involves a direct individual client to service provider model, more and more occupational therapists and occupational therapy assistants are beginning to serve clients at the group and population level (i.e., organization, community). When providing interventions other than in a one-to-one model, the occupational therapist and occupational therapist assistant are seen as agents who help others to support client engagement in occupations rather than as those who personally provide that support. Often, they use education and consultation as interventions. When occupational therapists and occupational therapy assistants are collaborating with clients to provide services at the group or population level, an important point to recognize is that although interventions may be directed to a group or population (i.e., organization, community), the individuals within those entities are the ones who are being evaluated and served. The wants, needs, occupational risks or problems, and performance patterns and skills of individuals within the group or population (i.e., organization, community) are evaluated as an aggregate, and information is compiled to determine group or population occupational issues and solutions.

A client-centered approach is used throughout the Framework. The Framework incorporates the value of client-centered evaluation and intervention by recognizing from the outset that all interventions must be focused on client priorities. The very nature of engagement in occupation—which is internally motivated, is individually defined, and requires active participation by the client—means that the client must be an active participant in the process. Clients identify what occupations and activities are important to them and determine the degree of engagement in each occupation. However, in some circumstances the client's ability to provide a description of the perceived or desired occupations or activity may be limited because of either the nature of the client's problems (e.g., autism, dementia) or the stage of development (e.g., infants). When this occurs, the occupational therapist and occupational therapy assistant must then take a broader view of the client and seek input from others such as family or significant others who would have knowledge and insight into the client's desires. By involving the family or significant others, the occupational therapist and assistant can better understand the client's history, developmental stage, and current contexts. Inclusion of others in these circumstances allows the client to be represented in intervention planning and implementation.

The entire process of service delivery begins with a collaborative relationship with the client. The collaborative relationship continues throughout the process and affects all phases of the process. The central importance of this collaboration is noted in Figure 3.

The Framework is based on the belief that the occupational therapist, occupational therapy assistant, and the client bring unique resources to the Framework process. Occupational therapists and occupational therapy assistants bring knowledge about how engagement in occupation affects health and performance. They also bring knowledge about disease and disability and couple this information with their clinical reasoning and theoretical perspectives to critically observe, analyze, describe, and interpret human performance. Therapists and assistants combine their knowledge and skills to modify the factors that influence engagement in occupation to improve and support performance. Clients bring knowledge about their life experiences and their hopes and dreams for the future. Clients share their priorities, which are based on what is important to them, and collaborate with the therapist and assistant in directing the intervention process to those priorities.

"Engagement in occupation" is viewed as the overarching outcome of the occupational therapy process. The Framework emphasizes occupational therapy's unique contribution to health by identifying "engagement in occupation to support participation" as the end objective of the occupational therapy process. The profession recognizes that in some areas of practice (e.g., acute rehabilitation, hand therapy) occupational therapy intervention may focus primarily on performance skills or on client factors (i.e., body functions, body structures) that will enable engagement in occupations later in the continuum of care.

Evaluation Process

The evaluation process sets the stage for all that follows. Because occupational therapy is concerned with performance in daily life and how performance affects engagement in occupations to support participation, the evaluation process is

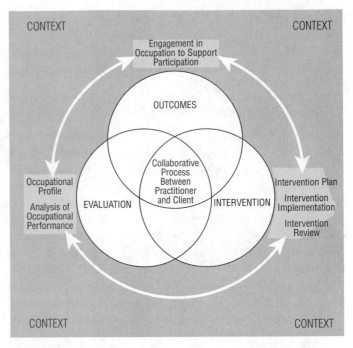

Figure 3. Framework Collaborative Process Model. Illustration of the framework emphasizing client–practitioner interactive relationship and interactive nature of the service delivery process.

focused on finding out what the client wants and needs to do and on identifying those factors that act as supports or barriers to performance. During the evaluation process, this information is paired with the occupational therapist's knowledge about human performance and the effect that illness, disability, and engagement in occupation have on performance. The occupational therapist considers performance skills, performance patterns, context, activity demands, and client factors and determines how each influences performance. The occupational therapist's skilled observation, use of specific assessments, and interpretation of results leads to a clear delineation of the problems and probable causes. The occupational therapy assistant may contribute to the evaluation process based on established competencies and under the supervision of an occupational therapist.

During the evaluation, a collaborative relationship with the client is established that continues throughout the entire occupational therapy process. The evaluation process is divided into two substeps, the first of which is the occupational profile—the initial step during which the client's needs, problems, and concerns about occupations and daily life activity performance are identified and priorities and values ascertained. The client's background and history in reference to engagement in occupations and in activities are also explored. The second substep of the evaluation process, analysis of occupational performance, focuses on more specifically identifying occupational performance issues and evaluating selected factors that support and hinder performance. Although each subsection is described separately and sequentially, in actuality, information pertinent to both subsections may be gathered during either one. The client's input is central in this process, and the client's priorities guide choices and decisions made during the process of evaluation.

Occupational Profile

An occupational profile is defined as information that describes the client's occupational history and experiences, patterns of daily living, interests, values, and needs. The profile is designed to gain an understanding of the client's perspective and background. Using a client-centered approach, information is gathered to understand what is currently important and meaningful to the client (what he or she wants and needs to do) and to identify past experiences and interests that may assist in the understanding of current issues and problems. During the process of collecting this information, the client's priorities and desired targeted outcomes that will lead to engagement in occupation to support participation in life are also identified. Only clients can identify the occupations that give meaning to their lives and select the goals and priorities that are important to them. Valuing and respecting the client's input helps to foster client involvement and can more efficiently guide interventions.

Information about the occupational profile is collected at the beginning of contact with the client. However, additional information is collected over time throughout the process, refined, and reflected in changes subsequently made to targeted outcomes.

Process. The theories and frames of reference that the occupational therapist selects to guide his or her reasoning will influence the information that is collected during the occupational profile. Scientific knowledge and evidence about diagnostic conditions and occupational performance problems is used to guide information gathering.

The process of completing the occupational profile will vary depending on the setting and the client. The information gathered in the profile may be obtained both formally and informally and may be completed in one session or over a much longer period while working with the client. Obtaining information through both formal interview and casual conversation is a way of beginning to establish a therapeutic relationship with the client. Ideally, the information obtained through the occupational profile will lead to a more individualized approach in the evaluation, intervention planning, and intervention implementation stages.

Specifically, the following information is collected:

- Who is the client (individual, caregiver, group, population)?
- Why is the client seeking service, and what are the client's current concerns relative to engaging in occupations and in daily life activities?

- What areas of occupation are successful, and what areas are causing problems or risks? (see Figure 1)
- What contexts support engagement in desired occupations, and what contexts are inhibiting engagement?
- What is the client's occupational history (i.e., life experiences, values, interests, previous patterns of engagement in occupations and in daily life activities, the meanings associated with them)?
- What are the client's priorities and desired targeted outcomes (see Appendix, Table 9)?
  - Occupational performance
  - Client satisfaction
  - Role competence
  - Adaptation
  - Health and wellness
  - Prevention
  - Quality of life

After profile data are collected, the therapist reviews the information and develops a working hypothesis regarding possible reasons for identified problems and concerns and identifies the client's strengths and weaknesses. Outcome measures are preliminarily selected.

Analysis of Occupational Performance

Occupational performance is defined as the ability to carry out activities of daily life, including activities in the areas of occupation: activities of daily living (ADL) [also called basic activities of daily living (BADL) and personal activities of daily living (PADL)], instrumental activities of daily living (IADL), education, work, play, leisure, and social participation. Occupational performance results in the accomplishment of the selected occupation or activity and occurs through a dynamic transaction among the client, the context, and the activity. Improving or developing skills and patterns in occupational performance leads to engagement in one or more occupations (adapted in part from Law et al., 1996, p. 16).

When occupational performance is analyzed, the performance skills and patterns used in performance are identified, and other aspects of engaging in occupation that affect skills and patterns (e.g., client factors, activity demands, context or contexts) are evaluated. The analysis process identifies facilitators as well as barriers in various aspects of engagement in occupations and in daily life activities. Analyzing occupational performance requires an understanding of the complex and dynamic interaction among performance skills, performance patterns, context or contexts, activity demands, and client factors rather than of any one factor alone.

The information gathered during the occupational profile about the client's needs, problems, and priorities guides decisions during the analysis of occupational performance. The profile information directs the therapist's selection of the specific occupations or activities that need to be further analyzed and influences the selection of specific assessments that are used during the analysis process.

Process. Using available evidence and all aspects of clinical reasoning (scientific, narrative, pragmatic, ethical), the therapist selects one or more frames of reference to guide further collection of evaluation information. The following actions are taken:

- Synthesize information from the occupational profile to focus on specific areas of occupation and their contexts that need to be addressed.
- Observe the client's performance in desired occupations and activities, noting effectiveness of the performance skills and performance patterns. May select and use specific assessments to measure performance skills and patterns as appropriate.
- Select assessments, as needed, to identify and measure more specifically context or contexts, activity demands, and client factors that may be influencing performance skills and performance patterns.
- Interpret the assessment data to identify what supports performance and what hinders performance.
- Develop and refine hypotheses about the client's occupational performance strengths and weaknesses.
- Create goals in collaboration with the client that address the desired targeted outcomes. Confirm outcome measure to be used.
- Delineate potential intervention approach or approaches based on best practice and evidence.

Intervention Process

The intervention process is divided into three substeps: intervention plan, intervention implementation, and intervention review. During the intervention process, information from the evaluation step is integrated with theory, frames of reference, and evidence and is coupled with clinical reasoning to develop a plan and carry it out. The plan guides the actions of the occupational therapist and occupational therapy assistant and is based on the client's priorities. Interventions are carried out to address performance skills, patterns, context or contexts, activity demands, and client factors that are hindering performance. Periodic reviews throughout the process allow for revisions in the plan and actions. Again, collaboration with the client is vital in this section of the process to ensure effectiveness and success. All interventions are ultimately directed toward achieving the overarching outcome of engagement in occupation to support participation.

Intervention Plan

An intervention plan is defined as a plan that is developed based on the results of the evaluation process and describes selected occupational therapy approaches and types of interventions to reach the client's identified targeted outcomes. An intervention plan is developed collaboratively with the client (including, in some cases, family or significant others) and is based on the client's goals and priorities.

The design of the intervention plan is directed by

- the client's goals, values, and beliefs;
- the health and well-being of the client;
- the client's performance skills and performance patterns, as they are influenced by the interaction among the context or contexts, activity demands, and client factors; and
- the setting or circumstance in which the intervention is provided (e.g., caregiver expectations, organization's purpose, payer's requirements, or applicable regulations).

Interventions are designed to foster engagement in occupations and in activities to support participation in life. The selection and design of the intervention plan and goals are directed toward addressing the client's current and potential problems related to engagement in occupations or in activities.

Process. Intervention planning includes the following steps:

1. Develop the plan. The occupational therapist develops the plan. The occupational therapy assistant, based on established competencies and under the supervision of the occupational therapist, may contribute to the plan's development. The plan includes the following:
   - Objective and measurable goals with a timeframe
   - Occupational therapy intervention approach or approaches based on theory and evidence (see Appendix, Table 7).
     - Create or promote
     - Establish or restore
     - Maintain
     - Modify
     - Prevent
   - Mechanisms for service delivery
     - Who will provide intervention
     - Types of interventions
     - Frequency and duration of service
2. Consider potential discharge needs and plans.
3. Select outcome measures.
4. Make recommendation or referral to others as needed.

Intervention Implementation

Intervention is the process of putting the plan into action. Intervention implementation is defined as the skilled process of effecting change in the client's occupational performance, leading to engagement in occupations or in activities to support participation. Intervention implementation is a collaborative process among the client and the occupational therapist and assistant.

Interventions may be focused on changing the context or contexts, activity demands, client factors, performance skills, or performance patterns. Occupational therapists and occupational therapy assistants recognize that change in one factor may influence other factors. All factors that affect performance are interrelated and influence one another in a continuous dynamic process that results in performance in desired areas of occupation. Because of this dynamic interrelationship, dynamic assessment continues throughout the implementation process.

Process. Intervention implementation includes the following steps:

1. Determine and carry out the type of occupational therapy intervention or interventions to be used (see Appendix, Table 8).
   - Therapeutic use of self
   - Therapeutic use of occupations or activities
     - Occupation-based activity
     - Purposeful activity
     - Preparatory methods
   - Consultation process
   - Education process
2. Monitor client's response to interventions based on ongoing assessment and reassessment.

Intervention Review

Intervention review is defined as a continuous process for reevaluating and reviewing the intervention plan, the effectiveness of its delivery, and the progress toward targeted outcomes. This process includes collaboration with the client (including, in some cases, family, significant others, and other service providers). Reevaluation and review may lead to change in the intervention plan. The intervention review process may be carried out differently in a variety of settings.

Process. The intervention review includes the following steps:

1. Reevaluate the plan and how it is carried out with the client relative to achieving targeted outcomes.
2. Modify the plan as needed.
3. Determine the need for continuation, discontinuation, or referral.

Outcomes Process

Outcomes are defined as important dimensions of health that are attributed to interventions, including ability to function, health perceptions, and satisfaction with care (adapted from Request for Planning Ideas, 2001). The important dimension of health that occupational therapists and occupational therapy assistants target as the profession's overarching outcome is "engagement in occupation to support participation." The two concepts included in this outcome are defined as follows:

- Engagement in occupation—The commitment made to performance in occupations or activities as the result

of self-choice, motivation, and meaning, and includes the objective and subjective aspects of carrying out occupations and activities that are meaningful and purposeful to the person.
- Participation—"involvement in a life situation" (WHO, 2001, p. 10).

Engagement in occupation to support participation is the broad outcome of intervention that is designed to foster performance in desired and needed occupations or activities. When clients are actively involved in carrying out occupations or daily life activities that they find purposeful and meaningful in home and community settings, participation is a natural outcome. Less broad and more specific outcomes of occupational therapy intervention (see Appendix, Table 9) are multidimensional and support the end result of engagement in occupation to support participation.

In targeting engagement in occupation to support participation as the broad, overarching outcome of the occupational therapy intervention process, the profession underscores its belief that health and well-being are holistic and that they are developed and maintained through active engagement in occupation.

The focus on outcomes is interwoven throughout the process of service delivery within occupational therapy. During the evaluation phase of the process, the client's initial targeted outcomes regarding desired engagement in occupation or daily life activities are identified. As further analysis of occupational performance and development of the treatment plan take place, targeted outcomes are further refined. During intervention implementation and reevaluation, targeted outcomes may be modified based on changing needs, contexts, and performance abilities. Outcomes have numerous definitions and connotations for different clients, payers, regulators, and organizations. The specific outcomes chosen will vary by practice setting and will be influenced by the particular stakeholders in each setting.

Process. Implementation of the outcomes process includes the following steps:

1. Select types of outcomes and measures, including, but not limited to occupational performance, client satisfaction, adaptation, role competence, health and wellness, prevention, and quality of life.
   - Selection of outcome measures occurs early in the intervention process (see Evaluation Process, Occupational Profile section).
   - Outcome measures that are selected are valid, reliable, and appropriately sensitive to change in the client's occupational performance, and they match the targeted outcomes.
   - Selection of an outcome measure or instrument for a particular client should be congruent with client goals.

- Selection of an outcome measure should entail considering its actual or purported ability to predict future outcomes.
2. Measure and use outcomes.
   - Compare progress toward goal achievement to targeted outcomes throughout the intervention process.
   - Assess outcome results and use to make decisions about future direction of intervention (i.e., continue intervention, modify intervention, discontinue intervention, provide follow-up, refer to other services).

An Overview of the Occupational Therapy Practice Process

Table 10 in the Appendix summarizes the process that occurs during occupational therapy service delivery. The arrow placed between the Occupational Profile and Analysis of Occupational Performance evaluation substeps indicates the interactions between these two. However, a similar interaction occurs among all of the steps and substeps. The process is not linear but, instead, is fluid and dynamic, allowing the occupational therapist and occupational therapy assistant to operate with an ongoing focus on outcomes while continually reflecting and changing an overall plan to accommodate new developments and insights along the way.

Acknowledgments

The Commission on Practice (COP) would like to thank and acknowledge all those who participated in the review and comment process associated with the development of the *Occupational Therapy Practice Framework: Domain and Process*. The COP has found this process invaluable and enriching. Everyone's input has been carefully reviewed and considered. Often, small comments repeated by many can lead to significant discussion and change. The COP hopes that all those who contributed to this process will continue to do so for future documents and will encourage others to participate. The profession is richer for this process.

The COP would like to thank the following individuals for their significant contributions to the direction and final content of this document: Carolyn Baum, PhD, OTR, FAOTA; Elizabeth Crepeau, PhD, OTR, FAOTA; Patricia A. Crist, PhD, FAOTA; Winifred Dunn, PhD, OTR, FAOTA; Anne G. Fisher, PhD, OTR, FAOTA; Gail S. Fidler, OTR, FAOTA; Mary Foto, OT, FAOTA; Nedra Gillette, ScD (Hon), MEd, OTR, FAOTA; Jim Hinojosa, PhD, OT, FAOTA; Margo B. Holm, PhD, OTR, FAOTA; Gary Kielhofner, DrPH, OTR/L, FAOTA; Paula Kramer, PhD, OTR, FAOTA; Mary Law, PhD, OT(C); Linda T. Learnard, OTR/L; Anne Mosey, PhD, OTR, FAOTA; Penelope A. Moyers, Edd, OTR, FAOTA; David Nelson, PhD, OTR, FAOTA; Marta Pelczarski, OTR; Kathlyn L. Reed, PhD, OTR, FAOTA; Barbara Schell, PhD, OTR/L, FAOTA; Janette Schkade, PhD, OTR; Wendy Schoen; Carol Siebert, MS, OTR/L; V. Judith Thomas, MGA; Linda Kohlman Thomson, MOT, OT, OT(C), FAOTA; Amy L. Walsh, OTR/L; Wendy Wood, PhD, OTR, FAOTA; Boston University OT Students mentored by Karen Jacobs, Edd, OTR/L, CPE, FAOTA; and the University of Kansas Occupational Therapy Education Faculty.

Appendix

Table 1. Areas of Occupation

Various kinds of life activities in which people engage, including ADL, IADL, education, work, play, leisure, and social participation.

Activities of daily living (ADL)

Activities that are oriented toward taking care of one's own body (adapted from Rogers & Holm, 1994, pp. 181–202)—also called basic activities of daily living (BADL) or personal activities of daily living (PADL).

- **Bathing, showering**—Obtaining and using supplies; soaping, rinsing, and drying body parts; maintaining bathing position; and transferring to and from bathing positions.
- **Bowel and bladder management**—Includes complete intentional control of bowel movements and urinary bladder and, if necessary, use of equipment or agents for bladder control (Uniform Data System for Medical Rehabilitation [UDSMR], 1996, pp. III–20, III–24).
- **Dressing**—Selecting clothing and accessories appropriate to time of day, weather, and occasion; obtaining clothing from storage area; dressing and undressing in a sequential fashion; fastening and adjusting clothing and shoes; and applying and removing personal devices, prostheses, or orthoses.
- **Eating**—"The ability to keep and manipulate food/fluid in the mouth and swallow it" (O'Sullivan, 1995, p. 191) (AOTA, 2000, p. 629).
- **Feeding**—"The process of [setting up, arranging, and] bringing food [fluids] from the plate or cup to the mouth" (O'Sullivan, 1995, p. 191) (AOTA, 2000, p. 629).
- **Functional mobility**—Moving from one position or place to another (during performance of everyday activities), such as in-bed mobility, wheelchair mobility, transfers (wheelchair, bed, car, tub, toilet, tub/shower, chair, floor). Performing functional ambulation and transporting objects.
- **Personal device care**—Using, cleaning, and maintaining personal care items, such as hearing aids, contact lenses, glasses, orthotics, prosthetics, adaptive equipment, and contraceptive and sexual devices.
- **Personal hygiene and grooming**—Obtaining and using supplies; removing body hair (use of razors, tweezers, lotions, etc.); applying and removing cosmetics; washing, drying, combing, styling, brushing, and trimming hair; caring for nails (hands and feet); caring for skin, ears, eyes, and nose; applying deodorant; cleaning mouth; brushing and flossing teeth; or removing, cleaning, and reinserting dental orthotics and prosthetics.
- **Sexual activity**—Engagement in activities that result in sexual satisfaction.
- **Sleep/rest**—A period of inactivity in which one may or may not suspend consciousness.
- **Toilet hygiene**—Obtaining and using supplies; clothing management; maintaining toileting position; transferring to and from toileting position; cleaning body; and caring for menstrual and continence needs (including catheters, colostomies, and suppository management).

Instrumental activities of daily living (IADL)

Activities that are oriented toward interacting with the environment and that are often complex—generally optional in nature (i.e., may be delegated to another) (adapted from Rogers & Holm, 1994, pp. 181–202).

- **Care of others (including selecting and supervising caregivers)**—Arranging, supervising, or providing the care for others.
- **Care of pets**—Arranging, supervising, or providing the care for pets and service animals.
- **Child rearing**—Providing the care and supervision to support the developmental needs of a child.
- **Communication device use**—Using equipment or systems such as writing equipment, telephones, typewriters, computers, communication boards, call lights, emergency systems, braille writers, telecommunication devices for the deaf, and augmentative communication systems to send and receive information.
- **Community mobility**—Moving self in the community and using public or private transportation, such as driving, or accessing buses, taxi cabs, or other public transportation systems.
- **Financial management**—Using fiscal resources, including alternate methods of financial transaction and planning and using finances with long-term and short-term goals.
- **Health management and maintenance**—Developing, managing, and maintaining routines for health and wellness promotion, such as physical fitness, nutrition, decreasing health risk behaviors, and medication routines.
- **Home establishment and management**—Obtaining and maintaining personal and household possessions and environment (e.g., home, yard, garden, appliances, vehicles), including maintaining and repairing personal possessions (clothing and household items) and knowing how to seek help or whom to contact.
- **Meal preparation and cleanup**—Planning; preparing; serving well-balanced, nutritional meals; and cleaning up food and utensils after meals.
- **Safety procedures and emergency responses**—Knowing and performing preventive procedures to maintain a safe environment as well as recognizing sudden, unexpected hazardous situations and initiating emergency action to reduce the threat to health and safety.
- **Shopping**—Preparing shopping lists (grocery and other); selecting and purchasing items; selecting method of payment; and completing money transactions.

Education

Includes activities needed for being a student and participating in a learning environment.

- **Formal educational participation**—Including the categories of academic (e.g., math, reading, working on a degree), nonacademic (e.g., recess, lunchroom, hallway), extracurricular (e.g., sports, band, cheerleading, dances), and vocational (prevocational and vocational) participation.

Table 1. Areas of Occupation, Cont.

- Exploration of informal personal educational needs or interests (beyond formal education)—Identifying topics and methods for obtaining topic-related information or skills.
- Informal personal education participation—Participating in classes, programs, and activities that provide instruction/training in identified areas of interest.

Work

Includes activities needed for engaging in remunerative employment or volunteer activities (Mosey, 1996, p. 341).

- Employment interests and pursuits—Identifying and selecting work opportunities based on personal assets, limitations, likes, and dislikes relative to work (adapted from Mosey, 1996, p. 342).
- Employment seeking and acquisition—Identifying job opportunities, completing and submitting appropriate application materials, preparing for interviews, participating in interviews and following up afterward, discussing job benefits, and finalizing negotiations.
- Job performance—Including work habits, for example, attendance, punctuality, appropriate relationships with coworkers and supervisors, completion of assigned work, and compliance with the norms of the work setting (adapted from Mosey, 1996, p. 342).

- Retirement preparation and adjustment—Determining aptitudes, developing interests and skills, and selecting appropriate avocational pursuits.
- Volunteer exploration—Determining community causes, organizations, or opportunities for unpaid "work" in relationship to personal skills, interests, location, and time available.
- Volunteer participation—Performing unpaid "work" activities for the benefit of identified selected causes, organizations, or facilities.

Play

"Any spontaneous or organized activity that provides enjoyment, entertainment, amusement, or diversion" (Parham & Fazio, 1997, p. 252).

- Play exploration—Identifying appropriate play activities, which can include exploration play, practice play, pretend play, games with rules, constructive play, and symbolic play (adapted from Bergen, 1988, pp. 64–65).
- Play participation—Participating in play; maintaining a balance of play with other areas of occupation; and obtaining, using, and maintaining, toys, equipment, and supplies appropriately.

Leisure

"A nonobligatory activity that is intrinsically motivated and engaged in during discretionary time, that is, time not committed to obligatory occupations such as work, self-care, or sleep" (Parham & Fazio, 1997, p. 250).

- Leisure exploration—Identifying interests, skills, opportunities, and appropriate leisure activities.
- Leisure participation—Planning and participating in appropriate leisure activities; maintaining a balance of leisure activities with other areas of occupation; and obtaining, using, and maintaining equipment and supplies as appropriate.

Social participation

Activities associated with organized patterns of behavior that are characteristic and expected of an individual or an individual interacting with others within a given social system (adapted from Mosey, 1996, p. 340).

- Community—Activities that result in successful interaction at the community level (i.e., neighborhood, organizations, work, school).
- Family—"[Activities that result in] successful interaction in specific required and/or desired familial roles" (Mosey, 1996, p. 340).
- Peer, friend—Activities at different levels of intimacy, including engaging in desired sexual activity.

Note. Some of the terms used in this table are from, or adapted from, the rescinded *Uniform Terminology for Occupational Therapy—Third Edition* (AOTA, 1994, pp. 1047–1054).

Table 2. Performance Skills

Features of what one does, not what one has, related to observable elements of action that have implicit functional purposes (adapted from Fisher & Kielhofner, 1995, p. 113).

MOTOR SKILLS—skills in moving and interacting with task, objects, and environment (A. Fisher, personal communication, July 9, 2001).

- **Posture**—Relates to the stabilizing and aligning of one's body while moving in relation to task objects with which one must deal.

  Stabilizes—Maintains trunk control and balance while interacting with task objects such that there is no evidence of transient (i.e., quickly passing) propping or loss of balance that affects task performance.

  Aligns—Maintains an upright sitting or standing position, without evidence of a need to persistently prop during the task performance.

  Positions—Positions body, arms, or wheelchair in relation to task objects and in a manner that promotes the use of efficient arm movements during task performance.

- **Mobility**—Relates to moving the entire body or a body part in space as necessary when interacting with task objects.

  Walks—Ambulates on level surfaces and changes direction while walking without shuffling the feet, lurching, instability, or using external supports or assistive devices (e.g., cane, walker, wheelchair) during the task performance.

  Reaches—Extends, moves the arm (and when appropriate, the trunk) to effectively grasp or place task objects that are out of reach, including skillfully using a reacher to obtain task objects.

  Bends—Actively flexes, rotates, or twists the trunk in a manner and direction appropriate to the task.

- **Coordination**—Relates to using more than one body part to interact with task objects in a manner that supports task performance.

  Coordinates—Uses two or more body parts together to stabilize and manipulate task objects during bilateral motor tasks.

  Manipulates—Uses dexterous grasp-and-release patterns, isolated finger movements, and coordinated in-hand manipulation patterns when interacting with task objects.

  Flows—Uses smooth and fluid arm and hand movements when interacting with task objects.

- **Strength and effort**—Pertains to skills that require generation of muscle force appropriate for effective interaction with task objects.

  Moves—Pushes, pulls, or drags task objects along a supporting surface.

  Transports—Carries task objects from one place to another while walking, seated in a wheelchair, or using a walker.

  Lifts—Raises or hoists task objects, including lifting an object from one place to another, but without ambulating or moving from one place to another.

  Calibrates—Regulates or grades the force, speed, and extent of movement when interacting with task objects (e.g., not too much or too little).

  Grips—Pinches or grasps task objects with no "grip slips."

- **Energy**—Refers to sustained effort over the course of task performance.

  Endures—Persists and completes the task without obvious evidence of physical fatigue, pausing to rest, or stopping to "catch one's breath."

  Paces—Maintains a consistent and effective rate or tempo of performance throughout the steps of the entire task.

Process skills—"Skills…used in managing and modifying actions en route to the completion of daily life tasks" (Fisher & Kielhofner, 1995, p. 120).

- **Knowledge**—Refers to the ability to seek and use task-related knowledge.

  Chooses—Selects appropriate and necessary tools and materials for the task, including choosing the tools and materials that were specified for use prior to the initiation of the task.

  Uses—Uses tools and materials according to their intended purposes and in a reasonable or hygienic fashion, given their intrinsic properties and the availability (or lack of availability) of other objects.

  Handles—Supports, stabilizes, and holds tools and materials in an appropriate manner that protects them from damage, falling, or dropping.

  Heeds—Uses goal-directed task actions that are focused toward the completion of the specified task (i.e., the outcome originally agreed on or specified by another) without behavior that is driven or guided by environmental cues (i.e., "environmentally cued" behavior).

  Inquires—(a) Seeks needed verbal or written information by asking questions or reading directions or labels or (b) asks no unnecessary information questions (e.g., questions related to where materials are located or how a familiar task is performed).

- **Temporal organization**—Pertains to the beginning, logical ordering, continuation, and completion of the steps and action sequences of a task.

  Initiates—Starts or begins the next action or step without hesitation.

  Continues—Performs actions or action sequences of steps without unnecessary interruption such that once an action sequence is initiated, the individual continues on until the step is completed.

  Sequences—Performs steps in an effective or logical order for efficient use of time and energy and with an absence of (a) randomness in the ordering and/or (b) inappropriate repetition ("reordering") of steps.

  Terminates—Brings to completion single actions or single steps without perseveration, inappropriate persistence, or premature cessation.

- **Organizing space and objects**—Pertains to skills for organizing task spaces and task objects.

Table 2. Performance Skills, Cont.

Searches/locates—Looks for and locates tools and materials in a logical manner, including looking beyond the immediate environment (e.g., looking in, behind, on top of).

Gathers—Collects together needed or misplaced tools and materials, including (a) collecting located supplies into the workspace and (b) collecting and replacing materials that have spilled, fallen, or been misplaced.

Organizes—Logically positions or spatially arranges tools and materials in an orderly fashion (a) within a single workspace and (b) among multiple appropriate workspaces to facilitate ease of task performance.

Restores—(a) Puts away tools and materials in appropriate places, (b) restores immediate workspace to original condition (e.g., wiping surfaces clean), (c) closes and seals containers and coverings when indicated, and (d) twists or folds any plastic bags to seal.

Navigates—Modifies the movement pattern of the arm, body, or wheelchair to maneuver around obstacles that are encountered in the course of moving through space such that undesirable contact with obstacles (e.g., knocking over, bumping into) is avoided (includes maneuvering objects held in the hand around obstacles).

- **Adaptation**—Relates to the ability to anticipate, correct for, and benefit by learning from the consequences of errors that arise in the course of task performance.

Notices/responds—Responds appropriately to (a) nonverbal environmental/perceptual cues (i.e., movement, sound, smell, heat, moisture, texture, shape, consistency) that provide feedback with respect to task progression and (b) the spatial arrangement of objects to one another (e.g., aligning objects during stacking). Notices and, when indicated, makes an effective and efficient response.

Accommodates—Modifies his or her actions or the location of objects within the workspace in anticipation of or in response to problems that might arise.

The client anticipates or responds to problems effectively by (a) changing the method with which he or she is performing an action sequence, (b) changing the manner in which he or she interacts with or handles tools and materials already in the workspace, and (c) asking for assistance when appropriate or needed.

Adjusts—Changes working environments in anticipation of or in response to problems that might arise. The client anticipates or responds to problems effectively by making some change (a) between working environments by moving to a new workspace or bringing in or removing tools and materials from the present workspace or (b) in an environmental condition (e.g., turning on or off the tap, turning up or down the temperature).

Benefits—Anticipates and prevents undesirable circumstances or problems from recurring or persisting.

Communication/interaction skills—Refer to conveying intentions and needs and coordinating social behavior to act together with people (Forsyth & Kielhofner, 1999; Forsyth, Salamy, Simon, & Kielhofner, 1997; Kielhofner, 2002).

- **Physicality**—Pertains to using the physical body when communicating within an occupation.

Contacts—Makes physical contact with others.

Gazes—Uses eyes to communicate and interact with others.

Gestures—Uses movements of the body to indicate, demonstrate, or add emphasis.

Maneuvers—Moves one's body in relation to others.

Orients—Directs one's body in relation to others and/or occupational forms.

Postures—Assumes physical positions.

- **Information exchange**—Refers to giving and receiving information within an occupation.

Articulates—Produces clear, understandable speech.

Asserts—Directly expresses desires, refusals, and requests.

Asks—Requests factual or personal information.

Engages—Initiates interactions.

Expresses—Displays affect/attitude.

Modulates—Uses volume and inflection in speech.

Shares—Gives out factual or personal information.

Speaks—Makes oneself understood through use of words, phrases, and sentences.

Sustains—Keeps up speech for appropriate duration.

- **Relations**—Relates to maintaining appropriate relationships within an occupation.

Collaborates—Coordinates action with others toward a common end goal.

Conforms—Follows implicit and explicit social norms.

Focuses—Directs conversation and behavior to ongoing social action.

Relates—Assumes a manner of acting that tries to establish a rapport with others.

Respects—Accommodates to other people's reactions and requests.

Note. The Motor and Process Skills sections of this table were compiled from the following sources: Fisher (2001), Fisher and Kielhofner (1995)—updated by Fisher (2001). The Communication/Interaction Skills section of this table was compiled from the following sources: Forsyth and Kielhofner (1999); Forsyth, Salamy, Simon, and Kielhofner (1997); and Kielhofner (2002).

Table 3. Performance Patterns

Patterns of behavior related to daily life activities that are habitual or routine.

HABITS—"Automatic behavior that is integrated into more complex patterns that enable people to function on a day-to-day basis" (Neistadt & Crepeau, 1998, p. 869). Habits can either support or interfere with performance in areas of occupation.

Type of Habit	Examples
• Useful habits	
Habits that support performance in daily life and contribute to life satisfaction.	– Always put car keys in the same place so they can be found easily.
Habits that support ability to follow rhythms of daily life.	– Brush teeth every morning to maintain good oral hygiene.
• Impoverished habits	
Habits that are not established.	– Inconsistently remembering to look both ways before crossing the street.
Habits that need practice to improve.	– Inability to complete all steps of a self-care routine.
• Dominating habits	
Habits that are so demanding they interfere with daily life.	– Repetitive self-stimulation such as type occurring in autism.
	– Use of chemical substances, resulting in addiction.
Habits that satisfy a compulsive need for order.	– Neatly arranging forks on top of each other in silverware drawer.

ROUTINES—"Occupations with established sequences" (Christiansen & Baum, 1997, p. 6).

ROLES—"A set of behaviors that have some socially agreed upon function and for which there is an accepted code of norms" (Christiansen & Baum, 1997, p. 603).

Note. Information for Habits section of this table adapted from Dunn (2000, Fall).

Table 4. Context or Contexts

Context (including cultural, physical, social, personal, spiritual, temporal, and virtual) refers to a variety of interrelated conditions within and surrounding the client that influence performance.

Context	Definition	Example
Cultural	Customs, beliefs, activity patterns, behavior standards, and expectations accepted by the society of which the individual is a member. Includes political aspects, such as laws that affect access to resources and affirm personal rights. Also includes opportunities for education, employment, and economic support.	• Ethnicity, family, attitude, beliefs, values
Physical	Nonhuman aspects of contexts. Includes the accessibility to and performance within environments having natural terrain, plants, animals, buildings, furniture, objects, tools, or devices.	• Objects, built environment, natural environment, geographic terrain, sensory qualities of environment
Social	Availability and expectations of significant individuals, such as spouse, friends, and caregivers. Also includes larger social groups that are influential in establishing norms, role expectations, and social routines.	• Relationships with individuals, groups, or organizations; relationships with systems (political, economic, institutional)
Personal	"[F]eatures of the individual that are not part of a health condition or health status" (WHO, 2001, p. 17). Personal context includes age, gender, socio-economic status, and educational status.	• Twenty-five-year-old unemployed man with a high school diploma
Spiritual	The fundamental orientation of a person's life; that which inspires and motivates that individual.	• Essence of the person, greater or higher purpose, meaning, substance
Temporal	"Location of occupational performance in time" (Neistadt & Crepeau, 1998, p. 292).	• Stages of life, time of day, time of year, duration
Virtual	Environment in which communication occurs by means of airways or computers and an absence of physical contact.	• Realistic simulation of an environment, chat rooms, radio transmissions

Note. Some of the definitions for areas of context or contexts are from the rescinded *Uniform Terminology for Occupational Therapy—Third Edition* (AOTA, 1994).

Table 5. Activity Demands

The aspects of an activity, which include the objects, space, social demands, sequencing or timing, required actions, and required underlying body functions and body structure needed to carry out the activity.

Activity Demand Aspects	Definition	Examples
Objects and their properties	The tools, materials, and equipment used in the process of carrying out the activity	• Tools (scissors, dishes, shoes, volleyball) • Materials (paints, milk, lipstick) • Equipment (workbench, stove, basketball hoop) • Inherent properties (heavy, rough, sharp, colorful, loud, bitter tasting)
Space demands (relates to physical context)	The physical environmental requirements of the activity (e.g., size, arrangement, surface, lighting, temperature, noise, humidity, ventilation)	• Large open space outdoors required for a baseball game
Social demands (relates to social and cultural contexts)	The social structure and demands that may be required by the activity	• Rules of game • Expectations of other participants in activity (e.g., sharing of supplies)
Sequence and timing	The process used to carry out the activity (specific steps, sequence, timing requirements)	• Steps—to make tea: gather cup and tea bag, heat water, pour water into cup, etc. • Sequence—heat water before placing tea bag in water • Timing—leave tea bag to steep for 2 minutes
Required actions	The usual skills that would be required by any performer to carry out the activity. Motor, process, and communication inter-action skills should each be considered. The performance skills demanded by an activity will be correlated with the demands of the other activity aspects (i.e., objects, space)	• Gripping handlebar • Choosing a dress from closet • Answering a question
Required body functions	"The physiological functions of body systems (including psycho-logical functions)" (WHO, 2001, p. 10) that are required to sup-port the actions used to perform the activity.	• Mobility of joints • Level of consciousness
Required body structures	"Anatomical parts of the body such as organs, limbs, and their components [that support body function]" (WHO, 2001, p. 10) that are required to perform the activity.	• Number of hands • Number of eyes

Table 6. Client Factors

Those factors that reside within the client and that may affect performance in areas of occupation. Client factors include body functions and body structures. Knowledge about body functions and structures is considered when determining which functions and structures are needed to carry out an occupation/activity and how the body functions and structures may be changed as a result of engaging in an occupation/activity. Body functions are "the physiological functions of body systems (including psychological functions)" (WHO, 2001, p. 10). Body structures are "anatomical parts of the body such as organs, limbs and their components [that support body function]" (WHO, 2001, p. 10).

Client Factor	Selected Classifications From ICF and Occupational Therapy Examples
BODY FUNCTION CATEGORIES[a]	
Mental functions (affective, cognitive, perceptual)	
• Global mental functions	*Consciousness functions*—level of arousal, level of consciousness.
	Orientation functions—to person, place, time, self, and others.
	Sleep—amount and quality of sleep. *Note:* Sleep and sleep patterns are assessed in relation to how they affect ability to effectively engage in occupations and in daily life activities.
	Temperament and personality functions—conscientiousness, emotional stability, openness to experience. *Note:* These functions are assessed relative to their influence on the ability to engage in occupations and in daily life activities.
	Energy and drive functions—motivation, impulse control, interests, values.
• Specific mental functions	*Attention functions*—sustained attention, divided attention.
	Memory functions—retrospective memory, prospective memory.
	Perceptual functions—visuospatial perception, interpretation of sensory stimuli (tactile, visual, auditory, olfactory, gustatory).
	Thought functions—recognition, categorization, generalization, awareness of reality, logical/coherent thought, appropriate thought content.
	Higher-level cognitive functions—judgment, concept formation, time management, problem solving, decision-making.
	Mental functions of language—able to receive language and express self through spoken and written or sign language. *Note:* This function is assessed relative to its influence on the ability to engage in occupations and in daily life activities.
	Calculation functions—able to add or subtract. *Note:* These functions are assessed relative to their influence on the ability to engage in occupations and in daily life activities (e.g., making change when shopping).
	Mental functions of sequencing complex movement—motor planning.
	Psychomotor functions—appropriate range and regulation of motor response to psychological events.
	Emotional functions—appropriate range and regulation of emotions, self-control.
	Experience of self and time functions—body image, self-concept, self-esteem.
Sensory functions and pain	
• Seeing and related functions	*Seeing functions*—visual acuity, visual field functions.
• Hearing and vestibular functions	*Hearing function*—response to sound. *Note:* This function is assessed in terms of its presence or absence and its affect on engaging in occupations and in daily life activities.
	Vestibular function—balance.
• Additional sensory functions	*Taste function*—ability to discriminate tastes.
	Smell function—ability to discriminate smell.
	Proprioceptive function—kinesthesia, joint position sense.
	Touch functions—sensitivity to touch, ability to discriminate.
	Sensory functions related to temperature and other stimuli—sensitivity to temperature, sensitivity to pressure, ability to discriminate temperature and pressure.
• Pain	*Sensations of pain*—dull pain, stabbing pain.

Table 6. Client Factors, Cont.

Client Factor	Selected Classifications From ICF and Occupational Therapy Examples
Neuromusculoskeletal and movement-related functions • Functions of joints and bones	*Mobility of joint functions*—passive range of motion. *Stability of joint functions*—postural alignment. *Note:* This refers to physiological stability of the joint related to its structural integrity as compared to the motor skill of aligning the body while moving in relation to task objects. *Mobility of bone functions*—frozen scapula, movement of carpal bones.
• Muscle functions	*Muscle power functions*—strength. *Muscle tone functions*—degree of muscle tone (e.g., flaccidity, spasticity). *Muscle endurance functions*—endurance.
• Movement functions	*Motor reflex functions*—stretch reflex, asymmetrical tonic neck reflex. *Involuntary movement reaction functions*—righting reactions, supporting reactions. *Control of voluntary movement functions*—eye–hand coordination, bilateral integration, eye–foot coordination. *Involuntary movement functions*—tremors, tics, motor perseveration. *Gait pattern functions*—walking patterns and impairments, such as asymmetric gait, stiff gait. (*Note:* Gait patterns are assessed in relation to how they affect ability to engage in occupations and in daily life activities.)
Cardiovascular, hematological, immunological, and respiratory system function • Cardiovascular system function	*Blood pressure functions*—hypertension, hypotension, postural hypotension.
• Hematological and immunological system function	Occupational therapists and occupational therapy assistants have knowledge of these body functions and understand broadly the interaction that occurs between these functions and engagement in occupation to support participation. Some therapists may specialize in evaluating and intervening with a specific function as it is related to supporting performance and engagement in occupations and activities targeted for intervention.
• Respiratory system function	*Respiration functions*—rate, rhythm, and depth.
• Additional functions and sensations of the cardiovascular and respiratory systems	*Exercise tolerance functions*—physical endurance, aerobic capacity, stamina, and fatigability.
Voice and speech functions **Digestive, metabolic, and endocrine system function** • Digestive system function • Metabolic system and endocrine system function **Genitourinary and reproductive functions** • Urinary functions • Genital and reproductive functions	Occupational therapists and occupational therapy assistants have knowledge of these body functions and understand broadly the interaction that occurs between these functions and engagement in occupation to support participation. Some therapists may specialize in evaluating and intervening with a specific function as it is related to supporting performance and engagement in occupations and activities targeted for intervention.

Table 6. Client Factors, Cont.

Client Factor	Selected Classifications From ICF and Occupational Therapy Examples
Skin and related structure functions	
• Skin functions	*Protective functions of the skin*—presence or absence of wounds, cuts, or abrasions. *Repair function of the skin*—wound healing.
• Hair and nail functions	Occupational therapists and occupational therapy assistants have knowledge of these body functions and understand broadly the interaction that occurs between these functions and engagement in occupation to support participation. Some therapists may specialize in evaluating and intervening with a specific function as it is related to supporting performance and engagement in occupations and activities targeted for intervention.

Client Factor	Classifications (Classifications are not delineated in the Body Structure section of this table)
BODY STRUCTURE CATEGORIES[b] Structure of the nervous system The eye, ear, and related structures Structures involved in voice and speech Structures of the cardiovascular, immunological, and respiratory systems Structures related to the digestive, metabolic, and endocrine systems Structure related to the genitourinary and reproductive systems Structures related to movement Skin and related structures	Occupational therapists and occupational therapy assistants have knowledge of these body structures and understand broadly the interaction that occurs among these structures and engagement in occupation to support participation. Some therapists may specialize in evaluating and intervening with a specific structure as it is related to supporting performance and engagement in occupations and activities targeted for intervention.

Note. The reader is strongly encouraged to use *International Classification of Functioning, Disability and Health* (ICF) in collaboration with this table to provide for in-depth information with respect to classification in terms (inclusion and exclusion).

[a]Categories and classifications are adapted from the ICF (WHO, 2001). [b]Categories are from the ICF (WHO, 2001).

Table 7. Occupational Therapy Intervention Approaches

Specific strategies selected to direct the process of intervention that are based on the client's desired outcome, evaluation data, and evidence.

Approach	Focus of Intervention	Examples
Create, promote (health promotion)[a]—an intervention approach that does not assume a disability is present or that any factors would interfere with performance. This approach is designed to provide enriched contextual and activity experiences that will enhance performance for all persons in the natural contexts of life (adapted from Dunn, McClain, Brown, & Youngstrom, 1998, p. 534).	Performance skills	• Create a parenting class for first-time parents to teach child development information (performance skill).
	Performance patterns	• Promote handling stress by creating time-use routines with healthy clients (performance pattern).
	Context or contexts	• Create a variety of equipment available at public playgrounds to promote a diversity of sensory play experiences (context).
	Activity demands	• Promote the establishment of sufficient space to allow senior residents to participate in congregate cooking (activity demand).
	Client factors (body functions, body structures)	• Promote increased endurance in schoolchildren by having them ride bicycles to school (client factor: body function).
Establish, restore (remediation, restoration)[a]—an intervention approach designed to change client variables, to establish a skill or ability that has not yet developed, or to restore a skill or ability that has been impaired (adapted from Dunn et al., 1998, p. 533).	Performance skills	• Improve coping needed for changing workplace demands by improving assertiveness skills (performance skill).
	Performance patterns	• Establish morning routines needed to arrive at school or work on time (performance pattern).
	Client factors (body functions, body structures)	• Restore mobility needed for play activities (client factor: body function).
Maintain—an intervention approach designed to provide the supports that will allow clients to preserve their performance capabilities that they have regained, that continue to meet their occupational needs, or both. The assumption is that without continued maintenance intervention, performance would decrease, occupational needs would not be met, or both, thereby affecting health and quality of life.	Performance skills	• Maintain the ability to organize tools by providing a tool outline painted on a pegboard (performance skill).
	Performance patterns	• Maintain appropriate medication schedule by providing a timer (performance pattern).
	Context or contexts	• Maintain safe and independent access for persons with low vision by providing increased hallway lighting (context).
	Activity demands	• Maintain independent gardening for persons with arthritic hands by providing tools with modified grips (activity demand).
	Client factors (body functions, body structures)	• Maintain proper digestive system functions by developing a dining program (client factor: body function). • Maintain upper-extremity muscles necessary for independent wheelchair mobility by developing an after-school–based exercise program (client factor: body structure).
Modify (compensation, adaptation)[a]—an intervention approach directed at "finding ways to revise the current context or activity demands to support performance in the natural setting…[includes] compensatory techniques, including enhancing some features to provide cues, or reducing other features to reduce distractibility" (Dunn et al., 1998, p. 533).	Context or contexts	• Modify holiday celebration activities to exclude alcohol to support sobriety (context).
	Activity demands	• Modify office equipment (e.g., chair, computer station) to support individual employee body function and performance skill abilities (activity demand).
	Performance patterns	• Modify daily routines to provide consistency and predictability to support individual's cognitive ability (performance pattern).

Table 7. Occupational Therapy Intervention Approaches, cont.

Approach	Focus of Intervention	Examples
Prevent (disability prevention)[a]—an intervention approach designed to address clients with or without a disability who are at risk for occupational performance problems. This approach is designed to prevent the occurrence or evolution of barriers to performance in context. Interventions may be directed at client, context, or activity variables (adapted from Dunn et al., 1998, p. 534).	Performance skills	• Prevent poor posture when sitting for prolonged periods by providing a chair with proper back support (performance skill).
	Performance patterns	• Prevent the use of chemical substances by introducing self-initiated strategies to assist in remaining drug free (performance pattern).
	Context or contexts	• Prevent social isolation by suggesting participation in after-work group activities (context).
	Activity demands	• Prevent back injury by providing instruction in proper lifting techniques (activity demand).
	Client factors (body functions, body structures)	• Prevent increased blood pressure during homemaking activities by learning to monitor blood pressure in a cardiac exercise program (client factor: body function).
		• Prevent repetitive stress injury by suggesting that a wrist support splint be worn when typing (client factor: body structure).

[a]Parallel language used in Moyers (1999, p. 274).

Table 8. Types of Occupational Therapy Interventions

THERAPEUTIC USE OF SELF—A practitioner's planned use of his or her personality, insights, perceptions, and judgments as part of the therapeutic process (adapted from Punwar & Peloquin, 2000, p. 285).

THERAPEUTIC USE OF OCCUPATIONS AND ACTIVITIES[a]—Occupations and activities selected for specific clients that meet therapeutic goals. To use occupations/activities therapeutically, context or contexts, activity demands, and client factors all should be considered in relation to the client's therapeutic goals.

Occupation-based activity	*Purpose:* Allows clients to engage in actual occupations that are part of their own context and that match their goals. *Examples:* • Play on playground equipment during recess. • Purchase own groceries and prepare a meal. • Adapt the assembly line to achieve greater safety. • Put on clothes without assistance.
Purposeful activity	*Purpose:* Allows the client to engage in goal-directed behaviors or activities within a therapeutically designed context that lead to an occupation or occupations. *Examples:* • Practice vegetable slicing. • Practice drawing a straight line. • Practice safe ways to get in and out of a bathtub equipped with grab bars. • Role play to learn ways to manage anger.
Preparatory methods	*Purpose:* Prepares the client for occupational performance. Used in preparation for purposeful and occupation-based activities. *Examples:* • Sensory input to promote optimum response. • Physical agent modalities. • Orthotics/splinting (design, fabrication, application). • Exercise.

CONSULTATION PROCESS—A type of intervention in which practitioners use their knowledge and expertise to collaborate with the client. The collaborative process involves identifying the problem, creating possible solutions, trying solutions, and altering them as necessary for greater effectiveness. When providing consultation, the practitioner is not directly responsible for the outcome of the intervention (Dunn, 2000, p. 113).

EDUCATION PROCESS—An intervention process that involves the imparting of knowledge and information about occupation and activity and that does not result in the actual performance of the occupation/activity.

[a]Information adapted from Pedretti and Early (2001).

Table 9. Types of Outcomes

The examples listed specify how the broad outcome of engagement in occupation may be operationalized. The examples are not intended to be all-inclusive.

Outcome	Description
Occupational performance	The ability to carry out activities of daily life (areas of occupation). Occupational performance can be addressed in two different ways: • Improvement—used when a performance deficit is present, often as a result of an injury or disease process. This approach results in increased independence and function in ADL, IADL, education, work, play, leisure, or social participation. • Enhancement—used when a performance deficit is not currently present. This approach results in the development of performance skills and performance patterns that augment performance or prevent potential problems from developing in daily life occupations.
Client satisfaction	The client's affective response to his or her perceptions of the process and benefits of receiving occupational therapy services (adapted from Maciejewski, Kawiecki, & Rockwood, 1997).
Role competence	The ability to effectively meet the demand of roles in which the client engages.
Adaptation	"A change a person makes in his or her response approach when that person encounters an occupational challenge. This change is implemented when the individual's customary response approaches are found inadequate for producing some degree of mastery over the challenge" (Schultz & Schkade, 1997, p. 474).
Health and wellness	*Health*—"A complete state of physical, mental, and social well-being and not just the absence of disease or infirmity"(WHO, 1947, p. 29). *Wellness*—The condition of being in good health, including the appreciation and the enjoyment of health. Wellness is more than a lack of disease symptoms; it is a state of mental and physical balance and fitness (adapted from *Taber's Cyclopedic Medical Dictionary*, 1997, p. 2110).
Prevention	Promoting a healthy lifestyle at the individual, group, organizational, community (societal), and governmental or policy level (adapted from Brownson & Scaffa, 2001).
Quality of life	A person's dynamic appraisal of his or her life satisfactions (perceptions of progress toward one's goals), self-concept (the composite of beliefs and feelings about oneself), health and functioning (including health status, self-care capabilities, role competence), and socioeconomic factors (e.g., vocation, education, income) (adapted from Radomski, 1995; Zhan, 1992).

Note. ADL = activities of daily living; IADL = instrumental activities of daily living.

Table 10. Occupational Therapy Practice Framework Process Summary

Evaluation		Intervention			Outcomes
Occupational Profile ⟷	*Analysis of Occupational Performance*	*Intervention Plan*	*Intervention Implementation*	*Intervention Review*	*Engagement in Occupation to Support Participation*
• Who is the client? • Why is the client seeking services? • What occupations and activities are successful or are causing problems? • What contexts support or inhibit desired outcomes? • What is the client's occupational history? • What are the client's priorities and targeted outcomes?	• Synthesize information from the occupational profile. • Observe client's performance in desired occupation/activity. • Note the effectiveness of performance skills and patterns and select assessments to identify factors (context or contexts, activity demands, client factors) that may be influencing performance skills and patterns. • Interpret assessment data to identify facilitators and barriers to performance. • Develop and refine hypotheses about client's occupational performance strengths and weaknesses. • Collaborate with client to create goals that address targeted outcomes. • Delineate areas for intervention based on best practice and evidence.	• Develop plan that includes – objective and measurable goals with timeframe, – occupational therapy intervention approach based on theory and evidence, and – mechanisms for service delivery. • Consider discharge needs and plan. • Select outcome measures. • Make recommendation or referral to others as needed.	• Determine types of occupational therapy interventions to be used and carry them out. • Monitor client's response according to ongoing assessment and reassessment.	• Reevaluate plan relative to achieving targeted outcomes. • Modify plan as needed. • Determine need for continuation, discontinuation, or referral.	• Focus on outcomes as they relate to engagement in occupation to support participation. • Select outcome measures. • Measure and use outcomes.

← Continue to renegotiate intervention plans and targeted outcomes. →

← Ongoing interaction among evaluation, intervention, and outcomes occurs throughout the process. →

Glossary

A

Activities of daily living or ADL (an area of occupation)

Activities that are oriented toward taking care of one's own body (adapted from Rogers & Holm, 1994, pp. 181–202). (See Appendix, Table 1, for definitions of terms.) ADL is also referred to as basic activities of daily living (BADL) and personal activities of daily living (PADL).

- Bathing, showering
- Bowel and bladder management
- Dressing
- Eating
- Feeding
- Functional mobility
- Personal device care
- Personal hygiene and grooming
- Sexual activity
- Sleep/rest
- Toilet hygiene

Activity (activities)

A term that describes a class of human actions that are goal directed.

Activity demands

The aspects of an activity, which include the objects, space, social demands, sequencing or timing, required actions, and required underlying body functions and body structures needed to carry out the activity. (See Appendix, Table 5, for definitions of these aspects.)

Adaptation (as used as an outcome; see Appendix, Table 9)

"A change a person makes in his or her response approach when that person encounters an occupational challenge. This change is implemented when the individual's customary response approaches are found inadequate for producing some degree of mastery over the challenge" (Schultz & Schkade, 1997, p. 474).

Adaptation (as used as a performance skill; see Appendix, Table 2)

Relates to the ability to anticipate, correct for, and benefit by learning from the consequences of errors that arise in the course of task performance (Fisher, 2001; Fisher & Kielhofner, 1995—updated by Fisher [2001].

Areas of occupations

Various kinds of life activities in which people engage, including the following categories: ADL, IADL, education, work, play, leisure, and social participation. (See Appendix, Table 1, for definitions of terms.)

Assessment

"Shall be used to refer to specific tools or instruments that are used during the evaluation process" (AOTA, 1995, pp. 1072–1073).

B

Body functions (a client factor, including physical, cognitive, psychosocial aspects)

"The physiological functions of body systems (including psychological functions)" (WHO, 2001, p. 10). (See Appendix, Table 6, for categories.)

Body structures (a client factor)

"Anatomical parts of the body such as organs, limbs and their components [that support body function]" (WHO, 2001, p. 10). (See Appendix, Table 6, for categories.)

C

Client

(a) Individuals (including others involved in the individual's life who may also help or be served indirectly such as caregiver, teacher, parent, employer, spouse), (b) groups, or (c) populations (i.e., organizations, communities).

Client-centered approach

An orientation that honors the desires and priorities of clients in designing and implementing interventions (adapted from Dunn, 2000, p. 4).

Client factors

Those factors that reside within the client and that may affect performance in areas of occupation. Client factors include body functions and body structures. (See Appendix, Table 6, for categories.)

Client satisfaction

The client's affective response to his or her perceptions of the process and benefits of receiving occupational therapy services (adapted from Maciejewski, Kawiecki, & Rockwood, 1997, pp. 67–89).

Communication/interaction skills (a performance skill)

Refer to conveying intentions and needs as well as coordinating social behavior to act together with people (Forsyth & Kielhofner, 1999; Forsyth, Salamy, Simon, & Kielhofner, 1997; Kielhofner, 2002). (See Appendix, Table 2, for skills.)

Context or contexts

Refers to a variety of interrelated conditions within and surrounding the client that influence performance. Contexts include cultural, physical, social, personal, spiritual, temporal, and virtual. (See Appendix, Table 4, for definitions of terms.)

Cultural (a context)

"Customs, beliefs, activity patterns, behavior standards, and expectations accepted by the society of which the individual is a member. Includes political aspects, such as laws that affect access to resources and affirm personal rights. Also includes opportunities for education, employment, and economic support" (AOTA, 1994, p. 1054).

D

Dynamic assessment

Describes a process used during intervention implementation for testing the hypotheses generated through the evaluation process. Allows for evaluation of change and intervention effectiveness during intervention. Assesses the interactions among the person, environment, and activity to understand how the client learns and approaches activities. May lead to adjustments in intervention plan (adapted from Primeau & Ferguson, 1999, p. 503).

E

Education (an area of occupation)

Includes activities needed for being a student and participating in a learning environment. (See Appendix, Table 1, for definitions of terms.)

- Formal educational participation
- Informal personal educational needs or interests exploration (beyond formal education)
- Informal personal education participation

Engagement in occupation

This term recognizes the commitment made to performance in occupations or activities as the result of self-choice, motivation, and meaning and alludes to the objective and subjective aspects of being involved in and carrying out occupations and activities that are meaningful and purposeful to the person.

Evaluation

"Shall be used to refer to the process of obtaining and interpreting data necessary for intervention. This includes planning for and documenting the evaluation process and results" (AOTA, 1995, p. 1072).

G

Goals

"The result or achievement toward which effort is directed; aim; end" (*Random House Webster's College Dictionary*, 1995).

H

Habits (a performance pattern)

"Automatic behavior that is integrated into more complex patterns that enable people to function on a day-to-day basis…" (Neistadt & Crepeau, 1998, p. 869). Habits can either support or interfere with performance in areas of occupation. (See Appendix, Table 3, for descriptions of types of habits.)

Health

"A complete state of physical, mental, and social well-being and not just the absence of disease or infirmity" (WHO, 1947, p. 29).

Health status

A condition in which one successfully and satisfactorily performs occupations (adapted from McColl, Law, & Stewart, 1993, p. 5).

I

Identity

"A composite definition of the self and includes an interpersonal aspect (e.g., our roles and relationships, such as mother, wives, occupational therapists), an aspect of possibility or potential (who we *might* become), and a values aspect (that suggests importance and provides a stable basis for choices and decisions).… Identity can be viewed as the superordinate view of ourselves that includes both self-esteem and self-concept, but also importantly reflects and is influenced by the larger social world in which we find ourselves" (Christiansen, 1999, pp. 548–549) [see Chapter 42].

Independence

"Having adequate resources to accomplish everyday tasks" (Christiansen & Baum, 1997, p. 597). "The profession views independence as the ability to self-determine activity performance, regardless of who actually performs the activity" (AOTA, 1994, p. 1051).

Instrumental activities of daily living or IADL (an area of occupation)

Activities that are oriented toward interacting with the environment and that are often complex. IADL are generally optional in nature, that is, may be delegated to another (adapted from Rogers & Holm, 1994, pp. 181–202). (See Appendix, Table 1, for definitions of terms.)

- Care of others (including selecting and supervising caregivers)
- Care of pets
- Child rearing
- Communication device use
- Community mobility

- Financial management
- Health management and maintenance
- Home establishment and management
- Meal preparation and cleanup
- Safety procedures and emergency responses
- Shopping

Interests

"Disposition to find pleasure and satisfaction in occupations and the self-knowledge of our enjoyment of occupations" (Kielhofner, Borell, Burke, Helfrick, & Nygard, 1995, p. 47).

Intervention approaches

Specific strategies selected to direct the process of interventions that are based on the client's desired outcome, evaluation date, and evidence. (See Appendix, Table 7, for definitions of various occupational therapy intervention approaches.) The terms in parentheses indicate parallel language used in Moyers (1999, p. 274).

- Create/promote (health promotion)
- Establish/restore (remediation/restoration)
- Maintain
- Modify (compensation/adaptation)
- Prevent (disability prevention)

Intervention implementation

The skilled process of effecting change in the client's occupational performance leading to engagement in occupations or activities to support participation.

Intervention plan

An outline of selected approaches and types of interventions, which is based on the results of the evaluation process, developed to reach the client's identified targeted outcomes.

Intervention review

A continuous process for reevaluating and reviewing the intervention plan, the effectiveness of implementation, and the progress toward targeted outcomes.

Interventions

(See Appendix, Table 8, for definitions of the types of occupational therapy interventions.)

- Therapeutic use of self
- Therapeutic use of occupations/activities
- Consultation process
- Education process

L

Leisure (an area of occupation)

"A nonobligatory activity that is intrinsically motivated and engaged in during discretionary time, that is, time not committed to obligatory occupations such as work, self-care, or sleep" (Parham & Fazio, 1997, p. 250). (See Appendix, Table 1, for definitions of terms.)

- Leisure exploration
- Leisure participation

M

Motor skills (a performance skill)

Skills in moving and interacting with task, objects, and environment (A. Fisher, personal communication, July 9, 2001).

O

Occupation

"Activities…of everyday life, named, organized, and given value and meaning by individuals and a culture. Occupation is everything people do to occupy themselves, including looking after themselves…enjoying life…and contributing to the social and economic fabric of their communities…." (Law, Polatajko, Baptiste, & Townsend, 1997, p. 34).

Occupational performance

The ability to carry out activities of daily life. Includes activities in the areas of occupation: ADL (also called BADL and PADL), IADL, education, work, play, leisure, and social participation. Occupational performance is the accomplishment of the selected activity or occupation resulting from the dynamic transaction among the client, the context, and the activity. Improving or enabling skills and patterns in occupational performance leads to engagement in occupations or activities. (Adapted in part from Law et al., 1996, p. 16.)

Occupational profile

A profile that describes the client's occupational history, patterns of daily living, interests, values, and needs.

Outcomes

Important dimensions of health attributed to interventions, including ability to function, health perceptions, and satisfaction with care (adapted from Request for Planning Ideas, 2001).

P

Participation

"Involvement in a life situation" (WHO, 2001, p. 10).

Performance patterns

Patterns of behavior related to daily life activities that are habitual or routine. Performance patterns include habits and routines. (See Appendix, Table 3, for descriptions of terms.)

Performance skills

Features of what one does, not of what one has, related to observable elements of action that have implicit functional purposes (adapted from Fisher & Kielhofner, 1995, p. 113). Performance skills include motor skills, process skills, and communication/interaction skills. (See Appendix, Table 2, for definitions of skills.)

Personal (a context)

"Features of the individual that are not part of a health condition or health status" (WHO, 2001, p. 17). Personal context includes age, gender, socioeconomic status, and educational status.

Physical (a context)

"Nonhuman aspects of contexts. Includes the accessibility to and performance within environments having natural terrain, plants, animals, buildings, furniture, objects, tools, or devices" (AOTA, 1994, p. 1054).

Play (an area of occupation)

"Any spontaneous or organized activity that provides enjoyment, entertainment, amusement, or diversion" (Parham & Fazio, 1997, p. 252). (See Appendix, Table 1, for definitions of terms.)

- Play exploration
- Play participation

Prevention

Promoting a healthy lifestyle at the individual, group, organizational, community (societal), governmental/policy level (adapted from Brownson & Scaffa, 2001).

Process skills (a performance skill)

"Skills … used in managing and modifying actions en route to the completion of daily life tasks" (Fisher & Kielhofner, 1995, p. 120).

Purposeful activity

"An activity used in treatment that is goal directed and that the …[client] sees as meaningful or purposeful" (Low, 2002).

Q

Quality of life

A person's dynamic appraisal of his or her life satisfactions (perceptions of progress toward one's goals), self-concept (the composite of beliefs and feelings about oneself), health and functioning (including health status, self-care capabilities, and role competence), and socioeconomic factors (e.g., vocation, education, income) (adapted from Radomski, 1995; Zhan, 1992).

R

Reevaluation

A reassessment of the client's performance and goals to determine the type and amount of change.

Role competence

The ability to effectively meet the demand of roles in which the client engages.

Role(s)

"A set of behaviors that have some socially agreed upon function and for which there is an accepted code of norms" (Christiansen & Baum, 1997, p. 603).

Routines (a performance pattern)

"Occupations with established sequences" (Christiansen & Baum, 1997, p. 16).

S

Self-efficacy

"People's beliefs in their capabilities to organize and execute the courses of action required to deal with prospective situations" (Bandura, 1995, as cited in Rowe & Kahn, 1997, p. 437).

Social (a context)

"Availability and expectations of significant individuals, such as spouse, friends, and caregivers. Also includes larger social groups which are influential in establishing norms, role expectations, and social routines" (AOTA, 1994, p. 1054).

Social participation (an area of occupation)

"Organized patterns of behavior that are characteristic and expected of an individual in a given position within a social system" (Mosey, 1996, p. 340). (See Appendix, Table 1, for definitions of terms.)

- Community
- Family
- Peer, friend

Spiritual (a context)

The fundamental orientation of a person's life; that which inspires and motivates that individual.

T

Temporal (a context)

"Location of occupational performance in time" (Neistadt & Crepeau, 1998, p. 292).

V

Values

"A coherent set of convictions that assigns significance or standards to occupations, creating a strong disposition to perform accordingly" (Kielhofner, Borell, Burke, Helfrick, & Nygard, 1995, p. 46).

Virtual (a context)

Environment in which communication occurs by means of airways or computers and an absence of physical contact.

W

Wellness

The condition of being in good health, including the appreciation and the enjoyment of health. Wellness is more than a lack of disease symptoms; it is a state of mental and physical balance and fitness (*Taber's Cyclopedic Medical Dictionary*, 1997).

Work (an area of occupation)

Includes activities needed for engaging in remunerative employment or volunteer activities (Mosey, 1996, p. 341). (See Appendix, Table 1, for definitions of terms.)

- Employment interests and pursuits
- Employment seeking and acquisition
- Job performance
- Retirement preparation and adjustment
- Volunteer exploration
- Volunteer participation

References

American Occupational Therapy Association. (1994). Uniform terminology for occupational therapy—Third edition. *American Journal of Occupational Therapy, 48,* 1047–1054.

American Occupational Therapy Association. (1995). Clarification of the use of terms assessment and evaluation. *American Journal of Occupational Therapy, 49,* 1072–1073.

American Occupational Therapy Association. (2000). Specialized knowledge and skills for eating and feeding in occupational therapy practice. *American Journal of Occupational Therapy, 54,* 629–640.

Bergen, D. (Ed.). (1988). *Play as a medium for learning and development: A handbook of theory and practice.* Portsmouth, NH: Heinemann Educational Books.

Brownson, C. A., & Scaffa, M. E. (2001). Occupational therapy in the promotion of health and the prevention of disease and disability. *American Journal of Occupational Therapy, 55,* 656–660.

Christiansen, C. H. (1999). Defining lives: Occupation as identity—An essay on competence, coherence, and the creation of meaning, 1999 Eleanor Clarke Slagle lecture. *American Journal of Occupational Therapy, 53,* 547–558. Reprinted as Chapter 42.

Christiansen, C. H., & Baum, C. M. (Eds.). (1997). *Occupational therapy: Enabling function and well-being.* Thorofare, NJ: Slack.

Dunn, W. (2000, Fall). Habit: What's the brain got to do with it? *Occupational Therapy Journal of Research, 20* (Suppl. 1), 6S–20S.

Dunn, W. (2000). *Best practice in occupational therapy in community service with children and families.* Thorofare, NJ: Slack.

Dunn, W., McClain, L. H., Brown, C., & Youngstrom, M. J. (1998). The ecology of human performance. In M. E. Neistadt & E. B. Crepeau (Eds.), *Willard & Spackman's occupational therapy* (9th ed., pp. 525–535). Philadelphia: Lippincott Williams & Wilkins.

Fisher, A. G. (2001). *Assessment of motor and process skills, Vol. 1.* (User manual.) Ft. Collins, CO: Three Star Press.

Fisher, A., & Kielhofner, G. (1995). Skill in occupational performance. In G. Kielhofner (Ed.), *A model of human occupation: Theory and application* (2nd ed., pp. 113–128). Philadelphia: Lippincott Williams & Wilkins.

Forsyth, K., & Kielhofner, G. (1999). Validity of the assessment of communication of interaction skills. *British Journal of Occupational Therapy, 62,* 69–74.

Forsyth, K., Salamy, M., Simon, S., & Kielhofner, G. (1997). *Assessment of communication and interaction skills.* Chicago: University of Illinois, Model of Human Occupation Clearinghouse.

Kielhofner, G. (2002). Dimensions of doing. In G. Kielhofner (Ed.), *A model of human occupation: Theory and application* (3rd ed.). Philadelphia: Lippincott Williams & Wilkins.

Kielhofner, G., Borell, L., Burke, J., Helfrick, C., & Nygard, L. (1995). Volition subsystem. In G. Kielhofner (Ed.), *A model of human occupation: Theory and application* (2nd ed., pp. 39–62). Philadelphia: Lippincott Williams & Wilkins.

Law, M., Cooper, B., Strong, S., Stewart, D., Rigby, P., & Letts, L. (1996). Person-environment-occupation model: A transactive approach to occupational performance. *Canadian Journal of Occupational Therapy, 63,* 9–23.

Law, M., Polatajko, H., Baptiste, W., & Townsend, E. (1997). Core concepts of occupational therapy. In E. Townsend (Ed.), *Enabling occupation: An occupational therapy perspective* (pp. 29–56). Ottawa, ON: Canadian Association of Occupational Therapists.

Low, J. F. (2002). Historical and social foundations for practice. In C. A. Trombly & M. V. Radomski (Eds.), *Occupational therapy for physical dysfunction* (5th ed.; pp. 17–30). Philadelphia: Lippincott Williams & Wilkins.

Maciejewski, M., Kawiecki, J., & Rockwood, T. (1997). Satisfaction. In R. L. Kane (Ed.), *Understanding health-care outcomes research* (pp. 67–89). Gaithersburg, MD: Aspen.

McColl, M., Law, M. C., & Stewart, D. (1993). *Theoretical basis of occupational therapy.* Thorofare, NJ: Slack.

Mosey, A. C. (1981). *Occupational therapy: Configuration of a profession.* New York: Raven.

Mosey, A. C. (1996). *Applied scientific inquiry in the health professions: An epistemological orientation* (2nd ed.). Bethesda, MD: American Occupational Therapy Association.

Moyers, P. (1999). The guide to occupational therapy practice. *American Journal of Occupational Therapy, 53,* 247–322.

Neistadt, M. E., & Crepeau, E. B. (Eds.). (1998). *Willard & Spackman's occupational therapy* (9th ed.). Philadelphia: Lippincott Williams & Wilkins.

Parham, L. D., & Fazio, L. S. (Eds.). (1997). *Play in occupational therapy for children.* St. Louis, MO: Mosby.

Pedretti, L. W., & Early, M. B. (2001). Occupational performance and model of practice for physical dysfunction. In L. W. Pedretti & M. B. Early (Eds.), *Occupational therapy practice skills for physical dysfunction* (pp. 7–9). St. Louis, MO: Mosby.

Pierce, D. (2001). Untangling occupation and activity. *American Journal of Occupational Therapy, 55,* 138–146.

Primeau, L., & Ferguson, J. (1999). Occupational frame of reference. In P. Kramer & J. Hinojosa (Eds.), *Frames of reference for pediatric occupational therapy* (pp. 469–516). Philadelphia: Lippincott Williams & Wilkins.

Punwar, A. J., & Peloquin, S. M. (2000). *Occupational therapy principles and practice* (3rd ed.). Philadelphia: Lippincott Williams & Wilkins.

Radomski, M. V. (1995). There is more to life than putting on your pants. *American Journal of Occupational Therapy, 49,* 487–490.

Random House Webster's College Dictionary. (1995). New York: Random House.

Request for Planning Ideas for the Development of the Children's Health Outcomes Initiative, 66 Fed. Reg. 11296 (2001).

Rogers, J., & Holm, M. (1994). Assessment of self-care. In B. R. Bonder & M. B. Wagner (Eds.), *Functional performance in older adults* (pp. 181–202). Philadelphia: F. A. Davis.

Rowe, J. W., & Kahn, R. L. (1997). Successful aging. *Gerontologist, 37,* 433–440.

Schultz, S., & Schkade, J. (1997). Adaptation. In C. Christiansen & C. Baum (Eds.), *Occupational therapy: Enabling function and well-being* (p. 474). Thorofare, NJ: Slack.

Taber's Cyclopedic Medical Dictionary. (1997). Philadelphia: F. A. Davis.

Uniform Data System for Medical Rehabilitation (UDSMR). (1996). *Guide for the uniform data set for medical rehabilitation (including the FIM instrument).* Buffalo, NY: Author.

World Health Organization. (1947). Constitution of the World Health Organization. *Chronicle of the World Health Organization, 1*(1), 29–40.

World Health Organization. (2001). *International classification of functioning, disability, and health (ICF).* Geneva, Switzerland: Author.

Zhan, L. (1992). Quality of life: Conceptual and measurement issues. *Journal of Advanced Nursing, 17,* 795–800.

Bibliography

Accreditation Council for Occupational Therapy Education. (1999a). Glossary: Standards for an accredited educational program for the occupational therapist and occupational therapy assistant. *American Journal of Occupational Therapy, 53,* 590–591.

Accreditation Council for Occupational Therapy Education. (1999b). Standards for an accredited educational program for the occupational therapist. *American Journal of Occupational Therapy, 53,* 575–582.

Accreditation Council for Occupational Therapy Education. (1999c). Standards for an accredited educational program for the occupational therapy assistant. *American Journal of Occupational Therapy, 53,* 583–589.

American Occupational Therapy Association. (1995). Occupation: A position paper. *American Journal of Occupational Therapy, 49,* 1015–1018.

Baum, C. (1999, November 12–14). *At the core of our profession: Occupation-based practice* [overheads]. Presented at the AOTA Practice Conference, Reno, Nevada.

Blanche, E. I. (1999). *Play and process: The experience of play in the life of the adult.* Ann Arbor, MI: University of Michigan.

Borg, B., & Bruce, M. (1991). Assessing psychological performance factors. In C. H. Christiansen & C. M. Baum (Eds.), *Occupational therapy: Overcoming human performance deficits* (pp. 538–586). Thorofare, NJ: Slack.

Borst, M. J., & Nelson, D. L. (1993). Use of uniform terminology by occupational therapists. *American Journal of Occupational Therapy, 47,* 611–618.

Buckley, K. A., & Poole, S. E. (2000). Activity analysis. In J. Hinojosa & M. L. Blount (Eds.), *The texture of life: Purposeful activities in occupational therapy* (pp. 51–90). Bethesda, MD: American Occupational Therapy Association.

Canadian Association of Occupational Therapists. (1997). *Enabling occupation: An occupational therapy perspective.* Ottawa, ON: Author.

Christiansen, C. H. (1997). Acknowledging a spiritual dimension in occupational therapy practice. *American Journal of Occupational Therapy, 51,* 169–172.

Christiansen, C. H. (2000). The social importance of self-care intervention. In C. H. Christiansen (Ed.), *Ways of living: Self-care strategies for special needs* (2nd ed., pp. 1–11). Bethesda, MD: American Occupational Therapy Association.

Clark, F. A., Parham, D., Carlson, M. C., Frank, G., Jackson, J., Pierce, D., et al. (1991). Occupational science: Academic innovation in the service of occupational therapy's future. *American Journal of Occupational Therapy, 45,* 300–310.

Clark, F. A., Wood, W., & Larson, E. (1998). Occupational science: Occupational therapy's legacy for the 21st century. In M. E. Neistadt & E. B. Crepeau (Eds.), *Willard & Spackman's occupational therapy* (9th ed., pp. 13–21). Philadelphia: Lippincott Williams & Wilkins.

Culler, K. H. (1993). Occupational therapy performance areas: Home and family management. In H. L. Hopkins & H. D. Smith (Eds.), *Willard & Spackman's occupational therapy* (8th ed., pp. 207–269). Philadelphia: Lippincott Williams & Wilkins.

Dunn, W., Brown, C., & McGuigan, A. (1994). The ecology of human performance: A framework for considering the effect of context. *American Journal of Occupational Therapy, 48,* 595–607. Reprinted as Chapter 17.

Elenki, B. K., Hinojosa, J., Blount, M. L., & Blount, W. (2000). Perspectives. In J. Hinojosa & M. L. Blount (Eds.), *The texture of life: Purposeful activities in occupational therapy* (pp. 16–34). Bethesda, MD: American Occupational Therapy Association.

Gardner, H. (1999). *Intelligence reframed: Multiple intelligences for the 21st century.* New York: Basic Books.

Hill, J. (1993). Occupational therapy performance areas. In H. L. Hopkins & H. D. Smith (Eds.), *Willard & Spackman's occupational therapy* (8th ed., pp. 191–268). Philadelphia: Lippincott.

Hinojosa, J., & Blount, M. L. (2000). Purposeful activities within the context of occupational therapy. In J. Hinojosa & M. L. Blount (Eds.), *The texture of life: Purposeful activities in occupational therapy* (pp. 1–15). Bethesda, MD: American Occupational Therapy Association.

Holm, M. B., Rogers, J. C., & Stone, R. G. (1998). Treatment of performance contexts. In M. E. Neistadt & E. B. Crepeau (Eds.), *Willard & Spackman's occupational therapy* (9th ed., pp. 471–517). Philadelphia: Lippincott Williams & Wilkins.

Horsburgh, M. (1997). Toward an inclusive spirituality: Wholeness, interdependence, and waiting. *Disability and Rehabilitation, 19,* 398–406.

Intagliata, S. (1993). Rehabilitation centers. In H. L. Hopkins & H. D. Smith (Eds.), *Willard & Spackman's occupational therapy* (8th ed., pp. 784–789). Philadelphia: Lippincott.

Kane, R. L. (1997). Approaching the outcomes question. In R. L. Kane (Ed.), *Understanding health-care outcomes research* (pp. 1–15). Gaithersburg, MD: Aspen.

Kielhofner, G. (1992). Conceptual foundations of occupational therapy. Philadelphia: F. A. Davis.

Kielhofner, G. (1995). Habituation. In G. Kielhofner (Ed.), *A model of human occupation: Theory and application* (2nd ed., pp. 63–82). Philadelphia: Lippincott Williams & Wilkins.

Law, M. (1991). The environment: A focus for occupational therapy. *Canadian Journal of Occupational Therapy, 58,* 171–179.

Law, M. (1993). Evaluating activities of daily living: Directions for the future. *American Journal of Occupational Therapy, 47,* 233–237.

Law, M. (1998). Assessment in client-centered occupational therapy. In M. Law (Ed.), *Client-centered occupational therapy* (pp. 89–106). Thorofare, NJ: Slack.

Lifson, L. E., & Simon, R. I. (Eds.) (1998). *The mental health practitioner and the law: A comprehensive handbook.* Cambridge, MA: Harvard University Press.

Llorens, L. (1993). Activity analysis: Agreement between participants and observers on perceived factors and occupation components. *Occupational Therapy Journal of Research, 13,* 198–211.

Ludwig, F. M. (1993). Anne Cronin Mosey. In R. J. Miller & K. F. Walker (Eds.), *Perspectives on theory for the practice of occupational therapy* (pp. 41–63). Gaithersburg, MD: Aspen.

Mosey, A. C. (1981). Legitimate tools of occupational therapy. In A. Mosey (Ed.), *Occupational therapy: Configuration of a profession* (pp. 89–118). New York: Raven.

Mosey, A. C. (1986). *Psychosocial components of occupational therapy.* New York: Raven.

Nelson, D. L. (1988). Occupation: Form and performance. *American Journal of Occupational Therapy, 42,* 633–641.

Pierce, D. (1999, September). Putting occupation to work in occupational therapy curricula. *Education Special Interest Section Quarterly, 9*(3), 1–4.

Pollock, N., & McColl, M. A. (1998). Assessments in client-centered occupational therapy. In M. Law (Ed.), *Client-centered occupational therapy* (pp. 89–105). Thorofare, NJ: Slack.

Reed, K., & Sanderson, S. (1999). *Concepts of occupational therapy* (4th ed.). Philadelphia: Lippincott Williams & Wilkins.

Schell, B. B. (1998). Clinical reasoning: The basis of practice. In M. E. Neistadt & E. B. Crepeau (Eds.), *Willard & Spackman's occupational therapy* (9th ed., pp. 90–100). Philadelphia: Lippincott Williams & Wilkins.

Scherer, M. J., & Cushman, L. A. (1997). A functional approach to psychological and psychosocial factors and their assessment in rehabilitation. In S. S. Dittmar & G. E. Gresham (Eds.), *Functional assessment and outcomes measurement for the rehabilitation health professional* (pp. 57–67). Gaithersburg, MD: Aspen.

Trombly, C. (1993). The Issue Is—Anticipating the future: Assessment of occupational function. *American Journal of Occupational Therapy, 47,* 253–257.

Urbanowski, R., & Vargo, J. (1994). Spirituality, daily practice, and the occupational performance model. *Canadian Journal of Occupational Therapy, 61,* 88–94.

Watson, D. E. (1997). *Task analysis: An occupational performance approach.* Bethesda, MD: American Occupational Therapy Association.

Yerxa, E. J. (1980). Occupational therapy's role in creating a future climate of caring. *American Journal of Occupational Therapy, 34,* 529–534.

Background

Background of Uniform Terminology

The first edition of *Uniform Terminology* was titled the *Occupational Therapy Product Output Reporting System and Uniform Terminology for Reporting Occupational Therapy Services* (American Occupational Therapy Association [AOTA], 1979). It was approved by the Representative Assembly and published in 1979. It was originally developed in response to the Education for All Handicapped Children Act of 1975 (Public Law 94–142) and the Medicare-Medicaid Anti-Fraud and Abuse Amendments of 1977 (Public Law 95–142), which required the Secretary of the U.S. Department of Health and Human Services (DHHS) to establish regulations for uniform reporting systems for all departments in hospitals, including consistent terminology upon which to base reimbursement decisions. The AOTA developed the 1979 document to meet this requirement. However, the federal government's DHHS never adopted or implemented the system because of antitrust concerns related to price fixing. Occupational therapists and occupational therapy assistants, however, began to use the terminology outlined in this system, and some state governments incorporated it into their own payment reporting systems. This original document created consistent terminology that could be used in official documents, practice, and education.

The second edition of *Uniform Terminology for Occupational Therapy* (AOTA, 1989) was approved by the Representative Assembly and published in 1989. The document was organized somewhat differently. It was not designed to replace the "Product Output Reporting System" portion of the first edition but, rather, focused on delineating and defining only the occupational performance areas and occupational performance components that are addressed in occupational therapy direct services. Indirect services and the "Product Output Reporting System" were not revised or included in the second edition. The intent was to revise the document to reflect current areas of practice and to advance uniformity of definitions in the profession.

The last revision, *Uniform Terminology for Occupation-al Therapy—Third Edition* (UT-III, AOTA, 1994) was adopted by the Representative Assembly in 1994 and was "expanded to reflect current practice and to incorporate contextual aspects of performance" (p. 1047). The intended purpose of the document was "to provide a generic outline of the domain of concern of occupational therapy and … to create common terminology for the profession and to capture the essence of occupational therapy succinctly for others" (p. 1047).

Each revision reflects changes in current practice and provides consistent terminology that could be used by the profession. During each of the three revisions, the purpose of the document shifted slightly. Originally a document that responded to a federal requirement to develop a uniform reporting system, the document gradually shifted to describing and outlining the domain of concern of occupational therapy.

Development of the Occupational Therapy Practice Framework: Domain and Process

In the fall of 1998, the Commission on Practice (COP) began an extensive review process to solicit input from all levels of the profession with respect to the need for another revision of UT-III. The review process is a normal activity during which each official document can be updated and revised as needed. Themes of concern expressed by reviewers included the following:

- Terms defined in the document were unclear, inaccurate, or categorized improperly.
- Terms that should have been in the document were missing.
- Too much emphasis was placed on performance components.
- The concept of occupation was not included.
- Terms were used that were unfamiliar to external audiences (i.e., performance components, performance areas).
- Consideration should be given to using terminology proposed in the revision of *International Classification of Functioning, Disability and Health* (ICF).
- The document is being used inappropriately to design curricula.
- The role of theory application in clinical reasoning is being minimized by using UT-III as a recipe for practice.

The COP recognized that the practice environment had changed significantly since the last revision and that the profession's understanding of its core constructs and service delivery process had further evolved. The recently published *Guide to Occupational Therapy Practice* (Moyers, 1999) outlined many of these contemporary shifts, and the COP carefully reviewed this document. In light of these changes and the feedback received during the review process, the COP decided that practice needs had changed and that it was time to develop a different kind of document. The *Occupational Therapy Practice Framework: Domain and Process* was developed in response to these needs and changing conditions.

Relationship of the Framework to the Rescinded UT-III and the ICF

The Framework updates, revises, and incorporates the primary elements (performance areas, performance components, performance contexts) outlined in the rescinded UT-III. In some cases, the names of these elements were updated to reflect shifts in thinking and to create more obvious links with terminology outside of the profession. Feedback from the review indicated that the use of occupational therapy terminology often made it more difficult for others to understand what occupational therapy contributes. The ICF language is also seen as important to incorporate. The following chart shows how terminology has evolved by comparing terminology used in the Framework, the rescinded UT-III, and the ICF documents.

Comparison of Terms

Framework	Rescinded UT-III	ICF
Occupations—"activities…of everyday life, named, organized, and given value and meaning by individuals and a culture. Occupation is everything people do to occupy themselves, including looking after themselves… enjoying life…and contributing to the social and economic fabric of their communities…" (Law, Polatajko, Baptiste, & Townsend, 1997, p. 32).	Not addressed.	Not addressed.
Areas of occupation—various kinds of life activities in which people engage, including the following categories: ADL, IADL, education, work, play, leisure, and social participation.	**Performance areas** (pp. 1051–1052)— • Activities of daily living • Work and productive activities • Play or leisure activities	**Activities and participation**— • Activities—"execution of a task or action by an individual" (p. 10). • Participation—"involvement in a life situation" (p. 10). Examples of both: learning, task demands (routines), communication, mobility, self-care, domestic life, interpersonal interactions and relationships, major life areas, community, social and civic life. Activities and Participation examples from ICF overlap Areas of Occupation, Performance Skills, and Performance Patterns in the Framework.
Performance skills—features of what one does, not what one has, related to observable elements of action that have implicit functional purposes (adapted from Fisher & Kielhofner, 1995, p. 113). Performance skills include motor, process, and communication/interaction skills.	**Performance components**—sensorimotor components, cognitive interaction and cognitive components, as well as psychosocial skills and psychological components. These components consist of some performance skills and some client factors as presented in the Framework (pp. 1052–1054).	**Activities and participation**— • Activities—"execution of a task or action by an individual" (p. 10). • Participation—"involvement in a life situation" (p. 10). Examples of both: learning, task demands (routines), communication, mobility, self-care, domestic life, interpersonal interactions and relationships, major life areas, community, social and civic life. Activities and Participation examples from ICF overlap Areas of Occupation, Performance Skills, and Performance Patterns in the Framework.

Comparison of Terms, Cont.

Framework	Rescinded UT-III	ICF
Performance patterns—patterns of behavior related to daily life activities that are habitual or routine. Performance patterns include habits, routines, and roles.	Habits and routines not addressed. Roles listed as performance components (p. 1050).	**Activities and participation**— • **Activities**—"execution of a task or action by an individual" (p.10). • **Participation**—"involvement in a life situation" (p. 10). Examples of both: learning, task demands (routines), communication, mobility, self-care, domestic life, interpersonal interactions and relationships, major life areas, community, social and civic life. Activities and Participation examples from ICF overlap Areas of Occupation, Performance Skills, and Performance Patterns in the Framework.
Context or contexts—refers to a variety of interrelated conditions within and surrounding the client that influence performance. Context includes cultural, physical, social, personal, spiritual, temporal, and virtual contexts.	**Performance contexts** (p. 1054)— • Temporal aspects (chronological, developmental, life cycle, disability status) • Environment (physical, social, cultural)	**Contextual factors**—"represent the complete background of an individual's life and living. They include environmental factors and personal factors that may have an effect on the individual with a health condition and the individual's health and health-related states" (p. 16). • **Environmental factors**—"make up the physical, social and attitudinal environment in which people live and conduct their lives. The factors are external to individuals …" (p. 16). • **Personal factors**—"the particular background of an individual's life and living …" (p. 17) (e.g., gender, race, lifestyle, habits, social background, education, profession). Personal factors are not classified in ICF because they are not part of a health condition or health state, though they are recognized as having an effect on outcomes.
Activity demands—the aspects of an activity, which include the objects, space, social demands, sequencing or timing, required actions, and required underlying body functions and body structures needed to carry out the activity.	Not addressed.	Not addressed.
Client factors—those factors that reside within the client that may affect performance in areas of occupation. Client factors include the following: • **Body functions**—"the physiological functions of body systems (including psychological functions)" (WHO, 2001, p. 10). • **Body structures**—"anatomical parts of the body such as organs, limbs and their components [that support body function]" (WHO, 2001, p. 10).	Performance components—sensorimotor components, cognitive interaction and cognitive components, as well as psychosocial skills and psychological components. These components consist of some performance skills and some client factors as presented in the Framework (pp. 1052–1054).	• Body functions—"the physiological functions of body systems (including psychological functions)" (p. 10). • Body structures—"anatomical parts of the body such as organs, limbs and their components [that support body function]" (p. 10).

Framework	Rescinded UT-III	ICF
Outcomes—important dimensions of health attributed to interventions, including ability to function, health perceptions, and satisfaction with care (adapted from Request for Planning Ideas, 2001).	Not addressed.	Not addressed.

Note. UT-III = *Uniform Terminology for Occupational Therapy—Third Edition* (AOTA, 1994); ICF = *International Classification of Functioning, Disability, and Health* (WHO, 2001).

References

American Occupational Therapy Association. (1979). Uniform terminology for reporting occupational therapy services—First edition. *Occupational Therapy News, 35*(11), 1–8.

American Occupational Therapy Association. (1989). Uniform terminology for occupational therapy—Second edition. *American Journal of Occupational Therapy, 43,* 808–815.

American Occupational Therapy Association. (1994). Uniform terminology for occupational therapy—Third edition. *American Journal of Occupational Therapy, 48,* 1047–1054.

Education for all Handicapped Children Act. (1975). Pub. L. 94–142, 20 U.S.C. §1400 et seq.

Fisher, A., & Kielhofner, G. (1995). Skill in occupational performance. In G. Kielhofner (Ed.), *A model of human occupation: Theory and application* (2nd ed., pp. 113–128). Baltimore: Williams & Wilkins.

Law, M., Polatajko, H., Baptiste, W., & Townsend, E. (1997). Core concepts of occupational therapy. In E. Townsend (Ed.), *Enabling occupation: An occupational therapy perspective* (pp. 29–56). Ottawa, ON: Canadian Association of Occupational Therapists.

Medicare-Medicaid Anti-Fraud and Abuse Amendments. (1977). Pub. L. 95–142, 42 U.S.C. §1395(h).

Moyers, P. (1999). The guide to occupational therapy practice. *American Journal of Occupational Therapy, 53,* 247–322.

Request for Planning Ideas for the Development of the Children's Health Outcomes Initiative, 66 Fed. Reg. 11296 (2001).

World Health Organization. (2001). *International classification of functioning, disability, and health (ICF).* Geneva, Switzerland: Author.

Authors

The Commission on Practice:

Mary Jane Youngstrom, MS, OTR, FAOTA, Chairperson (1998–2002)

Sara Jane Brayman, PhD, OTR, FAOTA, Chairperson-Elect (2001–2002)

Paige Anthony, COTA

Mary Brinson, MS, OTR/L, FAOTA

Susan Brownrigg, OTR/L

Gloria Frolek Clark, MS, OTR/L, FAOTA

Susanne Smith Roley, MS, OTR

James Sellers, OTR/L

Nancy L. Van Slyke, EdD, OTR

Stacy M. Desmarais, MS, OTR/L, ASD Liaison

Jane Oldham, MOTS, Immediate-Past ASCOTA Liaison

Mary Vining Radomski, MA, OTR, FAOTA, SIS Liaison

Sarah D. Hertfelder, MEd, MOT, OTR, FAOTA, National Office Liaison

With contributions from

Deborah Lieberman, MHSA, OTR/L, FAOTA

for

The Commission on Practice

Mary Jane Youngstrom, MS, OTR, FAOTA, Chairperson

Adopted by the Representative Assembly 2002M29

This document replaces the *1994 Uniform Terminology for Occupational Therapy—Third Edition and Uniform Terminology—Third Edition: Application to Practice.*

Scope of Practice

Statement of Purpose

The purpose of this document is to define the scope of practice in occupational therapy in order to:

1. Delineate the domain of occupational therapy practice that directs the focus and actions of services provided by occupational therapists and occupational therapy assistants;

2. Delineate the dynamic process of occupational therapy evaluation and intervention services to achieve outcomes that support the participation of clients in their everyday life activities (occupations);

3. Describe the education and certification requirements to practice as an occupational therapist and occupational therapy assistant; and

4. Inform consumers, health-care providers, educators, the community, funding agencies, payers, referral sources, and policy makers regarding the scope of occupational therapy.

This appendix was previously published in the *American Journal of Occupational Therapy, 58,* 673–677. Copyright © 2004, American Occupational Therapy Association.

Introduction

The occupational therapy scope of practice is based on the American Occupational Therapy Association (AOTA) document *Occupational Therapy Practice Framework: Domain and Process* (AOTA, 2002 [see Appendix A]) and on the *Philosophical Base of Occupational Therapy* (see Appendix E), which states that "the understanding and use of occupations shall be at the central core of occupational therapy practice, education, and research" (AOTA, 2003a, Policy 1.11). Occupational therapy is a dynamic and evolving profession that is responsive to consumer needs and to emerging knowledge and research.

This scope of practice document is designed to support and be used in conjunction with the *Definition of Occupational Therapy Practice for the Model Practice Act* (AOTA, 2004a [see Appendix C]). While this scope of practice document helps support state laws and regulations that govern the practice of occupational therapy, it does not supersede those existing laws and other regulatory requirements. Occupational therapists and occupational therapy assistants are required to abide by statutes and regulations when providing occupational therapy services. State laws and other regulatory requirements typically include statements about educational requirements to practice occupational therapy, procedures to practice occupational therapy legally within the defined area of jurisdiction, the definition and scope of occupational therapy practice, and supervision requirements.

AOTA (1994) states that a referral is not "required for the provision of occupational therapy services" (p. 1034); however, a referral may be indicated by some state laws and other regulatory requirements. The AOTA 1994 document *Statement of Occupational Therapy Referral* states that "occupational therapists respond to requests for services, whatever their sources. They may accept and enter cases at their own professional discretion and based on their own level of competency" (p. 1034). Occupational therapy assistants provide services under the supervision of an occupational therapist. State laws and other regulatory requirements should be viewed as minimum criteria to practice occupational therapy. Ethical guidelines that ensure safe and effective delivery of occupational therapy services to clients always influence occupational therapy practice (AOTA, 2000).

Definition of Occupational Therapy

AOTA's *Definition of Occupational Therapy for the Model Practice Act* defines *occupational therapy* as:

> the therapeutic use of everyday life activities (occupations) with individuals or groups for the purpose of participation in roles and situations in home, school, workplace, community, and other settings. Occupational therapy services are provided for the purpose of promoting health and wellness and to those who have or are at risk for developing an illness, injury, disease, disorder, condition, impairment, disability, activity limitation, or participation restriction. Occupational therapy addresses the physical, cognitive, psychosocial, sensory, and other aspects of performance in a variety of contexts to support engagement in everyday life activities that affect health, well-being, and quality of life (AOTA, 2004a).

Scope of Practice—The Domain and Process

The scope of practice includes the domain and process of occupational therapy services. These concepts are intertwined with the *domain* defining the focus of occupational therapy (see Figure 1) and the *process* defining the delivery of occupational therapy (see Figure 2). The domain of occupational therapy is the everyday life activities (occupations) that people find meaningful and purposeful. Within this domain, occupational therapy services enable clients to engage (participate) in their everyday life activities in their desired roles, context, and life situations. Clients may be individuals, groups, communities, or populations. The occupations in which clients engage occur throughout the life span and include:

- Activities of daily living (self-care activities);
- Education (activities to participate as a learner in a learning environment);
- Instrumental activities of daily living (multistep activities to care for self and others, such as household management, financial management, and child care);
- Leisure (nonobligatory, discretionary, and intrinsically rewarding activities);
- Play (spontaneous and organized activities that promote pleasure, amusement, and diversion);
- Social participation (activities expected of individuals or individuals interacting with others); and
- Work (employment-related and volunteer activities).

Within this domain of practice, occupational therapists and occupational therapy assistants consider the repertoire of occupations in which the client engages, the performance skills and patterns the client uses, the contexts influencing

---

ENGAGEMENT IN OCCUPATION TO SUPPORT PARTICIPATION IN CONTEXT OR CONTEXTS

Performance in Areas of Occupation

Activities of Daily Living (ADL)*
Instrumental Activities of Daily Living (IADL)
Education
Work
Play
Leisure
Social Participation

Performance Skills	**Performance Patterns**
Motor Skills	Habits
Process Skills	Routines
Communication/Interaction Skills	Roles

Context	**Activity Demands**	**Client Factors**
Cultural	Objects Used and Their Properties	Body Functions
Physical	Space Demands	Body Structures
Social	Social Demands	
Personal	Sequencing and Timing	
Spiritual	Required Actions	
Temporal	Required Body Functions	
Virtual	Required Body Structures	

*Also referred to as basic activities of daily living (BADL) or personal activities of daily living (PADL).

Figure 1. Domain of Occupational Therapy. This figure represents the domain of occupational therapy and is included to allow readers to visualize the entire domain with all of its various aspects. No aspect is intended to be perceived as more important than another.

---

engagement, the features and demands of the activity, and the client's body functions and structures. Occupational therapists and occupational therapy assistants use their knowledge and skills to help clients "attain and resume daily life activities that support function and health" throughout the lifespan (AOTA, 2002, p. 610). Participation in activities and occupations that are meaningful to the client involves emotional, psychosocial, cognitive, and physical aspects of performance. This participation provides a means to enhance health, well-being, and life satisfaction.

The domain of occupational therapy practice complements the World Health Organization's (WHO) conceptualization of participation and health articulated in the *International Classification of Functioning, Disability, and Health* (ICF; WHO, 2001). Occupational therapy incorporates the basic constructs of ICF, including environment, participation, activities, and body structures and functions, when addressing the complexity and richness of occupations and occupational engagement.

The process of occupational therapy relates to service delivery (see Figure 2) and includes evaluating, intervening, and targeting outcomes. Occupation remains central to the occupational therapy process. It is client-centered, involving collaboration with the client throughout each aspect of service delivery. During the evaluation, the therapist develops an occupational profile; analyzes the client's ability to carry out everyday life activities; and determines the client's occupational needs, problems, and priorities for intervention. Evaluation and intervention may address one or more of the domains (see Figure 1) that influence occupational performance. Intervention includes planning and implementing occupational therapy services and involves therapeutic use of self, activities, and occupations, as well as consultation and education. The occupational therapist and occupational therapy assistant utilize occupation-based theories, frames of reference, evidence, and clinical reasoning to guide the intervention (AOTA, 2002).

The outcome of occupational therapy intervention is directed toward "engagement [of the client] in occupations that support participation in [daily life situations]" (AOTA, 2002, p. 618). Outcomes of the intervention determine future actions with the client. Outcomes include the client's occupational performance, role competence and adaptation, health and wellness, quality of life and satisfaction, and prevention initiatives (AOTA, 2002, p. 619).

Occupational Therapy Practice

Occupational therapists and occupational therapy assistants are experts at analyzing the performance skills and patterns necessary for people to engage in their everyday activities in the context in which those activities and occupations occur. The occupational therapist assumes responsibility for the delivery of all occupational therapy services and for the safety

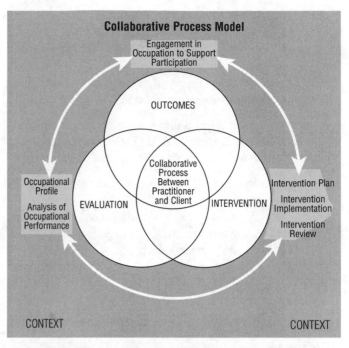

Figure 2. Illustration of the framework emphasizing client–practitioner interactive relationship and interactive nature of the service delivery process.

and effectiveness of occupational therapy services provided. The occupational therapy assistant delivers occupational therapy services under the supervision of and in partnership with the occupational therapist (AOTA, 2004b).

The practice of occupational therapy includes:

A. Strategies selected to direct the process of interventions, such as:

1. Establishment, remediation, or restoration of a skill or ability that has not yet developed or is impaired.
2. Compensation, modification, or adaptation of activity or environment to enhance performance.
3. Maintenance and enhancement of capabilities without which performance in everyday life activities would decline.
4. Health promotion and wellness to enable or enhance performance in everyday life activities.
5. Prevention of barriers to performance, including disability prevention.

B. Evaluation of factors affecting activities of daily living (ADL), instrumental activities of daily living (IADL), education, work, play, leisure, and social participation, including:

1. Client factors, including body functions (e.g., neuromuscular, sensory, visual, perceptual, cognitive) and body structures (e.g., cardiovascular, digestive, integumentary, genitourinary systems).

2. Habits, routines, roles, and behavior patterns.
3. Cultural, physical, environmental, social, and spiritual contexts and activity demands that affect performance.
4. Performance skills, including motor, process, and communication/interaction skills.

C. Interventions and procedures to promote or enhance safety and performance in ADL, IADL, education, work, play, leisure, and social participation, including:

1. Therapeutic use of occupations, exercises, and activities.
2. Training in self-care, self-management, home management, and community/work reintegration.
3. Development, remediation, or compensation of physical, cognitive, neuromuscular, sensory functions, and behavioral skills.
4. Therapeutic use of self, including one's personality, insights, perceptions, and judgments, as part of the therapeutic process.
5. Education and training of individuals, including family members, caregivers, and others.
6. Care coordination, case management, and transition services.
7. Consultative services to groups, programs, organizations, or communities.
8. Modification of environments (home, work, school, or community) and adaptation of processes, including the application of ergonomic principles.
9. Assessment, design, fabrication, application, fitting, and training in assistive technology, adaptive devices, and orthotic devices and training in the use of prosthetic devices.
10. Assessment, recommendation, and training in techniques to enhance functional mobility, including wheelchair management.
11. Driver rehabilitation and community mobility.
12. Management of feeding, eating, and swallowing to enable eating and feeding performance.
13. Application of physical agent modalities and use of a range of specific therapeutic procedures (e.g., wound care management; techniques to enhance sensory, perceptual, and cognitive processing; manual therapy techniques) to enhance performance skills (AOTA, 2004a).

Site of Intervention

Along the continuum of service, occupational therapy services may be provided to clients throughout the life span in a variety of settings. The settings may include, but are not limited to, the following:

- Institutional settings (inpatient) (e.g., acute rehabilitation, psychiatric hospital, community and specialty focused hospitals, nursing facilities, prisons);

- Outpatient settings (e.g., hospitals, clinics, medical and therapy offices);
- Home and community settings (e.g., home care, group homes, assisted living, schools, early intervention centers, day care centers, industry and business, hospice, sheltered workshops, wellness and fitness centers, community mental health facilities);
- Research facilities.

Education and Certification Requirements

To practice as an occupational therapist, the individual:

- Must have graduated from an occupational therapy program accredited by the Accreditation Council for Occupational Therapy Education (ACOTE®) or predecessor organizations, and
- Must have successfully completed a period of supervised fieldwork experience required by the recognized educational institution where the applicant met the academic requirements of an educational program for occupational therapists that is accredited by ACOTE® or predecessor organization (AOTA, 2003b, Policy 5.3).

To practice as an occupational therapy assistant, the individual:

- Must have graduated from an associate- or certificate-level occupational therapy assistant program accredited by ACOTE® or predecessor organizations, and
- Must have successfully completed a period of supervised fieldwork experience required by the recognized educational institution where the applicant met the academic requirements of an educational program for occupational therapy assistants that is accredited by ACOTE® or predecessor organizations (AOTA, 2003b, Policy 5.3).

AOTA supports licensure of qualified occupational therapists and occupational therapy assistants (AOTA, 2003b, Policy 5.3). State and other legislative or regulatory agencies may impose additional requirements to practice as an occupational therapist and occupational therapy assistant in their area of jurisdiction.

References

American Occupational Therapy Association. (1994). Statement of occupational therapy referral. *American Journal of Occupational Therapy, 48,* 1034.

American Occupational Therapy Association. (2000). Occupational therapy code of ethics. *American Journal of Occupational Therapy, 54,* 614–616.

American Occupational Therapy Association. (2002). Occupational therapy practice framework: Domain and process. *American Journal of Occupational Therapy, 56,* 609–639. Reprinted as Appendix A.

American Occupational Therapy Association. (2003a). Policy 1.11: The philosophical base of occupational therapy. In *Policy manual* (2003 ed.). Bethesda, MD: Author. Reprinted as Appendix E.

American Occupational Therapy Association. (2003b). Policy 5.3: Licensure. In *Policy manual* (2003 ed.). Bethesda, MD: Author.

American Occupational Therapy Association. (2004a). Definition of occupational therapy practice for the AOTA Model Practice Act. (Available from the State Affairs Group, American Occupational Therapy Association, 4720 Montgomery Lane, PO Box 31220, Bethesda, MD 20824-1220.) Reprinted as Appendix C.

American Occupational Therapy Association. (2004b). Guidelines for supervision, roles, and responsibilities during the delivery of occupational therapy services. *American Journal of Occupational Therapy, 58* (November/December).

World Health Organization. (2001). *International classification of functioning, disability, and health.* Geneva, Switzerland: Author.

Additional Reading

American Occupational Therapy Association. (1993). Occupational therapy roles. *American Journal of Occupational Therapy, 47,* 1087–1099.

American Occupational Therapy Association. (1994). Statement of occupational therapy referral. *American Journal of Occupational Therapy, 48,* 1034.

American Occupational Therapy Association. (1998). Guidelines to the occupational therapy code of ethics. *American Journal of Occupational Therapy, 2,* 881–884.

American Occupational Therapy Association. (1999). The guide to occupational therapy practice. *American Journal of Occupational Therapy, 53,* 247–322.

Moyers, P. (1999). The guide to occupational therapy practice. *American Journal of Occupational Therapy, 53,* 247–322.

Youngstrom, M. J. (2002). Introduction to the occupational therapy practice and framework: Domain and process. *OT Practice,* CE-1–CE-7.

Authors

The Commission on Practice:

Sara Jane Brayman, PhD, OTR/L, FAOTA, Chairperson

Gloria Frolek Clark, MS, OTR/L, FAOTA

Janet V. DeLany, DEd, OTR/L

Eileen R. Garza, PhD, OTR, ATP

Mary V. Radomski, MA, OTR/L, FAOTA

Ruth Ramsey, MS, OTR/L

Carol Siebert, MS, OTR/L

Kristi Voelkerding, BS, COTA/L

Patricia D. LaVesser, PhD, OTR/L, SIS Liaison

Lenna King, ASD Liaison

Deborah Lieberman, MHSA, OTR/L, FAOTA, AOTA Headquarters Liaison

for

The Commission on Practice

Sara Jane Brayman, PhD, OTR/L, FAOTA, Chairperson

Adopted by the Representative Assembly 2004C23

Definition of Occupational Therapy

AOTA's *Definition of Occupational Therapy for the Model Practice Act* defines *occupational therapy* as:

The therapeutic use of everyday life activities (occupations) with individuals or groups for the purpose of participation in roles and situations in home, school, workplace, community, and other settings. Occupational therapy services are provided for the purpose of promoting health and well-ness to those who have or are at risk for developing an illness, injury, disease, disorder, condition, impairment, disability, activity limitation, or participation restriction. Occupational therapy addresses the physical, cognitive, psychosocial, sensory, and other aspects of performance in a variety of contexts to support engagement in everyday life activities that affect health, well-being, and quality of life.

Address in Honor of Eleanor Clarke Slagle

ADOLF MEYER

It is a great privilege to have an opportunity to speak on this occasion, which honors a friend and long-time co-worker, our Mrs. Eleanor Clarke Slagle, as a person and as the personification of occupational therapy. Presidents and officers have come and gone, but for 20 years Mrs. Slagle has brought into the field just that kind of personality which proved highly fruitful and auspicious: she has been, not a dictator, not a boss, but a leader by example, a human being and human factor among human beings, a cultivator of human relationships, in gathering around herself co-workers and in making co-workers of the patients. Such is the human being Mrs. Slagle and what she means to us and to the thousands of patients who have been and are still reached by her and her pupils. And inseparable from this personal human side, there stands before us the nature and character of the product of her work and the spirit and philosophy her life and life-work exemplify, that which brings us together in this assembly and in this large and impressive organization.

This gathering and the work achieved by this body with Mrs. Slagle as the head worker are enough of a testimonial for a cause and its leading and stabilizing captain. Obviously Mrs. Slagle has had her ideal not only in perpetuating herself in a special role but in training a rank and file ever able to furnish timber for leadership from the ranks and in the ranks, and growth from the ranks.

For 20 years, from the beginning of our organization, Mrs. Slagle has, as treasurer and secretary, done that work of continuity which with changing presidents and changing topics represents the very constitution of this growing force in the ranks of dealing with those who, for a time and sometimes for good, are forced into that army that needs shelter and protection and among whom the work of restoring health and better ways of prevention and achievement of the handicapped brings care and cure.

In these days in which we are perhaps too much inclined to look upon leadership as a profession, and upon professional agitators as the reapers of honor and power, it is a tremendous satisfaction to see one of the chief workers completing 20 years in that office which personifies the very constitution of this body. Mrs. Slagle and Dr. Dunton have been the spirits in the ranks and from the ranks and for the ranks, not imposed managers, but the souls of the essence of the work, giving freely of their time and experience while carrying on the work itself.

In the great division of labor we need continuity and examples that survive the changes and are embodiments of the very essentials which only the best workers can perpetuate in steady growth, in stability of motion and promotion, those who see that ever new deals are fair deals, deals embodying the wisdom of those who do and actually work and never cease to grow and to create.

Growth and work and achievement and attainment are all a function of that one virtual commodity—time, that steady rhythm of day and night, of seasons and years, not a mere eternal return but eternal progression. No 2 days can be quite the same, and no 2 years; but there has to be an element of continuity and cohesion; and for this it takes those starting with enough personality, capable of maintaining themselves and of remaining forces and centers of growth. And as in the nature of humanity, generation follows generation, the young work beside the old and the old work beside the young, those capable of being the bearers of con-

This chapter was previously published in *Occupational Therapy in Mental Health, 5*(3), 109–113.

tinuity are few and rare and, we are glad to see, honored and sought as the very essence of progress.

Mrs. Slagle comes from the same source and soil that gave me my first opportunities and encouragement: the opportunity to realize the need for more, the need for growth, the opportunity to find similarly minded forces and the spirit of action that has to go with knowledge and vision to make it both fertile and practical: Illinois, large needs and large enterprises, a whole group of aspiring forces and engaging problems, needs in practice and needs in hospitals, close to Missouri, wanting to be shown and shown by actual work and performances. The educator, the social worker, and the physician were bound to get together. Miss Lathrop was one of the great links. As the great gardener Froebel in education and his pupil Grossman in the therapeutic training of psychopaths by work recognized the need of a setting for work and for therapy in sound use of time, so there was the shaping of an atmosphere of work and action at Kankakee, encouraged by the social spirit about Hull House, all working for the training by action and not only by word. The old ideal of the Middle Ages, pray and work, took real form in the union of one's best thought and work, and when we opened the Phipps Clinic for action, Miss Lathrop was able to lend us Mrs. Slagle as the model and instigator of workmanship in the service of therapy. That the greatest benefit for the sufferer was to come from the philosophy of time and its use and from the right person to exemplify it was natural in the pragmatic atmosphere of the middle west and Mrs. Slagle brought the fruit of experience to our new center. She started us and, like all good workers, inspired others, so that, when she was needed for more and more training of new forces, she left with us the workers who carried on while she was drawn into that field of training and teaching and organizing, that did so much in the emergencies of that international madness called war and again for the needs arising from the madness and the immaturity and blunderings even in peace. As a contributor to the philosophy of time and life, as a cultivator of life and health in activity, Mrs. Slagle has become a guide, philosopher, and friend of hundreds and hundreds, and as I said, the embodiment of example and principle. What she has added in the nearly 25 years since she came to help us is a proud record, a rare fulfillment of a life still growing and still progressing.

The demands of actual life and work where it is most needed have wrought a wonderful change in turning psychology from esoteric contemplation into the service of actual life. Real needs and real opportunities have led us into modern psychobiology and a science of human nature and behavior. And the basis of this modern psychobiology is not mere analysis and preaching of license, but a study and cultivation of the person and action. This is how the old principle of engaging patients in activity has become the basic setting of all modern therapy. Pathology is no longer a kind of gloating over what can be found at autopsy. It is the study of the mistakes and maladjustments, the failures of man to use his best sense and opportunities. Mistakes become damage and damage becomes disease and disease in turn has to be brought back to where it is treated as "poor work" to be replaced by good and helpful work. This is the role of occupational therapy, not merely making a lot of stereotyped articles but releasing or implanting and fostering action with the reward and joy of achievement. I heard Mrs. Slagle quote from a passage in the first paper I ever wrote on the treatment of nervous and mental disorders, addressed to the Chicago Pathological Society in February, 1893, nearly 45 years ago, in which I asked my colleagues for the discussion of the kind of work which could be expected from and recommended to American ladies. I do not know why I picked on the ladies; I suppose because the doctors present were all men and I felt I knew them. I said: 'Experience alone can give suggestions in this line.' I called it mental hygiene, foreshadowing what I now mean by "mind," the person in action, good or bad, helpful and effective or mere restlessness, often overactive only as the result of fatigue and mismanagement.

I should like to be able to voice adequately what so many of my patients have gained through Mrs. Slagle and her pupils and what it all means not only for the sufferer but also for the healthy of our time. When the development of machinery supersedes the driving power of necessity in the development of habits and possibilities of work, we turn to the ingenuity of those who know the creative possibilities available not only for the sick but for the rank and file of those with "time on their hands."

From reveling in thoughts of eternity, we now have the great task to inject again the joys of activity of the day so that we may make a return of the pleasure of the day's work an efficient competitor with the mere pleasure and glamour of night life. We are grateful to Mrs. Slagle and her pupils and co-workers for their devotion and skill and creative zeal and achievements in the furtherance of the joy and rewards of work and creation.

It must be a great satisfaction to Mrs. Slagle to see the onward march of what had but slender beginnings. There is a need of leisure for the spreading of the wisdom that has come from the wide experience under difficult conditions. As wisdom grows there comes the demand for a spreading into wider usefulness. Today we have come into a period of prostitution of the capacity and love for work to the service of the something and the somebody else of mere wages. We have more and more cause to search for the natural inducements to work and the opportunities for new creative principles. We have to study work for its own rewards and to honor and cherish it and to cultivate it so as to make it deserve the honor and joy. Working under the difficulties met by the psychiatric occupational worker should and will give us much material for a usable knowledge of the relation of person and work, worker and work, and worker and leadership.

What is the work one can love and live with and live on? What are the conditions of work that are needed if the worker is to love the work and to live on and through it?

I shall never forget the deplorable words of a Secretary of Labor in a discussion of immigration. He told us we needed some immigration to get labor to do the dirty work which no American parent would want his children to do.

We occupational workers know that there is no work that cannot be shaped so as to find its worker able to get satisfaction from the doing and the result.

In these days in which continuity of purpose seems overshadowed by doctrines of change and where leadership in a democratic sense threatens to be belittled and to degenerate in other lands into high-power dictatorships, it is a matter of great joy and cheer to see respect and honor brought to a leader of unusual modesty and gentleness.

In the midst of talk and reality of change we see careers of continuity of progress, of action and creativeness in the ranks, and as part of the ranks.

We see those natural and inspiring instances in which a rare individual becomes a live and effective example of ideas and ideals as the living and active person, and persons expressive of ideals.

And we are glad to see those persons who become living symbols of great movements and realizations, in the midst of the younger and the budding generations, sharing with them the experience of a lifetime and the spirit of everbudding youth.

It is the pride of democracy to cherish its leaders as parts of the ranks, as influence by example, and as recipients of recognition and of fellowship in the rank and file.

We like to see it brought home that a lifetime of work and service and devotion and leadership in a cause also finds its recognition, and recognition and esteem its expression.

The Philosophical Base of Occupational Therapy

Man is an active being whose development is influenced by the use of purposeful activity. Using their capacity for intrinsic motivation, human beings are able to influence their physical and mental health and their social and physical environment through purposeful activity. Human life includes a process of continuous adaptation. Adaptation is a change in function that promotes survival and self-actualization. Biological, psychological, and environmental factors may interrupt the adaptation process at any time throughout the lifecycle. Dysfunction may occur when adaptation is impaired. Purposeful activity facilitates the adaptive process.

Occupational therapy is based on the belief that purposeful activity (occupation), including its interpersonal and environmental components, may be used to prevent and mediate dysfunction, and to elicit maximum adaptation. Activity as used by the occupational therapist includes both an intrinsic and a therapeutic purpose.

This statement was adopted by the April 1979 Representative Assembly of The American Occupational Therapy Association, Inc. as Resolution C #531–79. The text can be noted below:

American Occupational Therapy Association. (1979). The philosophical base of occupational therapy. *American Journal of Occupational Therapy, 33,* 785.

American Occupational Therapy Association. (1979). Policy 1.11. The philosophical base of occupational therapy. In *Policy Manual of The American Occupational Therapy Association. Inc.* Rockville, MD: Author.

Core Values and Attitudes of Occupational Therapy Practice

Introduction

In 1985, the American Occupational Therapy Association (AOTA) funded the Professional and Technical Role Analysis Study (PATRA).This study had two purposes: to delineate the entry-level practice of OTRs and COTAs through a role analysis and to conduct a task inventory of what practitioners actually do. Knowledge, skills, and attitude statements were to be developed to provide a basis for the role analysis. The PATRA study completed the knowledge and skills statements. The Executive Board subsequently charged the Standards and Ethics Commission (SEC) to develop a statement that would describe the attitudes and values that undergird the profession of occupational therapy. The SEC wrote this document for use by AOTA members.

This appendix was previously published in the *American Journal of Occupational Therapy, 47,* 1085–1086. Copyright © 1993, American Occupational Therapy Association.

Prepared by Elizabeth Kanny, MA, OTR, for the Standards and Ethics Commission (Ruth A. Hansen, PhD, OTR, FAOTA, Chairperson). Approved by the Representative Assembly June 1993.

The list of terms used in this statement was originally constructed by the American Association of Colleges of Nursing (AACN) (1986). The PATRA committee analyzed the knowledge statements that the committee had written and selected those terms from the AACN list that best identified the values and attitudes of our profession. This list of terms was then forwarded to SEC by the PATRA Committee to use as the basis for the Core Values and Attitudes paper.

The development of this document is predicated on the assumption that the values of occupational therapy are evident in the official documents of AOTA. The official documents that were examined are: (a) *Dictionary Definition of Occupational Therapy* (AOTA, 1986), (b) *The Philosophical Base of Occupational Therapy* (AOTA, 1979) (reprinted as Appendix E), (c) *Essentials and Guidelines for an Accredited Educational Program for the Occupational Therapist* (AOTA, 1991a), (d) *Essentials and Guidelines for an Accredited Educational Program for the Occupational Therapy Assistant* (AOTA, 1991b), and (e) *Occupational Therapy Code of Ethics* (AOTA, 1988). It is further assumed that these documents are representative of the values and beliefs reflected in other occupational therapy literature.

A *value* is defined as a belief or an ideal to which an individual is committed. Values are an important part of the base or foundation of a profession. Ideally, these values are embraced by all members of the profession and are reflected in the members' interactions with those persons receiving services, colleagues, and society at large. Values have a central role in a profession and are developed and reinforced throughout an individual's life as a student and as a professional.

Actions and attitudes reflect the values of the individual. An attitude is the disposition to respond positively or negatively toward an object, person, concept, or situation. Thus, there is an assumption that all professional actions and interactions are rooted in certain core values and beliefs.

Seven Core Concepts

In this document, the core values and attitudes of occupational therapy are organized around seven basic concepts—altruism, equality, freedom, justice, dignity, truth, and prudence. How these core values and attitudes are expressed and implemented by occupational therapy practitioners may vary depending upon the environments and situations in which professional activity occurs.

Altruism is the unselfish concern for the welfare of others. This concept is reflected in actions and attitudes of commitment, caring, dedication, responsiveness, and understanding.

Equality requires that all individuals be perceived as having the same fundamental human rights and opportunities. This value is demonstrated by an attitude of fairness and impartiality. We believe that we should respect all individuals, keeping in mind that they may have values, beliefs, or lifestyles that are different from our own. Equality is practiced in the broad professional arena, but is particularly important in day-to-day interactions with those individuals receiving occupational therapy services.

Freedom allows the individual to exercise choice and to demonstrate independence, initiative, and self-direction. There is a need for all individuals to find a balance between autonomy and societal membership that is reflected in the choice of various patterns of interdependence with the human and nonhuman environment. We believe that individuals are internally and externally motivated toward action in a continuous process of adaptation throughout the life span. Purposeful activity plays a major role in developing and exercising self-direction, initiative, interdependence, and relatedness to the world. Activities verify the individual's ability to adapt, and they establish a satisfying balance between autonomy and societal membership. As professionals, we affirm the freedom of choice for each individual to pursue goals that have personal and social meaning.

Justice places value on the upholding of such moral and legal principles as fairness, equity, truthfulness, and objectivity. This means we aspire to provide occupational therapy services for all individuals who are in need of these services and that we will maintain a goal-directed and objective relationship with all those served. Practitioners must be knowledgeable about and have respect for the legal rights of individuals receiving occupational therapy services. In addition, the occupational therapy practitioner must understand and abide by the local, state, and federal laws governing professional practice.

Dignity emphasizes the importance of valuing the inherent worth and uniqueness of each person. This value is demonstrated by an attitude of empathy and respect for self and others. We believe that each individual is a unique combination of biologic endowment, sociocultural heritage, and life experiences. We view human beings holistically, respecting the unique interaction of the mind, body, and physical and social environment. We believe that dignity is nurtured and grows from the sense of competence and self-worth that is integrally linked to the person's ability to perform valued and relevant activities. In occupational therapy we emphasize the importance of dignity by helping the individual build on his or her unique attributes and resources.

Truth requires that we be faithful to facts and reality. Truthfulness or veracity is demonstrated by being accountable, honest, forthright, accurate, and authentic in our attitudes and actions. There is an obligation to be truthful with ourselves, those who receive services, colleagues, and society. One way that this is exhibited is through maintaining and upgrading professional competence. This happens, in part, through an unfaltering commitment to inquiry and learning, to self-understanding, and to the development of an interpersonal competence.

Prudence is the ability to govern and discipline oneself through the use of reason. To be prudent is to value judiciousness, discretion, vigilance, moderation, care, and circumspection in the management of one's affairs, to temper extremes, make judgments, and respond on the basis of intelligent reflection and rational thought.

Summary

Beliefs and values are those intrinsic concepts that underlie the core of the profession and the professional interactions of each practitioner. These values describe the profession's philosophy and provide the basis for defining purpose. The emphasis or priority that is given to each value may change as one's professional career evolves and as the unique characteristics of a situation unfold. This evolution of values is developmental in nature. Although we have basic values that cannot be violated, the degree to which certain values will take priority at a given time is influenced by the specifics of a situation and the environment in which it occurs. In one instance dignity may be a higher priority than truth; in another prudence may be chosen over freedom. As we process information and make decisions, the weight of the values that we hold may change. The practitioner faces dilemmas because of conflicting values and is required to engage in thoughtful deliberation to determine where the priority lies in a given situation.

The challenge for us all is to know our values, be able to make reasoned choices in situations of conflict, and be able to clearly articulate and defend our choices. At the same time, it is important that all members of the profession be committed to a set of common values. This mutual commitment to a set of beliefs and principles that govern our practice can provide a basis for clarifying expectations between the recipient and the provider of services. Shared values empower the profession and, in addition, build trust among ourselves and with others.

References

American Association of Colleges of Nursing. (1986). *Essentials of College and University Education for Professional Nursing. Final report.* Washington, DC: Author.

American Occupational Therapy Association. (1986, April). *Dictionary definition of occupational therapy.* Adopted and approved by the Representative Assembly to fulfill Resolution #596-83. (Available from AOTA, 1383 Piccard Drive, PO Box 1725, Rockville, MD 20849–1725.)

American Occupational Therapy Association. (1988). Occupational therapy code of ethics. *American Journal of Occupational Therapy, 42,* 795–796.

American Occupational Therapy Association. (1991a). Essentials and guidelines for an accredited educational program for the occupational therapist. *American Journal of Occupational Therapy, 45,* 1077–1084.

American Occupational Therapy Association. (1991b). Essentials and guidelines for an accredited educational program for the occupational therapy assistant. *American Journal of Occupational Therapy, 45,* 1085–1092.

American Occupational Therapy Association. (1979). The philosophical base of occupational therapy. *American Journal of Occupational Therapy, 33,* 785. (Reprinted as Appendix E.)

Lifestyle Performance Profile

The Lifestyle Performance Profile presents a structure for organizing and identifying performance skills and deficits within the context of an individual's sociocultural norms and characteristic patterns of responding to and managing life tasks. It offers a focus for describing sociocultural and environmental factors that can be tapped as resources to support the development of skills. It helps to delineate external forces that interfere with learning and require intervention. Because impaired performance is related to neuropsychological factors and interpersonal components as well as sociocultural ones, the assessment process must include the evaluation of these components. Specific concerns addressed in the Lifestyle Performance frame of reference are:

Skill and Skill Level, "Appropriate" Balance Determined By Age, Culture, and Biology

Self-Care and Maintenance	Self-Needs/Intrinsic Gratification	Service to Others
Self-Care: 　Washing 　Dressing 　Eating 　Toileting	Acknowledgment of own personal needs 　and interests	Role identity and responsibilities: 　Household and financial management 　Job-market role 　Support/care of dependents 　Student role
	Interests manifested	Family member role
	Interests actually pursued	
Self-maintenance: 　Food preparation 　Shopping 　Money management 　Transportation 　Daily schedule—time	Abilities and skills being used	Role/job demands and pressures Skills required
	Skill deficits	Existing skills
Care of: 　Living area 　Personal belongings	Intrinsic gratification values and 　attitudes	Skill deficits
Self support	External resources/barriers: 　Family/social	Appropriateness of role identity/responsibilities
Existing skills	Culture 　Economics 　Environment	Service values and attitudes
Skill deficits		External resources/barriers: 　Family/social 　Culture 　Economics 　Environment
Self-care values and attitudes External resources/barriers: 　Family/social 　Culture 　Economics 　Environment		

This appendix was originally published in S.C. Robertson, (Ed). (1988). *FOCUS: Skills for assessment and treatment*, pp. 3–38.

Skill and Skill Level, "Appropriate" Balance Determined By Age, Culture, and Biology, Cont.

Self-Care and Maintenance	Self-Needs/Intrinsic Gratification	Service to Others
Reciprocal Relationships		

Patterns of relating
Friends
Peers
Family
Groups
Intimacy
Interpersonal
Values
Expectation of self/others
Roles and responsibilities
Skills required
Existing skills/assets
Skill deficits
External resources
Family
Culture
Economics
Environment

Position Paper: Occupational Therapy and the Americans With Disabilities Act (ADA)

The American Occupational Therapy Association (AOTA) applauds the Americans With Disabilities Act (ADA) (Public Law 101–336) as landmark legislation passed by Congress to promote the integration of individuals with disabilities into the mainstream of society. Since its inception, the profession of occupational therapy has worked to foster independence in individuals with disabilities through the teaching and modification of independent living skills, work behaviors and skills, and compensatory strategies to minimize the limiting effect physical or mental impairments may have on the life of an individual.

The ADA prevents discrimination against individuals with disabilities by extending to them the same civil rights protection guaranteed under the law to individuals on the basis of race, creed, sex, national origin, and religion. Furthermore, the ADA provides comprehensive civil rights protection for individuals with disabilities in the areas of employment, public accommodations, transportation, state and local government services, and telecommunications, and the power to enforce these rights. The AOTA supports these mandates and urges all occupational therapy practitioners to embrace opportunities to empower individuals with disabilities in the following five areas specified by the ADA:

1. Employment
2. Public accommodations
3. State and local government
4. Public transportation
5. Telecommunications.

Employment

Historically, occupational therapy practitioners have played a significant role in assisting individuals with disabilities to enter into or return to the workforce. Under the employment provisions of the ADA, the occupational therapy practitioner continues to maintain a significant role in this area. Occupational therapy practitioners' understanding of everyday functional abilities and the demands that work places on individuals with disabilities enables them to assist consumers, employers, human resource professionals, risk and safety managers, occupational health personnel, and supervisors in developing reasonable accommodations to allow a person with a physical or mental disability access to the workforce.

Occupational therapy practitioners' training and expertise in the areas of job-site analysis, combined with their knowledge of work, human performance, and function, places them in a unique position to assist employers in implementing the ADA. The occupational therapist performs a job-site analysis to identify the essential and marginal functions of a job, and the job's environmental, cognitive, and psychological considerations. The job-site analysis provides a basis for the development of job descriptions written in specific functional terms. These job descriptions, based on the job-site analysis, become a working document that allows employers to provide accurate, job-specific information to job applicants and the human resources staff.

The occupational therapist may work as a consultant to teach human resources professionals how to use the functional job description as a tool during the interview process. Occupational therapy practitioners' education and understanding of sensorimotor, cognitive, psychosocial, and motor dysfunction, and how these affect the individual, place them in an excellent position to sensitize co-workers and supervisors to use proper disability etiquette to interact with, supervise, and work effectively with persons with disabilities. As consultants, occupational therapy practitioners may play a key role in dispelling the myths, misconceptions, stereotypes, and fears about disabilities found in the workplace.

To meet the new challenges presented to individuals with disabilities by the ADA's employment provisions, occupational therapists can work with employers to assess the occupational performance of individuals to determine their ability to perform the essential functions of a given job, with or without reasonable accommodations. Where accommodations are required to facilitate job performance, occupational therapists may recommend appropriate adaptive equipment, auxiliary aids, job restructuring, task adaptation, schedule changes, or work site or workstation modifications to enable these prospective or returning employees to perform the essential functions of their jobs.

Occupational therapy practitioners can play a key role in the employer's determination of whether an individual poses a direct threat to himself or herself or others in the workplace. Where a direct threat is found, occupational therapy practitioners can suggest reasonable accommodations to reduce the risk of harm. Employers, risk and safety managers, and human resources directors who wish to develop injury prevention programs that comply with the ADA will also benefit from the occupational therapist's consultation. This may include developing post-offer, job-related employee screenings and evaluations for high-risk injury positions.

Working in concert with individuals with disabilities, including work-related injuries, occupational therapy practitioners develop strategies to prepare the individual for employment. Through job-seeking skills training, clients are taught what to expect during the interview process, which reasonable accommodations to suggest and how to suggest them, and what their rights are during the application and interview process.

Public Accommodations

The occupational therapy practitioner facilitates compliance with the ADA's public accommodations provisions by working with architects, engineers, businesses, other professionals, and the consumer to determine the accessibility of places frequented by the general public and specified in the ADA, such as stores, theaters, health clubs, restaurants, hotels, office buildings, physicians' offices, and hospitals. Where inaccessible facilities, programs, goods, or services are identified, occupational therapy practitioners, on the basis of their knowledge of the functional abilities of individuals with disabilities, suggest adaptive equipment, auxiliary aids, policy changes, alternative methods of service provision, and environmental adaptations to make the facilities, programs, goods, or services accessible and usable. By promoting compliance with the ADA, the occupational therapy practitioner expands the individual's access to public accommodations in the mainstream of independent living.

State and Local Government Services

In the area of state and local services, the occupational therapy practitioner can consult with program staff from local governments to assist in integrating individuals with disabilities into the various services provided by the government agencies. For example, if a county provides a summer day camp for children through its parks department, an occupational therapy practitioner can develop a program to allow children with disabilities an equal opportunity to participate in the same camp program. Occupational therapy practitioners can also assist local governments to acquire auxiliary aids or adaptations needed to make other programs and services accessible to individuals with disabilities. Occupational therapy practitioners can serve as a resource for government task forces and departments providing consultation for ADA compliance in the areas of employment, accessibility, and communication.

Public Transportation

The ADA requires public transportation systems to provide more access to individuals with disabilities. On the basis of their knowledge of accessibility requirements, auxiliary aides, and functional mobility limitations of individuals, occupational therapy practitioners can assist public and private transportation system planners with providing access to buses, taxicabs, trains, airplanes, and subway systems. For example, occupational therapy practitioners can assist with making terminals accessible and suggesting that schedules be made available in alternative formats.

Telecommunications

The ADA's telecommunications provision requires the establishment of interstate and intrastate telecommunications relay services for individuals with hearing and speech impairments. Occupational therapy practitioners can assist telecommunications companies in assessing the need for information relay systems and can provide information about assistive device acquisition and training issues related to individuals with disabilities.

In summary, occupational therapy practitioners play a key role in educating the public as well as individuals with disabilities about their rights and responsibilities under the ADA. The occupational therapy practitioner's understanding of work and task analysis, knowledge of the functional limitations of disability, and experience with adaptive equipment provision and environmental adaptation places the practitioner in a unique position to serve as a resource in ADA-related matters. The AOTA supports the fundamental purposes of the ADA and encourages its members to assist the public in complying with its mandates to promote the entry of individuals with disabilities into the mainstream of independent living.

Reference

Americans With Disabilities Act of 1990 (Public Law 101-336), 42 U.S.C. § 12101.

Prepared by Barbara L. Kornblau, JD, OTR, DAAPM for The Commission on Practice (Jim Hinojosa, PhD, OTR, FAOTA, Chairperson).

Approved by the Representative Assembly June 1993.

This document was originally prepared as a White Paper (October 1991 to June 1993) for the American Occupational Therapy Association and was revised as a Position Paper for the Commission on Practice.

Position Paper: Broadening the Construct of Independence

We, the members of the occupational therapy profession, support the following expanded definition of independence: Independence is a self-directed state of being characterized by an individual's ability to participate in necessary and preferred occupations in a satisfying manner, irrespective of the amount or kind of external assistance desired or required.

We submit this Position Paper to embrace this broad definition and to support the view that:

- Self-determination is essential to achieving and maintaining independence;
- An individual's independence is unrelated to whether he or she performs the activities related to an occupation himself or herself, performs the activities in an adapted or modified environment, makes use of various devices or alternative strategies, or oversees activity completion by others;
- Independence is defined by the individual's culture and values, support systems, and ability to direct his or her life; and
- An individual's independence should not be based on pre-established criteria, perception of outside observers, or how independence is accomplished.

The occupational therapy profession is committed to a broad definition of independence for all members of society. We believe that an individual's self-directed state of independence strengthens the inclusion of all people into society as functional members, regardless of how they perform their chosen endeavors. In support of this view, occupational therapy practitioners are committed to supporting and training individuals in the use of a variety of strategies to increase their independent participation in their chosen occupations. Occupational therapy practitioners support a society that embraces an expanded definition of independence and that provides reasonable accommodations that allow individuals to have access to social, educational, recreational, and vocational opportunities.

Author

Jim Hinojosa, PhD, OT, FAOTA
for
The Commission on Practice
Mary Jane Youngstrom, MS, OTR, FAOTA—Chairperson

Adopted by the Representative Assembly 2002M40

This appendix was previously published in the *American Journal of Occupational Therapy, 56,* 660. Copyright © 2002, American Occupational Therapy Association.

Note: This document replaces the 1995 Position Paper, Broadening the Construct of Independence.

Index

health care
    business-driven, 399–400
    children, 574–576
    demands, 488
    efficiency, 531–532, 400
    environment and, 355–356
    excellence, 532–533
    financing, 400, 574
    holistic, 505–508
    management, 531–532
    trends, 423–424
help-seeking, patterns, 205
heredity, mental illness, 40
history, 1–2, 6–7, 55–56, 113–114
holding environment, 307
holistic frames of reference, 422
holistic health care, 505–508
home care, 387–393, 529
home management, 156
home space, 268
hope, 259
hospital-based models, 121–122, 179,
    400–401
hospitals, 7–8, 531–532
House of God, 541–542
humanism, 347, 527–530
human occupation, model of, 382
humanistic model, 119
humans
    involvement in tasks, 55
    meaning, 449–451
humor, 355
hypermobile behavior, 108
hypotheses, 77–84, 434, 514
hypothesis generation, 440

I

IADL. See instrumental activities of daily
    living
identity, 349–350, 582, 626
    adaptations, 416
    building, 417–418
    coherence and well-being, 417
    experience and, 414
    goals and occupational performance,
        415
    loss, 257
    occupation as, 409–420
    relationships with others and, 410–412
ideology, 581, 584
illness, 198, 205, 442
imbalance, 325
impairment, 549–550
impersonality, 400
inclusion, 305
    interactive strategies, 308–310
inclusive community, 177
independence, 449, 626
    construct, 599, 561
    functional, 448–449

independent living movement, 120–121,
    305
individual, role of, 349
individuality, 130–131
individualized transition planning (ITP)
    team, 176–177, 282
Individuals with Disabilities Education Act
    of 1990, 305
industrialization, 27, 29–34, 37, 457, 465
    postindustrial society, 340
Industrial Rehabilitation Act, 19
informant, 388
information, 341–342
injustice, 323–325
inpatient rehabilitation, occupational adapta-
    tion, 475
insanity, 36
instrumental activities of daily living (IADL),
    556, 612, 626–627
instrumentation, 436
intactness, 592–594
integration, 110, 510
intention, 246
interaction. See communication/interaction
interactional model, 304
interactive environment, 307
interactive reasoning, 442–443
interactive strategies, choice and inclusion,
    308–310
interests, 340, 627
*International Classification of Functioning,
    Disability, and Health* (ICF), 632
    Framework and, 633–635
interpersonal intelligence, 443
interpersonal relatedness, contact, linking,
    132, 299, 309
interpretation, 389, 391
interrelationships, 512
interventions, 605–606, 627, 640
    activities, 285
    approaches, 621–622, 627
    direct, 139
    implementation, 609–610, 627
    methods, 138–139
    plan, 609, 627
    play, 276–277
    prescribing, 89
    principles, 284
    process, 139–145, 609–610
    review, 610, 627
    site, 640
    strategies, culture and, 215–216
intrapersonal communication, 308
intuition, 406
invalid occupation, 12

J

job
    environment, 289–290
    essential functions, 293–294, 296
    marginal functions, 293
    see also occupation
Johnson, Eleanor, 13
Johnson, Susan Cox, 18–19
justice, 652

K

Keynes, John Maynard, 335
Keyser, Cassimir J., 28
Kidner, Thomas Bessell, 19–21, 461
kinetic behaviors, 197
Kirkbride, Thomas, 35
Kirkbride Plan, 37
knowing, being and, 265–266
knowledge, 82, 506, 516, 529, 545
    assessment, 428–430
    developing a comprehensive system,
        583–584
    ethics, 432–433
    options, 431–432
    translation to practice, 588–589

L

labor, maldistributed, 315
LaForce, Laura, 13
Lai, Lisa, 534
language and literacy, 66, 523
Lathrop, Julia, 12, 30
leadership, 503
legal issues, decision-making, 496–498
legislation, 288–299, 305, 461, 512, 521
    see also particular act, e.g., Americans
        with Disabilities Act
legitimate activities, 139
leisure, 156, 613, 627
Lewis, Steven, 552–553
liberationist approach, 423, 482–484
Licht, Sidney, 467
life events, interpretation, 412
life meaning, 412
    creating, 414–415
life-satisfaction, 412
life skills training, 564, 566
life stories, 414
lifestyle performance, 127–134
    application of, 132–133
    environment, 130–132
    model, 100
    principles, 129–130
    profile, 599, 655–656
lifeworld, 266
literature
    art of practice, 539–540
    flow, 239
local government services, 658

Locke, John, 44
Lorenz, Konrad, 331–333
Lu, Francis, 533
Luther, Jessie, 458

M

maintenance, 621
maladaptive responses, 316
management, 531–533
    case study, 533–534
    reimbursement and, 522
marginalization, 315, 324–325
marginal job functions, 293
Maslow, Abraham, 513
mature behavior, 108–109
McAfee, Larry, 550
Mead, George Herbert, 413
meaning
    finding, 260
    personal, 261–263
    source of, 246
meaningfulness, 142, 159–171, 451
    activity, 137
    time use, 316
mechanisms, 529
media, 455–456
    assumptions, 457
    selection, 456–457
Medicaid, 520
medical model, 505
Medicare, 520
medicine, 356, 516
    OT and, 520
    turn of the 20th century, 30
memory book, 156
mental functions, 618
mental health, 7
    ADA and, 290
    U.S., 547
mental illness, theories, 40
mental impairment, attitudes toward,
    292–293
mental problems, 19–21, 26
Merton, Robert, 512
method, 398–399, 455–456
    assumptions, 457
    selection, 456–457
Meyer, Adolph, 1, 12, 16, 30, 52–53, 61,
    71, 226, 599
    paper, 25–28, 645–647
Mill, John Stuart, 70–71
mind and body inextricably conjoined, 55
Mitchell, Weir, 41
models, 91–92, 116–122, 459
    function of, 128–129
    intervention process, 139–145
    occupational adaptation, 470–471
    of the patient, 434–435
    physical dysfunction, 160–161
    practice, 100

    see also Ecology of Human Performance;
    frameworks; *Occupational Therapy*
    Practice Framework
modification, 621
moral treatment, 2, 10–11, 35–42, 45, 519
    context and, 36–37
    crisis in, 40–41
    decline, 39–40, 48
    defined, 35–36
    expansion, 47
mortality, 343–344
Mosey, A. C., 537–538
motion study, 466–467
motivation, 429, 471, 489
    evidence-based practice, 569–570
motivational dimension, 141
motivational loss, 96
motor control and motor learning
    models, 120
motor impairments, 163–166
motor skills, 604, 614, 627
multiple tasks, 299
Murphy, Gardner, 81–82
Murphy, Robert, 547–548
Myers, Cordelia, 13

N

narrative, 250–251
narrative reasoning, 348, 367–375
national health care, 520
National Society for the Promotion of
    Occupational Therapy (NSPOT), 19,
    21–22, 71, 466–467
natural science of the human, 55
nature, appreciation of, 251
need, 80
    human, 331–337
    to be cared for, 352
nervous invalids, 17
neuromusculoskeletal functions, 619
neuropsychology, 557–558
new directions, 510
Newton, Isabel G., 7
normalcy, 205
Norristown State Hospital, 32–33
novices, 437–428
nurses, 9, 14, 49
nursing, 557
    occupation-based, 504

O

objective orientation, 86
occupation, 105, 159–168, 602, 627
    activities, 471–473
    asylum context, 38
    case, 153–157
    concept ownership, 123
    of daily living, 470
    defining, 114–115, 136–139

    design, 506, 587–597
    dimensions of, 580–595
    as end and means, 100–101, 149–158
    as ends, 151–152, 162–163
    healing power of, 1
    health and, 340–343
    justice, 178
    levels of, 161
    as means, 152–153, 163–168
    power of, 506
    practice context, 137–138
    purposes, 50–51
    role, 73
    science of, 91–92
    synthesis, 100
    therapy, 49
    as treatment, U.S. and Canada, 71–72
    see also activities
occupational adaptation, 103–111, 115,
    469–477
    framework, 105–107
    guide to practice, 471–474, 477
    illustrations, 474–476
    practice model, 470–471
    processes, 107–110
    theory, 104–105
occupational alienation, 323–324
occupational analysis, 461–462
occupational competence model, 551
occupational deprivation, 178, 313–318,
    324
    challenges, 316–317
    definition, 314
    human costs, 316
    identifying, 314–315
    maladaptive responses, 316
occupational director, 14, 16
occupational disruption, 314
occupational dysfunction, 314
occupational environment, 105–106, 109
occupational imbalance, 325
occupational injustice, 323–325
occupational justice, 317
    client-centered practice and, 319–329
    literature, 321–323
    theory, 322–323
    workshops, 321
occupational marginalization, 324–325
occupational performance, 627
    analysis of, 608–609
    enhancing, 383–385
    process, 609
occupational perspective, 317
occupational profile, 608–609, 627
    process, 608
occupational readiness, 423, 470, 472
occupational rights, 323
occupational science, 505–506, 579–585
    OT and, 579–580

surveillance zone, 268
symbolic interactionism, 413
symbolizing capacity, 377–378

T

task dimension, 141
task-oriented groups, 87
tasks, human involvement, 55
Taylor, Frederick Winslow, 531
teachers, 18, 423
teaching patients, 479–485
    approaches, 480–483
technology, 121, 178
    occupational deprivation and, 314
telecommunications, 658–659
tempo, 226–228
temporal, 628
temporality, 228–229
temporal adaptation, 174–175, 219–224
    case examples, 223–224
    conceptual framework, 220–222
    flow, 175
    implementation, 222–223
temporal context, 592–593
temporal dimension, 141
temporal environment, 284
tenacity, method of, 404
theory, 73, 514
    comprehensive, 91
    of experience, 44–45
    frameworks, 99–101
    practice and, 135–147
therapeutic climate, 470
    facilitating, 470–471
therapeutic employment, 372–374
therapeutic intervention, 192–193
therapeutic occupation, 138
    conceptual framework, 115–116
    models, 116–122
therapeutic power, 589–595
therapeutic process, 384–385
therapeutic progress, monitoring, 407
therapeutic rapport, 142
therapeutic relationship, 347–350
    elements of, 354–355
therapist approach, 423, 481–484
thinking, skill in, 436–437
third-party payment, 502, 523–524
threat, direct, 296
time
    consumed, 229
    health outcome, 231–232
    pressure, 299
    reclaimed, 229
    ruptured, 228
    studying, 230–231

time-use, 229–232
    methodologies, 230–231
    studies, 227, 229–230
Todd, Eli, 36, 38–39
tools of practice, 422, 552, 455–463, 589
top-down approach, 142, 153–155
touch, 355
Tracy, Susan Elizabeth, 8–10, 49
traditional thinking, 488–489
training, 16, 18–19
    standards, 520
transcendence, 244–245, 343
transition services, 284–285
transportation, 156
trauma, personal and social meaning,
    257–258
traumatic brain injury, occupational adapta-
    tion, 475
treatment
    identifying, 441
    individualizing, 442–443
    process, 82
    selection, 435–436
    whole person, 445
treatment activity, example, 424–425
truth, 652
Tuke, D. Hack, 48
Tuke, Samuel, 46–47
Tuke, William, 36, 45–47

U

understanding, 523–524
Uniform Terminology, 632
    Framework and, 633–635
    United States, 47–48, 71–72
    American character, 79
    21st millennium, 503, 543–548
Upham, Elizabeth G., 461
urbanization, 37, 459

V

values, 355, 441, 483, 523, 599, 651, 629
    conflicting, 33
    decision-making and, 495–496
    humanistic, 527–530
    meaning of, 510–511
    new directions and, 509–517
    professional, 496–497, 506, 516–517
    reimbursement vs., 501–502
    statement, 553
Vaux, Charles, 16
verbal persuasion, 291
verbal skills, 88
vicarious experience, 381
vicarious learning, 384
virtual, 629

virtual context, 178
vision, 514
vocational training, 12
vocational work, 156–157
volition, 131
Voltaire, 70
volunteer work, 156–157
volunteerism, 524

W

Wade, Beatrice D., 53–55
ward classes, 52
wartime aides, 13
well-being, 412, 417–418
    perceived self-efficacy and, 380–381
wellness, 629
    models, 121
White, Robert W., 87
wholeness, 440
wholism, 351
will, 246, 259
Williams, Frankwood, 13
Wilson, Susan Colson, 33
women, 14
women's work, 17
Woodward, Samuel, 41
woodworking, 459–460
work, 613, 629
    cure, 118
    latent consequences, 342–343
    simplification, 467
    spirituality and, 251
    see also occupation
working hypothesis, 430–431
workmanship, inferior, 53
work-related programs, 460–461
workshops, therapeutic, 31
workwoman, 47
World Health Organization, rehabilitation
    definition, 74
World War I, 12–15, 71–72, 459
    between the wars, 467
World War II, 520
worth, 355

Y

York Retreat, 46–47

About the Editor

Rita P. Fleming Cottrell, MA, OT/L, FAOTA, is a professor in the occupational therapy program at the University of Scranton, Scranton, PA. Ms. Cottrell received her baccalaureate and post-professional master's degrees in occupational therapy from New York University. She is currently a doctoral student in the occupational therapy program at New York University. Since 1987, Ms. Cottrell has held a number of academic positions at New York University, Dominican College, and other occupational therapy and occupational therapy assistant programs. Prior to entering academia, she worked as an occupational therapist in practice settings across the mental health continuum of care, from inpatient acute psychiatry to community day treatment and transitional living programs. She has published and presented nationally on the role of occupational therapy professional education, contemporary psychosocial occupational therapy practice, case management, disability rights, and social policy. She is Director of Research and Development for International Educational Resources (IER) and a course instructor for IER review courses for the NBCOT Certification Examination for the Occupational Therapist.

Ms. Cottrell is the editor of *Proactive Approaches in Psychosocial Occupational Therapy*; *Psychosocial Occupational Therapy: Proactive Approaches*; *Perspectives on Purposeful Activity: Foundation and Future of Occupational Therapy*; and the *National Occupational Therapy Certification Review and Study Guide*. She has also authored a number of journal articles and text chapters. A member of the American Occupational Therapy Association (AOTA), the World Federation of Occupational Therapy, the New York State Occupational Therapy Association, and numerous professional advocacy and consumer organizations, Ms. Cottrell serves on the editorial board of the *American Journal of Occupational Therapy* and *Occupational Therapy in Mental Health*.

Ms. Cottrell's professional experience in mental health practice, disability rights advocacy, and academia, along with her personal experience as a long-term caregiver for a beloved family member, has resulted in a strong, unwavering commitment to the inherent value of authentic occupational therapy. In addition, she is most interested in the promotion of occupational therapy to the public and to policymakers as the profession most suited to intervene holistically to meet societal needs. In 1994, Ms. Cottrell was awarded an AOTA "Award of Achievement" for her publications and contributions to the profession. She received the honor of being named an AOTA Fellow for innovation and leadership in education and advocacy in 2002.